Sande's

Commissioning Editor: *Sue Hodgson/Belinda Kuhn*
Development Editor: *Poppy Garraway*
Editorial Assistant: *Sam Crowe*
Project Manager: *Andrew Riley*
Design: *Charles Gray/Miles Hitchen*
Illustration Manager: *Bruce Hogarth*
Illustrator: *Antbits Ltd*
Marketing Manager (UK/USA): *Carla Holloway*

Sande's HIV/AIDS Medicine

Medical Management of AIDS 2012

Second Edition

Paul A. Volberding MD

Professor and Vice Chair, Department of Medicine, University of California San Francisco, Co-Director, UCSF-GIVI Center for AIDS Research, Chief, Medical Service, San Francisco Veterans Affairs Medical Center, San Francisco, CA, USA

Warner C. Greene MD, PhD

Director, Gladstone Institute of Virology and Immunology, President, Accordia Global Health Foundation, Nick and Sue Hellmann Distinguished Professor of Translational Medicine, Professor of Medicine, Microbiology and Immunology, University of California, San Francisco, San Francisco, CA, USA

Joep M. A. Lange MD, PhD

Professor of Medicine, Department of Global Health, Academic Medical Center, University of Amsterdam, Amsterdam Institute for Global Health and Development, Amsterdam, The Netherlands

Joel E. Gallant MD, MPH

Professor of Medicine and Epidemiology, Associate Director, Johns Hopkins AIDS Service, Division of Infectious Diseases, Department of Medicine, Johns Hopkins University School of Medicine, Baltimore, MD, USA

Nelson Sewankambo MBChB, M.Med FRCP

Principal, College of Health Sciences, Makerere University, Mulago Hospital, Kampala, Uganda

ELSEVIER
SAUNDERS

ELSEVIER
SAUNDERS

SAUNDERS is an imprint of Elsevier Inc.
© 2012, Elsevier Inc. All rights reserved.

First edition 2008

ISBN: 9781455706952

Transferred to Digital Printing in 2012

Contents

Contents

Preface

The rapid pace of change in HIV/AIDS management is an appropriate challenge to the ongoing revolution in medical publishing and information exchange. *Sande's HIV/AIDS Medicine: Medical Management of AIDS 2012* is a thorough revision of its predecessor, *Global AIDS Management*, published in 2007, now named in perpetual recognition of the pioneering efforts of Merle Sande, MD, one of the first edition's co-editors and a champion of AIDS care worldwide. The current book similarly addresses HIV management in the resource-rich "North" and that in the resource-constrained "South". Appreciating the challenge of medical care in both settings and the differing available resources, *Sande's HIV/AIDS Medicine* is now being offered in two overlapping but distinct versions. Each has content focused on the regional nature of disease and available resources and on an appropriate format of content, delivery mechanism, and cost.

This version of *Sande's HIV/AIDS Medicine* aimed at practitioners in settings with more abundant care resources is published in an ebook format operable across all common devices, and as a soft-bound book that is printed on demand to reduce environmental impact, reduce costs, and facilitate rapid updating. This version will be revised annually, allowing an unprecedented currency needed given the rapid developments in our scientific understanding of HIV pathogenesis and in our treatment options. We are particularly hoping that the ebook format will be widely used to move the very current and practical content of the book as close to the bedside as possible, increasing the impact of the book in improving HIV/AIDS care regardless of the multiple sites in which that care takes place. Electronic publishing combined with frequent revisions and a modest cost should help to ensure continuing wide use of this important textbook and day-to-day application in direct patient care.

While excited at the innovations in publication format, the editors of *Sande's HIV/AIDS Medicine* are equally proud of the book's content. Each editor has worked directly with chapter authors deeply expert in their field and focused on providing an authoritative yet clinically directed and practical review of a wide range of topics. The book begins with the fundamental underpinnings of HIV pathogenesis and epidemiology. It moves on to consider the treatment of HIV infection itself as well as the diagnosis and management of common co-morbidities, including the opportunistic diseases well known to be HIV induced, as well as conditions such as cardiovascular disease arising from the chronic disease that HIV infection has increasingly become in settings where early and continuous antiretroviral therapy is possible.

The editors applaud the vision of our publisher, Elsevier, in embracing this ground-breaking project and our authors in eagerly accepting the task of updating their contributions and adjusting them to the new publication format. We believe this will become the standard way textbooks will be distributed in the future and are excited that, once again, HIV and AIDS will lead the way.

Paul Volberding
Warner Greene
Joep Lange
Joel Gallant
Nelson Sewankambo
2012

Contributors

Frederick L. Altice, MD, MA
Professor of Medicine
Epidemiology and Public Health
Divisions of Infectious Diseases and Epidemiology
of Microbial Diseases
Yale University
New Haven, CT, USA

Andrew F. Angelino, MD
Associate Professor
Department of Psychiatry and Behavioral Sciences
Johns Hopkins University School of Medicine
Baltimore, MD, USA

Leyla Azis, MD
Fellow
Section of Infectious Diseases
Boston Medical Center
Boston, MA, USA

John G. Bartlett, MD
Professor of Medicine
Division of Infectious Diseases
Johns Hopkins University School of Medicine
Baltimore, MD, USA

Robert J. Blount, MD
Fellow, Pulmonary and Critical Care Medicine
Division of Pulmonary Medicine
University of California, San Francisco
San Francisco, CA, USA

R. Douglas Bruce, MD, MA, MSc
Assistant Professor of Medicine and Epidemiology
Divisions of Infectious Diseases and Epidemiology
of Microbial Diseases
Yale University
New Haven, CT, USA

Richard Chaisson, MD
Professor of Medicine, Epidemiology
and International Health
Johns Hopkins University School of Medicine
Baltimore, MD, USA

David B. Clifford, MD
Melba and Forest Seay Professor of
Neuropharmacology in Neurology
Departments of Neurology and Medicine
Washington University in St Louis
St Louis, MO, USA

Susa Coffey, MD
Associate Professor
Department of Medicine, Positive Health Program
University of California, San Francisco
San Francisco, CA, USA

David A. Cooper, MD, DSc
Director, The Kirby Institute for infection and immunity in society
University of New South Wales
Director, St Vincent's Centre for Applied Medical Research
St Vincent's Hospital
Sydney, NSW, Australia

Suzanne M. Crowe, MBBS, FRACP, MD
Head, Centre for Virology and Professor of Medicine
Burnet Institute and Monash University
Melbourne, Victoria, Australia

J. Lucian Davis, MD, MAS
Assistant Professor
Division of Pulmonary and Critical Care Medicine
University of California, San Francisco
San Francisco General Hospital
San Francisco, CA, USA

Kevin M. De Cock, MD, FRCP (UK), DTM&H
Director
Center for Global Health
Centers for Disease Control and Prevention
Atlanta, GA, USA

Douglas T. Dieterich
Professor of Medicine
Director of Continuing Medical Education,
Department of Medicine
Director of Outpatient Hepatology
Division of Liver Diseases
Mount Sinai School of Medicine
New York, NY, USA

Elizabeth H. Doby, MD
Pediatric Infectious Diseases Fellow
Department of Pediatrics, University of Utah
School of Medicine,
Salt Lake City, UT, USA

W. Lawrence Drew, MD, PhD
Professor Emeritus
Departments of Laboratory Medicine and Medicine
University of California, San Francisco
UCSF Medical Center at Mount Zion
San Francisco, CA, USA

James P. Dunn, MD
Associate Professor
The Wilmer Eye Institute
Johns Hopkins University School of Medicine
Baltimore, MD, USA

Jerrold J. Ellner, MD
Professor and Chief of Infectious Diseasee
Department of Medicine
Boston University and Boston Medical Center
Boston, MA, USA

Kim S. Erlich, MD
Consultant in Infectious Diseases
Associate Clinical Professor of Medicine
University of California, San Francisco
Daly City, CA, USA

Charles W. Flexner, MD
Professor, Medicine, and Pharmacology and Molecular Sciences,
and International Health
Bloomberg School of Public Health
Johns Hopkins University School of Medicine
Baltimore, MD, USA

Gerald Friedland, MD
Professor of Medicine and Epidemiology
Departments of Medicine and Epidemiology of
Microbial Diseases
Yale University School of Medicine
New Haven CT, USA
Adjunct Professor
Mailman School of Public Health
Columbia University
New York City, NY

Monica Gandhi, MD, MPH
Associate Professor
Department of Medicine, Division of HIV/AIDS
University of California, San Francisco
San Francisco, CA, USA

Trevor E. Gerntholtz, MD
Nephrologist and Director of Research
Chris Hani Baragwanath Hospital
Soweto, Johannesburg, South Africa

Clive M. Gray, MSc, PhD
Professor and Chair, Division of Immunology
Institute of Infectious Disease and Molecular Medicine
University of Cape Town
South Africa

Ruth M. Greenblatt, MD
Professor
Departments of Clinical Pharmacy, Medicine
Epidemiology and Biostatistics
University of California, San Francisco, Schools of
Pharmacy and Medicine
San Francisco, CA, USA

Warner C. Greene, MD, PhD
Director, Gladstone Institute of Virology and Immunology,
President, Accordia Global Health Foundation
Nick and Sue Hellmann Distinguished Professor
of Translational Medicine
Professor of Medicine, Microbiology and Immunology,
University of California, San Francisco
San Francisco, CA, USA

Deborah Greenspan, BDS, DSc
Leland A. and Gladys K. Barber Distinguished
Professor in Dentistry
Chair, Orofacial Sciences, School of Dentistry
University of California, San Francisco
San Francisco, CA, USA

John S. Greenspan, BSc, BDS, PhD, FRCPath,
FDS(RCSEng)
Distinguished Professor of Oral Pathology
Orofacial Sciences, School of Dentistry
Distinguished Professor
Pathology, School of Medicine
Associate Dean for Global Oral Health
School of Dentistry
Director, AIDS Research Institute
University of California, San Francisco
San Francisco, CA, USA

Carl Grunfeld, MD, PhD
Professor, Department of Medicine
University of California, San Francisco
Associate Chief of Staff for Research and Development, and
Chief, Division of Metabolism and Endocrinology
San Francisco Veterans Affairs Medical Center
San Francisco, CA, USA

Pamela Gumbi, PhD
Research Scientist
Division of Virology, Institute of Infectious Disease and Molecular
Medicine, University of Cape Town
Cape Town, South Africa

Guan-Zhu Han, BS
Graduate Student
Department of Ecology and Evolutionary Biology
University of Arizona
Tucson, AZ, USA

Laurence Huang, MD
Professor of Medicine
Department of Medicine
University of California, San Francisco School of Medicine
Chief, HIV/AIDS Chest Clinic
San Francisco General Hospital
San Francisco, CA, USA

Jula K. Inrig, MD, MHS
Assistant Professor of Medicine
Division of Nephrology
UT Southwestern Medical Center
Adjunct Associate of Medicine
Duke University Medical Center
Durham, NC, USA

Mark A. Jacobson, MD
Professor of Medicine
Positive Health Program
University of California, San Francisco
Medical Director
UCSF CTSI Clinical Research Center at San Francisco
General Hospital
San Francisco, CA, USA

Malcolm John
Associate Professor
UCSF School of Medicine
University of California, San Francisco
San Francisco, CA, USA

Edward C. Jones-López, MD, MS
Assistant Professor of Medicine
Section of Infectious Diseases
Boston University School of Medicine and Boston Medical Center
Boston, MA, USA

Salim S. Abdool Karim, MBChB, PhD
Director
Centre for the AIDS Programme of Research
in South Africa (CAPRISA)
University of KwaZulu-Natal
Doris Duke Medical Research Institute
Nelson R Mandela School of Medicine
Congella, South Africa

Anthony D. Kelleher, MBBS, PhD
Clinical Academic
HIV, Immunology and Infectious Diseases Clinical Services Unit
St Vincent's Hospital
Head, Immunovirology Laboratory
St Vincent's Centre for Applied Medical Research
St Vincent's Hospital
Head, Immunovirology and Pathogenesis Program
The Kirby Institute for infection and immunity in society
University of New South Wales
Sydney, NSW, Australia

Jerome H. Kim, MD
Project Manager, HIV Vaccines and
Chief, Laboratory of Molecular Virology and Pathogenesis
US Military HIV Research Program
Walter Reed Army Institute of Research
Silver Spring, MD, USA

Jeffrey D. Klausner, MD, MPH
Professor of Medicine and Global Health
Division of Infectious Diseases
Department of Medicine
University of California, Los Angeles
Los Angeles, CA, USA

Paul E. Klotman, BS MD
President and CEO
Baylor College of Medicine
Houston, TX USA

Jane E. Koehler, MA, MD
Professor of Medicine
Division of Infectious Diseases
University of California, San Francisco
San Francisco, CA, USA

Oliver Laeyendecker, MS, MBA
Sr. Research Associate
Laboratory of Immunoregulation
National Institute of Allergy and Infectious Diseases,
National Insitutes of Health
Instructor
Division of Infectious Diseases
Department of Medicine
Johns Hopkins University School of Medicine
Baltimore, MD, USA

Elysia Larson
Epidemiologist
Department of Epidemiology
Boston University
Boston, MA, USA

Simon Mallal, MBBS, FRACP, FRCPA
Director
Institute for Immunology and Infectious Diseases
Murdoch University
Murdoch, WA, Australia

Toby Maurer, MD
Professor of Clinical Dermatology
Department of Dermatology
University of California, San Francisco
San Francisco, CA, USA

Concepta Merry, FRCPI, PhD
Senior Lecturer, Global Health Trinity College
Dublin, Ireland
Infectious Diseases Institute Makerere University
Kampala, Uganda

Nelson L. Michael, MD, PhD
Director
US Military HIV Research Program
Walter Reed Army Institute of Research
Silver Spring, MD, USA

Rakesh K. Mishra, MD
Assistant Clinical Professor
Division of Cardiology, Department of Medicine
San Francisco Veterans Affairs Medical Center and
University of California, San Francisco
San Francisco, CA, USA

Ronald T. Mitsuyasu, MD
Professor of Medicine and Director
UCLA Center for Clinical AIDS Research and Education
Group Chair, AIDS Malignancy Consortium
Department of Medicine
University of California, Los Angeles
Los Angeles, CA, USA

Lynne M. Mofenson, MD
Chief, Pediatric, Adolescent and Maternal AIDS Branch
Center for Research for Mothers and Children
Eunice Kennedy Shriver National Institute of Child Health
and Human Development National Institutes of Health
Rockville, MD, USA

Pablo A. Moncado, MD
Postdoctoral Fellow, Internal Medicine
Infectious Diseases and Geographic Medicine
Stanford School of Medicine
Stanford, CA, USA
Departamento Medicina Interna, Division Infectologia
Fundación Valle del Lili
Cali, Colombia

Jose G. Montoya, MD
Associate Professor of Medicine
Department of Medicine and Division of Infectious
Diseases and Geographic Medicine
Stanford University School of Medicine
Stanford, CA
Director, Toxoplasma Serology Laboratory
Palo Alto Medical Foundation
Palo Alto, CA, USA

David Nolan, MBBS, FRACP, PhD
Consultant Physician and Associated Professor
Department of Clinical Immunology (Royal Perth Hospital), and,
Institute of Immunology and Infectious Disease
(Murdoch University)
Royal Perth Hospital and Murdoch University
Perth, WA, Australia

Chiadi U. Onyike, MD, MHS
Assistant Professor
Department of Psychiatry and Behavioral Sciences
Johns Hopkins University
Baltimore, MD, USA

Julie Overbaugh, PhD
Member
Division of Human Biology
Fred Hutchinson Cancer Research Center
Seattle, WA, USA

Kathleen R. Page, MD
Assistant Professor
Division of Infectious Diseases
Johns Hopkins University School of Medicine
Baltimore, MD, USA

Andrew T. Pavia, MD
George and Esther Gross Presidential
Professor and Chief
Division of Pediatric Infectious Diseases
Department of Pediatrics
University of Utah School of Medicine
Salt Lake City, UT, USA

B. Matija Peterlin, MD
Professor, Departments of Medicine and
Microbiology/Immunology
University of California, San Francisco
San Francisco, CA, USA

Marion G. Peters, MD
Professor of Medicine
Chief of Hepatology Research
Division of Gastroenterology
University of California, San Francisco
San Francisco, CA, USA

William G. Powderly, MD
Dean of Medicine
Professor of Medicine and Therapeutics
School of Medicine and Medical Sciences
University College Dublin
Dublin, Ireland

Thomas C. Quinn, MD, MSc
Associate Director for International Research, NIAID
Director, Johns Hopkins Center for Global Health
Professor of Medicine and Pathology
Johns Hopkins University School of Medicine
Baltimore, MD, USA

Mopo Radebe, BTech, MTech
PhD Candidate
Department of Paediatrics and Child Health
Nelson R. Mandela School of Medicine
University of KwaZulu-Natal
Durban, South Africa

Peter Reiss, MD, PhD
Professor of Medicine
Department of Global Health and Division
of Infectious Diseases
Amsterdam Institute for Global Health and Development
Academic Medical Center, University of Amsterdam
Amsterdam, The Netherlands

The Late Merle A. Sande, MD
Formerly Professor of Medicine
University of Washington School of Medicine
Formerly President, Academic Alliance for AIDS
Care and Prevention in Africa
Seattle, WA, USA

Monika Sarkar, MD
Gastroenterology Fellow
Department of Medicine, Division of Gastroenterology
University of California, San Francisco
San Francisco, CA, USA

Morris Schambelan, MD
Professor Emeritus of Medicine
Department of Medicine
University of California, San Francisco
San Francisco, CA, USA

Hanneke Schuitemaker, PhD
Professor in Virology
Department of Experimental Immunology
Academic Medical Center of the
University of Amsterdam
Amsterdam, The Netherlands

James C. Shepherd, MD PhD
Associate Director
CDC Botswana
Gaborone, Botswana

Thira Sirisanthana, MD
Professor of Medicine
National Research University Program
Chiang Mai University
Chiang Mai, Thailand

Matthew Stremlau, PhD
Postdoctoral Fellow
The Broad Institute
Cambridge, MA, USA

Khuanchai Supparatpinyo, MD
Professor of Medicine
Department of Medicine, Faculty of Medicine
Chiang Mai University
Chiang Mai, Thailand

Lynda A. Szczech, MD
Associate Professor of Medicine
Department of Medicine
Duke University School of Medicine
Durham, NC, USA

Steven A. Taylor, MD
Assistant Professor of Medicine
Department of Medicine
University of Texas Southwestern School of Medicine
Austin, TX, USA

Mengesha A. Teshome, MD
Research Patient Coordinator/Professional
Department of Neurology
Washington University in St Louis
St Louis, MI, USA

Glenn J. Treisman, MD, PhD
Professor of Psychiatry and Behavioral Sciences
Professor of Internal Medicine
Johns Hopkins University School of Medicine
Baltimore, MD, USA

Marie-Louise Vachon, MD, MSc
Division of Infectious Diseases
Centre Hospitalier de l'Université Laval
Quebec, Canada

Daniëlle van Manen
Post-Doctoral Fellow
Department of Experimental Immunology
Academica Medical Center of the University of Amsterdam
Amsterdam, The Netherlands

Angélique B. van 't Wout
Principal Investigator
Department of Experimental Immunology
Academica Medical Center of the University of Amsterdam
Amsterdam, The Netherlands

Paul A. Volberding, MD
Professor and Vice Chair, Department of Medicine
University of California San Francisco
Co-Director
UCSF-GIVI Center for AIDS Research
Chief, Medical Service, San Francisco
Veterans Affairs Medical Center
San Francisco, CA, USA

Mark A. Wainberg, PhD
Professor and Director
McGill University AIDS Centre
Lady Davis Institute
Jewish General Hospital
Montreal, Quebec, Canada

Bruce Walker, MD
Director
Ragon Institute of MGH, MIT and Harvard
Charlestown, MA, USA

Michael Worobey, BS, DPhil
Professor
Department of Ecology and Evolutionary Biology
University of Arizona
Tucson, AZ, USA

Gerasimos J. Zaharatos, MD, CM
Assistant Professor
Department of Medicine
Division of Infectious Diseases
McGill University AIDS Centre
Jewish General Hospital
Montreal, Quebec, Canada

Irum Zaidi, MPH
Epidemiologist
Division of Global HIV/AIDS
Centers for Disease Control and Prevention
Atlanta, GA
USA

Lycias Zembe, BSc, MSc, Med
PhD student
Clinical Laboratory Science, Division of Medical Virology
Institute of Infectious Diseases and Molecular Medicine
University of Cape Town
Cape Town, South Africa

Acknowledgments

We would like to thank Terry O'Donnell at the University of California, San Francisco and Poppy Garraway at Elsevier for their help in making this book a reality.

Section | 1 |

Epidemiology and biology of HIV infection

Chapter | 1 |

The global epidemiology of HIV/AIDS

Irum Zaidi, Kevin M. De Cock

OVERVIEW OF THE GLOBAL EPIDEMIC

There have been tremendous changes in the global HIV epidemic since the 1990s with declines in incident infections, increased coverage of antiretroviral therapy, stabilization or declines in HIV prevalence, reduction of mother-to-child transmission, and reduction in AIDS-related deaths. Many of these advances resulted from the dramatic increase in HIV program investments in low- and middle-income countries, which grew from US$1.4 billion in 2001 to US$15.9 billion in 2009. These resources have supported HIV treatment for over 6 million people worldwide [1].

Nonetheless, even with the recent stabilization of the global epidemic, HIV/AIDS has had devastating impact on lives worldwide and especially in sub-Saharan Africa. There were an estimated 33.3 million (31.4–35.3 million) people globally living with HIV at the end of 2009, a number that may continue to increase as incident cases continue to accrue and deaths to fall secondary to antiretroviral therapy. A decrease in new HIV infections has occurred, from an estimated 3.1 million (2.9–3.4 million) in 2001 to 2.6 million (2.3–2.8 million) in 2009 [1].

There is genetic, epidemiologic, and behavioral heterogeneity in the global HIV epidemic, with different regions disproportionately impacted by the virus. Generalized spread has occurred in sub-Saharan Africa while HIV/AIDS elsewhere has largely been restricted to key vulnerable populations (men who have sex with men, injecting drug users, and sex workers and their clients) [1].

Phylogenetically, two types of HIV are recognized, HIV-1 and HIV-2; within HIV-1 there are four groups, group M, group N, group O, and group P and within HIV-2, eight groups. HIV-1 group M is the predominant cause of the global epidemic and shows great genetic diversity with nine subtypes (A–D, F–H, J, and K) and at least 48 circulating recombinant forms. HIV-1 groups N, O, and P are rare and essentially restricted to persons from Central Africa. The single most common subtype of HIV-1 is subtype C, which affects nearly 17 million people in southern Africa, parts of East Africa, and Asia [2]. The number of HIV-2 infections globally is small and seems to be decreasing; most are associated with West Africa.

MEASUREMENT OF DISEASE

Methods for measuring HIV incidence and prevalence continue to evolve to more accurately measure disease burden [3]. The progression of the disease, late manifestation of symptoms, HIV testing behaviors, and antiretroviral therapy all challenge our ability to use epidemiologic and laboratory methods to measure HIV incidence and prevalence [4, 5].

Surveillance methods have drastically improved within the past decade. In low- and middle-income countries, sentinel surveillance among pregnant women attending antenatal clinics has been the cornerstone of efforts to estimate HIV prevalence in the general population. Pregnant women are by definition sexually active, give insight into prevalence trends in the general population, and are easy to survey since they access health services [6]. The coverage and quality of this surveillance approach has improved to provide more representative data [7].

Countries with generalized HIV epidemics, meaning that HIV transmission is sustained in the general population outside of core groups, have in addition been conducting periodic national household surveys to estimate national

HIV prevalence and collect behavioral information related to HIV acquisition and transmission. Arbitrarily, an HIV prevalence greater than 1% has sometimes been assumed to indicate generalized spread, although this assumption is unreliable. Several high-burden countries have now conducted more than one household survey, usually at approximately 5-year intervals, to monitor trends and measure impact of HIV programs. These national surveys are used to adjust prevalence levels from sentinel site surveillance in pregnant women to more accurately reflect those of the general population. Common experience has been that in relation to nationally representative household surveys, sentinel site surveillance based on pregnant women attending antenatal clinics has tended to overestimate HIV prevalence. This realization was key to UNAIDS and the World Health Organization (WHO) lowering global HIV estimates considerably in late 2007 [3].

Countries with low-level or concentrated epidemics conduct biological and behavioral surveys among high-risk populations, which include injection drug users, men who have sex with men, and male and female sex workers. New methods for accessing higher-risk populations that are often hard to reach continue to be validated [8]. Recently, countries with generalized epidemics have also been conducting biological and behavioral surveys among higher-risk populations that are disproportionately affected even in generalized epidemics. An important epidemiologic exercise has been estimating the respective population sizes of these high-risk groups, allowing estimates of their total numbers of HIV infections and contributions to overall HIV infection incidence, which is useful for allocation of resources for prevention of different modes of transmission.

In high-income, industrialized countries such as the United States and countries in Europe, which have concentrated epidemics, individual AIDS case reporting was for a long time the basis for monitoring epidemiologic trends. Because of the long incubation period between HIV infection and disease, AIDS case surveillance reflects patterns of HIV transmission that were prevalent several years earlier. With the advent of antiretroviral therapy the predictable progression to AIDS was interrupted, thus severely limiting the ability of AIDS data to give insight into HIV transmission patterns. As a result, the importance of HIV infection case reporting was considerably enhanced. Today, high-income countries with robust surveillance systems track both HIV and AIDS case reports, but both give incomplete information.

HIV case reports reflect HIV incidence imperfectly because they require HIV-infected persons to be tested and reported. AIDS case rates are affected by previous HIV incidence but also by the effectiveness of HIV diagnosis, access to antiretroviral therapy, and response to treatment. For as complete as possible an understanding of the HIV/AIDS epidemic, in addition to case reporting there is also a need for surveys and special studies. Surveys include behavioral and biologic studies in special groups such as men who have sex

with men, and special studies can address diverse issues such as access to and adherence to therapy or the spectrum of disease in people living with HIV.

Case reporting requires use of a standard case definition which is a surveillance tool, and not intended for clinical management of patients. For clinical purposes, staging systems can help assist clinicians define where individual patients lie on the spectrum of HIV-associated immunodeficiency and disease. Different case definitions have been used over time as understanding of HIV/AIDS and surveillance practices evolved, and taking account of local resources for investigation and reporting of cases.

The revised 2006 case definitions and staging system proposed by WHO provide standardized definitions for global use to improve patient management, patient monitoring, and surveillance [9, 10]. Four clinical stages and four immunological stages were established (Table 1.1a and 1.1b), reflecting the known decline in clinical status and CD4 cells with the progression of HIV disease. The surveillance definitions for HIV/AIDS were also revised to include three categories: HIV infection, advanced HIV disease, and AIDS (Box 1.1). Although a standard case definition for primary (acute) HIV infection is not established, identifying and reporting cases of primary infection may be important because these represent very recent infections. Symptomatic primary HIV infection presents one to four weeks after HIV acquisition and may include any of the following symptoms:

- Lymphadenopathy;
- Pharyngitis;
- Maculopapular rash;
- Orogenital or oesophageal ulcers;
- Menigoencephalitis;
- Lymphopenia (including low CD4); and
- Opportunistic infections.

These clinical conditions should not be confused with clinical staging criteria. Primary HIV infection can be diagnosed by recent HIV antibody development or by identifying HIV products (HIV-RNA or HIV-DNA and/or ultrasensitive HIV p24 antigen with a negative HIV antibody test).

Table 1.1a WHO clinical staging of established HIV infection	
HIV-ASSOCIATED SYMPTOMS	**WHO CLINICAL STAGE**
Asymptomatic	1
Mild symptoms	2
Advanced symptoms	3
Severe symptoms	4

Table 1.1b WHO immunological classification for established HIV infection

HIV-ASSOCIATED IMMUNODEFICIENCY	AGE-RELATED CD4 VALUES			
	< 11 mo (%)	12–35 mo (%)	36–59 mo (%)	≥ 5 yrs (per mm³)
None/not significant	> 35	> 30	> 25	> 500
Mild	30–35	25–30	20–25	350–499
Advanced	25–30	20–25	15–20	200–349
Severe	< 25	< 20	< 15	< 200 or < 15%

Box 1.1 **WHO case definition for HIV infection for reporting for adults and children**

1. **Adults, and children 18 months and older: Diagnosis of HIV infection is made with:**
   Positive HIV antibody testing (rapid or laboratory-based EIA). This is usually confirmed by a second HIV antibody test (rapid or laboratory-based EIA) relying on different antigens or on different operating characteristics.
   And/or
   Positive virological test for HIV or its components (HIV-RNA or HIV-DNA or ultrasensitive HIV p 24 antigen) confirmed by a second virological test obtained from a separate determination.

2. **Children younger than 18 months: Diagnosis of HIV infection is made with:**
   Positive virological test for HIV or its components (HIV-RNA or HIV-DNA or ultrasensitive HIV p 24 antigen) confirmed by a second virological test obtained from a separate determination taken more than 4 weeks after birth [1].
   Positive antibody testing is not recommended for definitive or confirmatory diagnosis of HIV infection in children until 18 months of age.
   WHO criteria for diagnosis of advanced HIV (including AIDS [2]) for reporting for adults and children

1. **Clinical criteria for diagnosis of advanced HIV in adults and children with documented HIV infection:**
   Presumptive or definitive diagnosis of any one stage 3 or stage 4 condition.

2. **Immunologic criteria for diagnosis of advanced HIV in adults and children ≥ 5 years, with documented HIV infection:**
   CD4 count less than 350/mm³ in an HIV-infected adult or child.

3. **Immunologic criteria for diagnosis of advanced HIV in a child <5 years of age with documented HIV infection:**
   %CD4 < 30 in those ≤11 months of age;
   %CD4 < 25 in those aged 12–35 months; and
   %CD4 < 20 in those aged 36–59 months.

[1]*Where access to virological testing in children less than 18 months is limited, confirmation of HIV infection can be obtained from repeat testing on the same specimen where laboratory quality assurance, including specimen handling is guaranteed.*
[2]AIDS in adults and children is defined as clinical diagnosis (presumptive or definitive) of any one stage 4 condition (as defined in annex 1); OR immunological criteria in adults and children ≥ 5 years with documented HIV infection first-ever documented CD4 count less than 200/mm³ or %CD4 <15; or in a child < 5 years with documented HIV infection first-ever documented CD4 of %CD4 < 25 in those infants ≤ 11 months of age; %CD4 < 20 in those aged 12–35 months, or %CD4 < 15 in those aged 35–59 months.
Note: AIDS case reporting is no longer required if HIV infection or advanced HIV infection is reported.

Countries with established national HIV case surveillance systems (mostly Western countries) use back-calculation methods or direct calculation to determine HIV prevalence and incidence [4, 11]. Other countries rely on epidemic models based on data from surveillance of key populations to estimate HIV prevalence and incidence and monitor trends [12].

HIV TRANSMISSION

HIV is transmitted from person to person through heterosexual and male-to-male sexual intercourse; through exposure to infected blood or blood products; and from mother to child, including through breastfeeding. Surveillance plays an important role in quantifying the proportional contribution of different modes of transmission to the overall epidemic in any country, allowing rational resource allocation for prevention, treatment, and care to different groups.

Sexual transmission

Most HIV infections are transmitted sexually, with heterosexual transmission being the dominant mode of transmission globally. As with all modes of transmission, infectiousness is determined by viral load: the higher the viral load, the more likely that transmission will occur. Other sexually transmitted infections, especially ulcerative conditions including HSV-2 infection, increase viral shedding in genital fluids and transmissibility [13]. Male circumcision is partially protective (approximately 50–60% efficacy) against heterosexual acquisition of HIV [14]. Although there is no definitive evidence that male circumcision protects against male-to-female transmission, indirect benefit to women will ultimately result from reduced HIV prevalence in men. The risk of HIV infection increases with the number of sex partners, and because of their high viral load, persons recently infected may contribute disproportionately to spread [15]. The highest rates of HIV infection are found in persons with the greatest rate of partner change such as sex workers. There is debate about the epidemiologic impact of concurrent versus sequential partnerships, the former suggested as establishing more efficient transmission networks. In the generalized epidemics of southern and eastern Africa, a substantial proportion of heterosexually transmitted infections occur in stable or long-term sero-discordant couples.

High rates of HIV infection are found among men who have sex with men almost everywhere they have been studied. Recognition that male-to-male sex occurs in virtually all countries, including in sub-Saharan Africa, is relatively recent, as is the documentation of high rates of HIV infection in men who have sex with men in societies suffering generalized HIV epidemics [16].

Mother-to-child transmission

HIV can be transmitted from mother to child *in utero*, around delivery, or after birth during breastfeeding. Prophylaxis or treatment with antiretroviral drugs has drastically reduced the vertical transmission rate, which without intervention ranges from about 15% in nonbreastfeeding women to 45% for those breastfeeding up to 24 months [17].

The great majority of HIV-infected women reside in sub-Saharan Africa where the overall HIV prevalence in women aged 15–24 was estimated at 3.4%; in 2009 there were an estimated 370,000 children newly infected with HIV, with the majority of these infections occurring in sub-Saharan Africa.

Injection drug use and exposure to contaminated blood

There are an estimated 15.9 million (11–21 million) injectors worldwide, and injection drug use is an increasing phenomenon globally that is extending into regions where it was previously not seen. Eastern Europe has the highest rates of injection drug use (Fig. 1.1), which is coupled with high rates of HIV among this population. Overall, there are an estimated 3 million HIV-positive drug injectors worldwide with the majority residing in China, Russia, and the United States [18].

Although HIV infection from exposure to contaminated blood and blood products was recognized early on as an important mode of transmission, transfusion safety initiatives have essentially eliminated or very greatly reduced the risk of acquiring HIV infection from contaminated blood. Although the risk of HIV transmission through needlestick injury is well understood (0.003 risk of transmission for uncomplicated needlesticks from an infected source), the relative contribution of such nosocomial events to overall numbers of HIV infections in high-burden settings has been difficult to quantify [19].

REGIONAL REVIEW

Sub-Saharan Africa

Although two-thirds of all HIV-infected persons reside in sub-Saharan Africa, this most heavily affected part of the world has seen substantial epidemiologic changes over the past 10 years, with a decrease in new HIV infections and deaths and stabilizing or declining HIV prevalence. Sub-Saharan Africa illustrates better than any other region the social, economic, demographic, and medical impact of HIV/AIDS which accounted for the unprecedented global health response.

Striking heterogeneity characterizes the sub-Saharan African epidemic, with the highest rates of infection in southern African countries, followed by countries in East, West, and Central Africa (Fig. 1.2). Twenty-five percent of all persons living with HIV in sub-Saharan Africa reside in South Africa. Although rates of infection are extremely high in neighboring countries, their small populations mean that absolute numbers of infected persons are limited. Nigeria, which has a much lower HIV prevalence than countries in southern Africa, accounts for 15% of Africans living with HIV, and countries of East Africa for one quarter [1].

Heterosexual transmission accounts for most of the HIV transmission in sub-Saharan Africa and women contribute approximately 60% of all HIV infections. Serial age and sex-specific prevalence shows women are infected at younger ages than men, presumably a reflection of older men with HIV having sex with younger women. A relatively recent

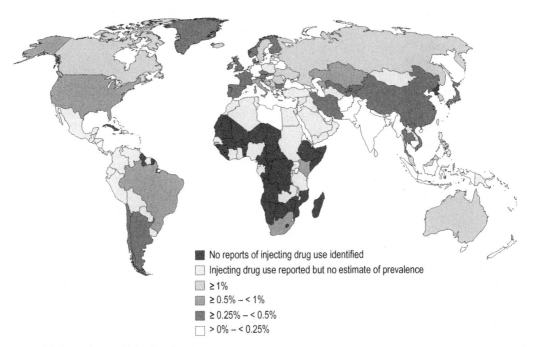

Figure 1.1 Global prevalence of injection drug use.
Reprinted from the Lancet. Mathers BM, Degenhardt L, Phillips B, et al. Global epidemiology of injecting drug use and HIV among people who inject drugs: a systematic review. Lancet 2010; 375:1014–1028. Copyright Elsevier 2010.

Legend (Figure 1.1):
- No reports of injecting drug use identified
- Injecting drug use reported but no estimate of prevalence
- ≥1%
- ≥0.5% – <1%
- ≥0.25% – <0.5%
- >0% – <0.25%

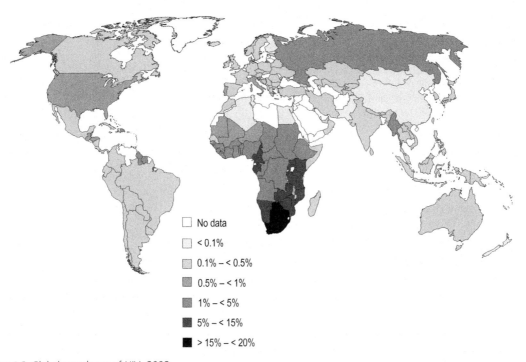

Legend (Figure 1.2):
- No data
- <0.1%
- 0.1% – <0.5%
- 0.5% – <1%
- 1% – <5%
- 5% – <15%
- >15% – <20%

Figure 1.2 Global prevalence of HIV, 2009.
From UNAIDS. Global report: UNAIDS report on the global AIDS epidemic 2010. With permission of UNAIDS/ONUSIDA 2010.

recognition is that sub-Saharan Africa also has an epidemic of HIV among men who have sex with men and that many of such men also have sexual relations with women. Most studies have shown higher HIV prevalence among men who have sex with men than among exclusively heterosexual males, in the range of approximately 12–30% [16].

Although approximately 70% of AIDS-related deaths worldwide occur in sub-Saharan Africa, AIDS-related mortality on the continent has declined with scale-up of antitretroviral therapy [1].

South

Countries in southern Africa have the highest rates of HIV in the world with the largest number of people living with HIV in South Africa, an estimated 5.6 million. Lack of male circumcision, high rates of HSV-2, intergenerational sex, and high rates of partner change consequent upon large-scale migration for work all likely contributed to generating and sustaining these severe epidemics. Swaziland has the highest adult HIV prevalence (25.9%) in the world. Botswana and Lesotho also have extremely high prevalence (24.8%, 23.6%), while HIV prevalence in Angola (2%) is very low compared to other countries within the sub-region [1]. The prolonged civil war in Angola seems to have had a protective effect against HIV by limiting travel and interactions with other countries in the region with higher HIV prevalence [20].

Incidence estimates suggest decreasing numbers of new infections since 2001 in almost all countries in southern Africa, with Botswana, Namibia, Swaziland, and Zimbabwe experiencing the greatest relative declines. Additionally, in Malawi, Namibia, Zambia, and Zimbabwe, measurement of sexual behaviors shows declines in the percent of people who had had sex by the age of 15–19 years, who had more than one partner in the past year, and who had more than one partner in the past and did not use condoms [21]. HIV prevalence is higher among young women than young men in most of the countries in the sub-region.

East

The HIV epidemic in East Africa shows sign of slowing and stabilization. Although adult HIV prevalence rates are lower in the sub-region than in southern Africa, ranging from 2.9% in Rwanda to 6.3% in Kenya, the actual number of people living with HIV is high given the large populations in East African countries [1]. Overall there may have been changes in HIV risk behaviors and likely reduced HIV incidence in countries such as Ethiopia, Kenya, and Tanzania, but patterns of change are diverse [21]. In Uganda, for example, there is concern that gains in HIV prevention achieved early on in the epidemic are being reversed [22]. While antenatal HIV prevalence has declined in Kenya in the early part of this century, the trend in antenatal HIV prevalence in Uganda has been upwards [22].

West

West Africa has considerable virologic diversity, with all subtypes and circulating recombinant forms found in this sub-region [2]. Nigeria has the largest HIV epidemic in the sub-region, with an estimated adult prevalence of 3.6% and 3.3 million persons living with HIV. Others countries with higher prevalence are Côte d'Ivoire, Ghana, and Togo, countries that have been closely linked by trade and movement of people. Most countries have either stabilizing or decreasing HIV epidemics, although Sierra Leone (1.1% in 2001 to 1.6% in 2009) and Gambia have shown increasing adult HIV prevalence (0.6 to 2.0% in Gambia).

HIV incidence estimates indicate slowing epidemics in many countries in the sub-region, with Côte d'Ivoire, Guinea-Bissau, and Ghana showing the greatest reduction in incident infections. With the reduction of incidence (and prevalence) in Guinea-Bissau and other countries with HIV-2, the overall prevalence of HIV-2 is also decreasing to less than one million infections worldwide [2]. Data from Côte d'Ivoire also illustrate a reduction in behaviors related to HIV transmission among men and women with decreasing HIV prevalence, including among young women 15–24 years attending antenatal clinics [21]. The lower prevalence of HIV infection in West Africa than in other sub-regions is likely to be due in part to high rates of male circumcision [23].

Central

Cameroon and the Democratic Republic of Congo (DRC) have the greatest HIV-1 genetic diversity in the world, with nearly all subtypes and CRF in these countries. HIV prevalence in this sub-region is stabilizing, with some countries experiencing a decrease in incident infections. Cameroon has the greatest number of persons infected (610,000), with an overall adult HIV prevalence of 5.3%. The Republic of Congo shows the lowest adult HIV prevalence, 3.4%. Incidence estimates in the region show decreasing new infections in the Central African Republic, Congo, and Gabon [1]. Data from surveillance in antenatal clinics in the DRC also illustrate declining prevalence among antenatal clinic attendees from 2004 to 2009 [24].

Europe

There were an estimated 2.2 million people living with HIV in WHO's European Region whose countries have HIV and AIDS case reporting systems of varying completeness. A total of 53,427 cases of HIV were diagnosed and reported from 49 of the 53 countries in the WHO European Region in 2009 (case surveillance data were not available from Austria, Monaco, Russia, and Turkey). There were a total of 6,568 AIDS cases reported in 2009 (Austria, Sweden, Monaco, Russia, and Turkey did not report) and 1,776 cases diagnosed with AIDS were reported to have died, almost half the AIDS-related deaths reported in 2008 [25]. The three sub-regions within Europe have differing epidemics, with Eastern Europe experiencing increasing HIV incidence related to injection drug use; HIV epidemics in the central and western sub-regions seem to be stable with HIV infection rates remaining similar over the past five years.

West

In 2009, 24,703 cases of HIV infection were newly diagnosed from 21 of 23 countries in the sub-region, a rate of 6.7 per 100,000. Seventy-two percent of cases diagnosed were among males and 10% of cases were in persons 15–24 years old. Nearly half (40%) of the cases diagnosed with HIV in 2009 resulted from heterosexual transmission, many of which were in persons originating from sub-Saharan Africa. The remaining cases diagnosed were among men who have sex with men (37%), among whom rates have consistently increased since 2004, and 4% were among injecting drug users in whom rates have been steadily declining. Less than 1% of cases were the result of perinatal transmission, transfusions, or nosocomial infections. A total of 4,361 AIDS cases were diagnosed in 2009 from 20 of 23 countries in the western sub-region, with an overall AIDS rate of 1.1 per 100,000 [25].

East

In 2009, 27,112 HIV cases were diagnosed and reported from 14 of the 15 countries in the eastern sub-region (Russia did not report, and the reported data therefore represent a serious underestimate of the sub-region's epidemic). Fewer than half the cases (41%) were among females and 14% among 15–24 year olds. Although 46% of cases diagnosed in 2009 identified heterosexual transmission as the mode of transmission, this may be an underestimate because of unrecognized or unreported sexual transmission from partners who inject drugs, such as in Georgia and Azerbaijan [25].

Overall, heterosexual transmission has increased since 2004 along with the overall rate of new HIV reports in the sub-region (11.3 per 100,000 in 2004 and 18.9 in 2009). Injection drug use accounted for 39% of reported cases while perinatal transmission and transmission among men who have sex with men accounted for less than 3% of the cases; perinatal transmission has doubled in the past two years, and male-to-male transmission has also increased although the reported numbers remain relatively small. In 2009, a total of 1803 AIDS cases were diagnosed from 13 of the 14 countries, with an overall AIDS rate of 1.3 per 100,000. Underreporting from countries in this sub-region is substantial and data presented are an underestimate [25].

Recent results from epidemic modeling suggest that the HIV epidemic in Russia (1% HIV prevalence in 2009)

has doubled since 2001, with most infections among drug injectors. HIV prevalence among high-risk populations in Moscow show elevated prevalence among injection drug users (15.6%), men who have sex with men (8.3%), and female sex workers (4.5%) [1]. With an estimated 1.8 million injection drug users in Russia, the HIV epidemic among this population is increasing and an important public health challenge since HIV-infected drug injectors can drive secondary transmission to sex partners and children as a result of mother-to-child transmission [18].

Central

A total of 1,612 cases of HIV were diagnosed in 2009 (all 14 countries reporting); a rate of 1.4 per 100,000. The majority of cases diagnosed were among males (80%) and 19% of the cases were in persons between 15 and 24 years of age. Of the cases reported with risk factor information (63%), one-third identified male-to-male sex as the mode of transmission, which represents a doubling since 2004. Heterosexual transmission remained relatively stable since 2004 (24% of cases) while injection drug use increased 157% since 2004 (8% of cases), though the absolute number of injection drug use cases remain small. A total of 404 AIDS cases were diagnosed in 2009 from 14 of the 15 countries in the central sub-region, with an overall AIDS rate of 0.3 per 100,000.

North America

United States

With an estimated 1.1 million people living with HIV, the United States is the most heavily affected country in the industrialized world [26, 27]. In the 40 states that have stable HIV reporting systems, the rate of HIV diagnoses was 17.4 per 100,000 in 2009 [27]. AIDS reporting from all 50 states shows an AIDS diagnosis rate of 11.2 per 100,000 in 2009. In 2008, the death rate of persons with HIV (the cause of death may or may not have been HIV-related) was 7.0 per 100,000 population, a rate that has been stable since 2006. Deaths in persons reported with AIDS were 5.3 per 100,000, a 7% annual decrease from 2006.

The overall rate of HIV diagnoses seems to have stabilized since 2006 with an estimated 42,000 diagnoses per year. Males account for 76% of HIV diagnoses, with a rate of 32.7 per 100,000, constant since 2006, while the rate of diagnoses among women has slightly decreased to 9.8 per 100,000 in 2009. There has been an increase in HIV diagnoses among younger age groups (15–19 and 20–24 years) as well as in the older age group of 55–59 years. HIV diagnoses among children less than 13 years due to perinatal transmission continued to decrease, with an estimated 131 children diagnosed in 2009, maintaining the precipitous decline in mother-to-child transmission of

Table 1.2 Diagnoses of HIV Infection among adults and adolescents, 2009—40 states and 5 US dependent areas

	No.	%
Transmission category		
Male-to-male sexual category	24,312	56.4
Injection drug use	4,172	9.7
Male-to-male sexual contact and IDU	1,157	2.7
Heterosexual contact[a]	13,257	31.0
Other[b]	75	0.2
Race/ethnicity		
American Indian/Alaska Native	91	0.04
Asian	293	1.2
Black/African American	10,135	42.0
Hispanic/Latino[c]	4,692	19.4
Native Hawaiian/Other Pacific Islander	22	0.1
White	8,613	35.7
Multiple races	287	1.2

Source: Centers of Disease Control and Prevention. HIV Surveillance Report, 2009; vol 21. http://www.cdc.gov/hiv/topics/surveillance/resources/reports. Published February 2011. Accessed April 9, 2011.
Note: Data include persons with a diagnosis of HIV infection regardless of stage of disease at diagnosis. All displayed data have been statistically adjusted to account for reporting delays and missing risk-factor Information, but not for incomplete reporting.
[a]Heterosexual contact with a person known to have, or to be at high risk for, HIV infection.
[b]Includes hemophilia, blood transfusion, perinatal exposure, and risk factor not reported or not identified.
[c]Hispanics/Latinos can be of any race.

HIV infections, their rate (7.2 per 100,000) was about nine times lower than that in African Americans; the lowest overall rate of reported HIV infections was in Asians (6.4 per 100,000) (Table 1.2). In 2008, 33% of people diagnosed with HIV also received an AIDS diagnosis within one year, indicating HIV is being diagnosed relatively late.

Canada

The HIV epidemic seems to be stable in Canada, with approximately 65,000 people estimated to be living with HIV. The majority of new infections are among men who have sex with men and heterosexuals from HIV endemic countries. The indigenous Aboriginal population is disproportionately affected [28].

Latin America and the Caribbean

Caribbean

There are an estimated 240,000 people living with HIV in the Caribbean region. With an estimated prevalence of HIV infection of 1%, the Caribbean is the second highest burdened region in the world. Overall, more women (53%) are estimated to be living with HIV than men, but this is greatly influenced by the epidemic in Haiti where 61% of infections are among women. The Bahamas has the highest estimated adult HIV prevalence in the region, 3.1%, although there has been a decrease in HIV prevalence among 15- to 24-year-old pregnant women in the past 10 years [1, 21]. Other countries in the region have less than 2% prevalence. Most countries in the Caribbean have concentrated epidemics with elevated HIV prevalence in key populations including sex workers and men who have sex with men [29]. Haiti stands out as an exception, having been affected earliest and demonstrating a predominantly heterosexual epidemic. AIDS-related deaths have decreased in the sub-region since 2001 by 37%, with an estimated 12,000 AIDS-related deaths in 2009 [1].

Central and South America

There are an estimated 1.4 million people living with HIV in Latin America, slightly higher than in 2001, with an estimated adult HIV prevalence of 0.5%. However, there has been a reduction in new infections since 2001, down to 92,000 new infections in 2009. Belize has the highest adult HIV prevalence (2.3%), with most countries having a prevalence below 1%. Over half of HIV-infected persons reside in three countries: Brazil, Argentina, and Columbia. In most of the countries in the sub-region HIV prevalence is slightly higher among young males than young females, with the exception of Belize and Guyana. Similar to the

HIV since the 1990s. Male-to-male sex accounted for over half of the new cases diagnosed in 2009 followed by heterosexual contact (31%) and injection drug use (Table 1.2).

Over half of HIV diagnoses in 2009 were among African Americans, with a rate of 66.6 per 100,000, the highest rate across all racial and ethnic groups. The second most highly affected group by race or ethnicity were Hispanics and Latinos who accounted for 17% of infections with a rate of 22.8 per 100,000. Although whites accounted for 28% of

Caribbean and North America, the epidemic is concentrated among high-risk populations.

HIV seroprevalence surveys in capital cities show elevated prevalence specifically among men who have sex with men and female sex workers. Georgetown, Guyana, has the highest HIV prevalence among female sex workers (16.6%), followed by San Salvador (4.1%). Prevalence among men who have sex with men is also higher than in the general population; in recent surveys their prevalence ranged from 20.3% in Santiago, Chile, to 4.2% in Nicaragua [1].

More data are also available on population size estimates for high-risk groups. For example, in El Salvador there are an estimated 12,500 men who have sex with men (3.4% of men) and 7000 female sex workers (1.4% of women)[30]. Triangulating the population size estimates for high-risk groups with their HIV prevalence estimates provides valuable insights into the risks and prevention needs of male and female partners and clients of sex workers.

Asia

Overall an estimated 4.9 million people are living with HIV in the Asia region, for an estimated stable HIV prevalence in adults of 0.4%. HIV incidence in Asia appears to have decreased slightly from 2001 to 360,000 new infections annually, with an estimated 300,000 total AIDS-related deaths in 2009. Overall more men are infected with HIV (66% of all infections) in this region, although HIV infections among women seem to be increasing. Thailand has the highest adult prevalence in the region, estimated at 1.3%, indicating about 520,000 persons living with HIV, lower than the 1.7% prevalence estimated for 2001. India accounts for almost half of all HIV infections in the region, with 2.4 million persons living with HIV, which represents an adult HIV prevalence of 0.3%. HIV infection in the region is primarily concentrated among high-risk groups including injection drug users, sex workers and their clients, and men who have sex with men, although there is great variation regionally in the contribution to the epidemic from specific risk groups [1].

South and Southeast Asia

HIV epidemics in this region of Asia are mainly among injection drug users, female sex workers, and their clients. Although HIV prevalence estimates remain low, the increase in the estimated numbers or persons living with HIV suggests there may be emerging, concentrated epidemics in countries like Bangladesh, Nepal, Pakistan, and the Philippines. Other countries, such as Cambodia, Myanmar, and Thailand exhibit decreasing HIV prevalence. In 2009, Cambodia had an estimated 0.5% adult HIV prevalence (56,000

adults living with HIV), which was lower than the 1.2% adult prevalence in 2001. AIDS-related deaths decreased by almost half in 2009 to 3100 deaths among adults and children. In contrast HIV prevalence has increased in Indonesia where there are now 300,000 adults living with HIV for a prevalence of 0.2%. Although the majority of infections are among high-risk groups, there are geographic differences and in the general population of Tanah Papau the prevalence was 2.4% [31]. Indonesia, like many other countries in the sub-region, has a high HIV prevalence among injection drug users in the capital city (52.4% in 2007), as do Thailand (38.7%, 2009), Myanmar (36.3%, 2008), Cambodia (24.4%, 2007), and Pakistan and Nepal (21%) [1].

East Asia

There are an estimated 770,000 persons living with HIV in the five countries of East Asia, with 96% of the infections in China, which represents an adult HIV prevalence of 0.1%, the highest in the sub-region. Although females only account for 32% of infections the proportion has been increasing since 2001, along with the overall increasing prevalence in China. The rate of new infections seems to be stabilizing, with an estimated 48,000 new infections in 2009. Modes of transmission have been changing over the years, with most recent estimates showing a small increase in the proportion of men who have sex with men infected. Given the vast size of China, there are important geographic variations, with six provinces carrying over 70% of the disease burden (Yunnan, Guangxi, Henan, Sichuan, Xinjiang, and Guangdong) [32]. Estimated AIDS-related deaths were 26,000 in 2009, suggesting a stabilization of mortality in recent years.

Central Asia and Middle East

In 2009 there were an estimated 60,000 people living with HIV in the Central Asia sub-region, with HIV prevalence apparently increasing among certain populations, especially injection drug users [33]. Adult HIV prevalence in 2009 was highest in Kyrgyzstan at 0.3% and lowest in Uzbekistan and Kazakhstan at 0.1%. There are an estimated 247,500 injection drug users in Central Asia, with HIV prevalence ranging from 17.6% in Dushanbe to 2.9% in Astana [18].

The HIV epidemic in the Middle East (including countries in North Africa) remains the lowest burdened in the world, concentrated among certain risk groups, primarily injection drug users and men who have sex with men [34]. Sudan has the highest prevalence in the sub-region, with an estimated 260,000 people living with HIV, which accounts for over half of the estimated 460,000 in the entire sub-region [1].

REFERENCES

[1] UNAIDS. Global Report: UNAIDS Report on the Global AIDS Epidemic 2010. http://www.unaids.org/globalreport/; Published November 2010 [accessed 09.04.11].

[2] Tebit D, Arts E. Tracking a century of global expansion and evolution of HIV to understand and to combat disease. Lancet Infect Dis 2011;11:45–56.

[3] Diaz T, Garcia-Calleja JM, Ghys P, Sabin K. Advances and future directions in HIV surveillance in low and middle income countries. Curr Opin HIV AIDS 2009;4:253–9.

[4] Karon JM, Song R, Brookmeyer R, et al. Estimating HIV incidence in the United States from HIV/AIDS surveillance data and biomarker HIV test results. Stat Med 2008;300:520–9.

[5] Hallett T. Estimating the HIV incidence rate: recent and future developments. Curr Opin HIV AIDS 2011;6:102–7.

[6] WHO/UNAIDS. Technical guidelines for conducting HIV sentinel serosurveys among pregnant women and other groups. Geneva: UNAIDS/WHO Working Group on Global HIV/AIDS and STI Surveillance; 2003. Available at: http://data.unaids.org/publications/irc-pub06/jc954-anc-serosurveys_guidelines_en.pdf.

[7] Garcia-Calleja JM, Jacobson J, Garg R, Thuy N, et al. Has the quality of serosurveillance in low- and middle-income countries improved since the last HIV estimates round in 2007? Status and trends through 2009. Sex Transm Infect 2010;86 (Suppl. 2):ii.35–ii.42.

[8] Johnston LG, Malekinejad M, Kendall C, et al. Implementation challenges to using respondent driven sampling methodology for HIV biological and behavioral surveillance: field experience in international settings. AIDS Behav 2008;12(Suppl. 4):S105–S130.

[9] World Health Organization. WHO case definitions of HIV for surveillance and revised clinical staging and immunological classification of HIV-related disease

in adults and children. Switzerland: World Health Organization; 2007.

[10] Centers for Disease Control and Prevention. Revised surveillance case definitions for HIV infection among adults, adolescents, and children aged <18 months and for HIV infection and AIDS among children aged 18 months to <13 years—United States, 2008. MMWR 2008;57(No. RR-10).

[11] Hall HI. Estimation of HIV incidence in the United States. JAMA 2008;300:520–9.

[12] Ghys P, Garnett G. The 2009 HIV and AIDS estimates and projections: methods, tools and analyses. Sex Transm Infect 2010;86(Suppl. 2).

[13] Boily MC, Baggaley RF, Wang L, et al. Heterosexual risk of HIV-1 infection per sexual act: systematic review and meta-analysis of observational studies. Lancet Infect Dis 2009;9:118–29.

[14] Gray RH, Kigozi G, Serwadda D, et al. Male circumcision for HIV prevention in men in Rakai, Uganda: a randomised trial. Lancet 2007;369:657–66.

[15] Miller WC, Rosenberg NE, Rutstein SE, Powers KA. Role of acute and early HIV infection in the sexual transmission of HIV. Curr Opin HIV AIDS 2010;5 (4):277–82.

[16] van Griensven F, van Wijngaarden JW, Baral S, Grulich AE. The global epidemic of HIV infection among men who have sex with men. Curr Opin HIV AIDS 2009;4:300–7.

[17] De Cock KM, Fowler MG, Mercier E, et al. Prevention of mother-to-child HIV transmission in resource-poor countries: translating research into policy and practice. JAMA 2000;283:1175–82.

[18] Mathers BM, Degenhardt L, Phillips B, et al. Global epidemiology of injecting drug use and HIV among people who inject drugs: a systematic review. Lancet 2008;372:1733–45.

[19] Bell DM. Occupational risk of human immunodeficiency virus infection in healthcare workers: an

overview. Curr Opin HIV AIDS 2011;6(2):102–7.

[20] Strand RT, Dias FL, Bergstrom S, Anderson S. Unexpected low prevalence of HIV among fertile women in Luanda, Angola. Does war prevent the spread of HIV. Int J STD AIDS 2007;18:467–71.

[21] The International Group on Analysis of Trends in HIV Prevalence and Behaviors in Young People in Countries Most Affected by HIV. Trends in HIV prevalence sexual behaviors in young people aged 15-24 years in countries most affected by HIV. Sex Transm Infect 2010;86:ii.72–ii.83.

[22] Kim AA, Hallett T, Stover J, et al. Estimating HIV incidence among adults in Kenya and Uganda: a systematic comparison of multiple methods. PLoS One 2011;6(3): e17535.

[23] Orroth KK, Freeman EE, Bakar R, et al. Understanding the differences between contrasting HIV epidemics in east and west Africa: results from a simulation model of the Four Cities Study. Sex Transm Infect 2007;83:i.5–i.16.

[24] Behets F, Edmonds A, Kitenge F, et al. Heterogeneous and decreasing HIV prevalence among women seeking antenatal care in Kinshasa, Democratic Republic of Congo. Int J Epidemiol 2010;39:1066–73.

[25] European Centre for Disease Prevention and Control/WHO Regional Office for Europe. HIV/AIDS surveillance in Europe 2009. Stockholm: European Centre for Disease Prevention and Control; 2010.

[26] Campsmith M, Rhodes P, Hall HI, Greene T. Undiagnosed HIV prevalence among adults and adolescents in the United States at the end of 2006. J Acquir Immune Defic Syndr 2010;53:619–24.

[27] Centers of Disease Control and Prevention. HIV Surveillance Report, 2009, vol. 21. Published February 2011. http://www.cdc.gov/hiv/topics/surveillance/resources/reports 2011 [accessed 09.04.11].

[28] Public Health Agency of Canada. HIV and AIDS in Canada. Surveillance Report to December 31, 2009. Surveillance and Risk Assessment Division, Centre for Communicable Diseases and Infection Control, Public Health Agency of Canada; 2010.

[29] Figueroa P. The HIV epidemic in the Caribbean: meeting the challenges of achieving universal access to prevention, treatment and care. West Indian Med J 2008;57 (3):195.

[30] Paz-Bailey G, Jacobson JO, Guardado ME, et al. How many men who have sex with men and female sex workers live in El Salvador? Using respondent-driven sampling and capture-recapture to estimate population sizes. Sex Transm Infect 2011; doi:10.1136/ sti.2010.045633.

[31] Yeane Irmanigrum S, Siahaan T, Ruslam P, et al. Risk Behavior and HIV Prevalence in Tanah Papua 2006: Results of the IBBS 2006 in Tanah Papua. BNPP Publication; 2006.

[32] Ministry of Health, People's Republic of China, Joint United Nations Programme on HIV/AIDS, World Health Organization. Estimates for the HIV/AIDS epidemic in China, Published May 31, 2010. Available at: http://www. unaids.org.cn/download/2009% 20China%20Estimation% 20Report-En.pdf; 2010.

[33] Thorne C, Ferencic N, Malyuta R, et al. Central Asia: hotspot in the worldwide epidemic. Lancet Infect Dis 2010;10:479–88.

[34] Abu-Raddad LJ, Hilmi N, Mumtaz G, et al. Epidemiology of HIV infection in the Middle East and North Africa. AIDS 2010;24 (Suppl. 2):S5–23.

Chapter | 2 |

The origins and diversification of HIV

Michael Worobey, Guan-Zhu Han

INTRODUCTION

Human immunodeficiency virus (HIV) is not one but several related viruses that have crossed into the human population on multiple occasions from non-human primate reservoir species in Africa. Only one such lineage, the "main" group of HIV type 1 (HIV-1 group M), has reached pandemic proportions; it accounts for more than 99% of the more than 40 million HIV infections and has a global distribution. The other HIVs, though relatively minor, hold important clues about the nature of the origins and diversification of this important group. This chapter will begin with a broad scope, surveying the primate lentivirus radiation and placing the various HIV groups within it. It will then focus specifically on the genesis of HIV-1 group M, summarizing when, where, and how this most important HIV variant originated, diversified, and spread around the world. An important goal of this chapter will be to bring into sharp relief the biological meaning and medical relevance of the various levels of HIV genetic diversity commonly recognized ("types," "groups," "subtypes," and so on). Understanding what such classifications do and do not represent is critical to any rational approach to exploiting knowledge about viral evolution in order to combat HIV/AIDS.

THE DEEP ROOTS OF HIV

Phylogenetic trees, reconstructed using the remarkably rich historical information stamped into the genomes of these viruses, have emerged as the pre-eminent tools for reconstructing the history of HIV and simian immunodeficiency virus (SIV). The genealogical patterns that emerge from phylogenies provide not only an invaluable historical record but also a window through which we can glimpse the medically relevant evolutionary and epidemiological processes that generated the patterns. Gene trees also offer a framework for systematizing the extensive genetic diversity of HIV and related viruses into a coherent classification scheme. With any organism's classification, however, there is a danger of becoming fixated on *pattern* rather than *process*, and HIV is no exception. Some of the potential pitfalls of doing so are discussed below.

AIDS was first recognized in the USA in the early 1980s [1], and the discovery of HIV followed soon after [2]. It is now clear, however, that HIV emerged decades earlier, from naturally infected primates on another continent [3]. Figure 2.1 illustrates the relationships between the different variants of HIV and related viruses that have been discovered in a large number of African monkeys and apes. To date, over 40 species of non-human primates have shown evidence of infection by SIV [4], every one of which is restricted in range to sub-Saharan Africa. Since the primate lentiviruses form a single, distinct clade on the mammalian lentivirus phylogeny, and given that no primates outside of Africa appear to be infected, SIV evidently had its origin in an African monkey at some point sufficiently deep in time to account for its spread throughout most of the continent, and into most of the (catarrhine) primate species there.

Unlike HIV, natural SIV infections generally cause little illness in their hosts and most are thought to be non-pathogenic. The low pathogenicity has been well documented in African green monkeys and sooty mangabeys. However, a recent breakthrough demonstrated that wild chimpanzees naturally infected with SIV do develop hallmarks of AIDS-like illness; SIV infection, as with HIV-1

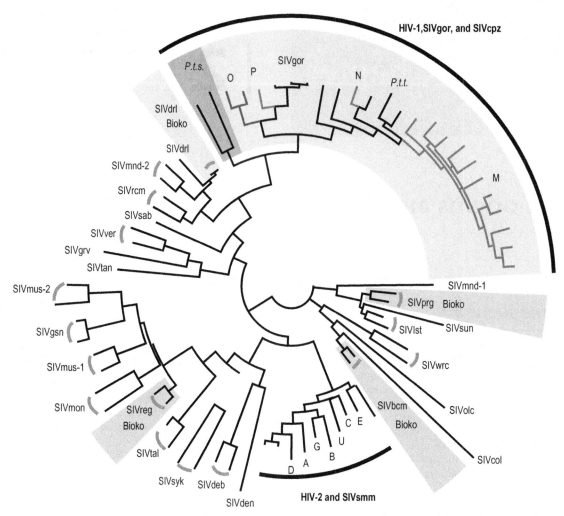

Figure 2.1 Maximum likelihood phylogenetic tree of SIV and HIV partial pol protein sequences. The sequences were downloaded from the Los Alamos National Laboratories HIV database (http://www.hiv.lanl.gov). The phylogenetic tree was reconstructed under the Jones-Taylor-Thornton (JTT) model of amino acid substitution with gamma distributed with invariant sites. SIVcpz strains recovered from *Pan troglodytes troglodytes* (*P.t.t.*) and SIVgor strains from Gorilla gorilla are lightly shaded, while those from *P. t. schweinfurthii* (*P.t.s.*) are darkly shaded. The SIV strains isolated from Bioko island are lightly shaded. The abbreviations and species names are as follows: SIVdrl, drill; SIVmnd-1 and SIVmnd-2, mandrill; SIVrcm, red-capped mangabey; SIVsab, green monkey; SIVgrv, grivet; SIVtan, tantalus monkey; SIVver, vervet monkey; SIVmus-1 and SIVmus-2, mustached guenon; SIVgsn, greater spot-nosed monkey; SIVmon, mona monkey; SIVreg, red-eared guenon; SIVtal, talapoin; SIVsyk, Sykes's monkey; SIVdeb, De Brazza's monkey; SIVden, Dent's mona; SIVbcm, black colobus monkey; SIVcol, colobus monkey; SIVolc, olive colobus; SIVwrc, western red colobus; SIVlst, L'Hoest's monkey; SIVsun, sun-tailed monkey; SIVprg, Preuss's guenon; SIVsmm, sooty mangabey; SIVcpz, common chimpanzee; SIVgor, gorilla.

and HIV-2 infection, is associated with progressive CD4 cell loss, lymphatic tissue destruction, and premature death [5]. *Pan troglodytes schweinfurthii* infected with SIV in Gombe National Park in Tanzania have a markedly higher death rate than non-infected animals [5].

The precise nature of the time scale of SIV evolution is still open to question. Initially, comparisons of primate and virus phylogenies led to suggestions that some SIVs have

co-diverged with their primate hosts, as the animals split into new species from their common ancestors. However, the pattern of closely related hosts having closely related viruses might be explained not by co-divergence but by cross-species transmission events occurring preferentially between closely related hosts [6]. For example, detailed phylogenetic analysis shows that recent cross-species transmission events, instead of ancient co-divergence, likely underlie the fact that three closely related hominoid primates (human, chimpanzees, and gorillas) harbor closely related lentiviruses [7]. Studies of genes involved in innate immunity, such as *APOBEC3G* [8], suggest just the sort of mechanism that could generate such a pattern of correspondence even if the viruses and their hosts did not co-diverge.

Hence, even at this advanced stage of the investigation of one of the most medically important pathogens, until recently there has been little agreement on whether its progenitors have been circulating in African primates for millions or just thousands of years. A recent study, however, revealed evidence for several SIV lineages endemic to Bioko Island, Equatorial Guinea. This island was isolated from Africa as sea level rose 10,000 to 12,000 years ago. Notably, each of Bioko's four SIV lineages is most closely related to a virus circulating in hosts of the same genus on the African mainland rather than to the SIVs of other Bioko species (Fig. 2.1). This phylogeographic approach established that SIV is ancient—at least 32,000 years old [9].

The discovery of an endogenous lentivirus in the genome of the gray mouse lemur (*Microcebus murinus*) also suggests a time scale of millions of years for primate lentiviruses [10]. On the other hand, molecular clock methods calibrated by using modern sequences make it hard to conceive of dates older than a few thousand years for the SIV MRCA [11, 12]. Extrapolations from the rapid short-term evolutionary rates observed in lentiviruses [13] suggest that, for SIV lineages that diverged more than even a few thousand years ago, the molecular evidence of shared ancestry ought to have become overwritten by a succession of nucleotide substitutions. Clearly, more work is still needed to resolve this conundrum, including developing new models of sequence evolution that incorporate the idiosyncrasies of RNA virus evolution. Nevertheless, it is now very clear that SIV is no newcomer; these viruses have almost certainly been circulating for tens of thousands of years at least, raising the obvious question: what changed within the past hundred years that allowed multiple SIV lineages to successfully establish themselves in the human population?

HIV/SIV NOMENCLATURE

Of the dozens of species with naturally occurring SIV, just three, the common chimpanzee (*Pan troglodytes*), the gorilla (*Gorilla gorilla*), and the sooty mangabey (*Cercocebus atys*), are the putative reservoirs of HIV. HIV type 1 (HIV-1) is the designation given to forms of the human virus linked to SIV from *P. troglodytes* (SIVcpz) and *G. gorilla* (SIVgor), while HIV type 2 (HIV-2) denotes human viruses related to the sooty mangabey virus (SIVsmm). Inspection of the SIV/HIV phylogenetic tree shows that, within both SIVcpz/SIVsmm and SIVsmm, more than one cross-species transmission event has occurred (Fig. 2.1). The key observation here is

that HIV lineages intermingle on the tree with SIV lineages. HIV-1 groups N and M are both more closely related to some of the SIVcpz viruses on the tree than they are to HIV-1 group O, whose lineage branched off the main trunk at an earlier point. In other words, HIV-1 group M shared a most recent common ancestor with a chimpanzee virus, not with HIV-1 group O. HIV-1 groups P and O are most closely related to SIVgor [7, 14]. Likewise, HIV-2 group E is the "sister" group to one SIVsmm strain, and HIV-2 group A is the sister group of another. If there had been only a single transmission from each reservoir species to humans, we would expect the human viruses to fall into single clusters (or monophyletic clades, in the jargon of phylogenetics)—one for HIV-1 and one for HIV-2. This is not the case.

Recombination, whereby genes from separate strains are combined into a new, chimeric viral genome within a dually infected host, complicates these phylogenetic inferences somewhat. For example, HIV-1 group N (or its SIV precursor), though closely related to HIV-1 group M in the *pol* region (Fig. 2.1), apparently arose from a recombination event [15]: some of its genome is much more distantly related to group M [16]. Such complications aside, the HIV lineages depicted in Fig. 2.1 are thought to have arisen from an independent cross-species transmission, and hence each of these groups is thought to be more closely related to either SIVcpz or SIVsmm than to the other groups in its type.

So, while the different *types* of HIV denote the different primate reservoirs that have served as sources of human infection, the various *groups* within each type represent putative independent introductions from primate to human. Within HIV-1, at least four such events are inferred, giving rise to HIV-1 groups M, O [17], N [15], and P [14]. Within HIV-2, eight independent transmissions are indicated, corresponding to HIV-2 groups A through H [3, 18]. Earlier studies of HIV-2 used the term *subtype* for these lineages, but this usage has given way to the use of the term *group* in order to bring HIV-2 nomenclature in line with the more widely cited (if slightly less logical) HIV-1 conventions [18]. The goal of the change was to emphasize the biological parallel between the different lineages of HIV-1 and HIV-2 that arose via unique zoonotic origins. In this sense, HIV nomenclature reflects rather well the evolutionary processes driving observed patterns of genetic diversity.

The term *subtype*, in turn, is used within HIV-1 group M. Each of the branches in the M group in Fig. 2.1 represents one of the recognized subtypes (A to D, F to H, J, K). Different subtypes dominate in different regions. For example, subtype B accounts for most infections in Europe and the Americas, subtype C predominates in southern African countries like South Africa, as well as in India, and subtype D is common in east Africa. The unfortunate fact that *subtypes* are nested within *groups*, rather than *types*, in this naming scheme, owes to the fact that the use of the term predates the discovery of HIV-1 group O, at which point the new designation of *group* had to be wedged between *type* and *subtype*. The system of naming HIVs and SIVs has thus evolved over time as the full diversity of natural SIV infections in African primates was revealed, and as new, distinct lineages of HIV have been discovered.

As hinted above, recombination plays a large role in the evolution of both SIV and HIV [19]. The existence of clear recombinants, with genomes that are mosaics of distinct lineages, has led to the introduction of a formal system for recognizing them [20]. These *circulating recombinant forms* (CRFs) represent virus populations that have diversified from a single, ancestral strain generated by recombination between two or more of the recognized M group subtypes [20]. The "missing" subtypes, E and I, have been re-classified as CRFs after detailed analysis of their genomes revealed that they had recombinant origins [20]. Some CRFs are the dominant HIV-1 group M strain in some locales (e.g. CRF01 in Thailand, CRF02 in Nigeria).

There is also abundant evidence of recombination among the SIVs of different primate species, and even between HIV-1 groups M and O [21]. Most notably, the progenitor of HIV-1, SIVcpz, turns out to be a recombinant between the SIVs of red-capped mangabeys and greater spot-nosed monkeys, two prey species of the chimpanzee [22]. All strains of HIV-1 are thus ultimately recombinant in origin, their genomes a mosaic of two monkey viruses, trafficked through an ape intermediary.

In summary, the primate lentivirus phylogenetic tree and the system of HIV nomenclature reflect some key evolutionary insights. First, SIVs are naturally found in a variety of sub-Saharan African primates and this region is hence the cradle of HIV. Second, despite the many primates infected, and frequent opportunities for human exposure, as far as is known SIV has only crossed successfully into humans from chimpanzees, gorillas, and sooty mangabeys, but has crossed multiple times from each, a curious pattern for which no definitive explanation has been proposed. Finally, the virus that first appeared on the medical world's radar in high-risk populations in the USA made an extraordinary journey there: from African monkeys, then to the apes that preyed upon them, then onto human beings in central Africa and beyond.

WHERE DID HIV ENTER THE HUMAN POPULATION?

Using the geographic distributions of the primate species that have spawned HIV variants it has been possible to infer, with remarkable precision, the specific areas in Africa where the various HIV-1 and HIV-2 groups originated. HIV-2 was the first to give up its secrets, and by the early 1990s it was clear that different groups of HIV-2 were independently derived from SIVsmm, the SIV variant endemic in the sooty mangabey monkeys of West Africa [23]. HIV-2 is endemic to the same region, and is only rarely detected elsewhere. Although HIV-2 accounts for relatively few infections compared with HIV-1, many more cross-species transmissions involving this virus have been detected, with eight groups (A–H) currently recognized. Only two of these, groups A and B, appear to have established themselves as endemic human infections. In all the other cases, the "group" is in fact composed of a single patient infected with an HIV-2 variant that is sufficiently genetically divergent from the others that it was likely acquired independently. Some or all of these may represent evolutionary "dead ends [24]." In some cases, the human virus bears a surprisingly close resemblance to SIVsmm, infecting free-living or pet sooty mangabeys from the same local area [24, 25], strong evidence of repeated independent cross-species transmission.

The geographical origins of HIV-1 have taken longer to piece together, but it now seems clear that all four HIV-1 groups, as well as SIVgor, form a monophyletic cluster with SIVcpz from *P. troglodytes troglodytes*, the "central" chimpanzee, whose range encompasses southern Cameroon, Central African Republic, Equatorial Guinea, Gabon, and the Republic of Congo (Congo-Brazzaville) [3, 16, 26, 27]. Although both the central chimpanzee and the "eastern" subspecies, *P. t. schweinfurthii*, are naturally infected with SIVcpz, the viruses recovered from the two chimpanzee lineages form distinct clades on the SIV phylogenetic tree (Fig. 2.1), indicating that they have been evolving in isolation for a considerable time.

While two instances of cross-species transmission from chimpanzees to humans (HIV-1 groups M and N) are unequivocally phylogenetically linked to the SIVcpz of the *P. t. troglodytes* chimpanzee, HIV-1 groups O and P fall within the radiation of SIVcpz strains but are mostly closed to SIVgor of *G. gorilla* (Fig. 2.1). It remains unclear whether gorillas were the immediate source of either or both of HIV-1 groups O and P. No known variant of HIV-1 has emerged from the eastern chimpanzee (dark shading in Fig. 2.1). HIV-1 groups N, O, and P are all endemic to Cameroon, within the range of *P. t. troglodytes*, and none have spread substantially beyond this presumptive region of origin. Group O exhibits about 0.4% prevalence in Cameroon [28], group N is exceedingly rare, with less than 10 infected individuals identified to date [29], and group P infections are also extremely rare, accounting for only 0.06% of HIV infections [30]. Despite the relative rarity of groups N and O, their pathogenic profile appears indistinguishable from group M's [28], an indication that *pathogenic* potential and *epidemic* behavior of AIDS viruses are not necessarily coupled [18]. Since group P was identified only recently, little is known on its pathogenic profile.

Given the very different properties of the four groups, M, O, N, and P, in terms of rate of spread through human host populations, it is tempting to speculate that their pathogenic properties may owe more to their common genetic heritage, as close relatives descended from SIVcpz, than to convergent evolutionary trajectories once they entered humans.

The discovery of the first rare variant of HIV-2 known to cause immunosuppression lends support to this notion [18], but future studies will be required to further clarify the ground rules of the evolution of HIV pathogenicity.

The geographical source of the main group of HIV-1 has been somewhat obscured by its global spread, but the available evidence links it to the same region. Group M falls soundly among the diverse viruses of the *P. t. troglodytes* chimpanzees—powerful evidence that it emerged from within their range [16]. By screening non-invasively collected fecal samples from the region, Beatrice Hahn and colleagues have identified several closely related SIVcpz strains from wild-living Cameroonian chimpanzees, viruses that are remarkably similar to group M, and which form a well-supported cluster with it on phylogenetic trees. These analyses pinpoint the probable source of the viruses that gave rise to the HIV-1 group M pandemic as being chimpanzees in southeastern Cameroon [31]. From there, the virus likely made its way, perhaps diffusing along the Sangha River and then down the Congo River, to Kinshasa [32]. While the fuse was evidently lit in rural southeastern Cameroon, the truly explosive growth of the pandemic was likely linked to its arrival in the region's largest city.

WHEN DID HIV ENTER THE HUMAN POPULATION?

It has been said that RNA viruses represent a "moving target," and the point is well taken. HIV has been measured directly and found to have an error rate as high as 10^{-4} mutations per site and two to three recombination events per genome per replication cycle. The high error rate of its reverse transcriptase, plus its high replication rate, mean that mutations rapidly arise and accumulate, making HIV one of the fastest evolving organisms in nature.

Generally, the longer the time span since two HIV sequences diverged from a common ancestor, the greater the number of nucleotide differences we expect when we compare their homologous gene sequences. Although different regions of the genome evolve at different rates [33], and a strict "molecular clock" is often rejected with HIV molecular data sets [13], this observation means that illuminating inferences about the timing of HIV evolution can often be culled from alignments of gene sequences.

Estimates of the time to the most recent common ancestor of each of the four most prevalent HIV groups have been inferred using phylogenetic trees and maximum likelihood and/or Bayesian statistical methods [13, 33, 34]. Behind the sophisticated mathematical models used for such inferences lies a simple concept: if viral nucleotide sequences diverge from each other by, say, 1% per year after they split from a common ancestor, then a pair of sequences that differ by, say, 30% must have diverged about 30 years ago. The tricks with HIV are (1) to correct for multiple changes at the same site—a particular concern with fast-evolving organisms, (2) to calibrate the "molecular clock," and (3) to account adequately for the inherent "sloppiness" of the clock and any potential methodological biases. Fortunately, we can calibrate the clock simply by watching HIV evolve in real time: samples collected over a span of several years will reveal the rate at which substitutions accrue, with early sampled sequences tending to have short branches (less change) and late-sampled sequences tending to have longer branch lengths (more change). As for dealing with the noisy phylogenetic signal, it is important to consider appropriate confidence intervals around estimated divergence dates. A recent study of HIV-1 group O, for example, estimated that its most recent common ancestor existed in 1920, but with a wide confidence interval (1890–1940) [33]. The estimate for group M is 1912 (1884–1924) [32], while those for HIV-2 groups A and B are 1940 (1924–1956) and 1945 (1931–1959), respectively [34]. And although the specter of unaccounted-for recombination biasing such estimates looms over such analyses [35], there is surprisingly little indication that it systematically affects divergence date inferences in one direction or the other [33].

Inferences from more or less contemporary sequences, though, are not the only source of information about historical landmarks in HIV evolution. Arguably the most important HIV-1 sequence published to date is that of ZR59, recovered from an archival blood sample taken from an adult male in 1959 in what is now the Democratic Republic of the Congo (DRC) [36]. Recently we recovered viral sequences (DRC60) from a Bouin's-fixed paraffin-embedded lymph node biopsy specimen obtained in 1960 from an adult female in Kinshasa (DRC) [32]. While ZR59 is basal to subtype D, DRC60 is closet to the ancestral node of subtype A/A1. The genetic distance between ZR59 and DRC60 showed not only that the main group of HIV-1 was already circulating in the human population at this early date but also, more importantly, that this group of viruses must have been circulating for some considerable time *before* this point. Relaxed molecular clock analyses with DRC60 and ZR59 date the MRCA of the M group to near the beginning of the twentieth century, right around the same time that sizeable cities first appeared in the region [32]. It seems likely that the rise of cities, plus the roads, railways, and steamboats that linked their inhabitants into large national and regional social fabrics, played a crucial role in allowing nascent HIVs to establish themselves in human populations at this time.

HIV/AIDS: COLLATERAL DAMAGE FROM UNSAFE MEDICAL PRACTICES?

The phylogenetic position of ZR59 and DRC60 sequences are, on their own, enough to argue convincingly against the controversial theory that HIV-1 group M had its origins in experimental polio vaccines allegedly prepared using SIV-contaminated chimpanzee tissue, then administered across central Africa in the late 1950s [37]. Perhaps more than any other modern human disease, AIDS has inspired impassioned debate about the circumstances surrounding its origins and spread, and the "Oral Polio Vaccine/AIDS" (OPV/AIDS) hypothesis has been one of the most controversial explanations. While the idea was worthy of careful consideration since—at least in later incarnations—it correctly implicated chimpanzees as the source of HIV-1 group M, several lines of evidence have argued strongly against it. First there is the "disconnect" between the inferred M group divergence date (around the turn of the 20th century) and the earliest use of the experimental vaccines (1957), a discrepancy in timing that, as explained in the next section, cannot be resolved by invoking a separate introduction for each subtype [38]. There is also the geographical evidence discussed above: all forms of HIV-1, including the M group, evidently evolved from a *P. t. troglodytes* SIVcpz-like ancestor. The chimpanzees implicated in the OPV/AIDS theory were collected from the Democratic Republic of the Congo. Such *P. t. schweinfurthii* chimpanzees, including ones collected near Kisangani, where the polio vaccine work was centered, are infected by a distant cousin of HIV-1 group M [27, 39], one that is not a plausible M group precursor.

The fact that SIVcpz is a recombinant of two monkey SIVs is also very telling since it puts the lie to the woolly notion that non-natural circumstances such as mass vaccinations are somehow required for the successful transmission of SIV from one species to the next [37]. In fact, the non-human primate SIVs tell a very different story, one where transmission between species is a common, perhaps even dominant, evolutionary process. Recombination events imply a history of cross-species transfers among not only chimpanzees, red-capped mangabeys, and greater spot-nosed monkeys [22] but also others, including green monkeys (*C. sabeus*). Cross-species transmission must also have introduced at least one of the two distinct mandrill SIVs (Fig. 2.1) [40]. Moreover, several species, including patas monkeys, yellow baboons, and chacma baboons, have acquired SIV from local African green monkeys with which they interact [41]. Despite claims to the contrary [37, 42], the phylogenetics of SIV and HIV indicate that primate lentiviruses have the capacity to cross species boundaries and establish new epidemics naturally. And the discovery that SIV in chimpanzees is pathogenic [5] is as clear a demonstration as one could ask for that neither vaccines nor injections are necessary to generate pathogenic lentiviruses.

It follows from this observation, and from the pre-1950 divergence dates for all the epidemic forms of HIV, that the rapid growth of unsterile injections in Africa beginning in the 1950s was not the key to the establishment of HIV, as has been proposed [42]. When considering the emergence of HIV, it is helpful to decompose the process into factors promoting the establishment of HIV as a human-to-human

infection, and those favoring the subsequent spread of a virus that has become established. A plethora of "dirty needles" may have helped *spread* HIV-2 groups A, B and HIV-1 groups M and O in Africa in the 1950s and later, but the *establishment* of each—the transmission of the ancestral SIV into the first human host, and the initial human-to-human transmission of each nascent HIV—appears to have occurred earlier. Iatrogenic infection is not currently the dominant mode of HIV transmission in sub-Saharan Africa [43, 44], and may never have been, but this is not to say that it is not a serious concern. Even if it accounts for only 5% of HIV incidence there, then there are presumably more medically infected HIV-positive Africans than there are HIV-positive Americans in the entire US epidemic. Such is the magnitude of the HIV/AIDS epidemic in the hardest hit region.

THE MEANING OF GENETIC DIVERSITY WITHIN HIV-1 GROUP M

Given the attention paid to them, it is of clear medical importance to understand the nature of the HIV-1 group M subtypes. Recognizing certain lineages as "subtypes" has certainly aided the tracking of epidemiologically important lineages across the globe [20]. But parsing the huge amount of genetic diversity within the main group of HIV-1 into subtypes has also imbued them with an undeserved status. Are they well-defined biological entities with intrinsic, medically meaningful properties? Is it a sound idea, for example, to pursue *subtype*-specific vaccines against different portions of global HIV-1 M variation (as opposed to broader or narrower phylogenetic criteria)? Answering such fundamental questions requires careful differentiation between pattern and process.

Figure 2.2 shows a phylogenetic tree encompassing the global diversity of group M strains. Below the tree are two schematic phylogenies showing the phylogenetic pattern observed when only sequences from outside of the group M epicenter are analyzed (left), versus the pattern obtained when sequences from the putative source population are added (right). The labels indicate recognized subtype/CRF designations. The crucial point here is that the subtypes within group M are artifacts of "founder" effects and biased sampling [38, 45]. The "subtypiness" of group M, with distinct clades separated by long internal branches reflective of independent evolutionary history, only arises on phylogenies reconstructed with sequences sampled *outside* of the central African source of the pandemic. When samples from the source population are included, the gaps between the subtypes fill in and largely disappear (lower right schematic). So do the subtypes [38].

The "source" population is represented in Figure 2.2 by HIV sequences sampled in the Democratic Republic of the Congo (DRC), the country with the most extensive

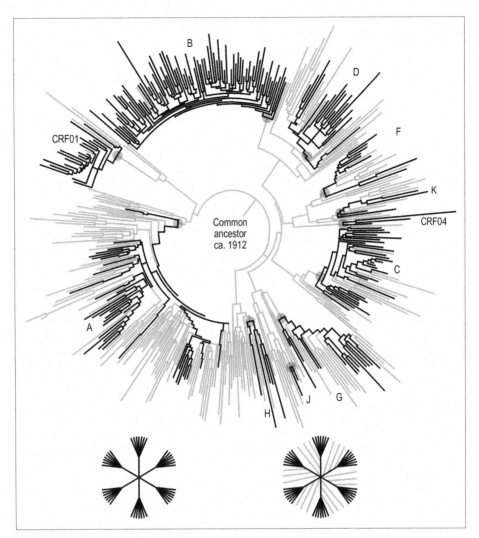

Figure 2.2 A maximum likelihood phylogenetic tree of HIV-1 group M (top) plus schematic representations of the M group subtypes (below). The phylogeny is courtesy of Andrew Rambaut and is based on partial *env* gene (V2–V5) sequences collected both within the Democratic Republic of the Congo (light branches) [38, 46] and outside the DRC (dark branches) (http://www.hiv.lanl.gov). The branches radiating from the center are drawn to scale. The ancestor of each subtype/CRF is marked with a circle. Several DRC strains fall basal to these points, and the much more extensive diversity of group M lineages encountered in the DRC indicates that this region has experienced a long, continuous epidemic.

M-group genetic diversity described to date [46] and the longest evidence of the presence of the virus [36]. It is the best sampled central African country [46], but whether its M group diversity is uniquely rich remains to be seen. M-group genetic diversity on the other side of the Congo River, in Brazzaville (Republic of Congo), is also extensive [47]. Although the sampling in the Congo–Brazzaville study was far less intensive, the same pattern emerges from the phylogenies: there is a preponderance of unclassifiable strains and strains that fell *basal* to the subtypes as defined

by global diversity. Describing such basal lineages as *members* of these subtypes misses the point. The subtypes only have meaning outside of this epicenter region, and these basal lineages already existed before the "birth" of the subtype (i.e. before some strain was exported out of the source region and began a chain of infections elsewhere, in relative isolation). The lack of a clear distinction between strains in this part of the group M phylogeny underscores the lack of intrinsic biological properties uniting members of a subtype (Fig. 2.3).

21

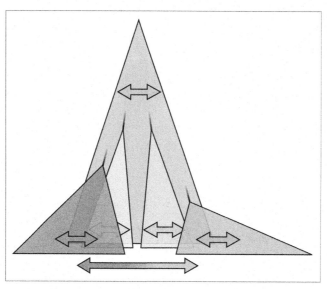

Figure 2.3 The processes underlying the phylogenetic patterns observed in HIV-1 group M. Time/divergence increases down the vertical axis; number of infected hosts is represented on the horizontal axis; arrows depict recombination. Several successful lineages (smaller triangles) trace their ancestry back to the source population (large triangle). This source population derives from a single infected host (apex), and has been evolving as a continuous epidemic; hence the lack of clear subtypes [29]. In addition to nucleotide substitution, recombination occurs regularly within all the populations (arrows) [26], but will be most conspicuous within the source with its full range of diversity, and between contemporary, divergent strains (bottom arrow). Early, complex recombinants reflect the special legacy of recombination in the ancestral zone where the most divergent strains have always co-circulated and recombined. Small triangles correspond both to subtypes and circulating recombinants forms (e.g. CRF02 in Nigeria). In each instance, a founder effect has occurred such that one strain has been exported outside the geographical range of the source population and has initiated an epidemic elsewhere.
(Adapted from Worobey M, The occurrence and impact of viral recombination, DPhil thesis, 2001: University of Oxford, UK.)

CONCLUSION

Although it is clear that it would be naïve to treat subtypes as "immunotypes," rational vaccine design (to highlight one important medical example) demands much more detailed information about the precise relationship between HIV genetic diversity and human biology. How many future HIV vaccines will be required to protect people in an HIV-diverse country like the DRC? One? Ten? Or is the notion of an effective, protective vaccine perhaps doomed to failure? We simply cannot say at the moment. In light of the fact that wild-type HIV-infected individuals are eventually unable to protect against even the most *local* level of phylogenetic diversity—the swarm of strains that replicate within their own bodies—we cannot currently rule out this sobering possibility. Without such fundamental knowledge about the consequences of HIV genetic variation, it is difficult to make informed decisions about how best to allocate research dollars among the different methods of control.

The rapid evolution of HIV has left behind a record of the virus's past, and reconstructing the circumstances of its origins and emergence has been a major triumph, one that has yielded key insights into the public health risks posed by SIV and HIV. A more difficult challenge still confronts us: fully discerning the medically relevant aspects of past, current, and future HIV genetic diversity and then translating such knowledge into successful therapeutic and preventive control measures. With many existing and potential medical approaches, there is an urgent need to come to grips not only with the remarkable diversity of currently circulating strains of HIV but also with the relentless onslaught of new genetic variation that will be generated by these viruses in future months, years, and decades.

On the other hand, and on a more positive note, many of the most effective or promising interventions in our current arsenal, including widespread antiretroviral therapy, counseling and testing, pre-exposure prophylaxis, circumcision, partner reduction efforts, microbical gels, and condom use, are ones that *do not* depend on a deep understanding of HIV genetic diversity. Indeed, many or all of these approaches can be expected to work about equally well across the entire range of HIV variation. It is conceivable that ardent prevention efforts based on these approaches will lead to the effective extirpation of HIV in many areas long before we have worked out HIV's evolutionary enigmas or developed clever vaccines that can surmount the challenges posed by the virus's genetic diversity.

REFERENCES

[1] Gottlieb MS, Schanker HM, Fan PT, et al. Pneumocystis pneumonia—Los Angeles. MMWR 1981;30:250–2.

[2] Barre-Sinoussi F, Chermann JC, Rey F, et al. Isolation of a T-lymphotrophic retrovirus from a patient at risk for acquired immune-deficiency syndrome (AIDS). Science 1983;220:868–71.

[3] Hahn BH, Shaw GM, DeCock KM, et al. AIDS—AIDS as a zoonosis: Scientific and public health implications. Science 2000;287:607–14.

[4] Bibollet-Ruche F, Bailes E, Gao F, et al. New simian immunodeficiency virus infecting De Brazza's monkeys (Cercopithecus neglectus): Evidence for a Cercopithecus monkey virus clade. J Virol 2004;78:7748–62.

[5] Keele BF, Jones JH, Terio KA, et al. Increased mortality and AIDS-like immunopathology in wild chimpanzees infected with SIVcpz. Nature 2009;460:515–19.

[6] Charleston MA, Robertson DL. Preferential host switching by primate lentiviruses can account for phylogenetic similarity with the primate phylogeny. Syst Biol 2002;51:528–35.

[7] Van Heuverswyn F, Li Y, Neel C, et al. Human immunodeficiency viruses: SIV infection in wild gorillas. Nature 2006;444:164.

[8] Turelli P, Trono D. Editing at the crossroad of innate and adaptive immunity. Science 2005;307:1061–5.

[9] Worobey M, Telfer P, Souquière S, et al. Island biogeography reveals the deep history of SIV. Science 2010;329:1487.

[10] Gifford RJ, Katzourakis A, Tristem M, et al. A transitional endogenous lentivirus from the genome of a basal primate and implications for lentivirus evolution. Proc Natl Acad Sci U S A 2008;105:20362–7.

[11] Sharp PM, Bailes E, Gao F, et al. Origins and evolution of AIDS viruses: estimating the time-scale. Biochem Soc Trans 2000;28:275–82.

[12] Wertheim JO, Worobey M. Dating the age of the SIV lineages that gave rise to HIV-1 and HIV-2. PLoS Comput Biol 2009;5: e1000377.

[13] Korber B, Muldoon M, Theiler J, et al. Timing the ancestor of the HIV-1 pandemic strains. Science 2000;288:1789–96.

[14] Plantier JC, Leoz M, Dickerson JE, et al. A new human immunodeficiency virus derived from gorillas. Nat Med 2009;15:871–2.

[15] Simon F, Mauclere P, Roques P, et al. Identification of a new human immunodeficiency virus type 1 distinct from group M and group O. Nat Med 1998;4:1032–7.

[16] Gao F, Bailes E, Robertson DL, et al. Origin of HIV-1 in the chimpanzee Pan troglodytes troglodytes. Nature 1999;397:436–41.

[17] Gurtler LG, Hauser PH, Eberle J, et al. A new subtype of human immunodeficiency virus type 1 (MVP-5180) from Cameroon. J Virol 1994;68:1581–5.

[18] Damond F, Worobey M, Campa P, et al. Identification of a highly divergent HIV type 2 and proposal for a change in HIV type 2 classification. AIDS Res Hum Retroviruses 2004;20:666–72.

[19] Peeters M. Recombinant HIV sequences: Their role in the global epidemic. In: Theoretical Biology and Biophysics Group, editors HIV sequence compendium. Los Alamos: Los Alamos National Laboratory; 2000. pp 39–54.

[20] Robertson DL, Anderson JP, Bradac JA, et al. HIV-1 nomenclature proposal. Science 2000;288:55–7.

[21] Takehisa J, Zekeng L, Ido E, et al. Human immunodeficiency virus type 1 intergroup (M/O) recombination in Cameroon. J Virol 1999;73:6810–20.

[22] Bailes E, Gao F, Bibollet-Ruche F, et al. Hybrid origin of SIV in chimpanzees. Science 2003;300:1713.

[23] Gao F, Yue L, White AT, et al. Human infection by genetically diverse SIVsm-related HIV-2 in West Africa. Nature 1992;358: 495–9.

[24] Chen ZW, Telfer P, Gettie A, et al. Genetic characterization of new west African simian immunodeficiency virus SIVsm: Geographic clustering of household-derived SIV strains with human immunodeficiency virus type 2 subtypes and genetically diverse viruses from a single feral sooty mangabey troop. J Virol 1996;70:3617–27.

[25] Chen ZW, Luckay A, Sodora DL, et al. Human immunodeficiency virus type 2 (HIV-2) seroprevalence and characterization of a distinct HIV-2 genetic subtype from the natural range of simian immunodeficiency virus-infected sooty mangabeys. J Virol 1997;71:3953–60.

[26] Santiago ML, Rodenburg CM, Kamenya S, et al. SIVcpz in wild chimpanzees. Science 2002;295:465.

[27] Worobey M, Santiago ML, Keele BF, et al. Origin of AIDS—Contaminated polio vaccine theory refuted. Nature 2004;428:820.

[28] Ayouba A, Mauclere P, Martin PMV, et al. HIV-1 group O infection in Cameroon, 1986–1998. Emerg Infect Dis 2001;7:466–7.

[29] Roques P, Robertson DL, Souquiere S, et al. Phylogenetic characteristics of three new HIV-1 N strains and implications for the origin of group N. AIDS 2004;18:1371–81.

[30] Vallari A, Holzmayer V, Harris B, et al. Confirmation of putative HIV-1 group P in Cameroon. J Virol 2011;85:1403–7.

[31] Keele BF, Van Heuverswyn F, Li Y, et al. Chimpanzee reservoirs of pandemic and non-pandemic HIV-1. Science 2006;313:523–6.

[32] Worobey M, Gemmel M, Teuwen DE, et al. Direct evidence of extensive diversity of HIV-1 in Kinshasa by 1960. Nature 2008;455:661–4.

[33] Lemey P, Pybus OG, Rambaut A, et al. The molecular population genetics of HIV-1 group O. Genetics 2004;167:1059–68.

[34] Lemey P, Pybus OG, Wang B, et al. Tracing the origin and history of the HIV-2 epidemic. Proc Natl Acad Sci U S A 2003;100:6588–92.

[35] Worobey M. A novel approach to detecting and measuring recombination: New insights into evolution in viruses, bacteria, and mitochondria. Mol Biol Evol 2001;18:1425–34.

[36] Zhu TF, Korber BT, Nahmias AJ, et al. An African HIV-1 sequence from 1959 and implications for the origin of the epidemic. Nature 1998;391:594–7.

[37] Hooper E. The River: A Journey Back to the Source of HIV and AIDS. London: Penguin; 1999.

[38] Rambaut A, Robertson DL, Pybus OG, et al. Human immunodeficiency virus—Phylogeny and the origin of HIV-1. Nature 2001;410:1047–8.

[39] Santiago ML, Lukasik M, Kamenya S, et al. Foci of endemic simian immunodeficiency virus infection in wild-living eastern chimpanzees (*Pan troglodytes schweinfurthii*). J Virol 2003;77:7545–62.

[40] Souquiere S, Bibollet-Ruche F, Robertson DL, et al. Wild Mandrillus sphinx are carriers of two types of lentivirus. J Virol 2001;75:7086–96.

[41] Bibollet–Ruche F, GalatLuong A, Cuny G, et al. Simian immunodeficiency virus infection in a patas monkey (*Erythrocebus patas*): Evidence for cross-species transmission from African green monkeys (*Cercopithecus aethiops sabaeus*) in the wild. J Gen Virol 1996;77:773–81.

[42] Marx PA, Alcabes PG, Drucker E. Serial human passage of simian immunodeficiency virus by unsterile injections and the emergence of epidemic human immunodeficiency virus in Africa. Philos Trans R Soc Lond Ser 2001;356:911–20.

[43] Schmid GP, Buve A, Mugyenyi P, et al. Transmission of HIV-1 infection in sub-Saharan Africa and effect of elimination of unsafe injections. Lancet 2004;363: 482–488.

[44] Walker PR, Worobey M, Rambaut A, et al. Sexual transmission of HIV in Africa. Other routes of infection are not the dominant contributor to the African epidemic. Nature 2003;422:679.

[45] Rambaut A, Posada D, Crandall KA, et al. The causes and consequences of HIV evolution. Nat Rev Genet 2004;5:52–61.

[46] Vidal N, Peeters M, Mulanga-Kabeya C, et al. Unprecedented degree of human immunodeficiency virus type 1 (HIV-1) group M genetic diversity in the Democratic Republic of Congo suggests that the HIV-1 pandemic originated in Central Africa. J Virol 2000;74:10498–507.

[47] Taniguchi Y, Takehisa J, Bikandou B, et al. Genetic subtypes of HIV type 1 based on the vpu/env sequences in the Republic of Congo. AIDS Res Hum Retroviruses 2002;18:79–83.

Chapter | 3 |

Molecular biology of HIV: implications for new therapies

Warner C. Greene, B. Matija Peterlin, Matthew H. Stremlau

Sharply curbing the expanding global HIV epidemic requires more effective approaches to decrease the horizontal and vertical spread of this pathogenic retrovirus coupled with the broader use of existing and likely new antiretroviral therapies. These interventions must be deployable in the developing world, where HIV is hitting the hardest. Understanding the dynamic interplay of HIV with its host at the molecular and cellular levels forms the foundation for success in this endeavor. In the following sections, we review our current understanding of the HIV life cycle, highlighting promising future points of attack.

HIV ENTRY

The 9-kilobase HIV RNA encodes nine genes, yielding 15 distinct proteins. Compared to other retroviruses, HIV is genetically complex. Investigations over the past several years yielded informative insights into the function of each of HIV's individual gene products, many of which could form potential targets for new therapies (Fig. 3.1). To productively infect a cellular target, HIV must introduce its genetic material into the cytoplasm of this cell. HIV entry requires the initial binding or attachment of the HIV envelope protein to (Env) CD4 receptors on the surface of target cells. The rational development of inhibitors of HIV attachment has been propelled by structural studies unraveling the "lock and key" assembly of trimeric gp120 Env spikes present on virions with CD4 receptors residing on the surface of the target cells [1]. The insertion of a key phenylalanine residue in the outer portion of the CD4 protein into a recessed pocket in gp120 produces a very high-affinity interaction of these two proteins.

BMS 488043 is a promising second-generation attachment inhibitor that blocks the insertion of this CD4 residue into this pocket of gp120. Protein-based approaches to interrupting the gp120–CD4 interaction are also being developed. Numerous studies have identified a handful of monoclonal antibodies against HIV-1 that neutralize primary isolates of HIV-1 *in vitro* and prevent infection in non-human primate models [2–4]. Although these antibodies clearly prevent infection in animal models, very high doses of the antibodies are required for clinical effects in HIV-infected patients. Other protein-based therapies include PRO 542, a tetravalent fusion protein containing the D1 and D2 domains of human CD4 and the heavy- and light-chain constant regions of human IgG2 [5, 6]. Phase I and II clinical trials revealed modest decreases in viral load in patients with advanced disease [7]. Another candidate is ibalizumab (formerly TNX-355), a humanized anti-CD4 IgG4 monoclonal antibody that specifically reacts with a conformational epitope in the D2 domain of CD4 induced by gp120 binding. This antibody blocks subsequent Env engagement of the HIV chemokine co-receptors [8]. The antibody showed beneficial activity relative to optimized background therapy in patients and has advanced to phase II clinical trials [9].

The second phase of HIV entry involves the engagement of the HIV co-receptors. The initial binding of trimeric gp120 to CD4 induces a conformational change in the envelope that promotes binding of the virion to a specific subset of chemokine co-receptors. These receptors contain seven membrane-spanning domains and normally help hematopoietic cells to migrate down specific chemokine gradients to sites of inflammation. Although these receptors signal through G proteins [10], such signaling is not required for HIV infection. Twelve different chemokine receptors function as HIV co-receptors

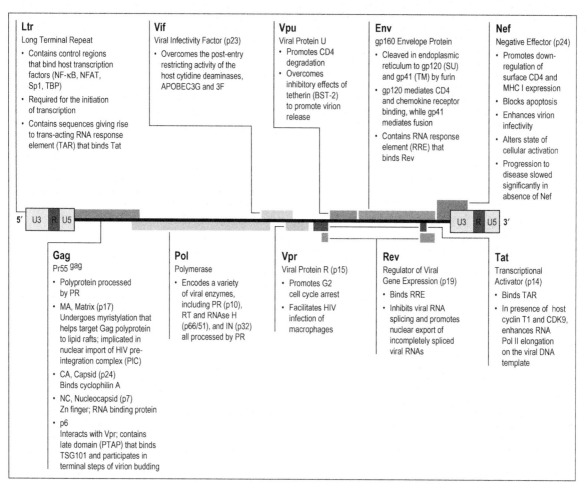

Figure 3.1 An overview of the organization of the ~9-kb genome of the HIV provirus and a summary of the functions of its nine genes encoding 15 different proteins.

in cultured cells, but only two, CCR5 and CXCR4, are normally used *in vivo* [10]. CCR5 binds macrophage-tropic, non-syncytium-inducing (R5-tropic) viruses, which are associated with mucosal and intravenous transmission of HIV infection. CXCR4 binds T-cell-tropic, syncytium-inducing (X4-tropic) viruses, which generally emerge only during the later stages of disease [11]. Utilization of CXCR4 is associated with accelerated disease progression but only occurs in about half of patients infected with HIV.

A naturally occurring deletion of 32 base pairs in the CCR5 gene [12, 13] is present in approximately 13% of individuals of northern European descent. This mutation gives rise to a truncated form of the CCR5 receptor that never reaches the cell surface. Emphasizing the key role of CCR5 in horizontal transmission, individuals homozygous for this CCR5 Δ32mutation (1–2% of the Caucasian population) are almost completely resistant to HIV infection [12, 13]. This "experiment of nature" propelled

pharmaceutical development of small molecules that prevent HIV interaction with CCR5. Within only 7 years after the discovery of HIV co-receptors, several small-molecule antagonists of CCR5 entered clinical use. Maraviroc (Selzentry) is a low-molecular-weight CCR5 antagonist used for treatment of HIV-infected persons harboring R5 viruses resistant to conventional drugs [14]. Treatment of therapy-naïve patients with Maraviroc is still being analyzed in clinical trials. TAK-220, another low-molecular-weight compound, targets a pocket between the transmembrane helices of CCR5, thereby altering the conformation of the receptor, and has advanced to phase I clinical trials [15]. Protein-based CCR5 inhibitors include PRO 140, a humanized mouse antibody that recognizes an epitope at the CCR5 N-terminus, which has entered phase II clinical trials [16]. Interest has also focused on using modified versions of the chemokine RANTES, a natural ligand for CCR5, to block HIV infection. A key unanswered concern is whether blockade of CCR5 will promote an earlier switch to CXCR4 co-receptor utilization by HIV. As noted, such a switch could lead to more rapid clinical deterioration since many more CD4 T cells express CXCR4 than CCR5.

Both CD4 and chemokine co-receptors for HIV are found disproportionately within lipid signaling rafts located within the cell membrane [17]. These cholesterol- and sphingolipid-enriched microdomains likely provide a better environment for membrane fusion possibly because HIV virions bud from such lipid rafts and acquire similar lipids [18]. Removing cholesterol from virions, producer cells, or target cells greatly decreases the infectivity of HIV [19]. Studies are under way exploring whether cholesterol-depleting compounds might be efficacious as topically applied microbicides to inhibit HIV transmission at mucosal surfaces. The development of effective microbicides would form an exceptionally valuable approach in efforts to prevent HIV transmission. Approximately 50 microbicide candidates are in different stages of development in the microbicide pipeline. Thus far, mostly non-specific microbicides, such as surfactants and polyanions, have completed phase III clinical testing, and none has demonstrated clear statistical evidence of protection [20]. Tenofovir, a nucleotide analogue reverse transcriptase inhibitor, is the most advanced clinical candidate. A 1% vaginal gel formulation of tenofovir reduced HIV acquisition by nearly 40% overall in the recently completed CAPRISA phase II trial in South African women [21].

The third phase of HIV entry is virion fusion. The binding of surface gp120, CD4, and the chemokine co-receptors generates a sharp conformational change in gp41, the second HIV envelope protein [22]. Assembled as a trimer on the virion membrane, this coiled-coil protein springs open, projecting three peptide fusion domains that "harpoon" the lipid bilayer of the target cell. The gp41 trimers then fold back on themselves, forming a hairpin structure. The recently approved T20 fusion inhibitor, enfuvirtide, prevents the formation of the hairpin structure essential for successful fusion. The fusion reaction leads to intracytoplasmic insertion of the HIV viral core [22].

HIV virions also enter cells by endocytosis. However, this form of entry does not lead to productive viral infection likely because the internalized virions are inactivated within acidified endosomes. However, a special form of endocytosis associated with facilitated infection of CD4 T cells has been described in dendritic cells. These cells normally process and present antigens to immune cells, and many dendritic cells express a specialized attachment receptor termed DC-SIGN [23] or closely related C-type lectin receptors. DC-SIGN binds HIV gp120 with high affinity but does not trigger the conformational changes in *env* required for fusion. Rather, virions bound to DC-SIGN may be internalized into a vesicular compartment that does not lead to viral inactivation. These vesicles containing viable HIV virions are transported back to the cell surface after the dendritic cell has matured and migrated to regional lymph nodes, where it engages T cells [24]. Indeed, these virus-laden vesicles may selectively accumulate at the immunological synapse formed between dendritic cells and CD4 T cells. Thus, dendritic cells expressing DC-SIGN or related C-type lectin receptors may act as "Trojan horses," facilitating the spread of HIV from mucosal surfaces to lymphatic organs in the absence of productive infection of the dendritic cell itself.

Recent studies describe an innate recognition pathway for HIV-1 in dendritic cells [25]. HIV-1 does not replicate in dendritic cells; however, this block can be overcome by the accessory protein Vpx from simian immunodeficiency virus (SIV_{mac}). When this block is bypassed, HIV-1 replaces dendritic cell activation and the production of type I interferons. HIV-1-mediated activation of dendritic cells induced virus-specific IFN-γ-producing T cells and caused proliferation of CD4 T cells. Activating the HIV-1 sensor in dendritic cells could potentially improve the effectiveness of current vaccine candidates.

EARLY CYTOPLASMIC EVENTS

HIV-1 contains an internal viral RNA–protein complex surrounded by a protein shell, termed the capsid core [26]. Upon viral fusion, the capsid core is released into the cytoplasm of the target cell. Although the ensuing stages are poorly understood, the capsid core is thought to undergo a controlled disassembly reaction. This process appears to involve phosphorylation of the matrix protein by a mitogen-activated protein (MAP) kinase [27] and additional actions of cyclophilin A [28] and the viral proteins Nef [29] and Vif [30]. Optimal stability of the capsid core appears to be critical for successful infection of the host cell. Mutations that alter the stability of the core, by rendering the particle either too stable or unstable, impair infection [31]. Thus, small molecules that perturb the structure and/or disassembly process may have therapeutic benefit. One recently identified candidate, PF-3450074 (PF74), appears to trigger premature uncoating of the capsid core, leading to an inability to successfully complete subsequent steps in the viral life cycle [32].

After the viral core is uncoated, the viral reverse transcription complex is liberated and begins the conversion of viral RNA into double-stranded DNA [33]. This complex includes the diploid viral RNA genome, $tRNA^{Lys}$ primer, reverse transcriptase, integrase, matrix, nucleocapsid, viral protein R (Vpr), and various host proteins. It docks with actin microfilaments [34]. This interaction, mediated by the phosphorylated matrix, is required for the commencement of efficient reverse transcription. A variety of nucleoside (AZT, ddI, ddC, and 3TC), nucleotide (tenofovir), and non-nucleoside (nevirapine) inhibitors of the HIV reverse transcriptase are widely used in the clinic. Indeed, targeting of the viral reverse transcriptase represents one of the most successful strategies for impairing HIV growth. Effective reverse transcription yields the HIV preintegration complex (PIC), composed of double-stranded viral cDNA, integrase, matrix, Vpr, reverse transcriptase, and the high mobility group DNA-binding protein HMGI(Y) [35]. The PIC may move toward the nucleus by sliding down microtubules [36, 37]. Adenovirus and herpes simplex virus 1 similarly dock to microtubules and use the microtubule-associated dynein molecular motor for cytoplasmic transport. This finding suggests that many viruses utilize these cytoskeletal structures for directional movement. Overexpression of FEZ1, a regulator of cytoskeletal transport, blocks both HIV-1 and murine leukemia virus infection at a step after reverse transcription [38]. Thus, overexpressed FEZ1 might disrupt normal virus trafficking.

At least two host proteins associate with the PIC and are important for its function. One is BAF-1 (barrier to autointegration factor-1), a small DNA-binding protein [39]. Removal of BAF-1 promotes the suicidal pathway of autointegration, which occurs when the 3'-ends of the reverse transcript attack sites within the viral DNA. The other host protein is LAP2α, a laminin-associated component of the nuclear envelope, which promotes productive PIC integration [40].

CROSSING THE NUCLEAR PORE

Unlike most animal retroviruses, HIV can infect nondividing cells, such as terminally differentiated macrophages [41]. This requires an ability of the viral PIC to cross intact nuclear membranes. With a Stokes radius of approximately ~28 nm, resembling the size of a ribosome [42], the PIC is about twice as large as the maximal diameter of the central aqueous channel of the nuclear pore. It seems likely that the 3-μm contour length of viral DNA must undergo significant compaction, and the import process must involve considerable molecular gymnastics.

One of the more controversial areas of HIV research involves the identification of key viral proteins that mediate the nuclear import of the PIC. Integrase [43], matrix [44], and Vpr [45] have each been implicated (Fig. 3.2). Because plus-strand synthesis is discontinuous in reverse transcription, a triple helical DNA domain or "DNA flap" that may bind a host protein containing a nuclear targeting signal is produced [46]. Matrix encodes a canonical nuclear localization signal that is recognized by the importins-α and -β, which are key components in the classical nuclear import pathway. However, recent studies questioned the contributions of the nuclear import signal in integrase as well as the DNA flap to the nuclear uptake of the PIC [47]. The HIV Vpr gene product [48] contains at least three noncanonical nuclear targeting signals. Vpr may bypass the importin system altogether, perhaps mediating the direct docking

of the PIC with one or more components of the nuclear pore complex. The multiple nuclear targeting signals within the PIC, which could involve yet-to-be-identified cellular factors, may also function in a cooperative manner or play larger roles individually in different target cells. For example, while Vpr is not needed for HIV infection of nondividing, resting T cells [49], it markedly enhances viral infection in nondividing macrophages [50]. The finding that both matrix [51] and Vpr [48] shuttle between the nucleus and cytoplasm likely ensures their availability for incorporation into new virions.

Host factors involved in nuclear import of the PIC also remain to be identified. One report implicated importin 7, one of a family of nuclear import receptors responsible for the uptake of ribosomal proteins and histones [52]. Another report suggested Nup98, a component of the nuclear pore complex, could be required for HIV-1 infection [53]. More recent work suggests small host RNAs, such as specific tRNAs, bind to the PIC and facilitate its entry into the nucleus [54]. However, the roles of these factors have yet to be conclusively demonstrated.

INTEGRATION

Once inside the nucleus, the viral PIC establishes a functional provirus (Fig. 3.2). Effective integration of the double-stranded viral DNA into the host chromosome is mediated by the HIV integrase, which binds the ends of the viral DNA [35]. The host proteins HMGI(Y) and barrier to autointegration (BAF) are required for efficient integration, although their precise functions remain unknown [55]. Integrase removes nucleotides from viral ends, producing a two-base recess and thereby correcting the ragged ends generated by the terminal transferase activity of reverse transcriptase [35]. It also catalyzes the subsequent joining reaction that establishes the HIV provirus within the chromosome. Recent studies indicate that HIV integration preferentially occurs in actively transcribed genes [56].

The search for integrase inhibitors has been slow. Only one integrase inhibitor, raltegravir (Isentress 1), is approved for clinical use [57]. Raltegravir, as well as similar compounds, selectively blocks DNA strand transfer activity and is therefore referred to as integrase strand transfer inhibitors (INSTIs). Resistance to raltegravir develops rapidly: a single mutation is sufficient to confer resistance [58].

One host factor required for HIV-1 integration is LEDGF/p75 (lens epithelium-derived growth factor), a nuclear transcriptional co-activator [59]. LEDGF/p75 binds tightly to HIV-1 integrase and appears to act as a chromatin-associated receptor for preintegration complexes [60, 61]. In cells devoid of endogenous LEDGF/p75 protein, both the levels of HIV-1 integration and their genomic distribution are significantly perturbed [62, 63].

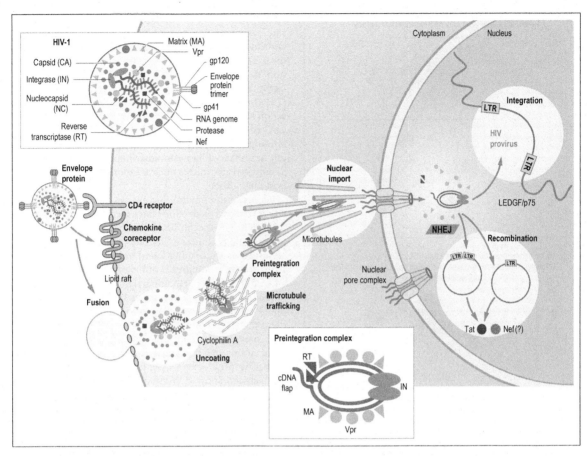

Figure 3.2 Schematic description of early events occurring after HIV infection of a susceptible target cell, interactions among gp120, CD4, and chemokine receptors (CCR5 or CXCR4) lead to gp41-mediated fusion followed by virion uncoating, reverse transcription of the RNA genome, nuclear import of the viral preintegration complex, and integration of the double-stranded viral cDNA into the host chromosome, thus establishing the HIV provirus.

Another host factor that seems to mediate the association of the preintegration complex with chromatin after nuclear entry is emerin, a component of the inner nuclear membrane [64]. The association of emerin with the PIC is mediated by BAF, and both proteins appear to cooperate to promote HIV integration into chromatin.

Not all PICs that enter the nucleus result in a functional provirus. The ends of the viral DNA may be joined to form a 2-LTR (long terminal repeat) circle or the viral genome may undergo homologous recombination yielding a single LTR circle. Finally, the viral DNA may autointegrate into itself, producing a rearranged circular structure. Although some circular forms may direct the synthesis of the transcriptional transactivator Tat and Nef, none produces infectious virus [65]. The nonhomologous end-joining system may form 2-LTR circles to protect the cell [66]. This system is responsible for rapid repair of double-strand breaks, which minimizes the number of free DNA ends within the cell, thereby preventing an apoptotic response. A single double-strand break detected within a cell is sufficient to induce G1 cell-cycle arrest. The ability of the free ends of the viral DNA to mimic such double-strand chromosomal breaks may contribute to the direct cytopathic effects observed with HIV.

TRANSCRIPTIONAL EVENTS

Integration can lead to latent or transcriptionally active forms of viral infection [67]. The chromosomal environment at the site of viral integration likely helps shape the provirus's transcriptional activity [68]. For example, proviral integration into repressed heterochromatin might favor the generation of latent proviruses (Fig. 3.3). In addition, the transcriptional status of HIV-1 is tightly coupled to the activation state of the cell. In resting T cells, nucleosomes adjacent to the HIV promoter (e.g., Nuc 1) bear the

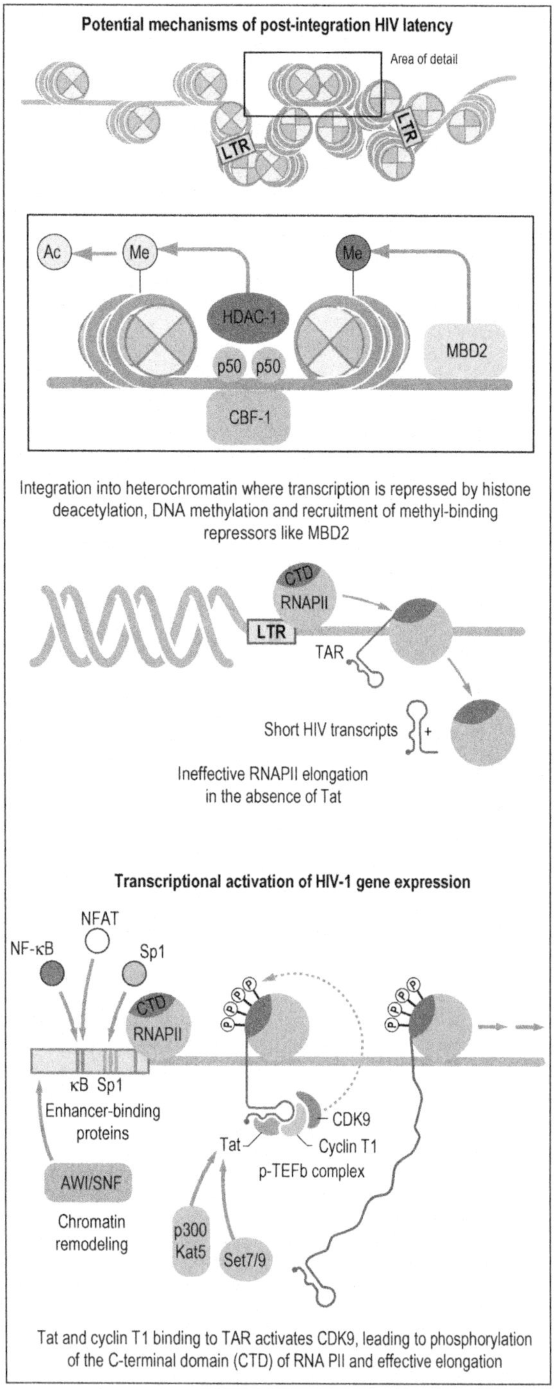

Potential mechanisms of post-integration HIV latency

Integration into heterochromatin where transcription is repressed by histone deacetylation, DNA methylation and recruitment of methyl-binding repressors like MBD2

Ineffective RNAPII elongation in the absence of Tat

Transcriptional activation of HIV-1 gene expression

Tat and cyclin T1 binding to TAR activates CDK9, leading to phosphorylation of the C-terminal domain (CTD) of RNA PII and effective elongation

Figure 3.3 A summary of two different mechanisms potentially underlying post-integration HIV latency contrasted with the central role of Tat in promoting productive infection of target cells.

characteristic marks of silent heterochromatin, such as lysine 9 trimethylated histone 3, heterochromatin protein 1, and low levels of histone acetylation [69]. Furthermore, the 5′ LTR of HIV can bind negative regulators of transcription, such as p50 homodimers (inactive form of nuclear factor κB, NF-κB) or the C-promoter binding factor 1 [70]. Both of these factors recruit histone deacetylases that act on Nuc1. Silencing is reinforced by methylation of two CpG islands and the subsequent binding of Methyl-CpG binding domain protein 2 (MDB2) [71, 72]. Finally, latency can be enhanced by post-transcriptional mechanisms, such as impaired HIV mRNA nuclear export and the expression of host micro-RNAs.

Because antiretroviral therapy can control, but not cure HIV infection, recent efforts have focused on the possibility that latent viruses can be reactivated and then purged by pharmacological manipulations. Three types of agents, all aimed at reactivating latent viruses, have been tested: T cell activators, inhibitors of histone-modifying enzymes, and inhibitors of DNA methylation [73]. Clinical trials have assessed T cell activators such as IL-2, IL-7, and antibodies specific to the T cell receptor CD3 subunit. Although these therapies transiently reduced the latent virus reservoir, patients generally experienced rapid viral rebound upon antiretroviral therapy cessation [74, 75]. In other studies, valproic acid, a weak inhibitor of histone deacetylase activity, showed some ability to decrease the pool of latently infected resting CD4 T cells; however, these effects have not been confirmed [76, 77]. *In vivo* studies have shown induction of transcriptionally repressed latent viruses using a combination of activators (e.g. the NF-κB inducer prostratin) in combination with inhibitors of histone deacetylation (e.g. valproic acid and suberoylanilide hydroxamic acid) and DNA methylation (e.g., 5-aza-2′-deoxycytidine) [71, 74, 78]. The combination of drugs aimed at purging latent reservoirs of virus may also activate endogenous retroelements. Thus, the benefits of reactivating latent proviruses must be weighed against the risk of retrotransposition-induced insertional mutagenesis.

In the host genome, the 5′ LTR functions like other eukaryotic transcriptional units. It contains downstream and upstream promoter elements, which include the initiator (Inr), TATA-box (T), and three Sp1 sites [79]. These regions help position the RNA polymerase II (RNAPII) at the site of initiation of transcription and assemble the pre-initiation complexes. Transcription begins, but the polymerase fails to elongate efficiently along the viral genome (Fig. 3.3). In the process, short nonpolyadenylated transcripts are synthesized, which are stable and persist in cells due to the formation of an RNA stem loop called the transactivation response (TAR) element [80]. Slightly upstream of the promoter is the transcriptional enhancer, in which HIV-1 binds NF-κB, nuclear factor of activated T cells (NFAT), and Ets family members [81]. NF-κB and NFAT relocalize to the nucleus after cellular activation. NF-κB is liberated from its cytoplasmic inhibitor, IκB, by stimulus-coupled phosphorylation, polyubiquitylation, and proteasomal degradation of the inhibitor [82]. NFAT is dephosphorylated by calcineurin (a reaction inhibited by cyclosporin A) and, after its nuclear import, assembles with AP1 to form the fully active transcriptional complex [83]. NF-κB, which is composed of p50 and p65 (RelA) subunits, increases both the rates of initiation and elongation of viral transcription [84]. Since NF-κB is activated after several antigen-specific and cytokine-mediated events, it can stimulate transcription of silent proviruses primarily through the recruitment of histone acetyltransferases that remodel Nuc1.

Tat is responsible for markedly increasing the rate of viral gene expression. With cyclin T1 (CycT1), it binds TAR and recruits the cellular cyclin-dependent kinase 9 (Cdk9) to the HIV LTR (Fig. 3.3) [85]. In the positive transcription elongation factor b (P-TEFb) complex, Cdk9 phosphorylates the C-terminal domain of RNAPII, which marks the transition from initiation to elongation of eukaryotic transcription [86]. Other targets of P-TEFb include negative transcription elongation factors (N-TEF), such as the DRB-sensitivity inducing (DSIF) and negative elongation (NELF) factors [86]. P-TEFb can be found in two distinct complexes, a small P-TEFb that contains only cdk9 and cyclin T, and a large P-TEFb that also contains 7SK small nuclear RNA and HEXIM1 (hexamethylene bisacetamide-induced protein 1).

In the absence of Tat, the HIV LTR functions as a very poor promoter because it so effectively binds these negative transcription factors *in vivo*. An arginine-rich motif (ARM) within Tat binds to the 5′ bulge region in TAR. A shorter ARM in cyclin T1, which is also called the Tat-TAR recognition motif (TRM), engages the central loop of TAR [85]. These regions form a high-affinity RNA-binding unit that is required for Tat transactivation. In the presence of the complex between Tat and P-TEFb, the RNAPII becomes a highly efficient elongating complex. Tat also recruits the SWI/SNF chromatin remodeling complex to the HIV promoter [87–89] to relieve the elongation block imposed by repressive nucleosomes.

Because murine CycT1 contains a cysteine at position 261, the complex between Tat and murine P-TEFb binds TAR weakly [90]. Thus, Tat transactivation is severely compromised in murine cells. Cdk9 also must be autophosphorylated on several serines and threonines near its C-terminus for productive interactions among Tat, P-TEFb, and TAR [91]. Additionally, basal levels of P-TEFb may be low in resting cells or only weakly active due to the interaction between P-TEFb and 7SK RNA [92].

Post-translational modifications of Tat, such as phosphorylation, methylation, and acetylation, modify its function and allow it to specifically interact with a wide array of cellular partners. For example, the lysine methyltransferase Set7/9 associates with the HIV promoter and monomethylates lysine 51, a highly conserved residue located in the RNA-binding domain of Tat [93]. Several histone-modifying enzymes, such as p300/CBP, also associate with Tat. These enzymes acetylate Tat at lysines 50 and 51, promoting the disassociation of Tat from the TAR RNA and leading to the start of transcriptional elongation [94–96].

EXPRESSION OF VIRAL GENES

Transcription of the viral genome results in more than a dozen different HIV-specific transcripts [97]. Some are processed cotranscriptionally and, in the absence of inhibitory RNA sequences (IRS), transported rapidly into the cytoplasm [98]. These multiply spliced transcripts encode Nef, Tat, and Rev, the "early" expressed genes of HIV. Other singly spliced or unspliced viral transcripts remain in the nucleus and are relatively stable. These viral transcripts encode the structural, enzymatic, and accessory proteins and represent viral genomic RNAs needed for the assembly of fully infectious virions.

Incomplete splicing likely results from suboptimal splice donor and acceptor sites in viral transcripts. In addition, the regulator of virion gene expression, Rev, may inhibit splicing by its interaction with alternate splicing factor/splicing factor 2 (ASF/SF2) [99] and its associated p32 protein [100].

Transport of the incompletely spliced viral transcripts to the cytoplasm depends on an adequate supply of Rev [98]. Rev is a small shuttling protein that binds a complex RNA stem loop termed the Rev response element (RRE), which is located in the *env* gene. Rev binds first with high affinity to a small region of the RRE termed the stem loop IIB (Fig. 3.4) [101]. This binding leads to the multimerization of Rev on the remainder of the RRE. In addition to a nuclear localization signal, Rev contains a leucine-rich nuclear export sequence (NES) [98]. Of note, the study of Rev was the catalyst for the identification of such NESs in many cellular proteins and of the complex formed between CRM-1/exportin-1 and this sequence [98].

Rev functions by binding directly to CRM-1, the main nuclear export receptor for host ribosomal and small nuclear RNAs [102]. In addition to CRM-1, Rev also uses several other co-factors for RNA export. These factors include Rab/hRIP [103], RanBP1 [104], Sam68 [105], and heterogeneous nuclear ribonucleoprotein A1 (hnRNP A1). Ran is a small guanine nucleotide–binding protein that switches between GTP- and GDP-bound states. RanGDP is found predominantly in the cytoplasm because RanGAP is expressed in this cellular compartment. Conversely, the Ran nucleotide exchange factor RCC1, which charges Ran with GTP, is expressed predominantly in the nucleus. The inverse nucleocytoplasmic gradients of RanGTP and RanGDP produced by the subcellular localization of these enzymes likely plays a major role in determining the directional transport of proteins into and out of the nucleus. Outbound cargo is only effectively loaded onto the CRM-1/exportin-1 in the presence of RanGTP. However, when the complex reaches

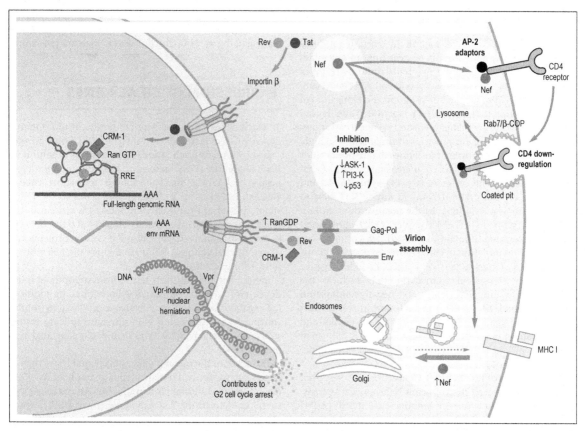

Figure 3.4 A summary of late events in the HIV-infected cell, culminating in the assembly of new infectious virions. Highlighted are the roles of various viral proteins in optimizing the intracellular environment for viral replication including, down-regulation of CD4 and MHC I and inhibition of apoptosis by Nef, and the induction of G2 cell-cycle arrest by Vpr. A key action of the HIV Rev protein in promoting nuclear export of incompletely spliced viral transcripts that encode the structural and enzymatic proteins as well as the viral genome of new virions is also illustrated.

the cytoplasm, GTP is hydrolyzed to GDP and the bound cargo is released. The opposite relationship regulates the nuclear import by importins-α and -β, where nuclear RanGTP stimulates cargo release [98].

For HIV infection to spread, a balance between splicing and transport of incompletely spliced viral mRNA species must be achieved. If splicing is too efficient, then only the multiply spliced transcripts appear in the cytoplasm. Although required, these regulatory proteins are insufficient to support full viral replication. However, if splicing is markedly impaired, adequate synthesis of Tat, Rev, and Nef will not occur. In many non-primate cells, HIV transcripts may be overly spliced, thus producing a block to viral replication in these hosts [106].

The HIV-1 RNA transcript contains a long 5′-untranslated region (UTR) leader. Consequently, the start codons for Gag translation are often preceded by nonproductive start and stop codons. This situation suggests that HIV-1 might contain an internal ribosome entry site (IRES) to initiate

translation [107]. Translation of the Gag–Pol polyprotein requires a ribosomal frameshift before the Gag stop codon and presumably host proteins to complete protein synthesis; however, the identities of these factors remain unknown.

REPLICATING NEW VIRUSES

In contrast to Tat and Rev, which act directly on viral RNA structures, Nef reshapes the environment of the infected cell to optimize viral replication (Fig. 3.4) [10]. The absence of Nef in infected monkeys and humans is associated with much slower clinical progression to AIDS [108, 109]. This increase in virulence caused by Nef appears to be associated with its ability to affect signaling cascades, including the activation of T cell antigen receptor [110], and to decrease the expression of CD4 on the cell surface [111, 112]. Nef also promotes the production and release of more infectious virions [113, 114]. Effects of Nef on the PI3-K signaling cascade—which involves the guanine nucleotide exchange factor Vav, the small GTPases Cdc42 and Rac1, and p21-activated kinase PAK—cause profound cytoskeletal rearrangments and alter downstream effector functions [115]. Indeed, Nef and viral structural proteins colocalize in lipid rafts [114, 116]. Two other HIV proteins assist Nef in down-regulating expression of CD4 [117]. Trimeric gp120 binds CD4 in the endoplasmic reticulum, slowing its export to the plasma membrane [118], and Vpu binds the cytoplasmic tail of CD4, promoting recruitment of TrCP and Skp1p (Fig. 3.5). These events target CD4 for ubiquitylation and proteasomal degradation before it reaches the cell surface [119].

Nef reduces immunological response to HIV infections directly and indirectly. In T cells, Nef activates the expression of FasL (CD95L), which induces apoptosis in bystander cells that express Fas [120], thereby killing cytotoxic T cells that could eliminate HIV-1-infected cells. It reduces the expression of MHC I determinants on the cell surface [121] (Fig. 3.4) and so decreases the immunological

visibility of infected cells to CD8 cytotoxic T cells. For rerouting MHC 1 to the lysosomes for degradation, Nef recruits the clatherin adaptor AP-1 and subsequently β-COP, to the cytoplasmic tail of MHC 1 [122–124]. However, Nef does not decrease the expression of HLA-C [125], so that natural killer cells cannot recognize and kill the infected cells.

Nef also inhibits apoptosis. It binds to and inhibits the intermediate apoptosis signal regulating kinase-1 (ASK-1) [126] that functions in the Fas and TNFR death signaling pathways and stimulates the phosphorylation of Bad leading to its sequestration by 14-3-3 proteins (Fig. 3.4) [127]. Nef also binds and inhibits p53 [128]. Via these different mechanisms, Nef prolongs the life of the infected cell, thereby optimizing viral replication.

Other viral proteins also participate in the modification of the environment in infected cells. Rev-dependent expression of Vpr induces the arrest of proliferating infected cells at the G2/M phase of the cell cycle [129]. Since the viral LTR is more active during G2, this arrest likely enhances viral gene expression [130]. These cell-cycle arresting properties

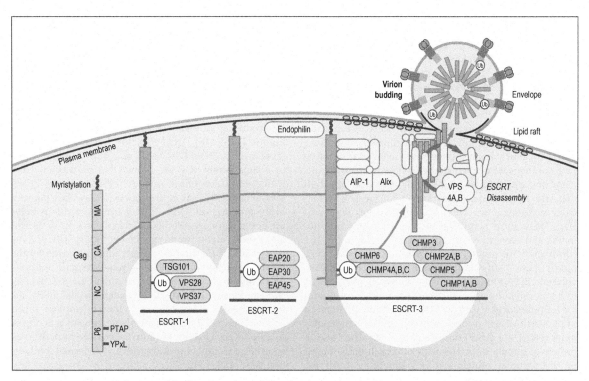

Figure 3.5 Late steps in the assembly of new virions and host factors in virion budding. Components of the endosomal sorting complex for transport (ESCRT) machinery, most notably TSG101, AIP/Alix, and Vps4, play critical roles in the terminal phases of virion budding. In infected cells, Gag redirects the ESCRT machinery to the plasma membrane and uses it to bud out from the cell. Ubiquitylation of cargo is usually involved in ESCRT function. Therefore, ubiquitylation of Gag likely facilitates its interaction with components of the ESCRT-1, ESCRT-2, and ESCRT-3 complexes. Several other host proteins not traditionally classified as part of the ESCRT machinery may also play a role in budding. For example, the endophilins are a family of proteins that induce membrane curvature. Endophilins, or similar proteins, may facilitate endocytic vesicle budding of the virus.

involve localized defects in the structure of the nuclear lamina that lead to dynamic, DNA-filled herniations that project from the nuclear envelope into the cytoplasm (Fig. 3.4) [131]. Intermittently, these herniations rupture, causing the mixing of soluble nuclear and cytoplasmic proteins.

ASSEMBLY AND BUDDING OF HIV VIRIONS

New virions are assembled at the plasma membrane (Fig. 3.5). Each virion consists of roughly 1,500 Gag and 100 Gag–Pol polyproteins [132], two copies of the viral RNA genome, and Vpr [133]. Several proteins participate in the assembly process, including Gag–Pol, and Gag polyproteins as well as Nef and Env. A human ATP-binding protein, HP68 (previously identified as an RNase L inhibitor), likely acts as a molecular chaperone, facilitating conformational changes in Gag needed for the assembly of these capsids [134]. The Gag polyproteins are subject to myristylation [135], and thus preferentially associate with cholesterol- and glycolipid-enriched membrane microdomains, often referred to as membrane rafts [136]. Virion budding occurs through these specialized regions in the lipid bilayer, yielding virions with cholesterol-rich membranes. This lipid composition likely favors release, stability, and fusion of virions with the subsequent target cell [18].

The process of retroviral budding usurps the endosomal sorting complex required for transport (ESCRT) machinery. This complex comprises of approximately 20 proteins that form four complexes and is responsible for sorting cargo proteins for delivery to the late endosome compartment or multivesicular bodies [137]. It is now apparent that HIV-1 makes specific contacts with the ESCRT machinery through two regions within the p6 region of Gag. These short peptide sequences are called late domains and serve to recruit the cellular proteins TSG101 (through PTAP motifs) and AIP-1/ALIX (through YPxL motifs) [138, 139]. Ubiquitylation of cargo is usually involved in ESCRT function, and the p6 protein also appears to be modified by ubiquitylation. The product of the tumor suppressor gene 101 or TSG101 binds the PTAP motif of p6 Gag and also recognizes ubiquitin through its ubiquitin enzyme 2 (UEV) domain [140, 141]. The TSG101 protein normally associates with other cellular proteins in the vacuolar protein-sorting pathway to form the ESCRT-1 complex that selects cargo for incorporation into the multivesicular body (MVB) [142]. The MVB is produced when surface patches on late endosomes bud away from the cytoplasm and fuse with lysosomes, releasing their contents for degradation within this organelle. In the case of HIV, TSG101 appears to be "hijacked" for the budding of virions into the extracellular space away from the cytoplasm. Several other host proteins not traditionally classified as part of the ESCRT pathway also likely play a role in budding. For example, endophilin belongs to a family of proteins that induce membrane curvature, thereby facilitating endocytic vesicle budding [143].

Although overexpression of the Gag binding domains of TSG101 and AIP/Alix potently inhibit spreading lentiviral infection in tissue culture, neither domain is viable as a therapeutic target. However, small molecules that interfere with the p6–TSG101 and p6–AIP/Alix interaction sites could have therapeutic benefits. As a first step towards this goal, PTAP peptide mimetics that competitively inhibit the p6–TSG101 interaction have been engineered; however, to be useful therapeutically, they need to be rendered cell permeable [144].

ANTIVIRAL HOST FACTORS

APOBEC3G

In primary CD4 T lymphocytes, Vif plays a key but poorly understood role in the assembly of infectious virions. In the absence of Vif, normal levels of virus are produced, but these virions are noninfectious, displaying an arrest at the level of reverse transcription in the subsequent target cell. Heterokaryon analyses involving the fusion of nonpermissive (requires Vif for viral growth) and permissive cells (support the growth of Vif-deficient viruses) revealed that Vif overcomes the effects of a natural inhibitor of HIV replication [145, 146]. This restriction factor was ultimately identified as APOBEC3G [147] and shown be a member of a large family of RNA editing/DNA mutator enzymes with cytidine deaminase activity. In the absence of Vif expression, APOBEC3G is incorporated into virus particles in the producer cell [148, 149]. When these virions infect the next target cells, APOBEC3G deaminates dC in the single-stranded minus strand viral DNA producing dU at these sites [150]. These viral DNAs are either degraded by the combined action of uracil N-glycosylase and apurinic-apyrimidinic endoculease or plus strand DNA is synthesized producing dG→dA hypermutations and likely the introduction of multiple stop codons in normally open reading frames. Vif circumvents these antiviral activities of APOBEC3G by targeting the antiviral enzyme for both accelerated degradation in proteasomes and decreased synthesis (Fig. 3.6) [148, 151, 152]. In terms of the accelerated degradation, Vif both binds to APOBEC3G and a specifc E3 ligase complex that mediates polyubiquitylation of APOBEC3G, marking it for proteasomal degradation [153]. These combined effects lead to the depletion of intracellular APOBEC3G in the virus-producing cell; thus, the enzyme is not available for virion incorporation.

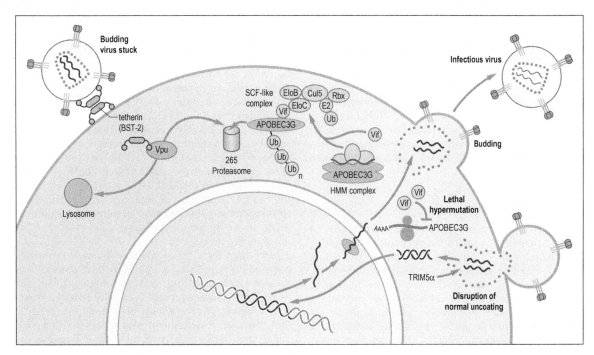

Figure 3.6 Host restriction factors block HIV-1 at various stages in its life cycle. TRIM5α targets the incoming viral capsid and disrupts the normal uncoating process. APOBEC3G, as well as other members of the APOBEC3 family, are incorporated into budding virions in the absence of Vif. Once in the target cell, APOBEC3 enzymes deaminate cytosine residues in the single-stranded minus-strand viral DNA, leading to lethal hypermutation. Vif overcomes the APOBEC3G block by both promoting polyubiquitylation and proteasome-mediated degradation of this enzyme and by partially blocking APOBEC3G translation. In the absence of Vpu, tetherin/BST-2 prevents the budding of HIV virions. Vpu antagonizes tetherin by promoting its degradation by the proteasome and lysosome.

The assembly of Vif with APOBEC3G and Vif-induced degradation of the antiretroviral enzyme provide an intriguing new target for antiviral drug development. The goal is to identify small molecules that would interfere with APOBEC3G degradation. The result would be to preserve the intracellular levels of the enzyme, making it available for incorporation into the virion and poised to unleash its potent DNA-mutating effects during the next round of reverse transcription. To this end, cell-based screens in which APOBEC3G is fused to a fluorescent protein and expressed in the presence of Vif have been devised [154, 155]. Although several compounds that display antiviral activity were identified by these screens, none has entered clinical trials.

TRIM5α

HIV fails to replicate in most nonhuman primate cells (chimpanzee and gibbon ape cells are notable exceptions). HIV entry occurs normally in these "nonpermissive" primate cells, but encounters a block prior to reverse transcription. The host restriction factor responsible for this block in nonhuman primate cells was identified as the tripartite

motif 5α protein, or TRIM5α [156]. TRIM5α derives its name from its tripartite motif that includes a zinc-binding ring finger, a B box domain that also binds zinc, and a coiled-coil region (SPRY domain). TRIM5α also contains a C-terminal B30.2/SPRY domain hypothesized to mediate protein–protein interactions. When levels of rhesus TRIM5α are decreased by RNA interference, HIV replication in these cells is greatly increased. In contrast to the inhibitory effects of rhesus TRIM5α, human TRIM5α only modestly impairs HIV replication.

The mechanism by which TRIM5α exerts its antiviral effect is not fully understood. TRIM5α targets intact or partially uncoated incoming viral cores [157–159]. It has been suggested that TRIM5α blocks HIV-1 infection by causing the cells to undergo rapid disassembly [160, 161] and/or by recruiting cellular proteasomal degradation machinery [162–165]. Interestingly, in some primate species (e.g., owl monkey), the C-terminal B30.2/SPRY domain has been replaced by cyclophilin A [166]. This "TRIM-Cyp" fusion protein potently inhibits HIV-1 infection. Indeed, fusion of cyclophilin A to the C-termini of several nonrestriction TRIM proteins also generated functional HIV-1 restriction factors.

With a greater understanding of how rhesus TRIM5α acts, it may be possible to develop small molecules that enhance the ability of human TRIM5α to associate with and restrict HIV-1. A single amino acid substitution greatly enhances the antiviral potency of human TRIM5α [167]. The binding of a small molecule could induce a conformational change that transforms human TRIM5α into a potent restriction factor. However, this poses a substantial challenge because most drugs are designed to disrupt an interaction or interfere with an enzymatic activity rather than elicit a gain-of-function interaction between two binding partners.

Tetherin

The most recently identified host restriction factor, tetherin (BST-2), inhibits viral replication by "tethering" mature virions on infected cell surfaces and preventing their release [168, 169]. HIV-1 escapes the tetherin block through the actions of its accessory protein Vpu. The mechanism by which Vpu antagonizes tetherin are not well understood; however, Vpu seems to sequester tetherin from the site of budding, reduce its surface expression, and promote its proteasomal degradation [170–172]. Tetherin is inducible by IFN-α, and high levels can suppress viral replication even in the presence of Vpu [173]. Therefore, enhancing tetherin expression by treatment with IFN-α represents a possible therapeutic approach. However, IFN-α treatment also has harmful consequences, such as contributing to the high levels of immune activation that drive progression toward AIDS. A more direct approach (e.g., identifying small molecules that interfere with the tetherin–Vpu interaction) may ultimately prove most useful as a therapeutic strategy.

SUMMARY AND PERSPECTIVE

The global AIDS pandemic continues to expand. Advances in antiretroviral therapies have slowed its advance in the industrialized world but due to limited availability have had less impact in the developing world. Because of its high rate of mutation, HIV is able to refine and optimize its interactions with various host proteins and pathways, thereby promoting its growth and spread. The virus ensures that the host cell survives until the viral replicative cycle is completed. Possibly even more damaging, HIV establishes stable latent forms that support the chronic nature of infection. Eradication of the virus appears unlikely until effective methods for purging these latent viral reservoirs are developed.

Basic science will clearly play a leading role in future attempts to solve the mysteries of viral latency and replication. A small-animal model that recapitulates the pathogenic mechanisms of HIV is sorely needed to study the mechanisms underlying viral cytopathicity. Such cell death is not only limited to infected targets but also involves uninfected bystander cells [174]. Murine cells do not support efficient assembly and/or release of Gag [175]. Currently, this defect represents a major impediment to the successful development of a rodent model of AIDS.

Proposed mechanisms for HIV killing of T cells include the formation of giant cell syncytia through the interactions of gp120 with CD4 and chemokine receptors [176]; the accumulation of unintegrated linear forms of viral DNA; the proapoptotic effects of the Tat [177], Nef [178], and Vpr [179] proteins; and the adverse effects conferred by the metabolic burden that HIV replication [180] places on the infected cell. Of note, expression of Nef alone as a transgene in mice recapitulates many of the clinical features of AIDS, including immunodeficiency and loss of CD4-infected cells [181].

Although CD4 T cells undergo a dramatic cytopathic response during infection, more than 95% of these cells are not productively infected. The mechanism of cell death in these bystander cells has eluded HIV researchers for many years. A recent study now shows that death of these bystander cells involves abortive HIV infection [182]. Drugs that block HIV entry or the early steps of reverse transcription prevent CD4 T cell death, while inhibitors of later events in the viral life cycle do not. Abortive infection appears to lead to the accumulation of incomplete reverse transcripts [182]. These cytoplasmic nucleic acids activate a host defense program that elicits a coordinated apoptotic and inflammatory response that ultimately leads to cell death.

Technical advances in recent years have vastly expanded our view of viral–host protein interactions. Genome-wide screens using libraries of small interfering RNA molecules have identified hundreds of new host cell factors required for HIV-1 replication. Three recent screens, which evaluated more than 20,000 genes, identified a total of 842 genes that reduce HIV-1 infection when knocked-down by RNA interference [183–185]. The lack of overlap between the three screens surprised many researchers in the HIV field. Therefore, caution must be used in interpreting the results. In addition to in vitro screens, molecular genetics are using genome-wide association studies to identify an even greater number of host factors. These studies involve large cohorts of HIV-infected individuals to identify human genetic differences that influence viral load and progression toward AIDS [186]. Although the role and relevance of these host factors to HIV-1 infection need to be confirmed, their identification vastly expands the number of potential targets for antiretroviral therapy.

Finally, future therapies will likely target viral proteins other than its enzymes, namely reverse transcriptase, protease, and integrase. Although only under preclinical evaluation, small chemicals capable of interfering with Tat transactivation [187] and Rev-dependent nuclear export of viral transcripts are under study [188]. As a proof of principle, dominant-negative mutants of Tat, Rev, and Gag proteins block viral replication [189]. By increasing the number of antiviral compounds available that target different steps in the viral replicative cycle and by ensuring that these drugs can be deployed in developing countries, we should be positioned better both to extend survival and to improve the quality of life for infected individuals and to inhibit the spread of AIDS.

ACKNOWLEDGMENTS

We thank Gary Howard and Stephen Ordway for editorial support, Robin Givens and Sue Cammack for administrative support, and the National Institutes of Health (R01 AI45234, R01 CA86814, P01 HD40543), the UCSF California AIDS Research Center (CC02-SF-002), and the J. David Gladstone Institutes for funding support.

REFERENCES

[1] Kwong PD, Wyatt R, Robinson J, et al. Structure of an HIV gp120 envelope glycoprotein in complex with the CD4 receptor and a neutralizing human antibody. Nature 1998;393(6686): 648–59.

[2] Pantophlet R, Burton DR. GP120: target for neutralizing HIV-1 antibodies. Annu Rev Immunol 2006;24:739–69.

[3] Scheid JF, Mouquet H, Feldhahn N, et al. Broad diversity of neutralizing antibodies isolated from memory B cells in HIV-infected individuals. Nature 2009;458(7238):636–40.

[4] Wu X, Yang ZY, Li Y, et al. Rational design of envelope identifies broadly neutralizing human monoclonal antibodies to HIV-1. Science 2010;329(5993):856–61.

[5] Jacobson JM, Israel RJ, Lowy I, et al. Treatment of advanced human immunodeficiency virus type 1 disease with the viral entry inhibitor PRO 542. Antimicrob Agents Chemother 2004;48(2):423–9.

[6] Jacobson JM, Lowy I, Fletcher CV, et al. Single-dose safety, pharmacology, and antiviral activity of the human immunodeficiency virus (HIV) type 1 entry inhibitor PRO 542 in HIV-infected adults. J Infect Dis 2000;182(1):326–9.

[7] Fletcher CV, DeVille JG, Samson PM, et al. Nonlinear pharmacokinetics of high-dose recombinant fusion protein CD4-IgG2 (PRO 542) observed in HIV-1-infected children. J Allergy Clin Immunol 2007;119(3):747–50.

[8] Kuritzkes DR, Jacobson J, Powderly WG, et al. Antiretroviral activity of the anti-CD4 monoclonal antibody TNX-355 in patients infected with HIV type 1. J Infect Dis 2004;189(2):286–91.

[9] Jacobson JM, Kuritzkes DR, Godofsky E, et al. Safety, pharmacokinetics, and antiretroviral activity of multiple doses of ibalizumab (formerly TNX-355), an anti-CD4 monoclonal antibody, in human immunodeficiency virus type 1-infected adults. Antimicrob Agents Chemother 2009;53(2):450–7.

[10] Doms RW, Trono D. The plasma membrane as a combat zone in the HIV battlefield. Genes Dev 2000;14 (21):2677–88.

[11] Scarlatti G, Tresoldi E, Bjorndal A, et al. In vivo evolution of HIV-1 co-receptor usage and sensitivity to chemokine-mediated suppression. Nat Med 1997;3(11):1259–65.

[12] Liu R, Paxton WA, Choe S, et al. Homozygous defect in HIV-1 coreceptor accounts for resistance of some multiply-exposed individuals to HIV-1 infection. Cell 1996;86 (3):367–77.

[13] Martinson JJ, Chapman NH, Rees DC, et al. Global distribution of the CCR5 gene 32-basepair deletion. Nat Genet 1997;16 (1):100–3.

[14] Perry CM. Maraviroc: a review of its use in the management of CCR5-tropic HIV-1 infection. Drugs 2010;70(9):1189–213.

[15] Imamura S, Ichikawa T, Nishikawa Y, et al. Discovery of a piperidine-4-carboxamide CCR5 antagonist (TAK-220) with highly potent Anti-HIV-1 activity. J Med Chem 2006;49(9):2784–93.

[16] Jacobson JM, Saag MS, Thompson MA, et al. Antiviral activity of single-dose PRO 140, a CCR5 monoclonal antibody, in HIV-infected adults. J Infect Dis 2008;198(9):1345–52.

[17] Kozak SL, Heard JM, Kabat D. Segregation of CD4 and CXCR4 into distinct lipid microdomains in T lymphocytes suggests a mechanism for membrane destabilization by human immunodeficiency virus. J Virol 2002;76(4):1802–15.

[18] Campbell SM, Crowe SM, Mak J. Lipid rafts and HIV-1: from viral entry to assembly of progeny virions. J Clin Virol 2001;22 (3):217–27.

[19] Liao Z, Cimakasky LM, Hampton R, et al. Lipid rafts and HIV pathogenesis: host membrane cholesterol is required for infection by HIV type 1. AIDS Res Hum Retroviruses 2001;17 (11):1009–19.

[20] Hladik F, Doncel GF. Preventing mucosal HIV transmission with topical microbicides: challenges and opportunities. Antiviral Res 2010;88(Suppl. 1):S3–9.

[21] Van Damme L, Ramjee G, Alary M, et al. Effectiveness of COL-1492, a nonoxynol-9 vaginal gel, on HIV-1 transmission in female sex workers: a randomised controlled trial. Lancet 2002;360(9338):971–7.

[22] Chan DC, Kim PS. HIV entry and its inhibition. Cell 1998;93(5):681–4.

[23] Geijtenbeek TB, Kwon DS, Torensma R, et al. DC-SIGN, a dendritic cell-specific HIV-1-binding protein that enhances trans-infection of T cells. Cell 2000;100 (5):587–97.

[24] Kwon DS, Gregorio G, Bitton N, et al. DC-SIGN-mediated internalization of HIV is required for trans-enhancement of T cell

infection. Immunity 2002;16 (1):135–44.

[25] Manel N, Hogstad B, Wang Y, et al. A cryptic sensor for HIV-1 activates antiviral innate immunity in dendritic cells. Nature 2010;467 (7312):214–17.

[26] Ganser-Pornillos BK, Yeager M, Sundquist WI. The structural biology of HIV assembly. Curr Opin Struct Biol 2008;18(2):203–17.

[27] Cartier C, Sivard P, Tranchat C, et al. Identification of three major phosphorylation sites within HIV-1 capsid. Role of phosphorylation during the early steps of infection. J Biol Chem 1999;274 (27):19434–40.

[28] Franke EK, Yuan HE, Luban J. Specific incorporation of cyclophilin A into HIV-1 virions. Nature 1994;372(6504):359–62.

[29] Schaeffer E, Geleziunas R, Greene WC. Human immunodeficiency virus type 1 Nef functions at the level of virus entry by enhancing cytoplasmic delivery of virions. J Virol 2001;75 (6):2993–3000.

[30] Ohagen A, Gabuzda D. Role of Vif in stability of the human immunodeficiency virus type 1 core. J Virol 2000;74(23):11055–66.

[31] Forshey BM, von Schwedler U, Sundquist WI, Aiken C. Formation of a human immunodeficiency virus type 1 core of optimal stability is crucial for viral replication. J Virol 2002;76(11):5667–77.

[32] Shi J, Zhou J, Shah VB, et al. Small-molecule inhibition of human immunodeficiency virus type 1 infection by virus capsid destabilization. J Virol 2011;85 (1):542–9.

[33] Karageorgos L, Li P, Burrell C. Characterization of HIV replication complexes early after cell-to-cell infection. AIDS Res Hum Retroviruses 1993;9(9):817–23.

[34] Bukrinskaya A, Brichacek B, Mann A, Stevenson M. Establishment of a functional human immunodeficiency virus type 1 (HIV-1) reverse transcription complex involves the cytoskeleton. J Exp Med 1998;188(11):2113–25.

[35] Miller MD, Farnet CM, Bushman FD. Human immunodeficiency virus type 1 preintegration complexes: studies of organization and composition. J Virol 1997;71(7):5382–90.

[36] McDonald D, Vodicka MA, Lucero G, et al. Visualization of the intracellular behavior of HIV in living cells. J Cell Biol 2002;159:441–52.

[37] Greber UF, Way M. A superhighway to virus infection. Cell 2006;124 (4):741–54.

[38] Naghavi MH, Hatziioannou T, Gao G, Goff SP. Overexpression of fasciculation and elongation protein zeta-1 (FEZ1) induces a post-entry block to retroviruses in cultured cells. Genes Dev 2005;19 (9):1105–15.

[39] Lee MS, Craigie R. A previously unidentified host protein protects retroviral DNA from autointegration. Proc Natl Acad Sci U S A 1998;95(4):1528–33.

[40] Suzuki Y, Yang H, Craigie R. LAP2alpha and BAF collaborate to organize the Moloney murine leukemia virus preintegration complex. EMBO J 2004;23 (23):4670–8.

[41] Weinberg JB, Matthews TJ, Cullen BR, Malim MH. Productive human immunodeficiency virus type 1 (HIV-1) infection of nonproliferating human monocytes. J Exp Med 1991;174 (6):1477–82.

[42] Pemberton LF, Blobel G, Rosenblum JS. Transport routes through the nuclear pore complex. Curr Opin Cell Biol 1998;10 (3):392–9.

[43] Gallay P, Hope T, Chin D, Trono D. HIV-1 infection of nondividing cells through the recognition of integrase by the importin/karyopherin pathway. Proc Natl Acad Sci U S A 1997;94(18):9825–30.

[44] Bukrinsky MI, Haggerty S, Dempsey MP, et al. A nuclear localization signal within HIV-1 matrix protein that governs infection of non-dividing cells. Nature 1993;365(6447):666–9.

[45] Heinzinger NK, Bukinsky MI, Haggerty SA, et al. The Vpr protein of human immunodeficiency virus type 1 influences nuclear localization of viral nucleic acids in nondividing host cells. Proc Natl Acad Sci U S A 1994;91 (15):7311–15.

[46] Zennou V, Petit C, Guetard D, et al. HIV-1 genome nuclear import is mediated by a central DNA flap. Cell 2000;101(2):173–85.

[47] Dvorin JD, Bell P, Maul GG, et al. Reassessment of the roles of integrase and the central DNA flap in human immunodeficiency virus type 1 nuclear import. J Virol 2002;76:12087–96.

[48] Sherman MP, de Noronha CM, Heusch MI, et al. Nucleocytoplasmic shuttling by human immunodeficiency virus type 1 Vpr. J Virol 2001;75 (3):1522–32.

[49] Eckstein DA, Sherman MP, Penn ML, et al. HIV-1 Vpr enhances viral burden by facilitating infection of tissue macrophages but not nondividing CD4+ T cells. J Exp Med 2001;194(10):1407–19.

[50] Vodicka MA, Koepp DM, Silver PA, Emerman M. HIV-1 Vpr interacts with the nuclear transport pathway to promote macrophage infection. Genes Dev 1998;12(2):175–85.

[51] Dupont S, Sharova N, DeHoratius C, et al. A novel nuclear export activity in HIV-1 matrix protein required for viral replication. Nature 1999;402 (6762):681–5.

[52] Fassati A, Gorlich D, Harrison I, et al. Nuclear import of HIV-1 intracellular reverse transcription complexes is mediated by importin 7. EMBO J 2003;22(14):3675–85.

[53] Ebina H, Aoki J, Hatta S, et al. Role of Nup98 in nuclear entry of human immunodeficiency virus type 1 cDNA. Microbes Infect 2004;6 (8):715–24.

[54] Zaitseva L, Myers R, Fassati A. tRNAs promote nuclear import of HIV-1 intracellular reverse transcription complexes. PLoS Biol 2006;4(10): e332.

[55] Chen H, Engelman A. The barrier-to-autointegration protein is a host factor for HIV type 1 integration. Proc Natl Acad Sci U S A 1998;95 (26):15270–4.

[56] Schroder AR, Shinn P, Chen H, et al. HIV-1 integration in the human genome favors active genes and local hotspots. Cell 2002;110 (4):521–9.

[57] Summa V, Petrocchi A, Bonelli F, et al. Discovery of raltegravir, a potent, selective orally bioavailable HIV-integrase inhibitor for the treatment of HIV-AIDS infection. J Med Chem 2008;51(18):5843–55.

[58] Marcelin AG, Ceccherini-Silberstein F, et al. Resistance to novel drug classes. Curr Opin HIV AIDS 2009;4(6):531–7.

[59] Cherepanov P, Maertens G, Proost P, et al. HIV-1 integrase forms stable tetramers and associates with LEDGF/p75 protein in human cells. J Biol Chem 2003;278(1):372–81.

[60] Maertens G, Cherepanov P, Pluymers W, et al. LEDGF/p75 is essential for nuclear and chromosomal targeting of HIV-1 integrase in human cells. J Biol Chem 2003;278 (35):33528–39.

[61] Llano M, Vanegas M, Fregoso O, et al. LEDGF/p75 determines cellular trafficking of diverse lentiviral but not murine oncoretroviral integrase proteins and is a component of functional lentiviral preintegration complexes. J Virol 2004;78 (17):9524–37.

[62] Ciuffi A, Llano M, Poeschla E, et al. A role for LEDGF/p75 in targeting HIV DNA integration. Nat Med 2005;11(12):1287–9.

[63] Shun MC, Raghavendra NK, Vandegraaff N, et al. LEDGF/p75 functions downstream from preintegration complex formation to effect gene-specific HIV-1 integration. Genes Dev 2007;21 (14):1767–78.

[64] Jacque JM, Stevenson M. The inner-nuclear-envelope protein emerin regulates HIV-1 infectivity. Nature 2006;441(7093):641–5.

[65] Wu Y, Marsh JW. Selective transcription and modulation of resting T cell activity by preintegrated HIV DNA. Science 2001;293(5534):1503–6.

[66] Li L, Olvera JM, Yoder KE, et al. Role of the non-homologous DNA end joining pathway in the early steps of retroviral infection. EMBO J 2001;20(12):3272–81.

[67] Adams M, Sharmeen L, Kimpton J, et al. Cellular latency in human immunodeficiency virus-infected individuals with high CD4 levels can be detected by the presence of promoter- proximal transcripts. Proc Natl Acad Sci U S A 1994;91 (9):3862–6.

[68] Jordan A, Defechereux P, Verdin E. The site of HIV-1 integration in the human genome determines basal transcriptional activity and response to Tat transactivation. EMBO J 2001;20(7):1726–38.

[69] Van Lint C, Emiliani S, Ott M, Verdin E. Transcriptional activation and chromatin remodeling of the HIV-1 promoter in response to histone acetylation. EMBO J 1996;15(5):1112–20.

[70] Marban C, Suzanne S, Dequiedt F, et al. Recruitment of chromatin-modifying enzymes by CTIP2 promotes HIV-1 transcriptional silencing. EMBO J 2007;26 (2):412–23.

[71] Blazkova J, Trejbalova K, Gondois-Rey F, et al. CpG methylation controls reactivation of HIV from latency. PLoS Pathog 2009;5(8): e1000554.

[72] Kauder SE, Bosque A, Lindqvist A, et al. Epigenetic regulation of HIV-1 latency by cytosine methylation. PLoS Pathog 2009;5(6):e1000495.

[73] Trono D, Van Lint C, Rouzioux C, et al. HIV persistence and the prospect of long-term drug-free remissions for HIV-infected individuals. Science 2010;329 (5988):174–80.

[74] Geeraert L, Kraus G, Pomerantz RJ. Hide-and-seek: the challenge of viral persistence in HIV-1 infection. Annu Rev Med 2008;59:487–501.

[75] Wang FX, Xu Y, Sullivan J, et al. IL-7 is a potent and proviral strain-specific inducer of latent HIV-1 cellular reservoirs of infected individuals on virally suppressive HAART. J Clin Invest 2005;115 (1):128–37.

[76] Lehrman G, Hogue IB, Palmer S, et al. Depletion of latent HIV-1 infection in vivo: a proof-of-concept study. Lancet 2005;366 (9485):549–55.

[77] Siliciano JD, Lai J, Callender M, et al. Stability of the latent reservoir for HIV-1 in patients receiving valproic acid. J Infect Dis 2007;195(6):833–6.

[78] Reuse S, Calao M, Kabeya K, et al. Synergistic activation of HIV-1 expression by deacetylase inhibitors and prostratin: implications for treatment of latent infection. PLoS One 2009;4(6):e6093.

[79] Taube R, Fujinaga K, Wimmer J, et al. Tat transactivation: a model for the regulation of eukaryotic transcriptional elongation. Virology 1999;264(2):245–53.

[80] Kao SY, Calman AF, Luciw PA, Peterlin BM. Anti-termination of transcription within the long terminal repeat of HIV-1 by tat gene product. Nature 1987;330 (6147):489–93.

[81] Jones KA, Peterlin BM. Control of RNA initiation and elongation at the HIV-1 promoter. Annu Rev Biochem 1994;63:717–43.

[82] Karin M, Ben-Neriah Y. Phosphorylation meets ubiquitination: the control of NF-[kappa]B activity. Annu Rev Immunol 2000;18:621–63.

[83] Crabtree GR. Generic signals and specific outcomes: signaling through Ca^{2+}, calcineurin, and NF-AT. Cell 1999;96(5):611–14.

[84] Barboric M, Nissen RM, Kanazawa S, et al. NF-kappaB binds P-TEFb to stimulate transcriptional elongation by RNA polymerase II. Mol Cell 2001;8(2):327–37.

[85] Wei P, Garber ME, Fang SM, et al. A novel CDK9-associated C-type cyclin interacts directly with HIV-1 Tat and mediates its high-affinity, loop-specific binding to TAR RNA. Cell 1998;92(4):451–62.

[86] Price DH. P-TEFb, a cyclin-dependent kinase controlling elongation by RNA polymerase II. Mol Cell Biol 2000;20(8):2629–34.

[87] Agbottah E, Deng L, Dannenberg LO, et al. Effect of SWI/SNF chromatin remodeling complex on HIV-1 Tat activated transcription. Retrovirology 2006;3:48.

[88] Mahmoudi T, Parra M, Vries RG, et al. The SWI/SNF chromatin-remodeling complex is a cofactor for Tat transactivation of the HIV promoter. J Biol Chem 2006;281 (29):19960–8.

[89] Treand C, du Chene I, Bres V, et al. Requirement for SWI/SNF chromatin-remodeling complex in Tat-mediated activation of the HIV-1 promoter. EMBO J 2006;25 (8):1690–9.

[90] Garber ME, Wei P, KewalRamani VN, et al. The interaction between HIV-1 Tat and human cyclin T1 requires zinc and a critical cysteine residue that is not conserved in the murine CycT1 protein. Genes Dev 1998;12 (22):3512–27.

[91] Garber ME, Mayall TP, Suess EM, et al. CDK9 autophosphorylation regulates high-affinity binding of the human immunodeficiency virus type 1 tat-P-TEFb complex to TAR RNA. Mol Cell Biol 2000;20 (18):6958–69.

[92] Yang Z, Zhu Q, Luo K, Zhou Q. The 7SK small nuclear RNA inhibits the CDK9/cyclin T1 kinase to control transcription. Nature 2001;414 (6861):317–22.

[93] Pagans S, Kauder SE, Kaehlcke K, et al. The cellular lysine methyltransferase Set7/9-KMT7 binds HIV-1 TAR RNA, monomethylates the viral transactivator Tat, and enhances HIV transcription. Cell Host Microbe 2010;7(3):234–44.

[94] Ott M, Schnolzer M, Garnica J, et al. Acetylation of the HIV-1 Tat protein by p300 is important for its transcriptional activity. Curr Biol 1999;9(24):1489–92.

[95] Kiernan RE, Vanhulle C, Schiltz L, et al. HIV-1 tat transcriptional activity is regulated by acetylation. EMBO J 1999;18(21):6106–18.

[96] Col E, Gilquin B, Caron C, Khochbin S. Tat-controlled protein acetylation. J Biol Chem 2002;277 (40):37955–60.

[97] Saltarelli MJ, Hadziyannis E, Hart CE, et al. Analysis of human immunodeficiency virus type 1 mRNA splicing patterns during disease progression in peripheral blood mononuclear cells from infected individuals. AIDS Res Hum Retroviruses 1996;12(15):1443–56.

[98] Cullen BR. Retroviruses as model systems for the study of nuclear RNA export pathways. Virology 1998;249 (2):203–10.

[99] Powell DM, Amaral MC, Wu JY, et al. HIV Rev-dependent binding of SF2/ASF to the Rev response element: possible role in Rev-mediated inhibition of HIV RNA splicing. Proc Natl Acad Sci U S A 1997;94(3):973–8.

[100] Luo Y, Yu H, Peterlin BM. Cellular protein modulates effects of human immunodeficiency virus type 1. Rev J Virol 1994;68(6):3850–6.

[101] Malim MH, Tiley LS, McCarn DF, et al. HIV-1 structural gene expression requires binding of the Rev trans-activator to its RNA target sequence. Cell 1990;60 (4):675–83.

[102] Farjot G, Sergeant A, Mikaelian I. A new nucleoporin-like protein interacts with both HIV-1 Rev nuclear export signal and CRM-1. J Biol Chem 1999;274 (24):17309–17.

[103] Bogerd HP, Fridell RA, Madore S, Cullen BR. Identification of a novel cellular cofactor for the Rev/Rex class of retroviral regulatory proteins. Cell 1995;82 (3):485–94.

[104] Zolotukhin AS, Felber BK. Mutations in the nuclear export signal of human ran-binding protein RanBP1 block the Rev-mediated posttranscriptional regulation of human immunodeficiency virus type 1. J Biol Chem 1997;272 (17):11356–60.

[105] Reddy TR, Xu W, Mau JK, et al. Inhibition of HIV replication by dominant negative mutants of Sam68, a functional homolog of HIV-1. Rev Nat Med 1999;5 (6):635–42.

[106] Malim MH, Cullen BR. Rev and the fate of pre-mRNA in the nucleus: implications for the regulation of RNA processing in eukaryotes. Mol Cell Biol 1993;13 (10):6180–9.

[107] Brasey A, Lopez-Lastra M, Ohlmann T, et al. The leader of human immunodeficiency virus type 1 genomic RNA harbors an internal ribosome entry segment that is active during the G2/M phase of the cell cycle. J Virol 2003;77(7):3939–49.

[108] Kestler 3rd HW, Ringler DJ, Mori K, et al. Importance of the nef gene for maintenance of high virus loads and for development of AIDS. Cell 1991;65(4):651–62.

[109] Deacon NJ, Tsykin A, Solomon A, et al. Genomic structure of an attenuated quasi species of HIV-1 from a blood transfusion donor

and recipients. Science 1995;270 (5238):988–91.

[110] Simmons A, Aluvihare V, McMichael A. Nef triggers a transcriptional program in T cells imitating single-signal T cell activation and inducing HIV virulence mediators. Immunity 2001;14(6):763–77.

[111] Khan IH, Sawai ET, Antonio E, et al. Role of the SH3-ligand domain of simian immunodeficiency virus Nef in interaction with Nef-associated kinase and simian AIDS in rhesus macaques. J Virol 1998;72 (7):5820–30.

[112] Glushakova S, Munch J, Carl S, et al. CD4 down-modulation by human immunodeficiency virus type 1 Nef correlates with the efficiency of viral replication and with CD4(+) T-cell depletion in human lymphoid tissue ex vivo. J Virol 2001;75(21):10113–17.

[113] Lama J, Mangasarian A, Trono D. Cell-surface expression of CD4 reduces HIV-1 infectivity by blocking Env incorporation in a Nef- and Vpu-inhibitable manner. Curr Biol 1999;9 (12):622–31.

[114] Zheng YH, Plemenitas A, Linnemann T, et al. Nef increases infectivity of HIV via lipid rafts. Curr Biol 2001;11(11):875–9.

[115] Geyer M, Fackler OT, Peterlin BM. Structure–function relationships in HIV-1 Nef. EMBO Rep 2001;2 (7):580–5.

[116] Wang JK, Kiyokawa E, Verdin E, Trono D. The Nef protein of HIV-1 associates with rafts and primes T cells for activation. Proc Natl Acad Sci U S A 2000;97(1):394–9.

[117] Chen BK, Gandhi RT, Baltimore D. CD4 down-modulation during infection of human T cells with human immunodeficiency virus type 1 involves independent activities of vpu, env, and nef. J Virol 1996;70(9):6044–53.

[118] Crise B, Buonocore L, Rose JK. CD4 is retained in the endoplasmic reticulum by the human immunodeficiency virus type 1 glycoprotein precursor. J Virol 1990;64(11):5585–93.

[119] Margottin F, Bour SP, Durand H, et al. A novel human WD protein,

h-beta TrCp, that interacts with HIV-1 Vpu connects CD4 to the ER degradation pathway through an F-box motif. Mol Cell 1998;1 (4):565–74.

[120] Xu XN, Laffert B, Screaton GR, et al. Induction of Fas ligand expression by HIV involves the interaction of Nef with the T cell receptor zeta chain. J Exp Med 1999;189 (9):1489–96.

[121] Collins KL, Chen BK, Kalams SA, et al. HIV-1 Nef protein protects infected primary cells against killing by cytotoxic T lymphocytes. Nature 1998;391(6665):397–401.

[122] Noviello CM, Benichou S, Guatelli JC. Cooperative binding of the class I major histocompatibility complex cytoplasmic domain and human immunodeficiency virus type 1 Nef to the endosomal AP-1 complex via its mu subunit. J Virol 2008;82 (3):1249–58.

[123] Roeth JF, Williams M, Kasper MR, et al. HIV-1 Nef disrupts MHC-I trafficking by recruiting AP-1 to the MHC-I cytoplasmic tail. J Cell Biol 2004;167(5):903–13.

[124] Schaefer MR, Wonderlich ER, Roeth JF, et al. HIV-1 Nef targets MHC-I and CD4 for degradation via a final common beta-COP-dependent pathway in T cells. PLoS Pathog 2008;4(8):e1000131.

[125] Le Gall S, Erdtmann L, Benichou S, et al. Nef interacts with the mu subunit of clathrin adaptor complexes and reveals a cryptic sorting signal in MHC I molecules. Immunity 1998;8(4):483–95.

[126] Geleziunas R, Xu W, Takeda K, et al. HIV-1 Nef inhibits ASK1-dependent death signalling providing a potential mechanism for protecting the infected host cell. Nature 2001;410 (6830):834–8.

[127] Wolf D, Witte V, Laffert B, et al. HIV-1 Nef associated PAK and PI3-kinases stimulate Akt-independent Bad-phosphorylation to induce anti-apoptotic signals. Nat Med 2001;7(11):1217–24.

[128] Greenway AL, McPhee DA, Allen K, et al. Human immunodeficiency virus type 1 Nef binds to tumor suppressor p53 and protects cells against p53-mediated apoptosis. J Virol 2002;76 (6):2692–702.

[129] Jowett JB, Planelles V, Poon B, et al. The human immunodeficiency virus type 1 vpr gene arrests infected T cells in the G2 + M phase of the cell cycle. J Virol 1995;69(10):6304–13.

[130] Goh WC, Rogel ME, Kinsey CM, et al. HIV-1 Vpr increases viral expression by manipulation of the cell cycle: a mechanism for selection of Vpr in vivo. Nat Med 1998;4(1):65–71.

[131] de Noronha CM, Sherman MP, Lin HW, et al. Dynamic disruptions in nuclear envelope architecture and integrity induced by HIV-1 Vpr. Science 2001;294 (5544):1105–8.

[132] Wilk T, Gross I, Gowen BE, et al. Organization of immature human immunodeficiency virus type 1. J Virol 2001;75(2):759–71.

[133] Freed EO. HIV-1 gag proteins: diverse functions in the virus life cycle. Virology 1998;251(1):1–15.

[134] Zimmerman C, Klein KC, Kiser PK, et al. Identification of a host protein essential for assembly of immature HIV-1 capsids. Nature 2002;415(6867):88–92.

[135] Gottlinger HG, Sodroski JG, Haseltine WA. Role of capsid precursor processing and myristoylation in morphogenesis and infectivity of human immunodeficiency virus type 1. Proc Natl Acad Sci U S A 1989;86 (15):5781–5.

[136] Ono A, Freed EO. Plasma membrane rafts play a critical role in HIV-1 assembly and release. Proc Natl Acad Sci U S A 2001;98 (24):13925–30.

[137] Morita E, Sundquist WI. Retrovirus budding. Annu Rev Cell Dev Biol 2004;20:395–425.

[138] Garnier L, Parent LJ, Rovinski B, et al. Identification of retroviral late domains as determinants of particle size. J Virol 1999;73 (3):2309–20.

[139] Strack B, Calistri A, Craig S, et al. AIP1/ALIX is a binding partner for HIV-1 p6 and EIAV p9 functioning in virus budding. Cell 2003;114 (6):689–99.

[140] Garrus JE, von Schwedler UK, Pornillos OW, et al. Tsg101 and the vacuolar protein sorting pathway are essential for HIV-1 budding. Cell 2001;107(1):55–65.

[141] VerPlank L, Bouamr F, LaGrassa TJ, et al. Tsg101, a homologue of ubiquitin-conjugating (E2) enzymes, binds the L domain in HIV type 1 Pr55(Gag). Proc Natl Acad Sci U S A 2001;98 (14):7724–9.

[142] Katzmann DJ, Babst M, Emr SD. Ubiquitin-dependent sorting into the multivesicular body pathway requires the function of a conserved endosomal protein sorting complex, ESCRT-I. Cell 2001;106(2):145–55.

[143] Farsad K, Ringstad N, Takei K, et al. Generation of high curvature membranes mediated by direct endophilin bilayer interactions. J Cell Biol 2001;155(2): 193–200.

[144] Liu F, Stephen AG, Waheed AA, et al. SAR by oxime-containing peptide libraries: application to Tsg101 ligand optimization. Chembiochem 2008;9 (12):2000–4.

[145] Simon JH, Gaddis NC, Fouchier RA, Malim MH. Evidence for a newly discovered cellular anti-HIV-1 phenotype. Nat Med 1998;4(12):1397–400.

[146] Madani N, Kabat D. An endogenous inhibitor of human immunodeficiency virus in human lymphocytes is overcome by the viral Vif protein. J Virol 1998;72:10251–5.

[147] Sheehy AM, Gaddis NC, Choi JD, Malim MH. Isolation of a human gene that inhibits HIV-1 infection and is suppressed by the viral Vif protein. Nature 2002;418:646–50.

[148] Stopak K, De Noronha C, Yonemoto W, Greene WC. HIV-1 Vif blocks the antiviral activity of APOBEC3G by impairing both its translation and intracellular stability. Mol Cell 2003;12:591–601.

[149] Yu Q, Konig R, Pillai S, et al. Single-strand specificity of APOBEC3G accounts for minus-strand deamination of the HIV genome. Nat Struct Mol Biol 2004;11:435–42.

[150] Mariani R, Chen D, Schrofelbauer B, et al. Species-

specific exclusion of APOBEC3G from HIV-1 virions by Vif. Cell 2003;114(1):21–31.

[151] Marin M, Rose KM, Kozak SL, Kabat D. HIV-1 Vif protein binds the editing enzyme APOBEC3G and induces its degradation. Nat Med 2003;9(11):1398–403.

[152] Sheehy AM, Gaddis NC, Malim MH. The antiretroviral enzyme APOBEC3G is degraded by the proteasome in response to HIV-1 Vif. Nat Med 2003;9 (11):1404–7.

[153] Yu X, Yu Y, Liu B, et al. Induction of APOBEC3G ubiquitination and degradation by an HIV-1 Vif-Cul5-SCF complex. Science 2003;302 (5647):1056–60.

[154] Nathans R, Cao H, Sharova N, et al. Small-molecule inhibition of HIV-1 Vif. Nat Biotechnol 2008;26 (10):1187–92.

[155] Cen S, Peng ZG, Li XY, et al. Small molecular compounds inhibit HIV-1 replication through specifically stabilizing APOBEC3G. J Biol Chem 2010;285(22):16546–52.

[156] Stremlau M, Owens CM, Perron MJ, et al. The cytoplasmic body component TRIM5alpha restricts HIV-1 infection in Old World monkeys. Nature 2004;427 (6977):848–53.

[157] Forshey BM, Shi J, Aiken C. Structural requirements for recognition of the human immunodeficiency virus type 1 core during host restriction in owl monkey cells. J Virol 2005;79 (2):869–75.

[158] Hatziioannou T, Cowan S, Von Schwedler UK, et al. Species-specific tropism determinants in the human immunodeficiency virus type 1 capsid. J Virol 2004;78 (11):6005–12.

[159] Owens CM, Song B, Perron MJ, et al. Binding and susceptibility to postentry restriction factors in monkey cells are specified by distinct regions of the human immunodeficiency virus type 1 capsid. J Virol 2004;78 (10):5423–37.

[160] Stremlau M, Perron M, Lee M, et al. Specific recognition and accelerated uncoating of retroviral capsids by the TRIM5alpha

restriction factor. Proc Natl Acad Sci U S A 2006;103 (14):5514–9.

[161] Perron MJ, Stremlau M, Lee M, et al. The human TRIM5alpha restriction factor mediates accelerated uncoating of the N-tropic murine leukemia virus capsid. J Virol 2007;81(5):2138–48.

[162] Anderson JL, Campbell EM, Wu X, et al. Proteasome inhibition reveals that a functional preintegration complex intermediate can be generated during restriction by diverse TRIM5 proteins. J Virol 2006;80 (19):9754–60.

[163] Campbell EM, Perez O, Anderson JL, Hope TJ. Visualization of a proteasome-independent intermediate during restriction of HIV-1 by rhesus TRIM5alpha. J Cell Biol 2008;180 (3):549–61.

[164] Rold CJ, Aiken C. Proteasomal degradation of TRIM5alpha during retrovirus restriction. PLoS Pathog 2008;4(5):e1000074.

[165] Wu X, Anderson JL, Campbell EM, et al. Proteasome inhibitors uncouple rhesus TRIM5alpha restriction of HIV-1 reverse transcription and infection. Proc Natl Acad Sci U S A 2006;103 (19):7465–70.

[166] Sayah DM, Sokolskaja E, Berthoux L, Luban J Cyclophilin A. retrotransposition into TRIM5 explains owl monkey resistance to HIV-1. Nature 2004;430 (6999):569–73.

[167] Stremlau M, Perron M, Welikala S, Sodroski J. Species-specific variation in the B30.2(SPRY) domain of TRIM5alpha determines the potency of human immunodeficiency virus restriction. J Virol 2005;79 (5):3139–45.

[168] Neil SJ, Zang T, Bieniasz PD. Tetherin inhibits retrovirus release and is antagonized by HIV-1 Vpu. Nature 2008;451(7177):425–30.

[169] Van Damme N, Goff D, Katsura C, et al. The interferon-induced protein BST-2 restricts HIV-1 release and is downregulated from the cell surface by the viral Vpu protein. Cell Host Microbe 2008;3 (4):245–52.

[170] Jouvenet N, Neil SJ, Zhadina M, et al. Broad-spectrum inhibition of retroviral and filoviral particle release by tetherin. J Virol 2009;83 (4):1837–44.

[171] Goffinet C, Allespach I, Homann S, et al. HIV-1 antagonism of CD317 is species specific and involves Vpu-mediated proteasomal degradation of the restriction factor. Cell Host Microbe 2009;5 (3):285–97.

[172] Mangeat B, Gers-Huber G, Lehmann M, et al. HIV-1 Vpu neutralizes the antiviral factor Tetherin/BST-2 by binding it and directing its beta-TrCP2-dependent degradation. PLoS Pathog 2009;5(9):e1000574.

[173] McNatt MW, Zang T, Hatziioannou T, et al. Species-specific activity of HIV-1 Vpu and positive selection of tetherin transmembrane domain variants. PLoS Pathog 2009;5(2):e1000300.

[174] Finkel TH, Tudor-Williams G, Banda NK, et al. Apoptosis occurs predominantly in bystander cells and not in productively infected cells of HIV- and SIV-infected lymph nodes. Nat Med 1995;1 (2):129–34.

[175] Bieniasz PD, Cullen BR. Multiple blocks to human immunodeficiency virus type 1 replication in rodent cells. J Virol 2000;74(21):9868–77.

[176] Kowalski M, Potz J, Basiripour L, et al. Functional regions of the envelope glycoprotein of human immunodeficiency virus type 1. Science 1987;237(4820):1351–5.

[177] Westendorp MO, Frank R, Ochsenbauer C, et al. Sensitization of T cells to CD95-mediated apoptosis by HIV-1 Tat and gp120. Nature 1995;375(6531):497–500.

[178] Baur AS, Sawai ET, Dazin P, et al. HIV-1 Nef leads to inhibition or activation of T cells depending on its intracellular localization. Immunity 1994;1(5):373–84.

[179] Stewart SA, Poon B, Jowett JB, Chen IS. Human immunodeficiency virus type 1 Vpr induces apoptosis following cell cycle arrest. J Virol 1997;71 (7):5579–92.

[180] Somasundaran M, Robinson HL. Unexpectedly high levels of HIV-1

RNA and protein synthesis in a cytocidal infection. Science 1988;242(4885):1554–7.

[181] Hanna Z, Kay DG, Rebai N, et al. Nef harbors a major determinant of pathogenicity for an AIDS-like disease induced by HIV-1 in transgenic mice. Cell 1998;95 (2):163–75.

[182] Doitsh G, Cavrois M, Lassen KG, et al. Abortive HIV infection mediates CD4 T cell depletion and inflammation in human lymphoid tissue. Cell 2010;143(5):789–801.

[183] Brass AL, Dykxhoorn DM, et al. Identification of host proteins required for HIV infection through a functional genomic screen. Science 2008;319(5865):921–6.

[184] Konig R, Zhou Y, Elleder D, et al. Global analysis of host–pathogen interactions that regulate early-stage HIV-1 replication. Cell 2008;135(1):49–60.

[185] Zhou H, Xu M, Huang Q, et al. Genome-scale RNAi screen for host factors required for HIV replication. Cell Host Microbe 2008;4(5):495–504.

[186] Fellay J, Shianna KV, Ge D, et al. A whole-genome association study of major determinants for host control of HIV-1. Science 2007;317(5840):944–7.

[187] Chao SH, Fujinaga K, Marion JE, et al. Flavopiridol inhibits P-TEFb and blocks HIV-1 replication. J Biol Chem 2000;275 (37):28345–8.

[188] Wolff B, Sanglier JJ, Wang Y. Leptomycin B is an inhibitor of nuclear export: inhibition of nucleo-cytoplasmic translocation of the human immunodeficiency virus type 1 (HIV-1) Rev protein and Rev-dependent mRNA. Chem Biol 1997;4(2):139–47.

[189] Meredith LW, Sivakumaran H, Major L, et al. Potent inhibition of HIV-1 replication by a Tat mutant. PLoS One 2009;4(11):e7769.

Chapter 4

The immune response to HIV

Clive M. Gray, Pamela Gumbi, Lycias Zembe, Mopo Radebe, Bruce Walker

INTRODUCTION

Most people in the world live in poverty-stricken conditions where they are continuously confronted with a plethora of pathogenic organisms—some successfully repelled, some resulting in clinically overt disease, and others resulting in persistent latent infection. The human immune system has evolved to combat these genetically diverse organisms, including viruses, bacteria, and protozoa, through genetically governed responses involving multiple receptors and ligands. Even with clinically overt or persistent infections, most people with an intact immune system ultimately survive most infections.

In marked contrast stands HIV infection. The spread of HIV-1 worldwide represents one of the great challenges to confront host immunity, since the key target is the CD4 T cell lymphocyte, infection and depletion of which severely undermines effective immune responses. As a result, most people who become infected and remain untreated will ultimately succumb to one or more of the large variety of infectious organisms that humans are confronted with on a daily basis. By 2010, there was an estimated 2.4–2.9 million people becoming newly infected with HIV, with 1.8 million dying of AIDS-related causes (http://www.unaids.org, 2011 Global Report).

The ultimate solution to the HIV epidemic relies on the development of an effective vaccine that can be delivered to those at risk. The ability to achieve this elusive goal will be facilitated by a comprehensive understanding of the key immune responses that contribute to protection from infection, or protection from disease progression in those who become infected. In this chapter, we will review the current state of knowledge of what is needed for an AIDS vaccine, first by comparison to effective immune clearance of acute viral infections (such as influenza, rotavirus, or respiratory syncytial virus) as well as acute viral infections followed by latent infection (herpes simplex virus or Epstein–Barr virus). This will allow a foundation for discussing why successful immune mechanisms are not functional in the majority of HIV-1-infected individuals. Much knowledge on the first immune events during acute HIV-1 infection has also accumulated, providing additional clues to the arms of immunity that are triggered upon first encounter with the virus. The field has been shaped by the hypothesis that the initial immune response to HIV infection is translatable to what would be expected or required from a vaccine. We will discuss clues as to what may constitute a protective immune response from disease progression in a small proportion of people who are HIV-1 infected, but can spontaneously contain viral replication to only a few RNA copies. Finally, we will discuss some of the failures and partial successes of recent vaccine trials, which have provided insight into the requirements for potential protective immune mechanisms.

GENERAL PRINCIPLES OF AN ANTIVIRAL IMMUNE RESPONSE

The degree to which pathogenic organisms establish productive infections is determined in part by the integrity of epithelial and mucosal cells: skin, respiratory tract, alimentary tract, urogenital tract, and conjunctiva. These regions serve as physical barriers between the exterior and internal environment and any abrasions or lesions will allow potential pathogenic organisms into either the blood or lymphatic circulation. Once these physical barriers have been transcended, there are two major categories of host immune responses, namely innate and acquired immunity.

The innate immune response represents the first line of defense, and serves to rapidly attenuate the impact of most infectious organisms. From an evolutionary perspective, innate immunity shares properties with lower vertebrate mechanisms of engulfment and phagocytosis and the response consists of specialized cells, such as macrophages, natural killer cells, dendritic cells, and polymorphonuclear leukocytes. Infectious organisms that survive the innate immune response, or residues from such a response, are dealt with by the specific acquired immune response.

Acquired immunity has three central tenets: *specificity*, recognition of protein structures via the interaction of receptors and ligands; *diversity*, variations in specificity, where multiple receptors interact with different protein structures; and *memory*, where different T and B cells that have been primed to antigens can be recalled at a subsequent point in time with a more rapid response.

What governs specificity and diversity of the adaptive immune response is the genetic make-up of the host, where genes encoding for the major histocompatibility complex (MHC), T cell receptors (TcR), and immunoglobulins (B cell receptors) dictate how and which regions of the pathogen are encountered by the immune system. The molecules encoded by these genes are central to specificity, diversity, and memory and constitute the internal composition of each individual and is collectively known as "self." An acquired immune response that results in the successful clearance of an invading organism can be understood by the exquisite difference in recognition between "self" and "non-self." The ultimate outcome of this process is preservation and survival of the species.

ACQUIRED IMMUNITY TO VIRAL INFECTIONS

The immune system consists of parallel blood and lymphatic circulations, ensuring that different cells participating in an immune response can migrate back and forth between non-lymphoid tissue and the different secondary lymphoid structures (such as the spleen and lymph nodes). Bone marrow is the primary lymphoid organ, where the precursors to all mature immunocompetent cells are derived as pluripotential progenitor cells. B and T cells develop into mature immunocompetent cells in the bone marrow and thymus, respectively. T cells that leave the thymus are "naïve" and have yet to encounter invading pathogens.

Lymph nodes are crucial for providing the correct microenvironment and anatomical structures required for initiating an immune response. The micro-anatomical arrangement of the lymph node enables T cells to encounter processed viral proteins presented by specialized antigen presenting cells, which initiates the adaptive immune response. In general terms, if the anatomical arrangement of lymphoid tissue disintegrates due to pathology, the impact will result in disrupted antigen presentation and loss of both B and T cell priming and the inability to provide protective immunity.

Movement of T cells from one lymphoid region to another allows both CD4 and CD8 T cells to encounter processed antigen in the paracortical region of the lymph node. After engaging and processing antigen in the peripheral tissue, dendritic cells will migrate to lymph nodes, where there is selection of reactive T cells through TcR engagement with viral peptides situated in the binding groove of the human leukocyte antigen molecules on the surface of the antigen presenting cells. This process results in multiple clones of expanded T cells, leading to diversity.

The MHC in humans is known as the human leukocyte antigen (HLA) system and is one of the most polymorphic proteins in the human population. The uniqueness of individuals is partly defined by HLA, where each person has a defined HLA type consisting of pairs of inherited genes. As the sole function of class I and II HLA is to present processed pathogen-derived peptides, or epitopes, to circulating T cells, possible aberrant T cell function and recognition of self, as in autoimmunity, will thus involve the HLA. HLA class I molecules are co-dominantly expressed on antigen presenting cells, and they play an important role in regulating the fitness of the immune system through a process of selecting and presenting immunogenic peptides to CD8 T cells by TcR recognition (Fig. 4.1A). HLA alleles are X-linked and inherited in pairs (heterozygous), and it is noteworthy that in HIV infection, individuals who are homozygous for one or more alleles (inheriting the same HLA allele from both parents) progress more rapidly to AIDS than heterozygotes [1]. Additionally, HLA-B is more polymorphic than HLA-A and HLA-C and the influence of HLA-B is known to have the strongest impact in HIV set point, which is strongly predictive of the rate of progression [2] when compared to HLA-A and HLA-C molecules [3, 4]. The manner by which epitopes are processed and bound by the HLA molecule is highly specific and governed by certain rules associated with the binding motif structures of each HLA and in the correct orientation will be recognized by activated CD8 cytotoxic T lymphocytes (Fig. 4.1A). Sequence changes can occur at anchor positions of targeted epitopes and reduce or interfere with peptide binding to the restricting HLA class I molecule. Moreover, amino acid changes within or immediately adjacent to CD8 T cell epitopes can impede intracellular antigen processing or directly modify the structural interaction between the epitope of HLA class I complex and the TcR of the corresponding CD8 T cells. The ability of viruses to acquire sequence mutations resulting in the loss of recognition by HIV-1-specific CD8 T cells poses a major hurdle for current vaccine efforts.

HLA class II molecules have a more restricted distribution and are expressed only on specific cell types and on T cells after activation. Classically, CD4 T cells provide

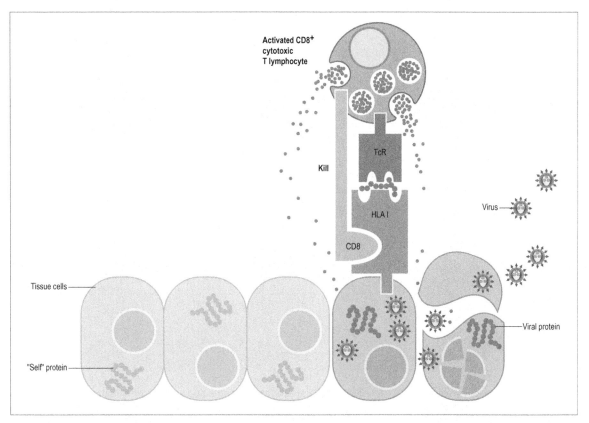

Figure 4.1A Cells infected by viruses or intracellular bacteria are detected and destroyed by CD8 cytotoxic T lymphocytes. CD8 cytotoxic T lymphocytes are activated in the secondary lymphoid organs and migrate to sites of inflammation where they scan cell surfaces with their T cell receptors (TcR) for recognition of foreign peptide antigens displayed on cell surface HLA class I molecules. HLA class I receptors are constitutively expressed on the surface of all cells except erythrocytes. CD8 cytotoxic T lymphocytes destroy target cells by releasing granzymes and perforin and cell-degrading molecules (with permission from Immunopaedia, http://www.immunopaedia.org).

"help" to the immune response by liberating a series of cytokines important for coordinating cellular activity and inducing activated B cells to become antibody-secreting plasma cells (Fig. 4.1B). First identified in murine models, the multitudinous number of cytokines have been organized into a network model of Th1, Th2, Treg, and Th17 cells. A Th1-type response consists of CD4 T cells liberating a profile of cytokines that direct T cell immunity and involves IL-1, IL-2, IL-6, IL-12, IL-15, TNF-α, and IFN-γ, for example. A Th-2-type response consists of CD4 T cells liberating a profile of cytokines that directs humoral immune responses and is involved in switching on B cell immunity. These cytokines include, among others, IL-4, IL-5, and IL-10. A Th17-type response consists of an IL-17A, IL-17F, and IL-22 profile and is involved in conferring protection against bacteria, fungi, and mycobacteria [5] and to play a role in mucosal defense in the gut. Tregs are $CD4^+CD25^{hi}FoxP3^+$ and have been shown to downregulate the activation and proliferation of T cells [5].

A balance exists between pro- and anti-inflammatory immune responses imparted by these CD4 subsets for maintaining the integrity and homeostatic balance of cells in the host. Recently, T helper follicular cells that are involved in the development of antibody-producing plasma cells in the germinal centers of lymphoid tissue have been described [6].

How do these cells fit together in healthy humans? CD8 T cells make up the smaller proportion of CD3 T cells and are involved in protecting the host from invading pathogens. These cells function by killing virally infected cells, which are marked by the surface expression of HLA class I molecules that present virus-derived epitopes that are typically 8-11 amino acids in length (as described above, Fig. 4.1A). These CD8 T cells function with the help of CD4 T helper cells. The killing potential of CD8 T cells is through either perforin/granzyme or Fas–Fas-L interactions and erupted and effete infected cells are engulfed and processed by dendritic cells; virally derived epitopes are presented via cross-presentation [7] by class II HLA

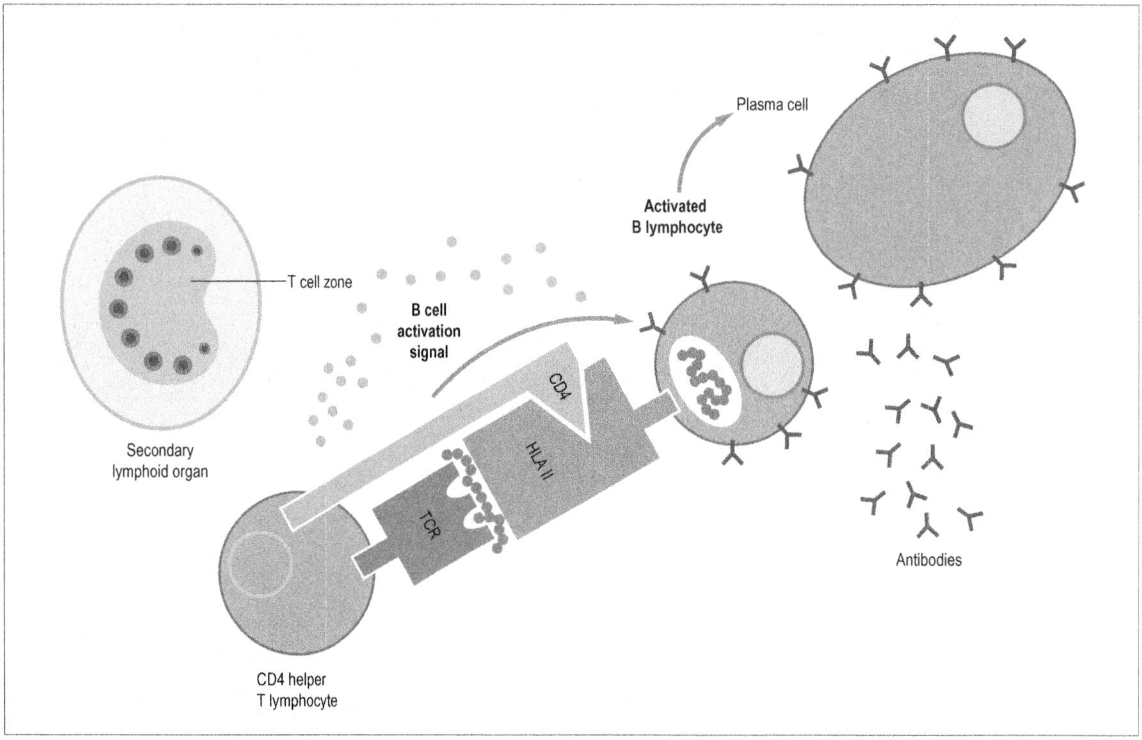

Figure 4.1B CD4 helper T lymphocytes stimulate B lymphocytes presenting peptide antigens associated with HLA class II receptors in the T cell zone of secondary lymphoid organs. The CD4 helper T lymphocyte provides activation signals to the B lymphocyte to proliferate and differentiate into antibody-secreting plasma cells. Memory B lymphocytes are also generated for long-term immunity (with permission from Immunopaedia, http://www.immunopaedia.org).

molecules and drive CD4 T cell responses. Typically most (99%) expanded viral antigen-specific T cell effector clones induced in the acute phase of infection will die through apoptosis as the immune response wanes, leaving a small residual population of T effector memory cells that migrate to non-lymphoid tissues or T central memory (TCM) cells that recirculate through the lymphatic system and blood circulation and can be rapidly reactivated upon secondary exposure to viral antigens.

IMMUNE RESPONSE TO HIV-1 INFECTION

The course of immunological events from the time of transmission can be divided into acute, early, and chronic phases of infection. The greatest challenges HIV presents to the immune system include the selective infection of CD4 T lymphocytes and the extensive viral genetic variability due to mutations.

Is HIV a disease of the mucosal immune system? A number of studies have highlighted the importance of the mucosa in HIV pathogenesis and it is now increasingly being recognized as a disease of the mucosal immune system [8], where vaginal and rectal mucosa are the predominant sites of HIV entry and the gut-associated lymphoid tissue (GALT) is the site of initial HIV replication. During the early phase of simian immunodeficiency virus (SIV) and HIV infection, there is a rapid and widespread massive depletion of activated mucosal CD4 T cells at mucosal sites and this occurs before significant depletion in blood and lymph nodes [9]. Recent evidence confirms that the level of CD4 T cell depletion is far higher than at first anticipated, with 60–80% of memory CD4 T cells depleted during early infection. Thus, within the first few weeks of HIV infection, the virus targets the mucosal immune system and dramatically depletes the CD4 T cells at this site. It has also been shown that HIV targeting of activated CD4 T cells in mucosal tissues persists throughout infection, and not just in acute infection as previously thought. Mucosal tissues are likely to be a major source of viral replication, persistence, and continual CD4 T cell loss in HIV-infected individuals. Reduced CD4 T cell frequencies during chronic HIV infection have also been shown in other mucosal sites such as rectal mucosa [10], male genital tract [11], female genital tract [9], and lung mucosa [12].

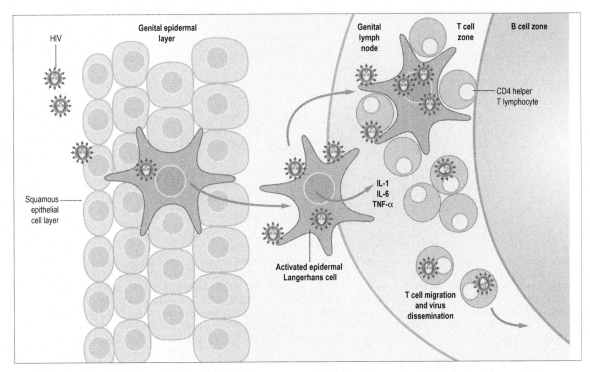

Figure 4.2 Epidermal Langerhans cells are a subset of dendritic cells found in the squamous epithelium of the female vagina and male inner foreskin and are the first immune cells to contact HIV during heterosexual contact. They express surface CD207 (langerin) that capture virus by binding to gp120 and induces internalization and degradation of virus. Activated cells migrate to draining lymph nodes for antigen presentation to CD4 T lymphocytes, which can also become infected by surface-bound virus. Langerhans cells also express CD4 and CCR5 and can become infected. Activated Langerhans cells produce pro-inflammatory cytokines IL-1, IL-6, and TNF-α that can cause fever in acute infection (with permission from Immunopaedia, http://www.immunopaedia.org).

Figure 4.2 shows some of the local factors in the mucosal microenvironment that may facilitate HIV replication in mucosal tissues independently from blood: (i) the localized cytokine milieu; (ii) differing inflammatory signals; and (iii) the presence of different immune cell types in these distinct compartments. These factors highlight mucosal sites as critically important in the context of not only understanding HIV pathogenesis but also in terms of being able to possibly dampen or correct the imbalance of proinflammatory signals in potential therapeutic or preventive modalities.

During acute HIV infection, there appears to be a hierarchy of systemic immune responses that occur. Figure 4.3 shows a composite schema of the known sequence of immunological responses that occur during infection. After viral transmission (1), where there appears to be a selection of single strain variants at the mucosa [13], there is dissemination (2) of the virus to the lymphoid tissue [14] during the acute phase of infection. Within days after viral transmission, viremia peaks and the downward slope is thought to be a result of a robust cellular immune response leading to initial control (3) of virus [15]. Natural history studies have shown that viral set point is achieved within 6 months of infection and is

prognostic of disease outcome, where high levels of viremia are associated with a more rapid course of infection leading to AIDS. It is noteworthy that seroconversion (4), by the detection of anti-Gag binding antibodies, occurs after peak viremia and that detection of neutralizing antibodies occurs only after approximately 3 months post transmission.

In addition to virus-specific CD8 T cells, CD4 T cells appear to be critical for immune control. Animal models of chronic viral infections established that virus-specific CD4 T cells play an essential role in maintenance of effective immunity (reviewed in Day and Walker [16]), and the immune response to HIV appears to follow these same requirements. The detection of enhanced proliferation of anti-HIV-specific CD4 T cells in individuals who maintain long-term control of HIV replication [17] and in patients treated for acute infection with potent antiretroviral therapy [17–19] suggest that the function of these cells is central to influencing viral set point and for controlling virus. As discussed, a large number of CD4 T cells are infected in the gut and that the bulk of the CD4 T cell pool resides within lymphoid tissue around the gastrointestinal tract. Direct killing of CCR5 CD4 T cells within the gut [20, 21] and memory CD4 cells in multiple tissues [22]

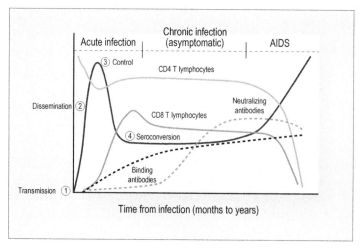

Figure 4.3 A typical immune response to untreated HIV infection shows a rapid increase in viremia in the acute phase, which declines to a set point. A decline in CD4 T cells coincides with the increase in viral load. HIV-specific CD8 cytotoxic T lymphocyte responses reduce the viral load and an increase in CD4 T cells is observed. HIV-specific binding antibodies appear after the reduction of viremia, but antibodies are detectable by ELISA only later in acute infection. During chronic infection, CD4 T cells decline slowly and viral load remains stable. Neutralizing antibodies begin to appear around 3 months post infection. Continued HIV replication and immune evasion exhausts the immune system, leading to opportunistic infection and AIDS in most infected people, albeit with varying lengths of time (with permission from Immunopaedia, http://www.immunopaedia.org).

by HIV has been postulated as the main mechanism for CD4 T cell depletion during SIV infection in monkeys, and extrapolations to HIV-induced depletion of CD4 T cells within the human gut have also been made [23]. Figure 4.4 shows the potential scenario of microbial translocation from the gut lumen. Studies of HIV/AIDS pathogenesis have long-focused on the role of CD4 T-cell depletion as a key marker of disease progression [24]. The pathogenesis of HIV infection is now characterized by CD4 T cell immunodeficiency in the context of generalized immune activation and dysregulation, with massive memory CD4 T cell infection and depletion during acute infection. This is followed by gradual loss of remaining CD4 T cells caused by persistent immune hyperactivation. Activation of CD4 T cells results in increased target cells for the virus, excessive apoptosis of uninfected T cells, generalized immune dysfunction, and impaired ability to control HIV replication.

In addition to cellular immune responses that emerge rapidly after HIV transmission, active humoral immunity is apparent by the increased titers of anti-Gag antibodies, which are used diagnostically to assess seroconversion. Functional antibodies are those that can block or neutralize HIV entry into CD4-bearing cells and such neutralizing antibodies mainly target the highly variable V3 loop, the CD4 binding domain, and the more conserved gp41 transmembrane protein of HIV-1. Although high titers of neutralizing antibodies can completely prevent infection in animal models, the role of these responses in viral containment following infection in humans remains uncertain. During acute infection, these responses appear following the initial drop in viremia, and experimental depletion of B cells in

monkeys during acute SIV infection led to delayed emergence of neutralizing antibodies and no change in early viral kinetics [25]. Additionally, passive transfer of neutralizing antibodies in monkeys can protect against intravenous and mucosal challenge of SIV [26]. Thus it is clear that neutralizing antibodies are important for prevention of viral infection, but perhaps less clear once HIV-1 infection has become established. Recent comprehensive longitudinal studies of autologous neutralizing antibody responses following acute infection indicate a significant antiviral effect of these responses, in that the viral inhibitory capacity is of sufficient magnitude to completely replace circulating neutralization-sensitive virus with successive populations of neutralization-resistant virus [33].

WHY THE IMMUNE RESPONSE FAILS TO CONTROL HIV

From our discussion so far, HIV infection provokes a burst of immune activity that results in potent targeted cytotoxic-T lymphocyte (CTL) responses, CD4 T cell function, and the induction of antibodies. These immunological components have been found to be central role-players in effective clearance of many other viral infections, but fail to clear HIV-1 infection without exception. Why is HIV neither eliminated nor effectively contained following infection?

A number of possibilities exist. First, it is important to understand from a virological perspective that HIV-1 establishes persistent infection by infecting CD4-bearing cells

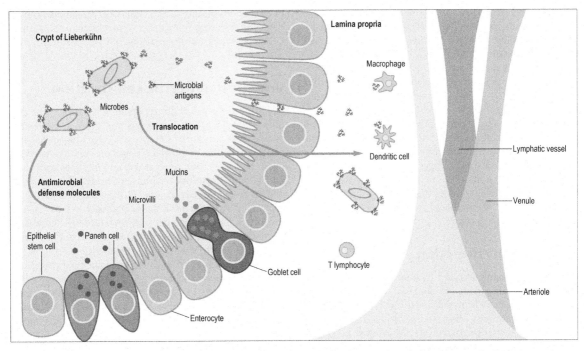

Figure 4.4 Activation of the mucosal immune system due to HIV replication in CD4 T helper lymphocytes in the lamina propria leads to the production of pro-inflammatory cytokines. This can cause a disruption of gut epithelial cell development, most notably resulting in villous atrophy and increased gut permeability to microbes and microbial antigens. The consequences of this are malabsorption of nutrients due to reduced absorptive surface area and further stimulation of mucosal immune cells that can enhance HIV replication (with permission from Immunopaedia, http://www.immunopaedia.org).

and integrates into the host genome as provirus. Both primary and secondary lymphoid tissues are targets for seeding by HIV soon after transmission and the anatomical structures within lymph nodes, spleen, and bone marrow are affected by the presence of virus. Consequently, from an immunological perspective, the persistence of antigen directly within the secondary lymphoid structures will influence T and B cell clonality and drive cells into a hyperactivated state. As discussed earlier, the high rate of HIV mutability, due to the error-prone nature of reverse transcriptase, in response to specific B and T cell reactivity, leads to immune escape and contributes to viral persistence within the host.

It is also important to understand that almost 30 years after AIDS was first identified, the critical immune functions that control HIV replication remain to be defined. A simplistic view has been that strong CD8 T cell responses, together with strong neutralizing antibodies and virus-specific CD4 T cells, would lead to control of viremia. The breadth and magnitude of CD8 T cell responses do not correlate with control of viremia, at least as measured by IFN-γ responses. Although neutralizing antibodies are detectable, there is no simple relationship between these and viremia. Even virus-specific CD4 T cells, which seem critical for maintenance of effective cellular and humoral immune responses in animal models of chronic infection, can be found in some persons with progressive infection. Thus the mechanisms that

account for a lack of long-term control of HIV infection are probably complex. The following are some of the factors for which there is now experimental evidence suggesting that they may participate in the ultimate lack of ability to control HIV replication.

Escape from neutralizing antibodies

Despite gradual broadening of the neutralizing antibody response following acute infection, it does not become sufficiently broad to neutralize the next population of virus to arise [27, 28], and the neutralizing antibody responses forever lag behind the evolution of the envelope gene. The relevance of neutralization antibody escape in loss of overall control of viremia is open to debate as escape has also been observed in HIV-infected individuals who persistently control viremia [29, 30].

Escape from CD8 T cell control

Studies in acute HIV infection have shown that mutations in the HIV genome occurs rapidly, resulting in viral escape from specific CD8 T cell recognition. During the course of infection the HIV-1 pathogen encodes numerous potentially immunogenic determinants; yet, CD8 T cells only recognize and respond to a minute fraction of potential viral epitopes. These CD8 T cells responses can be classified as immunodominant, co-dominant, and subdominant, depending on their relative contribution to the overall magnitude of HIV-1-specific CD8 T cell responses in a given individual. Data from both human and animal models indicate that during acute infection, highly effective HIV-1-specific CD8 T cells are narrowly directed against selected epitopes and do so in a hierarchal order [31]. This may suggest that the hierarchy of HIV-1-specific CD8 T-cell responses in acute infection may be crucial for the effectiveness of the immune response in chronic infection [31, 32]. Mutations within targeted epitopes [33, 34] can also abrogate established CD8 T cell responses, as can mutations in flanking residues that impair normal antigen processing. Both of these lead to loss of recognition by established T cell responses.

CD8 T cell dysfunction

Defects in differentiation and maturation of CTL [35–37] may result in impaired *in vivo* function, and may relate to lack of CD4 T cells help that is critical for maintenance of effective immunity. Most studies to date have defined CD8 T cell responses based on the ability to secrete IFN-γ, which based on animal model data may be the last effector response to be lost by CD8 T cells [38]. While T cells, in particular CD8 T cells, have the ability to carry out many functions in response to antigens including cytotoxicity, release of IFN-γ, TNF-α, and MIP-1β, for example, many previous studies on HIV-specific T cell responses focused on measuring one or two functions of these cells. The advancement in flow cytometry recently has allowed the measurement of multiple T cell functions, including degranulation (CD107a mobilization), cytokines (for example IFN-γ, IL-2, and TNF-α) and chemokine production (for example, MIP-1β) [39] to determine whether it is the quality of HIV-specific T cell response rather than frequency or breadth that is the important factor in HIV disease progression. Interestingly such studies have found out that non-progression [39] or elite control [40] in HIV infection is associated with maintenance of high levels of polyfunctional CD8 T cells. Other studies further dissected polyfunctionality and demonstrated that it is the up-regulation of perforin, a cytolytic enzyme, that is associated with control in HIV infection [41]. Recent data indicate a functional impairment in the ability of CD8 T cells to proliferate to viral antigens in persons with progressive disease that is maintained in persons with non-progressing infection [36], and present in the earliest stages of acute infection when viral load is rapidly declining [42].

Impaired CD4 T cell responses

The composition of functionally distinct subsets of virus-specific CD4 T cells, including IL-2- and IL-2/IFN-γ-secreting HIV-1-specific CD4 T cells, may be critical [43–45], as may cell killing by CD8 T cells [46]. Infection of a subset

of CD8 T cells that are CD4^{dim} following activation has been demonstrated, suggesting that infection of this population of CD8 T cells may contribute to loss of CD8 T cell function *in vivo* [47, 48].

Impaired dendritic cell function

Dendritic cells (DCs) are reported to be among the first cells with which HIV-1 interacts and through expression of a diverse array of receptors and signaling molecules, DC's capture and process HIV-1, and present associated antigens to T cells. DCs serve as crucial links between innate and adaptive immune responses through expression of pattern-recognition receptors (PRRs) such as Toll-like receptors (TLRs) and intracellular pathogen sensors, which trigger specific signaling pathways that lead to host defense. There are also recent studies in the SIV model and in a small human clinical trial suggesting impaired induction of immune responses in chronic infection, which may be related to the impaired function of DC during viral infection. These studies [49], in which adoptive transfer of *in vitro* matured DCs loaded with inactivated virus led to a decrease in set point viremia and increase in virus-specific immune responses, need to be confirmed by additional groups, but suggest that there is impairment in the inductive phase of the immune response.

Lymphoid structure degeneration

After infection, HIV-1 resides within the germinal centers of the lymph nodes, spleen, tonsils, and thymus and exists, in the main, as whole virus on the surface of follicular dendritic cells (FDCs) in the lymph node. As a result, the normal function of FDC in presenting antigen may be overridden. Viral transmission is thought to be cell-associated and productive infection most likely takes place in lymphoid structures in close proximity to the cervix and rectum, where DCs from the newly infected individual migrate from the cervical region to lymph nodes elsewhere in the body. Complete virus is most likely carried on DCs by dendritic cell-specific intercellular adhesion molecule-3-grabbing non-integrin (DC-SIGN), which aids in transmission to T cells [50] in the lymph nodes distal to the point of viral transmission. Although there are no clear data relating the dissolution of the lymph node architecture with persistence of virus, and ongoing immune responses, it may be hypothesized that destruction of the platform used to initiate immune responses leads to an overall failure in T cell priming to new antigens. Evidence from regenerated lymphoid structures after successful antiretroviral treatment supports this notion [51].

Other concomitant infections

The extent to which the ability to control HIV may be impaired by other concomitant infections is a particularly relevant question for those areas where the epidemic is currently most rapidly expanding. In many regions of the world, co-infections with *Mycobacterium tuberculosis* (mTB) [52] and other co-viral infections are predominant, and the impact of co-infections on host immunity to HIV is also relatively unknown. Herpes simplex virus type 2 (HSV-2) infection, for example, results in a persistent localized inflammatory response in the dermis below the healed lesion, consisting of HSV-2-specific CD4 T cells that express CCR5 or CXCR4, which are important HIV co-receptors. [53] Furthermore, HSV-2 suppressive therapy was shown to significantly reduce plasma viral loads and reduce genital tract HIV shedding in HIV-infected women co-infected with HSV-2 [54].

Human papilloma virus (HPV) infection of the cervix may influence HIV pathogenesis by inducing the production of immune and inflammatory factors that enhance HIV expression [55]. A meta-analysis was recently performed on 39 different studies that reported the effect of genital tract infections on the detection of HIV shedding in the genital tract [56]. In this meta-analysis, HIV-1 detection in the genital tract was increased most substantially by urethritis and cervicitis. Cervical discharge or mucopus, gonorrhoea, chlamydial infection, and vulvovaginal candidiasis were also significantly associated with HIV shedding. Alternatively, some studies have shown that there may be beneficial protective effects of HIV co-infection with GB virus C (GBV-C) [57], where protection may result from the induction of different chemokines that have anti-HIV properties. However, the mortality rates within cohort studies in populations of mine workers in southern Africa who are co-infected with mTB and HIV suggest that co-bacterial infections are anything but protective [58, 59].

EVIDENCE FOR CORRELATES OF PROTECTION TO HIV-1 INFECTION

Even though HIV-1 infection establishes persistence and undermines immunity, there are a small number of people who are infected but are clinically healthy and can control viremia to extraordinarily low levels: to less than 50 copies/mL plasma. Additionally, there are also individuals who have frequent high-risk sexual encounters and who have a high probability of being exposed to HIV, but remain uninfected. These two cohorts of individuals may provide clues to which factors of host immunity correlate with delayed disease or possible protection from infection [57]. Identity of these immune factors is important for providing clues to protective immunity and for devising successful vaccine strategies. Several cohort studies, including those of highly exposed persistently seronegative (HEPS) sex workers, occupationally exposed healthcare workers, and uninfected babies born to HIV-infected mothers, have reported evidence for systemic and mucosal

cytotoxic T cell activity and chemokine receptor mutations as significant markers associating with their seronegative status. Less well-associated factors such as chemokine production, HLA alleles/haplotypes, helper T cell responses, humoral responses, and soluble inhibitory factors have been described, but less uniformly. Evidence for mucosal HIV-specific IgA antibodies in HEPS individuals also provide evidence for possible protective roles of local antibody responses—although these studies often have examined small numbers of individuals [60].

A more recent exploration of defining which immune factors correlate with protection, or attenuation of disease in HIV-infected individuals, has been to identify human genes with polymorphic variants that influence the outcome of HIV-1 exposure or infection. Several AIDS-restricting genes (ARG) have been identified within the human genome that are related to either resistance or acceleration of disease (reviewed by O'Brien and Nelson [61]). Unbiased assessment of genes involved in viral control in HIV-infected people, using a whole genome association strategy, have strongly associated specific HLA genes, most notably *HLA-B*57-01*, with viral set point.

PROSPECTS FOR VACCINES

A vaccine is of paramount importance to develop and implement as a public health option in many regions of the globe where HIV-1 incidence rates are extremely high. If a preventive vaccine can lower the rate of secondary viral transmission, this will have a significant effect of mitigating the epidemic. Although successful vaccines have been implemented for diseases such as smallpox, polio, measles, and hepatitis B, replicating these designs for HIV-1 may not be appropriate. Persistence of HIV leading to chronic infection and the continuous viral evolution in the infected host, to evade antibody and CTL responses, needs to be accounted for. It is known, for example, that chronic persistence of antigen leads to diminished central memory T cells, and the inability of the immune system to mount an effective secondary response [62]. Thus a vaccine would be required to enhance the pool of central memory, either in a preventive nature or as a therapeutic option. Development of therapeutic vaccines is extremely relevant for the large numbers of HIV-1-infected individuals, where the aim would be to redirect immunity under the cover of antiretroviral therapy to effectively contain infection.

There is no doubt that a successful preventive vaccine will need to evoke aspects of innate, cellular, and humoral immunity. As the major determining factor of disease progression in an individual is viremia and the level of infectiousness is proportional to the magnitude of the viral load in plasma, genital tract secretions, and breast-milk, a vaccine capable of controlling viral replication would potentially lower the rate of disease progression and secondary transmission. Typically a phase IIb test-of-concept or III efficacy vaccine trial measures the candidate vaccine relative to a placebo control arm. The primary end-point measurement is lower incidence in the vaccine arm, although it is more likely that a secondary end-point will be levels of viremia at a specific time post infection and the time to set point. The recently halted STEP study, which was a double-blind phase II test-of-concept trial in 3,000 HIV seronegative volunteers in North America, the Caribbean, South America, and Australia receiving three injections of an adenovirus vector (MRKAd5) containing subtype B *gag/pol/nef* genes, failed to show efficacy and made no impact on levels of viremia at 3 months after vaccination in those who became infected [63]. Early follow-up showed that the vaccine arm may have been deleterious and hinted at promoting infection, but over longer-term follow-up, the number of infections per study arm became non-significant. The one factor associated with infection was whether men were circumcised [63], with the uncircumcised male being more susceptible. Whether this has to do with epidermal Langerhans cells in the foreskin that can trap virus (Fig. 4.2) is open to question. A companion trial in South Africa, the Phambili trial, showed a HIV infectivity pattern similar to that of the STEP study, with the major difference being that more women than men were enrolled and thus the enhanced infectivity in the vaccine arm in this trial was not related to circumcision status [64]. In contrast to the failure of the STEP and Phambili studies to show vaccine efficacy was the modest success of the prime boost phase III RV144 trial in Thailand [65]. This trial consisted of priming with a recombinant canarypox vector vaccine (ALVAC-HIV vCP1521) plus two booster doses of a recombinant glycoprotein 120 subunit (AIDSVAX B/E) in 16,402 HIV-1 seronegative men and women in Thailand. The recombinant gp120 immunogen alone showed no efficacy in a large earlier trial in Thailand [66], but when combined with the ALVAC product as a boost, showed a 31.2% efficacy using a modified intent-to-treat analysis [65].

Through the combined analyses of the STEP/Phambili and RV144 trial results, there will hopefully be insight into immune responses that are, and are not, important for vaccine efficacy. However, what clues do we have so far of the kind of immune response that will be required from a vaccine? The immune responses detected in monkeys as well as those detected in HEPS individuals and long-term non-progressors suggest that an effective HIV vaccine will need to elicit neutralizing antibodies, CD4 T cell responses, and CTL [52]. As discussed, since the major route of viral transmission is through mucosal barriers, and that HIV may be regarded as a disease of mucosal immunity, it will be crucial to elicit mucosal vaccine-induced immunity and not only systemic immunity. One feature of a vaccine-induced response is the elicitation of long-lived memory CD4 and CD8 T cells that can be rapidly recalled

in the event of a subsequent exposure or infection with HIV-1. The aim of an HIV vaccine response would be to generate pools of vaccine-specific long-lived central memory CD8 T cells. As discussed above, the persistence of antigen upon HIV infection compromises the development of central memory CD8 T cells, whereas the transient nature of vaccine-related antigens would create a more favorable environment for induction of central memory.

Other vaccine candidates are either in early clinical trials or in the pipeline of development (http://www.iavi.org, http://www.hvtn.org, http://www.chavi.org, and http://www.cavd.org). Whatever the eventual mechanisms leading to successful vaccine immunity, mucosal responses that can neutralize or contain HIV at the point of entry will need to be elicited, to cater for the genetic heterogeneity of HIV-1 across the globe, and to generate long-term memory. Notwithstanding these challenging scientific issues, uniform access of a stable vaccine to all individuals at an affordable cost is a social and political challenge that needs to be addressed in tandem with scientific development.

CONCLUSION

HIV infection elicits robust cellular and humoral immune responses, but the vast majority of persons ultimately fail to control viremia and progress to AIDS. Although progress has been made in understanding the reasons for ultimate lack of control, there are critical gaps in our knowledge that need to be resolved to facilitate rational vaccine design, and to guide immunotherapeutic interventions. Among these are the critical ratios of humoral and cellular immune responses, the critical viral antigens to target, the means to induce broadly cross-reactive protective immunity to the multiple strains currently fueling the global epidemics, and vaccine vector systems that are able to elicit potent antiviral immune responses. Great strides have been made recently in the detection, isolation, and crystallization of broadly neutralizing antibodies [67–70] and the design of candidate immunogens based on the structures of these antibody molecules.

With a modestly successful vaccine strategy and learning from trial failures, as well as major scientific advances in the structure and function of broadly neutralizing antibodies, there is reason for optimism. Emerging data also suggest that HIV may not be infinitely mutable, but that there are predictable mutations that occur within given residues when they come under immune selection pressure. Whether this knowledge can lead to the refinement of a vaccine strategy that would provide sufficient protection against circulating viruses remains to be determined. In the meantime, HIV will remain the most significant infectious disease of our generation, and will continue to extract a disproportionate toll on those most marginalized and disenfranchised in each society.

REFERENCES

[1] Carrington M, Nelson GW, Martin MP, et al. HLA and HIV-1: heterozygote advantage and B*35-Cw*04 disadvantage. Science 1999;283:1748–52.

[2] Mellors JW, Rinaldo Jr. CR, Gupta P, et al. Prognosis in HIV-1 infection predicted by the quantity of virus in plasma. Science 1996;272:1167–70.

[3] Goulder PJ, Watkins DI. Impact of MHC class I diversity on immune control of immunodeficiency virus replication. Nature Rev Immunol 2008;8:619–30.

[4] Kiepiela P, Leslie AJ, Honeyborne I, et al. Dominant influence of HLA-B in mediating the potential co-evolution of HIV and HLA. Nature 2004;432:769–75.

[5] Prendergast A, Prado JG, Kang YH, et al. HIV-1 infection is characterized by profound depletion of CD161+ Th17 cells and gradual decline in regulatory T cells. AIDS 2010;24:491–502.

[6] Batten M, Ramamoorthi N, Kljavin NM, et al. IL-27 supports germinal center function by enhancing IL-21 production and the function of T follicular helper cells. J Exp Med 2010;207(13):2895–906.

[7] Melief CJ. Mini-review: Regulation of cytotoxic T lymphocyte responses by dendritic cells: peaceful coexistence of cross-priming and direct priming? Eur J Immunol 2003;33:2645–54.

[8] Derdeyn CA, Silvestri G. Viral and host factors in the pathogenesis of HIV infection. Curr Opin Immunol 2005;17:366–73.

[9] Veazey RS, Marx PA, Lackner AA. Vaginal CD4+ T cells express high levels of CCR5 and are rapidly depleted in simian immunodeficiency virus infection. J Infect Dis 2003;187:769–76.

[10] Critchfield JW, Young DH, Hayes TL, et al. Magnitude and complexity of rectal mucosa HIV-1-specific CD8+ T-cell responses during chronic infection reflect clinical status. PLoS One 2008;3:e3577.

[11] Politch JA, Mayer KH, Anderson DJ. Depletion of CD4+ T cells in semen during HIV infection and their restoration following antiretroviral therapy. J Acquir Immune Defic Syndr 2009;50:283–9.

[12] Vajdy M, Veazey R, Tham I, et al. Early immunologic events in mucosal and systemic lymphoid tissues after intrarectal inoculation with simian immunodeficiency virus. J Infect Dis 2001;184:1007–14.

[13] Keele BF, Giorgi EE, Salazar-Gonzalez JF, et al. Identification and characterization of transmitted and early founder virus envelopes in primary HIV-1 infection. Proc Natl Acad Sci U S A 2008;105:7552–7.

[14] Gray CM, Mlotshwa M, Riou C, et al. Human immunodeficiency virus-specific gamma interferon enzyme-linked immunospot assay responses targeting specific regions of the proteome during primary subtype c infection are poor predictors of the course of viremia and set point. J Virol 2009;83:470–8.

[15] Kemal KS, Burger H, Mayers D, et al. HIV-1 drug resistance in variants from the female genital tract and plasma. J Infect Dis 2007;195:535–45.

[16] Day CL, Walker BD. Progress in defining CD4 helper cell responses in chronic viral infections. J Exp Med 2003;198:1773–7.

[17] Rosenberg ES, Billingsley JM, Caliendo AM, et al. Vigorous HIV-1-specific CD4+ T cell responses associated with control of viremia. Science 1997;278:1447–50.

[18] Malhotra U, Berrey MM, Huang Y, et al. Effect of combination antiretroviral therapy on T-cell immunity in acute human immunodeficiency virus type 1 infection. J Infect Dis 2000;181:121–31.

[19] Oxenius A, Price DA, Easterbrook PJ, et al. Early highly active antiretroviral therapy for acute HIV-1 infection preserves immune function of CD8+ and CD4+ T lymphocytes. Proc Natl Acad Sci U S A 2000;97:3382–7.

[20] Veazey RS, Lackner AA. HIV swiftly guts the immune system. Nat Med 2005;11:469–70.

[21] Li Q, Duan L, Estes JD, et al. Peak SIV replication in resting memory CD4+ T cells depletes gut lamina propria CD4+ T cells. Nature 2005;434:1148–52.

[22] Mattapallil JJ, Douek DC, Hill B, et al. Massive infection and loss of memory CD4+ T cells in multiple tissues during acute SIV infection. Nature 2005;434:1093–7.

[23] Mehandru S, Poles MA, Tenner-Racz K, et al. Primary HIV-1 infection is associated with preferential depletion of CD4+ T lymphocytes from effector sites in the gastrointestinal tract. J Exp Med 2004;200:761–70.

[24] Sodora DL, Silvestri G. HIV, mucosal tissues, and T helper 17 cells: where we come from, where we are, and where we go from here. Curr Opin HIV AIDS 2010;5:111–13.

[25] Schmitz JE, Kuroda MJ, Santra S, et al. Effect of humoral immune responses on controlling viremia during primary infection of rhesus monkeys with simian immunodeficiency virus. J Virol 2003;77:2165–73.

[26] Mascola JR, Stiegler G, VanCott TC, et al. Protection of macaques against vaginal transmission of a pathogenic HIV-1/SIV chimeric virus by passive infusion of neutralizing antibodies. Nat Med 2000;6:207–10.

[27] Richman DD, Wrin T, Little SJ, Petropoulos CJ. Rapid evolution of the neutralizing antibody response to HIV type 1 infection. Proc Natl Acad Sci U S A 2003;100:4144–9.

[28] Wei X, Decker JM, Wang S, et al. Antibody neutralization and escape by HIV-1. Nature 2003;422:307–12.

[29] Bradney AP, Scheer S, Crawford JM, et al. Neutralization escape in human immunodeficiency virus type 1-infected long-term nonprogressors. J Infect Dis 1999;179:1264–7.

[30] Montefiori DC, Altfeld M, Lee PK, et al. Viremia control despite escape from a rapid and potent autologous

neutralizing antibody response after therapy cessation in an HIV-1-infected individual. J Immunol 2003;170:3906–14.

[31] Streeck H, Jolin JS, Qi Y, et al. Human immunodeficiency virus type 1-specific CD8+ T-cell responses during primary infection are major determinants of the viral set point and loss of CD4+ T cells. J Virol 2009;83:7641–8.

[32] Allen TM, O'Connor DH, Jing P, et al. Tat-specific cytotoxic T lymphocytes select for SIV escape variants during resolution of primary viraemia. Nature 2000;407:386–90.

[33] Yokomaku Y, Miura H, Tomiyama H, et al. Impaired processing and presentation of cytotoxic-T-lymphocyte (CTL) epitopes are major escape mechanisms from CTL immune pressure in human immunodeficiency virus type 1 infection. J Virol 2004;78:1324–32.

[34] Kimura Y, Gushima T, Rawale S, et al. Escape mutations alter proteasome processing of major histocompatibility complex class I-restricted epitopes in persistent hepatitis C virus infection. J Virol 2005;79:4870–6.

[35] Champagne P, Ogg GS, King AS, et al. Skewed maturation of memory HIV-specific CD8 T lymphocytes. Nature 2001;410:106–11.

[36] Migueles SA, Laborico AC, Shupert WL, et al. HIV-specific CD8+ T cell proliferation is coupled to perforin expression and is maintained in nonprogressors. Nat Immunol 2002;3:1061–8.

[37] Appay V, Dunbar PR, Callan M, et al. Memory CD8+ T cells vary in differentiation phenotype in different persistent virus infections. Nat Med 2002;8:379–85.

[38] Wherry EJ, Blattman JN, Murali-Krishna K, et al. Viral persistence alters CD8 T-cell immunodominance and tissue distribution and results in distinct stages of functional impairment. J Virol 2003;77:4911–27.

[39] Betts MR, Nason MC, West SM, et al. HIV nonprogressors preferentially maintain highly functional HIV-specific CD8+ T cells. Blood 2006;107:4781–9.

[40] Owen RE, Heitman JW, Hirschkorn DF, et al. HIV+ elite controllers have low HIV-specific T-cell activation yet maintain strong, polyfunctional T-cell responses. AIDS 2010;24:1095–105.

[41] Hersperger AR, Pereyra F, Nason M, et al. Perforin expression directly ex vivo by HIV-specific CD8+ T-cells is a correlate of HIV elite control. PLoS Pathog 2010;6:e1000917.

[42] Lichterfeld M, Kaufmann DE, Yu XG, et al. Loss of HIV-1-specific CD8+ T cell proliferation after acute HIV-1 infection and restoration by vaccine-induced HIV-1-specific CD4+ T cells. J Exp Med 2004;200:701–12.

[43] Boaz MJ, Waters A, Murad S, et al. Presence of HIV-1 Gag-specific IFN-gamma+IL-2+ and CD28+IL-2+ CD4 T cell responses is associated with nonprogression in HIV-1 infection. J Immunol 2002;169:676–85.

[44] Iyasere C, Tilton JC, Johnson AJ, et al. Diminished proliferation of human immunodeficiency virus-specific CD4+ T cells is associated with diminished interleukin-2 (IL-2) production and is recovered by exogenous IL-2. J Virol 2003;77:10900–9.

[45] Harari A, Petitpierre S, Vallelian F, Pantaleo G. Skewed representation of functionally distinct populations of virus-specific CD4 T cells in HIV-1-infected subjects with progressive disease: changes after antiretroviral therapy. Blood 2004;103:966–72.

[46] Boritz E, Palmer BE, Wilson CC. Human immunodeficiency virus type 1 (HIV-1)-specific CD4+ T cells that proliferate in vitro detected in samples from most viremic subjects and inversely associated with plasma HIV-1 levels. J Virol 2004;78:12638–46.

[47] Cochrane A, Imlach S, Leen C, et al. High levels of human immunodeficiency virus infection of CD8 lymphocytes expressing CD4 in vivo. J Virol 2004;78:9862–71.

[48] Zloza A, Sullivan YB, Connick E, et al. CD8+ T cells that express CD4 on their surface (CD4dimCD8bright T cells) recognize an antigen-specific target, are detected in vivo, and can be productively infected by T-tropic HIV. Blood 2003;102:2156–64.

[49] Lu W, Wu X, Lu Y, et al. Therapeutic dendritic-cell vaccine for simian AIDS. Nat Med 2003;9:27–32.

[50] Arrighi JF, Pion M, Garcia E, et al. DC-SIGN-mediated infectious synapse formation enhances X4 HIV-1 transmission from dendritic cells to T cells. J Exp Med 2004;200:1279–88.

[51] Gray CM, Lawrence J, Ranheim EA, et al. Highly active antiretroviral therapy results in HIV type 1 suppression in lymph nodes, increased pools of naive T cells, decreased pools of activated T cells, and diminished frequencies of peripheral activated HIV type 1-specific CD8+ T cells. AIDS Res Hum Retroviruses 2000;16:1357–69.

[52] Kaufmann SH, McMichael AJ. Annulling a dangerous liaison: vaccination strategies against AIDS and tuberculosis. Nat Med 2005;11:S33–S44.

[53] Zhu J, Hladik F, Woodward A, et al. Persistence of HIV-1 receptor-positive cells after HSV-2 reactivation is a potential mechanism for increased HIV-1 acquisition. Nat Med 2009;15:886–92.

[54] Anderson BL, Cu-Uvin S. Determinants of HIV shedding in the lower genital tract of women. Curr Infect Dis Rep 2008;10:505–11.

[55] Smith JS, Moses S, Hudgens MG, et al. Increased risk of HIV acquisition among Kenyan men with human papillomavirus infection. J Infect Dis 2010;201:1677–85.

[56] Johnson LF, Lewis DA. The effect of genital tract infections on HIV-1 shedding in the genital tract: a systematic review and meta-analysis. Sex Transm Dis 2008;35:946–59.

[57] Kulkarni PS, Butera ST, Duerr AC. Resistance to HIV-1 infection: lessons learned from studies of highly exposed persistently seronegative (HEPS) individuals. AIDS Rev 2003;5:87–103.

[58] Day JH, Grant AD, Fielding KL, et al. Does tuberculosis increase HIV load? J Infect Dis 2004; 190:1677–84.

[59] Corbett EL, Charalambous S, Moloi VM, et al. Human immunodeficiency virus and the prevalence of undiagnosed tuberculosis in African gold miners. Am J Respir Crit Care Med 2004;170:673–9.

[60] Kaul R, Plummer F, Clerici M, et al. Mucosal IgA in exposed, uninfected subjects: evidence for a role in protection against HIV infection. AIDS 2001;15:431–2.

[61] O'Brien SJ, Nelson GW. Human genes that limit AIDS. Nat Genet 2004;36:565–74.

[62] Garber DA, Silvestri G, Feinberg MB. Prospects for an AIDS vaccine: three big questions, no easy answers. Lancet Infect Dis 2004;4:397–413.

[63] Buchbinder SP, Mehrotra DV, Duerr A, et al. Efficacy assessment of a cell-mediated immunity HIV-1 vaccine (the Step Study): a double-blind, randomised, placebo-controlled, test-of-concept trial. Lancet 2008;372:1881–93.

[64] Gray G, Buchbinder S, Duerr A. Overview of STEP and Phambili trial results: two phase IIb test-of-concept studies investigating the efficacy of MRK adenovirus type 5 gag/pol/nef subtype B HIV vaccine. Curr Opin HIV AIDS 2010;5:357–61.

[65] Rerks-Ngarm S, Pitisuttithum P, Nitayaphan S, et al. Vaccination with ALVAC and AIDSVAX to prevent HIV-1 infection in Thailand. N Engl J Med 2009;361:2209–20.

[66] Pitisuttithum P, Gilbert P, Gurwith M, et al. Randomized, double-blind, placebo-controlled efficacy trial of a bivalent recombinant glycoprotein 120 HIV-1 vaccine among injection drug users in Bangkok, Thailand. J Infect Dis 2006;194:1661–71.

[67] Pancera M, McLellan JS, Wu X, et al. Crystal structure of PG16 and chimeric dissection with somatically related PG9: structure–function analysis of two quaternary-specific antibodies that effectively neutralize HIV-1. J Virol 2010;84:8098–110.

[68] Wu X, Yang ZY, Li Y, et al. Rational design of envelope identifies broadly neutralizing human monoclonal antibodies to HIV-1. Science 2010;329:856–61.

[69] Zhou T, Georgiev I, Wu X, et al. Structural basis for broad and potent neutralization of HIV-1 by antibody VRC01. Science 2010;329:811–17.

[70] Walker LM, Phogat SK, Chan-Hui PY, et al. Broad and potent neutralizing antibodies from an African donor reveal a new HIV-1 vaccine target. Science 2009;326 (5950):285–9.

Chapter 5

Viral and host determinants of HIV-1 disease progression

Daniëlle van Manen, Angélique B. van 't Wout, Hanneke Schuitemaker

INTRODUCTION

The clinical course of HIV-1 infection can be highly variable, with extremes of disease progression within 12 months after seroconversion or continuous asymptomatic infection for more than 20 years. The loss of CD4 T cells is one of the hallmarks of HIV-1 infection, which in the absence of combination antiviral therapy ultimately leads to immunodeficiency. The mechanism by which CD4 T cells are lost is still under debate, but the vital role of virus-driven chronic immune activation and increased cell turnover is now well accepted. A high and persistent level of virus replication seems to be the driving force. The high variability in the clinical course of HIV-1 infection is therefore determined by the level of HIV-1 load, which itself is determined by the interplay between viral and host (genetic) factors. In this chapter, we will discuss these factors and their effect on HIV-1 load and disease progression in the natural course of infection.

SPECIFIC (ADAPTIVE) ANTIVIRAL IMMUNE RESPONSE

Humoral immune response

Upon infection with HIV-1, both cellular and humoral immune responses are mounted against the virus. The humoral immune response initially consists mainly of binding antibodies. Only after a few weeks to months, neutralizing antibodies emerge [1, 2]. The importance of neutralizing antibodies in controlling infection was indicated in SIV-infected macaques by B cell depletion [3–5], albeit not in all studies [6]. Moreover, passive transfer of three broadly neutralizing antibodies resulted in a delay in viral rebound after cessation of antiretroviral therapy in acutely HIV-1-infected individuals [7]. However, HIV-1 can escape from neutralizing antibodies and a neutralization-resistant phenotype is associated with changes in the viral envelope [2, 8–10]. The existence of this escape mechanism was first demonstrated in macaques [11] and in a laboratory worker who became accidentally infected with the neutralization-sensitive HIV-1 variant IIIB and in whom a neutralization-resistant IIIB-related variant evolved [12]. A major component of the viral escape mechanism is the increase and repositioning of glycans, the so-called glycan shield [1, 2]. Glycans are strategically positioned and repositioned continuously throughout infection, in a way that minimally affects the interaction of the envelope with the receptor molecules on the cell surface, but maximally hinders the binding of neutralizing antibodies [2]. Additionally, elongation of variable loops in Env has been associated with neutralization resistance [9, 10, 13, 14].

Despite the rapid escape of HIV-1, the neutralizing antibody response was initially still considered to be important because escape from humoral immunity was thought to coincide with a loss of viral fitness [15], which would give rise to a lower viral load set point and hence an ameliorated disease course. However, later studies found that escape from neutralizing antibodies did not coincide with a reduction in replication fitness [16]. In recent years, interest has increased for broadly neutralizing antibodies. These antibodies can neutralize HIV-1 variants from different subtypes and are therefore considered to be directed against conserved epitopes. Based on this it was hypothesized that escape from these broadly neutralizing antibodies would be extremely difficult for the virus and would come at an extreme fitness cost. Surprisingly, escape from autologous serum with broadly neutralizing antibodies occurred rapidly and was also not associated with a loss in viral replication fitness [10]. This is most likely because escape is not associated with mutations in the epitope itself, but rather with the above-mentioned changes in the viral envelope, being an increased number of glycans and an increased length of the variable loops that may occlude the antibody epitope. In agreement with the rapid escape, the presence of even broadly neutralizing activity in serum was not associated with a prolonged asymptomatic course of infection [17, 18].

Cellular immune response: cytotoxic T lymphocytes

HIV-1 specific cellular immune responses, mediated by cytotoxic and helper T lymphocytes, emerge very rapidly after infection [19–21]. Several observations have suggested that HIV-1 specific CD8 cytotoxic T cells (CTLs) contribute to the control of HIV infection. Strong CTL responses are often observed in long-term asymptomatic HIV-1-infected individuals but diminish with progression to AIDS [22]. It cannot be excluded, however, that these preserved CTL responses are a consequence, rather than a cause, of prolonged asymptomatic survival. Experimental depletion of CD8 T cells in SIV-infected macaques led to the loss of control of acute infection and to increased viral load in chronic infection [23, 24]. Later studies showed, however, that CD4 T cells under these conditions started to proliferate, providing the virus with an excellent opportunity to replicate, which may explain the rise in viral load [25].

Finally, the quality of T cell responses early in infection was not associated with AIDS-free survival [26]. As for neutralizing humoral immunity, this lack of effect of CTLs may be due to viral escape. Escape mutations in even a single epitope may lead to loss of immune control by CTLs [27]. Viruses with CTL escape mutations can be rapidly selected and overtake the viral quasispecies in as little as 6 weeks after first emergence [28]. The rapid selection of these escape variants is in fact the strongest argument that CTLs are effective *in vivo*. The impact of certain CTL escape mutations on viral fitness [29, 30] was also demonstrated by complete reversal of the escape mutation to the wild-type sequence upon transmission to a new individual [31]. The selective pressure of CTLs is such that at a population level, the virus strains circulating in a population have adapted to the most common human leukocyte antigen (HLA) types in that population [32, 33]. The complex influence of HLA on HIV-1 disease course will be discussed later in the section on host polymorphisms. Mutations outside CTL epitopes have also been described to influence CTL function, by affecting antigen processing and presentation [34].

Cellular immune response: helper T lymphocytes

The functioning of HIV-1-specific CTL depends on the presence of functional CD4 helper T cells. The presence of CD4 helper T cells that proliferate and produce both IL-2 and IFN-γ in response to HIV-specific peptide pools early in infection are not predictive for prolonged AIDS-free survival [35]. However, during the course of infection, the loss of these helper T cells, together with the loss of all functional CD4 T cells, causes a less efficient immune response, thus allowing opportunistic infections to bypass the immune system, finally resulting in disease progression and AIDS. In mouse models it was demonstrated that the presence of CD4 T cells during priming of CTLs is essential for the maintenance of immunological memory after the acute infection phase, whereas their continuous presence was not required for CTL expansion [36, 37]. It can thus be envisioned that with the loss of CD4 T cells during HIV-1 infection no efficient new CD8 T cell memory is generated in later phases of the infection.

CHRONIC IMMUNE ACTIVATION AND CD4 T CELL LOSS

Depletion of CD4 T cells, which is preceded by a loss of proliferative responses to polyclonal stimuli [38] and recall antigens [39], is one of the major characteristics of HIV-1 infection [40]. The fact that HIV-1 uses CD4 as a cellular entry receptor together with the observation that CD4 T cells are specifically lost in HIV-1 infection led to the logical conclusion that virus-mediated killing of target cells was the main cause for this cell loss. However, the frequency of infected cells in peripheral blood in the chronic phase of infection is too low to account for the ongoing depletion of CD4 T cells by viral infection [41, 42]. Several converging lines of evidence now suggest that hyperactivation of the immune system in response to chronic HIV-1 infection may be the culprit [43]. Hyperactivation is responsible for an increased naive T cell turnover, leading ultimately to the exhaustion of the naive T cell compartment, which then cannot compensate for the enhanced death of memory CD4 T cells into which the activated CD4 T cells mature. Indeed, the level of immune activation was found to be at least as good a predictor of disease progression as the level of viral replication [44, 45]. Additional evidence came from the comparison of SIV infection in sooty mangabeys and African green monkeys on the one hand and in Asian macaque species on the other [46]. SIV infection in Asian macaques generally leads to high virus loads, declining CD4 T cell numbers, and disease within 2 years [47]. Sooty mangabeys and African green monkeys can both be infected with SIV and despite overt viral replication these animals have stable CD4 counts and do not progress to disease [48, 49]. The stable CD4 counts in the presence of high viral load is in line with the assumption that virus-mediated killing has no large effect on total CD4 T cell numbers. Despite the high viral load, these animals show no evidence of hyperactivation of their immune system as observed in SIV-infected macaques and HIV-1-infected humans [49]. This suggests that although the increased turnover of naive T cells in HIV-1-infected individuals is virus driven, the responsiveness is determined by host factors. More recently it was demonstrated that the initial immune response against the virus was similar in both the non-pathogenic and pathogenic macaque model. Interestingly, this initial response was then down-regulated only in the non-pathogenic macaque model but not in the pathogenic SIV macaque model [50–52]. The underlying mechanism for the differential regulation of the immune response needs to be elucidated. It has been suggested that at least two populations of CD4 T cells are important in mediating this immune response: Th17 cells, defined by the secretion of cytokine IL-17, which are thought to be critical in the defense against bacterial and fungal pathogens, and regulatory T cells (Tregs), expressing FoxP3, which are able to induce tolerance against self-antigens and prevent autoimmunity. The pro-inflammatory Th17 cells and immunoregulatory Tregs have antagonistic effector functions; a shift in this balance might be critical in the outcome of HIV disease. Indeed, the loss of Th17/Treg balance was associated with chronic immune activation and pathogenic SIV infection in non-human primates [53]. The mechanisms responsible for selective Th17/Treg imbalance during pathogenic infection are as yet undefined.

CD4 depletion in the gut

In both the SIV macaque model and in HIV-1-infected humans it was demonstrated that already during the phase of primary infection a massive depletion of CD4 T cells occurs in all tissues, including the gut-associated lymphoid tissues (GALT) where more than 80% of T cells reside [54–57]. This depletion of lymphocytes from the GALT occurs within days and seems to be irreversible [58]. It was shown that HIV-1 infection and depletion in the acute phase was not restricted to activated memory cells as also a high frequency of infected resting CD4 T cells could be demonstrated [59, 60]. The unique capacity of HIV-1 to replicate in non-dividing cells is in agreement with this observation [61]. Recently it has been reported that Th17 cells are preferentially lost from the GI tract. Importantly, this loss is observed in HIV-1 infection and pathogenic SIV infection of rhesus macaques, but not in non-pathogenic SIV infection of sooty mangabeys [62, 63].

VIRAL FACTORS THAT INFLUENCE VIRAL LOAD: BIOLOGICAL PHENOTYPE

HIV-1 can vary with respect to biological properties such as replication rate, cell tropism, co-receptor use, and neutralization sensitivity. The use of different co-receptors by HIV-1 is a general phenomenon for viruses from all different subtypes and circulating recombinant forms (CRFs), although quantitative differences in the prevalence of HIV-1 variants that can use the CXC chemokine receptor 4 (CXCR4-using variants) among subtypes exist. Virus variants with different biological properties dominate in different phases of infection. New infections are generally established by HIV-1 variants that use CD4 and additionally the CC chemokine receptor 5 (CCR5) as a co-receptor (R5 variants) [64–68]. Even if both R5 and CXCR4-using variants are present in the donor, most often only the R5 variants are detected in the recipient [65, 66, 69]. With progression of disease, a shift in the viral quasispecies toward more rapidly replicating T cell-tropic R5 variants is observed [64]. In the natural course of approximately half of HIV-1 subtype B-infected individuals this is associated with the appearance of CXCR4-using HIV-1 variants prior to AIDS diagnosis [70]. CXCR4-using variants are associated with an accelerated CD4 T cell decline and a more rapid disease progression [71, 72]. The accelerated loss of CD4 T cells after appearance of CXCR4-using variants can be explained from the fact that naïve T cells express CXCR4 but not CCR5, while memory cells express both CXCR4 and CCR5 [73]. This co-receptor expression pattern makes naïve T cells a unique target cell population for CXCR4-using variants. Indeed, clonal virus isolation from naïve T cells resulted in predominantly CXCR4-using variants, whereas both R5 and CXCR4-using biological virus clones could be obtained from the memory T cells from the same individuals [74]. It can be envisaged that infection and subsequent virus-mediated killing of naïve T cells by CXCR4-using virus variants directly interferes with T cell ontogeny as the infected and killed naïve T cell will no longer give rise to a daughter cell population. Considering the potential beneficial effect of an expanded target cell population and the limited number of amino acid substitutions in V3 that is sufficient to confer CXCR4-using capability to R5 variants, it is puzzling that CXCR4-using variants emerge prior to AIDS diagnosis in only a proportion of infected individuals [75, 76]. It has been hypothesized that the absence of CXCR4-using variants early in HIV-1 infection may be due to their higher vulnerability to the host adaptive immune responses, in particular neutralizing antibodies. The fact that these variants appear more frequently after the initial decline of CD4 T cells indeed suggests that they may represent a peculiar, congenic form of opportunistic infection. The first appearing CXCR4-using variants are more sensitive to neutralizing antibodies directed against the CD4 binding site than their coexisting R5 variants [77]. Moreover, a conserved neutralization epitope, designated D19, is invariably cryptic in R5 variants of different genetic subtypes, but it is consistently exposed in CXCR4-using variants, rendering such variants sensitive to neutralization by a specific antibody [78].

Evolution of co-receptor use

Phylogenetic analyses of HIV-1 envelope sequences have shown that CXCR4-using variants directly evolve from R5 variants, after which the CXCR4-using and R5 viruses coexist within the same individual [79, 80]. After the first appearance of CXCR4-using variants, both R5 and CXCR4-using variants continuously evolve away from the common ancestor and each other. However, this is only evident for the *env* gene as CXCR4-using and R5 virus populations cannot be distinguished on the basis of *gag* sequences due to frequent recombination events outside the *env* gene [81]. In general, the first CXCR4-using variants can still use CCR5 on primary cells, albeit it far less efficiently [82]. Recent studies have shown that failure of maraviroc, a small molecule CCR5 antagonist, is caused by the presence of R5 variants that can use maraviroc-bound CCR5 for entry [83] or by the presence of CXCR4-using variants, which upon closer inspection were existent pretherapy [84, 85]. The continued evolution of CXCR4-using and R5 variants is also evident from changes in their biological properties over time. Early CXCR4-using variants are more sensitive to the inhibitory effect of co-receptor antagonists AMD3100 and T22 than late-stage-obtained CXCR4-using variants [82]. In analogy, late-stage R5 variants from individuals who never developed CXCR4-using variants are less sensitive to inhibition by the natural ligand of CCR5, RANTES [86]. The co-receptor inhibitor resistance of R5 and CXCR4-using variants is correlated with the immune status of the host. Although the exact mechanism of resistance remains to be established, the observation is suggestive for selection of HIV-1 variants that use their co-receptor with increasing efficiency as the infection progresses. In a recent study we have observed that viruses with this late-stage phenotype can be transmitted to a new host after which evolution continued [87]. So, while R5 variants are preferentially transmitted over CXCR4-using variants, there does not seem to be a preferential transmission phenotype within R5 variants. The fact that HIV-1 envelope is changing at a population level over calendar time is in line with this observation [88].

Viral accessory genes

The HIV-1 genome encodes for three structural proteins (Gag, Pol, and Env), two regulatory proteins (Tat and Rev) and four accessory proteins: Vpr, Vpu, Nef, and Vif. Initially the function of the accessory genes was not clear

and they are dispensable for viral replication in some cell types. It is believed that their main function is dedicated to mechanisms to escape or manipulate adaptive and innate immunity. Here we describe how Vpr, Vpu, Nef, and Vif each suppress the antiviral activity of specific host cell factors.

Nef

In the SIV macaque model it was demonstrated that inoculation with SIV that lacked the *Nef* gene resulted in infection but not disease progression [89]. A cohort of individuals in Sydney infected with HIV-1 from the same source and classified as long-term non-progressors, all carried a ΔNef HIV-1 variant [90], although some have ultimately progressed to AIDS-defining events [91]. Multiple Nef activities are known, which are mostly genetically separable and make use of distinct elements located throughout the Nef molecule. Nef alters the intracellular trafficking of important immune molecules, such as class I and II major histocompatibility complex proteins (MHC-I, MHC-II), CD4, and DC-SIGN [92–95]. Down-regulation of MHC-I proteins on the surface of the cell by Nef protects HIV-infected cells from recognition and killing by CTLs, while Nef-dependent CD4 removal enables optimal release of infectious virions. More directly, Nef also triggers apoptotic pathways, affecting survival of bystander CD4 T cells [96]. Furthermore, Nef promotes the induction of cellular transcription factors that can elevate viral replication [97] and Nef intersects with the macrophage CD40L signaling pathway to promote infectivity [98]. Recently it has been reported that Nef can transfer from infected cells into B cells, leading to impaired class switching [99]. Thus, Nef supports viral replication via both direct and indirect mechanisms.

Vif

The HIV-1 protein Vif is essential for viral replication by counteracting the effects of apolipoprotein B mRNA editing enzyme, catalytic polypeptide-like (APOBEC) 3 G and APOBEC3F, mediators of one aspect of the innate immunity, a potent cellular defense system against retroviral infection [100, 101]. APOBEC3F and APOBEC3G are members of the APOBEC superfamily of cytosine deaminases which, in the absence of Vif, are incorporated into the virion. During reverse transcription of the viral genome in a new cell, they deaminate cytidine to uracil, inducing lethal G-to-A hypermutation in the viral DNA [102, 103]. Vif can bind both APOBEC3F and APOBEC3G and redirect it by ubiquitination to degradation in the proteasome, thereby preventing the viral DNA from mutation [104, 105]. More recently it was reported that the expression of truncated or misfolded viral proteins due to APOBEC3G editing enhances the recognition of HIV-1-infected cells by CTLs, linking the innate and adaptive immune responses [106].

Vpr

Monkeys infected with SIV without Vpr function had severely attenuated infections with much lower viral burden and no evidence of disease progression [107], confirming the role of Vpr in viral pathogenesis. Multiple functions of the viral protein Vpr have been reported. First, Vpr has been shown to interact with cellular factors leading to the inhibition of host cell proliferation by a G2 cell cycle arrest of infected cells [108], although the virological role remains unclear. Vpr also has a nuclear localization signal and facilitates nuclear localization of the viral pre-integration complex [109, 110]. By interaction of Vpr with various transcriptional factors on the LTR promoter, the viral protein induces HIV-1 viral gene transcription [111]. Additionally, Vpr causes cell death by inducing apoptosis [112].

Vpu

Two distinct functions have been associated with the viral protein U (Vpu). Vpu down-regulates CD4 cell surface expression by targeting CD4 for degradation in the endoplasmic reticulum of infected cells [113]. Vpu is also known to enhance efficient viral particle release, by antagonizing the action of tetherin [114, 115]. Tetherin is a transmembrane protein that blocks the release of budding HIV-1 virions by directly anchoring the viral particle to the surface of the cell. The retained virions are internalized by endocytosis and subsequently degraded.

HOST FACTORS THAT INFLUENCE HIV-1 ACQUISITION AND DISEASE PROGRESSION

Several host factors that influence the clinical course of HIV-1 infection have been identified. Initially, these host genetic factors were discovered in candidate gene studies (see Table 5.1), in which gene variants that were already known or suspected to play a role in HIV-1 pathogenesis and immune regulation were tested for association with HIV-1 infection and/or disease progression. Examples of these are genes that encode proteins necessary for HIV-1 entry in a cell or for efficient replication and propagation of the virus. In addition, variations in innate and adaptive immune-regulatory genes and in specific viral-restriction genes have been studied for association with HIV-1 disease. Of these, the HLA genes are discussed in more detail below. The variants that were identified in most of these candidate gene studies turned out to have large effects on disease risk, even in small cohorts (see Table 5.1) and most have been reviewed extensively before [116–118]. In the case of CCR5, this has even resulted in the development of new antiviral strategies to block CCR5 in HIV-1-infected individuals, as uninfected individuals without CCR5 function (i.e. those homozygous for the 32 base pair deletion in CCR5) show no overt clinical symptoms.

The more recent genome-wide association studies (GWAS) offer a hypothesis-free analysis of the genome to find novel factors influencing HIV-1 infection and disease course. GWAS are a tool to examine the complete genome of different individuals to determine variation between individuals, mostly at the level of single DNA mutations, the so-called single-nucleotide polymorphisms (SNPs). Associations between these SNPs and HIV-1 susceptibility or HIV-1 disease course and thus identification of genes essential to HIV-1 and of gene variants present in healthy individuals that affect HIV-1 may ultimately lead to new prevention strategies and therapies, similar to the development of CCR5 antagonists.

Human leukocyte antigens

The HLA genes map to chromosome 6 and form one of the most polymorphic regions in the human genome. HLA class I loci, HLA-A, B, and C all encode for a large number of different alleles. Each individual expresses two HLA-A, two HLA-B, and two HLA-C alleles on the surface of all their cells. These HLA molecules present viral antigens to CD8 T cells, thereby initiating a cytotoxic T cell response. Due to the large variation that is created by six different HLA molecules, a large diversity of viral peptides that supports potent immunity can be presented. Homozygosity for HLA alleles reduces the repertoire that can be presented to the immune system, thereby limiting the number of epitopes recognized by CTLs. Indeed, homozygosity has been associated with faster disease progression [119, 120]. Moreover, certain class I alleles have been implicated in the variable clinical course of HIV-1 infection. HLA-B*27 [27] and B*57 are consistently associated with effective control of HIV-1 and delayed disease progression, albeit that this association is not absolute [29, 30]. HLA-B*5701 has been associated with long-term non-progression in Caucasian populations [121, 122], while the closely related HLA-B*5703 is associated with delayed disease progression after HIV-1 infection in individuals from African descent [123, 124]. This was confirmed in a GWAS in African Americans [125]. Additionally, HLA-B*57 seems to be associated with control of HIV-1 already early in infection as the prevalence of this allele was significantly lower in individuals with symptomatic acute infection, when compared to a chronically infected population [126]. HLA-B*27 and HLA-B*57 restricted CTL select for HIV-1 variants that have escape mutations in certain epitopes in more conserved regions that come at a relatively high fitness cost to the virus. This is supported by the observation that escape mutations in some epitopes that are restricted by HLA-B*57 immediately revert to wild-type sequences after transmission to a non-HLA-B*57 individual [31]. Interestingly, HIV-1

Table 5.1 Host factors that influence HIV-1 acquisition and disease progression discovered by candidate gene studies

HOST FACTOR	FUNCTION	POLYMORPHISM	EFFECT ON GENE	EFFECT ON HIV	EVIDENCE	REFERENCES
Chemokine receptors						
CCR5	Viral co-receptor	32 bp deletion	Truncation, no membrane expression	Protection from HIV-1 infection	Strong	[148–150]
				Delayed disease progression	Strong	[148, 151, 152]
		m303	Truncation, no membrane expression	Protection from HIV-1 infection	Strong	[153]
		CCR5P1	Increased expression	Accelerated disease progression	Strong	[154]
CCR2	Viral co-receptor	V64I	Interaction with CXCR4	Delayed disease progression	Strong	[155–158]
CCR2+CCR5	Viral co-receptor	HHE haplotype	Increased CCR5 expression	Accelerated disease progression	Strong	[154, 159]
DARC	Trans-receptor	-46 C	Decreased expression	Susceptibility to HIV-1 infection	Controversial	[160–162]
				Delayed disease progression	Controversial	[160–164]
CXCR6	Secondary co-receptor	rs2234358		Delayed disease progression	Weak	[165]
CXCR1	Il 8 receptor	Haplotype Ha		Delayed disease progression	Weak	[166]
CX3CR1	Secondary co-receptor	V249I		Accelerated or delayed disease progression	Controversial	[167–170]
		T280M		Accelerated disease progression	Controversial	[167–172]
Chemokine ligands						
CCL5	CCR5 ligand	-403 G/A, -28 G/C, In1.1 C haplotype	Influences expression	Accelerated or delayed disease progression	Controversial	[173–177]
CCL3L1	CCR5 ligand	Low copy number	Decreased expression	Susceptibility to HIV-1 infection	Controversial	[178–181]
				Accelerated disease progression	Controversial	[179–182]
CXCL12	CXCR4 ligand	3'A		Accelerated or delayed disease progression	Controversial	[183–186]

Interleukins						
IL4	Immune regulation	-589	Increased expression	Increased or decreased CXCR4-emergence	Controversial	[187, 188]
				Delayed disease progression	Controversial	[187–189]
IL10	Immune regulation	5'-A	Decreased expression	Susceptibility to HIV-1 infection	Strong	[190]
				Accelerated disease progression	Strong	[190]
Toll-like receptors						
TLR4	PAMP recognition	1063A/G		High viral load	Weak	[191]
TLR7	PAMP recognition	Gln11Leu		Accelerated disease progression	Weak	[192]
TLR9	PAMP recognition	1635A/G		Accelerated or delayed disease progression	Controversial	[191, 193, 194]
HIV dependency factors						
TSG101	Viral budding	-183 T/C and 181A/C		Accelerated or delayed CD4 T cell decline and viral load	Controversial	[195, 196]
HIV restriction factors						
TRIM5α	Uncoating	H43Y	Decreased activity	Accelerated disease progression	Controversial	[197–200]
		R136Q	Decreased activity	Protection from HIV-1 infection	Controversial	[199, 201]
PPIA	Uncoating	1604A/G		Accelerated CD4 T cell decline	Controversial	[195, 202, 203]
		1650 C/G		Accelerated or delayed disease progression	Controversial	[195, 202, 203]
APOBEC3G	Deamination	H186R		Accelerated disease progression in Africans	Controversial	[204, 205]
		C40693T		Susceptibility to HIV-1 infection	Weak	[206]

Continued

Table 5.1 Host factors that influence HIV-1 acquisition and disease progression discovered by candidate gene studies—cont'd

HOST FACTOR	FUNCTION	POLYMORPHISM	EFFECT ON GENE	EFFECT ON HIV	EVIDENCE	REFERENCES
Human leukocyte antigens						
All HLA types	Ag recognition	Homozygosity	Decreased recognition	Accelerated disease progression	Strong	[119, 120]
HLA-B*27	Ag recognition		Protective epitope recognition	Delayed disease progression	Strong	[27]
HLA-B*57	Ag recognition		Protective epitope recognition	Delayed disease progression	Strong	[29, 30, 121, 122, 125, 126, 128, 207]
HLA-B*35Px	Ag recognition		Protective epitope recognition	Accelerated disease progression	Strong	[120]
HLA-C	Ag recognition	rs9264942	Increased expression	Delayed disease progression	Strong	[128, 129]
NK receptors, KIR						
KIR3DS1	NK activity		Increased activity	Decreased viral load set point		[208]
				Protection from HIV-1 infection		[209]
KIR3DS1 + HLA-B Bw4-80I	NK activity		Increased activity	Delayed disease progression		[210, 211]
HLA-B Bw4-80I and/or HLA-B*57				Protection from HIV-1 infection		[212]

variants of HLA-B*57-typed individuals with a typical disease course had additional mutations that compensated for the fitness cost associated with the mutations in CTL epitopes. These compensatory mutations were not observed in HLA-B*57-typed long-term non-progressors [29]. Another mechanism for HLA-B*57-related control involves induction of strong CTL responses against the escaped epitopes [127].

HLA-B*35Px, a subgroup of HLA-B*35 based on peptide-binding properties, is associated with a more benign disease course after HIV-1 infection [120], for which the underlying mechanism is not fully clear. While it seems that HLA-B is most frequently implicated in the course of HIV-1 disease, a GWAS revealed genetic variation in the HLA-C gene region to be associated with viral control and slower progression to AIDS [128, 129], confirming earlier data [130]. The protective allele of this polymorphism is associated with high HLA-C cell surface expression, possibly through affecting a 3'UTR miRNA binding site that can degrade or repress translation of the HLA-C gene [129, 131].

GENOME-WIDE ASSOCIATION STUDIES

To date, the disease-associated phenotypes that have been used in the search for novel host genetic factors involved in HIV pathogenesis are largely overlapping and correlated with each other. The first reported GWAS performed in the EURO-CHAVI cohort used two phenotypes: HIV RNA viral load at set point, with viral load set point defined as the steady-state viral load after the acute phase of the primary HIV-1 infection, or extrapolated time to a CD4 count < 350 cells/mm^3 [128]. In the EURO-CHAVI cohort two loci were genome-wide significantly ($p < 5 \times 10^{-8}$) associated with viral load set point. One of these loci is tagged by SNP rs2395029 near the HLA complex 5 gene (HCP5), a gene localized within the MHC class I region. SNP rs2395029 is in nearly absolute linkage disequilibrium (LD) with HLA-B*57, whose protective effect was known already, as discussed above [121, 122]. The other locus is tagged by SNP rs9264942, located 35 kb upstream of HLA-C.

This first GWAS additionally identified variants in the zinc ribbon domain-containing protein 1 (ZNRD1) to be associated with progression to CD4 count < 350 cells/mm^3. Dalmasso et al. [132] also used viral load as a disease phenotype in their GWAS, but evaluated plasma HIV-RNA and cellular HIV-DNA levels during primary infection rather than at set point. Most of the variants strongly associated with HIV-RNA and HIV-DNA levels were localized in the MHC region, including rs2395029 in the HCP5 region. Limou et al. [133] and Le Clerc et al. [134] looked for genetic associations with extreme phenotypes in HIV-1

infection in long-term non-progressors (LTNPs) and rapid progressors (RP), in the genomics of resistance to immunodeficiency virus (GRIV) cohort. The non-progression GRIV GWAS identified mainly associations between the clinical course of infection and genetic variation in chromosome 6 and could confirm both the HCP5 and the ZNRD1 locus identified by the EURO-CHAVI cohort. The analysis of RP revealed several interesting loci, but these need to be replicated in other cohorts. Viral load was also used as a phenotype in the multinational HIV controllers study. A large cohort was divided into HIV-1 controllers, who are able to control viral load after infection to levels < 50 copies of viral RNA/ml plasma, and HIV-1 progressors, those who failed to ever control viremia. Over 300 SNPs that were genome-wide significantly associated with viral load were identified and all were located within the MHC gene region. Specific amino acids in the HLA-B peptide binding groove (associated with rs2395029 HCP5 SNP), as well as an independent HLA-C effect (associated with rs9264942 HLA-C SNP), were found to be associated with the capacity to control HIV-1 [135].

A multi-stage GWAS in US seroconverters compared RP, moderate progressors, and LTNPs, followed by replication of interesting signals in another cohort [136]. Variation upstream of PROX1, a negative regulator of IFN-γ expression in T cells, was associated with slower progression to AIDS. Another GWAS amongst US seroconverters identified a cluster of SNPs in the gene PARD3B to be associated with a delayed survival time to AIDS [137]. One of the variants in this cluster could be confirmed in two European cohorts of rapid progressors.

The majority of GWAS performed have focused on populations from European descent. The first published GWAS on a non-European population searched for associations with viral load at set point in African Americans [125]. Although no loci were genome-wide significantly associated with viral load at set point, one of the strongest associations was a SNP tagging the HLA-B*5703 allele. This confirms the important association between HLA-B*57 and viral load variation, both in African Americans and in individuals of European ancestry.

In a mother-to-child transmission cohort in Malawi, in which HIV-uninfected children and HIV-infected infants from HIV-infected mothers are compared, several regions were identified to be potentially associated with vertical transmission of HIV-1. However, these findings still need further examination and replication [138].

A linkage analysis in a cohort of SIV-infected macaques [139] revealed MHC class I markers and an unknown X chromosomal locus to be associated with progression to AIDS. The association between the signal on the X chromosome and AIDS progression could be replicated in a cohort of HIV-1-infected patients.

Two studies performed a genetic association analysis of *in vitro* susceptibility to HIV-1 infection in lymphoblastoid B cell lines from a family cohort (CEPH) [140] and in primary monocyte-derived macrophages [141]. The first study identified the LY6 gene family and the SNP in LY6 subsequently turned out to be associated with accelerated disease progression in one of two cohorts of HIV-1-infected patients. In the second study we observed a strong association between a SNP intronic of DYRK1A and *in vitro* HIV-1 replication in monocyte-derived macrophages. This SNP appeared to be associated with HIV-1 disease progression *in vivo* in two independent cohort studies.

GENOME-WIDE siRNA, cDNA AND GENE-EXPRESSION SCREENS ON HIV-1 REPLICATION

Genome-wide scanning of RNA for more than 20,000 human proteins has been performed to identify genes required for HIV-1 replication. Three studies used siRNA transfection to knock down gene expression [142–144] and one study used short hairpin RNA transduction for gene silencing [145]. These four studies identified over 1,000 proteins that may be required for optimal viral replication. However, only three genes were identified in all four studies [146]. These were mediator complex subunit 6 (MED6), which is involved in transcription of RNA polymerase II-dependent genes, mediator complex subunit 7 (MED7), which is required for efficient transcription of Sp1, and v-rel reticuloendotheliosis viral oncogene homolog A (RELA), which is part of the NF-κB complex. The minimal overlap in outcome of these studies may be caused by differences in cell types used for analysis and the steps in

the replication cycle of HIV-1 that were studied. Interestingly, several genes that were identified to be involved in HIV-1 replication could be grouped in pathways or categories of genes, such as nuclear import and export, transcription factors, components of the NF-κB complex, and kinases. In another approach, a cDNA library representing 15,000 unique genes was used to find novel factors that when overexpressed could enhance HIV-1 infection [147]. The mixed lineage kinase 3 (MLK3) was identified as one of the strongest enhancers of HIV-1 replication, confirmed by RNAi gene expression silencing.

CONCLUSION

As is clear from the above, the clinical course of HIV-1 infection is influenced by many host genetic factors as well as viral factors. This is logical from the point of view that the genome of HIV-1 only encodes a limited number of proteins, rendering it dependent on cellular proteins for replication. On the other hand, HIV-1 needs to protect itself from the host's innate and adaptive antiviral defense mechanisms in order to persist. Multiple interactions between viral proteins and host cellular factors have been observed, and may be pursued for the design of new antiviral therapies. As described, polymorphisms in several host factors have been identified and some variants have now been convincingly associated with disease progression in several cohorts. However, it will require meta-analyses to complete and validate the identification of host genetic factors that are associated with disease course.

REFERENCES

[1] Richman DD, Wrin T, Little SJ, et al. Rapid evolution of the neutralizing antibody response to HIV type 1 infection. Proc Natl Acad Sci U S A 2003;7:4144–9.

[2] Wei X, Decker JM, Wang S, et al. Antibody neutralization and escape by HIV-1. Nature 2003;6929:307–12.

[3] Johnson WE, Lifson JD, Lang SM, et al. Importance of B-cell responses for immunological control of variant strains of simian immunodeficiency virus. J Virol 2003;1:375–81.

[4] Schmitz JE, Kuroda MJ, Santra S, et al. Effect of humoral immune responses on controlling viremia during primary infection of rhesus monkeys with simian

immunodeficiency virus. J Virol 2003;3:2165–73.

[5] Miller CJ, Genesca M, Abel K, et al. Antiviral antibodies are necessary for control of simian immunodeficiency virus replication. J Virol 2007;10:5024–35.

[6] Gaufin T, Gautam R, Kasheta M, et al. Limited ability of humoral immune responses in control of viremia during infection with SIVsmmD215 strain. Blood 2009;18:4250–61.

[7] Trkola A, Kuster H, Rusert P, et al. Delay of HIV-1 rebound after cessation of antiretroviral therapy through passive transfer of human neutralizing antibodies. Nat Med 2005;6:593–4.

[8] McKeating JA, Gow J, Goudsmit J, et al. Characterization of HIV-1 neutralization escape mutants. AIDS 1989;777–84.

[9] Bunnik EM, Pisas L, van Nuenen AC, et al. Autologous neutralizing humoral immunity and evolution of the viral envelope in the course of subtype B human immunodeficiency virus type 1 infection. J Virol 2008;16:7932–41.

[10] van Gils MJ, Bunnik EM, Burger JA, et al. Rapid escape from preserved cross-reactive neutralizing humoral immunity without loss of viral fitness in HIV-1-infected progressors and long-term nonprogressors. J Virol 2010;7:3576–85.

[11] Chackerian B, Rudensey LM, Overbaugh J. Specific N-linked and O-linked glycosylation modifications in the envelope V1 domain of simian immunodeficiency virus variants that evolve in the host alter recognition by neutralizing antibodies. J Virol 1997;10:7719–27.

[12] Beaumont T, van Nuenen A, Broersen S, et al. Reversal of HIV-1 IIIB towards a neutralization resistant phenotype in an accidentally infected laboratory worker with a progressive clinical course. J Virol 2001;5:2246–52.

[13] Rong R, Bibollet-Ruche F, Mulenga J, et al. Role of V1V2 and other human immunodeficiency virus type 1 envelope domains in resistance to autologous neutralization during clade C infection. J Virol 2007;3:1350–9.

[14] Sagar M, Wu X, Lee S, et al. Human immunodeficiency virus type 1 V1-V2 envelope loop sequences expand and add glycosylation sites over the course of infection, and these modifications affect antibody neutralization sensitivity. J Virol 2006;19:9586–98.

[15] Moore JP, Ho DD. HIV-1 neutralization: the consequences of viral adaptation to growth on transformed T cells. AIDS 1995; S117–36.

[16] Quakkelaar ED, Bunnik EM, van Alphen FP, et al. Escape of human immunodeficiency virus type 1 from broadly neutralizing antibodies is not associated with a reduction of viral replicative capacity in vitro. Virology 2007;2:447–53.

[17] Euler Z, van Gils MJ, Bunnik EM, et al. Cross-reactive neutralizing humoral immunity does not protect from HIV type 1 disease progression. J Infect Dis 2010;7:1045–53.

[18] Piantadosi A, Panteleeff D, Blish CA, et al. Breadth of neutralizing antibody response to human immunodeficiency virus type 1 is affected by factors early in infection but does not influence disease progression. J Virol 2009;19:10269–74.

[19] Borrow P, Lewicki H, Hahn BH, et al. Virus-specific CD8+ cytotoxic T-lymphocyte activity associated with control of viremia in primary human immunodeficiency virus type 1 infection. J Virol 1994;68 (9):6103–10.

[20] Harari A, Rizzardi GP, Ellefsen K, et al. Analysis of HIV-1- and CMV-specific memory CD4 T-cell responses during primary and chronic infection. Blood 2002;4:1381–7.

[21] Koup RA, Safrit JT, Cao Y, et al. Temporal associations of cellular immune responses with the initial control of viremia in primary human immunodeficiency virus type 1 syndrome. J Virol 1994;68 (7):4650–5.

[22] Klein MR, Van Baalen CA, Holwerda AM, et al. Kinetics of Gag-specific CTL responses during the clinical course of HIV-1 infection: a longitudinal analysis of rapid progressors and long-term asymptomatics. J Exp Med 1995;181(4):1365–72.

[23] Jin X, Bauer DE, Tuttleton SE, et al. Dramatic rise in plasma viremia after CD8(+) T cell depletion in simian immunodeficiency virus-infected macaques. J Exp Med 1999;6:991–8.

[24] Schmitz JE, Kuroda MJ, Santra S, et al. Control of viremia in simian immunodeficiency virus infection by CD8+ lymphocytes. Science 1999;283(5403):857–60.

[25] Mueller YM, Do DH, Boyer JD, et al. CD8+ cell depletion of SHIV89.6P-infected macaques induces CD4+ T cell proliferation that contributes to increased viral loads. J Immunol 2009;8:5006–12.

[26] Schellens IM, Borghans JA, Jansen CA, et al. Abundance of early functional HIV-specific CD8+ T cells does not predict AIDS-free survival time. PLoS ONE 2008;7:e2745.

[27] Goulder PJ, Phillips RE, Colbert RA, et al. Late escape from an immunodominant cytotoxic T-lymphocyte response associated with progression to AIDS. Nat Med 1997;2:212–7.

[28] Borrow P, Lewicki H, Wei X, et al. Antiviral pressure exerted by HIV-1 specific cytotoxic T lymphocytes (CTLs) during primary infection demonstrated by rapid selection of CTL escape virus. Nat Med 1997;3 (2):205–11.

[29] Navis M, Schellens I, van Baarle D, et al. Viral replication capacity as a correlate of HLA B57/B5801-associated nonprogressive HIV-1 infection. J Immunol 2007;5:3133–43.

[30] Migueles SA, Laborico AC, Imamichi H, et al. The differential ability of HLA B*5701+ long-term nonprogressors and progressors to restrict human immunodeficiency virus replication is not caused by loss of recognition of autologous viral gag sequences. J Virol 2003;12:6889–98.

[31] Leslie AJ, Pfafferott KJ, Chetty P, et al. HIV evolution: CTL escape mutation and reversion after transmission. Nat Med 2004;3:282–9.

[32] Leslie A, Kavanagh D, Honeyborne I, et al. Transmission and accumulation of CTL escape variants drive negative associations between HIV polymorphisms and HLA. J Exp Med 2005;6:891–902.

[33] Kawashima Y, Pfafferott K, Frater J, et al. Adaptation of HIV-1 to human leukocyte antigen class I. Nature 2009;7238:641–5.

[34] Allen TM, Altfeld M, Yu XG, et al. Selection, transmission, and reversion of an antigen-processing cytotoxic T-lymphocyte escape mutation in human immunodeficiency virus type 1 infection. J Virol 2004;13:7069–78.

[35] Jansen CA, De CI, Hooibrink B, et al. Prognostic value of HIV-1 Gag-specific CD4+ T-cell responses for progression to AIDS analyzed in a prospective cohort study. Blood 2006;4:1427–33.

[36] Janssen EM, Lemmens EE, Wolfe T, et al. CD4+ T cells are required for secondary expansion and memory in CD8+ T lymphocytes. Nature 2003;6925:852–6.

[37] Sun JC, Williams MA, Bevan MJ. CD4+ T cells are required for the maintenance, not programming, of memory CD8+ T cells after acute infection. Nat Immunol 2004;9:927–33.

[38] Meyaard L, Otto SA, Hooibrink B, et al. Quantitative analysis of CD4+ T cell function in the course of human immunodeficiency virus infection: decline of both naive and memory alloreactive T cells. J Clin Invest 1994;94(5):1947–52.

[39] Wahren B, Morfeldt-Månson L, Biberfeld G, et al. Characteristics of the specific cell-mediated immune response in human immunodeficiency virus infection. J Virol 1987;61(6):2017–23.

[40] Lane HC, Depper JL, Greene WC, et al. Qualitative analysis of immune function in patients with the acquired immunodeficiency syndrome. N Engl J Med 1985;313 (2):79–84.

[41] Douek DC, Brenchley JM, Betts MR, et al. HIV preferentially infects HIV-specific CD4+ T cells. Nature 2002;417(6884):95–8.

[42] Haase AT. Population biology of HIV-1 infection: viral and CD4$^+$ T cell demographics and dynamics in lymphatic tissues. Ann Rev Immunol 1999;17:625–56.

[43] Silvestri G, Feinberg MB. Turnover of lymphocytes and conceptual paradigms in HIV infection. J Clin Invest 2003;6:821–4.

[44] Giorgi JV, Hultin LE, McKeating JA, et al. Shorter survival in advanced human immunodeficiency virus type 1 infection is more closely associated with T lymphocyte activation than with plasma virus burden or virus chemokine coreceptor usage. J Infect Dis 1999;179(4):859–70.

[45] Hazenberg MD, Otto SA, van Benthem BH, et al. Persistent immune activation in HIV-1 infection is associated with progression to AIDS. AIDS 2003;13:1881–8.

[46] Silvestri G, Fedanov A, Germon S, et al. Divergent host responses during primary simian immunodeficiency virus SIVsm infection of natural sooty mangabey and nonnatural rhesus macaque hosts. J Virol 2005;7:4043–54.

[47] Hirsch VM, Fuerst TR, Sutter G, et al. Patterns of viral replication correlate with outcome in simian immunodeficiency virus (SIV)-infected macaques: effect of prior immunization with a trivalent SIV vaccine in modified vaccinia virus Ankara. J Virol 1996;6:3741–52.

[48] Broussard SR, Staprans SI, White R, et al. Simian immunodeficiency virus replicates to high levels in naturally infected African green monkeys without inducing immunologic or neurologic disease. J Virol 2001;5:2262–75.

[49] Silvestri G, Sodora DL, Koup RA, et al. Nonpathogenic SIV infection of sooty mangabeys is characterized by limited bystander immunopathology despite chronic high-level viremia. Immunity 2003;3:441–52.

[50] Kornfeld C, Ploquin MJ, Pandrea I, et al. Antiinflammatory profiles during primary SIV infection in African green monkeys are associated with protection against AIDS. J Clin Invest 2005;4:1082–91.

[51] Jacquelin B, Mayau V, Targat B, et al. Nonpathogenic SIV infection of African green monkeys induces a strong but rapidly controlled type I IFN response. J Clin Invest 2009;12:3544–55.

[52] Bosinger SE, Li Q, Gordon SN, et al. Global genomic analysis reveals rapid control of a robust innate response in SIV-infected sooty mangabeys. J Clin Invest 2009;12:3556–72.

[53] Favre D, Lederer S, Kanwar B, et al. Critical loss of the balance between Th17 and T regulatory cell populations in pathogenic SIV infection. PLoS Pathog 2009;2: e1000295.

[54] Brenchley JM, Schacker TW, Ruff LE, et al. CD4+ T cell depletion during all stages of HIV disease occurs predominantly in the gastrointestinal tract. J Exp Med 2004;6:749–59.

[55] Mehandru S, Poles MA, Tenner-Racz K, et al. Primary HIV-1 infection is associated with preferential depletion of CD4+ T lymphocytes from effector sites in the gastrointestinal tract. J Exp Med 2004;6:761–70.

[56] Schneider T, Jahn HU, Schmidt W, et al. Loss of CD4 T lymphocytes in patients infected with human immunodeficiency virus type 1 is more pronounced in the duodenal mucosa than in the peripheral blood. Berlin Diarrhea/Wasting Syndrome Study Group. Gut 1995;4:524–9.

[57] Veazey RS, DeMaria M, Chalifoux LV, et al. Gastrointestinal tract as a major site of CD4+ T cell depletion and viral replication in SIV infection. Science 1998;5362:427–31.

[58] Guadalupe M, Reay E, Sankaran S, et al. Severe CD4+ T-cell depletion in gut lymphoid tissue during primary human immunodeficiency virus type 1 infection and substantial delay in restoration following highly active antiretroviral therapy. J Virol 2003;21:11708–17.

[59] Li Q, Duan L, Estes JD, et al. Peak SIV replication in resting memory CD4+ T cells depletes gut lamina propria CD4+ T cells. Nature 2005;7037:1148–52.

[60] Mattapallil JJ, Douek DC, Hill B, et al. Massive infection and loss of memory CD4+ T cells in multiple tissues during acute SIV infection. Nature 2005;7037:1093–7.

[61] Unutmaz D, KewalRamani VN, Marmon S, et al. Cytokine signals are sufficient for HIV-1 infection of resting human T lymphocytes. J Exp Med 1999;11:1735–46.

[62] Raffatellu M, Santos RL, Verhoeven DE, et al. Simian immunodeficiency virus-induced mucosal interleukin-17 deficiency promotes Salmonella dissemination from the gut. Nat Med 2008;4:421–8.

[63] Brenchley JM, Paiardini M, Knox KS, et al. Differential Th17 CD4 T-cell depletion in pathogenic and nonpathogenic lentiviral infections. Blood 2008;7:2826–35.

[64] Schuitemaker H, Koot M, Kootstra NA, et al. Biological phenotype of human immunodeficiency virus type 1 clones at different stages of infection: progression of disease is associated with a shift from monocytotropic to T-cell-tropic virus populations. J Virol 1992;66 (3):1354–60.

[65] Van 't Wout AB, Kootstra NA, Mulder-Kampinga GA, et al. Macrophage-tropic variants initiate human immunodeficiency

virus type 1 infection after sexual, parenteral, and vertical transmission. J Clin Invest 1994;5:2060–7.

[66] Zhu T, Mo H, Wang N, et al. Genotypic and phenotypic characterization of HIV-1 in patients with primary infection. Science 1993;5125:1179–81.

[67] Keele BF, Giorgi EE, Salazar-Gonzalez JF, et al. Identification and characterization of transmitted and early founder virus envelopes in primary HIV-1 infection. Proc Natl Acad Sci U S A 2008;21:7552–7.

[68] Salazar-Gonzalez JF, Bailes E, Pham KT, et al. Deciphering human immunodeficiency virus type 1 transmission and early envelope diversification by single-genome amplification and sequencing. J Virol 2008;8:3952–70.

[69] Long EM, Rainwater SM, Lavreys L, et al. HIV type 1 variants transmitted to women in Kenya require the CCR5 coreceptor for entry, regardless of the genetic complexity of the infecting virus. AIDS Res Hum Retroviruses 2002;8:567–76.

[70] Koot M, Vos AHV, Keet RPM, et al. HIV-1 biological phenotype in long-term infected individuals, evaluated with an MT-2 cocultivation assay. AIDS 1992;6 (1):49–54.

[71] Bozzette SA, McCutchan JA, Spector SA, et al. A cross-sectional comparison of persons with syncytium- and non-synctium inducing human immunodeficiency virus. J Infect Dis 1993;168(6):1374–9.

[72] Koot M, Keet IPM, Vos AHV, et al. Prognostic value of human immunodeficiency virus type 1 biological phenotype for rate of CD4$^+$ cell depletion and progression to AIDS. Ann Intern Med 1993;681–8.

[73] Bleul CC, Wu L, Hoxie JA, et al. The HIV coreceptors CXCR4 and CCR5 are differentially expressed and regulated on human T lymphocytes. Proc Natl Acad Sci U S A 1997;1925–30.

[74] Blaak H, Van 't Wout AB, Brouwer M, et al. In vivo HIV-1

infection of CD45RA$^+$CD4$^+$ T cells is established primarily by syncytium-inducing variants and correlates with the rate of CD4$^+$ T cell decline. Proc Natl Acad Sci U S A 2000;1269–74.

[75] De Jong JJ, De Ronde A, Keulen W, et al. Minimal requirements for the human immunodeficiency virus type 1 V3 domain to support the syncytium-inducing phenotype: analysis by single amino acid substitution. J Virol 1992;6777–80.

[76] Pastore C, Nedellec R, Ramos A, et al. Human immunodeficiency virus type 1 coreceptor switching: V1/V2 gain-of-fitness mutations compensate for V3 loss-of-fitness mutations. J Virol 2006;2:750–8.

[77] Bunnik EM, Quakkelaar ED, van Nuenen AC, et al. Increased neutralization sensitivity of recently emerged CXCR4-using human immunodeficiency virus type 1 strains compared to coexisting CCR5-using variants from the same patient. J Virol 2007;2:525–31.

[78] Lusso P, Earl PL, Sironi F, et al. Cryptic nature of a conserved, CD4-inducible V3 loop neutralization epitope in the native envelope glycoprotein oligomer of CCR5-restricted, but not CXCR4-using, primary human immunodeficiency virus type 1 strains. J Virol 2005;11:6957–68.

[79] van Rij RP, Blaak H, Visser JA, et al. Differential coreceptor expression allows for independent evolution of non-syncytium-inducing and syncytium-inducing HIV-1. J Clin Invest 2000;1039–52.

[80] Van 't Wout AB, Blaak H, Ran LJ, et al. Evolution of syncytium inducing and non-syncytium inducing biological virus clones in relation to replication kinetics during the course of HIV-1 infection. J Virol 1998;6:5099–107.

[81] van Rij RP, Worobey M, Visser JA, et al. Evolution of R5 and X4 human immunodeficiency virus type 1 gag sequences in vivo: evidence for recombination. Virology 2003;1:451–9.

[82] Stalmeijer EH, van Rij RP, Boeser-Nunnink B, et al. In vivo evolution

of X4 human immunodeficiency virus type 1 variants in the natural course of infection coincides with decreasing sensitivity to CXCR4 antagonists. J Virol 2004;6:2722–8.

[83] Westby M, Smith-Burchnell C, Mori J, et al. Reduced maximal inhibition in phenotypic susceptibility assays indicates that viral strains resistant to the CCR5 antagonist maraviroc utilize inhibitor-bound receptor for entry. J Virol 2007;5:2359–71.

[84] Westby M, Lewis M, Whitcomb J, et al. Emergence of CXCR4-using human immunodeficiency virus type 1 (HIV-1) variants in a minority of HIV-1-infected patients following treatment with the CCR5 antagonist maraviroc is from a pretreatment CXCR4-using virus reservoir. J Virol 2006;10:4909–20.

[85] Fatkenheuer G, Nelson M, Lazzarin A, et al. Subgroup analyses of maraviroc in previously treated R5 HIV-1 infection. N Engl J Med 2008;14:1442–55.

[86] Koning FA, Kwa D, Boeser-Nunnink B, et al. Decreasing sensitivity to RANTES neutralization of CC chemokine receptor 5-using, non-syncytium-inducing virus variants in the course of human immunodeficiency virus type 1 infection. J Infect Dis 2003;6:864–72.

[87] Edo-Matas D, Rachinger A, Setiawan LC, et al. The evolution of human immunodeficiency virus type-1 (HIV-1) envelope molecular properties and coreceptor use at all stages of infection in an HIV-1 donor-recipient pair. Virology 2011.

[88] Bunnik EM, Euler Z, Welkers MR, et al. Adaptation of HIV-1 envelope gp120 to humoral immunity at a population level. Nat Med 2010;9:995–7.

[89] Kestler III HW, Ringler DJ, Mori K, et al. Importance of the nef gene for maintenance of high virus loads and for development of AIDS. Cell 1991;4:651–62.

[90] Deacon NJ, Tsykin A, Solomon A, et al. Genomic structure of an attenuated quasi species of HIV-1 from a blood transfusion donor

and recipients. Science 1995;988–91.

[91] Gorry PR, McPhee DA, Verity E, et al. Pathogenicity and immunogenicity of attenuated, nef-deleted HIV-1 strains in vivo. Retrovirology 2007;66.

[92] Garcia JV, Miller AD. Serine phosphorylation-independent downregulation of cell-surface CD4 by nef. Nature 1991;508–11.

[93] Schwartz O, Maréchal V, Le Gall S, et al. Endocytosis of major histocompatibility complex class I molecules is induced by the HIV-1 nef protein. Nature Med 1996;338–42.

[94] Sol-Foulon N, Moris A, Nobile C, et al. HIV-1 Nef-induced upregulation of DC-SIGN in dendritic cells promotes lymphocyte clustering and viral spread. Immunity 2002;1:145–55.

[95] Stumptner-Cuvelette P, Morchoisne S, Dugast M, et al. HIV-1 Nef impairs MHC class II antigen presentation and surface expression. Proc Natl Acad Sci U S A 2001;21:12144–9.

[96] Lenassi M, Cagney G, Liao M, et al. HIV Nef is secreted in exosomes and triggers apoptosis in bystander CD4+ T cells. Traffic 2010;1:110–22.

[97] Manninen A, Huotari P, Hiipakka M, et al. Activation of NFAT-dependent gene expression by Nef: conservation among divergent Nef alleles, dependence on SH3 binding and membrane association, and cooperation with protein kinase C-theta. J Virol 2001;6:3034–7.

[98] Swingler S, Brichacek B, Jacque JM, et al. HIV-1 Nef intersects the macrophage CD40L signalling pathway to promote resting-cell infection. Nature 2003;6945:213–9.

[99] Xu W, Santini PA, Sullivan JS, et al. HIV-1 evades virus-specific IgG2 and IgA responses by targeting systemic and intestinal B cells via long-range intercellular conduits. Nat Immunol 2009;9:1008–17.

[100] Sheehy AM, Gaddis NC, Choi JD, et al. Isolation of a human gene that inhibits HIV-1 infection and is suppressed by the viral Vif protein. Nature 2002;6898:646–50.

[101] Zheng YH, Irwin D, Kurosu T, et al. Human APOBEC3F is another host factor that blocks human immunodeficiency virus type 1 replication. J Virol 2004;11:6073–6.

[102] Mangeat B, Turelli P, Caron G, et al. Broad antiretroviral defence by human APOBEC3G through lethal editing of nascent reverse transcripts. Nature 2003;6944:99–103.

[103] Zhang H, Yang B, Pomerantz RJ, et al. The cytidine deaminase CEM15 induces hypermutation in newly synthesized HIV-1 DNA. Nature 2003;6944:94–8.

[104] Marin M, Rose KM, Kozak SL, et al. HIV-1 Vif protein binds the editing enzyme APOBEC3G and induces its degradation. Nat Med 2003;11:1398–403.

[105] Sheehy AM, Gaddis NC, Malim MH. The antiretroviral enzyme APOBEC3G is degraded by the proteasome in response to HIV-1 Vif. Nat Med 2003;11:1404–7.

[106] Casartelli N, Guivel-Benhassine F, Bouziat R, et al. The antiviral factor APOBEC3G improves CTL recognition of cultured HIV-infected T cells. J Exp Med 2010;1:39–49.

[107] Gibbs JS, Lackner AA, Lang SM, et al. Progression to AIDS in the absence of a gene for vpr or vpx. J Virol 1995;4:2378–83.

[108] He J, Choe S, Walker R, et al. Human immunodeficiency virus type 1 viral protein R (Vpr) arrests cells in the G2 phase of the cell cycle by inhibiting p34cdc2 activity. J Virol 1995;11: 6705–11.

[109] Heinzinger NK, Bukrinsky MI, Haggerty SA, et al. The vpr protein of human immunodeficiency virus type 1 influences nuclear localization of viral nucleic acids in nondividing cells. Proc Natl Acad Sci U S A 1994;7311–15.

[110] Popov S, Rexach M, Zybarth G, et al. Viral protein R regulates nuclear import of the HIV-1 pre-integration complex. EMBO J 1998;4:909–17.

[111] Felzien LK, Woffendin C, Hottiger MO, et al. HIV transcriptional activation by the accessoty protein, Vpr, is mediated by the p300 co-activator. Proc Natl Acad Sci U S A 1998;5281–6.

[112] Stewart SA, Poon B, Jowett JB, et al. Human immunodeficiency virus type 1 Vpr induces apoptosis following cell cycle arrest. J Virol 1997;7:5579–92.

[113] Margottin F, Bour SP, Durand H, et al. A novel human WD protein, h-beta TrCp, that interacts with HIV-1 Vpu connects CD4 to the ER degradation pathway through an F-box motif. Mol Cell 1998;4:565–74.

[114] Neil SJ, Zang T, Bieniasz PD. Tetherin inhibits retrovirus release and is antagonized by HIV-1 Vpu. Nature 2008;7177:425–30.

[115] Van DN, Goff D, Katsura C, et al. The interferon-induced protein BST-2 restricts HIV-1 release and is downregulated from the cell surface by the viral Vpu protein. Cell Host Microbe 2008;4:245–52.

[116] O'Brien SJ, Nelson GW. Human genes that limit AIDS. Nat Genet 2004;6:565–74.

[117] Lama J, Planelles V. Host factors influencing susceptibility to HIV infection and AIDS progression. Retrovirology 2007;52.

[118] Fellay J. Host genetics influences on HIV type-1 disease. Antivir Ther 2009;6:731–8.

[119] Tang J, Costello C, Keet IPM, et al. HLA Class I homozygosity accelerates disease progression in human immunodeficiency virus type 1 infection. AIDS Res Hum Retrovir 1999;317–24.

[120] Carrington M, Nelson GW, Martin MP, et al. HLA and HIV-1: heterozygote advantage and B*35-Cw*04 disadvantage. Science 1999;1748–52.

[121] Kaslow RA, Carrington M, Apple R, et al. Influence of combinations of human major histocompatibility complex genes in the course of HIV-1 infection. Nat Med 1996;405–11.

[122] Migueles SA, Sabbaghian MS, Shupert WL, et al. HLA B*5701 is highly associated with restriction of virus replication in a subgroup of HIV-infected long term nonprogressors. Proc Natl Acad Sci U S A 2000;6:2709–14.

[123] Costello C, Tang J, Rivers C, et al. HLA-B*5703 independently associated with slower HIV-1 disease progression in Rwandan women. AIDS 1999;14:1990–1.

[124] Shrestha S, Aissani B, Song W, et al. Host genetics and HIV-1 viral load set-point in African-Americans. AIDS 2009;6:673–7.

[125] Pelak K, Goldstein DB, Walley NM, et al. Host determinants of HIV-1 control in African Americans. J Infect Dis 2010;8:1141–9.

[126] Altfeld M, Addo MM, Rosenberg ES, et al. Influence of HLA-B57 on clinical presentation and viral control during acute HIV-1 infection. AIDS 2003;18:2581–91.

[127] Miura T, Brockman MA, Schneidewind A, et al. HLA-B57/B*5801 human immunodeficiency virus type 1 elite controllers select for rare gag variants associated with reduced viral replication capacity and strong cytotoxic T-lymphocyte [corrected]. recognition. J Virol 2009;6:2743–55.

[128] Fellay J, Shianna KV, Ge D, et al. A whole-genome association study of major determinants for host control of HIV-1. Science 2007;5840:944–7.

[129] Thomas R, Apps R, Qi Y, et al. HLA-C cell surface expression and control of HIV/AIDS correlate with a variant upstream of HLA-C. Nat Genet 2009;12:1290–4.

[130] Kiepiela P, Leslie AJ, Honeyborne I, et al. Dominant influence of HLA-B in mediating the potential co-evolution of HIV and HLA. Nature 2004;7018:769–75.

[131] Kulkarni S, Savan R, Qi Y, et al. Differential microRNA regulation of HLA-C expression and its association with HIV control. Nature 2011;7344:495–8.

[132] Dalmasso C, Carpentier W, Meyer L, et al. Distinct genetic loci control plasma HIV-RNA and cellular HIV-DNA levels in HIV-1 infection: the ANRS Genome Wide Association 01 study. PLoS ONE 2008;12:e3907.

[133] Limou S, Le Clerc S, Coulonges C, et al. Genomewide association study of an AIDS-nonprogression cohort emphasizes the role played by HLA genes (ANRS Genomewide Association Study 02). J Infect Dis 2009;3:419–26.

[134] Le Clerc S, Limou S, Coulonges C, et al. Genomewide association study of a rapid progression cohort identifies new susceptibility alleles for AIDS (ANRS Genomewide Association Study 03). J Infect Dis 2009;8:1194–1201.

[135] Pereyra F, Jia X, McLaren PJ, et al. The major genetic determinants of HIV-1 control affect HLA class I peptide presentation. Science 2010;6010:1551–7.

[136] Herbeck JT, Gottlieb GS, Winkler CA, et al. Multistage genomewide association study identifies a locus at 1q41 associated with rate of HIV-1 disease progression to clinical AIDS. J Infect Dis 2010;4:618–26.

[137] Troyer JL, Nelson GW, Lautenberger JA, et al. Genome-wide association study implicates PARD3B-based AIDS restriction. J Infect Dis 2011;203 (10):1491–502.

[138] Joubert BR, Lange EM, Franceschini N, et al. A whole genome association study of mother-to-child transmission of HIV in Malawi. Genome Med 2010;3:17.

[139] Siddiqui RA, Sauermann U, Altmuller J, et al. X chromosomal variation is associated with slow progression to AIDS in HIV-1-infected women. Am J Hum Genet 2009;2:228–39.

[140] Loeuillet C, Deutsch S, Ciuffi A, et al. In vitro whole-genome analysis identifies a susceptibility locus for HIV-1. PLoS Biol 2008;2:e32.

[141] Bol SM, Moerland PD, Limou S, et al. Genome-wide association study identifies single nucleotide polymorphism in DYRK1A associated with replication of HIV-1 in monocyte-derived macrophages. PLoS ONE 2011;2:e17190.

[142] Brass AL, Dykxhoorn DM, Benita Y, et al. Identification of host proteins required for HIV infection through a functional genomic screen. Science 2008;5865:921–6.

[143] König R, Zhou Y, Elleder D, et al. Global analysis of host–pathogen interactions that regulate early-stage HIV-1 replication. Cell 2008;1:49–60.

[144] Zhou H, Xu M, Huang Q, et al. Genome-scale RNAi screen for host factors required for HIV replication. Cell Host Microbe 2008;5:495–504.

[145] Yeung ML, Houzet L, Yedavalli VS, et al. A genome-wide short hairpin RNA screening of jurkat T-cells for human proteins contributing to productive HIV-1 replication. J Biol Chem 2009;29:19463–73.

[146] Bushman FD, Malani N, Fernandes J, et al. Host cell factors in HIV replication: meta-analysis of genome-wide studies. PLoS Pathog 2009;5:e1000437.

[147] Nguyen DG, Yin H, Zhou Y, et al. Identification of novel therapeutic targets for HIV infection through functional genomic cDNA screening. Virology 2007;1:16–25.

[148] Dean M, Carrington M, Winkler C, et al. Genetic restriction of HIV-1 infection and progression to AIDS by a deletion allele of the CKR5 structural gene. Science 1996;1856–62.

[149] Liu R, Paxton WA, Choe S, et al. Homozygous defect in HIV-1 coreceptor accounts for resistance of some multiply-exposed individuals to HIV-1 infection. Cell 1996;3:367–77.

[150] Samson M, Libert F, Doranz BJ, et al. Resistance to HIV-1 infection in caucasian individuals bearing mutant alleles of the CCR-5 chemokine receptor gene. Nature 1996;722–5.

[151] Rappaport J, Cho YY, Hendel H, et al. 32 bp CCR-5 gene deletion and resistance to fast progression in HIV-1 infected heterozygotes. Lancet 1997;9056:922–3.

[152] De Roda Husman AM, Koot M, Cornelissen M, et al. Association between CCR5 genotype and the clinical course of HIV-1 infection. Ann Intern Med 1997;882–90.

[153] Quillent C, Oberlin E, Braun J, et al. HIV-1-resistance phenotype conferred by combination of two separate inherited mutations of CCR5 gene. Lancet 1998;14–8.

[154] Martin MP, Dean M, Smith MW, et al. Genetic acceleration of AIDS progression by a promotor variant of CCR5. Science 1998;1907–11.

[155] Smith MW, Dean M, Carrington M, et al. Contrasting genetic influence of CCR2 and CCR5 variants on HIV-1 infection and disease progression. Science 1997;959–65.

[156] Ioannidis JPA, O'Brien TR, Rosenberg PS, et al. Genetic effects on HIV disease progression. Nat Med 1998;536.

[157] Kostrikis LG, Huang Y, Moore JP, et al. A chemokine receptor CCR2 allele delays HIV-1 disease progression and is associated with a CCR5 promotor mutation. Nat Med 1998;350–3.

[158] van Rij RP, De Roda Husman AM, Brouwer M, et al. Role of CCR2 genotype in the clinical course of syncytium-inducing (SI) or non-SI human immunodeficiency virus type 1 infection and in the time to conversion to SI virus variants. J Infect Dis 1998;1806–11.

[159] McDermott DH, Zimmerman PA, Guignard F, et al. CCR5 promotor polymorphism and HIV-1 disease progression. Lancet 1998;866–70.

[160] He W, Neil S, Kulkarni H, et al. Duffy antigen receptor for chemokines mediates trans-infection of HIV-1 from red blood cells to target cells and affects HIV-AIDS susceptibility. Cell Host Microbe 2008;1:52–62.

[161] Walley NM, Julg B, Dickson SP, et al. The Duffy antigen receptor for chemokines null promoter variant does not influence HIV-1 acquisition or disease progression. Cell Host Microbe 2009;5:408–10.

[162] Winkler CA, An P, Johnson R, et al. Expression of Duffy antigen receptor for chemokines (DARC) has no effect on HIV-1 acquisition or progression to AIDS in African Americans. Cell Host Microbe 2009;5:411–3.

[163] Horne KC, Li X, Jacobson LP, et al. Duffy antigen polymorphisms do not alter progression of HIV in African Americans in the MACS cohort. Cell Host Microbe 2009;5:415–7.

[164] Julg B, Reddy S, van der Stok M, et al. Lack of Duffy antigen receptor for chemokines: no influence on HIV disease progression in an African treatment-naive population. Cell Host Microbe 2009; 5:413–5.

[165] Limou S, Coulonges C, Herbeck JT, et al. Multiple-cohort genetic association study reveals CXCR6 as a new chemokine receptor involved in long-term nonprogression to AIDS. J Infect Dis 2010;6:908–15.

[166] Vasilescu A, Terashima Y, Enomoto M, et al. A haplotype of the human CXCR1 gene protective against rapid disease progression in HIV-1+ patients. Proc Natl Acad Sci U S A 2007;9:3354–9.

[167] Faure S, Meyer L, Costagliola D, et al. Rapid progression to AIDS in HIV+ individuals with a structural variant of the chemokine receptor CX3CR1. Science 2000;2274–7.

[168] Singh KK, Hughes MD, Chen J, et al. Genetic polymorphisms in CX3CR1 predict HIV-1 disease progression in children independently of CD4+ lymphocyte count and HIV-1 RNA load. J Infect Dis 2005;11:1971–80.

[169] Vidal F, Vilades C, Domingo P, et al. Spanish HIV-1-infected long-term nonprogressors of more than 15 years have an increased frequency of the CX3CR1 249I variant allele. J Acquir Immune Defic Syndr 2005;5:527–31.

[170] Hendel H, Winkler C, An P, et al. Validation of genetic case-control studies in AIDS and application to the CX3CR1 polymorphism. J Acquir Immune Defic Syndr 2001;5:507–11.

[171] Kwa D, Boeser-Nunnink B, Schuitemaker H. Lack of evidence for an association between a polymorphism in CX3CR1 and the clinical course of HIV infection or virus phenotype evolution. AIDS 2003;759–61.

[172] McDermott DH, Colla JS, Kleeberger CA, et al. Genetic polymorphism in CX3CR1 and risk of HIV disease. Science 2000;2031.

[173] Liu H, Chao D, Nakayama EE, et al. Polymorphism in RANTES chemokine promoter affects HIV-1 disease progression. Proc Natl Acad Sci U S A 1999;8:4581–5.

[174] McDermott DH, Beecroft MJ, Kleeberger CA, et al. Chemokine RANTES promotor polymorphism affects risk of both HIV infection and disease progression in the Multicenter AIDS Cohort Study. AIDS 2000;2671–8.

[175] Gonzalez E, Dhanda R, Bamshad M, et al. Global survey of genetic variation in CCR5, RANTES and MIP1a: impact on the epidemiology of the HIV-1 pandemic. Proc Natl Acad Sci U S A 2001;5199–204.

[176] Duggal P, Winkler CA, An P, et al. The effect of RANTES chemokine genetic variants on early HIV-1 plasma RNA among African American injection drug users. J Acquir Immune Defic Syndr 2005;5:584–9.

[177] An P, Nelson GW, Wang L, et al. Modulating influence on HIV/AIDS by interacting RANTES gene variants. Proc Natl Acad Sci U S A 2002;15:10002–7.

[178] Gonzalez E, Kulkarni H, Bolivar H, et al. The influence of CCL3L1 gene-containing segmental duplications on HIV-1/AIDS susceptibility. Science 2005;5714:1434–40.

[179] Bhattacharya T, Stanton J, Kim EY, et al. CCL3L1 and HIV/AIDS susceptibility. Nat Med 2009;10:1112–15.

[180] Field SF, Howson JM, Maier LM, et al. Experimental aspects of copy number variant assays at CCL3L1. Nat Med 2009;10:1115–7.

[181] Urban TJ, Weintrob AC, Fellay J, et al. CCL3L1 and HIV/AIDS susceptibility. Nat Med 2009;10:1110–12.

[182] Dolan MJ, Kulkarni H, Camargo JF, et al. CCL3L1 and CCR5 influence cell-mediated immunity and affect HIV-AIDS pathogenesis via viral entry-independent mechanisms. Nat Immunol 2007; 12:1324–36.

[183] Winkler C, Modi W, Smith MW, et al. Genetic restriction of AIDS pathogenesis by an SDF-1 chemokine gene variant. Science 1998;389–93.

[184] Mummidi S, Ahuja SS, Gonzalez E, et al. Genealogy of the CCR5 locus and chemokine system gene variants associated with altered rates of HIV-1 disease progression. Nat Med 1998;786–93.

[185] van Rij RP, Broersen S, Goudsmit J, et al. The role of a stromal cell-derived factor-1 chemokine gene variant in the clinical course of HIV-1 infection. AIDS 1998;F85–F90.

[186] Ioannidis JP, Rosenberg PS, Goedert JJ, et al. Effects of CCR5-Delta32, CCR2-64I, and SDF-1 3′A alleles on HIV-1 disease progression: an international meta-analysis of individual-patient data. Ann Intern Med 2001;9:782–95.

[187] Nakayama EE, Meyer L, Iwamoto A, et al. Protective effect of interleukin-4–589T polymorphism on human immunodeficiency virus type 1 disease progression: relationship with virus load. J Infect Dis 2002;8:1183–6.

[188] Kwa D, van Rij RP, Boeser-Nunnink B, et al. Association between an interleukin-4 promoter polymorphism and the acquisition of CXCR4 using human immunodeficiency virus type 1 variants. AIDS 2003;981–5.

[189] Wichukchinda N, Nakayama EE, Rojanawiwat A, et al. Protective effects of IL4-589T and RANTES-28G on HIV-1 disease progression in infected Thai females. AIDS 2006;2:189–96.

[190] Shin HD, Winkler C, Stephens JC, et al. Genetic restriction of HIV-1 pathogenesis to AIDS by promotor alleles of IL10. Proc Natl Acad Sci U S A 2000;14467–72.

[191] Pine SO, McElrath MJ, Bochud PY. Polymorphisms in toll-like receptor 4 and toll-like receptor 9 influence viral load in a seroincident cohort of HIV-1-infected individuals. AIDS 2009;18:2387–95.

[192] Oh DY, Baumann K, Hamouda O, et al. A frequent functional toll-like receptor 7 polymorphism is associated with accelerated HIV-1 disease progression. AIDS 2009;3:297–307.

[193] Bochud PY, Hersberger M, Taffe P, et al. Polymorphisms in Toll-like receptor 9 influence the clinical course of HIV-1 infection. AIDS 2007;4:441–6.

[194] Soriano-Sarabia N, Vallejo A, Ramirez-Lorca R, et al. Influence of the Toll-like receptor 9 1635A/G polymorphism on the CD4 count, HIV viral load, and clinical progression. J Acquir Immune Defic Syndr 2008;2:128–35.

[195] Bleiber G, May M, Martinez R, et al. Use of a combined ex vivo/in vivo population approach for screening of human genes involved in the human immunodeficiency virus type 1 life cycle for variants influencing disease progression. J Virol 2005;20:12674–80.

[196] Bashirova AA, Bleiber G, Qi Y, et al. Consistent effects of TSG101 genetic variability on multiple outcomes of exposure to human immunodeficiency virus type 1. J Virol 2006;14:6757–63.

[197] Goldschmidt V, Bleiber G, May M, et al. Role of common human TRIM5alpha variants in HIV-1 disease progression. Retrovirology 2006;54.

[198] Nakayama EE, Carpentier W, Costagliola D, et al. Wild type and H43Y variant of human TRIM5alpha show similar anti-human immunodeficiency virus type 1 activity both in vivo and in vitro. Immunogenetics 2007;6:511–5.

[199] Speelmon EC, Livingston-Rosanoff D, Li SS, et al. Genetic association of the antiviral restriction factor TRIM5alpha with human immunodeficiency virus type 1 infection. J Virol 2006;5:2463–71.

[200] van Manen D, Rits MA, Beugeling C, et al. The effect of Trim5 polymorphisms on the clinical course of HIV-1 infection. PLoS Pathog 2008;2:e18.

[201] Javanbakht H, An P, Gold B, et al. Effects of human TRIM5alpha polymorphisms on antiretroviral function and susceptibility to human immunodeficiency virus infection. Virology 2006;1:15–27.

[202] An P, Wang LH, Hutcheson-Dilks H, et al. Regulatory polymorphisms in the cyclophilin A gene, PPIA, accelerate progression to AIDS. PLoS Pathog 2007;6:e88.

[203] Rits MA, van Dort KA, Kootstra NA. Polymorphisms in the regulatory region of the Cyclophilin A gene influence the susceptibility for HIV-1 infection. PLoS ONE 2008;12:e3975.

[204] An P, Bleiber G, Duggal P, et al. APOBEC3G genetic variants and their influence on the progression to AIDS. J Virol 2004;20:11070–6.

[205] Do H, Vasilescu A, Diop G, et al. Exhaustive genotyping of the CEM15 (APOBEC3G) gene and absence of association with AIDS progression in a French cohort. J Infect Dis 2005;2:159–63.

[206] Valcke HS, Bernard NF, Bruneau J, et al. APOBEC3G genetic variants and their association with risk of HIV infection in highly exposed Caucasians. AIDS 2006;15:1984–6.

[207] Fellay J, Ge D, Shianna KV, et al. Common genetic variation and the control of HIV-1 in humans. PLoS Genet 2009;12:e1000791.

[208] Barbour JD, Sriram U, Caillier SJ, et al. Synergy or independence? Deciphering the interaction of HLA Class I and NK cell KIR alleles in early HIV-1 disease progression. PLoS Pathog 2007;4:e43.

[209] Boulet S, Kleyman M, Kim JY, et al. A combined genotype of KIR3DL1 high expressing alleles and HLA-B*57 is associated with a reduced risk of HIV infection. AIDS 2008;12:1487–91.

[210] Martin MP, Gao X, Lee JH, et al. Epistatic interaction between KIR3DS1 and HLA-B delays the progression to AIDS. Nat Genet 2002;4:429–34.

[211] Alter G, Martin MP, Teigen N, et al. Differential natural killer cell-mediated inhibition of HIV-1 replication based on distinct KIR/HLA subtypes. J Exp Med 2007;12:3027–36.

[212] Boulet S, Sharafi S, Simic N, et al. Increased proportion of KIR3DS1 homozygotes in HIV-exposed uninfected individuals. AIDS 2008;5:595–9.

Chapter | 6 |

Acute HIV infection

Anthony D. Kelleher, David A. Cooper

INTRODUCTION

Although HIV infection is a chronic progressive infection, it is well recognized that the initial stages of the infection are characterized by an acute viral syndrome. Despite this illness often being mild and under-diagnosed, increasing understanding of the links between pathophysiology and clinical manifestations has provided insights into the earliest interactions between host and virus. The virological and immunological events that immediately follow HIV infection are highly dynamic and there is increasing evidence these events impact on long-term outcome of the infection and rates of disease progression. The clinical presentation of initial infection is variously referred to as acute HIV infection, primary infection illness, acute retroviral syndrome, or seroconversion illness. Although there is variation in the clinical manifestations, there are distinct characteristics associated with this illness. The diagnosis of acute HIV infection is based on a combination of clinical acumen and characteristic findings on a range of laboratory tests. Although there are theoretical arguments supporting the value of therapeutic intervention at this stage of the disease its clinical benefit is yet to be definitively demonstrated. However, the identification of this condition has the potential to impact upon both the care of an individual patient and upon the health of a population by early institution of interventions limiting spread of the infection.

PATHOPHYSIOLOGY

By the time a patient presents with clinical manifestations of acute HIV infection, even in those with negative or indeterminate serology, a whole series of virological and immunological events have already occurred (Fig. 6.1). The so-called window period, despite being apparently silent on diagnostic tests, is neither immunologically nor virologically silent. Insight into many of these earliest events has been gained from animal models such as SIV infection of rhesus macaques as these events are impossible to study in humans for a range of practical and ethical reasons.

Most infections occur at mucosal membranes. After crossing epithelial barriers, the initial cells infected by virus are both dendritic cells and CD4 T cells that populate the mucosal tissues of the genitourinary and/or colonic mucosa. Dendritic cells are capable of harboring and transporting the virus to lymphoid tissue with or without being productively infected [1]. However, whether infected or just transporting the virus, these cells are capable of transferring virus to multiple CD4 T cells as they fulfill their normal role of antigen presentation to T cells. This interaction simultaneously triggers an immune response consisting of both T cell (involving activation of both CD4 and CD8 T cells) and antibody responses while facilitating infection of responding CD4 T cells. This process drives preferential infection and subsequent death of HIV-specific CD4 T cells, resulting in the early deletion of these critical cells from the host's immune response to the virus [2]. After infection of lymphoid tissue there is subsequent, rapid dissemination of the virus to multiple tissues including the central nervous system.

CD4 T cell responses

As with any primary immune response, the adaptive immune response takes time to develop. The virus replicates relatively unchecked during this period. Plasma viremia is detectable and viral load increases exponentially (Fig. 6.1). At primary infection in SIV-macaque models

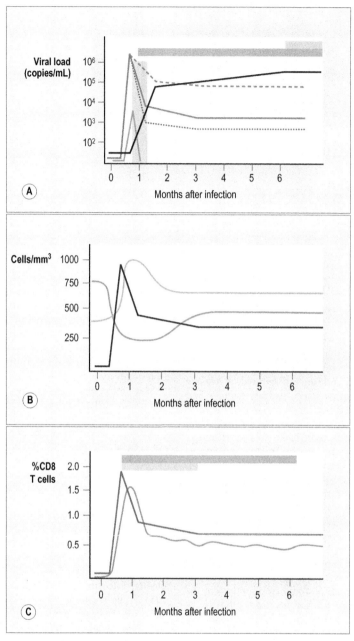

Figure 6.1 Dynamics of virological and immunological events during acute infection and their relationship to diagnostic readouts. (A) Green lines show the changes in plasma viral load measured in RNA copies/mL of plasma. The solid green line shows a typical viral load time course and outcome; the dashed green line shows viral load time course with a likely poor long-term outcome, and the dotted green line shows the time course of the patient likely to have a good prognosis. The blue-gray shaded area indicates the onset and offset of clinical manifestations. The blue line shows the typical time course of p24 antigen detection. The magenta line shows the time course of development of HIV antibodies. The horizontal gray box shows the period during which a typical EIA will be positive. The purple box shows the timing at which a detuned EIA will become positive. (B) Typical time course of CD4 and CD8 T cell counts in peripheral blood. The blue line is the CD4 T cell count; the yellow line is the CD8 T cell count. A typical viral load curve is shown for reference (green line). (C) The yellow line shows a representative antigen specific CD8 CTL response as measured by response to a single immuno-dominant epitope. The horizontal boxes show the typical time course of HIV-specific CD4 T cell responses and the blue horizontal bar shows the presence of CD4 T cells capable of proliferation and production of IL-2. The gray box shows time course of cells capable of producing IFN-γ.

there is massive infection and depletion of CD4 T cells, particularly those at tissue sites such as lymphoid tissue, gut, and genitourinary tracts [3, 4]. Similar processes appear to be occurring in humans early in HIV infection [5, 6]. This depletion in tissues is reflected in a reduction in CD4 T cell count in peripheral blood.

In humans, HIV-specific CD4 T cell responses are detectable early in infection [7, 8]. Initially, these consist of cells capable of producing both IL-2 and IFN-γ and of proliferating in response to HIV antigens, but these cells rapidly lose their ability to proliferate and produce IL-2 in the majority of patients (Fig. 6.1 C) [7, 9, 10]. The exception appears to be in those individuals that control virus replication. In the remainder of patients HIV-specific CD4 T cells are detectable, but consist almost entirely of cells capable of producing IFN-γ without proliferative or IL-2-producing capacity (Fig. 6.1 C). This depletion occurs in both peripheral blood and tissues.

T cells homing to peripheral lymphoid tissue such as the gut and genitourinary tracts preferentially express the chemokine receptor CCR5. The preferential depletion of these cells may be due to selective infection and cytolysis due to a heightened susceptibility to infection by the virus strain associated with transmission [11, 12]. Preferential infection of CD4 T cells specifically responding to HIV infection results in loss of these cells and almost certainly accounts for the pathognomic phenomenon of anergy to HIV antigens seen later in HIV infection [2]. Therapy initiated early can preserve this responsiveness and may limit the depletion from and support the repopulation of these cells at mucosal sites [5, 6].

CD8 T cell responses

In contrast to the decrease in CD4 T cell numbers, CD8 T cell numbers rise dramatically during acute infection (Fig. 6.1B). This increase consists almost entirely of activated T cells [13]. Many of these activated, proliferating, and expanding cells are cytotoxic T cells (CTL) specifically targeted to HIV (Fig. 6.1 C) [14, 15]. Their ability to lyse infected targets and prevent infection of new cells is thought to limit viral expansion, halting the exponential increase in plasma viral load that follows initial infection and to at least partially determine the eventual viral set point. While CD8 CTL are detectable, a second set of CD8 T cells capable of suppressing viral replication through secretion of a range of soluble factors, including MIP1-α, MIP1-β, RANTES, and an as yet unidentified cytokine called CAF, is also detectable during acute HIV-infection [16]. Deliberate depletion of CD8 T cells from SIV-infected macaques at primary infection results in increases of viral load set point and accounts for more rapid disease progression [17].

In peripheral blood, HIV-specific CD8 T cells are among the first immune responses detectable, usually during the clinical presentation of acute infection. In macaques, SIV-specific CD8 T cells can be detected within 8 days of infection [18]. The initial response is usually highly focused on a limited number of high-avidity epitopes. The response broadens with time. Responses to a range of HIV proteins, including regulatory and accessory proteins such as Tat and Nef, are present [19, 20].

CD8 CTL responses place pressure on the virus. Adaptive evolution of the virus to these responses occurs early, allowing selection of immune escape variants capable of evading CTL responses within several weeks of infection [21, 22].

Antibody responses

Although antibodies to various HIV proteins, particularly p24 and envelope proteins, are detectable soon after infection, most of these antibodies play no clear role in control of infection. The majority of the antibody response is to internal proteins. Of the antibodies directed at the envelope proteins, the overwhelming majority are not neutralizing in nature [23]. Neutralizing antibodies, capable of preventing viral entry and therefore new infection, are slow to arise and are usually detectable not less than 4–8 weeks after infection [24]. When neutralizing antibodies do occur they place pressure on the virus. The virus responds to this pressure, rapidly adapting through the generation of escape variants [25, 26]. New rounds of neutralizing antibodies are also delayed in their development.

Innate immune responses

The role of innate immune responses in primary infection is still not clearly understood. Dendritic cells play a role in the transport of virus to lymphoid tissue, and can act as a "Trojan horse," transmitting captured virus to CD4 T cells, assisting in the dissemination of infection. However, dendritic cells play a critical role in the control of infection as they are essential for cross-priming and induction of CD8 CTL responses as well as CD4 T cell responses [1]. While myeloid dendritic cell numbers are maintained, plasmacytoid dendritic cell numbers are depleted during primary infection [27].

Natural killer (NK) cells are a significant component of the innate immune response in the early control of viral infections. NK cells increase in number during acute HIV infection prior to seroconversion and before significant CD8 T cell responses are evident [28]. However, as viral replication increases, NK cell responses become impaired [29].

Immune and virological outcomes at resolution of primary infection

Upon onset of these HIV-specific immune responses viral load declines. CD4 T cell counts partially recover but do not return to normal levels. CD8 T cell numbers drop but remain elevated well above the normal range (Fig. 6.1).

These changes maintain a reversed CD4:CD8 T cell ratio, despite partial normalization of CD4 T cell counts. Markers of immune activation particularly those expressed on the surface of CD8 T cells (e.g. CD38), remain substantially increased. Plasma viral load reaches a steady state or set point approximately 3–6 months post-infection [30]. This level reflects a balance between the pathogenicity and replication fitness of the virus and the effectiveness of the host's initial immune response. This level predicts long-term disease outcome (Fig. 6.1) [31].

Virus

Initial infection in the overwhelming majority of cases occurs with the virus using the CCR5 co-receptor. This chemokine receptor is expressed preferentially on monocytes, dendritic cells, and memory CD4 T cells. Viral tropism for CCR5 is determined by the amino acid sequence of specific regions of Env. The observation of almost exclusive CCR5 co-receptor tropism in viruses isolated early in infection strongly suggests selection of viral strains from within the transmitting host's multiple quasispecies by the process of transmission.

Furthermore, the virus appears highly homogenous, shortly after transmission. Two factors may contribute to homogeneity of transmitted strains. The first is the concept of a molecular sieve, where the process of transmission selects for the variants most capable of transmission from among the swarm of quasispecies in the transmitting host. Certain envelope variants appear to have an advantage during the transmission process. The selection of CCR5 tropic variants is the clearest example. More recently, in subtype C virus, variants carrying *env* sequences with shorter V1–V4 intervals and reduced numbers of glycosylation sites appear to be preferentially transmitted [32]. This molecular sieve is most obvious in heterosexual transmission where the majority of transmissions are by a single viral quasispecies that is most often not the dominant quasispecies in the transmitting host. The restrictions on transmission are less stringent when they occur in men who have sex with men, in the presence of intercurrent sexually transmitted infections, and in intravenous drug users where a larger proportion of transmissions involve multiple quasispecies [33–35]. These observations suggest that intact mucosal surfaces impose a strong selection pressure on the virus.

Additionally, homogeneity of transmitted strains may be contributed to by rapid viral adaptation to its new host post-transmission. Post-transmission, the virus tends to revert from mutations that were advantageous in the original host towards wild type. This process of reversion affects both drug resistance and immune escape mutations [36, 37]. The rate of reversion inversely correlates with the fitness cost to the virus in its new host with reversion of non-advantageous mutations in the new host occurring very quickly.

Despite these processes, a range of adaptive mutations within the transmitted virus may be maintained. Horizontal and vertical transmission of both drug resistance mutations and immune escape mutations are well documented [38, 39]. However, thereafter, mutations reflecting adaptation to the new host also occur rapidly with mutations allowing escape from both CTL and neutralizing antibody pressure arising rapidly [21, 22, 26]. The virus adapts to the altered pressures placed upon it, with selection of the most replication-competent variants occurring rapidly. Variation can occur in all genes. The reasons for differences in the rate of variation relate to varying levels of gene plasticity and differences in the pressures applied.

Co-infection and superinfection

As explained above, simultaneous co-infection with several quasispecies occur in a significant minority of cases especially in the presence of impaired mucosal barriers. In addition superinfection with a second virus within the first 2 years post initial infection has been reported with increasing frequency, at least in non-B subtype infections. Superinfection, in B subtype infections, appears rare or at least uncommon [40–42]; however, in areas where microepidemics of different subtypes intersect, superinfection appears more common [43, 44]. The presence of more than one viral quasispecies may be advantageous to the virus, allowing it to evolve more quickly within a host through recombination events.

CLINICAL MANIFESTATIONS

The rate of recognition of the clinical manifestations of primary infection varies markedly. An acute illness associated with recent infection with HIV-1 can be identified in the majority of individuals with reported rates ranging from 50 to 90% [45–48]. Initial descriptions described the illness as resembling infectious mononucleosis, with the major manifestations being fever, pharyngitis, and adenopathy [45], but further studies have demonstrated that using this triad alone to describe the clinical manifestations is restrictive [48]. Symptoms associated with initial infection and subsequent seroconversion can vary from completely absent through to an acute debilitating illness requiring hospitalization. The rate of identification is dependent on high levels of clinical suspicion, experience with making the diagnosis, the availability of medical resources, and suspicion on the part of the patient. Although the overwhelming majority of reports of this illness have been in the context of the developed world with subtype B infections, similar manifestations have been reported with other viral subtypes in developing world settings. Similarly, although most reported series also arise from cohorts where the major mode of transmission is sexual, similar prevalence of symptomatic illness and similar clinical manifestations have been reported in intravenous drug users [9, 49]. In adults, clinical manifestations and severity are not dependent on age, sex, race, or geographical factors. Although no concurrent studies have been performed, a study in a US population showed that 49% sought medical attention for symptoms [50], while up to 44% of African women took some time off work due to primary infection symptoms [51]. Although published reports are sparse, similar manifestations are seen in adolescents [52].

The time from exposure to illness is typically 2–4 weeks (range: 6–42 days) [45–48], but there are rare, isolated reports of delayed seroconversion of up to 12 months postexposure. The acute illness typically lasts approximately 3 weeks and is of rapid onset. In the main, the symptoms are self-limiting. However, up to 20% of cases can require hospitalization or be associated with the presence of opportunistic infections like candidiasis, herpes zoster, cryptococcosis, and *Pneumocystis jiroveci* pneumonia. The likelihood of primary infection being complicated by an opportunistic infection is related to the extent of CD4 T cell depression [53].

The main clinical manifestations are fever, pharyngitis, adenopathy, rash, myalgia or arthralgia, headaches, and fatigue or asthenia. The pharyngitis is non-exudative and the tonsils are not coated. The rash is classically maculopapular, symmetrical with lesions 0.5–1 cm in diameter affecting face and or trunk, but may also affect the hands including the palms. Other manifestations include mouth ulcers and gastrointestinal upset including diarrhea, odynophagia, anorexia, abdominal pain, and vomiting. Headaches can be associated with retro-orbital pain exacerbated by movement of the eyes and meningitic or encephalitic symptoms and signs. Lymphadenopathy tends to be more common in the cervical region but can affect axillary and inguinal regions [45–48, 53].

The originally described triad of dominant manifestations—fever, pharyngitis, and lymphadenopathy—occurs in a significant minority of patients. Although fever is the most common manifestation, it occurs in less than three-quarters of patients. In the absence of a typical mononucleosis-like presentation, fever is most commonly associated with headache, oral ulceration, and/or abdominal pain. In the absence of fever the most common manifestations are pharyngitis, lethargy, myalgia, rash, headache, and adenopathy [48]. Lymphadenopathy may be slow to resolve, persisting well after the resolution of other manifestations.

Clinical presentations are reasonably nonspecific and not easily distinguishable from other viral illnesses on clinical grounds alone. However, this constellation of symptoms in those at risk should trigger consideration of primary infection illness in the differential diagnosis and should initiate laboratory investigation including HIV serology.

The severity of the illness appears to impact on long-term outcome, with greater severity predicting more rapid progression to disease. More rapid CD4 T cell count declines have been documented in those who present to a physician [54]. The presence of candidiasis, neurological involvement, or a prolonged illness lasting more than 14 days is associated with a worse prognosis [48].

Co-infection with other viruses, such as cytomegalovirus (CMV), or other sexually transmitted infections (STIs), occurs. These co-infections can make the clinical presentation more complicated [55]. Co-infection with other viruses such as herpes viruses, hepatitis B or C virus, or other STIs such as chlamydia or syphilis must be considered in the diagnostic work-up.

As stated, race, mode of acquisition, or viral subtype does not appear to impact upon the severity of the illness. Pre-existing impaired immune responses, as demonstrated by low pre-existing CD4 T cell count, low CD4:CD8 T cell ratios, or impaired delayed-type hypersensitivity reactions, are associated with increased risk of a symptomatic illness, as is transmission from an index case with advanced HIV disease [56, 57].

DIAGNOSIS

Clinical suspicion, based upon recognition of the constellation of clinical signs detailed in the previous section, combined with knowledge of possible exposure to the virus in the previous 2–8 weeks, plus laboratory confirmation of recent HIV infection, are the cornerstones of diagnosis. For these reasons, the diagnosis should always be considered in individuals presenting with apparently nonspecific symptoms if they belong to a risk group for HIV infection. The differential diagnosis of primary HIV-1 infection includes other viral infections, particularly with herpes viruses, such as Epstein–Barr virus (EBV) and CMV, but also includes other viral illnesses and STIs, particularly syphilis. Usually, the confirmation or exclusion of the diagnosis of acute HIV infection in the laboratory is straightforward. Therefore, the critical step in the process is the consideration of the diagnosis as a possibility.

Early diagnosis has advantages for both the individual and the population. It allows institution of therapies in the context of a relatively intact immune system. Furthermore, effective therapy reduces viral load and therefore viral turnover, markedly limiting the rate at which virus mutants arise, allowing adaptation to either drug pressure or immune responses. As the severity of the illness has implications for long-term outcome, it may influence decisions regarding timing of institution of therapy. Early initiation of risk-modification counseling limits the potential for transmission, particularly as transmission probability increases with high viral loads such as those that characterize primary infection [58–60]. However, the effectiveness of this intervention will depend upon the stage of the epidemic and the extent to which transmission is to casual partners [61]. The identification and early diagnosis of primary HIV infection is an essential component of the "Test and Treat" strategies that have been proposed as a mechanism of limiting or in the best-case scenario stalling the epidemic. This strategy relies on very early diagnosis of large proportions of all new infections in a population and the rapid institution of antiretroviral therapy (ART) to reduce viral load, thereby reducing or eliminating transmission of the virus. While modeling of this concept has provided encouraging results, this strategy requires substantial implementation research to provide evidence for practicality and effectiveness [62].

LABORATORY TESTING AND DIAGNOSIS

Although nucleic acid testing is playing a greater role in the diagnosis and management of acute HIV infection, serology is still the mainstay of diagnosis. The relative susceptibility of nucleic acid testing to false-negative results as a result of sequence variation, particularly across different viral subtypes, still prevents these tests becoming the mainstay of diagnosis.

The routine detection of primary infection relies on the generation of antibodies to the virus. As these take a finite period to develop, there is an unavoidable window period after infection when these tests will be negative, even in the presence of established infection (Fig. 6.1). The length of this period is, to some extent, dependent upon the sensitivity of the test used. In general, those assays where the viral proteins are derived from viral lysates alone are less sensitive than those in which lysates are supplemented by recombinant proteins or peptides. The window period can be further shortened by detection of virus directly, through either protein-based assays for the detection of p24 protein or nucleic acid testing based on the detection of either proviral DNA or viral RNA (Fig. 6.1). However, even these tests will be negative for up to 2 weeks following infection [63]. The sequential development of positive results initially on nucleic acid tests and then on various serological tests has been used to formally divide the period of primary infection into stages called Fiebig stages [63].

Criteria for diagnosis of HIV-1 infection vary from country to country but the diagnosis in the laboratory of acute HIV infection is dependent upon either an evolving pattern of antibody production or a new positive test in the presence of a documented recent negative test.

Serology

A range of tests for detecting antibodies that will make the diagnosis of HIV infection are available. These include a variety of enzyme immunoassay (EIA)-type technologies and immunoblotting. These now include a variety of "point of care"

testing platforms that can also employ fluids other than blood, including saliva. In general these rapid tests have lower specificity and sensitivity than the standard laboratory-based tests. This type of test may have a role in diagnosis, particularly in the absence of formal laboratory support in resource-poor settings [64]. In addition these rapid tests may also increase the overall coverage of HIV testing as a significant minority of people tested for HIV never return to receive their test results; however, in low prevalence populations, tests with even high specificity, if used alone, will result in substantial numbers of false-positive results [65].

As is typical of immune responses to infection anti-HIV IgM antibodies precede the development of IgG antibodies. However, detection of IgM antibodies alone is not routinely used in the diagnosis of recent HIV infection because of unacceptable rates of false-positive results. Antibodies are usually detectable by EIA or Western blot within 2 weeks of infection; however, the length of this window period varies depending on the diagnostic kit used (Fig. 6.1).

Immunoblotting demonstrates that antibodies develop in typical and predictable patterns (Fig. 6.2). This knowledge can be used for early identification of likely seroconverters triggering other testing to support the diagnosis of early or acute HIV infection. These tests include direct detection of virus (see below). Antibodies to p24 or Env are typically the earliest antibodies detectable with virtually all sera being positive 2 weeks or more after the onset of the acute illness. Antibodies to other proteins develop sequentially with a fully positive Western blot present by 3 months after infection. However, individuals identified soon after exposure may have negative EIA and negative or indeterminate immunoblot results at the time of their first blood draw. Definitive serological diagnosis then depends on tracking responses over time until diagnostic criteria are fulfilled. Laboratories interested in studying acute infection have developed algorithms for the rapid detection and confirmation of these cases (Fig. 6.3).

Importantly, highly suppressive ART commenced early in the course of acute HIV infection can change the pattern of antibody development, resulting in freezing antibody development at the stage at which therapy was commenced [66]. This can cause diagnostic difficulties; however, upon interruption of therapy and subsequent increases in viral load, antibody responses develop rapidly to a fully positive immunoblot pattern.

Detuned serology and other testing to detect recent infection

In the absence of a developing antibody pattern, diagnosis of early infection is usually dependent upon the availability of recently negative serology. However, a range of serological techniques that can indicate recent infection are becoming available. These techniques are based on the

Figure 6.2 Development of HIV antibodies over time, following infection. Sequential immunoblots performed on serum samples from a typical seroconverter showing characteristic pattern of antibodies to various HIV proteins at acute infection.

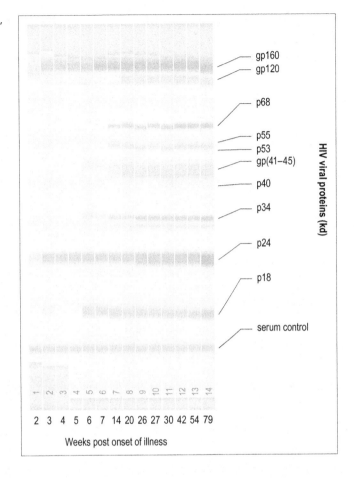

Figure 6.3 An example of a "flat" diagnostic algorithm for rapid identification of true acute infection cases. A barrage of diagnostic tests is set up in parallel, allowing for faster turnaround times, but this is a more expensive strategy and is usually only adopted in reference laboratories with an interest in primary infection.

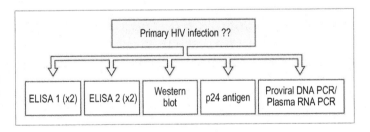

observation that both the intensity and the affinity of the antibodies increase over time. The best known of these techniques is the "detuned" EIA. In these assays, the sensitivity of a standard EIA is deliberately compromised through increasing the dilution of the sera tested and reducing incubation times. In these compromised EIA, sera from individuals with fully established infection still produce a positive response, but sera from those with recent infection will give a negative response and therefore "detune." The period over which recent infection can be detected by detuned EIAs varies from test to test, but in general these assays detect infections within the past 6 months (Figs 6.1, 6.4) [64].

However, this assay performs with quite different characteristics in non-B subtype viruses, limiting its utility outside the developed world [67]. More recent developments with IgG capture EIAs may have overcome some of these problems [68, 69]. Other methodologies for detecting recent infection depend on the affinity maturation of antibodies to particular epitopes or detection of development of p24

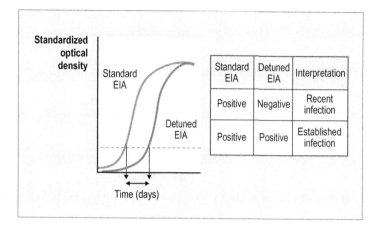

Figure 6.4 Relative performance of a standard diagnostic EIA and a detuned EIA. The detuned EIA will become positive several months later than the standard highly optimized and sensitive diagnostic EIA. In the interval shown by the double-headed arrow, the diagnosis of a recent infection can be made by the discrepant results between the two tests.

antibodies of a particular isotype [70]. However, the performance of these tests on non-B subtypes has not been assessed. Another mechanism of diagnosing early infection employs an algorithm that takes into account the characteristic patterns in development of individual bands and intensities of bands upon Western blot. This simple algorithm appears to have greater specificity for recent infection than detuned testing. The further development of this type of test will aid with collection of epidemiologic data on rates of new infections, rates of disease progression, and early diagnosis for individuals.

Detection of virus

The main role of direct viral detection in the diagnosis of primary infection is in reducing the window period in those with negative or indeterminate serological testing. The ability to directly detect viral components p24 or nucleic acid (plasma RNA or proviral DNA) supports the likely diagnosis of HIV infection.

p24 Antigen detection

This test employs EIA technology. The test is highly specific and, although not sensitive in chronic disease, is characteristically transiently positive early in acute infection in those with negative or very early antibody responses. The test is usually positive 3–6 days prior to a sensitive antibody EIA (Fig. 6.1) [63].

Many commercially available tests now combine antibody and antigen detection in a single EIA. These kits offer significant advantages in screening for positive diagnoses, especially at primary infection. Subsequent testing will reveal whether the positive result is driven by the presence of antigen or antibody. The majority of the latest generation of p24 antigen tests ("4th generation kits") perform well with non-B clade isolates [71].

Nucleic acid testing

Detection of proviral DNA by polymerase chain reaction (PCR) techniques is a sensitive and specific way of diagnosing HIV infection and is a very useful adjunct test in the context of primary infection in those with negative or indeterminate serology. The test is often positive up to 2 days prior to the p24 antibody test (Fig. 6.1); however, it works less efficiently in non-subtype B infections. The other major use of this test is for the early diagnosis of mother-to-child transmission, as maternal antibodies make the use of serological strategies for neonatal diagnosis problematical. Viral RNA can be used as an alternative, but care must used when choosing the correct test as many of the standard viral load tests used for monitoring of infection and response to therapy have a low but problematical false-positive rate in true seronegatives. Therefore, the viral load detected must be > 5000 copies/mL on two separate occasions before the diagnosis can be made with certainty. Used in this way, the test usually first becomes positive about the same time as the p24 antigen. Alternative qualitative RNA detection kits have been developed for screening of blood donations and can be used to screen pooled samples. These give positive readouts at lower RNA levels and therefore reduce the window period further but are not currently approved for use in routine diagnosis [63]. As with the proviral DNA test, RNA tests are susceptible to false-negative results in variant strains.

Viral load during primary infection

Following diagnosis, the patient is usually monitored using standard surrogate markers of disease progression, viral load, and CD4 T cell count. A low nadir CD4 cell count and higher viral load at 2–4 months, but not peak viral load, is associated with a poorer prognosis [54, 72], while rapid falls in viral load are associated with a better prognosis. Set point viral load is attained between 3 and 6 months post-infection [30], and the higher this level, the worse the prognosis. Cervical and semen HIV viral loads mirror plasma viral loads with high levels during primary infection before a set point is reached [73, 74]. This would contribute to the reported increase in transmission risk during primary HIV infection [59].

Drug resistance testing

Drug resistance can be determined either phenotypically or genotypically. The determination of drug resistance at primary infection is generally recommended by expert panels and can serve two purposes. First, it can serve as a public health surveillance mechanism providing information regarding population rates of transmission of drug-resistant variants. Second, it provides important information for the individual if therapeutic intervention is being considered. Rates of transmitted resistance vary markedly between populations [75]. In the absence of drug pressure, some of these mutations revert over time, while some, particularly those that are compensated by secondary mutations or those that do not significantly impact on viral fitness, tend to be maintained. The impact of these transmitted mutations on long-term outcome is still to be determined, but theoretically, they will compromise response to ART.

Transmitted resistance mutations may behave differently from those in an individual stopping therapy where there is often rapid outgrowth of wild-type or reversion variants. Mutations may be maintained post-transmission for much longer periods than after withdrawal of therapy. While the M184V 3TC mutation often reverts rapidly and the T215Y AZT mutation partially reverts to 215 S/C/D, others, particularly the K103N mutation, may be maintained for long periods of time [76].

MANAGEMENT

Once the definitive diagnosis is made, it must be communicated to the patient in a clear and supportive manner. The patient must fully understand the diagnosis and appreciate the need to adopt safe practices that minimize further spread of the infection. There is evidence that earlier diagnosis if linked to effective counseling services can modify behavior and reduce transmission at a time of high viral load and therefore the likely probability of transmission per unsafe event [77]. Therapy of primary infection is supportive. The initiation of ART during acute infection is suggested by a range of treatment guidelines, but usually only in the context of clinical trial. Although there are theoretical reasons to support this approach, there are still no definitive data from controlled clinical trials which demonstrate that combination antiretroviral chemotherapy has a positive effect on long-term clinical outcome [78]. Although the first randomized trial of zidovudine monotherapy at primary infection suggested a therapeutic benefit in the short term, longer-term follow-up suggested this effect was diluted with time [79, 80]. Some studies suggest that initiating early, transient therapy during acute HIV infection slows the rate of disease progression and delays the need for long-term ART [81, 82]. Combination ART is definitely effective in improving both CD4 T cell count and viral load, compared with untreated historical controls, while those patients are on treatment. However, the long-term advantage of these regimens has not been demonstrated and in general CD4 T cell counts and viral load return to similar set points as those untreated individuals upon cessation of therapy [78]. Other therapeutic approaches such as structured treatment interruptions and short-course therapy lasting up to 12 months have been advocated after apparent success in selected individuals. However, randomized clinical trials have demonstrated that structured treatment interruptions are detrimental to individuals compared to constant ART and should be avoided [83]. There are significant amounts of data suggesting improvements or maintenance of various functional HIV-specific immune responses mediated by both CD4 and CD8 T cells; however, the impact of these changes on long-term outcome are unclear at this time [7, 8].

The presumed benefits of early intervention with suppressive ART include reduction in viral load resulting in reduction of transmission and preservation of the immune system preventing depletion of CD4 T cells. Although there has been fairly universal acceptance of initiation of therapy for those diagnosed during acute infection, attitudes of physicians are becoming more conservative, driven by the lack of efficacy data and the cumulative toxicities of ART regimens. Recent data suggest that adverse events, including gastrointestinal upsets, lipodystrophy, and mood disorders, are recorded in 51% of individuals treated, with only 75% achieving good viral load control [84]. The first randomized clinical trial of combined ART commenced at primary infection (SPARTAC) will provide insight into whether early treatment of limited duration (3 months or 1 year) in patients with PHI can influence long-term CD4 T cell decline and disease progression [82]. This trial is complete and the preliminary results were released in late 2011. Hopefully, this study will give some definitive guidance on therapeutic intervention during primary infection.

CONCLUSION

Primary infection is a dynamic process. To a significant degree, long-term outcomes of the natural history of HIV infection are determined by the pathophysiological events occurring during this period. Identification of patients during acute infection allows for ideal management of the infection from its earliest stages and has the potential to significantly impact further spread of the epidemic through early institution of risk-reduction strategies.

REFERENCES

[1] Rinaldo Jr CR, Piazza P. Virus infection of dendritic cells: portal for host invasion and host defense. Trends Microbiol 2004;12 (7):337–45.

[2] Douek DC, Brenchley JM, Betts MR, et al. HIV preferentially infects HIV-specific CD4+ T cells. Nature 2002;417(6884):95–8.

[3] Couedel-Courteille A, Pretet JL, Barget N, et al. Delayed viral replication and CD4(+) T cell depletion in the rectosigmoid mucosa of macaques during primary rectal SIV infection. Virology 2003;316(2):290–301.

[4] Veazey RS, DeMaria M, Chalifoux LV, et al. Gastrointestinal tract as a major site of CD4+ T cell depletion and viral replication in SIV infection. Science 1998;280 (5362):427–31.

[5] Guadalupe M, Reay E, Sankaran S, et al. Severe CD4+ T-cell depletion in gut lymphoid tissue during primary human immunodeficiency virus type 1 infection and substantial delay in restoration following highly active antiretroviral therapy. J Virol 2003;77(21):11708–17.

[6] Mehandru S, Poles MA, Tenner-Racz K, et al. Primary HIV-1 infection is associated with preferential depletion of CD4+ T lymphocytes from effector sites in the gastrointestinal tract. J Exp Med 2004;200(6):761–70.

[7] Oxenius A, Price DA, Easterbrook PJ, et al. Early highly active antiretroviral therapy for acute HIV-1 infection preserves immune function of CD8+ and CD4+ T lymphocytes. Proc Natl Acad Sci U S A 2000;97(7):3382–7.

[8] Rosenberg ES, Billingsley JM, Caliendo AM, et al. Vigorous HIV-1-specific CD4+ T cell responses associated with control of viremia. Science 1997;278(5342):1447–50.

[9] Routy JP, Vanhems P, Rouleau D, et al. Comparison of clinical features of acute HIV-1 infection in patients infected sexually or through injection drug use. The Investigators of the Quebec Primary HIV Infection Study. J Acquir Immune Defic Syndr 2000;24(5):425–32.

[10] Younes SA, Yassine-Diab B, Dumont AR, et al. HIV-1 viremia prevents the establishment of interleukin 2-producing HIV-specific memory CD4+ T cells endowed with proliferative capacity. J Exp Med 2003;198 (12):1909–22.

[11] Zaunders JJ, Kaufmann GR, Cunningham PH, et al. Increased turnover of CCR5+ and redistribution of CCR5- CD4 T lymphocytes during primary human immunodeficiency virus type 1 infection. J Infect Dis 2001;183(5):736–43.

[12] Zaunders JJ, Moutouh-de Parseval L, Kitada S, et al. Polyclonal proliferation and apoptosis of CCR5+ T lymphocytes during primary human immunodeficiency virus type 1 infection: regulation by interleukin (IL)-2, IL-15, and Bcl-2. J Infect Dis 2003;187(11):735–47.

[13] Zaunders J, Carr A, McNally L, et al. Effects of primary HIV-1 infection on subsets of CD4+ and CD8+ T lymphocytes. AIDS 1995;9 (6):561–6.

[14] Pantaleo G, Demarest JF, Soudeyns H, et al. Major expansion of CD8+ T cells with a predominant V beta usage during the primary immune response to HIV. Nature 1994;370(6489):463–7.

[15] Wilson JD, Ogg GS, Allen RL, et al. Direct visualization of HIV-1-specific cytotoxic T lymphocytes during primary infection. AIDS 2000;14(3):225–33.

[16] Mackewicz CE, Yang LC, Lifson JD, Levy JA. Non-cytolytic CD8 T-cell anti-HIV responses in primary HIV-1 infection. Lancet 1994;344 (8938):1671–3.

[17] Jin X, Bauer DE, Tuttleton SE, et al. Dramatic rise in plasma viremia after CD8(+) T cell depletion in simian immunodeficiency virus-infected macaques. J Exp Med 1999;189(6):991–8.

[18] Reimann KA, Tenner-Racz K, Racz P, et al. Immunopathogenic events in acute infection of rhesus monkeys with simian immunodeficiency virus of macaques. J Virol 1994;68 (4):2362–70.

[19] Cao J, McNevin J, Holte S, et al. Comprehensive analysis of human immunodeficiency virus type 1 (HIV-1)-specific gamma interferon-secreting CD8+ T cells in primary HIV-1 infection. J Virol 2003;77 (12):6867–78.

[20] Lichterfeld M, Yu XG, Cohen D, et al. HIV-1 Nef is preferentially recognized by CD8 T cells in primary HIV-1 infection despite a relatively high degree of genetic diversity. AIDS 2004;18 (10):1383–92.

[21] Borrow P, Lewicki H, Wei X, et al. Antiviral pressure exerted by HIV-1-specific cytotoxic T lymphocytes (CTLs) during primary infection demonstrated by rapid selection of CTL escape virus. Nat Med 1997;3 (2):205–11.

[22] Price DA, Goulder PJ, Klenerman P, et al. Positive selection of HIV-1 cytotoxic T lymphocyte escape variants during primary infection. Proc Natl Acad Sci U S A 1997;94 (5):1890–5.

[23] Burton DR. A vaccine for HIV type 1: the antibody perspective. Proc Natl Acad Sci U S A 1997;94 (19):10018–23.

[24] Richman DD, Wrin T, Little SJ, Petropoulos CJ. Rapid evolution of the neutralizing antibody response to HIV type 1 infection. Proc Natl Acad Sci U S A 2003;100 (7):4144–9.

[25] Arendrup M, Nielsen C, Hansen JE, et al. Autologous HIV-1 neutralizing antibodies: emergence of neutralization-resistant escape virus and subsequent development of escape virus neutralizing antibodies. J Acquir Immune Defic Syndr 1992;5(3):303–7.

[26] Desrosiers RC. Escape from neutralizing antibody responses by sequence variation in the SIV envelope. 7th Annual Conference of the Australian Society for HIV Medicine, 1995.

[27] Pacanowski J, Kahi S, Baillet M, et al. Reduced blood CD123+ (lymphoid)

and CD11c+ (myeloid) dendritic cell numbers in primary HIV-1 infection. Blood 2001;98 (10):3016–21.

[28] Alter G, Teigen N, Ahern R, et al. Evolution of innate and adaptive effector cell functions during acute HIV-1 infection. J Infect Dis 2007;195(10):1452–60.

[29] Alter G, Teigen N, Davis BT, et al. Sequential deregulation of NK cell subset distribution and function starting in acute HIV-1 infection. Blood 2005;106(10):3366–9.

[30] Kaufmann GR, Cunningham P, Kelleher AD, et al. Patterns of viral dynamics during primary human immunodeficiency virus type 1 infection. The Sydney Primary HIV Infection Study Group. J Infect Dis 1998;178(6):1812–15.

[31] Mellors JW, Kingsley LA, Rinaldo Jr CR, et al. Quantitation of HIV-1 RNA in plasma predicts outcome after seroconversion. Ann Intern Med 1995;122(8):573–9.

[32] Derdeyn CA, Decker JM, Bibollet-Ruche F, et al. Envelope-constrained neutralization-sensitive HIV-1 after heterosexual transmission. Science 2004;303(5666):2019–22.

[33] Bar KJ, Li H, Chamberland A, et al. Wide variation in the multiplicity of HIV-1 infection among injection drug users. J Virol 2010;84 (12):6241–7.

[34] Fischer W, Ganusov VV, Giorgi EE, et al. Transmission of single HIV-1 genomes and dynamics of early immune escape revealed by ultra-deep sequencing. PLoS One 2010;5 (8):e12303.

[35] Li H, Bar KJ, Wang S, et al. High multiplicity infection by HIV-1 in men who have sex with men. PLoS Pathog 2010;6(5): e1000890.

[36] Allen TM, Altfeld M, Yu XG, et al. Selection, transmission, and reversion of an antigen-processing cytotoxic T-lymphocyte escape mutation in human immunodeficiency virus type 1 infection. J Virol 2004;78 (13):7069–78.

[37] Friedrich TC, Dodds EJ, Yant LJ, et al. Reversion of CTL escape-variant immunodeficiency viruses in vivo. Nat Med 2004;10 (3):275–81.

[38] Goulder PJ, Brander C, Tang Y, et al. Evolution and transmission of stable CTL escape mutations in HIV infection. Nature 2001;412 (6844):334–8.

[39] Leslie AJ, Pfafferott KJ, Chetty P, et al. HIV evolution: CTL escape mutation and reversion after transmission. Nat Med 2004;10 (3):282–9.

[40] Altfeld M, Allen TM, Yu XG, et al. HIV-1 superinfection despite broad CD8+ T-cell responses containing replication of the primary virus. Nature 2002;420 (6914):434–9.

[41] Smith DM, Wong JK, Hightower GK, et al. Incidence of HIV superinfection following primary infection. JAMA 2004;292 (10):1177–8.

[42] Yerly S, Jost S, Monnat M, et al. HIV-1 co/super-infection in intravenous drug users. AIDS 2004;18 (10):1413–21.

[43] Ritola K, Pilcher CD, Fiscus SA, et al. Multiple V1/V2 env variants are frequently present during primary infection with human immunodeficiency virus type 1. J Virol 2004;78(20):11208–18.

[44] Sagar M, Lavreys L, Baeten JM, et al. Infection with multiple human immunodeficiency virus type 1 variants is associated with faster disease progression. J Virol 2003;77 (23):12921–6.

[45] Cooper DA, Gold J, Maclean P, et al. Acute AIDS retrovirus infection. Definition of a clinical illness associated with seroconversion. Lancet 1985;1(8428):537–40.

[46] de Wolf F, Lange JM, Bakker M, et al. Influenza-like syndrome in homosexual men: a prospective diagnostic study. J R Coll Gen Pract 1988;38(315):443–5.

[47] Tindall B, Barker S, Donovan B, et al. Characterization of the acute clinical illness associated with human immunodeficiency virus infection. Arch Intern Med 1988;148(4):945–9.

[48] Vanhems P, Allard R, Cooper DA, et al. Acute human immunodeficiency virus type 1 disease as a mononucleosis-like illness: is the diagnosis too restrictive? Clin Infect Dis 1997;24 (5):965–70.

[49] Montessori V, Rouleau D, Raboud J, et al. Clinical characteristics of primary HIV infection in injection drug users. AIDS 2000;14 (12):1868–70.

[50] Celum CL, Buchbinder SP, Donnell D, et al. Early human immunodeficiency virus (HIV) infection in the HIV Network for Prevention Trials Vaccine Preparedness Cohort: risk behaviors, symptoms, and early plasma and genital tract virus load. J Infect Dis 2001;183(1):23–35.

[51] Lavreys L, Thompson ML, Martin Jr. HL, et al. Primary human immunodeficiency virus type 1 infection: clinical manifestations among women in Mombasa, Kenya. Clin Infect Dis 2000;30(3):486–90.

[52] Aggarwal M, Rein J. Acute human immunodeficiency virus syndrome in an adolescent. Pediatrics 2003;112(4):e323.

[53] Carr A, Cooper DA. Primary HIV infection. In: Sande MA, Volberding PA, editors. The Medical Management of AIDS. Philadelphia: Saunders; 1999, pp. 67–78.

[54] Schacker TW, Hughes JP, Shea T, et al. Biological and virologic characteristics of primary HIV infection. Ann Intern Med 1998;128 (8):613–20.

[55] Bonetti A, Weber R, Vogt MW, et al. Co-infection with human immunodeficiency virus-type 1 (HIV-1) and in two intravenous drug users. Ann Intern Med 1989;111(4):293–6.

[56] Marion SA, Schechter MT, Weaver MS, et al. Evidence that prior immune dysfunction predisposes to human immunodeficiency virus infection in homosexual men. J Acquir Immune Defic Syndr 1989;2 (2):178–86.

[57] Ward JW, Bush TJ, Perkins HA, et al. The natural history of transfusion-associated infection with human immunodeficiency virus. Factors influencing the rate of progression to disease. N Engl J Med 1989;321 (14):947–52.

[58] Chakraborty H, Sen PK, Helms RW, et al. Viral burden in genital secretions determines male-to-female sexual transmission of HIV-1: a probabilistic empiric model. AIDS 2001;15(5):621–7.

[59] Gray RH, Wawer MJ, Brookmeyer R, et al. Probability of HIV-1 transmission per coital act in monogamous, heterosexual, HIV-1-discordant couples in Rakai, Uganda. Lancet 2001;357 (9263):1149–53.

[60] Quinn TC, Wawer MJ, Sewankambo N, et al. Viral load and heterosexual transmission of human immunodeficiency virus type 1. Rakai Project Study Group. N Engl J Med 2000;342(13):921–9.

[61] Xiridou M, Geskus R, de Wit J, et al. Primary HIV infection as source of HIV transmission within steady and casual partnerships among homosexual men. AIDS 2004;18 (9):1311–20.

[62] Hamlyn E, Jones V, Porter K, Fidler S. Antiretroviral treatment of primary HIV infection to reduce onward transmission. Curr Opin HIV AIDS 2010;5(4):283–90.

[63] Fiebig EW, Wright DJ, Rawal BD, et al. Dynamics of HIV viremia and antibody seroconversion in plasma donors: implications for diagnosis and staging of primary HIV infection. AIDS 2003;17 (13):1871–9.

[64] Respess RA, Rayfield MA, Dondero TJ. Laboratory testing and rapid HIV assays: applications for HIV surveillance in hard-to-reach populations. AIDS 2001;15(Suppl. 3):S49–59.

[65] Roberts KJ, Grusky O, Swanson AN. Outcomes of blood and oral fluid rapid HIV testing: a literature review, 2000-2006. AIDS Patient Care STDS 2007;21(9):621–37.

[66] Zaunders JJ, Cunningham PH, Kelleher AD, et al. Potent antiretroviral therapy of primary human immunodeficiency virus type 1 (HIV-1) infection: partial normalization of T lymphocyte subsets and limited reduction of HIV-1 DNA despite clearance of plasma viremia. J Infect Dis 1999;180(2):320–9.

[67] Young CL, Hu DJ, Byers R, et al. Evaluation of a sensitive/less sensitive testing algorithm using the bioMérieux Vironostika-LS assay for detecting recent HIV-1 subtype B' or E infection in Thailand. AIDS Res Hum Retroviruses 2003;19 (6):481–6.

[68] Dobbs T, Kennedy S, Pau CP, et al. Performance characteristics of the immunoglobulin G-capture BED-enzyme immunoassay, an assay to detect recent human immunodeficiency virus type 1 seroconversion. J Clin Microbiol 2004;42(6):2623–8.

[69] Hu DJ, Vanichseni S, Mock PA, et al. HIV type 1 incidence estimates by detection of recent infection from a cross-sectional sampling of injection drug users in Bangkok: use of the IgG capture BED enzyme immunoassay. AIDS Res Hum Retroviruses 2003;19(9):727–30.

[70] Wilson KM, Johnson EI, Croom HA, et al. Incidence immunoassay for distinguishing recent from established HIV-1 infection in therapy-naive populations. AIDS 2004;18(17):2253–9.

[71] Weber B, Thorstensson R, Tanprasert S, et al. Reduction of the diagnostic window in three cases of human immunodeficiency-1 subtype E primary infection with fourth-generation HIV screening assays. Vox Sang 2003;85(2):73–9.

[72] Kaufmann GR, Cunningham P, Zaunders J, et al. Impact of early HIV-1 RNA and T-lymphocyte dynamics during primary HIV-1 infection on the subsequent course of HIV-1 RNA levels and CD4+ T-lymphocyte counts in the first year of HIV-1 infection. Sydney Primary HIV Infection Study Group. J Acquir Immune Defic Syndr 1999;22 (5):437–44.

[73] Morrison CS, Demers K, Kwok C, et al. Plasma and cervical viral loads among Ugandan and Zimbabwean women during acute and early HIV-1 infection. AIDS 2010;24 (4):573–82.

[74] Pilcher CD, Joaki G, Hoffman IF, et al. Amplified transmission of HIV-1: comparison of HIV-1 concentrations in semen and blood during acute and chronic infection. AIDS 2007;21(13):1723–30.

[75] Ammaranond P, Cunningham P, Oelrichs R, et al. Rates of transmission of antiretroviral drug resistant strains of HIV-1. J Clin Virol 2003;26(2):153–61.

[76] Barbour JD, Hecht FM, Wrin T, et al. Persistence of primary drug resistance among recently HIV-1 infected adults. AIDS 2004;18(12): 1683–9.

[77] Pilcher CD, Fiscus SA, Nguyen TQ, et al. Detection of acute infections during HIV testing in North Carolina. N Engl J Med 2005;352(18): 1873–83.

[78] Smith DE, Walker BD, Cooper DA, et al. Is antiretroviral treatment of primary HIV infection clinically justified on the basis of current evidence? AIDS 2004;18(5): 709–18.

[79] Kinloch-De Loes S, Hirschel BJ, Hoen B, et al. A controlled trial of zidovudine in primary human immunodeficiency virus infection. N Engl J Med 1995;333(7): 408–13.

[80] Lindback S, Vizzard J, Cooper DA, Gaines H. Long-term prognosis following zidovudine monotherapy in primary human immunodeficiency virus type 1 infection. J Infect Dis 1999;179 (6):1549–52.

[81] Bell SK, Little SJ, Rosenberg ES. Clinical management of acute HIV infection: best practice remains unknown. J Infect Dis 2010; 202(Suppl. 2):S278–88.

[82] Fidler S, Fox J, Touloumi G, et al. Slower CD4 cell decline following cessation of a 3 month course of HAART in primary HIV infection: findings from an observational cohort. AIDS 2007;21 (10):1283–91.

[83] El-Sadr WM, Lundgren JD, Neaton JD, et al. CD4+ count-guided interruption of antiretroviral treatment. N Engl J Med 2006;355 (22):2283–96.

[84] Schiffer V, Deveau C, Meyer L, et al. Recent changes in the management of primary HIV-1 infection: results from the French PRIMO cohort. HIV Med 2004;5(5):326–33.

Chapter | 7 |

Biology of HIV-1 transmission

Julie Overbaugh

INTRODUCTION

HIV-1 has spread rapidly around the globe, and in some parts of sub-Saharan Africa infects up to one-third of adults aged 15–49. Indeed, the effects of HIV-1 have been most devastating in the developing world: of the estimated 2.6 million new infections occurring each year, nearly 70% take place there (http://www.unaids.org). While there remains continued spread of HIV-1 globally, recent estimates suggest that the number of new infections are decreasing; there were ∼20% fewer infections in 2009 than in 1999 (http://www.unaids.org).

HIV-1 can be transmitted sexually, from mothers to their infants, and via contaminated blood. Globally, heterosexual transmission accounts for the vast majority of new cases of HIV-1 infection, and the epidemic has had similar impact on men and women, with cases in women on the rise [1]. Since sexually infected women who become pregnant can in turn transmit the virus to their infants (called vertical transmission), preventing sexual transmission is viewed as key to slowing the HIV-1 pandemic.

Despite the remarkable spread of HIV, the risk of transmission per exposure is low; estimates are on the order of 0.1% per contact for heterosexual transmission. The per-contact risk is higher (∼1%) for male-to-male sexual transmission, and for blood exposures via contaminated needles (called parenteral transmission) [2]. These numbers may underestimate the risk for persons who have other endogenous or exogenous risk factors that increase their susceptibility, as host factors of the source partner as well as those of the exposed individual are known to alter transmission risk. Certain features of the virus may also influence its fitness for transmission. Thus, the per-contact risk should be considered an average estimate that may be much higher (or lower) in certain circumstances, as discussed below [3].

HIV-1 can be transmitted from an infected mother to her infant *in utero*, during delivery, or through breastfeeding [4, 5]. In the absence of any interventions to reduce transmission, approximately one-third of infants born to HIV-1-infected mothers will become infected. In breastfeeding populations, the risk of HIV-1 infection is almost double the risk in non-breastfeeding populations. While it may seem reasonable to therefore recommend against breastfeeding for all HIV-1-infected mothers, this must be balanced with the potential for increased mortality due to other infectious diseases, which can often occur in regions where access to clean water is limited. Fortunately, mother-to-child transmission of HIV-1 can be lowered considerably by antiviral treatment. In developed countries where state-of-the-art treatment is available, and HIV-1 infected mothers do not breastfeed, transmission is as low as 1–2%. There is also increasing access to antivirals to prevent mother-to-child transmission in developing countries, leading to decreased transmission rates.

FACTORS IN THE INFECTING PARTNER THAT DETERMINE THE LIKELIHOOD OF TRANSMISSION

Higher virus levels in the infecting host (also called index case or source partner) are correlated with infection [2]. This is perhaps unsurprising, as one might expect that exposure to a higher dose of virus would increase the likelihood of transmission. In most studies, viral levels have been defined by measuring systemic HIV-1 RNA in plasma, even though plasma may not be the major bodily fluid to which the person is exposed to during sexual contact. These findings could therefore reflect the fact that the levels of virus in blood plasma are correlated with the viral levels in other body fluids, such as genital secretions. Indeed, one recent study provided direct evidence that genital virus levels predict HIV-1 transmission, and this was true even after accounting for plasma virus levels [6]. The presence of sexually transmitted diseases (STDs) has been shown to increase risk of transmission. Many STDs increase genital HIV-1 levels, which could in turn increase risk by increasing HIV-1 exposure.

Virus levels are highest during acute (primary) HIV-1 infection, before the virus is contained by the host, and this is thought to be the time when a person is most infectious [2]. Viral levels drop after primary infection resolves, and then slowly and steadily increase over time. Thus, the advanced stage of HIV-1 infection, when CD4 counts are low, is also a time when a person is potentially highly infectious [3].

There are several risk factors common to both vertical transmission and sexual transmission, including the levels of plasma virus in the index case [2, 4]. In the case of vertical transmission, it has been shown that the levels of maternal breast-milk virus and genital virus correlate with the risk of infant infection. Poor breast health in a breastfeeding mother, particularly mastitis, increases infant risk of infection.

Premature birth has been associated with increased infant HIV-1 infection, which could reflect an increased risk of premature birth for infants infected *in utero*, rather than prematurity leading to a greater chance of HIV-1 infection. A prolonged duration of ruptured membranes is associated with increased transmission, whereas cesarean-section birth is associated with decreased risk. Presumably, these associations reflect the fact that during transit through the birth canal, the infant may be exposed to HIV-1 in both blood and genital secretions.

FACTORS IN VIRAL SELECTION

HIV-1 is highly genetically variable and it continually evolves and adapts in the infected host [7]. HIV-1 seems to undergo a selective bottleneck during transmission because very few viruses are apparently transmitted from one host to another. It is possible that this bottleneck is at least partially a result of stochastic events that reflect the low frequency at which HIV-1 is transmitted. But it may also indicate that there is selection for particular variants with certain properties. The major lines of evidence to support selective transmission include the observations that (1) the early virus population is often genetically less diverse than the source-virus population; and (2) viruses present early in infection tend to infect cells using one particular co-receptor (CCR5).

Many studies of the past two decades have shown that the virus population early in infection, which is presumably very similar to the virus that was transmitted, is genetically more homogeneous than the virus population that is present during chronic infection [8]. The viral sequences present during the early stages of infection are often remarkably homogeneous, which suggest that a single virus was transmitted. This transmitted viral sequences, which can only be inferred from the sequence detected weeks later when HIV-1 reaches high enough levels to detect, has recently been dubbed a founder virus. However, studies in women first suggested that multiple viral sequences are sometimes transmitted, and this has now been observed in other populations and linked to the presence of biological cofactors such as other STDs [8]. Even in cases where the virus is genetically heterogeneous early in infection, it is generally less diverse than what would be expected during chronic infection, suggesting that only a subset of variants are successfully transmitted. More recent detailed studies of viruses in both the index case and their newly infected partner (transmission pairs) near the time of HIV-1 acquisition provide direct evidence for this transmission bottleneck [9]. However, in some situations it is possible that the limited diversity of transmitted strains indicates that the source partners harbored a virus population of limited diversity, perhaps because they transmitted during their primary infection, which is a time of high infectivity.

No matter what the complexity of the viral genotype, the viruses present within the first few months after infection almost invariably require the CCR5 co-receptor for entry (these are called R5 viruses) [10]; CCR5 is one of two major HIV-1 co-receptors (the other being CXCR4), and the co-receptor, along with the CD4 receptor, is critical for HIV-1 entry into cells. The observation that most recently transmitted viruses are R5 viruses suggests that CCR5 variants are favored for transmission. This apparent selection for R5 viruses occurs during all routes of transmission, including sexual, vertical, and parenteral routes. In support of this model, it has been shown that individuals who do not express cell surface CCR5 due to a specific genetic polymorphism are less susceptible to HIV infection (see also below).

Despite the fact that transmitted viruses share a common co-receptor requirement, the viruses transmitted from different individuals are quite genetically distinct. This diversity has made vaccine development a daunting prospect. Thus, there has been considerable interest in defining common features among transmitted viral strains. Signature sequence characteristics have been noted among viruses present early in infection, at least in some populations [8], and they may provide insights into which biological properties of viruses increase their fitness for transmission. Many studies have attempted to identify biological characteristics that confer the selective advantage for transmitted HIV-1 variants, but none have identified a clear biological phenotype common to all transmitted strains that may explain their selection.

ENDOGENOUS HOST FACTORS

Host genetics

Multiple host genetic polymorphisms have been linked to HIV-1 susceptibility [11–13]. The mutations that have been identified derive largely from targeted studies focused on genes that code for host factors known to be critical for HIV-1 replication. For example, many studies have focused on allelic variation within co-receptor genes, or genes coding for ligands that bind the HIV-1 co-receptors (e.g. CCL5/RANTES for CCR5 and CXCL12/SDF1 for CXCR4) and thus potentially compete for HIV-1 entry. Therefore, alterations in the expression or function of the proteins encoded by these genes could impact HIV-1 replication at the cellular level. Overall, studies of host genetic factors have provided a somewhat complex view of the effects of host genetics on HIV-1 transmission, as consistent results have not always been found across studies. This may partially be due to the complexity of the interactions between the different alleles, as well as differences in allele frequency and other factors in the populations examined. Moreover, with many of the mutations it is unclear whether they actually affect protein levels or function, or whether they were detected because they are genetically linked to other mutations in nearby genes, which play a more direct role in transmission.

Some studies have found clear and consistent evidence for a direct association between host genetics and HIV-1 susceptibility. This is the case with CCR5, where an inactivating genetic mutation (Δ32), which is present in a small fraction of Caucasians, has been associated with reduced susceptibility to HIV-1 infection in high-risk individuals with the homozygous Δ32 CCR5 allele. Lymphocytes and macrophages from these individuals are not permissive to replication of R5 viruses, providing biological support for the observed associations. However, this mutation is not found in Africans, and therefore is not a modulating risk factor for the African epidemic. Thus, although the Δ32 CCR5 mutation can have pronounced effects on HIV-1 susceptibility for an exposed individual, it has had limited global impact on HIV-1 spread.

A variety of other mutations in CCR5, found particularly in the promoter region, also appear to affect HIV-1 susceptibility. In addition, single nucleotide polymorphisms (SNPs) in several genes that encode chemokines or cytokines have been linked to HIV-1 susceptibility. In some cases, a particular haplotype, one that includes several SNPs, has been associated with susceptibility. The biological mechanism of action of most of these mutations, alone or in combination, remains to be elucidated.

Genetic variations in loci encoding molecules that play a role in acquired immunity have also been associated with HIV-1 transmission risk. Several studies suggest that human leukocyte antigen (HLA) allele concordance between the index case and the uninfected partner may increase the risk of transmission. HLA proteins are acquired on the virus as it buds from the host cell, and it has been postulated that discordance of HLA may mark the infectious virus as more immunologically foreign, and thus decrease transmission. Genes involved in innate immunity—the killer cell-immunoglobulin-like receptor (KIR) genes that bind to HLA proteins and modulate natural killer (NK) cell activity—have also been implicated in HIV-1 susceptibility. NK cells play a central role in the initial antiviral response. Both allelic differences and expression differences in KIR have been implicated in HIV susceptibility, although these findings are somewhat preliminary [11].

To date, host genes identified as risk factors for HIV-1 acquisition have primarily been uncovered because these genes/proteins were known to play a role in HIV-1 biology. It is possible that a more global genomic approach, which would sample a larger number of genes independently of whether they have an established link to HIV-1 replication or immunity, could yield a much longer list of polymorphisms involved in HIV-1 susceptibility. Indeed, there is considerable interest in these genome-wide approaches to studying HIV resistance in individuals who are HIV-1 negative despite being highly exposed to HIV-1 [12]. It is thought that examining a large group of highly exposed HIV-1 negative individuals may reveal other host genes important in HIV-1 susceptibility. However, identifying such cohorts is complicated because HIV-1 transmission is a somewhat rare event that can be influenced by many other factors, making it hard to truly define those who are more resistant to infection versus those who are simply beating the odds.

EXOGENOUS HOST FACTORS

STDs, female hormones, male circumcision

Sexually transmitted diseases are a major risk factor for HIV-1 infection, and both ulcerative and non-ulcerative STDs have been shown to increase susceptibility to HIV-1 [2,14]. These include a variety of specific sexually acquired infections, both viral (e.g. herpes simplex virus type 2, HSV-2) and bacterial (e.g. *Neisseria gonorrhoeae* and *Treponema pallidum*). It is likely that these STDs enhance susceptibility in part by increasing the number of activated T lymphocytes, which are targets for HIV-1 infection, at mucosal surfaces. In addition, some may disrupt mucosal integrity, providing access to T lymphocytes and other potential target cells in the submucosa.

The estimates of the effect of STDs on the risk of HIV-1 infection vary from study to study, but are likely to be in the range of two- to fivefold. Given the high prevalence of STDs in many parts of the world, the overall impact of STDs on HIV-1 spread is therefore potentially significant.

One of the STDs most commonly associated with increased HIV-1 infection is HSV-2, which can be treated with suppressive therapies such as daily acyclovir. However, studies evaluating the impact of treatment for HSV-2 on HIV-1 acquisition did not show any benefit [15]. This was true whether HSV-2 was treated in the HIV-1-infected partner (to attempt to reduce infectiousness) or in the HIV-1-exposed partner.

Three landmark studies have shown that male circumcision reduce the risk of HIV-1 acquisition in men by ~60% (e.g [16] http://www.who.int/hiv/topics/malecircumcision/en/index.html). The precise mechanism of protection is unknown but there are several plausible biological explanations including the fact that the foreskin may contain potential HIV-1 target cells and/or that tears in the foreskin could provide a portal of entry for HIV-1. There is also some evidence that circumcision may help reduce the risk of other STDs. Thus, the long-term benefit of circumcision for men may be even greater given the interplay of STDs and HIV-1 infection, and because the benefit of circumcision accrues over a lifetime.

Unfortunately, there is no evidence to suggest a protective effect of male circumcision on transmission from infected men to their female partners, but a long-term reduction of HIV prevalence in men may nonetheless benefit women by reducing their exposure. For women, several studies have shown that the use of hormonal contraceptives increases their risk of acquiring the virus. However, the association between use of hormonal contraceptives and HIV-1 susceptibility has not been observed in all studies, particularly those in which there is not frequent monitoring to permit good estimates of the time of infection. Thus, there is no clear consensus on the extent of risk to women that results from use of hormonal contraceptives [17].

EARLY TARGET CELLS AND INITIAL VIRUS–HOST DYNAMICS

At least two molecules are required for HIV-1 entry into cells: CD4, plus a multiple-membrane-spanning chemokine receptor, such as CCR5 or CXCR4 [7, 10]. Because CD4 is required for virus binding, the host range of HIV-1 is largely restricted to CD4 cells, which include a subset of T lymphocytes (T-helper cells), cells of the monocyte lineage, and dendritic cells. Each of these cells is therefore a potential target for initial HIV-1 infection, and there is some evidence to support a role for each in early infection. However, as much of this information derives from either animal or culture model systems, each of which has limitations, the initial target cell for HIV-1 infection in a new host is not known.

Studies using a SIV/macaque model of HIV-1 transmission showed that CD4 T lymphocytes are among the first target cells of SIV infection [18]. These findings imply that

CD4 T lymphocytes are important either in the initial infection event and/or in subsequent dissemination of the virus from the mucosal site of entry. There is local expansion of virus that preceded dissemination of SIV to the lymph nodes and periphery, at which point infection is irrevocably underway. Dendritic cells (DCs) are thought to play a role, possibly facilitating infection of the CD4 lymphocytes, and/or enhancing virus spread [19]. DCs express CD4 and, depending on their maturation state, may express HIV-1 co-receptor(s). Immature DCs express CCR5 and can be infected by HIV-1 *in vitro*, whereas mature DCs cannot. More importantly, both immature and mature DCs have been shown to capture HIV-1 and transfer it to CD4 T lymphocytes *in vitro*. Thus, one plausible model of HIV-1 transmission is that DCs positioned just below the mucosal epithelium capture HIV-1 and facilitate its transfer to lymphocytes, where the virus rapidly replicates and amplifies. Indeed, in the macaque model studies, virus dissemination to the draining lymph node has been shown to occur within 1 to 2 days after vaginal inoculation, and DCs have been implicated. During the initial stages of virus amplification, the gut-associated lymphoid tissue is a major site of virus replication, leading to considerable damage due to CD4 lymphocyte cell killing.

There is uncertainty over whether any of the models of HIV-1 transmission reflect reality, which stems from our inability to study the earliest events in HIV-1 infection. Generally, infection cannot be detected, at least using non-invasive methods, for several weeks after the initial transmission, at which time the virus has become well established throughout the host tissues. Thus, the earliest events that lead to successful HIV-1 transmission have simply not been studied. The studies conducted in the macaque model have employed a very high inoculum, and viruses that are unlikely to represent those typically transmitted between humans. Thus, it is hard to know how well these models mimic HIV-1 transmission. Remarkably, it is not even clear whether the virus that is transmitted is cell-free (extracellular, free virus) or cell-associated. Without good knowledge of the precise molecular interactions that govern initial infection, the design of interventions to target them is particularly challenging.

SUPERINFECTION

Re-infection by HIV-1 from another source partner

More and more data have been accumulating to suggest that transmission of HIV-1 occurs in the face of pre-existing HIV-1 infection [20]. The first definitive evidence for superinfection came from some intensively monitored subjects who were part of various trials or studies. In these cases, one virus was detected over several visits, and then a second virus, which differed more than would be expected by *de novo* variation, emerged in the virus population. One case presented particularly compelling evidence for superinfection: after the person had engaged in high-risk behavior on holiday, a second strain was detected that was characteristic of those circulating in the region where the subject had vacationed [21]. However, many of these cases were somewhat unusual because the subjects had had treatment interruptions, or showed evidence of a less virulent initial virus, in some cases because it had acquired drug-resistance mutations, presumably in a treated source partner prior to transmission.

Subsequent studies suggested that re-infections are almost as common as initial infections, and that they occur in the face of high levels of replication of the first virus [20]. This suggests that re-infection can occur even when the host already harbors a virus that is highly fit and well established. Of concern is the fact that re-infections appear to be occurring in some cases at a time when immune responses have had adequate time to develop to the first infection, but before immune function is completely compromised later in infection. Indeed, several studies have shown that individuals who became superinfected had immune responses to their first infection similar to responses of individuals who were not superinfected. Nonetheless, these responses did not protect them from a second HIV-1 infection [20]. These findings suggest that a vaccine will have to elicit anti-HIV-1 immune responses that are better than those that are generated to a naturally occurring HIV-1 infection.

PREVENTING HIV-1 TRANSMISSION

A highly effective vaccine would be the best method for significantly impacting HIV-1 spread and thus is the Holy Grail of HIV-1 prevention efforts. However, vaccine trials have met with only modest success [18] and an effective HIV-1 vaccine is not likely to become available any time in the near future. In the meantime, much of HIV-1 prevention has focused on educational efforts to reduce risk behaviors and consequent exposure. Increasing attention has been focused on the potential benefit of antivirals in preventing HIV-1 spread, including the use of these drugs in both the HIV-1-infected and HIV-1-uninfected partner. Providing antiretroviral drugs to HIV-1-exposed individuals

to prevent their infection is a concept similar to providing anti-malarial drugs to individuals in areas with high malaria burden. This prophylaxis approach was first successfully used in children exposed to maternal HIV-1. Several recent studies now support the use of this approach in adults exposed to HIV-1 through heterosexual contact [22, 23]. Importantly, antiviral prophylaxis was shown to provide protection whether it was taken orally as a daily medication or used topically as a vaginal microbicide. Protection was linked to adherence in using the medications and encouraging adherence will be critical in implementing these exciting new prevention approaches.

There is also considerable interest in the potential benefits of antiviral treatment of infected individuals in reducing virus spread. These treatments reduce source virus levels and treatment of infected mothers has been repeatedly shown to reduce transmission to their infants. Thus, treatment may not only benefit the infected individual but also can have an effect at the population level. It is currently unclear whether provision of drugs to HIV-1-infected or to HIV-1-uninfected, highly-exposed individuals would provide the most benefit in slowing the global spread of HIV-1, and this is a critical consideration given the limited resources available for antiviral treatment.

As a result of the findings of recent clinical trials, we now have several new effective approaches for preventing HIV transmission, including male circumcision and antiviral prophylaxis. Broad implementation of these prevention tools represents the next significant challenge, as these methods are seemingly more complex than other known effective methods, such as the use of condoms. Designing new, targeted approaches to prevent HIV transmission is also a challenge, given our rather limited understanding of the initial events in HIV-1 transmission. Critical aspects of transmission, such as the precise source of the virus and initial target cells for infection, are not known. Thus, a better understanding of the factors that drive transmission of HIV-1 may lead to novel approaches that can be added to the growing list of effective prevention tools.

ACKNOWLEDGMENTS

I thank Jared Baeten and Scott McClelland for their input.

REFERENCES

[1] Quinn TC, Overbaugh J. HIV/AIDS in women: an expanding epidemic. Science 2005;308:1582–3.

[2] Baeten JM, Overbaugh J. Measuring the infectiousness of persons with HIV-1: opportunities for preventing sexual HIV-1 transmission. Curr HIV Res 2003;1:69–86.

[3] Boily MC, Baggaley RF, Wang L, et al. Heterosexual risk of HIV-1 infection per sexual act: systematic review and meta-analysis of observational studies. Lancet Infect Dis 2009;9:118–29.

[4] John-Stewart G, Mbori-Ngacha D, ekpini R, et al. Breast-feeding and transmission of HIV-1. J Acquir Immune Defic Syndr 2004;35:196–202.

[5] Aldrovandi GM, Kuhn L. What infants and breasts can teach us about natural protection from HIV infection. J Infect Dis 2010;202 (Suppl. 3):S366–70.

[6] Baeten JM, Kahle E, Lingappa JR, et al. Genital HIV-1 RNA levels predict risk of heterosexual HIV-1 transmission. Sci Transl Med 2011;3(77):77ra29.

[7] Overbaugh J, Bangham CR. Selection forces and constraints on retroviral sequence variation. Science 2001;292:1106–9.

[8] Sagar M. HIV-1 transmission biology: selection and characteristics of infecting viruses. J Infect Dis 2010;202(Suppl. 2): S289–96.

[9] Derdeyn CA, Decker JM, Bibollet-Ruche F, et al. Envelope-constrained neutralization-sensitive HIV-1 after heterosexual transmission. Science 2004;303:2019–22.

[10] Margolis L, Shattock R. Selective transmission of CCR5-utilizing HIV-1: the 'gatekeeper' problem resolved? Nat Rev Microbiol 2006;4:312–17.

[11] Carrington M, Martin MP, van Bergen J. KIR-HLA intercourse in HIV disease. Trends Microbiol 2008;16:620–7.

[12] Lederman MM, Alter G, Daskalakis DC, et al. Determinants of protection among HIV-exposed seronegative persons: an overview. J Infect Dis 2010;202(Suppl. 3): S333–8.

[13] Kaslow RA, Dorak T, Tang JJ. Influence of host genetic variation on susceptibility to HIV type 1 infection. J Infect Dis 2005;191: S68–77.

[14] Fleming DT, Wasserheit JN. From epidemiological synergy to public health policy and practice: the contribution of other sexually transmitted diseases to sexual transmission of HIV infection. Sex Transm Infect 1999;75:3–17.

[15] Celum C, Wald A, Hughes J, et al. Effect of aciclovir on HIV-1 acquisition in herpes simplex virus 2 seropositive women and men who have sex with men: a randomised, double-blind, placebo-controlled trial. Lancet 2008;371:2109–19.

[16] Bailey RC, Moses S, Parker CB, et al. Male circumcision for HIV prevention in young men in Kisumu, Kenya: a randomised controlled trial. Lancet 2007;369:643–56.

[17] Blish CA, Baeten JM. Hormonal contraception and HIV-1 transmission. Am J Reprod Immunol 2011;65: 302–27.

[18] Haase AT. Early events in sexual transmission of HIV and SIV and opportunities for interventions. Annu Rev Med 2011;62:127–39.

[19] Pope M, Haase AT. Transmission, acute HIV-1 infection and the quest for strategies to prevent infection. Nat Med 2003;9: 847–52.

[20] Chohan BH, Piantadosi A, Overbaugh J. HIV-1 superinfection and its implications for vaccine design. Curr HIV Res 2010.

[21] Jost S, Bernard MC, Kaiser L, et al. A patient with HIV-1 superinfection. N Engl J Med 2002;347:731–6.

[22] Abdool Karim SS, Abdool Karim Q. Antiretroviral; prophylaxis: a defining moment is HIV control. Lancet 2011;15 July online.

Section | 2 |

Prevention, diagnosis, and treatment of HIV infection

Chapter | 8 |

The design of a global HIV vaccine[1]

Jerome H. Kim, Nelson L. Michael

Since our first knowledge of the HIV-1 epidemic in 1981 it is estimated that over 80 million persons have contracted the disease. In 2010 the United Nations Joint Programme on AIDS estimated a total of 33 million people living with HIV infection and 14,000 new infections per day—the majority of these infections occurring in resource-constrained settings where access to appropriate care and treatment is limited [1]. In sub-Saharan Africa HIV/AIDS is the leading cause of death and has reduced economic growth, caused social disruption, and loss of productivity.

It is possible, however, using available public health measures to significantly reduce the rates of infection. In a setting where the predominant route of infection was through commercial sex workers, Thailand dramatically slowed its HIV-1 epidemic by instituting a 100% condom campaign [2]. However, it has proven difficult to translate success in Thailand to other countries, as the characteristics of local epidemics, drug use, customs, sexual practices, funding, and perhaps viral subtypes have proved difficult to overcome.

For these reasons, since the discovery of the etiologic agent of HIV-1 in 1984, development of a vaccine has been a high priority. A number of approaches have been tested in efficacy trials [3–7], and one was recently found to have modest efficacy [7]. At the same time, efforts at prevention, care, and treatment have appeared to reduce the global burden of infection [1], and efficacy testing of both vaginal microbicides and pre-exposure chemoprophylaxis has recently been shown to prevent infection when used. However, as a public health tool, vaccines have the advantage of not requiring action on the part of the individual (except for vaccination itself). As a part of a comprehensive program of HIV prevention, an effective HIV-1 vaccine would still have a powerful impact on the epidemic, and modeling has suggested that a vaccine with efficacy as low as 30% ($\pm$ antiretroviral introduction) would be cost-effective and could reduce the epidemic r_0 to less than 1 [8].

HIV BIOLOGY

HIV-1 is a lentivirus, as are simian immunodeficiency virus (SIV), feline immunodeficiency virus, visna, equine infectious anemia virus, and bovine immunodeficiency virus. The HIV-1 capsid is surrounded by host cell membrane and 20–75 viral envelope spikes (gp120/gp41). The capsid holds two positive strand viral RNA genomes, tRNA, and reverse transcriptase. Viral entry occurs after a high-affinity interaction between CD4 and the gp120 envelope (Env) spike, causing a conformational change and exposure of a co-receptor binding site (CXCR4 or CCR5 most commonly) [9–11]. Interaction with the co-receptor initiates a further set of rapid conformational changes, resulting in apposition of the viral and host cell membranes and, ultimately, fusion. Membrane fusion is followed by entry of the capsid protein into the cytoplasm, release of the viral RNA and associated reverse transcriptase, reverse transcription, and integration of the viral DNA into the host cell DNA.

Once HIV-1 infects CD4 T cells, virions are formed at a rate of 10^8–10^9 per day. Infected CD4 T cells have a half-life of 1–2 days [12]. HIV-1 does not always result in lytic infection of the host cell. Latently infected, quiescent cells become a reservoir of infection; cell division is accompanied by bursts of viremia, some cell death, but also incidental replication of virus integrated in the host DNA by homeostatic proliferation [13, 14] (reviewed in Trono et al. [15]).

[1]The views expressed in this chapter are those of the authors and do not reflect the official views of the Departments of the Army or Defense.

Two features and related implications of HIV biology deserve to be highlighted with regard to vaccines. The first, which will be described more fully later, is ability of the virus to generate genotypic diversity through its rate of replication, intrinsic error-prone replication, and frequent recombination. Practically this means that the virus rapidly evades or "escapes" from incipient humoral and cellular immune responses [16–18]. More broadly, however, it suggests that it may be necessary to develop multiple "subtype"-specific vaccines or vaccine(s) capable of tackling the issue of subtypes and regional epidemic diversity. The second feature is the speed with which the post-infection events occur; after a "take" the virus spreads rapidly to regional then systemic lymphatic tissue, most prominently the gut-associated lymphoid tissue (GALT). Taken together with the profound and persistent depletion of the GALT and the early establishment of latently infected cells, the prevention of acquisition, if it is possible, may need to occur before productive infection is established—in the earliest phases of virus interaction with the host [17].

PATHOGENESIS OF ACUTE HIV-1 INFECTION

Acute HIV-1 infection, well described in rhesus macaques and less precisely known in humans, is the front line for HIV-1 vaccines. The mechanisms of viral "take" in the vaginal, urethral, glans, or rectal mucosa will need to be opposed by humoral or cellular effectors that can prevent the infection of CD4 targets, eliminate CD4 infected targets (without becoming infected), or prevent the infection of secondary CD4 targets. The relative contribution of these early infection scenarios and mechanisms *in vivo* is not known, so the study of acute HIV-1 infection and in particular the impact of vaccine-induced immune responses on these pathogenetic events is critical to successful vaccine development.

In the earliest stages of HIV infection, days–weeks after initial exposure in man, HIV-1 initiates massive infection and depletion of the GALT; home to roughly 70% of CD4 T cells [19–21]. In SIV vaccine challenge models, preservation of gut T central memory CD4 cells is correlated with improved survival. Integrin $\alpha_4\beta_7$, which appears to bind to the V2 loop of HIV-1 Env and to up-regulate virus production, also directs homing of CD4 T cells to gut and genital mucosa through its ligand MADCAM-1, which is expressed on mucosal epithelial cells [22, 23]. Interestingly, the infusion of a rhesus-mouse hybrid monoclonal antibody (MAb) prior to high-dose intravenous (IV) challenge results in significant reduction in plasma viremia and latent virus pools [24]. Whether human vaccines can induce responses that interfere with $\alpha_4\beta_7$ and whether this will affect acquisition of infection remain unknown.

FEATURES OF TRANSMITTED VIRUSES

Within a chronically infected individual HIV-1 exists as a quasispecies, or swarm, with hundreds or thousands of different variants. Diversity is generated through two mechanisms. First, the HIV RT is error prone (3×10^{-5} bases) and lacks a proof-reading function. Second, the virus is capable of recombination (7–30 crossovers per genome) during reverse transcription. Practically this means that, given the rate of HIV replication in chronic infection, thousands of mutant progeny might be generated every day (reviewed in Taylor and Hammer [25]).

However, studies suggest that transmitted viruses have unique features and are not necessarily representative of the quasispecies in the transmitting individual. That the most commonly recognized sequences in the quasispecies are not necessarily the transmitted/founder (T/F) isolate argues that there is "selection" for certain characteristics. It was early found that the vast majority of transmitted isolates utilized the CCR5 co-receptor. Transmitted Envs tend to be shorter and less glycosylated than "chronic" Env [26–29], but this finding has not been universal [30]. Several groups have reported that T/F viruses have shorter V1V2 loops, and it was recently found that the T/F Envs have a greater affinity for $\alpha_4\beta_7$ [31]. T/F strains may be able to use cells with lower CCR5 or CD4 density [31, 32], and are more susceptible to CCR5 inhibitors.

In addition several studies have shown that the typical infectious event in genital mucosal transmission involves a single T/F virus 80–90% of the time, while intrarectal mucosal transmission may involve single T/F 60–80% of the time [31, 33–35]. In transmission cases the founding viruses often resemble ancestral sequences more than the other members of the donor quasispecies [36], suggesting again that there are unique features of transmitting viruses that, in the relatively uncommon event of mucosal transmission, are associated with productive infection. These features of T/F envelopes suggest that there may be a brief window of opportunity, influenced by stochastic events not yet defined, where the individual infecting virus may be uniquely susceptible to innate or adaptive immune effector mechanisms that may limit subsequent events in pathogenesis that lead to local, then systemic, infection [37].

CHALLENGES TO HIV VACCINE DEVELOPMENT

What makes an HIV vaccine different?

Historically, vaccines have been developed for infections where the natural immune response controls the initial infection and prevents further infection of the host. This does not hold for HIV-1. The host immune response does not eliminate infection or control progressive disease, and in fact, participates in its persistence. The host immune response does not prevent superinfection (this is how recombinants develop). Practically this means that there is no proof of concept from natural infection that informs vaccine development; there is no protective (against acquisition) natural immune response that a vaccine should mimic. An empiric approach to vaccine testing, informed by clues from basic and translational research, would be a traditional response. A positive signal (i.e. protection) would then provide: (1) additional direction or clues; (2) potential or actual correlates of risk/protection [38, 39]; (3) a representative animal model; and (4) a basis upon which to build further informed (but still empirical) testing.

Thirty years into the epidemic, the challenges to the identification and development of HIV vaccine immunogens remain profound. Three issues deserve particular attention: (1) subtype diversity; (2) animal models; and (3) defining protective immune responses.

Subtype diversity

HIV-1 diversity is one of the greatest challenges to the development of an effective vaccine and is manifest virologically by the intrinsic error rate of reverse transcriptase and frequent intragenic recombination and at a population level by the diversity of subtypes, recombinant forms, and rapid and continuous evolution within infected hosts. From the time of the initial zoonotic transmission events of HIV (early twentieth century), three main groups are recognized: M (major), O (outlier), and N (non-major, non-outlier). A fourth group, designated P, related to a gorilla SIV, has also been described. There are regionally prominent subtypes that are geographically based and differ from each other by roughly 25–35% (intraperson variation typically is <10% and intrasubtype diversity is 15–20%)—the nine current subtypes and 50+ circulating recombinant forms (CRFs) underscore the complexity of the global epidemic [25]. In general, subtype B predominates in North America and Europe, subtype C in southern Africa and India, subtype A in East Africa, CRF01_AE in Southeast Asia, and CRF02_AG in West Africa. There are other regions with a mixture of subtypes, and some areas, such as East Africa, where ~50% of strains are unique recombinant forms (URFs), found (thus far) in only a single infected individual. Also subtype diversity is increasingly recognized in Europe and the USA; an HIV vaccine that targets only a single subtype may have limited utility in many parts of the world.

Animal models

Non-human primates (NHP) models of infection and challenge have been evolving rapidly in recent years (reviewed in Genesca et al. [40]). In the absence of a validated animal model (i.e. mirroring what is seen in terms of human

protection) it may be important to look at the parallels between the human and NHP infection models. We consider NHP first because many of the other issues are impacted by data from NHP studies, and appreciation of the strengths and weaknesses of the model are critical to this discussion. There are two types of virus: SIV and chimeric SIV-HIV (SHIV). Within SIV there are two different sources of challenge and inserts, SIVmac251 (SIVmac239 is a clone) and SIVsmE660. There are three principal challenge models: intravenous, intrarectal, and intravaginal. All are powered to achieve infection relatively quickly, and not with the frequency of infection/challenge seen with human intrarectal and intravaginal infection.

Vaccination with recombinant Ad5 (Merck) HIV vaccine followed by simian-human immunodeficiency viruses (SHIV) intravenous challenge was associated with reduction in post-infection viral load [41], but did not predict the outcome of the Step trial where the challenge was intrarectal. The SHIV used in those studies, SHIV89.6P, targeted CXCR4$^+$ cells and was therefore not a good mimic of acute HIV infection *in vivo*. When the challenge was SIVmac251, no benefit was seen [42]. Whether IV challenge with an X4/R5 tropic virus was an appropriate model for screening of candidate vaccines underscores the difficulties faced by NHP studies in the absence of human correlates. Alternatively, SHIV162P3 has been used to demonstrate the efficacy of various subunit HIV Env vaccines [43, 44] and to establish potential correlates of protection. These studies await confirmation in human efficacy testing, which will inform vaccine development and confirm the animal model/virus challenge.

In humans, the viral quasispecies in an infected person is broad (10–15%) and the T/F virus is usually (except in acute infection) a minority member of that quasispecies. In NHP studies, the challenge stocks are more narrow in distribution and are based largely upon SIVmac251 or SIVsmE660 (an alternative SIVdelta670 is not widely used). While it is possible to establish challenge conditions where the number of T/F viruses [45, 46] approximates the human condition, the chances of acquiring infection after a single intrarectal or intravaginal challenge still exceed the probability seen in humans [45, 46]. Since it has long been established in vaccinology that large challenge inocula can overcome vaccines of known efficacy, the impact of the high per challenge infection rate is unknown.

The use of low-dose mucosal SIV challenge has, however, demonstrated acquisition effects similar to that of the Thai HIV vaccine trial [47, 48], and refinements to the NHP model including penile challenge are being developed. One of the vaccines showing a protective effect in NHP is the Vaccine Research Center (VRC) DNA/recombinant adenovirus type 5; it is in phase IIb clinical testing now (HVTN505) and the outcome will inform and refine the NHP model [48]. SHIVs are the only way to test HIV Env vaccines and may be the principal test for new constructs utilizing "mosaic" antigens [49, 50]. The use of new SHIV constructs (SHIV SF162P3/4) and pathogenic SHIVs [51] will provide new insights and may extend the utility of the NHP model in conjunction with advances in human HIV vaccine design.

Defining protective immune responses

Which immune response(s) protects against HIV infection? Unfortunately the answer is unknown. Perhaps the recently completed RV144 trial will provide a correlate of risk that can be incorporated into the testing of future candidates. In the absence of correlate, empirically derived target immunogenicity that can be tested in efficacy trials in humans provides the most systematic (if expensive) approach. It is known from NHP studies that HIVIG and broadly neutralizing antibody (BNAb) can protect animals from intravaginal SHIV challenge. Interestingly, an ADCC null mutation of the Fc chain of the b12 BNAb reduces its ability to protect against infection, suggesting that neutralization works in concert with other humoral effector mechanisms *in vivo* to achieve an optimal effect [52, 53]. HIV-1-infected persons have recently been the source of a number of BNAbs [54–56] that neutralize 70–90% of all tested viral isolates. These BNAbs have high rates of VH gene mutation (12–30%) and abnormally long HCDR3 regions, so whether BNAbs can be elicited by vaccination is unknown. Also, BNAbs were isolated from persons with chronic progressive infection, implying that these antibodies were a response to chronic infection but did not control it [54–56].

Whether T cell responses, in the absence of antibody can protect against infection is not known [57]. Depletion of B cells did not affect NHP control of an intravenous SIV challenge, though depletion of CD8 T cells did [58, 59]. It is an assumption that the induction of non-neutralizing (and certainly non-broadly neutralizing) antibody may provide *de facto* evidence that T cell responses are sufficient to protect against infection. The premise of vaccines inducing primarily cellular immune responses (CMI vaccines) was that, while sterilizing immunity might be achieved by BNAb, CMI vaccines might reduce post-infection viral load [60–63] after high-dose intravenous (or mucosa) challenge. More recent studies have suggested that some "CMI" vaccines, such as DNA/Ad5, are capable of inducing antibody at the same level as seen in the Thai HIV vaccine trial and might still protect against infection by SIVsmE660 in low-dose mucosal challenge [48, 64].

Two other sources of information on what might constitute protective immune responses are found in special cases: those persons who, despite repetitive exposure remain uninfected (highly exposed persistently seronegative, HEPS) and those HIV-infected persons whose immune systems appear to nearly completely control viral replication (long-term nonprogressors, elite controllers, EC). It appears the HEPS groups manifest some level of HIV-specific cellular response [65–67]. Both cellular (proliferation) and IgA-mediated HIV neutralization were implicated as protecting HEPS against HIV infection in Kenyan CSW [68]. Among EC strong, polyfunctional, and broad HIV-specific cellular immune responses are associated with persistent, highly suppressive control of HIV infection [69, 70]. Similarly, strong cellular immune responses against SIV associated with post-infection viral load control are reported with both attenuated SIV vectors and replicating CMV-SIV vaccines [60, 61, 71].

Correlates from monkey studies

One of the advantages of a NHP model that is validated against the human model is that it may be possible to use a laboratory measure of immunogenicity/protection in monkeys that will reliably predict protection in humans. In the absence of a validated model, it is still possible to glean from NHP studies at least supportive evidence for advancing products to human efficacy trials.

How much antibody is enough? While protection from intravenous or high-dose intravaginal SHIV challenge required relatively high levels of NAb, polyclonal HIV$^+$ sera, or 1b12 [72, 73], lower doses appear to be necessary for prevention of acquisition using a low-dose intravaginal challenge [72, 74], but even these levels may exceed that seen in human HIV vaccine efficacy trials.

Using a NAb-sensitive SHIV (SF162P4) it was possible to prevent infection via intravaginal challenge using a homologous protein administered intramuscularly (IM) or IM and intranasally [44]. Protection appeared to correlate with NAb levels against SHIVSF162P4. Priming with alphavirus (Venezuelan equine encephalitis) viral vector encoding SF162P4 Env and boosting with a gp140ΔV2 homologous Env (MF59 adjuvant) protected NHP against an intrarectal SHIVSF162P4 challenge. Analogously, protection correlated with NAb to the challenge strain, but was also correlated with total Env binding antibody and pre-challenge avidity [43]. An HIV-ADA-based, DNA prime and MVA boost also protected NHP against intrarectal challenge with SHIVSF162P3 (not neutralization sensitive), and acquisition was inversely correlated with avidity to natural (but not monomeric or trimeric) ADA [75]. Letvin et al. have also reported that, after DNA (SIVmac251) prime and recombinant Ad5 boosting (SIVmac251), protection against intrarectal E660 challenge was correlated with low levels of NAb to E660 in a human PBMC assay and to a lesser degree in pseudovirus TZM-bl neutralization assays [48]. CD4 Env-specific responses were also correlated with protection against acquisition [48]. Whether the same correlations will hold in human studies is unknown. A DNA prime/rAd5 (subtype A, B, C) phase IIb study is currently under way, and has recently been changed to evaluate HIV-1 acquisition (HVTN505).

A replicating CMV-SIV vaccine has been shown to substantially reduce post-infection viral load in an SIVmac239 intrarectal challenge, occasionally to undetectable levels, with CD8 T effector memory (Tem) cells being the immune response correlated with viral load, and more recent data suggest that this vaccine may protect against acquisition as well in a low-dose intrarectal challenge [60].

HUMAN HIV VACCINE TRIALS

HIV/AIDS was first recognized syndromically in 1981. The virus was identified in 1984, and the first efficacy tests of HIV vaccines began in 1998. From a theoretical perspective, many have ruled out the use of whole inactivated and live attenuated vaccines, though preclinical work continues. Historically, the initial focus was upon Env subunit vaccines, such as the AIDSVAX B/B' protein tested in Vax004 that induced binding and type-specific antibody. This was followed by live recombinant prime–protein boost vaccines that appeared to increase cellular responses and to provide similar levels of antibody; an example is the ALVAC-HIV (canarypox) vCP1521 plus AIDSVAX B/E tested in Thailand (RV144). Interest then focused upon recombinant, replication deficient adenovirus type 5 vaccines, alone and with a DNA prime (the Merck rAd5 and the VRC DNA/rAd5 vaccines), which appeared to induce greater IFN-γ ELISpot positivity than canarypox vectors.

In this section we will first review the vaccines that have undergone efficacy testing and then proceed to a discussion of vaccines under development by class. We will conclude with a brief look at the future landscape of HIV vaccine development holds.

Human efficacy trials

Production of subunit Env proteins was centered initially on laboratory-grown viruses that are CXCR4-tropic. Both gp160 and gp120 proteins were prepared [76–86], and eventually two bivalent vaccines from VaxGen were tested in phase III trials. AIDSVAX B/B' contained gp120 from the laboratory-adapted strain MN and the primary isolate GNE8. Vax004 tested AIDSVAX B/B in 5,403 men who have sex with men (MSM) and high-risk women in the USA, Canada, and Europe. Infection rates among the 3,598 vaccine and 1,805 placebo recipients were similar at 6.7 and 7.0%, respectively [4]. Vax003 utilized the AIDSVAX B/E vaccine, consisting of the gp120 Env from the laboratory-adapted HIVMN and the primary isolate CM244 (designated A244). A total of 2,546 Thai injection drug users (IDUs) were enrolled into Vax003. Vaccine efficacy was estimated at 0.1% (95% CI, −30.8% to 23.8%) [6]. Further non-prespecified analyses of Vax004 antibody-directed cell-mediated viral inhibition (ADCVI) showed an inverse correlation between ADCVI levels and HIV acquisition. This effect was influenced by Fcγ IIa and IIIa polymorphisms [87]. More recently, Gilbert et al. reported low levels of neutralizing antibody against Tier 2 isolates in Vax 004 [88].

The Step (HVTN 502) and Phambili (HVTN 503) vaccine trials were the first human efficacy trials to explore whether the Merck recombinant adenovirus type 5 HIV vaccine, which induced strong IFN-γ ELISpot CMI responses, could prevent infection or reduce post-infection viremia. The Merck vaccine was composed of replication-incompetent Ad5 (MRKrAd5 HIV-1) expressing HIV-1 clade B *gag, pol,* and *nef.* The Step study enrolled predominantly high-risk populations including MSM and high-risk heterosexual women in North and South America and Australia, and heterosexual women and men in the Caribbean [3, 89]. The Phambili study enrolled heterosexual men and women in South Africa [5]. HVTN 502 was unexpectedly terminated for futility involving the study primary endpoints, virtually all of which were in MSM. Moreover, in subjects with pre-existing Ad5-specific neutralizing antibody titers, a greater number of HIV-1 infections occurred in vaccine than in placebo recipients. The biological basis for this observation remains unclear. Post-hoc multivariate analysis further suggested that the greatest increased risk was in men who had pre-existing Ad5-specific neutralizing antibodies and who were uncircumcised [90].

Though the Step and Phambili trials were stopped for futility, the trials suggested that the intravenous SHIV NHP challenge model (with the SHIVs tested) could be misleading and inadequate for evaluating T cell vaccines. While the MRKrAd5 vaccine generated more consistent Gag ELISpot than canarypox-based regimens, this did not appear to be sufficient to protect against infection. The SIVmac251 model did predict that the MRKrAd5 vaccine would not control viral load; it, however, did not predict the observed effect on acquisition [42]. An important lesson of the MRKrAd5 vaccine trials is that immunity to vectors should be evaluated in future clinical studies [91].

The Thai phase III HIV vaccine trial (RV144) of ALVAC-HIV and AIDSVAX gp120 B/E prime–boost showed modest protection (modified intent to treat, mITT) against acquisition of HIV infection in a community (low) risk population in Thailand with a 42-month vaccine efficacy of 31.2% [7]. AIDSVAX gp120 B/E had shown no efficacy in a previous phase III trial in Thai IDUs [6]. There was no effect on early post-infection HIV-1 RNA viral load or CD4 count. A combined analysis of previous phase I and II ALVAC-HIV and gp120 prime–boost studies showed a VE of 50% at roughly 12–24 months post vaccination, a difference that was not statistically significant. Similar to RV144 the results also showed no effect on viral load [92].

While a VE of 31% at 42 months is not sufficient for licensure, it does provide an important proof-of-principle—a safe and effective HIV vaccine is possible. Two findings that did not achieve statistical significance in the prespecified analysis are worthy of emphasis. The first observation was that those with the lowest baseline risk (incidence 0.23/100 person-years) had a VE of 40%, while those with the highest baseline risk (incidence 0.36/100 person-years) had a VE of 3.7%. The second important observation was that VE appeared to decrease with time; at month 12 of the study it was 60% and fell to 44% by month 18. If early VE of 60% could be extended with boosting, it would have important implications for vaccine development.

The NIAID Vaccine Research Center has developed a DNA–rAd5 prime–boost regimen that is currently in phase IIb efficacy testing (HVTN 505) among circumcised MSM who are Ad5 seronegative [93–95]. These subtype A/B/C vaccines were tested in three phase IIa trials, IAVI V001, HVTN 204, and RV172, and found to be safe and immunogenic [96, 97]. Pre-existing Ad5-NABs did not appear to affect the frequency or magnitude of T cell responses with this prime–boost vaccine.

HIV vaccine concepts

A partial list of current HIV vaccine trials is provided in Table 8.1. Part of the difficulty in describing the landscape of HIV vaccines has been the use of two or more different vaccines within a vaccination protocol. The *prime–boost concept* utilizes a DNA or viral vector prime with a boost of peptides/protein or different viral vector. Such an approach often avoids the problems inherent to the repetitive use of viral vectors—vector-specific immune responses that may limit the immunogenicity of the vaccine insert. In this section we will describe vaccines of interest, individually and in prime–boost combinations. Importantly, the prime–boost concept only has utility where the efficacy gained by two different vaccines is sufficiently large to justify the complications imposed by the use of two products.

Subunit vaccines

Since the failure of the AIDSVAX B/B' and B/E vaccines to prevent HIV infection in MSM and IDUs, respectively [4, 6], much work has been done to try to improve Env subunit design to induce broadly neutralizing antibodies. These approaches fall into three categories: (1) creating "native" Env trimers, simulating the mature Env trimer on virus particles [98–100]; (2) improving Env conformation by deletion of loops (V2) [101, 102], alteration of glycosylation, or epitope masking [101, 103, 104]; (3) presenting of epitopes exposed by ligand CD4 binding [105]. These approaches are confounded by the poor immunogenicity of conserved epitopes that are shielded by glycosylation [18, 106], appear only briefly [107], or are sterically or entropically impaired [108, 109]. In general these modifications have, as pure subunit vaccines and also in prime–boost configuration with viral vector or DNA prime, yielded some NAb against homologous viruses or easy-to-neutralize Tier 1 HIV but have not generated broadly neutralizing Ab (summarized in Mascola and Montefiori [110]).

DNA and viral vectors

Live recombinant vaccines are viral vector-based products including the canarypox (ALVAC), modified vaccinia Ankara (MVA), and adenovirus vaccines. These can be used individually or combined with other vaccines in prime–boost mode, to elicit cellular and humoral responses.

The pox viruses (canarypox, fowlpox, vaccinia, and MVA) have been studied alone and paired with a variety of different Env subunits (gp120, gp140, gp160). In addition to a vaccinia-vectored HIV vaccine, several groups have studied attenuated versions of vaccinia in the form of modified vaccinia Ankara (MVA) and NYVAC. An MVA containing subtype A inserts was found in phase II trials in Africa to be non-immunogenic, but subsequent trials using MVAs containing B, C, and CRF01 inserts showed elicited responses dominated by CD4 T cell responses [111–118]. Although strong anti-vector responses have been found, it is still possible to boost responses with additional doses of MVA [117].

DNA priming followed by Env boosting has generated some NAb but no BNAb [119]. Similarly, DNA has been used to prime MVA and adenovirus vaccines. HIV-1 neutralizing antibody was augmented by priming with gp160 recombinant vaccinia and boosting with rgp160 in vaccinia-naive adults. DNA/MVA gave strong IFN-γ ELISpot in a study conducted by the Karolinska Institute [120]. Similarly, DNA prime with a NYVAC boost induced polyfunctional and long-lasting T cell responses [121–123]. DNA/rAd5-induced binding antibody and HIV-specific T cell responses were detected in 63% of vaccinees. ELISpot responses for DNA prime with low-dose (63%) or high-dose (60%) rAd5 were similar—positive responses were predominantly to Env peptides, followed by Pol or Gag, regardless of the immunization regimen. The high-dose rAd5 boost had the highest frequency of responders to all three antigens tested (Env, Gag, or Pol), while responses were approximately equal for the other immunization groups for two antigens (20–26%) [97]. These studies are the basis for the ongoing HVTN 505 trial [93, 96, 97, 124].

The future

For the canarypox plus gp120 prime–boost combination, a series of phase IIb trials is anticipated in Thailand and South Africa to attempt to extend the durability and magnitude of the protective responses to levels consistent with public health value. Studies to determine whether an immunologic correlate of risk (or protection) exists in RV144 have been conducted; if that correlate of risk can be validated in humans and NHPs, it may accelerate the development of future HIV vaccine candidates. In addition, as a proof of concept, rapid adaptive design trials focused around the pox–protein prime–boost concept could be executed in order to more efficiently obtain information about potential correlates [125].

Table 8.1 List of phase II–III HIV vaccine trials

	START DATE	VACCINE STRATEGY	CANDIDATE VACCINES	VOLUNTEERS (N)	TRIAL SITES	CLADE	STATUS	REFERENCE OR CLINICALTRIALS.GOV IDENTIFIER
Phase III								
RV 144	October 2003	Canarypox vector prime and protein boost	ALVAC-HIV vCP1521, AIDSVAXgp 120 B/E	16,403	Thailand	B/E	Ongoing	Rerks-Ngarm S, Pitisuttithum P, Nitayaphan S, et al, Vaccination with ALVAC and AIDSVAX to prevent HIV-1 infection in Thailand, N Engl J Med 2009; 361:2209–2220.
VAX 003	March 1999	Protein	AIDSVAX B/E	2,500	Thailand	B/E	Completed	Pitisuttithum P, Gilbert P, Gurwith M, et al, Randomized, double-blind, placebo-controlled efficacy trial of a bivalent recombinant glycoprotein 120 HIV-1 vaccine among injection drug users in Bangkok, Thailand, J Infect Dis 2006; 194:1661–1671.
VAX 004	June 1998	Protein	AIDVAX B/B	5,400	USA, Canada, Puerto Rico, Netherlands	B	Completed	Flynn NM, Forthal DN, Harro CD, et al, Placebo-controlled phase 3 trial of a recombinant glycoprotein 120 vaccine to prevent HIV-1 infection, J Infect Dis 2005; 191:654–665.
Phase IIb								
Step Study: HVTN 502, Merck 023	July 2005	Adenovirus vector	MRKrAd5 HIV-1 Gaf/ Pol/Nef	3,000	USA, Canada, Peru, Dominican Republic, Haiti, Puerto Rico, Australia	B	Suspended	Buchbinder SP, Mehrotra DV, Duerr A, et al, Efficacy assessment of a cell-mediated immunity HIV-1 vaccine (the Step Study): a double-blind, randomised, placebo-controlled, test-of-concept trial, Lancet 2008; 372:1881–1893.

Continued

Table 8.1 List of phase II–III HIV vaccine trials—cont'd

	START DATE	VACCINE STRATEGY	CANDIDATE VACCINES	VOLUNTEERS (M)	TRIAL SITES	CLADE	STATUS	REFERENCE OR CLINICALTRIALS.GOV IDENTIFIER
Phase IIb—cont'd								
Phambili Study: HVTN 502	February 2007	Adenovirus vector	MRKrAd5 HIV-1 Gag/Pol/Nef	3,000	South Africa	B	Suspended	NCT00413725
PAVE 100	June 2007	Plasmid DNA prime and adenovirus vector boost	VRC-HIVDNA0 16-00-VP, VRC-HIVADV0 14-00-VP	—	USA	—	Withdrawn before enrollment	NCT00498056
Phase IIa								
HVTN 205	January 2009	Plasmid DNA prime and vaccinia virus vector boost	pGA2/JS7 DNA, MVA/HIV62	225	USA, Peru, South Africa	B	Ongoing	NCT00820846
IAVI 010	April 2003	Vaccinia virus vector with/without DNA plasmid primer	DNA, HIVA, MVA, HIVA	111	Kenya, UK	A	Completed	Peters BS, Jaoko W, Vardas E, et al, Studies of a prophylactic HIV-1 vaccine candidate based on modified vaccinia virus Ankara (MVA) with and without DNA priming: effects of dosage and route on safety and immunogenicity, Vaccine 2007; 25:2120–2127.
Phase II								
ANRSVAC 18	September 2004	Protein (lipopeptides)	LIPO-5	156	France	B	Completed	NCT00121758
TaMoVac 01	June 2010	Plasmid DNA prime and vaccinia virus vector boost	HIVIS, DNA, MVA-CMDR	120	Tanzania	Multiple	Due to start June 2010	Barkari M, personal communication 2010.

Trial	Date	Strategy	Vaccine	N	Country	Clade	Status	Reference
AVEG201	December 1992	Comparison of two recombinant proteins	rgp120, HIV-1 SF-2, MN rgp120	296	USA	B	Completed	McElrath MJ, Corey L, Montefiori D, et al, A phase II study of two HIV type 1 envelope vaccines, comparing their immunogenicity in populations at risk for acquiring HIV type 1 infection, AIDS Res Hum Retroviruses 2000; 16:907–919.
AVEG202, HIVNET 014	May 1997	Canarypox vector prime with/without recombinant gp120 protein boost	ALVAC-HIV MN120TMG strain (vCP205), rgp120, HIV 1SF-2	420	USA	B	Completed	Belshe RB, Stevens C, Gorse GJ, et al, Safety and immunogenicity of a canarypox-vectored human immunodeficiency virus type 1 vaccine with or without gp120: a phase 2 study in higher- and lower-risk volunteers, J Infect Dis 2001; 183:1343–1352.
HIVNET 026	June 2000	Canarypox vector prime with/without recombinant gp120 protein boost	ALVAC vCP1452, MN rgp120	200	Brazil, Haiti, Peru, Trinidad and Tobago	B	Completed	Cleghorn F, Pape JW, Schechter M, et al, Lessons from a multisite international trial in the Caribbean and South America of an HIV-1 canarypox vaccine (ALVAC-HIV vCP1452) with or without boosting with MN rgp120, J Acquir Immune Defic Syndr 2007; 46:222–230.
HVTN 203	December 2000	Canarypox vector prime with/without recombinant gp120 protein boost	ALVAC vCP1452, AIDSVAX B/B	330	USA	B	Completed	Russell ND, Graham BS, Keefer MC, et al, Phase 2 study of an HIV-1 canarypox vaccine (vCP1452) alone and in combination with rgp120: negative results fail to trigger a phase 3 correlates trial, J Acquir Immune Defic Syndr 2007; 44:203–212.

Continued

Table 8.1 List of phase II–III HIV vaccine trials—cont'd

Phase II—cont'd

	START DATE	VACCINE STRATEGY	CANDIDATE VACCINES	VOLUNTEERS (M)	TRIAL SITES	CLADE	STATUS	REFERENCE OR CLINICALTRIALS.GOV IDENTIFIER
HVTN 204	September 2005	Plasmid DNA prime and adenovirus vector boost	VRC-HIVDNA0 16-00-VP, VRC-HIVADV0 14-00-VP	480	USA	B	Completed	NCT00125970
HVTN 505	July 2009	Plasmid DNA prime and adenovirus vector boost	VRC-HIVDNA0 16-00-VP, VRC-HIVADV0 14-00-VP	Estimated 1350	USA	Multiple	Ongoing	NCT00865566
IAVI A002	November 2005	Plasmid DNA prime and adenovirus vector boost	tgAAC09	84	Zambia, Uganda, South Africa	C	Completed	NCT000888446
IAVI V002	2007	Plasmid DNA prime and adenovirus vector boost	VRC-HIVDNA0 16-00-VP, VRC-HIVADV0 14-00-VP	300	Kenya, Uganda, Zambia, Rwanda	Multiple	Withdrawn before enrollment	NCT00415649

Reprinted from The Lancet Infectious Diseases 10, Ross et al, Progress towards development of an HIV vaccine: report of the AIDS Vaccine 2009 Conference; 305–316. Copyright 2010. With permission from Elsevier.

A number of other vaccine concepts have not yet been tested in humans. These include virus-like particles (VLP), live attenuated HIV, or replication competent viral vectors (as opposed to attenuated vectors such as MVA or NYVAC). The early adeno-associated virus [126, 127] vectors were not sufficiently immunogenic. Data should be available soon on alphavirus-based vaccines (Sindbis and Venezuelan equine encephalitis). Other concepts such as rare serotype adenoviruses, and vaccines containing mosaic inserts are planned for human clinical trials in the near future [49, 50, 128, 129].

REFERENCES

[1] UNAIDS. UNAIDS Report on the Global AIDS Epidemic 2010; Geneva: Joint United Nations Programme on HIV/AIDS; 2010. Available from: http://www.unaids.org/globalreport/ [accessed 11.02.11].

[2] Nelson KE, Celentano DD, Eiumtrakol S, et al. Changes in sexual behavior and a decline in HIV infection among young men in Thailand. N Engl J Med 1996;335 (5): 297–303.

[3] Buchbinder SP, Mehrotra DV, Duerr A, et al. Efficacy assessment of a cell-mediated immunity HIV-1 vaccine (the Step Study): a double-blind, randomised, placebo-controlled, test-of-concept trial. Lancet 2008;372(9653): 1881–93.

[4] Flynn NM, Forthal DN, Harro CD, et al. Placebo-controlled phase 3 trial of a recombinant glycoprotein 120 vaccine to prevent HIV-1 infection. J Infect Dis 2005;191(5): 654–65.

[5] Gray G, Buchbinder S, Duerr A. Overview of STEP and Phambili trial results: two phase IIb test-of-concept studies investigating the efficacy of MRK adenovirus type 5 gag/pol/nef subtype B HIV vaccine. Curr Opin HIV AIDS 2010;5:357–61.

[6] Pitisuttithum P, Gilbert P, Gurwith M, et al. Randomized, double-blind, placebo-controlled efficacy trial of a bivalent recombinant glycoprotein 120 HIV-1 vaccine among injection drug users in Bangkok, Thailand. J Infect Dis 2006;194: 1661–71.

[7] Rerks-Ngarm S, Pitisuttithum P, Nitayaphan S, et al. Vaccination with ALVAC and AIDSVAX to prevent HIV-1 infection in Thailand. N Engl J Med 2009;361 (23):2209–20.

[8] Stover J, Bollinger L, Hecht R, et al. Impact of an AIDS vaccine in developing countries: a new model and initial results. Health Aff 2007;26(4):1147–58.

[9] Cocchi F, DeVico AL, Garzino-Demo A, et al. Identification of RANTES, MIP-1 alpha, and MIP-1 beta as the major HIV-suppressive factors produced by CD8[+] T cells. Science 1995;270(5243): 1811–15.

[10] Feng Y, Broder CC, Kennedy PE, Berger EA. HIV-1 entry cofactor: functional cDNA cloning of a seven-transmembrane, G protein-coupled receptor. Science 1996;272(5263):872–7.

[11] Deng H, Liu R, Ellmeier W, et al. Identification of a major co-receptor for primary isolates of HIV-1. Nature 1996;381 (6584):661–6.

[12] Ho DD, Neumann AU, Perelson AS, et al. Rapid turnover of plasma virions and CD4 lymphocytes in HIV-1 infection. Nature 1995;373(6510): 123–6.

[13] Chun TW, Carruth L, Finzi D, et al. Quantification of latent tissue reservoirs and total body viral load in HIV-1 infection. Nature 1997;387(6629):183–8.

[14] Chun TW, Engel D, Berrey MM, et al. Early establishment of a pool of latently infected, resting CD4($^{+}$) T cells during primary HIV-1 infection. Proc Natl Acad Sci U S A 1998;95(15):8869–73.

[15] Trono D, Van Lint C, Rouzioux C, et al. HIV persistence and the prospect of long-term drug-free remissions for HIV-infected individuals. Science 2010;329 (5988):174–80.

[16] Goonetilleke N, Liu MK, Salazar-Gonzalez JF, et al. The first T cell response to transmitted/founder virus contributes to the control of acute viremia in HIV-1 infection. J Exp Med 2009;206(6):1253–72.

[17] McMichael AJ, Borrow P, Tomaras GD, et al. The immune response during acute HIV-1 infection: clues for vaccine development. Nat Rev Immunol 2010;10(1):11–23.

[18] Wei X, Decker JM, Wang S, et al. Antibody neutralization and escape by HIV-1. Nature 2003;422 (6929):307–12.

[19] Guadalupe M, Reay E, Sankaran S, et al. Severe CD4[+] T-cell depletion in gut lymphoid tissue during primary human immunodeficiency virus type 1 infection and substantial delay in restoration following highly active antiretroviral therapy. J Virol 2003;77(21):11708–17.

[20] Li Q, Duan L, Estes JD, et al. Peak SIV replication in resting memory CD4[+] T cells depletes gut lamina propria CD4[+] T cells. Nature 2005;434(7037):1148–52.

[21] Mattapallil JJ, Douek DC, Hill B, et al. Massive infection and loss of memory CD4[+] T cells in multiple tissues during acute SIV infection. Nature 2005;434(7037):1093–7.

[22] Arthos J, Cicala C, Martinelli E, et al. HIV-1 envelope protein binds to and signals through integrin alpha4beta7, the gut mucosal homing receptor for peripheral T cells. Nat Immunol 2008;9(3): 301–9.

[23] Cicala C, Martinelli E, McNally JP, et al. The integrin alpha4beta7 forms a complex with cell-surface CD4 and defines a T-cell subset that is highly susceptible to infection by HIV-1. Proc Natl Acad Sci U S A 2009;106 (49):20877–82.

[24] Ansari AA, Reimann KA, Mayne AE, et al. Blocking of $\alpha_4\beta_7$ gut-homing integrin during acute infection leads to decreased plasma and

gastrointestinal tissue viral loads in simian immunodeficiency virus-infected rhesus macaques. J Immunol 2011;186(2):1044–59.

[25] Taylor BS, Hammer SM. The challenge of HIV-1 subtype diversity. N Engl J Med 2008;359 (18):1965–6.

[26] Chohan B, Lang D, Sagar M, et al. Selection for human immunodeficiency virus type 1 envelope glycosylation variants with shorter V1-V2 loop sequences occurs during transmission of certain genetic subtypes and may impact viral RNA levels. J Virol 2005;79(10):6528–31.

[27] Derdeyn CA, Decker JM, Bibollet-Ruche F, et al. Envelope-constrained neutralization-sensitive HIV-1 after heterosexual transmission. Science 2004;303 (5666):2019–22.

[28] Rong R, Bibollet-Ruche F, Mulenga J, et al. Role of V1V2 and other human immunodeficiency virus type 1 envelope domains in resistance to autologous neutralization during clade C infection. J Virol 2007;81 (3):1350–9.

[29] Sagar M. HIV-1 transmission biology: selection and characteristics of infecting viruses. J Infect Dis 2010;202(Suppl. 2): S289–96.

[30] Liu Y, Curlin ME, Diem K, et al. Env length and N-linked glycosylation following transmission of human immunodeficiency virus Type 1 subtype B viruses. Virology 2008;374(2):229–33.

[31] Nawaz F, Cicala C, Van Ryk D, et al. The genotype of early-transmitting HIV gp120s promotes $\alpha(4)\beta(7)$-reactivity, revealing $\alpha(4)\beta(7)^{+}$/CD4^{+} T cells as key targets in mucosal transmission. PLoS Pathog 2011;7(2):e1001301.

[32] Cicala C, Arthos J, Fauci AS. HIV-1 envelope, integrins and co-receptor use in mucosal transmission of HIV. J Transl Med 2011;9(Suppl. 1):S2.

[33] Haaland RE, Hawkins PA, Salazar-Gonzalez J, et al. Inflammatory genital infections mitigate a severe genetic bottleneck in heterosexual transmission of subtype A and C HIV-1. PLoS Pathog 2009;5(1): e1000274.

[34] Keele BF, Giorgi EE, Salazar-Gonzalez JF, et al. Identification and characterization of transmitted and early founder virus envelopes in primary HIV-1 infection. Proc Natl Acad Sci U S A 2008;105(21):7552–7.

[35] Salazar-Gonzalez JF, Salazar MG, Keele BF, et al. Genetic identity, biological phenotype, and evolutionary pathways of transmitted/founder viruses in acute and early HIV-1 infection. J Exp Med 2009;206(6):1273–89.

[36] Sagar M, Laeyendecker O, Lee S, et al. Selection of HIV variants with signature genotypic characteristics during heterosexual transmission. J Infect Dis 2009;199(4):580–9.

[37] Haase AT. Targeting early infection to prevent HIV-1 mucosal transmission. Nature 2010;464 (7286):217–23.

[38] Qin L, Gilbert PB, Corey L, et al. A framework for assessing immunological correlates of protection in vaccine trials. J Infect Dis 2007;196(9):1304–12.

[39] Plotkin SA. Vaccines: correlates of vaccine-induced immunity. Clin Infect Dis 2008;47(3):401–9.

[40] Genesca M, Miller CJ. Use of nonhuman primate models to develop mucosal AIDS vaccines. Curr HIV/AIDS Rep 2010;7 (1):19–27.

[41] Shiver JW, Fu TM, Chen L, et al. Replication-incompetent adenoviral vaccine vector elicits effective anti-immunodeficiency-virus immunity. Nature 2002;415 (6869):331–5.

[42] Watkins DI, Burton DR, Kallas EG, et al. Nonhuman primate models and the failure of the Merck HIV-1 vaccine in humans. Nat Med 2008;14(6):617–21.

[43] Barnett SW, Burke B, Sun Y, et al. Antibody-mediated protection against mucosal simian-human immunodeficiency virus challenge of macaques immunized with alphavirus replicon particles and boosted with trimeric envelope glycoprotein in MF59 adjuvant. J Virol 2010;84(12):5975–85.

[44] Barnett SW, Srivastava IK, Kan E, et al. Protection of macaques against vaginal SHIV challenge by systemic or mucosal and systemic

vaccinations with HIV-envelope. AIDS 2008;22(3):339–48.

[45] Liu J, Keele BF, Li H, et al. Low-dose mucosal simian immunodeficiency virus infection restricts early replication kinetics and transmitted virus variants in rhesus monkeys. J Virol 2010;84 (19):10406–12.

[46] Stone M, Keele BF, Ma ZM, et al. A limited number of simian immunodeficiency virus (SIV) env variants are transmitted to rhesus macaques vaginally inoculated with SIVmac251. J Virol 2010;84 (14):7083–95.

[47] Barouch DH, Liu J, Li H, et al. Vaccine protection against acquisition of neutralization-resistant SIV challenges in rhesus monkeys Nature 2012;482:89–93.

[48] Letvin NL, Rao SS, Montefiori DC, et al. Immune and genetic correlates of vaccine protection against SIVsmE660 mucosal infection in rhesus monkeys. Sci Transl Med 2011;3:1–11.

[49] Barouch DH, O'Brien KL, Simmons NL, et al. Mosaic HIV-1 vaccines expand the breadth and depth of cellular immune responses in rhesus monkeys. Nat Med 2010;16(3):319–23.

[50] Santra S, Liao HX, Zhang R, et al. Mosaic vaccines elicit CD8^{+} T lymphocyte responses that confer enhanced immune coverage of diverse HIV strains in monkeys. Nat Med 2010;16(3): 324–8.

[51] Siddappa NB, Song R, Kramer VG, et al. Neutralization-sensitive R5-tropic simian-human immunodeficiency virus SHIV-2873Nip, which carries env isolated from an infant with a recent HIV clade C infection. J Virol 2009;83(3):1422–32.

[52] Hessell AJ, Hangartner L, Hunter M, et al. Fc receptor but not complement binding is important in antibody protection against HIV. Nature 2007;449 (7158):101–4.

[53] Mascola JR, Stiegler G, VanCott TC, et al. Protection of macaques against vaginal transmission of a pathogenic HIV-1/SIV chimeric virus by passive infusion of

neutralizing antibodies. Nat Med 2000;6:207–10.

[54] Scheid JF, Mouquet H, Feldhahn N, et al. Broad diversity of neutralizing antibodies isolated from memory B cells in HIV-infected individuals. Nature 2009;458(7238):636–40.

[55] Walker LM, Phogat SK, Chan-Hui PY, et al. Broad and potent neutralizing antibodies from an African donor reveal a new HIV-1 vaccine target. Science 2009;326 (5950):285–9.

[56] Wu X, Yang ZY, Li Y, et al. Rational design of envelope identifies broadly neutralizing human monoclonal antibodies to HIV-1. Science 2010;329 (5993):856–61.

[57] Korber BT, Letvin NL, Haynes BF. T-cell vaccine strategies for human immunodeficiency virus, the virus with a thousand faces. J Virol 2009;83(17):8300–14.

[58] Gaufin T, Gautam R, Kasheta M, et al. Limited ability of humoral immune responses in control of viremia during infection with SIVsmmD215 strain. Blood 2009;113(18):4250–61.

[59] Schmitz JE, Kuroda MJ, Santra S, et al. Effect of humoral immune responses on controlling viremia during primary infection of rhesus monkeys with simian immunodeficiency virus. J Virol 2003;77(3):2165–73.

[60] Hansen SG, Vieville C, Whizin N, et al. Effector memory T cell responses are associated with protection of rhesus monkeys from mucosal simian immunodeficiency virus challenge. Nat Med 2009;15(3):293–9.

[61] Nilsson C, Makitalo B, Thorstensson R, et al. Live attenuated simian immunodeficiency virus (SIV)mac in macaques can induce protection against mucosal infection with SIVsm. AIDS 1998;12 (17):2261–70.

[62] Wyand MS, Manson K, Montefiori DC, et al. Protection by live, attenuated simian immunodeficiency virus against heterologous challenge. J Virol 1999;73:8356–63.

[63] Yeh WW, Jaru-Ampornpan P, Nevidomskyte D, et al. Partial protection of Simian immunodeficiency virus (SIV)-infected rhesus monkeys against superinfection with a heterologous SIV isolate. J Virol 2009;83 (6):2686–96.

[64] Robinson H, Lai L, Montefiori D, et al. Preclinical studies on DNA/MVA vaccines: co-expressed GM-CSF, a strong adjuvant for prevention of infection. AIDS Vaccine 2010. paper # 79LB.

[65] Kaul R, Plummer FA, Kimani J, et al. HIV-1-specific mucosal CD8+ lymphocyte responses in the cervix of HIV-1-resistant prostitutes in Nairobi. J Immunol 2000;164 (3):1602–11.

[66] Rowland-Jones S, Sutton J, Ariyoshi K, et al. HIV-specific cytotoxic T-cells in HIV-exposed but uninfected Gambian women. Nat Med 1995;1(1):59–64.

[67] Rowland-Jones SL, Dong T, Fowke KR, et al. Cytotoxic T cell responses to multiple conserved HIV epitopes in HIV-resistant prostitutes in Nairobi. J Clin Invest 1998;102(9):1758–65.

[68] Hirbod T, Kaul R, Reichard C, et al. HIV-neutralizing immunoglobulin A and HIV-specific proliferation are independently associated with reduced HIV acquisition in Kenyan sex workers. AIDS 2008;22 (6):727–35.

[69] Kosmrlj A, Read EL, Qi Y, et al. Effects of thymic selection of the T-cell repertoire on HLA class I-associated control of HIV infection. Nature 2010;465(7296): 350–4.

[70] Mouquet H, Scheid JF, Zoller MJ, et al. Polyreactivity increases the apparent affinity of anti-HIV antibodies by heteroligation. Nature 2010;467(7315): 591–5.

[71] Johnson RP, Glickman RL, Yang JQ, et al. Induction of vigorous cytotoxic T-lymphocyte responses by live attenuated simian immunodeficiency virus. J Virol 1997;71(10): 7711–18.

[72] Hessell AJ, Poignard P, Hunter M, et al. Effective, low-titer antibody protection against low-dose repeated mucosal SHIV challenge in macaques. Nat Med 2009;15 (8):951–4.

[73] Mascola JR, Lewis MG, Stiegler G, et al. Protection of macaques against pathogenic simian/human immunodeficiency virus 89.6PD by passive transfer of neutralizing antibodies. J Virol 1999;73 (5):4009–18.

[74] Hessell AJ, Rakasz EG, Poignard P, et al. Broadly neutralizing human anti-HIV antibody 2G12 is effective in protection against mucosal SHIV challenge even at low serum neutralizing titers. PLoS Pathog 2009;5(5):e1000433.

[75] Zhao J, Lai L, Amara RR, et al. Preclinical studies of human immunodeficiency virus/AIDS vaccines: inverse correlation between avidity of anti-Env antibodies and peak postchallenge viremia. J Virol 2009;83 (9):4102–11.

[76] Belshe RB, Graham BS, Keefer MC, et al. Neutralizing antibodies to HIV-1 in seronegative volunteers immunized with recombinant gp120 from the MN strain of HIV-1. NIAID AIDS Vaccine Clinical Trials Network. JAMA 1994;272 (6):475–80.

[77] Dolin R, Graham BS, Greenberg SB, et al. The safety and immunogenicity of a human immunodeficiency virus type 1 (HIV-1) recombinant gp160 candidate vaccine in humans. NIAID AIDS Vaccine Clinical Trials Network. Ann Intern Med 1991;114(2):119–27.

[78] Gorse GJ, Corey L, Patel GB, et al. HIV-1MN recombinant glycoprotein 160 vaccine-induced cellular and humoral immunity boosted by HIV-1MN recombinant glycoprotein 120 vaccine. National Institute of Allergy and Infectious Diseases AIDS Vaccine Evaluation Group. AIDS Res Hum Retroviruses 1999;15(2):115–32.

[79] Gorse GJ, McElrath MJ, Matthews TJ, et al. Modulation of immunologic responses to HIV-1MN recombinant gp160 vaccine by dose and schedule of administration. National Institute of Allergy and Infectious Diseases AIDS Vaccine Evaluation Group. Vaccine 1998;16(5):493–506.

[80] Keefer MC, Graham BS, Belshe RB, et al. Studies of high doses of a human immunodeficiency virus type 1 recombinant glycoprotein 160 candidate vaccine in HIV type 1-seronegative humans. The AIDS Vaccine Clinical Trials Network. AIDS Res Hum Retroviruses 1994;10(12):1713–23.

[81] Nitayaphan S, Khamboonruang C, Sirisophana N, et al. A phase I/II trial of HIV SF2 gp120/MF59 vaccine in seronegative Thais. Vaccine 2000;18:1448–55.

[82] Pitisuttithum P, Nitayaphan S, Thongcharoen P, et al. Safety and immunogenicity of combinations of recombinant subtype E and B human immunodeficiency virus type 1 envelope glycoprotein 120 vaccines in healthy Thai adults. J Infect Dis 2003;188(2):219–27.

[83] Schwartz DH, Gorse G, Clements ML, et al. Induction of HIV-1-neutralising and syncytium-inhibiting antibodies in uninfected recipients of HIV-1IIIB rgp120 subunit vaccine. Lancet 1993;342 (8863):69–73.

[84] Evans TG, McElrath MJ, Matthews T, et al. QS-21 promotes an adjuvant effect allowing for reduced antigen dose during HIV-1 envelope subunit immunization in humans. Vaccine 2001;19(15–16):2080–91.

[85] McElrath MJ, Corey L, Montefiori D, et al. A phase II study of two HIV type 1 envelope vaccines, comparing their immunogenicity in populations at risk for acquiring HIV type 1 infection. AIDS Vaccine Evaluation Group. AIDS Res Hum Retroviruses 2000;16(9): 907–19.

[86] Kovacs JA, Vasudevachari MB, Easter M, et al. Induction of humoral and cell-mediated anti-human immunodeficiency virus (HIV) responses in HIV sero-negative volunteers by immunization with recombinant gp160. J Clin Invest 1993;92 (2):919–28.

[87] Forthal DN, Gilbert PB, Landucci G, Phan T. Recombinant gp120 vaccine-induced antibodies inhibit clinical strains of HIV-1 in the presence of Fc receptor-bearing effector cells and correlate inversely with HIV infection rate. J Immunol 2007;178 (10):6596–603.

[88] Gilbert P, Wang M, Wrin T, et al. Magnitude and breadth of a nonprotective neutralizing antibody response in an efficacy trial of a candidate HIV-1 gp120 vaccine. J Infect Dis 2010;202 (4):595–605.

[89] McElrath MJ, De Rosa SC, Moodie Z, et al. HIV-1 vaccine-induced immunity in the test-of-concept Step Study: a case-cohort analysis. Lancet 2008;372 (9653):1894–905.

[90] D'Souza MP, Frahm N. Adenovirus 5 serotype vector-specific immunity and HIV-1 infection: a tale of T cells and antibodies. AIDS 2010;24(6):803–9.

[91] Priddy FH, Brown D, Kublin J, et al. Safety and immunogenicity of a replication-incompetent adenovirus type 5 HIV-1 clade B gag/pol/nef vaccine in healthy adults. Clin Infect Dis 2008;46 (11):1769–81.

[92] Lee D, Graham BS, Chiu YL, et al. Breakthrough infections during phase 1 and 2 prime-boost HIV-1 vaccine trials with canarypox vectors (ALVAC) and booster dose of recombinant gp120 or gp160. J Infect Dis 2004;190(5):903–7.

[93] Catanzaro AT, Koup RA, Roederer M, et al. Phase 1 safety and immunogenicity evaluation of a multiclade HIV-1 candidate vaccine delivered by a replication-defective recombinant adenovirus vector. J Infect Dis 2006;194:1638–49.

[94] Catanzaro AT, Roederer M, Koup RA, et al. Phase I clinical evaluation of a six-plasmid multiclade HIV-1 DNA candidate vaccine. Vaccine 2007;25 (20):4085–92.

[95] Graham BS, Koup RA, Roederer M, et al. Phase 1 safety and immunogenicity evaluation of a multiclade HIV-1 DNA candidate vaccine. J Infect Dis 2006;194:1650–60.

[96] Jaoko W, Karita E, Kayitenkore K, et al. Safety and immunogenicity study of Multiclade HIV-1 adenoviral vector vaccine alone or as boost following a multiclade HIV-1 DNA vaccine in Africa. PLoS One 2010;5(9):e12873.

[97] Kibuuka H, Kimutai R, Maboko L, et al. A phase I/II study of a multiclade HIV-1 DNA plasmid prime and recombinant Adenovirus-type 5 boost vaccine in HIV uninfected East Africans. J Infect Dis 2010;201(4):600–7.

[98] Binley JM, Sanders RW, Clas B, et al. A recombinant human immunodeficiency virus type 1 envelope glycoprotein complex stabilized by an intermolecular disulfide bond between the gp120 and gp41 subunits is an antigenic mimic of the trimeric virion-associated structure. J Virol 2000;74(2):627–43.

[99] Earl PL, Sugiura W, Montefiori DC, et al. Immunogenicity and protective efficacy of oligomeric human immunodeficiency virus type 1 gp140. J Virol 2001;75 (2):645–53.

[100] Yang X, Wyatt R, Sodroski J. Improved elicitation of neutralizing antibodies against primary human immunodeficiency viruses by soluble stabilized envelope glycoprotein trimers. J Virol 2001;75(3):1165–71.

[101] Cherpelis S, Shrivastava I, Gettie A, et al. DNA vaccination with the human immunodeficiency virus type 1 SF162DeltaV2 envelope elicits immune responses that offer partial protection from simian/human immunodeficiency virus infection to CD8($^+$) T-cell-depleted rhesus macaques. J Virol 2001;75(3):1547–50.

[102] Derby NR, Kraft Z, Kan E, et al. Antibody responses elicited in macaques immunized with human immunodeficiency virus type 1 (HIV-1) SF162-derived gp140 envelope immunogens: comparison with those elicited

during homologous simian/ human immunodeficiency virus SHIVSF162P4 and heterologous HIV-1 infection. J Virol 2006;80:8745–62.

[103] Reitter JN, Means RE, Desrosiers RC. A role for carbohydrates in immune evasion in AIDS. Nat Med 1998;4 (6):679–84.

[104] Srivastava IK, VanDorsten K, Vojtech L, et al. Changes in the immunogenic properties of soluble gp140 human immunodeficiency virus envelope constructs upon partial deletion of the second hypervariable region. J Virol 2003;77(4):2310–20.

[105] Fouts TR, Binley JM, Trkola A, et al. Neutralization of the human immunodeficiency virus type 1 primary isolate JR-FL by human monoclonal antibodies correlates with antibody binding to the oligomeric form of the envelope glycoprotein complex. J Virol 1997;71(4):2779–85.

[106] Binley JM, Ban YE, Crooks ET, et al. Role of complex carbohydrates in human immunodeficiency virus type 1 infection and resistance to antibody neutralization. J Virol 2010;84(11):5637–55.

[107] Frey G, Peng H, Rits-Volloch S, et al. A fusion-intermediate state of HIV-1 gp41 targeted by broadly neutralizing antibodies. Proc Natl Acad Sci U S A 2008;105 (10):3739–44.

[108] Kwong PD, Doyle ML, Casper DJ, et al. HIV-1 evades antibody-mediated neutralization through conformational masking of receptor-binding sites. Nature 2002;420(6916):678–82.

[109] Schief WR, Ban YE, Stamatatos L. Challenges for structure-based HIV vaccine design. Curr Opin HIV AIDS 2009;4(5):431–40.

[110] Mascola JR, Montefiori DC. The role of antibodies in HIV vaccines. Annu Rev Immunol 2010;28:413–44.

[111] Cebere I, Dorrell L, McShane H, et al. Phase I clinical trial safety of DNA- and modified virus Ankara-vectored human immunodeficiency virus type 1 (HIV-1) vaccines administered alone and in a prime-boost regime to healthy HIV-1-uninfected volunteers. Vaccine 2006;24 (4):417–25.

[112] Goonetilleke N, Moore S, Dally L, et al. Induction of multifunctional human immunodeficiency virus type 1 (HIV-1)-specific T cells capable of proliferation in healthy subjects by using a prime-boost regimen of DNA- and modified vaccinia virus Ankara-vectored vaccines expressing HIV-1 Gag coupled to CD8$^+$ T-cell epitopes. J Virol 2006;80(10):4717–28.

[113] Guimaraes-Walker A, Mackie N, McCormack S, et al. Lessons from IAVI-006, a phase I clinical trial to evaluate the safety and immunogenicity of the pTHr.HIVA DNA and MVA.HIVA vaccines in a prime-boost strategy to induce HIV-1 specific T-cell responses in healthy volunteers. Vaccine 2008;26(51):6671–7.

[114] Jaoko W, Nakwagala FN, Anzala O, et al. Safety and immunogenicity of recombinant low-dosage HIV-1 A vaccine candidates vectored by plasmid pTHr DNA or modified vaccinia virus Ankara (MVA) in humans in East Africa. Vaccine 2008;26(22):2788–95.

[115] Peters BS, Jaoko W, Vardas E, et al. Studies of a prophylactic HIV-1 vaccine candidate based on modified vaccinia virus Ankara (MVA) with and without DNA priming: effects of dosage and route on safety and immunogenicity. Vaccine 2007;25(11):2120–7.

[116] Ramanathan VD, Kumar M, Mahalingam J, et al. A Phase 1 study to evaluate the safety and immunogenicity of a recombinant HIV type 1 subtype C-modified vaccinia Ankara virus vaccine candidate in Indian volunteers. AIDS Res Hum Retroviruses 2009;25(11):1107–16.

[117] Currier JR, Ngauy V, de Souza MS, et al. Phase I safety and immunogenicity evaluation of MVA-CMDR, a multigenic, recombinant modified vaccinia Ankara-HIV-1 vaccine candidate. PLoS One 2010;5(11):e13983.

[118] Goepfert PA, Elizaga ML, Sato A, et al. Phase 1 safety and immunogenicity testing of DNA and recombinant modified vaccinia Ankara vaccines expressing HIV-1 virus-like particles. J Infect Dis 2011;203 (5):610–19.

[119] Wang S, Kennedy JS, West K, et al. Cross-subtype antibody and cellular immune responses induced by a polyvalent DNA prime-protein boost HIV-1 vaccine in healthy human volunteers. Vaccine 2008;26 (31):3947–57.

[120] Sandstrom E, Nilsson C, Hejdeman B, et al. Broad immunogenicity of a multigene, multiclade HIV-1 DNA vaccine boosted with heterologous HIV-1 recombinant modified vaccinia virus Ankara. J Infect Dis 2008;198 (10):1482–90.

[121] Bart PA, Goodall R, Barber T, et al. EV01: a phase I trial in healthy HIV negative volunteers to evaluate a clade C HIV vaccine, NYVAC-C undertaken by the EuroVacc Consortium. Vaccine 2008;26 (25):3153–61.

[122] Harari A, Bart PA, Stohr W, et al. An HIV-1 clade C DNA prime, NYVAC boost vaccine regimen induces reliable, polyfunctional, and long-lasting T cell responses. J Exp Med 2008;205 (1):63–77.

[123] McCormack S, Stohr W, Barber T, et al. EV02: a Phase I trial to compare the safety and immunogenicity of HIV DNA-C prime-NYVAC-C boost to NYVAC-C alone. Vaccine 2008;26 (25):3162–74.

[124] McCoy K, Tatsis N, Korioth-Schmitz B, et al. Effect of preexisting immunity to adenovirus human serotype 5 antigens on the immune responses of nonhuman primates to vaccine regimens based on human- or chimpanzee-derived adenovirus vectors. J Virol 2007;81 (12):6594–604.

[125] Corey L, Nabel GJ, Dieffenbach C, et al. HIV-1 vaccines and adaptive trial designs. Sci Transl Med 2011;3(79) 79 ps13.

[126] Mehendale S, van Lunzen J, Clumeck N, et al. A phase 1 study to evaluate the safety and immunogenicity of a recombinant HIV type 1 subtype C adeno-associated virus vaccine. AIDS Res Hum Retroviruses 2008;24 (6):873–80.

[127] Vardas E, Kaleebu P, Bekker LG, et al. A phase 2 study to evaluate the safety and immunogenicity of a recombinant HIV type 1 vaccine based on adeno-associated virus. AIDS Res Hum Retroviruses 2010;26(8):933–42.

[128] Fischer W, Perkins S, Theiler J, et al. Polyvalent vaccines for optimal coverage of potential T-cell epitopes in global HIV-1 variants. Nat Med 2007;13 (1):100–6.

[129] Rolland M, Carlson JM, Manocheewa S, et al. Amino-acid co-variation in HIV-1 Gag subtype C: HLA-mediated selection pressure and compensatory dynamics. PLoS One 2010;5(9)pii: e12463.

Chapter | 9 |

HIV prevention

Salim S. Abdool Karim

INTRODUCTION

One of the greatest challenges facing the world today is the control of the human immunodeficiency virus (HIV) epidemic. At the end of 2009 an estimated 33.3 million people were living with HIV [1]. While intravenous drug use is the major route of transmission in several countries, sexual transmission is the dominant mode of HIV spread globally, with a concomitant epidemic in infants born to HIV-infected mothers. Although many regions and countries are showing signs of declining or stabilizing epidemics, some countries still have unacceptably high HIV prevalence and incidence rates. In contrast to the first two decades of the HIV pandemic, today women comprise about half of all adults living with HIV/AIDS globally [1]. In sub-Saharan Africa, young women aged 15–24 years are as much as eight times more likely than men to be HIV-infected.

HIV prevention focuses, on the one hand, on reducing the likelihood of and vulnerability to infection in those who are currently uninfected and, on the other hand, on reducing the risk of transmission from those who are currently infected with HIV. The latter is an important new opportunity for enhancing prevention efforts through integration of prevention programs into the health services which are scaling up AIDS treatment and the prevention of mother-to-child transmission (MTCT).

Significant advances in HIV prevention have been achieved in the past three decades. This chapter summarizes the known existing HIV prevention options and describes the new HIV prevention strategies currently under development.

PREVENTING SEXUAL TRANSMISSION (BOX 9.1)

Reducing sexual transmission, especially heterosexual transmission, of HIV is critical to altering the current epidemic trajectory in many parts of the world. Prevention of sexual transmission can be achieved through reduction in the number of discordant sexual acts and/or reduction of the probability of HIV transmission in discordant sexual acts [2].

There is no risk of sexually acquired HIV infection among individuals who practice sexual abstinence or lifelong mutual monogamy. Serial monogamy, where there are multiple sequential individual short-lived monogamous partnerships, is associated with an increased risk of HIV, but not to the same extent as the increase in risk of transmission emanating from multiple concurrent sexual partnerships [3]. Reduction in the number of concurrent sexual partnerships and the use of condoms are key components of HIV prevention messages, widely promoted as part of "ABCCC" campaigns promoting Abstinence, Be faithful, Condomize, Counseling and testing, and Circumcision.

Abstinence

Abstinence is a HIV prevention strategy promoted primarily for adolescents and entails either delaying sexual initiation or practicing "secondary abstinence," which is a prolonged period without sexual activity amongst those frequency, and number of people with overlapping partnerships strongly influence this association [6–8]. The link between concurrent relationships and HIV risk is particularly relevant in sexual partnering between younger women and older men [9], which is a major factor in HIV spread in southern Africa.

Condoms

Condoms are inexpensive and relatively easy to use and provide protection against acquisition and transmission of HIV, a wide range of other sexually transmitted infections, and pregnancy. When used correctly and consistently, the latex male condom is highly effective in preventing the sexual transmission of HIV. Although numerous studies conducted over the past decade have demonstrated the steady increase in acceptability and use of male condoms [4, 10], a review of HIV risk studies [11] estimates that only about 20% of adolescents use male condoms consistently.

To be effective as a prevention option and to impact on the growth of the epidemic, access to condoms, especially female condoms, needs to be drastically scaled-up. In addition, barriers to condom use need to be addressed; some of the most common being: the widespread perception that condoms reduce sexual pleasure and that suggesting the use of condoms represents self-acknowledgment of HIV infection or a lack of trust in the partner [12, 13]. Some studies have found that young people may also associate condom use with promiscuity and sexually transmitted infections including HIV/AIDS [14]. In the context of a marital relationship or stable partnership where pregnancy is desired, or where subordination of women limits their ability to negotiate safer sex practices, attempts to introduce or promote condom use have had limited success.

who have previously been sexually active [4]. The impact of abstinence on HIV prevention appears to be limited, with short-lived success despite the widespread implementation of abstinence messages. In settings where the epidemic is generalized and probability of infection is high because of high disease burden, postponement of sexual initiation in women simply delays the age of infection, but does not in itself reduce rates of infection [5]. Regardless, abstinence remains an important component of HIV prevention in youth, especially targeting delaying sexual debut.

Be faithful

Individuals with multiple partners may face an increased HIV risk due to overlapping sexual relationships, although gender and other factors such as overlap duration, sexual

Counseling and testing

HIV counseling and testing has been shown to be both efficacious in reducing risky sexual behaviors [15] and cost-effective as a prevention intervention [16]. Knowledge of HIV status is an important gateway for targeted prevention and care efforts. It creates an opportunity for addressing prevention efforts along a continuum that includes those uninfected who are at high risk of getting infected, those recently infected, those with established infection but asymptomatic, those who have advancing HIV disease, and those on antiretroviral treatment. However, large numbers of people, especially in sub-Saharan Africa, are unaware of their HIV status [17]. A study in the USA has shown that individuals who are unaware of their HIV infection are 3.5 times more likely to transmit the virus to others than those who know about their infection [18].

Medical male circumcision

Medical male circumcision is a proven HIV prevention option for men [19], reducing the risk of female-to-male transmission of HIV by up to 60%. Although this prevention option took some time to be incorporated in the HIV prevention package, widespread use of medical male circumcision to reduce HIV risk is fast gaining momentum, particularly in sub-Saharan African countries. For example, in Kenya and Botswana, policies to have 80% of 0- to 49-year-old HIV-uninfected males circumcised by 2013 and 2014, respectively, have been approved [20]. It is estimated by mathematical modeling that widespread implementation of male circumcision could avert between 2 and 3 million HIV infections in sub-Saharan Africa [21]. While women do not gain a direct benefit from circumcision of men, they derive an indirect benefit over time as fewer men become infected with HIV. Medical male circumcision of HIV-infected men does not seem to reduce the risk of HIV acquisition in their female partners. Similarly, medical male circumcision does not demonstrate protection against HIV transmission in men who have sex with men (MSMs).

STD screening and treatment

An estimated 340 million new cases of curable sexually transmitted infections occurred globally in the 15–49 years old age group in 1999 [22]. HIV transmission and acquisition during heterosexual intercourse is enhanced in the presence of sexually transmitted infections, particularly ulcerative infections such as syphilis, chancroid, and herpes simplex type 2 virus infection [23, 24]. Despite the promising 42% reduction in HIV incidence rates observed in a randomized controlled trial conducted in Tanzania following treatment of sexually transmitted infections [25], other similar studies have failed to replicate these results [26]. Notwithstanding the inconsistent findings from these trials, the significant sexual and reproductive health challenge posed by the high burden of curable sexually transmitted infections needs to be addressed in any HIV prevention effort.

Antiretroviral microbicides for prevention of male-to-female transmission

The search for a female-controlled prevention option has been ongoing since 1990 [27]. In 2010, the CAPRISA 004 trial showed that an antiretroviral drug, formulated as a topical vaginal gel, prevents male-to-female transmission of HIV. In this trial, tenofovir gel, used before and after sex, reduced HIV acquisition by 39% [28].This trial has contributed to the growing body of randomized control trial-based evidence for preventing HIV sexual transmission (Fig. 9.1). It is anticipated that a licensed product will be available by 2014. Although tenofovir gel will not provide complete protection against HIV, it still has the potential to have an enormous public health benefit. In South Africa alone, this new prevention technology could avert an estimated 1.3 million new HIV infections and 800,000 AIDS deaths over the next 20 years [29].

Figure 9.1 Randomized controlled trial evidence-based effective strategies for preventing sexual transmission of HIV infection.

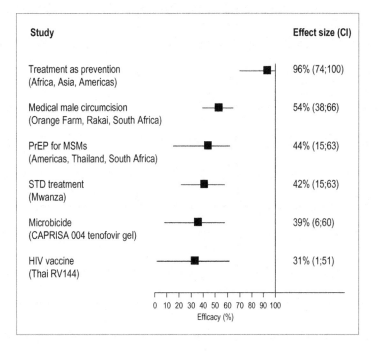

Despite the optimism that a licensed vaginal microbicide will be available soon, widespread implementation of microbicides as an HIV prevention option faces several challenges. Firstly, because the microbicides in the most advanced stage of development are mostly antiretroviral drugs that are also being used for AIDS treatment, there are concerns about the potential for drug resistance development. Regular HIV testing will most likely need to accompany the implementation of microbicides to minimize the potential of drug resistance development. Microbicides will also only work if they are widely accepted and used consistently by women. In clinical trial settings high levels of adherence have been achievable. However, the same may not pertain to "real world" settings where microbicides are likely to be implemented in under-developed public healthcare facilities without adequate attention to adherence support. Strategies for ensuring long-term adherence to microbicides will be essential if they are to succeed as a HIV prevention option. Concerns have been raised about the potential for risk compensation/behavioral disinhibition and careful attention will need to be paid to messaging if microbicides are implemented to ensure existing risk reduction behavior messaging is not undermined.

The development of microbicides for rectal use has gathered momentum recently but remains several years away. In addition to new formulations and delivery devices, future microbicide development is likely to focus on a combination of antiretroviral drugs and combinations of antiretroviral agents with contraceptives.

Oral antiretroviral pre-exposure prophylaxis for prevention of male-to-male transmission

Oral antiretroviral drugs used as pre-exposure prophylaxis (PrEP) have recently been shown to successfully reduce the risk of sexually transmitted HIV. The iPrEX trial showed that Truvada (a combination of tenofovir and emtricitabine) taken daily reduced HIV acquisition by 44% in men who have sex with men [30].

Since Truvada is already a licensed antiretroviral drug for AIDS treatment, its widespread implementation as HIV prevention among men who have sex with men began in 2011. Based on the results of the iPrEX study, the Centers for Disease Control and Prevention and other US Public Health Service agencies have issued guidance on the use of PrEP among MSMs at high risk for HIV acquisition in the United States as part of a comprehensive set of HIV prevention services [31].

However, oral PrEP has not yet been shown to be effective in other at-risk populations. A trial assessing the efficacy of Truvada as PrEP in women was prematurely halted in April 2011 [32] as it was considered futile to continue the trial following an interim analysis that showed

no protection against HIV infection. Several trials in discordant couples, women, and injecting drug users are still ongoing.

If successful, scale up of PrEP will require integration into existing HIV prevention services, which currently need to be strengthened, especially in Africa, where the need is greatest. Similar to microbicides, implementation of PrEP will require long-term follow-up and surveillance for monitoring adverse events, adherence, drug resistance, impact of drug resistance on later AIDS treatment, and risk compensation/behavioral disinhibition. The potential contribution of PrEP to drug resistance may not be as severe as originally thought. Mathematical modeling of the impact of antiretroviral therapy and PrEP combined on HIV transmission and drug resistance has shown that while prevalence of drug resistance is anticipated to increase to a median of 9% after 10 years of antiretroviral therapy (ART) and PrEP rollout, most of the new drug resistance is anticipated to be from ART of HIV-infected patients rather than PrEP[33] in HIV-uninfected people.

"Treatment for prevention" strategy

In addition to using antiretroviral drugs in HIV-uninfected people to prevent transmission of HIV, antiretroviral therapy has been shown to reduce infectiousness of an HIV-infected individual, thereby limiting the risk of onward viral transmission [34]. In the HPTN 052 trial [35], ART initiated in patients with CD4 counts between 350 and 550 cells/mm^3 reduced HIV incidence in their HIV-uninfected partners by 96% compared to patients where ART was deferred to the point at which the patient's CD4 count dropped below 250 cells/mm^3.

The rationale for this strategy stems from studies of discordant couples that demonstrate a strong relationship between viral load and the probability of HIV transmission [2]. A prospective cohort analysis among discordant heterosexual African couples showed that HIV transmission was rare in those on ART. In this study, the majority of HIV transmissions (70%) occurred when plasma HIV concentrations exceeded 50,000 copies/mL [36].

There are many challenges in implementing this approach: the difficulty in identifying HIV-infected people who are asymptomatic; the lack of health service capacity to increase the numbers of patients on treatment (especially in Africa, where the HIV burden is greatest); and financial constraints already hampering availability of AIDS treatment to those who need it for therapeutic reasons. Various approaches to implementing treatment for prevention are being developed and investigated. Several clinical trials for evaluating the community-level effectiveness of various strategies for HIV testing and initiation of ART for preventing transmission of HIV are currently underway. The scale-up of and increasing access to HIV counseling and testing and antiretroviral drugs has created a new opportunity for integrating prevention and care. According to a mathematical model with extreme assumptions, the "test and treat" strategy, where all individuals who test HIV-infected are immediately initiated on ART, irrespective of CD4 count, could lead to a substantial prevention benefit [37].

Integration of behavioral prevention programs into AIDS treatment services (prevention for positives)

Differentiated from generalized prevention, which targets everyone at risk for HIV as well as those who are HIV-infected but have not yet undergone HIV testing, positive prevention focuses on addressing continued high-risk practices for HIV transmission among people who know they are HIV-infected. Clinic-delivered positive prevention interventions have been most successful when integrated into routine clinical services. The Clinician-Initiated HIV Risk Reduction Intervention for HIV-Positive Persons, known as the Options Project, is one such example, where prevention was effectively integrated into care services by clinicians [38]. Two separate meta-analyses of randomized controlled trials have shown that interventions targeting HIV-infected individuals are efficacious in reducing unprotected sex and acquisition of sexually transmitted diseases [39, 40].

PREVENTING MOTHER-TO-CHILD TRANSMISSION (BOX 9.1)

Since the discovery in 1994 that the antiretroviral drug azidothymidine (AZT) could reduce MTCT of HIV from 25.5 to 8.3%, substantial progress has been made in this prevention area. The number of infants infected by their mothers continues to decline in most countries and in 2009 an estimated 370,000 children contracted HIV from their mothers, a decrease of almost 25% in 5 years [1].

Reduction in unwanted pregnancy in HIV-infected women is an important component of efforts to reduce the number of children acquiring HIV. MTCT of HIV occurs in the intrauterine period, during labor and delivery, and postnatally through breastfeeding. Prevention strategies for reducing MTCT have been targeted at these time points and include a combination of antiretroviral drugs, changes in obstetric practices, and alternatives to breastfeeding.

Antiretroviral drugs: The simplest and most affordable regimen for preventing MTCT is HIVNET 012, which uses a single dose of nevirapine for the mother and a single dose of nevirapine for the newborn. However, one of the biggest concerns with using this regimen has been nevirapine resistance. The single-dose nevirapine regimen

has since been superseded by trials testing combination antiretrovirals. The most effective therapy is a combination of three antiretroviral drugs taken during pregnancy and breastfeeding [41].

Obstetric practices: Cesarean delivery reduces MTCT by 80% compared to vaginal, although it is not a sustainable option in developing countries with high HIV prevalences as the health services would be unable to cope with the additional burden of additional cesarean sections and sepsis rates following cesarean section may be unacceptable.

Breastfeeding: Total avoidance of breastfeeding is the most effective mechanism for preventing breastfeeding transmission. In some resource-constrained settings the use of formula feeding to reduce MTCT is precluded due to the lack of clean running water. In these instances women should be advised to exclusively breastfeed and abruptly wean their infant or, if they have regular access to antiretroviral drugs, they should exclusively breastfeed for the first 6 months and then introduce mix feeding until the infant is able to have a safe diet without breastmilk [42]. Recent data from the HPTN 046 trial demonstrated that providing infants with daily nevirapine for up to 6 months lowered risk of breastfeeding MTCT by more than 50% compared to a placebo by age 6 months [43].

MTCT rates below 1% can be readily attained with effective implementation of existing MTCT prevention strategies and MTCT has been virtually eliminated in high-income countries. In 2009, UNAIDS made a call for the virtual elimination of MTCT in low- and middle-income countries by 2015, an accomplishment that can only be possible if 90% of pregnant women are reached with services matching WHO guidelines, HIV incidence is reduced by 50%, the need for family planning is met, and breastfeeding is restricted to 12 months [1].

PREVENTING BLOOD-BORNE TRANSMISSION (BOX 9.1)

Transmission of HIV through exposure to infected blood can occur through transfusion of blood and blood products, through sharing of needles and syringes among injecting drug users and through inadvertent nosocomial transmission (e.g. through needlestick injuries) in healthcare settings.

Harm reduction for injection drug users

Globally, there are approximately 15.9 million injecting drug users, 3 million of whom are HIV-infected. Although the majority of injecting drug users reside in low- and middle-income countries, especially in Eastern Europe, East and Southeast Asia, and Latin America, new epidemics of injecting drug use are also emerging in sub-Saharan Africa [44]. Although injection drug use is distinct from sexual intercourse as a mode of transmission, the two routes are frequently linked epidemiologically. Injection drug users are often young and sexually active, potentially exposing their sexual partners, children, and fetuses to the virus. In addition, injection drug use is common in the commercial sex industry.

There is substantial evidence that HIV epidemics among injecting drug users can be prevented, stabilized, and even reversed. The WHO, United Nations Office on Drugs and Crime (UNODC), and UNAIDS recommend the following nine activities be included in a comprehensive package for the prevention, treatment and care of HIV among injecting drug users:

(1) Needle and syringe programs;
(2) Opioid substitution therapy and other drug dependence treatment;
(3) HIV testing and counseling;
(4) Antiretroviral therapy for drug users living with HIV;
(5) Prevention and treatment of sexually transmitted infections;
(6) Condom promotion;
(7) Targeted information, education, and communication for injecting drug users and their sexual partners;
(8) Vaccination, diagnosis, and treatment of viral hepatitis; and
(9) Prevention, diagnosis, and treatment of tuberculosis [44].

Despite access to HIV prevention services, including harm-reduction programs having increased substantially in many countries, a systematic review of global, regional, and national coverage has shown that HIV prevention, treatment, and care services for people who inject drugs remains suboptimal [45]. In 2009 the median coverage of HIV prevention services for injecting drug users was estimated to be 32% [44].

HIV screening of the blood supply for safe transfusions

Notable progress has been made worldwide in improving the safety of national blood supplies. The creation of nationally coordinated blood transfusion services and introduction of a range of policies and procedures, with a particular focus on HIV screening of donated blood for detecting antibodies to HIV, the reduction of unnecessary transfusions, and development of improved donor screening and deferral techniques have helped to virtually eliminate the risk of transmitting HIV through donated blood in high-income countries. The use of the newer-generation p24 antigen assays and polymerase chain reaction for detecting viral RNA in blood donors who may be in the window period for HIV infection is a further strategy used to reduce the risk of transfusing infected blood. However, there are significant variations in the extent and quality of blood screening, and recipients of blood transfusions in some countries remain at risk of acquiring HIV.

Universal precautions and nosocomial transmission

Healthcare workers exposed to blood and body fluids have a low but measurable risk of occupational infection with HIV. In a review of transmission probability estimates, infectivity following a needlestick exposure was estimated to range from 0 to 2.38% (weighted mean, 0.23%) [46]. While international guidelines recommend the use of relatively inexpensive auto-disable syringes as the "equipment of choice" for helping prevent HIV transmission in healthcare settings, only 38% of low- and middle-income countries were using such syringes in their national vaccine programs in 2004 [47]. Risk of exposure to blood or other body fluids can be significantly lowered through healthcare workers' adherence to "universal precautions," which involves the routine use of gloves and other protective gear to prevent occupational exposures, safe disposal of sharps, and timely administration of a four-week prophylactic course of antiretroviral prophylaxis following exposure.

Antiretrovirals for post-exposure prophylaxis

Following exposure to HIV, there is a small "window of opportunity" to use ART to prevent systemic infection. This strategy, known as post-exposure prophylaxis (PEP), has been shown to prevent both occupational [48] and non-occupational exposure [49]. However, the effectiveness of PEP in preventing the establishment of HIV infection depends on a number of factors, including route and dose of exposure, efficacy of drug(s) used, interval between exposure and initiation of drug(s), and level of adherence to the drug [48, 49]. The current consensus is that combination ART should be initiated as soon as possible after exposure, and continued for at least four weeks [50]. To minimize the possibility of behavioral disinhibition among individuals receiving PEP for sexual or drug-use exposures, it is recommended that PEP provision be accompanied by behavioral counseling following a potential sexual exposure to HIV [51].

HIV PREVENTION STRATEGIES UNDER DEVELOPMENT

Vaccines

Although a safe, effective, preventive HIV vaccine would provide the best method for controlling the HIV pandemic, its successful development has, to date, eluded scientists.

Clinical trials of candidate HIV vaccines have been underway since 1987 but only a few products have reached late-stage clinical trial testing. Both the bivalent, recombinant gp120 vaccine (AIDSVAX) and Merck's adenovirus serotype 5 (Ad5)-based vaccine candidate (MRKAd5) failed to show protection against HIV. In fact, the latter trial may have enhanced the risk of HIV infection, especially in those with pre-existing immunity to the adenovirus-5 vector. In 2009, however, results from the Thai RV144 trial provided the first indication that a vaccine could prevent HIV infection. This trial tested a prime–boost combination of a canarypox vector vaccine (ALVAC HIV) and gp120 protein (AIDSVAX B/E) and showed that vaccine recipients had a 31% lower rate of HIV infection than those receiving the placebo [52]. Interestingly, the RV144 trial showed evidence of HIV prevention but no evidence of viral suppression and further studies for better understanding these results are underway. While this trial produced promising results, the vaccine is not being considered for implementation due to its suboptimal efficacy.

There are several other AIDS vaccine candidates in the clinical pipeline and nearly all are devised to elicit cell-mediated immunity, a strategy that has so far proved disappointing. In 2009, the isolation of two new broadly neutralizing antibodies, PG9 and PG16 [53], capable of targeting a wide spectrum of HIV variants, has reinvigorated the enthusiasm for broadly neutralizing antibodies and the role they could play in the development of a vaccine against HIV. Several more broadly neutralizing antibodies have also since been isolated.

Vaccine development is severely hampered by the lack of any immune correlate that has been shown to prevent viral infection or clear initial viral infection. The human immune system generally fails to spontaneously clear HIV infection and so there is no natural immune process for the vaccine candidates to mimic. It is, however, believed that approaches aimed at eliciting both humoral and cell-mediated immunity are most promising to prevent or at least control retroviral infection.

Combination prevention

A single HIV prevention intervention is unlikely to be able to alter the epidemic trajectory as HIV epidemics in communities are complex and comprise a mosaic of different risk factors and different routes of transmission. Hence, the proposal that a mix of behavioral, biomedical, and structural HIV prevention actions could alter the course of the HIV epidemic has arisen. The combination of HIV prevention interventions needed will vary depending on cultural context, the population targeted, and the stage of the epidemic. Studies are now being developed to assess whether the epidemic can be slowed or stopped at a community level through high coverage of a combination of existing prevention strategies.

CONCLUSION

The most recent estimates from UNAIDS indicate that approximately 7,100 people become infected with HIV daily and for every person initiated on treatment, two new infections occur. In the meantime, several countries have achieved substantial reductions in HIV incidence, in many instances without a clear reason to explain this outcome.

Providing treatment for everyone who needs it is at present unsustainable. New approaches for extending treatment for both its life-saving potential and its prevention benefit need to be developed. Substantial progress has been made in the development of HIV vaccines; results from the Thai RV144 trial and the identification of new anti-HIV antibodies with broadly neutralizing potential has injected new enthusiasm into this field which has suffered several setbacks in the past. An AIDS vaccine remains an important hope for the control of HIV/AIDS, but its realization is still several years away.

None of the existing HIV prevention strategies or technologies will, in isolation, be able to solve the AIDS pandemic. Rather, a synergistic combination of effective prevention strategies such as behavior change, HIV testing, circumcision, and widespread access to male and female condoms will be needed at high levels of coverage. At the same time, AIDS treatment and prevention needs to be integrated, to take advantage of "treatment for prevention" strategies, effective microbicides, or oral PrEP. Combining the recently identified benefits of antiretrovirals either as prophylaxis in HIV-uninfected people or as "treatment for prevention" in HIV-infected people with interventions like medical male circumcision and condom promotion could create the synergy necessary to turn the tide against HIV. With the addition of antiretroviral drugs to the prevention arsenal, stopping the HIV epidemic is now within our grasp.

REFERENCES

[1] UNAIDS. UNAIDS Report on the Global AIDS Epidemic 2010. Geneva: Joint United Nations Programme on HIV/AIDS; 2010. Available from: http://www.unaids.org/globalreport/ [accessed 11.02.11].

[2] Gray RH, Wawer MJ, Brookmeyer R, et al. Probability of HIV-1 transmission per coital act in monogamous, heterosexual, HIV-1-discordant couples in Rakai, Uganda. Lancet 2001;357 (9263):1149–53.

[3] Morris M, Kretzschmar M. Concurrent partnerships and the spread of HIV. AIDS 1997;11:641–8.

[4] Cleland J, Ali MM. Sexual abstinence, contraception, and condom use by young African women: a secondary analysis of survey data. Lancet 2006;368 (9549):1788–93.

[5] Pettifor AE, Rees HV, Kleinschmidt I, et al. Young people's sexual health in South Africa: HIV prevalence and sexual behaviors from a nationally representative household survey. AIDS 2005;19(14):1525–34.

[6] Nnko S, Boerma JT, Urassa M, et al. Secretive females or swaggering males? An assessment of the quality of sexual partnership reporting in rural Tanzania. Soc Sci Med 2004;59 (2):299–310.

[7] Lurie M, Rosenthal S. Concurrent partnerships as a driver of the HIV epidemic in sub-Saharan Africa? The evidence is limited. AIDS Behav 2010;14(1):17–24.

[8] Morris M, Epstein H, Wawer M, Jones JH. Timing is everything: international variations in historical sexual partnership concurrency and HIV prevalence. PLoS ONE 2010;5 (11):1706–28.

[9] Gregson S, Nyamukapa CA, Garnett GP, et al. Sexual mixing patterns and sex-differentials in teenage exposure to HIV infection in rural Zimbabwe. Lancet 2002;359 (9321):1896–903.

[10] DHS. Demographic Health Survey website 2005. http://www.measuredhs.com/.

[11] Eaton L, Flisher AJ, Aaro LE. Unsafe sexual behaviour in South African youth. Soc Sci Med 2003;56 (1):149–65.

[12] Rosengard C, Adler NE, Gurvey JE, et al. Protective role of health values in adolescents' future intentions to use condoms. J Adolesc Health 2001;29(3):200–7.

[13] Worth D. Sexual decision-making and AIDS: why condom promotion among vulnerable women is likely to fail. Stud Fam Plann 1989;20(6 Pt 1):297–307.

[14] Reddy P, Meyer-Weitz A, van den Borne B, Kok G. Determinants of condom-use behaviour among STD clinic attenders in South Africa. Int J STD AIDS 2000;11 (8):521–30.

[15] The Voluntary HIV-1 Counseling, and Testing Efficacy Study Group. Efficacy of voluntary HIV-1 counselling and testing in individuals and couples in Kenya, Tanzania, and Trinidada: a randomised trial. Lancet 2000;356:103–12.

[16] Sweat M, Gregorich S, Sangiwa G, et al. Cost-effectiveness of voluntary HIV-1 counselling and testing in reducing sexual transmission of HIV-1 in Kenya and Tanzania. Lancet 2000;356:113–21.

[17] Shisana O, Rehle T, Simbayi LC, et al. South African National HIV Prevalence, HIV Incidence, Behaviour and Communication Survey. Cape Town: Human Sciences Research Council Press; 2005.

[18] Marks G, Crepaz N, Janssen RS. Estimating sexual transmission of HIV from persons aware and unaware that they are infected with the virus in the USA. AIDS 2006;20 (10):1447–50.

[19] Siegfried N, Muller M, Deeks J, et al. HIV and male circumcision—a systematic review with assessment of the quality of studies. Lancet Infect Dis 2005;5(3):165–73.

[20] WHO, UNAIDS. Progress in male circumcision scale-up. country implementation update, December 2009. Geneva: Switzerland; 2009.

Available from: http://malecircumcision.org/documents/MC_country_update_web.pdf [accessed 11.02.11].

[21] Williams BG, Lloyd-Smith JO, Gouws E, et al. The potential impact of male circumcision on HIV in Sub-Saharan Africa. PLoS Med 2006;3 (7):e262.

[22] WHO. Global Prevalence and Incidence of Selected Curable Sexually Transmitted Infections: Overview and Estimates, Available from: http://www.who.int/docstore/hiv/GRSTI/who_hiv_aids_2001.02.pdf; 2001.

[23] Cohen MS. Sexually transmitted diseases enhance HIV transmission: no longer a hypothesis. Lancet 1998;351(Suppl. 3):5–7.

[24] Fleming DT, Wasserheit JN. From epidemiological synergy to public health policy and practice: the contribution of other sexually transmitted diseases to sexual transmission of HIV infection. Sex Transm Infect 1999;75(1):3–17.

[25] Grosskurth H, Mosha F, Todd J, et al. Impact of improved treatment of sexually transmitted diseases on HIV infection in rural Tanzania: randomised controlled trial. Lancet 1995;346(8974):530–6.

[26] Padian NS, McCoy SI, Balkus JE, Wasserheit JN. Weighing the gold in the gold standard: challenges in HIV prevention research. AIDS 2010;24 (5):621–35.

[27] Stein ZA. HIV prevention: the need for methods women can use. Am J Public Health 1990;80(4):460–2.

[28] Abdool Karim Q, Abdool Karim SS, et al. Effectiveness and safety of tenofovir gel, an antiretroviral microbicide, for the prevention of HIV infection in women. Science 2010;329:1168–74.

[29] Williams BG, Abdool Karim SS, Gouws E, Abdool Karim Q. Potential impact of tenofovir gel on the HIV epidemic in South Africa. XVIII International AIDS Conference. Vienna, Austria; 2010.

[30] Grant RM, Lama JR, Anderson PL, et al. Preexposure chemoprophylaxis for HIV

prevention in men who have sex with men. N Engl J Med 2010;363 (27):2587–99.

[31] Centers for Disease Control and Prevention. Interim guidance: preexposure prophylaxis for the prevention of HIV infection in men who have sex with men. MMWR Morb Mortal Wkly Rep 2011;60 (3):65–8.

[32] FHI . FHI Statement on the FEM-PrEP HIV Prevention Study [cited 2011 18 April 2011]. Available from: http://minilicious.wordpress.com/2011/04/18/fhi-statement-on-the-fem-prep-hiv-prevention-study/; 2011.

[33] Abbas U, Glaubius R, Mubayi A, et al. Predicting the Impact of ART and PrEP with Overlapping Regimens on HIV Transmission and Drug Resistance in South Africa [abstract #98LB]. 18th Conference on Retroviruses and Opportunistic Infections. Boston, Massachusetts; 2011.

[34] Quinn TC, Wawer MJ, Sewankambo N, et al. Viral load and heterosexual transmission of human immunodeficiency virus type 1. N Engl J Med 2000;342(13):921–9.

[35] HIV Prevention Trials Network . Press release: Initiation of Antiretroviral Treatment Protects Uninfected Sexual Partners from HIV Infection (HPTN Study 052) [cited 2011 13 May]. Available from: http://www.hptn.org/web%20documents/PressReleases/HPTN052PressReleaseFINAL5_12_118am.pdf; 2011.

[36] Donnell D, Baeten JM, Kiarie J, et al. Heterosexual HIV-1 transmission after initiation of antiretroviral therapy: a prospective cohort analysis. Lancet 2010;375 (9731):2092–8.

[37] Granich RM, Gilks CF, Dye C, et al. Universal voluntary HIV testing with immediate antiretroviral therapy as a strategy for elimination of HIV transmission: a mathematical model. Lancet 2009;373(9657):48–57.

[38] Fisher JD, Cornman DH, Osborn CY, et al. Clinician-initiated HIV risk reduction intervention for HIV-positive persons: Formative Research, Acceptability, and Fidelity

of the Options Project. J Acquir Immune Defic Syndr 2004;37 (Suppl. 2):S78–87.

[39] Crepaz N, Lyle C, Wolitski R, et al. Do prevention interventions reduce HIV risk behaviours among people living with HIV? A meta-analytic review of controlled trials. AIDS 2006;20:143–57.

[40] Kennedy CE, Medley AM, Sweat MD, O'Reilly KR. Behavioural interventions for HIV positive prevention in developing countries: a systematic review and meta-analysis. Bull World Health Organ 2010;88(8):615–23.

[41] The Kesho Bora Study Group . Triple antiretroviral compared with zidovudine and single-dose nevirapine prophylaxis during pregnancy and breastfeeding for prevention of mother-to-child transmission of HIV-1 (Kesho Bora study): a randomised controlled trial. Lancet Infect Dis 2011;11 (3):171–80.

[42] WHO. Antiretroviral Drugs for Treating Pregnant Women and Preventing HIV infection in Infants. Recommendations for a Public Health Approach. Geneva, Switzerland: World Health Organisation; 2010.

[43] Coovadia H, Brown E, Maldonado Y, et al. HPTN 046: Efficacy of extended daily infant nvp through age 6 months compared to 6 weeks for postnatal PMTCT of HIV through breastfeeding [Paper 123LB]. 18th Conference of Retroviruses and Opportunistic Infections. Boston, Massachusetts; 2011.

[44] UNAIDS. HIV Prevention among Injecting Drug Users. Geveva, Switzerland: UNAIDS; 2009. Available from: http://data.unaids.org/pub/InformationNote/2009/20090518_hiv_prevention_among_idus_final_en.pdf [accessed 01.03.11].

[45] Mathers BM, Degenhardt L, Ali H, et al. HIV prevention, treatment, and care services for people who inject drugs: a systematic review of global, regional, and national coverage. Lancet 2010;375 (9719):1014–28.

[46] Baggaley RF, Boily MC, White RG, Alary M. Risk of HIV-1 transmission for parenteral exposure and blood transfusion: a systematic review and meta-analysis. AIDS 2006;20 (6):805–12.

[47] WHO. The Safety of Immunization Practices Improves over Last Five Years, but Challenges Remain. Geneva, Switzerland: World Health Organisation; 2005.

[48] Cardo DM, Culver DH, Ciesielski CA, et al. A case-control study of HIV seroconversion in health care workers after percutaneous exposure. Centers for Disease Control and Prevention Needlestick Surveillance Group. N Engl J Med 1997;337 (21):1485–90.

[49] Smith DK, Grohskopf LA, Black RJ, et al. Antiretroviral postexposure prophylaxis after sexual, injection-drug use, or other nonoccupational exposure to HIV in the United States: recommendations from the U.S. Department of Health and Human Services. MMWR Recomm Rep 2005;54(RR-2):1–20.

[50] Panlilio AL, Cardo DM, Grohskopf LA, et al. Updated U.S. Public Health Service guidelines for the management of occupational exposures to HIV and recommendations for postexposure prophylaxis. MMWR Recomm Rep 2005;54(RR-9):1–17.

[51] Martin JN, Roland ME, Neilands TB, et al. Use of postexposure prophylaxis against HIV infection following sexual exposure does not lead to increases in high-risk behavior. AIDS 2004;18 (5):787–92.

[52] Rerks-Ngarm S, Pitisuttithum P, Nitayaphan S, et al. Vaccination with ALVAC and AIDSVAX to prevent HIV-1 infection in Thailand. N Engl J Med 2009;361 (23):2209–20.

[53] Pancera M, McLellan JS, Wu X, et al. Crystal structure of PG16 and chimeric dissection with somatically related PG9: structure–function analysis of two quaternary-specific antibodies that effectively neutralize HIV-1. J Virol 2010;84 (16):8098–110.

Chapter | 10 |

Laboratory testing for HIV infection

James C. Shepherd, Oliver Laeyendecker, Thomas C. Quinn

INTRODUCTION

In the 30 years since HIV infection was first recognized it has spurred the development of a number of laboratory tests to aid in the diagnosis and management of the disease. The use of these tests has become well established in America and Europe and there are a number of up-to-date reviews of HIV laboratory testing available for these areas [1]. There is less experience with using laboratory testing in the developing world where HIV subtypes may be different, host responses to the virus may vary, and technical and financial resources may be limited. Much experience has been gained since 2005 with the expansion of testing and treatment programs in sub-Saharan Africa and Asia. In this chapter, laboratory tests for the diagnosis and management of HIV infection are described with an emphasis on those in use or applicable to resource-limited settings.

Initially, tests for the diagnosis of HIV infection, including tests of body fluids other than blood, and tests for incident versus prevalent infections, are described. Next, tests that measure the robustness of the immune system, including relatively simple tests for measuring CD4 T cells are described. Tests that measure the amount of virus present in an individual for diagnosis, prognosis, and monitoring of therapy are then presented. Finally, an overview of tests that detect drug resistance mutations in HIV are also described. A brief additional section on two tests (HLA-B5701 testing and HIV tropism testing) has been included. None of these tests are valuable without accurate quality control procedures for validating the results being generated. Pricing[1] for each

of the test kits are shown when possible but do not reflect technician costs, which vary greatly by country and by region. Significant price reductions for some reagents have been negotiated by the World Health Organization (WHO) and the Clinton Foundation (http://www.clintonfoundation.org) in order to make these tests more affordable.

DIAGNOSTIC TESTING

During, or shortly after, the clinical presentation of acute retroviral infection, IgM antibodies to Gag (p17, p24, p55) and Env (gp41,120,160) first appear [2]. This response seems similar throughout the world, regardless of HIV subtype or host population [3]. The appearance of the IgM response is followed weeks to months later by IgG antibodies to Gag and Env epitopes and later still to viral enzymes and regulatory proteins. The time to first detectable IgG seroconversion by enzyme immunoassay in most studies in Europe and America is 2 weeks with a median of 3–4 weeks [2]. Almost all newly HIV-infected individuals will have detectable IgG by 6 months.

Currently the most established tests for detecting HIV infection rely on an enzyme-linked immunoabsorbent assay (ELISA) as an initial screening test (cost US\$1–1.50 per test). This method involves coating a solid surface such as the plastic of a 96 well plate with antigen and using this as an affinity matrix for IgG present in a serum sample. First-generation ELISA used crude lysates of HIV as antigen, followed by second- and third-generation tests using increasingly refined recombinant preparations of HIV proteins to coat the plastic. Current fourth-generation tests use a combination of IgG antibody capture by the immobilized recombinant antigen and HIV antigen capture by immobilized antibody simultaneously in the same reaction to

---

[1]Prices are quoted from UNAIDS, UNICEF, WHO, MSF—sources and prices of selected drugs and diagnostics for people living with HIV/AIDS; http://www.unaids.org/en/in+focus June 2004.

increase sensitivity [4]. The consequent reduction in the "window period," particularly in developing world areas where incident infection is frequent, is important for reducing the number of false-negative results.

The mechanics of ELISA lend themselves to high throughput, rapid testing with automation and thus is the preferred screening test in the developed world. The US FDA and the WHO have validated a number of these assays for use worldwide (see http://www.fda.gov/cber/products/testkits/htm; http://www.who.int/diagnostics_laboratory/evaluations/hiv/en). The ELISA has also been evaluated in less developed countries with a variety of HIV subtypes and similar results for accuracy have been obtained [3, 5]. The cost–benefit analysis of frequency of HIV testing will depend on the background risk of the population and the background incidence in the population but in developed countries testing is rarely recommended more frequently than annually.

Despite high specificity, the use of ELISA in populations where the prevalence of disease is low will lead to a high proportion of positive results being false. Thus, the preferred testing strategy in the developed world is to confirm positive or indeterminate (an intermediate colorimetric reaction) results in the ELISA with a second test, Western blot. This uses a similar concept to ELISA but the immobilized antigens are first separated by size through SDS-PAGE electrophoresis and then bound to a solid medium. Antibody reactivity to different-sized proteins of HIV can be determined. The criteria for a Western blot positive test vary depending on the manufacturer of the test kit and the fluid being tested. In general, sera with antibodies reactive to gp120 and gp160 plus either gp41 or p24 must be present to confirm a positive ELISA [2]. Western blots require significant time and resources and are costly (US$11 per test),

and therefore are not suited to many parts of the world where the prevalence of HIV is high.

A test that has worked well in resource-poor areas is the rapid HIV test. There are several of these approved for use by both the FDA and the WHO. The basic method requires spotting of whole blood or serum/plasma on a test strip with HIV antigen prebound (http://www.cdc.gov/hiv/rapid_testing). Lateral chromatography of the antibodies within the test strip and reaction with the immobilized HIV proteins is revealed colorimetrically in a "pregnancy test" fashion within minutes. These tests have higher than 99% sensitivity and specificity when combined with a confirmatory test such as Western blot in the developed world or a second rapid test in the developing world [6]. The lack of sample preparation, ease of storage, simple visual readout, speed, and cost (US$0.47–1.30) make these tests attractive for use all over the world and they have been evaluated in a number of African countries where their sensitivity and specificity profiles have been comparable with results in Europe and America [5, 7, 8]. A number of algorithms (Fig. 10.1) have been developed for confirmation of rapid testing results without resorting to ELISA or Western blotting and these have been validated in different resource-poor settings [9].

Other screening strategies for HIV infection have tested for the presence of antibodies in fluids other than blood. Levels of IgG are much lower in urine than in plasma but a highly sensitive screening test for urine, similar to ELISA, has a reported sensitivity of 99% and a specificity of 94% and is FDA approved [10]. A positive result should be confirmed with a standard serological ELISA. Saliva contains much higher concentrations of IgA and IgG than blood and there is an FDA-approved collection method involving soaking a pad in the mouth and then testing the

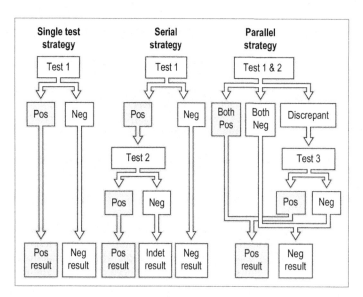

Figure 10.1 Testing algorithm for use with rapid testing. Pos, positive; Neg, negative; Indet, indeterminate.

adsorbed antibodies in a standard ELISA/Western blot system, which is extremely sensitive and specific [11]. An ELISA test for IgG in cervico-vaginal secretions is available. The principal benefit of these approaches lies in their convenience for the patient and the lessened risk of needle-stick injury to the tester, but their reliance on ELISA for screening or confirmation make them less adaptable to the developing world.

Vertical transmission of HIV presents a particular diagnostic challenge as placentally transfered maternal antibodies can persist in the neonate for as long as 18 months post-partum [12]. Nucleic acid testing (DNA or RNA) provides the most sensitive method for diagnosing HIV in an infant. At 4–6 weeks, most infants can be diagnosed using these methods.

For epidemiological purposes, it is important to measure the incidence of HIV infection in populations. Recently, chronically infected individuals can be differentiated by biological changes that occur as the immune system responds over time to the infection [13]. The evolution of the immune response is shown in Figure 10.2. There is a window period of approximately 3 weeks, where HIV RNA can be detected but an antibody response to the virus is not detectable. During the initial development of the humoral response, the strength of binding and concentration of antibody specific for HIV increases with time. There is also a switching of the class of antibody to the virus. An epidemiological tool for determining incidence rates from cross-sectional population sampling exploit these biologic differences between incident and chronically infected individuals. Currently the only commercially available assay is the BED-capture EIA (BED-CEIA), though many groups have developed their own assays [14]. Polymerase chain reaction (PCR) of pooled blood samples for detecting viral RNA positive samples before antibody has developed has been pioneered in North Carolina, USA, and may be the most sensitive

and specific method for detecting incident infection in at-risk populations, but requires surveys in excess of 50,000 individuals [15]. It has not been tested in resource-poor areas but may be rapidly adaptable to Eastern Europe or China where PCR technology is already available. For all cross-sectional incidence approaches, sample sizes in the thousands are needed with an accurate knowledge of factors associated with misclassification.

Laboratory diagnosis of HIV-2 is frequently necessary depending on geographical area, travel, and exposure history. Infection with HIV-2 is prevalent in West Africa and in many cases, HIV-1-infected people are also infected with HIV-2, although it is rare in the rest of the world. The virus is less transmissible, replicates more slowly, and causes a slower rate of T cell decline and there are few standardized tests useful for management. The diagnostic testing methodology for HIV-2 is identical to that for HIV-1, except that the serological tests are specific for antibodies against HIV-2 proteins. Currently there is one commercially available assay for HIV-2 Western blot testing (HIVBlot 2.2-Genelabs) but no viral load test. However, HIV-2 viral load data can be generated by real-time RT-PCR using primers specific for HIV-2 [16]. There are rapid test kits and diagnostic ELISA tests available specifically for HIV-2 and one test available for diagnosis of both HIV-1 and HIV-2 simultaneously [17,18], although 20–30% of HIV-1 ELISA tests do not detect antibodies to HIV-2 [1].

MONITORING PATIENT HEALTH

Tests for estimating T lymphocytes

Monitoring of the health of the immune system is accomplished with estimates of the number of CD4 T cells circulating in a person's bloodstream. This is the most

Figure 10.2 Biological changes that occur early in HIV infection. HIV virus in blood increases and falls to a viral set point (RNA, orange line); concentration of antibody specific to HIV increases (Ab, light blue line). The binding strength of antibody specific to HIV antigen increases and plateaus (Ab binding strength, dark blue line); switching of antibody isotype occurs with the temporal appearance of IgG$_3$ specific to HIV (anti-p24 IgG$_3$, green line).

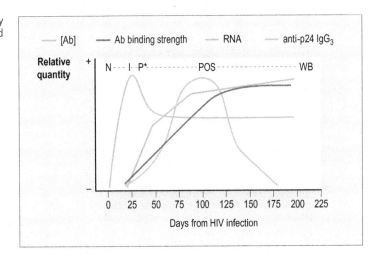

reliable prognostic test available [19] and is the primary means of deciding need for anti-viral treatment. Tests of CD8 T cells are valuable for measuring anti-HIV cytolytic activity as a research tool but their number has not been found to correlate with clinical outcome.

The value of a CD4 determination at any particular time point is approximate, with wide confidence intervals. Thus, the utility of testing is mainly in observing trends. The recommended interval of testing is 3–6 months (see DHHS, WHO guidelines) although some national treatment programs, notably Malawi, have scaled up without widespread CD4 testing. A result markedly different from prior results should be repeated. In addition, many factors other than HIV-1 influence the CD4 count, including diurnal variation, intercurrent illness, corticosteroid use, idiopathic lymphocytopenia, and splenectomy [1]. Of significance in some parts of the world, most notably Brazil and Haiti, is the interaction between HIV-1 and HTLV-1 co-infection. In these patients the true level of immunosuppression is more accurately represented by a CD4 T cell value half as high as that actually measured [20]. The CD4 T cell fraction of total lymphocytes, expressed as a CD4 percentage, is sometimes used to account for variation in the total number of T cells but this has not been found to correlate as accurately with risk for opportunistic infection as the absolute count [21]. The total lymphocyte count has been used with some success in resource-poor areas as a surrogate for T-cell counting, although the sensitivity of this strategy was found to be low in a cohort in Uganda [22].

The standard method in America and Europe for measuring CD4 T cells is by flow cytometry. This requires a fresh blood sample and antibody reagents specific for CD4 and CD8 that are labeled with fluorescent molecules. The number of labeled cells present is counted by flow of individual cells past a fluorescence detector. This is expensive, both in equipment and in reagents (US$6–20 per test), and requires frequent calibration of the machine. A variation on standard flow cytometry for CD4 counting is leukogating. The primary advantage of leukogating is the ability to do the analysis in a single reaction with a lowered cost of reagents (<US$4 per test) but still requires an expensive flow cytometer for detection. For medium throughput applications, a microflow method that is more portable and uses smaller volumes has been developed (Guava Technologies). Lower throughput methods such as FACSCount (Becton-Dickinson) and PointCare (Beckman Coulter) give automated, absolute, or absolute plus percentage CD4 counts, respectively, making the PointCare machine more useful for pediatric monitoring. Alternative, low throughput (<10 samples per day) methods that have been developed specifically for resource-limited laboratories are Cyto-Spheres (Beckman Coulter) (US$4–8 per test) and Dynabeads (Dynal Biotech) (US$3–5 per test). The former uses latex beads coated with anti-CD4 monoclonal antibody to "rosette"

CD4 lymphocytes that can then be counted in a hematocytometer by light microscopy. The latter uses magnetic beads that are coated with anti-CD4 antibody to purify CD4 lymphocytes from whole blood using a magnet. A newer test, the PIMA POC CD4 Counter (Clondial Gmbh), consists of a disposable test cartridge containing dried reagents. All of these "low-tech" methods correlate well with flow cytometry both in Europe and in the developing world [23].

Routine laboratory testing

Most of this chapter describes in detail the laboratory testing unique to the diagnosis and management of HIV. However, there are a number of routine screening tests that should be repeated at intervals during the management of HIV infection and these are summarized in Table 10.1 for a North American setting. It should be remembered that the normal parameters for most of these tests have been developed in North American and European populations and will need to be adjusted to local population norms. In addition, the differences in prevalence of opportunistic pathogens in different parts of the world (TB, HBV vs HCV, *cryptococcosis* vs toxoplasmosis, etc.) create different imperatives for screening.

MONITORING VIRAL REPLICATION

Viral load testing

Assays that detect the virus itself have been developed for two purposes—to detect incident infection earlier than possible with antibody testing and, more frequently, to monitor antiretroviral therapy (ART). Antigen capture assays that detect p24, an early viral antigen, have been evaluated for early diagnosis and monitoring of therapy and have been incorporated into the strategy of antibody/antigen detection in the fourth-generation ELISA [4]. As a screening tool in developed countries for early infection it has not been as popular as the STARHS technique or more sensitive nucleic acid detection methods. Limited evidence has suggested that p24 quantification (US$10 per test) may potentially replace nucleic acid quantification as a measure of viral load [24]. In the developing world the reliance of p24 detection on ELISA-type technology has hampered its widespread use for monitoring of therapy, although it has been successfully used to reduce the "window period" in subtype E infections in a research study [25]. There is evidence that although the specificity of p24 testing is close to 100% the sensitivity in non-subtype B infections can be quite low [26].

Much more widely used are tests that detect and measure viral nucleic acid in blood and other body fluids. The most

Table 10.1 Pocket guide to adult HIV/AIDS treatment, January 2010

TEST	COMMENT
HIV serology	Sensitivity and specificity standard serology is >99% False positives: human error False negatives: usually "window period" Acute HIV: HIV RNA level >10,000 copies/mL; confirm seroconversion Rapid tests: confirm positives
CD4	Reproducibility: 95% CI = 30% False high levels—splenectomy (use CD4%) concurrent HTLV-1 Repeat every 3–6 months %—CD4 >500 = >29%, 200–500 = 14–28%, <200 = <14%
HIV viral load	Reproducibility: 95% CI = 0.3 $\log_{10}$ copies/mL or 50% Repeat every 3–4 months Repeat at 2–6 weeks after starting or changing ART, then every 3–4 months
CBC	Repeat every 3–6 months; more frequently as indicated Macrocytosis with AZT and d4T
Chemical profile	Include LFT and renal function Repeat LFT with all Pls and NNRTIs, ETOH, and hepatitis Repeat renal function with IDV and TDF
Hepatitis screen	Anti-HCV, anti-HAV anti-HbsAg (if prior vaccine) or anti-HBcAg Abnormal LFT: get anti-HCV and HBsAg Positive anti-HCV: get quantitative HCV Neg anti-HBs: vaccinate for HBV Pos HBsAg or anti-HCV: get LFTs Neg anti-HAV: HAV vaccine routine
Fasting lipid profile and glucose	Patient at risk Baseline for ART; repeat at 3–6 months and then yearly
Toxoplasma IgG	10–15% positive in USA If negative repeat when symptomatic or when CD4 < 100
PPD	Indicated if no history of TB or prior positive PPD Induration >5 mm is indication for INH × 9 months
PAP smear	Baseline, at 6 months and then annual; if "inadequate"—repeat; if atypia—refer to gynecologist
Chest X-ray	Indicated with pulmonary sx, positive PPD or history of chest disease; some do baseline X-ray routinely
Urinary NAAT for gonorrhea and chlamydia	"Consider" in sexually active patients Repeat at 6–12-month intervals depending on risk
HLA-B 5701 test	Screening for ABC treatment
Tropism assay	If plan to use CCR5 antagonist (MVC)
VDRL	Baseline and repeat annually in sexually active patients Confirm positives with FTA-ABS
Renal screen	Urinalysis and creatinine If ≥1+ proteinuria or elevated creatinine: quantify urine protein and do renal ultrasound
G6PD level	Consider: most susceptible are men of African, Mediterranean, Asian, or Sephardic Jewish descent. If positive, avoid oxidant drugs dapsone and primaquine; ? sulfonamide

commonly used of these in the developed world is reverse-transcriptase polymerase chain reaction (RT-PCR) of viral RNA isolated from plasma (US$20–100 per test). Viral RNA is extracted and transcribed to single-stranded DNA and amplified by PCR. There is an ultrasensitive version of this test that can reliably measure virus as low as 50 RNA copies/mL in plasma as well as a standard version with sensitivity to 400 RNA copies/mL. There are tests in development that can measure virus at levels as low as 20 copies/mL. Sensitivity for diagnosis is excellent but specificity is significantly lower than serology and therefore these tests are not routinely recommended for primary screening, except for acute HIV infection [27]. The level of viral replication is very high during acute HIV infection and can be used for diagnosis of early HIV infection, particularly if the assay consistently reports an elevated viral load of at least 100,000 copies/mL. Values below 10,000 copies/mL are to be viewed with suspicion in the diagnosis of acute HIV [28]. Another proven technology frequently used for the quantification of HIV viral loads is branched DNA (bDNA). In this method, HIV RNA is captured by one set of immobilized oligonucleotides and detected by a second set. Amplification of the target is achieved by hybridizing with a successive set of probes attached to a signaling enzyme. A third and newer viral load testing methodology is NASBA (nucleic-acid sequence-based amplification). The Nuclisens EasyQ (bioMérieux) combined proprietary NASBA with real-time detection using molecular beacons in a single step.

The principal use of viral load monitoring is in monitoring of therapy. It is well established in Europe and America that those individuals with higher viral loads progress to AIDS more rapidly than those with lower viral loads [19]. It is also well established in developing world practice that the most sensitive test for detecting failure of ART is viral load. Thus, the very first sign that the virus is no longer completely susceptible to the antiretroviral drugs administered is a rising viral load rather than a falling CD4 cell count. Initial therapy should result in a 10-fold decrease in viral load within 1 week of initiating therapy and a 100-fold decline by 4 weeks [1]. Successfully treated patients should have a viral load below the limit of detection by an ultrasensitive test at 3 months. Reasons for declines in viral loads less dramatic than these after initiation of ART may be poor adherence with therapy or viral resistance to drugs. The standard error of viral load measurement is approximately 0.3 log copies/mL so any change in viral load less than this is not considered significant.

Current practice guidelines (Department of Health and Social Services, USA, http://www.aidsinfo.nih.gov) recommend a baseline viral load followed by regular measurements every 3 months, regardless of whether the patient is on therapy or not. This allows a rapid response to the emergence of resistant virus in individuals already on drug therapy, and initiation of therapy in those with a rising viral load and a falling CD4 count. It has been observed that

viral RNA detection by PCR behaves slightly differently to RNA detection by branched-chain DNA methods. The low cut-off for sensitivity is 50 copies/mL with PCR-based methods and 75 copies/mL with bDNA methods. Often a persistently positive result at the very low range of PCR will be below detection by bDNA. The clinical significance of these differences is unclear as patients with a persistent but very low level of viremia do not appear to collect resistance mutations [29].

Evidence that the RT-PCR-, bDNA-, and NASBA-based measurements are adaptable to non-subtype B HIV-1 is limited but current studies suggest that bDNA-based measurements may be the most reliable with subtypes A through G [30]. Of the PCR-based tests, the Roche Amplicor version 1.5 demonstrated good reproducibility. Nevertheless, the requirements for an antiseptic, dust-free environment, constant electricity, pure water, and significant equipment expenditure make viral nucleic acid detection one of the hardest tests to introduce into resource-poor laboratories. For these reasons, as well as cost, most resource-limited treatment programs have chosen to scale-up without any viral load testing and rely on immunological or clinical signs and symptoms to detect failure of ART. However, monitoring by clinical symptoms and signs or by only immunologic changes has been shown to be inaccurate in assessing those who are failing treatment [31]. There remains an urgent need for development of viral detection methods that are useful clinically but do not require delicate equipment or distilled water. Detection of viral DNA is extremely sensitive and DNA is a more stable molecule than RNA, but there are limited data on the correlation between circulating pro-viral DNA and viral replication.

Monitoring drug resistance mutations

The final cornerstone of laboratory monitoring of HIV is drug resistance testing. The importance of this is growing as the prevalence of HIV strains resistant to ART grows and the transmission of drug-resistant strains increases. Current estimates in the USA put the frequency of new infections caused by viruses with at least one major drug resistance mutation at around 10–25% [32]. This figure may be reached in the developing world as antiretrovirals are increasingly used, although levels of adherence have been sufficiently high to limit widespread drug resistance so far. The exception is common NNRTI resistance as a result of single-dose nevirapine use for prevention of vertical transmission, which is well documented [33]. The indications for resistance testing are growing from the original FDA-approved indications for rational drug selection in a patient on ART who has had either a less than satisfactory response to a new regimen or a rising viral load on an established regimen [33]. It is now recommended by many authorities for patients with new or chronic infections prior to selection of their first ART regimen (DHHS, http://www.aidsinfo.nih.gov/guidelines; IAS-USA, http://www.iasusa.org). It is proposed by WHO to monitor treatment of naïve individuals by country and regional sampling to detect the rate of drug-resistant viral transmission in different geographical areas of the developing world and respond accordingly (http://www.who.int/hiv/).

The cheapest and most commonly used test of resistant mutations is genotypic (US$100–150 per test), as opposed to the more time-consuming and laborious phenotypic testing (US$800–1000 per test). Genotyping involves amplification of the reverse transcriptase and protease genes by RT-PCR from the circulating swarm of viral RNA and DNA sequencing of the major products of the amplification. Currently there are two FDA-approved assays for the genotypic assessment for resistant virus (Trugene by Visible Genetics and ViroSeq by Applied Biosystems)[34, 35]. The mutations are reported as amino acid substitutions at specific numbered codons and the interpretation of drug susceptibility is aided by computer algorithms using rules generated from past data, most of which have been generated from sequencing of subtype B [33]. The test requires a viral load of at least 500 copies/mL and in most cases unless the selecting drug is present or recently withdrawn, the predominant species detected will be wild-type virus, which tends to outgrow mutated virus. Indeed, recent evidence suggests that transmitted drug-resistant virus may revert to wild type over time in the absence of drug selection pressure [36]. The extraction of viral RNA, amplification by RT-PCR, and sequencing of amplified products and their analysis, requires a laboratory with stable electricity, clean water, a highly trained staff, a dedicated laboratory manager, and initial investment in instrumentation of well over US$100,000.

The phenotyping assay also involves an initial amplification of the reverse transcriptase and protease genes, which are then cloned into an HIV pseudotyping vector that is then grown in the presence of permissive tissue culture cells and drug. The results are easier to interpret for single agents—the virus either grows efficiently in the drug's presence or not, but combinations of drugs in a phenotypic assay are still being evaluated [37]. The reliance on tissue culture imposes the rigors of sterility upon a laboratory and this may limit its attractiveness to resource-limited sites.

There is a pressing need for more information on mutations and mutational pathways in HIV-1 subtypes other than B and correlations between codon substitutions and phenotypic changes in drug susceptibility [38]. As more HIV-infected people are treated all over the world these data will become invaluable for guiding therapeutic decisions. The Stanford-IAS website (http://hivdb.stanford.edu) is a valuable and growing resource for this information.

Tests for treatment selection

Two new tests have been introduced since this chapter was last written. One, a test of the host genetics, detects the presence or absence of *Human Lymphocyte Antigen* allele (*HLA*) *B5701* (Labcorp, $100). A negative test for *HLAB5701* has a 100% negative predictive value for abacavir hypersensitivity reactions and testing is recommended before initiation of abacavir. *HLAB5701* is present in about 10% of Caucasians but is present in less than 1% of Africans [39]. The other new test detects viral tropism (either CCR5-tropic, CXCR4-tropic, or dual/mixed), which measures the HIV co-receptor molecule preference on CD4 T cells. The only current FDA-approved entry inhibitors are CCR5 antagonists and the indication for tropism testing is in preparation for use of one of these drugs. If CXCR4-tropic virus is present, then current entry inhibitors are contraindicated. The test is expensive (Trofile, Monogram Biosciences; $2000), takes several weeks, and has limited the widespread use of entry inhibitors up to now. There is evidence that, despite subtype differences in co-receptor tropism, entry inhibitors may be valuable in resource-limited settings but their cost and the cost of tropism testing has limited their use.

QUALITY ASSURANCE AND QUALITY CONTROL

As with all clinically useful tests, QA/QC is crucial. The accuracy of the results of all the tests described here are highly dependent upon the level of training of the technical staff and the maintenance and calibration of the equipment. In addition, the reproducibility of testing must be assured. Thus all labs performing laboratory monitoring for HIV diagnosis and management should be part of a network where each site can check their results against a panel of standards validated at other sites. In addition, there should be a mechanism whereby "low-tech" tests can be compared with "high-tech" gold standard tests at suitable intervals. Biological standards can be purchased commercially. Standards for testing in the USA are determined by the College of American Pathology (http://www.cap.org). The WHO is facilitating the establishment of an electronic data monitoring system for QA/QC of resource-poor laboratories.

REFERENCES

[1] Bartlett JG, Gallant JE. Medical Management of HIV Infection. Baltimore, MD: Johns Hopkins Medicine Health Publishing Business Group; 2010.

[2] Mylonakis E, Paliou M, Lally M, et al. Laboratory testing for infection with the human immunodeficiency virus: established and novel approaches. Am J Med 2000;109:568–76.

[3] Beelaert G, Vercauteren G, Fransen K, et al. Comparative evaluation of eight commercial enzyme linked immunosorbent assays and 14 simple assays for detection of antibodies to HIV. J Virol Methods 2002;105:197–206.

[4] Weber B, Meier T, Enders G. Fourth generation human immunodeficiency virus (HIV) screening assays with an improved sensitivity for p24 antigen close the second diagnostic window in primary HIV infection. J Clin Virol 2002;25:357–9.

[5] Makuwa M, Souquiere S, Niangui MT, et al. Reliability of rapid diagnostic tests for HIV variant infection. J Virol Methods 2002;103:183–90.

[6] Urassa W, Nozohoor S, Jaffer S, et al. Evaluation of an alternative confirmatory strategy for the diagnosis of HIV infection in Dar Es Salaam, Tanzania, based on simple rapid assays. J Virol Methods 2002;100:115–20.

[7] Solomon SS, Pulimi S, Rodriguez II, et al. Dried blood spots are an acceptable and useful HIV surveillance tool in a remote developing world setting. Int J STD AIDS 2004;15:658–61.

[8] Phili R, Vardas E. Evaluation of a rapid human immunodeficiency virus test at two community clinics in Kwazulu-Natal. S Afr Med J 2002;92:818–21.

[9] Wright RJ, Stringer JS. Rapid testing strategies for HIV-1 serodiagnosis in high-prevalence African settings. Am J Prev Med 2004;27:42–8.

[10] Urnovitz HB, Sturge JC, Gottfried TD, et al. Urine antibody tests: new insights into the dynamics of HIV-1 infection. Clin Chem 1999;45:1602–13.

[11] de Morgado Moura Machedo JE, Kayita J, Bakaki P, et al. IgA antibodies to human immunodeficiency virus in serum, saliva and urine for early diagnosis of immunodeficiency virus infection in Ugandan infants. Pediatr Infect Dis J 2003;22:193–5.

[12] Committee on Pediatric AIDS. Identification and care of HIV-exposed and HIV-infected infants, children and adolescents in faster care. Pediatrics 2000;106:149–53.

[13] Busch MP, Pilcher CD, Mastro TD, et al. WHO Working Group on HIV Incidence Assays. Beyond detuning: 10 years of progress and new challenges in the development and application of assays for HIV incidence estimation. AIDS 2010;24 (18):2763–71.

[14] Guy R, Gold J, Calleja JM, Kim AA, et al., WHO Working Group on HIV Incidence Assays. Accuracy of serological assays for detection of recent infection with HIV and estimation of population incidence: a systematic review. Lancet Infect Dis 2009;9(12):747–59. Review. Erratum in Lancet Infect Dis 2010;10(2):82.

[15] Pilcher CD, Fiscus SA, Nguyen TQ, et al. Detection of acute infections during HIV testing in North Carolina. N Engl J Med 2005;352:1873–83.

[16] Ruelle J, Mukadi BK, Schutten M, et al. Quantitative real-time PCR on Lightcycler for the detection of human immunodeficiency virus type 2 (HIV-2). J Virol Methods 2004;117:67–74.

[17] Parekh BS, Pau CP, Granade TC, et al. Oligomeric nature of transmembrane glycoproteins of HIV-2: procedures for their efficient dissociation and preparation of Western blots for diagnosis. AIDS 1991;5:1009–13.

[18] Holguin A. Evaluation of three rapid tests for detection of antibodies to HIV-1 non-B subtypes. J Virol Methods 2004;115:105–7.

[19] Mellors JW, Munoz A, Giorgi JV, et al. Plasma viral load and CD4+ lymphocytes as prognostic markers of HIV-1 infection. Ann Intern Med 1997;126:946–54.

[20] Schechter M, Harrison LH, Halsey NA, et al. Coinfection with human T-cell lymphotropic virus type I and HIV in Brazil. Impact on markers of HIV disease progression. JAMA 1994;271:353–7.

[21] Gebo KA, Gallant JE, Keruly JC, et al. Absolute CD4 vs. CD4 percentage for predicting the risk of opportunistic illness in HIV infection. J Acquir Immune Defic Syndr 2004;36:1028–33.

[22] Kamya MR, Semitala FC, Quinn TC, et al. Total lymphocyte count of 1200 is not a sensitive predictor of CD4 lymphocyte count among patients with HIV disease in Kampala, Uganda. Afr Health Sci 2004;4:94–101.

[23] Didier JM, Kazatchkine MD, Demouchy C, et al. Comparative assessment of five alternative methods for CD4+ T-lymphocyte enumeration for implementation in developing countries. J Acquir Immune Defic Syndr 2001;26:193–5.

[24] Sterling TR, Hoover DR, Astemborski J, et al. Heat-denatured human immunodeficiency virus type 1 protein 24 antigen: prognostic value in adults with early-stage disease. J Infect Dis 2002;186:1181–5.

[25] Weber B, Thorstensson R, Tanprasert S, et al. Reduction of the diagnostic window in three cases of human immunodeficiency-1 subtype E primary infection with fourth-generation HIV screening assays. Vox Sang 2003;85:73–9.

[26] Burgisser P, Vernazza P, Flepp M, et al. Performance of five different assays for the quantification of viral load in persons infected with various subtypes of HIV-1. Swiss HIV Cohort Study. J Acquir Immune Defic Syndr 2000;23:138–44.

[27] Daar ES, Little S, Pitt J, et al. Diagnosis of primary HIV-1 infection. Los Angeles County

Primary HIV Infection Recruitment Network. Ann Intern Med 2001;134:25–9.

[28] Rich JD, Merriman NA, Mylonakis E, et al. Misdiagnosis of HIV infection by HIV-1 plasma viral load testing: a case series. Ann Intern Med 1999;130:37–9.

[29] Kieffer TL, Finucane MM, Nettles RE, et al. Genotypic analysis of HIV-1 drug resistance at the limit of detection: virus production without evolution in treated adults with undetectable HIV loads. J Infect Dis 2004;189:1452–65.

[30] Elbeik T, Alvord WG, Trichavaroj R, et al. Comparative analysis of HIV-1 viral load assays on subtype quantification: Bayer Versant HIV-1 RNA 3.0 versus Roche Amplicor HIV-1 Monitor version 1.5. J Acquir Immune Defic Syndr 2002;29:330–9.

[31] Reynolds SJ, Nakigozi G, Newell K, et al. Failure of immunologic criteria to appropriately identify antiretroviral treatment failure in Uganda. AIDS 2009;23 (6):697–700.

[32] Little SJ, Holte S, Routy JP, et al. Antiretroviral-drug resistance among patients recently infected with HIV. N Engl J Med 2002;347:385–94.

[33] Hirsch MS, Brun-Vezinet F, Clotet B, et al. Antiretroviral drug resistance testing in adults infected with human immunodeficiency virus type 1: 2003 recommendations of an International AIDS Society-USA Panel. Clin Infect Dis 2003;37:113–28.

[34] Eshleman SH, Hoover DR, Chen S, et al. Resistance after single-dose nevirapine prophylaxis emerges in a high proportion of Malawian newborns. AIDS 2005;19: 2167–9.

[35] Tong CY, Mullen J, Kulasegaram R, et al. Genotyping of B and non-B subtypes of human immunodeficiency virus type 1. J Clin Microbiol 2005;43:4623–7.

[36] Gandhi RT, Wurcel A, Rosenberg ES, et al. Progressive reversion of human immunodeficiency virus type 1 resistance mutations in vivo after transmission of a multiply drug-resistant virus. Clin Infect Dis 2003;37:1693–8.

[37] Hachiya A, Matsuoka-Aizawa S, Tsuchiya K, et al. "All-in-One Assay", a direct phenotypic anti-human immunodeficiency virus type 1 drug resistance assay for three-drug combination therapies that takes into consideration in vivo drug concentrations. J Virol Methods 2003;111:43–53.

[38] Visco-Comandini U, Balotta C. Genotypic resistance tests for the management of the HIV-infected patient with non-B viral isolates. Scand J Infect Dis 2003;106: S75–9.

[39] Johnson VA, Brun-Vézinet F, Clotet B, et al. Drug resistance mutations in HIV-1. HIV Therapy 2003;8:36.

Chapter | 11 |

Overview of antiretroviral therapy

Susa Coffey, Paul A. Volberding

INTRODUCTION

Antiretroviral (ARV) therapy (ART) is one of the most dramatic examples of successful drug development in the history of medicine. While current ART cannot eradicate HIV infection, it can reduce HIV replication to extremely low levels and allow the restoration of immune function to safe (though perhaps not normal) levels in the vast majority of treated persons. It thus can make possible the recovery and maintenance of health in a previously progressive and uniformly fatal syndrome. ART can, furthermore, reduce HIV transmission and even prevent initial infection. The obvious benefits of ART realized in wealthy economies are also seen in resource-limited areas in which treatment increasingly is being made available.

Success in ART is not difficult, but does require substantial resources and the careful application of principles learned from clinical trials and from treatment program development. Drugs that form potent multi-agent regimens must be continuously available and affordable. Laboratory assays must be available to diagnose HIV infection and, ideally, to stage the illness and monitor treatment response and toxicity. Also important are assays used to detect ARV resistance both to improve initial response and to adjust regimens that have lost effectiveness. Effective ART also requires access to healthcare providers—physicians and others—sufficiently trained to diagnose infection, to select appropriate drug combinations and to initiate them at the appropriate stage in HIV disease, and to identify treatment failure. Providers must be expert in educating patients in medication adherence and in managing ARV toxicity and drug interactions. They must also be able to adjust regimens to maintain viral suppression despite drug resistance.

This chapter will provide a brief review of the biology of HIV therapy and the essential questions of ARV management including the design and timing of initial combination regimens and of secondary or salvage therapy. It will summarize current ARV drugs with respect to common toxicities, resistance patterns, and drug interactions, but will defer to other chapters that deal with many of these topics in much more detail.

The central goal of HIV therapy is maximal suppression of viral replication in order to allow immune recovery, and to prevent the selection of drug resistance mutations [1–3]. Successful ART must durably restore or maintain immune competence and the control of infections and malignancies that characterize the AIDS syndrome. Beyond that, ART should enhance and extend the healthy life span of treated individuals.

In the resource-rich world, the availability of newer ARV medications and new classes of ARVs has made it possible to achieve virologic suppression even in most patients infected with HIV resistant to multiple ARV agents or entire drug classes [4–6]. For those patients in whom therapy does not fully suppress viremia, ART can still dramatically slow disease progression [7, 8]. While ART does improve immune function and reduce morbidity and mortality associated with HIV (most strikingly in those with lower CD4 counts), control of HIV viremia unfortunately may not result in complete normalization of immune function or complete reversal of the inflammatory state associated with HIV; this is an area of active study [9–11].

THE NATURAL HISTORY OF HIV INFECTION

Untreated HIV infection results in persisting and relatively constant levels of viremia and a progressive immune attrition reflected most obviously, but only in part, by a decline in the numbers of circulating CD4 T lymphocytes [12, 13]. The rate of CD4 cell loss varies widely among infected individuals but averages 60–80 cells/mm^3 annually [14, 15]. Constitutional symptoms and serious infections and malignancies arise with immune attrition, particularly when the peripheral CD4 count falls below 200 cells/mm^3. Many with initial, or acute, primary HIV infection have a 1- to 2-week clinical illness [16, 17]. Following recovery from any symptoms of this acute phase of HIV infection, most are asymptomatic until much later in the disease course [18]. With progressing disease, some experience constitutional signs and symptoms—chronic or recurring fevers, malaise, weight loss, or other evidence of chronic inflammation. Advanced HIV disease, also termed AIDS, when the CD4 count is below 200/mm^3, is punctuated by opportunistic infections and malignancies that range from treatable inconveniences to rapidly fatal and irreversible acute illnesses. While the risk of AIDS-related conditions increases sharply with declining CD4 counts, some illnesses associated with HIV and AIDS may occur at high CD4 levels (e.g. tuberculosis, non-Hodgkin lymphoma). Additionally, a number of so-called "non-AIDS" complications, such as "non-AIDS" malignancies, and cardiovascular, liver, kidney, and neurocognitive disease, may occur at relatively high CD4 counts [11, 19–25]. A number of these complications appear to be associated with persistent immune activation and inflammation present in untreated persons with HIV infection, even at high CD4 counts, and are incompletely reversed by ART [26, 27]. Some researchers have suggested that HIV infection results in what may be considered an acceleration of the normal aging process [26, 27]. While some individuals progress from initial infection to death in as little as 12 months, most are relatively stable for a number of years. A very small number of HIV-infected individuals maintain control of HIV without medications and may survive many years with no apparent ill health [28].

HIV disease is staged by the CD4 count, with numbers above 500/mm^3 considered in the normal range, while those below 200/mm^3 [3] indicate advanced disease or AIDS. As the risk of specific opportunistic diseases correlates closely with the CD4 count, this test is of particular value in patient management. By contrast, levels of HIV viremia are less predictive of disease stage, but may correlate with the rate of disease progression, and may indicate treatment failure.

THE HIV LIFE CYCLE

Reviewed in detail elsewhere, a brief summary of the HIV life cycle focused on targets of existing drugs can help in considering ARV regimen design. These targets will be considered early, middle, or late in the life cycle, corresponding to currently approved ARV drugs blocking cell entry, reverse transcription, integration, or HIV protease processing.

Early targets in the HIV life cycle

After the viral surface glycoprotein gp120 and the cell surface protein CD4 interact in attachment [29], the CD4 changes its conformation to allow the engagement into this complex of a second cell surface protein, the co-receptor, whose natural function is to act as a chemokine receptor, either CCR5 or CXCR4 [30, 31]. The CD4–gp120–chemokine receptor complex in turn activates the viral gp41, which uncoils, inserts a fusion protein into the cell surface membrane, recoils while tethered to the cell, and approximates the viral and cell membranes, resulting in their fusion [32]. The CCR5 chemokine co-receptor is the target of one ARV class, the CCR5 antagonist. It is the first class directed at a human target. The currently available agent is maraviroc; others are in development. The tethered uncoiled gp41 is the target of the fusion inhibitor enfuvirtide. These "early" acting drugs can actually prevent cellular HIV infection, in contrast to other available ARV drugs.

Middle targets in the HIV life cycle

Following membrane fusion, the viral core enters and uncoats in the target cell cytoplasm where the viral genes encoded on the single-strand HIV RNA genome are reverse transcribed into a dual-strand DNA copy [33]. The enzyme that facilitates this, reverse transcriptase, is the target of many ARV drugs, some structural analogs of normal nucleosides or nucleotides [34, 35]. Other drugs that block this enzyme, the non-nucleosides, bind to the enzyme's active site, but have a chemical structure that does not resemble nucleosides [36, 37]. Reverse transcriptase inhibitors of both types only act following cellular infection by HIV. By convention, the nucleosides (or nucleotides)—like reverse transcriptase drugs—are called the NRTIs while the non-nucleoside agents are called the NNRTIs.

After reverse transcription, the dual-stranded HIV DNA virus is incorporated into the host cell's DNA via a process mediated by the viral enzyme integrase. Integrase inhibitors target this enzyme [38]. Raltegravir is the first available integrase inhibitor; others are in development.

Late targets in the HIV life cycle

As the new HIV virion forms inside the cell and then buds into the extracellular environment, trimming of the structural or *gag*-related proteins by HIV protease is necessary for full infectivity. HIV protease inhibitors (PIs) target that enzyme. Most PIs typically are used in combination with low-dose ritonavir. Ritonavir is itself a PI, but in current practice is used only as a pharmacokinetic enhancer of the co-administered PI, to increase plasma levels of that PI and allow added potency and convenience [39]. The co-administration of low-dose ritonavir is commonly called "boosting." A ritonavir-boosted PI is counted as a single drug as the ritonavir dosage is sub-therapeutic.

Potential drug targets in the late life cycle events include *gag* protein maturation [40] and *vif* [41], a viral gene that appears to act by inhibiting innate cellular antiretroviral factors.

COMPONENTS OF ARV REGIMENS

Achieving treatment goals through suppressing HIV replication to the lowest possible levels requires the simultaneous use of multiple ARV drugs. Most initial ARV regimens consist of a dual NRTI "backbone" and a third or "cornerstone" drug [2, 3]. Typically, the "cornerstone" drug is an NNRTI, a PI (usually boosted by low-dose ritonavir), or an integrase inhibitor. Alternative approaches, e.g. regimens composed of three NRTIs, a PI and an NNRTI without NRTIs, or boosted-PI monotherapy, have been attempted but generally have been less potent [42–44]. These are not currently a preferred option for most patients, though additional studies are underway. Each drug in a typical triple-drug combination must be considered on its own in terms of potency, convenience, and toxicity, but the entire regimen must be similarly considered. Designing an optimum regimen must be individualized for each patient. These factors are discussed in greater detail later in this chapter.

Summarizing each ARV drug and all possible regimens of choice is beyond the scope of this review, although Tables 11.1 and 11.2 offer a brief overview of commonly used agents and regimens. Excellent summaries of current ART information are included in guidelines published by national and international organizations. In the United States, both the DHHS [3] and the IAS-USA [2] guidelines are frequently updated. The DHHS guidelines are an especially extensive information resource for many aspects of drug potency, toxicity, and interactions. The IAS-USA also publishes updated guidelines of ARV resistance testing [45], which are extremely useful for planning treatment. Other chapters in this book address HIV biology and important ARV treatment issues including drug toxicity, drug resistance, adherence, and drug interactions. These chapters should be consulted for this crucial information.

AN OVERVIEW OF COMMON COMPONENTS OF ARV REGIMENS

Initial ARV regimens typically comprise a dual NRTI "backbone" and a third or "cornerstone" drug [2, 3].

NRTIs

Of all possible two-drug NRTI combinations, several are commonly prescribed, while others are to be avoided and yet others can be useful in specific situations affected by prior toxicity or drug resistance. Preferred combinations are co-formulations of two drugs in a single pill, with either lamivudine or emtricitabine as one of the agents. Co-formulation increases convenience and potentially improves medication adherence [46]. NRTIs as a class may cause lipoatrophy and lactic acidosis, though the risk of these varies widely with specific NRTIs.

Lamivudine (3TC) and emtricitabine (FTC)

Lamivudine and emtricitabine are closely related NRTIs and can be used interchangeably. One or the other typically is included in a dual NRTI backbone. They are very well tolerated, though emtricitabine may cause patchy hyperpigmentation, particularly in dark-skinned individuals. A single mutation, M184V, confers high-level HIV resistance to 3TC and FTC. Both NRTIs are also active against hepatitis B virus (HBV) but in persons with HBV co-infection, should not be used without other HBV-active drugs because HBV resistance commonly develops [47].

Dual NRTI backbones: co-formulations

Tenofovir (TDF) plus emtricitabine (FTC)

This is a potent and convenient one pill, once daily backbone, and is recommended by US [2, 3] and European guidelines [48] as the preferred NRTI combination for most patients. It also is co-formulated with efavirenz as a three-drug combination tablet. Tenofovir usually is well tolerated in short-term use but has been associated with renal toxicity; renal function should be monitored [49]. Questions of potential bone toxicity are under investigation [50, 51]. Tenofovir has interactions, especially with atazanavir (whose levels decrease) and didanosine (whose levels increase). When used with didanosine, increases in CD4 counts may be dampened; this combination should be avoided [52]. Both tenofovir and emtricitabine are active against hepatitis B virus, and in persons with HIV–HBV co-infection this combination is recommended as part of the anti-HIV regimen to co-treat HBV infection (although emtricitabine is not approved for this indication).

The HIV resistance pattern of tenofovir includes a K65R mutation that can lead to cross-resistance with some other drugs in this class. This mutation is rare if either a thymidine analog, or a potent "cornerstone" drug is co-administered [53]. Thymidine analog mutations (TAMs) may decrease the potency of tenofovir.

Abacavir (ABC) plus lamivudine (3TC)

This one pill, once daily co-formulation, also has had extensive clinical application [54]. Abacavir is a potent non-thymidine NRTI with no significant drug interactions. It is well tolerated in long-term use but may cause an occasionally severe hypersensitivity reaction in early use

Table 11.1 Antiretroviral drugs in common use

DRUG CLASS	GENERIC DRUG NAME	COMMON ABBREVIATION	DOSE IN COMMON FORMULATION	DOSING IN ADULTS	COMMENTS
Nucleoside/nucleotide reverse transcriptase inhibitor (NRTI)	Potential class adverse effects: lipoatrophy (especially D4T, ZDV), lactic acidosis Dosage must be adjusted in persons with renal impairment (abacavir is an exception)				
	Lamivudine	3TC	150-, 300-mg tabs (also available in two fixed dose combinations, one with ZDV, one with ABC and one with both ABC and ZDV in resource-limited settings (RLS), available in various generic co-formulations)	300 mg once daily or 150 mg b.i.d.	May be used interchangeably with FTC; a recommended agent for NRTI backbones. Well tolerated. Low genetic barrier to resistance. Active against hepatitis B (HBV) but resistance quickly develops if used as HBV monotherapy. In persons with HIV/HBV co-infection, should be used along with TDF or another HBV therapy, and as part of fully suppressive anti-HIV ART regimen. HBV may flare if discontinued
	Emtricitabine	FTC	200-mg caps (also available in two fixed dose combinations, one with TDF, and one with both TDF and EFV)	200 mg once daily	May be used interchangeably with 3TC; a recommended agent for NRTI backbones. Low genetic barrier to resistance. Well tolerated. May cause hyperpigmentation, especially in dark-skinned persons. Active against HBV—see 3TC for cautions
	Tenofovir	TDF	150-, 200-, 250-, 300-mg tabs Also oral powder (also available in three fixed dose combinations, one with FTC, one with both FTC and EFV, and one with both FTC and RPV)	300 mg once daily	A recommended agent for NRTI backbones (with FTC or 3TC). May cause renal toxicity. Active against hepatitis B, and hepatitis B may flare if discontinued. Combination of TDF + ddl may impair CD4 recovery; may have reduced potency

Drug		Formulation	Dose	Notes
Abacavir	ABC	300-mg tabs (also available in two fixed dose combinations, one with 3TC, and one with both 3TC and ZDV)	300 mg b.i.d. or 600 mg once daily	Can cause rash; also systemic hypersensitivity reaction in persons at risk (HLA B5701 positive) that can be fatal if drug not stopped or if it is reinitiated after initial reaction. Screen for HLA B5701 before treatment. May increase risk of myocardial infarction. May be less potent than TDF in persons with pretreatment HIV RNA >100,000 copies/mL
Zidovudine	ZDV, AZT	100-mg caps, 300-mg tabs (also available in two fixed dose combinations; one with 3TC, another with both 3TC and ABC; in RLS, available in various generic co-formulations)	300 mg b.i.d.	Common adverse effects: anemia, macrocytosis, fatigue, nausea, lipoatrophy. Must be used b.i.d. Should not be used with d4T
Stavudine	d4T	15-, 20-, 30-, 40-mg caps (in RLS, available in various generic co-formulations)	40 mg b.i.d. if >60 kg; 30 mg b.i.d. if <60 kg	Common adverse effects: peripheral neuropathy, lipoatrophy, lactic acidosis, pancreatitis; more common when used with ddl. Should not be used with ZDV
Didanosine	ddl	125-, 200-, 250-, 400-mg enteric-coated caps (in RLS, available in various genetic formulations)	400 mg once daily if >60 kg; 250 mg once daily if <60 kg or if used with TDF	Taken ½ hour before or 2 hours after a meal. See caution with d4T. Reduce dose when used with tenofovir. May increase risk of myocardial infarction. Inferior efficacy in several ART combinations. Combination of TDF + ddl may impair CD4 recovery
Non-nucleoside reverse transcriptase inhibitor (NNRTI)				Adverse effects: rash (usually transient but may be severe, including Stevens–Johnson syndrome) Many drug–drug interactions. Low genetic barrier to resistance (especially EFV, NVP, RPV), extensive cross-resistance

Continued

Table 11.1 Antiretroviral drugs in common use—cont'd

DRUG CLASS	GENERIC DRUG NAME	COMMON ABBREVIATION	DOSE IN COMMON FORMULATION	DOSING IN ADULTS	COMMENTS
	Efavirenz	EFV	50-, 200-mg caps; 600-mg tabs (also available in a fixed dose combination, with FTC and TDF)	600 mg once daily	Low genetic barrier to resistance. Common adverse effects: vivid dreams, sleep disturbance, dizziness, mood perturbation, usually transient; hyperlipidemia. Can cause teratogenicity. Take on empty stomach, usually at bedtime
	Nevirapine	NVP	Immediate release (IR): 200-mg tabs (in RLS, available in various generic co-formulations) Extended release (XR): 400-mg tabs	200 mg once daily for first 14 days, then 200 mg b.i.d. (IR) or 400 mg once daily (XR)	Low genetic barrier to resistance. Can cause hepatotoxicity, especially in those with higher pretreatment HIV CD4 counts ($>$250 cells/mm^3 in women, $>$400 cells/mm^3 in men) or chronic liver disease; occasionally fatal
	Etravirine	ETR	100-, 200-mg tabs	200 mg b.i.d.	Usually used in advanced lines of therapy. Effective against some HIV strains with NNRTI resistance; resistance testing should guide use
	Rilpivirine	RPV	25-mg tabs (also available in a fixed dose combination, with FTC and TDF)	25 mg once daily	Low genetic barrier to resistance. For use in initial therapy. Compared with EFV: higher rate of virologic failure in patients with baseline HIV RNA $>$100,000 copies/mL; more resistance in those with virologic failure; fewer adverse effects
Protease inhibitor (PI)	Potential class adverse effects: dyslipidemia, fat distribution abnormalities, hyperglycemia, nausea, diarrhea, hepatotoxicity, possible cardiovascular risk. Many drug–drug interactions. High genetic barrier to resistance (RTV-boosted PIs) RTV boosting: low-dose ritonavir can be co-administered with most PIs as a pharmacokinetic "booster"; some PIs require ritonavir boosting, and interactions with some other drugs may require that ritonavir be used				

Drug	Abbreviation	Formulations	Dosing	Comments
Atazanavir	ATV	100-, 150-, 200, 300–mg caps	• 300 mg once daily with RTV 100 mg once daily. • 400 mg once daily (without RTV)	Usually well tolerated; little lipid or GI effect. Causes elevated indirect bilirubin levels. Must be boosted by ritonavir when used with tenofovir. Gastric acid lowering medications (especially proton pump inhibitors) interfere with absorption
Darunavir	DRV	75-, 150-, 400-, 600-mg tabs	• 600 mg b.i.d. with RTV 100 mg b.i.d. • If no DRV resistance mutations, 800 mg once daily with ritonavir 100 mg once daily	Usually potent in HIV moderately resistant to other drugs in PI class. May cause rash
Fosamprenavir	FPV, f-APV	700-mg tabs	• 1400 mg once daily with RTV 200 mg once daily. • 700 mg b.i.d. with 100 mg RTV b.i.d. • 1400 mg b.i.d. (without RTV)	May cause rash, GI disorders, hyperlipidemia
Indinavir	IDV	100-, 200-, 333-, 400-mg caps	• 800 mg b.i.d. with RTV 100–200 mg b.i.d.	Adverse effects common: hyperbilirubinemia, retinoid-like effects, renal stones, GI disorders, metabolic abnormalities. Should be taken with extra hydration
Lopinavir/ritonavir	LPV/rtv	200-mg LPV/50-mg RTV tabs, 100-mg LPV/25-mg RTV tabs	• 400/100 mg b.i.d. • If treatment naïve, may give 800/200 mg once daily.	Can cause GI disorders, hyperlipidemia, cardiac conduction abnormalities. Increase to 500/125 mg b.i.d. if combined with EFV or NVP
Nelfinavir	NFV	250-, 625-mg tabs	• 1250 mg b.i.d.	Diarrhea is common. Less potent than RTV-boosted PIs

Continued

Table 11.1 Antiretroviral drugs in common use—cont'd

DRUG CLASS	GENERIC DRUG NAME	COMMON ABBREVIATION	DOSE IN COMMON FORMULATION	DOSING IN ADULTS	COMMENTS
	Ritonavir	RTV	100-mg tabs or caps	• 100–200 mg once daily—b.i.d. as boost for other PI (dosage depends on the specific PI).	Used as pharmacokinetic booster for several other PIs; not used as sole PI (because GI disorders, hyperlipidemia are common). Many drug–drug interactions
	Saquinavir	SQV	500-mg tabs, 200-mg caps	• 1000 mg b.i.d. with RTV 100 mg b.i.d.	May cause GI disorders, hyperlipidemias, cardiac conduction abnormalities
	Tipranavir	TPV	250-mg caps	• 500 mg once daily with 200 mg RTV	Approved only in salvage therapy. Must be ritonavir boosted. Can cause hepatotoxicity, GI disorders, hyperlipidemia, rash. Not for use in patients with moderate/severe hepatic insufficiency
Integrase inhibitor	Raltegravir	RAL	400-mg tabs	• 400 mg b.i.d.	Low genetic barrier to resistance. Few recognized adverse effects or drug–drug interactions (rifampin is an exception). Limited data in combination with NRTIs other than TDF/FTC
CCR5 antagonist	Maraviroc	MVC	150-, 300-mg tabs	• Dosage depends on co-administered ARVs and other medications	Only effective in patients with exclusive CCR5 tropism; must test tropism before giving maraviroc. Limited data in combination with NRTIs other than ZDV and 3TC. MVC levels may be affected by co-administered medications
Fusion inhibitor	Enfuvirtide	T-20	Vial of 108 mg lyophilized powder reconstituted with 1.1 mL sterile water	• 90 mg s.q. b.i.d.	Commonly causes injection site reactions

Table 11.2 Common antiretroviral regimens using FDC backbones for initial therapy

REGIMEN	ADVANTAGES	DISADVANTAGES OF THE REGIMEN[a]
NRTI backbone: TDF+FTC		**NRTI considerations**
[TDF+FTC]+EFV	All once daily in one combination pill. Extensive data demonstrating efficacy. Per US guidelines, a recommended regimen for initial therapy	Two drugs with low resistance barrier. Avoid EFV in first trimester of pregnancy or in women who may become pregnant
[TDF+FTC]+NVP	Low pill burden (2 pills). NVP effective in preventing HIV transmission in pregnant women. Can be once daily (with NVP XR formulation)	Two drugs with low resistance barrier
[TDF+FTC]+RPV	All once daily in one combination pill Low incidence of adverse effects	Two drugs with low resistance barrier. Compared with [TDF+FTC]+EFV, higher rate of virologic failure in those with baseline HIV RNA >100,000 copies/mL; more resistance in those with virologic failure. Little information available on interactions with other drugs
[TDF+FTC]+ATV/rtv	All once daily, low pill burden (3 pills). Per US guidelines, a recommended regimen for initial therapy	
[TDF+FTC]+DRV/rtv	Can be once daily if no DRV-associated resistance mutations. Per US guidelines, a recommended regimen for initial therapy	
[TDF+FTC]+LPV/rtv	Can be once daily	More pills and greater risk of adverse effects than in recommended combinations
[TDF+FTC]+SQV/rtv		No once daily option. More pills and greater risk of adverse effects than in recommended combinations
[TDF+FTC]+FPV/rtv	Can be once daily in initial therapy	More pills and greater risk of adverse effects than in recommended combinations
[TDF+FTC]+IDV/rtv		No once daily option. Likely has greater toxicity than other regimens
[TDF+FTC]+NFV		No once daily option. More pills and greater risk of adverse effects than in recommended combinations
[TDF+FTC]+RAL	Well tolerated. Few drug–drug interactions. Per US guidelines, a recommended regimen for initial therapy	Two drugs with low resistance barrier; RAL is b.i.d.
[TDF+FTC]+MVC		MVC effective only against CCR5 tropic virus; tropism testing must be done before starting MVC. Limited experience with this combination. MVC is b.i.d.

Continued

Table 11.2 Common antiretroviral regimens using FDC backbones for initial therapy—cont'd

REGIMEN	ADVANTAGES	DISADVANTAGES OF THE REGIMEN[a]
NRTI backbone: TDF+FTC		**NRTI considerations**
NRTI backbone: ABC+3TC		ABC+3TC (compared to TDF+FTC) may have higher rates of early virologic failure in patients with baseline viral load >100,000 copies/mL
[ABC+3TC]+EFV	All once daily, low pill burden (2 pills). Substantial data show efficacy	Two drugs with low resistance barrier. Both ABC and EFV can cause rash. Avoid EFV in first trimester of pregnancy or in women who may become pregnant
[ABC+3TC]+NVP	Low pill burden (3 pills). Can be once daily (with NVP XR formulation)	Two drugs with low resistance barrier. Both ABC and NVP can cause rash
[ABC+3TC]+ATV/rtv	All once daily, low pill burden (3 pills)	
[ABC+3TC]+ATV	All once daily; avoids RTV. Low pill burden (3 pills)	Lower genetic barrier to resistance than ATV/rtv
[ABC+3TC]+LPV/rtv	Can be once daily if no LPV/rtv resistance	See Table 11.1 for LPV/rtv considerations. More pills; greater risk of adverse effects than in recommended combinations, especially with once daily dosing
[ABC+3TC]+SQV/rtv		No once daily option. More pills and greater risk of adverse effects than in recommended combinations
[ABC+3TC]+FPV/rtv	Can be once daily in initial therapy	Both ABC and FPV can cause rash. More pills and greater risk of adverse effects than in recommended combinations
[ABC+3TC]+DRV/rtv	Can be once daily if no DRV resistance	Both ABC and DRV can cause rash
[ABC+3TC]+IDV/rtv		No once daily option. Likely has greater toxicity than other regimens
[ABC+3TC]+NFV		No once daily option. More pills and greater risk of adverse effects than in recommended combinations
[ABC+3TC]+RAL	Few drug–drug interactions. Low pill burden (3 pills)	Limited clinical experience with this combination. RAL is b.i.d. Two drugs with low resistance barrier
[ABC+3TC]+MVC		MVC effective only against CCR5 tropic virus; tropism testing must be done before starting MVC. MVC is b.i.d. Limited experience with this combination
NRTI backbone: ZDV+3TC		ZDV may have greater toxicity than TDF or ABC, may have lower CD4 increases than TDF/FTC or ABC/3TC. ZDV is b.i.d. AZT/3TC is the preferred NRTI backbone in pregnant women

Table 11.2 Common antiretroviral regimens using FDC backbones for initial therapy—cont'd

REGIMEN	ADVANTAGES	DISADVANTAGES OF THE REGIMEN[a]
NRTI backbone: TDF+FTC		**NRTI considerations**
[ZDV+3TC]+EFV		Two drugs with low resistance barrier. ZDV+3TC is b.i.d., EFV is once daily. Avoid EFV in first trimester of pregnancy or in women who may become pregnant
[ZDV+3TC]+NVP	All b.i.d. A preferred regimen for preventing mother-to-child transmission in pregnant women	Two drugs with low resistance barrier. No once daily option
[ZDV+3TC]+ATV/rtv		ZDV+3TC is b.i.d.
[ZDV+3TC]+DRV/rtv		ZDV+3TC is b.i.d.
[ZDV+3TC]+LPV/rtv	A preferred regimen for preventing mother-to-child transmission in pregnant women	No once daily option. More pills and greater risk of adverse effects than in recommended combinations
[ZDV+3TC]+SQV/rtv		No once daily option. More pills and greater risk of adverse effects than in recommended combinations
[ZDV+3TC]+FPV/rtv		No once daily option. More pills and greater risk of adverse effects than in recommended combinations
[ZDV+3TC]+IDV/rtv		No once daily option. Likely has greater toxicity than other regimens
[ZDV+3TC]+NFV	Effective in preventing mother-to-child transmission in pregnant women	No once daily option. More pills and greater risk of adverse effects than in recommended combinations
[ZDV+3TC]+RAL	All b.i.d. Few drug–drug interactions	
[ZDV+3TC]+MVC	All b.i.d.	MVC effective only against CCR5 tropic virus; tropism testing must be done before starting MVC. No once daily option
[ZDV+3TC+ABC]	Low pill burden—one pill b.i.d.	Less potent than regimens with NNRTI or PI component

[a]See Table 11.1 for disadvantages of individual ARVs.
Many combinations for initial ART can be constructed using available agents. Each has potential advantages and disadvantages, and the selection of ARV regimens should be individualized. Combinations that have a high degree of efficacy, safety, tolerability, and convenience include those listed above, all of which are recommended by current US and European guidelines (note that alternative combinations may be indicated for the individual patient).

characterized by fever, rash, malaise, and, in extreme cases where the drug is continued or reintroduced, circulatory collapse and death [55]. Hypersensitivity to abacavir is closely associated with HLA B*5701, and genetic screening for this allele should be done before treatment with abacavir, and those testing positive should not be given abacavir [3, 56]. Abacavir has been associated with adverse cardiovascular effects in some studies but not others; the possibility of cardiovascular toxicity remains under investigation [57, 58]. In patients with high pre-treatment HIV viral loads (>100,000 copies/mL) one study found that regimens containing abacavir–lamivudine were not as effective in suppressing HIV viremia as those with tenofovir–emtricitabine; this result has not been found consistently [59]. As mentioned above, lamivudine should not be used in persons with HBV infection without other HBV-active drugs because HBV resistance commonly develops. Drug resistance patterns with abacavir are similar to tenofovir with a K65R mutation, but also seen is the L74V mutation. TAMs may decrease the potency of abacavir.

Zidovudine (ZDV) plus lamivudine (3TC)

This combination was the first to be co-formulated and has had extensive use. It must be used twice daily. Zidovudine can cause anemia, sometimes of severe grade. It also may cause nausea, fatigue, facial and peripheral fat loss (lipoatrophy), and other symptomatic adverse effects. Because of toxicity concerns, zidovudine is not recommended in the resource-rich world unless other options are not possible; however, it still is commonly used in resource-constrained areas. For treatment of pregnant women, though, zidovudine remains the preferred NRTI, as it has been extensively studied in the prevention of perinatal HIV transmission [60]. This combination has minimal interactions with other ARV drugs. Zidovudine's resistance barrier is fairly broad. As mentioned above, lamivudine should not be used in persons with HBV without other HBV-active drugs because HBV resistance commonly develops.

Comments on other NRTIs

Stavudine (d4T)

This thymidine analog was used extensively in the past but long-term toxicities sharply limit its use. It is strongly associated with peripheral lipoatrophy, peripheral neuropathy, and lactic acidosis. The risk of these toxicities is compounded when stavudine is used with didanosine, and this combination is contraindicated. In the resource-rich world, stavudine is not recommended unless other ARVs cannot be used [2, 3]. Stavudine has been widely used in generic formulations in resource-constrained settings due to low cost, but there, too, toxicities may be severe, and WHO guidelines recommend the use of alternative NRTIs, if possible [61].

Didanosine (ddI)

Didanosine is a NRTI used once daily in an enteric-coated formulation. It may have significant adverse effects in longer-term use, and is not currently recommended if other NRTIs are available. Toxicities include peripheral neuropathy, pancreatitis, lipoatrophy, and lactic acidosis, especially if used with stavudine; this combination is contraindicated, particularly in pregnant women [3, 62].

Combination with tenofovir increases the risk of toxicity due to didanosine (dose adjustment of didanosine is required); additionally, various ART regimens that contain this NRTI backbone have had elevated rates of virologic failure, and (in patients with virologic suppression) poor CD4 increases [52, 63].

Cornerstone agents

Non-nucleoside RTIs

All NNRTIs may cause rash (occasionally severe, including Stevens–Johnson syndrome), and have interactions with many other medications, including other ARVs. Efavirenz and nevirapine have low genetic barriers to resistance, and single mutations can convey cross-class resistance.

Efavirenz (EFV)

Efavirenz is a potent, once daily NNRTI and is the preferred "third agent" in many initial ARV triple-drug regimens [2, 3, 48]. It is available in a co-formulation with tenofovir and emtricitabine. Short-term toxicity is usually temporary and typically does not require treatment interruption. Most common early adverse effects are central nervous system (CNS) symptoms, including vivid dreams and neuropsychiatric symptoms. Efavirenz usually is well tolerated in the long term. The resistance pattern of efavirenz overlaps that of other drugs in this class. Even single mutations, especially K103N and Y181 C or I, commonly lead to high-level resistance to nevirapine, and additional NNRTI resistance mutations accumulate with time spent on a failing regimen. The long serum half-life of efavirenz, on the other hand, may allow durable activity and limited resistance selection even with compromised adherence [64]. Importantly, because of reports of neural tube defects in infants of women exposed to efavirenz during early pregnancy, efavirenz is contraindicated in the first trimester of pregnancy and should be avoided if possible in women who may become pregnant while taking the drug [60]. If efavirenz is used, women should be fully informed about the need for effective contraception.

Nevirapine (NVP)

Nevirapine is similar in many respects to efavirenz, but may be somewhat less potent. The original formulation typically is dosed twice daily; an extended release tablet for once-daily dosing is also available. Its short-term toxicity includes rash (potentially severe) [65] but not the CNS side effects of efavirenz. Nevirapine, however, may cause an uncommon but occasionally severe or even fatal hepatic hypersensitivity reaction in the early weeks of treatment. In some studies, this has been more common in women and in those with higher CD4 counts at nevirapine initiation (women with CD4 >250 cells/mm^3, men with CD4 >400 cells/mm^3) [66], and nevirapine should not be started in these individuals unless expected benefits outweigh risks. Nevirapine resistance overlaps that of efavirenz. Nevirapine is extensively used worldwide in co-formulated regimens, and also is widely used during pregnancy, where it reduces risk of HIV transmission to the infant.

Other NNRTIs

Etravirine (ETR)

Etravirine is a newer NNRTI that is active against certain strains of HIV with resistance to efavirenz or nevirapine (resistance testing should be done to guide appropriate use).

Rilpivirine (RPV)

In 2011, rilpivirine was licensed for use in initial ARV regimens in adults. It is dosed once daily. It appears to be less effective than efavirenz in achieving virologic suppression in patients with high pretreatment HIV RNA (>100,000 copies/mL), but is associated with fewer adverse effects [67].

Other NNRTIs are in development.

Protease inhibitors (PIs)

Most PIs may be pharmacologically enhanced with the co-administration of low-dose ritonavir, and some PIs require such boosting to achieve therapeutic levels. Ritonavir-boosted PIs generally are the preferred PIs for most patients. Ritonavir boosting typically adds both potency and convenience, enabling less frequent administration and fewer pills per dose, but it may add adverse effects or drug–drug interactions. As a class, PIs have been associated with both short-term and persisting gastrointestinal (GI) distress, as well as metabolic disorders such as hyperlipidemia and insulin resistance. The incidence of these varies with the particular PI. PIs interact with many other medications, including other ARVs, usually via inhibition of hepatic cytochrome p450 isoenzymes. Ritonavir-boosted PIs have a broad genetic resistance barrier. Each has a characteristic set of induced mutations, described more fully in the chapter on ARV drug resistance.

Atazanavir (ATZ)

Atazanavir is administered once daily, typically in initial therapy, and may be used with or without ritonavir. Ritonavir boosting improves drug levels without substantially increased toxicity [68]. In resource-rich areas, atazanavir–ritonavir is a recommended PI for initial ART [2, 3, 48]. It usually is well tolerated, and has fewer GI and lipid effects than other PIs [69]. It commonly causes indirect hyperbilirubinemia and sometimes icterus or jaundice. While this is not a true hepatotoxicity, it may concern patients, and they should be appropriately informed. Unboosted atazanavir should not be used with tenofovir, as its levels are reduced by that NRTI, and absorption may be reduced by the concurrent use of medications that suppress gastric acid [3].

Darunavir (DRV)

Darunavir must be given with ritonavir boosting. Darunavir–ritonavir is used in both initial and salvage regimens, and is active against HIV with moderate resistance to other PI agents. It may be given once daily in persons whose HIV has no resistance to darunavir (twice daily in others). In resource-rich areas, it is a recommended PI for initial ART [2, 3, 48]. It is relatively well tolerated but may cause GI disturbance and hyperlipidemia [70].

Other PIs

Lopinavir (LPV)/ritonavir (RTV)

This co-formulated PI (the only one in this class) can be used once or twice daily in initial therapy. It is potent but is associated with moderate GI complaints and can increase adverse lipid profiles [69–72]. It has been associated with an increased risk of cardiovascular events [57]. It is potent and has a broad resistance barrier and may be used in initial therapy or in appropriate salvage regimens. It is the recommended PI for use in pregnant women [60].

Other PIs are in less common current use than those discussed above, but each can have a place in individualized ARV regimens.

Fosamprenavir (FPV) may be administered with or without ritonavir boosting. In initial therapy, boosted fosamprenavir may be given once or twice daily [73].

Saquinavir (SQV) in its current formulation is given twice daily and must be used with low-dose ritonavir [72]. It is relatively well tolerated and may be used in initial therapy or in appropriate salvage regimens.

Nelfinavir (NFV) is unique among the PIs in that it may not be ritonavir boosted and is thus used alone. It is less potent than boosted PIs [74]. This, and the fact that it commonly causes diarrhea, has limited its use except in ritonavir-intolerant patients and during pregnancy, where it is considered quite safe [60].

Indinavir (IDV) is rarely used because of toxicities. It can cause hyperglycemia and renal disease [75]. More common side effects include renal stones due to precipitated excreted drug and retinoid-like cutaneous reactions [76]. Boosted indinavir must be used twice daily, and unboosted indinavir must be used every 8 hours.

Tipranavir (TPV) is used to treat appropriate strains of PI-resistant HIV. It must be co-administered with a relatively high dosage of ritonavir, and may cause more GI and liver toxicity than other PIs. It must be refrigerated.

Integrase inhibitors

Raltegravir (RAL) is the only currently available integrase inhibitor. It is potent against susceptible HIV strains, and has few recognized adverse effects [77]. It may be used in initial therapy or in salvage regimens. Raltegravir must be given twice daily [78]. It has a relatively low barrier to resistance.

Other integrase inhibitors are in development.

CCR5 antagonists

Maraviroc (MVC) is the available agent in this class. It is active only against HIV that uses the CCR5 co-receptor exclusively, and testing for co-receptor tropism must be done in order to determine whether treatment with this agent is appropriate. It must be given twice daily, and its dosage must be adjusted according to co-administered medicines. It initially was used primarily as a component of salvage therapy but has been studied in initial therapy [79, 80]. Maraviroc has been less widely used in clinical practice than other classes. It has few recognized adverse effects, but long-term safety data are lacking. Resistance to maraviroc has been described but is not well characterized. Virologic nonresponse to maraviroc typically is due to the presence of viral tropism the CXCR4 co-receptor.

Other coreceptor antagonists are in development.

Fusion inhibitors

Enfuvirtide (ENF, T-20) is given subcutaneously twice daily and commonly causes bothersome reactions at the injection site. It is active against HIV with resistance to the other classes of ARVs and has been used in salvage regimens [81, 82]. Since newer classes of oral ARVs have become available to treat ARV-resistant HIV, the need for enfuvirtide has declined.

CLINICAL APPLICATION OF ART

Successful management of HIV infection requires the prescription of a potent ARV drug combination at an appropriate point in the disease course. This regimen must be taken correctly and continuously for many years (lifelong), to suppress this chronic and non-curable infection. The design of an ARV regimen is relatively straightforward with initial therapy (unless there is baseline resistance), but may become much more complex if treatment fails and drug resistance develops, or the patient develops unexpected or severe side effects or drug interactions.

ARV regimen design

The choice of a specific ARV regimen is an absolutely crucial one, because a good choice, individualized for that person's needs and concerns, can result in disease recovery and durable benefit (Table 11.2). Amongst potential regimens that have appropriate potency (e.g. chosen with resistance test and CD4 and viral load results in mind), the choice for the specific patient should consider factors such as his/her wishes for once- or twice-daily treatment, and other health conditions (e.g. hepatitis B, which may require co-treatment, or hyperlipidemia, which may be worsened by certain ARVs). The possibility of pregnancy should be considered in all women of reproductive age (e.g. to avoid efavirenz). Also, the patient's concern for specific side effects should be elicited. For example, some patients are less willing to tolerate the neuropsychiatric side effects associated with efavirenz while others may not tolerate diarrhea, even if mild, which can complicate some PIs. All possible drug interactions, both within the ARV regimen and with any other prescribed or non-prescribed drugs, must also be considered and, when possible, avoided. Ideally, all ARV agents in a regimen can be used simultaneously without restrictions on food or fluid intake.

Pretreatment assessment

Testing for presence of pre-existing genetic ARV resistance mutations should ideally be done before ART, and results should be considered in the design of the ARV regimen. If abacavir is being considered, screening for HLA B*5701 should be done (abacavir is contraindicated if positive for this allele); if maraviroc is considered, tropism testing must be done (maraviroc is contraindicated if CXCR4 is present); if integrase inhibitor resistance is possible, specific testing for integrase resistance mutations should be obtained.

Chronic health problems that may be exacerbated during ARV therapy such as hyperlipidemia or hyperglycemia should be diagnosed and appropriately managed. Also, a thorough medication history is required as ARV drugs may lead to adverse interactions (e.g. acid blocking medications decrease the absorption of atazanavir). The drug history should include non-prescription and illicit agents, and herbal remedies. Underlying factors that might affect drug absorption or metabolism should be assessed at baseline, especially renal and hepatic function. Guidelines for ARV use in the setting of chronic kidney disease are available [83].

Optimal timing of initial ARV therapy

ARV therapy of very recently acquired HIV infection is of uncertain benefit, and the appropriate subject of ongoing clinical trials [84, 85]. Chronic HIV infection—generally defined as beginning about 12 months after exposure—should be treated well before the onset of opportunistic infections or malignancies. In asymptomatic individuals, treatment is guided by CD4 T lymphocyte counts and, to a lesser degree, plasma viral loads.

The optimal CD4 threshold at which to start ART in asymptomatic persons is not clearly known, but based on recent studies, US and international guidelines generally have moved toward earlier treatment. While immunologic and clinical recovery is expected even when ARV use is delayed until late disease stages, immune restoration may be less robust in those cases and life expectancy may be significantly shorter [5, 6, 9–11, 20, 21, 86]. As a strategy, earlier treatment is based on an increasing understanding of the ongoing damage caused by HIV across the spectrum of CD4 counts, and of the long-term consequences of untreated HIV, including chronic immune activation and inflammation, and coincides with the availability of safer and more convenient ARV options [87]. An additional possible benefit of earlier ART is reduction in HIV transmission to others [88–90].

US and European guidelines strongly recommend ARV initiation if the CD4 count is <350 cells/mm^3, with the urgency of ART increasing as the CD4 declines further [2, 3, 48]. US guidelines also recommend ART in those with CD4 counts 350–500 cells/mm^3 [2, 3]. In persons with high CD4 counts (e.g. >500 cells/mm^3), ART initiation is of unproven benefit but is the subject of investigation [3, 18, 91]. Current US DHHS guidelines state that 50% of their experts favor ART initiation in those with CD4 >500 cells/mm^3 [3]. Some experts advocate treating all infected persons as soon as they are diagnosed, for possible individual as well as public health benefits [92, 93]. ART is strongly recommended in certain groups of patients regardless of CD4 count, such as pregnant women, those with hepatitis B when the hepatitis requires treatment, and those with HIV-associated nephropathy. In resource-limited settings, the WHO recommends ART when the CD4 count is ≤350 cells/mm^3 or clinical stage 3 or 4 disease is present [61].

In advanced-stage HIV disease, opportunistic infections (OIs) or cancers may require immediate management, before ART. Optimal timing of ART initiation in persons with an OI is not precisely known, but data available thus far suggest that for most OIs (including tuberculosis), starting ART soon after the start of treatment of the OI improves survival, though the incidence of immune reconstitution inflammatory reactions may be higher (an exception may be CNS infections such as cryptococcal meningitis, in which appropriate infection-specific treatment should be well established before ART initiation) [13, 94, 95]. Patients may have other conditions that affect the timing or choice of ARVs, e.g. pregnancy or hepatitis B infection.

Patients should be fully informed before ARV medications are first prescribed. Patient counseling should include information on potential drug side effects, the importance of excellent and continuous medication adherence, and the need for ongoing safe behaviors to prevent HIV transmission. The patient initiating ART should have access to sources knowledgeable in ARV use should questions or concerns arise.

Monitoring ART

There are no definitive standards for laboratory monitoring of ARV therapy. Most would check the viral load within several weeks of treatment initiation to assess initial virologic response and assess prescription adherence. At the same time, side effects can be discussed as they contribute to longer-term non-adherence and may be reduced by regimen alteration or symptomatic treatment. Laboratory testing shortly after ARV initiation is also useful for detecting drug toxicity. Early adverse effects of ARV drugs include hepatotoxicity, dyslipidemias, hyperbilirubinemia, and anemia. The frequency of toxicity monitoring should be driven by the specific agents used and individual patient considerations, and, of course, any interval clinical signs or symptoms.

The goal of initial ART, reducing plasma viral load below assay detection limits, is commonly achieved within 12 weeks, but may require 24 weeks of treatment, especially if the pre-treatment baseline viral load was extremely high [96]. Non-adherence should be suspected if the plasma viral load fails to fall quickly, or if it plateaus above detection levels. Prolonged viremia in the face of ARV exposure will result in drug resistance selection, limiting the possibility of successful ART.

The frequency of clinical and laboratory monitoring in patients with undetectable plasma HIV titers is variable. Many practitioners ask patients to be seen every 3 to 4 months if all is going well. With very stable patients, this interval can gradually be extended, but usually to no longer than every 6 months. Each visit should address potential drug toxicity and problems specific to HIV disease. Medication adherence should be assessed and reinforced at each visit, as should safe HIV transmission risk behaviors.

In resource-constrained settings, laboratory tests may not be available, and clinical recovery is used to guide treatment decisions, with or without CD4 counts. HIV viral load testing, although more expensive, is fundamentally important in identifying virologic failure, and lack of access to this testing increases the risk that treatment failure will not be detected until high levels of ARV resistance have been selected. Appropriate laboratory tests should be done if toxicity is suspected.

VIROLOGIC FAILURE

Current ARV regimens are sufficiently potent to suppress viremia in almost all patients (although low-level viremia (<200 copies/mm) may be present, and does not necessarily signify virologic failure) [3]. If virologic suppression does not happen, possible causes should be examined. The most common reason for failure of initial ART is poor medication adherence [46, 97]. Non-adherence can be intermittent or nearly continuous. It can involve the entire regimen or only selected agents. Non-adherence can be seen with the first doses prescribed or can occur at any later point, even after prolonged periods of excellent adherence. It may reflect a lack of appropriate baseline counseling, the onset of drug side effects, or interval substance or alcohol misuse. It also may represent "treatment fatigue."

Another possible cause of ART failure is preexisting HIV resistance—either because the patient was infected at baseline with HIV already harboring drug resistance or because he/she had developed resistance on a prior ARV regimen (including ARVs given to prevent perinatal HIV transmission). The risk of treatment failure due to resistance can be reduced with baseline resistance testing, if available. Alternatively, there may be inadequate ARV exposure due to malabsorption or drug interactions. The former is rare, but drug interactions are common and should be avoided by a careful baseline drug history, again including non-prescription products. Of non-ARV drugs, interactions threatening ARV response are most common with gastric acid blockers, especially the potent proton pump inhibitors and with antituberculosis therapy, where rifamycin interactions with protease inhibitors are common [3].

Regardless of the cause, ARV drug resistance often accompanies virologic failure, and certain mutations in each of the ARV classes cause extensive cross-resistance within the class. Resistance testing should be performed in every case of insufficient suppression or rebound, if possible. Virologic failure of the first or even second regimen should prompt an immediate reattempt to again suppress viremia below detection limits. As dictated by circumstances, this may involve adherence support or a change of one or more drugs to reduce side effects or to correct for resistance mutations. Resuppression in early failure typically is straightforward if non-adherence is the cause and can be corrected. Virologic failure with multiple resistance mutations is much more difficult to reverse.

Specific management approaches in virologic failure

Non-adherence to prescribed regimen

A crucial question is whether the patient stopped all medications or stopped only selected drugs. Also key are whether non-adherence was intermittent or continuous, and whether it was triggered by side effects or inconvenience. Finally and critically, it must be determined whether non-adherence resulted in resistance selection. Absent intolerance or resistance, the ARV regimen originally prescribed can be continued if adherence can be re-established, and if significant resistance mutations have not yet been selected. In all cases, the need for rigorous adherence should be stressed along with practical advice on how this can be achieved.

Toxicity to selected drugs

ARV side effects range in severity from minor inconveniences to life-threatening (see Chapter 14 for an expanded discussion). Some are transient, others continue over time. Some can be ameliorated with other medications while others are not treatable, and an alternative ARV must be substituted.

Serious side effects that require permanent avoidance of the offending drug include hypersensitivity reactions to abacavir and idiosyncratic nevirapine hepatotoxicity. On the other hand, in most cases the early CNS side effects with efavirenz or rashes with efavirenz or nevirapine are temporary and the drugs can be continued. In some cases additional medications can be used to control adverse effects. For example, zidovudine-associated anemia can be reversed at least partially by recombinant erythropoietin and hyperlipidemias can be controlled, although often only partially, with diet, exercise, or statins. In these cases, the ARV causing the side effect can either be replaced with one not having the toxicity or can be continued, along with additional medication to treat the adverse effect. Toxicity that is chronic and potentially irreversible includes stavudine-associated peripheral lipoatrophy or neuropathy. With these, the offending ARV should be replaced with an appropriate alternative.

It is important to consider the impact of "minor" but chronic treatment side effects. Over time, these can lead to non-adherence. Patients should be asked specifically about the impact of bothersome low-level gastrointestinal, CNS, or other toxicity. If present, changing to other drugs should be considered.

TOPICS IN "LATE" SALVAGE ARV THERAPY

Each case of "late failure" is unique in terms of prior drugs used, toxicity experienced, and drug resistance patterns seen, so broad generalizations are inescapable (and thus of limited practical value) in suggesting management strategies. Given the availability of agents in new ARV classes and additional ARVs in older classes, it is possible to achieve virologic suppression in the great majority of patients with ARV-resistant virus; thus in nearly all cases a new drug regimen should be designed for maximal suppression. If viral suppression is not possible with available ARVs, continued therapy is usually preferred to full discontinuation.

Adding a new drug to a "failing" regimen

In patients with ongoing viremia and resistance to multiple drugs, adding a single new ARV, whether of a new and non-cross-resistant class (as with an integrase inhibitor or CCR5 antagonist), or with less cross-resistance, like the PI darunavir, is of limited value. Unless a new ARV can be used with at least one, or preferably two, other active agents, its introduction is rapidly followed by drug resistance selection. Guidelines, therefore, suggest the earlier use of such new agents to improve the likelihood of resuppression of viremia with more durable clinical benefits [2, 3].

ARV TREATMENT APPROACHES IN RESOURCE-CONSTRAINED SETTINGS

There is no difference in the goals of ART in resource-limited settings, but the access to drugs and monitoring tests may necessitate very different choices. The availability of ARV regimens in many countries is severely limited by cost issues, often consisting primarily of generic fixed-dose combinations. Secondary regimens are even more constrained. In many countries, stavudine continues to be used even though neuropathy and lipoatrophy are common and international guidelines recommend against its use [61]. Important drugs like PIs are too expensive for common use. Initial regimens often are NNRTI based and PIs may not be available for salvage. Treatment of common co-infections, especially tuberculosis, also may pose problems in ART because of interactions between antimicrobials (particularly rifampicins) and PIs or NNRTIs.

Laboratory tests may also be unavailable in many settings. CD4 testing is more widely available than HIV viral load testing and resistance tests are generally unavailable. While clinical criteria can be used to initiate ART, this approach may lead to late treatment of many individuals. Current WHO Guidelines recommend ARV initiation when the CD4 falls to or below 350 cells/mm^3, and in anyone with advanced HIV disease (WHO stage 3 or 4) regardless of CD4 count [61]. Clinical and/or CD4 improvements are then followed as evidence of treatment benefit and ART is continued unless either suggests treatment failure. HIV viral load testing is of clear utility in identifying and managing treatment failure, and should be done, if possible, if ART failure is suspected. Appropriate laboratory tests should be done if toxicity is suspected.

Each element of this discussion is changing rapidly as more international funding for HIV care is reaching many countries most affected by the HIV epidemic.

ARVs as pre-exposure prophylaxis

Recent studies have examined the use of ARV medications in HIV-uninfected individuals to prevent HIV infection through sexual exposure. One study found that pre-exposure prophylaxis (PrEP) using daily oral tenofovir + emtricitabine reduced the risk of HIV in high-risk men who have sex with men [98] and another showed that tenofovir vaginal gel, used pericoitally, reduced the rate of HIV infection in heterosexual women [99]. On the other hand, preliminary results of another clinical trial using daily oral tenofovir + emtricitabine in HIV-uninfected heterosexual women did not show evidence of protection [100]. In each study, participants were also given other risk-reduction interventions, including counseling, condom provision, and STD testing and treatment. Additional studies of these and other prevention strategies using ARVs are under way.

REFERENCES

[1] Bartlett JA, Fath MJ, Demasi R, et al. An updated systematic overview of triple combination therapy in antiretroviral-naive HIV-infected adults. AIDS 2006;20(16): 2051–64.

[2] Thompson MA, Aberg JA, Cahn P, et al. Antiretroviral treatment of adult HIV infection: 2010 recommendations of the International AIDS Society-USA panel. JAMA 2010;304(3):321–33.

[3] US Department of Health and Human Services. Guidelines for the use of antiretroviral agents in HIV-1-infected adults and adolescents.

[4] Mocroft A, Phillips AN, Gatel l J, et al. and for the EuroSIDA Study Group. Normalisation of CD4 counts in patients with HIV-1 infection and maximum virological suppression who are taking combination antiretroviral therapy: an observational cohort study. Lancet 2007;370:407–13.

[5] Kaufmann GR, Perrin L, Pantaleo G, et al. CD4 T-lymphocyte recovery in individuals with advanced HIV-1 infection receiving potent antiretroviral therapy GR for 4 years: the Swiss HIV Cohort Study. Arch Intern Med 2003;163:2187–95.

[6] Kelley CF, Kitchen CM, Hunt PW, et al. Incomplete peripheral CD4 (+) cell count restoration in HIV-infected patients receiving long-term antiretroviral treatment. Clin Infect Dis 2009;48:787–94.

[7] Raffanti SP, Fusco JS, Sherrill BH, et al. Effect of persistent moderate viremia on disease progression during HIV therapy. J Acquir Immune Defic Syndr 2004;37:1147–54.

[8] Hejdeman B, Lenkei R, Leandersson AC, et al. Clinical and immunological benefits from highly active antiretroviral therapy in spite of limited viral load reduction in HIV type 1 infection. AIDS Res Hum Retroviruses 2001;17:277–86.

[9] The Antiretroviral Therapy Cohort Collaboration. Life expectancy of individuals on combination antiretroviral therapy in high-income countries: a collaborative analysis of 14 cohort studies. Lancet 2008;372:293–9.

[10] Bhaskaran K, Hamouda O, Sannes M, et al. Changes in the risk of death after HIV seroconversion compared with mortality in the general population. JAMA 2008;300:51–9.

[11] Lohse N, Hansen AB, Pedersen G, et al. Survival of persons with and without HIV infection in Denmark, 1995–2005. Ann Intern Med 2007;146:87–95.

[12] Pantaleo G, Graziosi C, Fauci AS. New concepts in the immunopathogenesis of human immunodeficiency virus infection. N Engl J Med 1993;328:327–35.

[13] Zolopa A, Andersen J, Powderly W, et al. Early antiretroviral therapy reduces AIDS progression/death in individuals with acute opportunistic infections: a multicenter randomized strategy trial. PLoS One 2009;4(5):e5575. Epub 2009 May 18.

[14] Soriano V, Castilla J, Gomez-Cano M, et al. The decline in CD4 T lymphocytes as a function of the duration of HIV infection, age at seroconversion, and viral load. J Infect 1998;36:307–11.

[15] Deeks SG, Kitchen CM, Liu L, et al. Immune activation set point during early HIV infection predicts subsequent CD4+ T-cell changes independent of viral load. Blood 2004;104:942–7.

[16] Rosenberg E, Cotton D. Primary HIV infection and the acute retroviral syndrome. AIDS Clin Care 1997;9(19):23–5.

[17] Schacker T, Hughes J, Shea T, et al. Biological and virological characteristics of primary HIV infection. Ann Intern Med 1998;128:613–20.

[18] Bacchetti P, Moss AR. Incubation period of AIDS in San Francisco. Nature 1989;338:251–3.

[19] Strategies for Management of Antiretroviral Therapy (SMART) Study Group. CD4 count-guided interruption of antiretroviral CD4 treatment. N Engl J Med 2006;355:2283–96.

[20] Smith C. Factors associated with specific causes of death amongst HIV-positive individuals in the D:A:D Study. AIDS 2010;24 (10):1537–48.

[21] Mocroft A, Reiss P, Gasiorowski J, et al. Serious fatal and nonfatal non-AIDS-defining illnesses in Europe. J Acquir Immune Defic Syndr 2010;55(2):262–70.

[22] Weber R, Sabin CA, Friis-Moller N, et al. Liver-related deaths in persons infected with the human immunodeficiency virus: the D:A:D study. Arch Intern Med 2006;166(15):1632–41.

[23] Bedimo RJ, McGinnis KA, Dunlap M, et al. Incidence of non-AIDS-defining malignancies in HIV-infected versus noninfected patients in the HAART era: impact of immunosuppression. J Acquir Immune Defic Syndr 2009;52 (2):203–8.

[24] Guiguet M, Boué F, Cadranel J, et al. Effect of immunodeficiency, HIV viral load, and antiretroviral therapy on the risk of individual malignancies (FHDH-ANRS CO4): a prospective cohort study. Lancet Oncol 2009;10(12):1152–9.

[25] Bhaskaran K, Mussini C, Antinori A, et al. Changes in the incidence and predictors of human immunodeficiency virus-associated dementia in the era of highly active antiretroviral therapy. Ann Neurol 2008;63 (2):213–21.

[26] Deeks SG, Phillips AN. HIV infection, antiretroviral treatment, ageing, and non-AIDS related morbidity. BMJ 2009;338:a3172.

[27] Reiss P. The art of managing human immunodeficiency virus infection: a balancing act. Clin Infect Dis 2009;49:1602–4.

[28] Saag M, Deeks S. How do HIV elite controllers do what they do? Clin Infect Dis 2010;51 (2):239–41.

[29] Wang HG, Williams RE, Lin PF. A novel class of HIV-1 inhibitors that targets the viral envelope and inhibits CD4 receptor binding. Curr Pharm 2004;10:1785–93.

[30] Berger EA, Murphy PM, Farber JM. Chemokine receptors as HIV-1 coreceptors: roles in viral entry, tropism, and disease. Annu Rev Immunol 1999;17:657–700.

[31] Carrington M, Dean M, Martin MP, O'Brien SJ. Genetics of HIV-1 infection: chemokine receptor CCR5 polymorphism and its consequences. Hum Mol Genet 1999;8:1939–45.

[32] Chen CH, Matthews TJ, McDanal CB, et al. A molecular clasp in the human immunodeficiency virus (HIV) type 1 TM protein determines the anti-HIV activity of gp41 derivatives: implication for viral fusion. J Virol 1995;69:3771–7.

[33] Gomez C, Hope TJ. The ins and outs of HIV replication. Cell Microbiol 2005;7:621–6.

[34] Gotte M. Inhibition of HIV-1 reverse transcription: basic principles of drug action and resistance. Expert Rev Anti Infect Ther 2004;2:707–16.

[35] Sharma PL, Nurpeisov V, Hernandez-Santiago B, et al. Nucleoside inhibitors of human immunodeficiency virus type 1 reverse transcriptase. Curr Top Med Chem 2004;4:895–919.

[36] Sluis-Cremer N, Temiz NA, Bahar I. Conformational changes in HIV-1 reverse transcriptase induced by nonnucleoside reverse transcriptase inhibitor binding. Curr HIV Res 2004; 2:323–32.

[37] Tronchet JM, Seman M. Nonnucleoside inhibitors of HIV-1 reverse transcriptase: from the biology of reverse transcription to molecular design. Curr Top Med Chem 2003;3:1496–511.

[38] McColl DJ, Chen X. Strand transfer inhibitors of HIV-1 integrase: bringing IN a new era of antiretroviral therapy. Antiviral Res 2010;85(1):101–18.

[39] Scott JD. Simplifying the treatment of HIV infection with ritonavir-boosted protease inhibitors in antiretroviral-experienced patients. Am J Health Syst Pharm 2005;62:809–15.

[40] Martin DE, Blum R, Wilton J, et al. Safety and pharmacokinetics of bevirimat (PA-457), a novel inhibitor of human immunodeficiency virus maturation, in healthy volunteers. Antimicrob Agents Chemother 2007;51(9):3063–6.

[41] Stopak K, Greene WC. Protecting APOBEC3G: a potential new target for HIV drug discovery. Curr Opin Investig Drugs 2005;6:141–7.

[42] Gulick RM, Ribaudo HJ, Shikuma CM, et al. Triple-nucleoside regimens versus efavirenz-containing regimens for the initial treatment of HIV-1 infection. N Engl J Med 2004;350:1850–61.

[43] Riddler SA, Haubrich R, DiRienzo AG, et al. Class-sparing regimens for initial treatment of HIV-1 infection. N Engl J Med 2008;358(20):2095–106.

[44] Pérez-Valero I, Arribas JR. Protease inhibitor monotherapy. Curr Opin Infect Dis 2011;24(1):7–11.

[45] Johnson VA, Brun-Vézine FT, Clotet B, et al. Update of the drug resistance mutations in HIV-1: December 2010. Top HIV Med 2010;18(5):156–63.

[46] Bartlett JA. Addressing the challenges of adherence. J Acquir Immune Defic Syndr 2002;29: S2–10.

[47] Benhamou Y, Bochet M, Thibault V, et al. Long-term incidence of hepatitis B virus resistance to lamivudine in human immunodeficiency virus-infected patients. Hepatology 1999;30 (5):1302–6.

[48] European AIDS Clinical Society. Guidelines. Clinical Management and Treatment of HIV Infected Adults in Europe. Version 5-2. November 2009.

[49] Cooper RD, Wiebe N, Smith N, et al. Systematic review and meta-analysis: renal safety of tenofovir disoproxil fumarate in HIV-infected patients. Clin Infect Dis 2010;51(5):496–505.

[50] McComsey G, Kitch D, Daar E, et al. Bone and limb fat outcomes of ACTG A5224a, a substudy of ACTG A5202: A prospective, randomized, partially blinded Phase III trial of ABC/3TC or TDF/FTC with EFV or ATV/r for initial treatment of HIV-1 infection, In: 17th Conference on Retroviruses and Opportunistic Infections; 2010. San Francisco, CA; February 16–19, Abstract 106LB.

[51] Stellbrink HJ, Orkin C, Arribas JR, et al. Comparison of changes in bone density and turnover with abacavir-lamivudine versus tenofovir-emtricitabine in HIV-infected adults: 48-week results from the ASSERT study. Clin Infect Dis 2010;51(8):963–72.

[52] Barrios A, Rendon A, Negredo E, et al. Paradoxical CD4+ T-cell decline in HIV-infected patients with complete virus suppression taking tenofovir and didanosine. AIDS 2005;19:569–75.

[53] Perez-Elias MJ, Moreno S, Gutierrez C, et al. High virological failure rate in HIV patients after switching to a regimen with two nucleoside reverse transcriptase inhibitors plus tenofovir. AIDS 2005;19:695–8.

[54] Moyle GJ, DeJesus E, Cahn P, et al. Abacavir once or twice daily combined with once-daily lamivudine and efavirenz for the treatment of antiretroviral-naive HIV-infected adults: results of the Ziagen Once Daily in Antiretroviral Combination Study. J Acquir Immune Defic Syndr 2005;38:417–25.

[55] Hewitt RG. Abacavir hypersensitivity reaction. Clin Infect Dis 2002;34:1137–42.

[56] Mallal S, Phillips E, Carosi G, et al. HLA-B*5701 screening for hypersensitivity to abacavir. N Engl J Med 2008;358(6):568–79.

[57] Worm SW, Sabin C, Weber R, et al. Risk of myocardial infarction in patients with HIV infection exposed to specific individual antiretroviral drugs from the 3 major drug classes: the data collection on adverse events of anti-HIV drugs (D:A:D) study. J Infect Dis 2010;201(3):318–30.

[58] Ding X, Andraca-Carrera E, Cooper C, et al. No association of myocardial infarction with ABC use: an FDA meta-analysis, In: 18th Conference on Retroviruses and Opportunistic Infections. Boston, MA; 2011 February 27–March 2, Abstract 808.

[59] Sax PE, Tierney C, Collier AC, et al. Abacavir-lamivudine versus tenofovir-emtricitabine for initial HIV-1 therapy. N Engl J Med 2009;361(23):2230–40.

[60] U.S. Department of Health and Human Services. Recommendations for use of antiretroviral drugs in pregnant HIV-1-infected women for maternal health and interventions to reduce perinatal HIV transmission in the United States. May 24, 2010.

[61] World Health Organization . Antiretroviral therapy for HIV infection in adults and adolescents. Recommendations for a public health approach. 2010.

[62] Anon. d4T plus ddI: warning for pregnant women. AIDS Treat News 2001;358:8.

[63] Maitland D, Moyle G, Hand J, et al. Early virologic failure in HIV-1 infected subjects on didanosine/tenofovir/efavirenz: 12-week results from a randomized trial. AIDS 2005;19:1183–8.

[64] Bangsberg D, Weiser S, Guzman D, et al. 95% adherence is not necessary for viral suppression in less than 400 copies/mL in the majority of individuals on NNRTI regimens, In: 12th Conference on Retroviruses and Opportunistic Infections. Boston, MA; 22–25 February, 2005.

[65] Metry DW, Lahart CJ, Farmer KL, et al. Stevens–Johnson syndrome caused by the antiretroviral drug nevirapine. J Am Acad Dermatol 2001;44:S354–S357.

[66] Boehringer Ingelheim . Dear Health Care Professional Letter: Clarification of risk factors for severe, life-threatening and fatal hepatotoxicity with VIRAMUNE (nevirapine). February 2004.

[67] Cohen C, Molina JM, Cahn P, et al. Pooled week 48 efficacy and safety results from ECHO and THRIVE, two double-blind, randomised, phase III trials comparing TMC278 versus efavirenz in treatment-naive, HIV-1-infected patients, In: Program and abstracts of the XVIII International AIDS Conference; 2010. Vienna; July 18–23, Abstract THLBB206.

[68] Malan DR, Krantz E, David N, et al. Efficacy and safety of atazanavir, with or without ritonavir, as part of once-daily highly active antiretroviral therapy regimens in antiretroviral-naive patients. J Acquir Immune Defic Syndr 2008;47(2):161–7.

[69] Molina JM, Andrade-Villanueva J, Echevarria J, et al. Once-daily atazanavir/ritonavir compared with twice-daily lopinavir/ritonavir, each in combination with tenofovir and emtricitabine, for management of antiretroviral-naive HIV-1-infected patients: 96-week efficacy and safety

results of the CASTLE study. J Acquir Immune Defic Syndr 2010;53(3):323–32.

[70] Ortiz R, Dejesus E, Khanlou H, et al. Efficacy and safety of once-daily darunavir/ritonavir versus lopinavir/ritonavir in treatment-naive HIV-1-infected patients at week 48. AIDS 2008;22 (12):1389–97.

[71] Kaplan SS, Hicks CB. Safety and antiviral activity of lopinavir/ritonavir-based therapy in human immunodeficiency virus type 1 (HIV-1) infection. J Antimicrob Chemother 2005;56:273–6.

[72] Walmsley S, Avihingsanon A, Slim J, et al. Gemini: a noninferiority study of saquinavir/ritonavir versus lopinavir/ritonavir as initial HIV-1 therapy in adults. J Acquir Immune Defic Syndr 2009;50(4):367–74.

[73] Eron Jr. J, Yeni P, Gathe Jr. J, et al. The KLEAN study of fosamprenavir-ritonavir versus lopinavir-ritonavir, each in combination with abacavir-lamivudine, for initial treatment of HIV infection over 48 weeks: a randomised non-inferiority trial. Lancet 2006;368(9534): 476–82.

[74] Walmsley S, Bernstein B, King M, et al. Lopinavir–ritonavir versus nelfinavir for the initial treatment of HIV infection. N Engl J Med 2002;346:2039–46.

[75] Olyaei AJ, deMattos AM, Bennett WM. Renal toxicity of protease inhibitors. Curr Opin Nephrol Hypertens 2000;9:473–6.

[76] Garcia-Silva J, Almagro M, Pena-Penabad C, et al. Indinavir-induced retinoid-like effects: incidence, clinical features and management. Drug Saf 2002;25:993–1003.

[77] Lennox JL, Dejesus E, Berger DS, et al. Raltegravir versus efavirenz regimens in treatment-naive HIV-1-infected patients: 96-week efficacy, durability, subgroup, safety, and metabolic analyses. J Acquir Immune Defic Syndr 2010;55(1):39–48.

[78] Eron J, Rockstroh J, Reynes J, et al. QDMRK, a phase III study of the safety and efficacy of once daily vs twice daily RAL in combination therapy for treatment-naïve HIV-infected patients, In: 18th Conference on Retroviruses and Opportunistic Infections; 2011. Boston, MA; February 27–March 2, Abstract 150LB.

[79] Gulick RM, Jacob Lalezari J, Goodrich J, et al. Maraviroc for previously treated patients with R5 HIV-1 infection. N Engl J Med 2008;359:1429–41.

[80] Cooper DA, Heera J, Goodrich J, et al. Maraviroc versus efavirenz, both in combination with zidovudine-lamivudine, for the treatment of antiretroviral-naive subjects with CCR5-tropic HIV-1 infection. J Infect Dis 2010;201 (6):803–13.

[81] Lalezari JP, Henry K, O'Hearn M, et al. Enfuvirtide, an HIV-1 fusion inhibitor, for drug-resistant HIV infection in North and South America. N Engl J Med 2003;348:2175–85.

[82] Lazzarin A, Clotet B, Cooper D, et al. Efficacy of enfuvirtide in patients infected with drug-resistant HIV-1 in Europe and Australia. N Engl J Med 2003;348:2186–95.

[83] Gupta SK, Eustace JA, Wunston JA, et al. Guidelines for the management of chronic kidney disease in HIV-infected patients: recommendations of the HIV Medicine Association of the Infectious Diseases Society of America. Clin Infect Dis 2005;40:1559–85.

[84] Strain MC, Little SJ, Daar ES, et al. Effect of treatment, during primary infection, on establishment and clearance of cellular reservoirs of HIV-1. J Infect Dis 2005;191:1410–18.

[85] Kaufmann DE, Lichterfeld M, Altfeld M, et al. Limited durability of viral control following treated acute HIV infection. PLoS Med 2004;1:e36.

[86] Garcia F, De Lazzari E, Plana M, et al. Long-term CD4+ T-cell response to highly active antiretroviral therapy according to baseline CD4+ T-cell count. J Acquir Immune Defic Syndr 2004;36:702–13.

[87] Willig JH, Abroms S, Westfall AO, et al. Increased regimen durability in the era of once-daily fixed-dose combination antiretroviral therapy. AIDS 2008;22 (15):1951–60.

[88] Montaner JS, Lima VD, Barrios R, et al. Association of highly active antiretroviral therapy coverage, population viral load, and yearly new HIV diagnoses in British Columbia, Canada: a population-based study. Lancet 2010;376 (9740):532–9.

[89] Granich RM, Gilks CF, Dye C, et al. Universal voluntary HIV testing with immediate antiretroviral therapy as a strategy for elimination of HIV transmission: a mathematical model. Lancet 2009;373(9657):48–57.

[90] National Institute of Allergy and Infectious Diseases. Treating HIV-infected people with antiretrovirals protects partners from infection findings result from NIH-funded International Study, NIH News. Available at: http://www.niaid.nih. gov/news/newsreleases/2011/ Pages/HPTN052.aspx; May 12, 2011 [accessed 23.05.11.].

[91] Sterne JA, May M, Costagliola D, et al. Timing of initiation of antiretroviral therapy in AIDS-free HIV-1-infected patients: a collaborative analysis of 18 HIV cohort studies. Lancet 2009;373 (9672):1352–63.

[92] Lima VD, Johnston K, Hogg RS, et al. Expanded access to highly active antiretroviral therapy: a potentially powerful strategy to curb the growth of the HIV epidemic. J Infect Dis 2008;198 (1):59–67.

[93] Charlebois ED, Havlir DV. "A bird in the hand…": A commentary on the test and treat approach for HIV. Comment on "Comparative effectiveness of HIV testing and treatment in highly endemic regions". Arch Intern Med 2010;170 (15):1354–6.

[94] Abdool Karim SS, Naidoo K, Grobler A, et al. Timing of initiation of antiretroviral drugs during tuberculosis therapy. N Engl J Med 2010;362 (8):697–706.

[95] Severe P, Juste MA, Ambroise A, et al. Early versus standard antiretroviral therapy for HIV-infected adults in Haiti. N Engl J Med 2010;363 (3):257–65.

[96] Lepri AC, Miller V, Phillips AN, et al. The virological response to highly active antiretroviral therapy over the first 24 weeks of therapy according to the pre-therapy viral load and the weeks 4–8 viral load. AIDS 2001;15:47–54.

[97] Nieuwkerk PT, Oort FJ. Self-reported adherence to antiretroviral therapy for HIV-1 infection and virologic treatment response: a meta-analysis. J Acquir Immune Defic Syndr 2005;38:445–8.

[98] Grant RM, Lama JR, Anderson PL, et al. iPrEx Study Team. Preexposure chemoprophylaxis for HIV prevention in men who have sex with men. N Engl J Med 2010;363(27):2587–99.

[99] Karim QA SSA, Frohlich JA, et al. Effectiveness and safety of tenofovir gel, an antiretroviral microbicide, for the prevention of HIV infection in women. Science 2010;329 (5996):1168–74.

[100] FHI . FHI Statement on the FEM-PrEP HIV Prevention Study, Available at: http://www.fhi.org/en/AboutFHI/Media/Releases/FEM-PrEP_statement041811.htm; April 18, 2011 [accessed 23.05.11.].

Chapter | 12 |

Development and transmission of HIV drug resistance

Mark A. Wainberg, Gerasimos J. Zaharatos

INTRODUCTION

HIV-1 drug resistance has emerged as a major problem that limits the effectiveness of antiviral drugs in treatment regimens. Many studies have shown that the development and transmission of drug-resistant HIV-1 is largely a consequence of incompletely suppressive antiretroviral regimens; HIV-1 drug resistance can significantly diminish the effectiveness and duration of benefit associated with combination therapy for the treatment of HIV/AIDS [1–6]. Resistance-conferring mutations in each of the HIV-1 reverse transcriptase (*RT*), protease (*PR*), and integrase (*IN*) genes may precede the initiation of therapy due to each of spontaneous mutagenesis and the spread of resistant viruses by sexual and other means. However, it is also generally believed that multiple drug mutations to any single or combination of antiretroviral agents (ARVs) are required in order to produce clinical resistance to most ARVs and that these are in fact selected following residual viral replication in the presence of incompletely suppressive drug regimens [7–9].

In the case of the protease inhibitors (PIs) [10–12], and most nucleoside analog reverse transcriptase inhibitors (NRTIs), the development of progressive high-level phenotypic drug resistance follows the accumulation of primary resistance-conferring mutations in each of the HIV-1 *PR* and *RT* genes [13–15]. Non-nucleoside reverse transcriptase inhibitors (NNRTIs) have low genetic barriers for the development of drug resistance and, frequently, a single primary drug resistance mutation to any one NNRTI may be sufficient to confer high-level phenotypic drug resistance to this entire class of ARVs [16, 17]. Raltegravir is the only currently approved integrase strand transfer inhibitor (INSTI) and has an intermediate genetic barrier for

resistance, since an accumulation of two or more mutations in *IN* are generally required in order for this compound to lose its antiviral efficacy [18, 19].

Furthermore, differences have also been reported in regard to the development and evolution of antiretroviral drug resistance between subtype B HIV-1 and several group M non-B subtypes. Non-B subtypes, e.g. subtype C HIV-1 variants, are known to possess naturally occurring polymorphisms at several *RT* and *PR* codons that are implicated in drug resistance [20, 21]. In some studies, the presence of these polymorphisms did not significantly reduce susceptibility to ARVs in phenotypic resistance assays or limit the effectiveness of an initial antiretroviral therapy regimen for a period of up to 18 months [20, 22]. However, it has also been suggested that polymorphisms at resistance positions may sometimes facilitate selection of novel pathways leading to drug resistance, especially with incompletely suppressive antiretroviral regimens [20]. This, in turn, may have important clinical implications with respect to choice of effective antiretroviral therapy (ART). This warrants increased genotypic surveillance on a worldwide basis, as the prevalence of non-B HIV-1 infection is increasing rapidly.

As illustrated in Figures 12.1–12.5, it has been possible to select numerous drug resistance mutations for all licensed ARVs and investigational agents such as some HIV-1 entry inhibitors [5, 6, 23]. In view of the hypervariability of HIV-1 and the inability of many current antiretroviral combinations to completely suppress viral replication, especially in patients with prior treatment failure, it is essential that new anti-HIV drug discovery initiatives focus on the identification of new therapeutic targets and the development of ARVs with more robust genetic barriers for resistance and a broader spectrum of activity against drug-resistant HIV-1 variants.

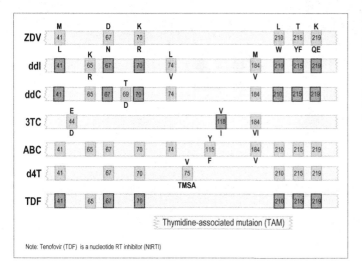

Figure 12.1 Common NRTI mutations associated with HIV drug resistance. The letter designation at the top of a box refers to the amino acid that is present in the wild-type sequence of RT. The letters at the bottom refer to substitutions associated with drug resistance. Sometimes, several different amino acid changes at the same codon can confer drug resistance, as for example both Y and F in the case of position 215.

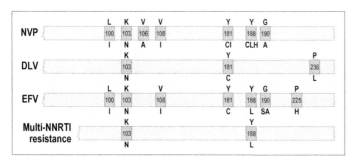

Figure 12.2 Common NNRTI mutations associated with HIV drug resistance. The letter designation at the top of a box refers to the amino acid that is present in the wild-type sequence of RT. The letters at the bottom refer to substitutions associated with drug resistance. Sometimes, several different amino acid changes at the same codon can confer drug resistance, as for example both C and I in the case of position 181. The novel NNRTI, etravirine (ETR) can often be used to treat individuals whose viruses contain mutations associated with resistance to either NVP or EFV. However, the signature mutation that is apparently responsible for resistance against both ETR as well as rilpivirine (RPV), the most recently approved member of the NNRTI family, is E138K. In all likelihood, the E138K mutation will have the ability to also confer cross-resistance to both NVP and EFV, thereby eliminating the likelihood for the successful use of NNRTIs in therapy. Accordingly, it is important that efforts be made to prevent the E138K mutation from arising and from being transmitted.

GENERATION OF HIV-1 DRUG RESISTANCE

Resistance mutations to ARVs may arise spontaneously as a result of the error-prone replication of HIV-1 and, in addition, are selected both *in vitro* and *in vivo* by pharmacological pressure [24–26]. The high rate of spontaneous mutation in HIV-1 has been largely attributed to the absence of a 3′-5′exonuclease proof-reading mechanism. Sequence analyses of HIV-1 DNA have detected several types of mutations including base substitutions, additions, and deletions [24]. The frequency of spontaneous mutation for HIV-1 varies considerably as a result of differences

among viral strains studied *in vitro* [27]. Overall mutation rates for wild-type laboratory strains of HIV-1 have been reported to range from 97×10^{-4} to 200×10^{-4} per nucleotide for the HXB2 clonal variant of HIV-1 to as high as 800×10^{-4} per nucleotide for the HIV-1 NY5 strain [24, 27].

In addition to the low fidelity of DNA synthesis by HIV-1 RT, other interdependent factors that affect rates of HIV mutagenesis include RT processivity, viral replication capacity, viral pool size, and availability of target cells for infection [28–31]. It follows that an alteration in any or a combination of these factors might influence the development of HIV drug resistance. There are also data showing that thymidine analog mutations (TAMs) in RT can significantly increase the likelihood of further mutational HIV-1

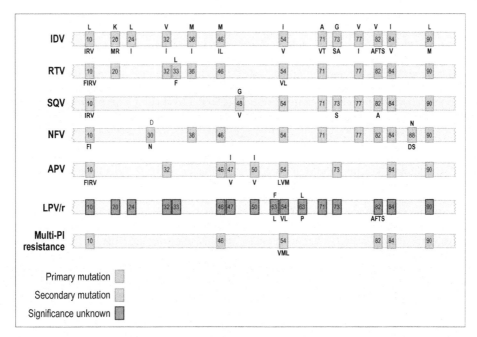

Figure 12.3 Common PR mutations associated with HIV drug resistance. The letter designation at the top of a box refers to the amino acid that is present in the wild-type sequence of PR. The letters at the bottom refer to substitutions associated with drug resistance. Sometimes, several different amino acid changes at the same codon can confer drug resistance, as for example both I and L in the case of position [46]. Resistance to darunanavir and tipranavir involve multiple combinations of the above mutations, and both these drugs have a higher genetic barrier for resistance then other members of the PI family of drugs.

Figure 12.4 Mutations in the envelope gene associated with resistance to enfuvirtide (T20, Fuzeon).

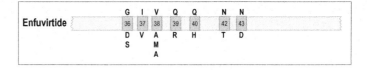

Figure 12.5 Primary mutations in the integrase gene associated with resistance to raltegravir. The development of clinically significant resistance to raltegravir requires the presence of one of the mutations in this Figure together with other secondary mutations that, together with a primary mutation, will increase the level of resistance while also causing an increase in viral repliative capacity.

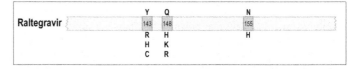

distributions and evolution of drug resistance; furthermore, this can happen in the presence or absence of concomitantly administered NRTIs [32, 33].

INHIBITORS OF REVERSE TRANSCRIPTASE

The RT enzyme is encoded by the HIV *pol* gene and is responsible for the transcription of double-stranded proviral DNA from viral genomic RNA. Two categories of drugs have been developed to block RT; these are NRTIs that act to arrest DNA chain elongation by acting as competitive inhibitors of RT and NNRTIs that act as non-competitive antagonists of enzyme activity by binding to the catalytic site of RT. NRTIs are administered to patients as precursor compounds that are phosphorylated to their active triphosphate form by cellular enzymes. These compounds lack a 3′ hydroxyl group (OH) necessary for elongation of viral DNA. These analogs can compete effectively with normal deoxynucleotide triphosphate (dNTP) substrates for binding to RT and incorporation into viral DNA [34, 35].

NNRTI antiviral activity involves the binding of these non-competitive inhibitors to a hydrophobic pocket close to the catalytic site of RT [36, 37]. NNRTI inhibition reduces the catalytic rate of polymerization without affecting nucleotide binding or nucleotide-induced conformational change [38]. NNRTIs are particularly active at template positions at which the RT enzyme naturally pauses. NNRTIs do not seem to influence the competition between dideoxynucleotide triphosphates (ddNTPs) and the naturally occurring dNTPs for insertion into the growing proviral DNA chain [39].

Both types of RT inhibitors have been shown to successfully diminish plasma viral burden in HIV-1-infected subjects. However, monotherapy with all drugs has led to drug resistance. Patients who receive combinations of three or more drugs are less likely to develop resistance, since these "cocktails" can suppress viral replication with much greater efficiency than single drugs or two drugs in combination. Although mutagenesis is less likely to happen in this circumstance, it can still occur, and the emergence of drug-resistant breakthrough viruses has been demonstrated in patients receiving highly active ART [40, 41]. Furthermore, the persistence of reservoirs of latently infected cells represents another major impediment to currently used anti-HIV chemotherapy [42]. Replication of HIV might resume once therapy is stopped or interrupted and, therefore, eradication of a latent reservoir of 10^5 cells might take as long as 60 years, a goal that is not practical with currently available drugs and technology [42, 43].

Resistance to 3TC ((-)-2', 3'-dideoxy-3'-thiacytidine, lamivudine) and emtricitabine (FTC) can develop quickly, whereas resistance to other NRTIs will commonly appear only after about 6 months of non-suppressive therapy. Phenotypic resistance is detected by comparing the IC_{50} (or drug concentration capable of blocking viral replication by 50%) of pretreatment viral isolates with those obtained after therapy. Thus, higher IC_{50} values obtained after months or years of treatment can reflect a loss in viral susceptibility to ARVs. Selective polymerase chain reaction (PCR) analysis of the *RT* genome confirms that the number of mutations associated with drug resistance usually increases concomitantly with increases in IC_{50} values.

Mutations associated with drug resistance have been reported in response to the use of any single NRTI or NNRTI [44]. However, not all drugs elicit the same mutagenic response; sensitivity and resistance patterns must be considered on an individual drug basis. For example, patients on 3TC monotherapy may develop high-level, i.e. 1000-fold resistance within weeks, whereas 6 months or more are often required in order for sensitivity to ZDV to drop by 50- to 100-fold. In contrast, HIV may appear to remain partially sensitive, even after prolonged monotherapy, to several other commonly used nucleoside analogs: ddI (didanosine), d4T (stavudine), and ABC (abacavir). Of the latter, only ABC is commonly used in Western countries today, although the use of d4T, which is often toxic, continues in many developing country settings, mainly because it

is inexpensive. In the case of ZDV, increases in IC_{50} below threefold are regarded as non-significant, while 10-to 50-fold increases usually represent partial resistance, and increases above 50-fold denote high-level resistance.

Patient resistance to nucleoside analogs can often develop independently of the dose of drug that is administered. Tissue culture data have shown that HIV-1 resistance can be easily demonstrated against each of NRTIs, NNRTIs, and PIs, by gradually increasing the concentration of compound in the tissue culture medium [45, 46]. Cell lines are especially useful in this regard, since HIV replication occurs very efficiently in such hosts. Tissue culture selection provides an effective pre-clinical means of studying HIV mutagenesis, especially since the same resistance-conferring mutations that arise in cell culture are usually predictive of those that will appear clinically. Owing to the high turnover and mutation rate of HIV-1, the retroviral quasispecies will also include defective virions and singly mutated drug-resistant variants that are present prior to commencement of therapy. Multiply mutated variants appear later, because it requires time to accumulate multiple mutations within a single viral genome. Therefore, multiply mutated viruses are not commonly found in the retroviral pool of untreated patients. An exception to this involves cases of new infection with drug-resistant viruses transmitted from extensively treated individuals. Patients with advanced infection have a higher viral load and a broader range of quasispecies than newly infected individuals. Such patients are often immunosuppressed and may also have diminished ability to immunologically control viral replication, possibly leading to more rapid development of drug resistance.

Site-directed mutagenesis has shown that a variety of *RT* mutations encode HIV resistance to both NRTIs and NNRTIs. Crystallographic and biochemical data have demonstrated that mutations conferring resistance to NNRTIs are found in the peptide residues that make contact with these compounds within their binding pocket [36, 37].

Resistance-encoding mutations to NRTIs are found in different regions of the RT enzyme, probably due to the complexities of nucleoside incorporation, which involve several distinct steps. These mutations can decrease RT susceptibility to nucleoside analogs. A summary of primary *RT* mutations has been published [44].

It has also been shown that a family of insertion and deletion mutations between codons 67 and 70 can cause resistance to a variety of NRTIs including ZDV, 3TC, ddI, ddC, and d4T. Usually, these insertion mutations confer multidrug resistance (MDR) when present in a ZDV-resistant background. Another less frequently observed resistance mutation, K65R, has been shown to be associated with prior treatment with ABC- and tenofovir (TDF)-containing regimens and results in reduced antiviral susceptibility to both of these agents. Hence, resistance to these ARVs can develop via genetic pathways involving either the TAMs or K65R as hallmark drug resistance mutations [47]. In recent years, the proportion of geno-typed clinical samples containing K65R has increased from less than 1 to almost 4%, reflecting the increased use of TDF in first-line treatment regimens in developed countries.

Diminished sensitivity to NNRTIs appears quickly both in culture selection protocols and in patients [36, 48]. NNRTIs share a common binding site, and mutations that encode NNRTI resistance are located within the binding pocket that makes drug contact [36, 37, 39–46, 48–53]. This explains the finding that extensive cross-resistance is observed among several approved NNRTIs. A substitution at codon 181 (tyrosine to cysteine) (Y181C) is a common mutation that encodes cross-resistance among many NNRTIs [49, 54, 55]. Replacement of Y181 by a serine or histidine also con-ferred HIV resistance to NNRTIs [56]. A mutation at amino acid 236 (proline to leucine) (P236L), conferring resistance to a particular class of NNRTIs that include delavirdine, can also diminish resistance to nevirapine (NVP) and efavirenz (EFV), particularly if a Y181C mutation is also present in the same virus [57]. Other important substitutions are Y188C and Y188H and can also confer NNRTI resistance.

Another drug resistance mutation, namely K103N (ly-sine to asparagine), is commonly observed and is respon-sible for reduced susceptibility to many approved NNRTIs including efavirenz and nevirapine [49, 54, 55]. Substitution of K103N results in alteration of interactions between NNRTIs and RT. The K103N mutation shows syn-ergy with Y181C in regard to resistance to NNRTIs, unlike antagonistic interactions involving Y181C and P236L [55]. Recently, a mutation at position E138K was shown to en-code resistance against a newer NNRTI termed etravirine that has been shown to be effective in second-line thera-peutic regimens [58]. This E138K mutation also seems to be associated with resistance to rilpivirine, a novel NNRTI that is currently undergoing advanced clinical trials for po-tential use in first-line therapy in association with NRTIs.

Resistance to NNRTIs is also observed in cell-free enzyme assays [52, 54, 59–61]. Both Y181I and Y188L mediate de-creased sensitivity to NNRTIs without affecting either sub-strate recognition or catalytic efficiency, supporting the idea that resistance to NNRTIs is attributable to diminished ability of these drugs to be bound by RT.

In recent years, a new member of the NNRTI family, etra-virine (ETV), has been approved for use in patients with pre-existing resistance against NVP and EFV. ETV possesses excellent activity against viruses containing the K103N and T181C mutations, among others, that are associated with resistance against first-generation NNRTIs [62, 63]. How-ever, the activity of ETV may be compromised by other mu-tations such as E138K, although it remains to be determined whether this mutation will appear to signifi-cant extent in patients who fail ETV-containing ARV regi-mens [64]. Several drug companies are now trying to develop novel NNRTIs that will hopefully have a higher ge-netic barrier for resistance than either NVP or EFV for use in first-line ARV regimens. Several such compounds are now being studied in clinical trials.

PROTEASE INHIBITORS

Drug-resistant viruses have been observed in the case of all PIs developed to date [65–67]. In addition, some strains of HIV have displayed cross-resistance to a variety of PIs after either clinical use or *in vitro* drug exposure [65–67]. In gen-eral, the patterns of mutations observed with PIs are more complex than those observed with RT antagonists. First, a greater number of mutations within the *PR* gene are re-quired for resistance to occur. This is especially true for both darunavir and tipranavir, that almost always require a greater accumulation of the resistant mutations listed in Figure 12.3 in order for resistance to occur, than would be the case for any other member of the PI family of drugs. There is also greater variability, among PIs, in temporal pat-terns of appearance of different mutations and the manner in which different combinations of mutations can give rise to phenotypic resistance. These data suggest that the PR en-zyme can adapt more easily than RT to pressures exerted by antiviral drugs. At least 40 mutations in *PR* have been iden-tified as responsible for resistance to PIs [65–67].

Certain of the mutations within the *PR* gene are more im-portant than others and can confer resistance, virtually on their own, to at least certain PIs [65–67]. One mutation, in particular, D30N, is probably unique to nelfinavir (NFV), a potent HIV PI. However, a variety of other mutations may confer cross-resistance among multiple drugs within the PI family. In addition, wide arrays of secondary mutations that, when combined with primary mutations, can cause in-creased levels of resistance to occur have been observed. On the other hand, the presence of certain of these secondary mu-tations on their own may not lead to drug resistance, and, in this context, some of these amino acid changes should be considered to represent naturally occurring polymorphisms. In addition, it should be noted that resistance to PIs can also result from mutations within the substrates of the PR enzyme, i.e. the gag and gag-pol precursor proteins of HIV. A variety of studies have now shown that mutations at cleavage sites within these substrates can be responsible for drug resistance, both in tissue culture and in treated patients. However, the full clinical significance of cleavage site mutations in regard to PR resistance is not understood.

FUSION AND ENTRY INHIBITORS

A single fusion inhibitor and a single entry inhibitor have been approved for use in clinical practice. The fusion inhib-itor is the polypeptide enfuvirtide (ENF), which is admin-istered subcutaneously. The entry inhibitor is maraviroc (MVC), which is orally bioavailable.

ENF is a 36 amino acid synthetic peptide that structurally mimics the heptad repeat 2 (HR2) region of gp41. It also inhibits the association of HR2 with the heptad repeat (HR1) of the same protein. This action impedes the formation of a six-helix bundle that mediates the fusion of the HIV envelope and cell membrane. ENF is generally reserved for highly experienced patients who have failed all other therapies and is used in association with an optimized background ARV regimen [68].

Mutations at positions 36–45 (GIVQQQNNLL) of the HR1 region are extremely important in the development of resistance. Even a single amino acid substitution can cause a significant reduction in drug susceptibility. As a result, ENF is considered to have a low genetic barrier for resistance. The emergence of mutations at amino acids 36–45 was detected in 94% (205/218) of viruses from patients experiencing virological failure while taking ENF in each of two clinical trials. The most frequent mutations were at positions 38 (47.7%, 104/218; most often V38A), 43 (30.7%, 58/218; most often N43D), and 36 (26.6%, 58/218; most often G36D) [68–70].

MVC is a CCR5 co-receptor inhibitor. It binds to the CCR5 co-receptor of the susceptible host cell. By doing so, it prevents the HIV-1 gp120 protein from interacting with the CCR5 co-receptor, resulting in blockage of viral entry. The results of the MOTIVATE trials showed that MVC can be effective in the treatment of advanced HIV disease, when combined with other ARVs, in patients whose viruses were CCR5-tropic. MVC seems not to be effective against viruses that are tropic for the CXCR4 co-receptor. Its use is limited to patients who have a laboratory assay that confirms that their virus is CCR5-tropic. Most testing for MVC eligibility is now conducted by sequencing of the HIV-1 *env* gene, although a phenotypic test is also available for this purpose [71, 72].

Resistance to MVC is associated with both a complex array of mutations in the V3 loop that do not cause cross-resistance to ENF as well a pre-existing minority populations of CXCR4-tropic viruses that may became predominant after treatment with MVC [73, 74].

Resistance to MVC can also be attributed to viruses of dual and/or mixed tropism in regard to CCR5 and CXCR4. It has also been demonstrated that certain CCR5-tropic variants may rarely be able to use complexes between MVC and CCR5 receptors to gain entry into cells. Recently, MVC had also been approved for use in treatment-naïve patients.

ANTIRETROVIRAL DRUG RESISTANCE IN NON-B SUBTYPES OF HIV-1 GROUP M

Genotypic divergence of *pol* gene sequences between different HIV-1 subtypes is only beginning to be investigated, although the RT and PR enzymes are the main targets of ART [75–79]. Group O and HIV-2 viruses carry natural polymorphisms Y181C and Y181I that confer intrinsic resistance to NNRTIs [80–82]. Subtype F isolates, showing 11% nucleotide sequence variation from subtype B and group M viruses, have also been reported to have reduced

sensitivity to some NNRTIs while retaining susceptibility to others such as nevirapine and delavirdine, NRTIs, and PIs [83–85]. In contrast, the drug sensitivity of subtype C isolates from treatment-naïve patients in Zimbabwe was reported to be similar to that of subtype B isolates [84]. Recent studies conducted with Ethiopian subtype C clinical isolates showed natural resistance to NNRTIs in one case and resistance to ZDV in another, due to natural polymorphisms at positions G190A and K70R, respectively [86]. Another study reported no differences in drug susceptibility among subtypes A, B, C, and E; subtype D viruses showed reduced susceptibility due to rapid growth kinetics [87]. High prevalence (i.e. 94%) of a valine polymorphism (GTG) at position 106 in RT from subtype C HIV-1 clinical isolates has also been reported [88]. In tissue culture experiments, selection of subtype C with efavirenz (EFV) was associated with development of high-level (i.e. 100- to 1000-fold) phenotypic resistance to all NNRTIs. This was a consequence of a V106M mutation that arose in place of the V106A substitution that is more commonly seen with subtype B viruses [88]. This V106M mutation conferred broad cross-resistance to all currently approved NNRTIs and was selected on the basis of differential codon usage at position 106 in RT, due to redundancy in the genetic code.

Genotypic diversity and drug resistance may be particularly relevant in establishing treatment strategies against African and Asian strains. First, since many antiviral drugs have been designed based on sequences of subtype B RT and PR enzymes, and drug resistance profiles, if not responses, may be different for non-B viral strains. Second, drug resistance may develop more rapidly in resource-poor countries where only suboptimal therapeutic regimens are often available. Global phenotypic and genotypic monitoring programs of non-B subtypes is warranted so as not to jeopardize the outcome of recently introduced antiretroviral strategies [89].

TRANSMISSION OF HIV DRUG RESISTANCE

As stated, highly active ART, including drugs that inhibit the RT and PR enzymes of HIV-1, has resulted in declining morbidity and mortality [90]. The failure to completely suppress viral replication allows for the development of genotypic changes in HIV-1 that confer resistance to each of the major classes of antiretroviral drugs [91–93]. Cumulative data now indicate that viruses containing single drug-resistance mutations can be transmitted to approximately 10–15% of newly infected persons in Western countries in which ARVs have been available for many years, with transmission of dual- and triple-class MDR observed in 3–5% of cases [94–97].

There is concern that the transmission of MDR viruses in primary HIV-1 infection (PHI) may limit future therapeutic options. Treatment failure has been observed in several individuals harboring MDR infections [97–99]. Some reports have shown an impaired fitness of transmitted MDR variants compared with wild-type infections acquired in PHI [100], and the mutations that were transmitted in such patients persisted in the absence of treatment [100]. This persistence differs from the rapid outgrowth of WT viruses in established infections upon treatment interruption, due to the selective growth advantage and fitness of WT variants [100–102]. Taken together, these findings suggest that archival WT viruses may not exist in MDR infections transmitted during PHI.

Several reports have also documented cases of intersubtype superinfection (A/E and B) in recently infected injection drug users (IDUs) [103, 104]. Other studies have failed to confirm superinfection following IDU exposure, suggesting that superinfection is a relatively rare event [105, 106]. Several subsequent reports demonstrated superinfection in subtype B infections. In one case, a WT superinfection arose following a primary MDR infection [107, 108].

It is important to assess the virological consequences of transmission of drug-resistant variants in primary infection, as well as the time to disappearance of resistant virus in those patients not initially treated.

Genotypic analysis indicates that a single dominant HIV-1 species can persist for more than 2 years in circulating plasma and peripheral blood mononuclear cells (PBMCs), regardless of route of transmission. Resistant and MDR infections can persist for 2–7 years following PHI.

Superinfection with a second MDR strain in a patient originally infected with an MDR strain from an identified source partner has also been described [109]. Despite a rapid decline in plasma viremia suggestive of an effective immune response, this patient was susceptible to a second infection, which occurred concomitantly with a dramatic rise in viral load. Other subtype B superinfections have also been described, as well as intersubtype A/E and B superinfections [103, 104, 108, 110, 111]. Most of the superinfections described have occurred in the first year following initial infection.

Many have attributed superinfection to co-infection during primary infection. Two longitudinal studies involving IDU populations ($n = 37$ in both studies) indicated that superinfection is a rare phenomenon not observed during 1–12 years of follow-up spanning 215 and 1,072 total years of exposure [107, 108]. However, it is not known whether any patients were recruited within the first year of HIV-1 exposure in these studies. In the case of the MDR infections cited above, identification of the source partner of infection argues against co-infection [109].

Findings of HIV-1 superinfection are a matter of concern insofar as such results challenge the assumption that immune responses can protect against reinfection. Of course, the impaired viral fitness of the initial MDR infection described above may be a factor in permitting superinfection. The initial MDR strain showed a 13-fold impaired replicative

capacity from a WT variant strain from the isolated source partner following a treatment interruption. Fitness considerations may also have been important in a WT superinfection of an initial MDR infection and cases of subtype B superinfection following A/E infections that elicited low-level viremia [103, 104].

In newly infected individuals, multi-mutated viruses conferring MDR may represent a new determinant of virological outcome. Persistence of MDR in the absence of treatment raises serious issues regarding HIV-1 management. For recently infected MDR patients, drug resistance analysis and viral fitness may provide useful information in regard to ultimate therapeutic strategies.

It is interesting to note that the presence of the M184V mutation in reverse transcriptase, associated with high-level resistance to 3TC, seems to have been associated with the persistence of low viral load. In two PHI cases, rebounds to a high level of plasma viremia occurred only at times when the M184V mutation in RT could no longer be detected. A third PHI patient maintained low plasma viremia over 5 years, and his virus also contained the M184V mutation throughout this time. In an additional individual, high viral loads were present at times after primary infection despite the M184V mutation, but virus could only be isolated from this individual in co-culture experiments after loss of the M184V mutation [109]. These data are consistent with previous findings on loss of fitness conferred by the M184V mutation in reverse transcriptase, alongside multiple other pleiotropic effects, including diminished processivity, diminished rates of nucleotide excision, and diminished rates of initiation of reverse transcription [112–114].

Other studies suggest that MDR infections have impaired replicative capacity, leading to more efficient antiviral immune responses [115–118]. A relative absence of genotypic changes in these viruses over time further supports the concept of expansion of predominant MDR quasispecies during primary infection. Recombination events can also occur in this period. It is also important to point out that the replication fitness of a given virus versus its transmission fitness may represent two very different concepts.

ART, by reducing HIV-1 replication, has been shown not only to impact significantly on morbidity and mortality but also to reduce the spread of HIV-1 [119, 120]. Treatment effectiveness is hampered by the development of drug-resistant (DR) strains, leading to virological failure [121]. The transmissibility of DR strains is not fully understood and may differ from that of wild-type [74] strains for at least two reasons. One is the relative fitness of DR strains compared with WT in the absence of therapy. Second is the degree to which partially active therapies can reduce viral load in persons harboring resistant viruses [122, 123]. As a consequence of widespread use of ART in North America, the transmission of DR strains in recently infected individuals increased from 3.8% in 1996 to 14% in 2000. Such an increase of primary DR is of public health concern, since a clear association between DR and early treatment failure has been reported [97]. However, several groups in Europe and Australia have reported a recent stable or decreasing trend in DR transmission for RT and/or PI [124, 125], and have attributed this decline to the widespread use of suppressive triple ARV regimens since 1996. This presupposes that transmission of DR variants may have previously been more common due to the widespread use of suboptimal therapy or even monotherapy regimes prior to 1996 and the likelihood that these suboptimal regimens may have been selected for drug resistance mutations with very high frequency [125].

CONCLUSION

The accumulation of specific resistance-conferring mutations is associated with the development of phenotypic resistance to anti-HIV drugs which can significantly diminish the effectiveness and longevity of ART. Cross-resistance among drugs of the same class also occurs frequently and is most problematic with NNRTIs due to their lower genetic barrier for rapid selection of drug resistance compared to other classes of ARVs. There are now also data indicating that cross-resistance amongst NRTIs may be more widespread than initially thought [126]. Furthermore, the emergence of new drug resistance mutations is helping to establish new mutant distributions with additional pathways for developing cross-resistance to ARVs [127]. These new patterns of cross-resistance, together with increasing transmission

of MDR HIV-1 variants, are problematic and can seriously limit the number of effective treatment options that are available for long-term management of HIV infection.

Additional strategies, in addition to new drug discovery programs, are urgently required to help curb the development of drug-resistant HIV-1. The best approach is to use non-toxic drugs in combination to suppress viral replication to as great an extent as is possible. If effective drugs are not available for reasons of resistance and/or availability, consideration could be given to the maintenance of specific fitness-attenuating drug resistance mutations [127, 128]. The M184V substitution in *RT* has been extensively studied in this regard because of its ability to impair viral replication capacity while limiting the development of subsequent drug resistance mutations in HIV-1 *RT*, e.g. TAMs and the Q151M multidrug complex resistance mutation associated with use of AZT and d4T [129, 130]. Of course, restricted evolution of drug resistance may also result from other alterations of *RT* function by M184V [112]. One recent study has shown that viruses containing the M184V mutation are detected less frequently than viruses containing other mutations associated with drug resistance in newly infected hosts [114], perhaps because M184V compromises viral replicative capacity. Further work on these and other topics is needed to improve our understanding of HIV drug resistance in the context of clinical relevance, successful antiviral chemotherapy, and likelihood of transmission of drug-resistant viruses [131].

REFERENCES

[1] Quiros-Roldan E, Signorini S, Castelli F, et al. Analysis of HIV-1 mutation patterns in patients failing antiretroviral therapy. J Clin Lab Anal 2001;15:43–6.

[2] Rousseau MN, Vergne L, Montes B, et al. Patterns of resistance mutations to antiretroviral drugs in extensively treated HIV-1-infected patients with failure of highly active antiretroviral therapy. J Acquir Immune Defic Syndr 2001;26:36–43.

[3] Winters MA, Baxter JD, Mayers DL, et al. Frequency of antiretroviral drug resistance mutations in HIV-1 strains from patients failing triple drug regimens: The Terry Beirn Community Programs for Clinical Research on AIDS. Antivir Ther 2000;5:57–63.

[4] Lorenzi P, Opravil M, Hirschel B, et al. Impact of drug resistance mutations on virologic response to salvage therapy. Swiss HIV Cohort Study. AIDS 1999;13:F17–F21.

[5] D'Aquila RT, Schapiro JM, Brun-Vezinet F, et al. Drug resistance mutations in HIV-1. Top HIV Med 2002;10:21–5.

[6] Yeni PG, Hammer SM, Carpenter CC, et al. Antiretroviral treatment for adult HIV infection in 2002: updated recommendations of the International AIDS Society-USA Panel. JAMA 2002;288:222–35.

[7] de Jong MD, Schuurman R, Lange JM, Boucher CA. Replication of a pre-existing resistant HIV-1 subpopulation in vivo after introduction of a strong selective

drug pressure. Antivir Ther 1996;1:33–41.

[8] Mayers DL. Prevalence and incidence of resistance to zidovudine and other antiretroviral drugs. Am J Med 1997;102:70–5.

[9] Balotta C, Berlusconi A, Pan A, et al. Prevalence of transmitted nucleoside analogue-resistant HIV-1 strains and pre-existing mutations in pol reverse transcriptase and protease region: outcome after treatment in recently infected individuals. Antivir Ther 2000;5:7–14.

[10] Molla A, Korneyeva M, Gao Q, et al. Ordered accumulation of mutations in HIV protease confers resistance to ritonavir. Nat Med 1996;2:760–6.

[11] Condra JH. Virological and clinical implications of resistance to HIV-1 protease inhibitors. Drug Resist Updat 1998;1:292–9.

[12] Deeks SG. Failure of HIV-1 protease inhibitors to fully suppress viral replication. Implications for salvage therapy. Adv Exp Med Biol 1999;458:175–82.

[13] Frost SD, Nijhuis M, Schuurman R, et al. Evolution of lamivudine resistance in human immunodeficiency virus type 1-infected individuals: the relative roles of drift and selection. J Virol 2000;74:6262–8.

[14] Gotte M, Wainberg MA. Biochemical mechanisms involved in overcoming HIV resistance to nucleoside inhibitors of reverse transcriptase. Drug Resist Updat 2000;3:30–8.

[15] Loveday C. International perspectives on antiretroviral resistance. Nucleoside reverse transcriptase inhibitor resistance. J Acquir Immune Defic Syndr 2001;26(Suppl 1):S10–S24.

[16] Deeks SG. International perspectives on antiretroviral resistance. Nonnucleoside reverse transcriptase inhibitor resistance. J Acquir Immune Defic Syndr 2001;26:S25–S33.

[17] Bacheler L, Jeffrey S, Hanna G, et al. Genotypic correlates of phenotypic resistance to efavirenz in virus isolates from patients failing nonnucleoside reverse transcriptase inhibitor therapy. J Virol 2001;75:4999–5008.

[18] Ferns RB, Kirk S, Bennett J, et al. The dynamics of appearance and disappearance of HIV-1 integrase mutations during and after withdrawal of raltegravir therapy. AIDS 2009;23:2159–64.

[19] Fransen S, Gupta S, Danovich R, et al. Loss of raltegravir susceptibility by human immunodeficiency virus type 1 is conferred via multiple nonoverlapping genetic pathways. J Virol 2009;83:11440–6.

[20] Holguin A, Soriano V. Resistance to antiretroviral agents in individuals with HIV-1 non-B subtypes. HIV Clin Trials 2002;3:403–11.

[21] Kantor R, Zijenah LS, Shafer RW, et al. HIV-1 subtype C reverse transcriptase and protease genotypes in Zimbabwean patients failing antiretroviral therapy. AIDS Res Hum Retroviruses 2002;18:1407–13.

[22] Alexander CS, Montessori V, Wynhoven B, et al. Prevalence and response to antiretroviral therapy of non-B subtypes of HIV in antiretroviral-naive individuals in British Columbia. Antivir Ther 2002;7:31–5.

[23] Wei X, Decker JM, Liu H, et al. Emergence of resistant human immunodeficiency virus type 1 in patients receiving fusion inhibitor (T-20) monotherapy. Antimicrob Agents Chemother 2002;46:1896–905.

[24] Roberts JD, Bebenek K, Kunkel TA. The accuracy of reverse transcriptase from HIV-1. Science 1988;242:1171–3.

[25] Preston BD, Dougherty JP. Mechanisms of retroviral mutation. Trends Microbiol 1996;4:16–21.

[26] Menendez-Arias L. Molecular basis of fidelity of DNA synthesis and nucleotide specificity of retroviral reverse transcriptases. Prog Nucleic Acid Res Mol Biol 2002;71:91–147.

[27] Rezende LF, Drosopoulos WC, Prasad VR. The influence of 3TC resistance mutation M184I on the fidelity and error specificity of human immunodeficiency virus type 1 reverse transcriptase. Nucleic Acids Res 1998;26:3066–72.

[28] Coffin JM. HIV population dynamics in vivo: implications for genetic variation, pathogenesis, and therapy. Science 1995;267:483–9.

[29] Drosopoulos WC, Rezende LF, Wainberg MA, et al. Virtues of being faithful: can we limit the genetic variation in human immunodeficiency virus? J Mol Med 1998;76:604–12.

[30] Colgrove R, Japour A. A combinatorial ledge: reverse transcriptase fidelity, total body viral burden, and the implications of multiple-drug HIV therapy for the evolution of antiviral resistance. Antiviral Res 1999;41:45–56.

[31] Overbaugh J, Bangham CR. Selection forces and constraints on retroviral sequence variation. Science 2001;292:1106–9.

[32] Mansky LM. HIV mutagenesis and the evolution of antiretroviral drug resistance. Drug Resist Updat 2002;5:219–23.

[33] Mansky LM, Le Rouzic E, Benichou S, Gajary LC. Influence of reverse transcriptase variants, drugs, and Vpr on human immunodeficiency virus type 1 mutant frequencies. J Virol 2003;77:2071–80.

[34] Furman PA, Fyfe JA, St Clair MH, et al. Phosphorylation of 3'-azido-3'-deoxythymidine and selective interaction of the 5'-triphosphate with human immunodeficiency virus reverse transcriptase. Proc Natl Acad Sci U S A 1986;83:8333–7.

[35] Hart GJ, Orr DC, Penn CR, et al. Effects of (-)-2'-deoxy-3'-thiacytidine (3TC) 5'-triphosphate on human immunodeficiency virus reverse transcriptase and mammalian DNA polymerases alpha, beta, and gamma. Antimicrob Agents Chemother 1992;36:1688–94.

[36] Ding J, Das K, Moereels H, et al. Structure of HIV-1 RT/TIBO R 86183 complex reveals similarity in the binding of diverse nonnucleoside inhibitors. Nat Struct Biol 1995;2:407–15.

[37] Wu JC, Warren TC, Adams J, et al. A novel dipyridodiazepinone inhibitor of HIV-1 reverse transcriptase acts through a nonsubstrate binding site. Biochemistry 1991;30:2022–6.

[38] Spence RA, Kati WM, Anderson KS, et al. Mechanism of inhibition of HIV-1 reverse transcriptase by nonnucleoside inhibitors. Science 1995;267:988–93.

[39] Gu Z, Quan Y, Li Z, et al. Effects of non-nucleoside inhibitors of human immunodeficiency virus type 1 in cell-free recombinant reverse transcriptase assays. J Biol Chem 1995;270:31046–51.

[40] Gunthard HF, Wong JK, Ignacio CC, et al. Human immunodeficiency virus

replication and genotypic resistance in blood and lymph nodes after a year of potent antiretroviral therapy. J Virol 1998;72:2422–8.

[41] Palmer S, Shafer RW, Merigan TC. Highly drug-resistant HIV-1 clinical isolates are cross-resistant to many antiretroviral compounds in current clinical development. AIDS 1999;13:661–7.

[42] Finzi D, Blankson J, Siliciano JD, et al. Latent infection of CD4+ T cells provides a mechanism for lifelong persistence of HIV-1, even in patients on effective combination therapy. Nat Med 1999;5:512–7.

[43] Wong JK, Hezareh M, Gunthard HF, et al. Recovery of replication-competent HIV despite prolonged suppression of plasma viremia. Science 1997;278:1291–5.

[44] Schinazi R, Larder B, Mellors J. Mutations in retroviral genes associated in drug resistance. Intl Antiviral News 1997;5:129–42.

[45] ACTG Virology Manual for HIV Laboratories. NAIDS, National Institutes for Allergy and Infectious Disease.

[46] Japour AJ, Mayers DL, Johnson VA, et al. Standardized peripheral blood mononuclear cell culture assay for determination of drug susceptibilities of clinical human immunodeficiency virus type 1 isolates. The RV-43 Study Group, the AIDS Clinical Trials Group Virology Committee Resistance Working Group. Antimicrob Agents Chemother 1993;37:1095–101.

[47] Winston A, Mandalia S, Pillay D, et al. The prevalence and determinants of the K65R mutation in HIV-1 reverse transcriptase in tenofovir-naive patients. AIDS 2002;16:2087–9.

[48] Montaner JSG, Reiss P, Cooper D, et al. for the INCAS Study Group. A randomized, double-blinded trial comparing combinations of nevirapine, didanosine and zidovudine for HIV-infected patients—The INCAS Trial. JAMA 1998;279:930–7.

[49] Richman D, Shih CK, Lowy I, et al. Human immunodeficiency virus type 1 mutants resistant to nonnucleoside inhibitors of reverse transcriptase arise in tissue culture. Proc Natl Acad Sci U S A 1991;88:11241–5.

[50] Vandamme AM, Debyser Z, Pauwels R, et al. Characterization of HIV-1 strains isolated from patients treated with TIBO R82913. AIDS Res Hum Retroviruses 1994;10:39–46.

[51] Chong KT, Pagano PJ, Hinshaw RR. Bisheteroarylpiperazine reverse transcriptase inhibitor in combination with 3′-azido-3′-deoxythymidine or 2′,3′-dideoxycytidine synergistically inhibits human immunodeficiency virus type 1 replication in vitro. Antimicrob Agents Chemother 1994;38:288–93.

[52] Esnouf R, Ren J, Ross C, et al. Mechanism of inhibition of HIV-1 reverse transcriptase by non-nucleoside inhibitors. Nat Struct Biol 1995;2:303–8.

[53] Fletcher RS, Arion D, Borkow G, et al. Synergistic inhibition of HIV-1 reverse transcriptase DNA polymerase activity and virus replication in vitro by combinations of carboxanilide nonnucleoside compounds. Biochemistry 1995;34 (32):10106–12.

[54] Byrnes VW, Sardana VV, Schleif WA, et al. Comprehensive mutant enzyme and viral variant assessment of human immunodeficiency virus type 1 reverse transcriptase resistance to nonnucleoside inhibitors. Antimicrob Agents Chemother 1993;37:1576–9.

[55] Balzarini J, Karlsson A, Perez-Perez MJ, et al. Treatment of human immunodeficiency virus type 1 (HIV-1)-infected cells with combinations of HIV-1-specific inhibitors results in a different resistance pattern than does treatment with single-drug therapy. J Virol 1993;67:5353–9.

[56] Sardana VV, Emini EA, Gotlib L, et al. Functional analysis of HIV-1 reverse transcriptase amino acids involved in resistance to multiple nonnucleoside inhibitors. J Biol Chem 1992;267:17526–30.

[57] Dueweke TJ, Pushkarskaya T, Poppe SM, et al. A mutation in reverse transcriptase of bis (heteroaryl)piperazine-resistant human immunodeficiency virus type 1 that confers increased sensitivity to other nonnucleoside inhibitors. Proc Natl Acad Sci U S A 1993;90:4713–7.

[58] Asahchop EL, Oliveira M, Wainberg MA, et al. Characterization of the E138K resistance mutation in HIV-1 reverse transcriptase conferring susceptibility to etravirine in B and non-B HIV-1 subtypes. Antimicrob Agents Chemother 2011;55 (2):600–7.

[59] Jonckheere H, Taymans JM, Balzarini J, et al. Resistance of HIV-1 reverse transcriptase against [2′,5′-bis-O-(tert-butyldimethylsilyl)-3′-spiro-5″-(4″-amino-1″,2″- oxathiole-2″,2″-dioxide)] (TSAO) derivatives is determined by the mutation Glu138->Lys on the p51 subunit. J Biol Chem 1994;269:25255–8.

[60] Loya S, Bakhanashvili M, Tal R, et al. Enzymatic properties of two mutants of reverse transcriptase of human immunodeficiency virus type 1 (tyrosine 181->isoleucine and tyrosine 188->leucine), resistant to nonnucleoside inhibitors. AIDS Res Hum Retroviruses 1994;10:939–46.

[61] Boyer PL, Currens MJ, McMahon JB, et al. Analysis of nonnucleoside drug-resistant variants of human immunodeficiency virus type 1 reverse transcriptase. J Virol 1993;67(4):2412–20.

[62] Andries K, Azijn H, Thielemans T, et al. TMC125, a novel next-generation nonnucleoside reverse transcriptase inhibitor active against nonnucleoside reverse transcriptase inhibitor-resistant human immunodeficiency virus type 1. Antimicrob Agents Chemother 2004;48:4680–6.

[63] Vingerhoets J, Azijn H, Fransen E, et al. TMC125 displays a high genetic barrier to the development of resistance: evidence from

in vitro selection experiments. J Virol 2005;79:12773–82.

[64] Asahchop EL, Oliveira M, Wainberg MA, et al. Characterization of the E138K resistance mutation in HIV-1 reverse transcriptase conferring susceptibility to etravirine in B and non-B HIV-1 subtypes. Antimicrob Agents Chemother 2011;55 (2):600–7.

[65] Condra JH. Virological and clinical implications of resistance to HIV-1 protease inhibitors. Drug Resist Updat 1998;1(5):292–9.

[66] Deeks SG. Failure of HIV-1 protease inhibitors to fully suppress viral replication. Implications for salvage therapy. Adv Exp Med Biol 1999;458:175–82.

[67] Murphy R. New antiretroviral drugs part I: PIs. AIDS Clin Care 1999;11:35–7.

[68] Reeves JD, Lee FH, Miamidian JL, et al. Enfuvirtide resistance mutations: impact on human immunodeficiency virus envelope function, entry inhibitor sensitivity, and virus neutralization. J Virol 2005;79 (8):4991–9.

[69] Sista PR, Melby T, Davison D, et al. Characterization of determinants of genotypic and phenotypic resistance to enfuvirtide in baseline and on-treatment HIV-1 isolates. AIDS 2004;18(13):1787–94.

[70] Lu J, Sista P, Giguel F, et al. Relative replicative fitness of human immunodeficiency virus type 1 mutants resistant to enfuvirtide (T-20). J Virol 2004;78 (9):4628–37.

[71] Swenson LC, Mo T, Dong WW, et al. Deep sequencing to infer HIV-1 co-receptor usage: application to three clinical trials of maraviroc in treatment-experienced patients. J Infect Dis 2011;203(2):237–45.

[72] Gulick RM, Lalezari J, Goodrich J, et al. Maraviroc for previously treated patients with R5 HIV-1 infection. N Engl J Med 2008;359 (14):1429–41.

[73] Cho MW, Lee MK, Carney MC, et al. Identification of determinants on a dualtropic human immunodeficiency virus

type 1 envelope glycoprotein that confer usage of CXCR4. J Virol 1998;72(3):2509–15.

[74] Nabatov AA, Pollakis G, Linnemann T, et al. Intrapatient alterations in the human immunodeficiency virus type 1 gp120 V1V2 and V3 regions differentially modulate coreceptor usage, virus inhibition by CC/CXC chemokines, soluble CD4, and the b12 and 2G12 monoclonal antibodies. J Virol 2004;78 (1):524–30.

[75] Vanden Haesevelde M, Decourt JL, De Leys RJ, et al. Genomic cloning and complete sequence analysis of a highly divergent African human immunodeficiency virus isolate. J Virol 1994;68(3):1586–96.

[76] Cornelissen M, van den Burg R, Zorgdrager F, et al. Pol gene diversity of five human immunodeficiency virus type 1 subtypes: evidence for naturally occurring mutations that contribute to drug resistance, limited recombination patterns, and common ancestry for subtypes B and D. J Virol 1997;71 (9):6348–58.

[77] Gao Q, Gu Z, Salomon H, et al. Generation of multiple drug resistance by sequential in vitro passage of the human immunodeficiency virus type 1. Arch Virol 1994;136(1–2):111–22.

[78] Shafer RW, Winters MA, Palmer S, Merigan TC. Multiple concurrent reverse transcriptase and protease mutations and multidrug resistance of HIV-1 isolates from heavily treated patients. Ann Intern Med 1998;128(11):906–11.

[79] Becker-Pergola G, Kataaha P, Johnston-Dow L, et al. Analysis of HIV type 1 protease and reverse transcriptase in antiretroviral drug-naive Ugandan adults. AIDS Res Hum Retroviruses 2000;16 (8):807–13.

[80] Descamps D, Collin G, Loussert-Ajaka I, et al. HIV-1 group O sensitivity to antiretroviral drugs. AIDS 1995;9(8):977–8.

[81] Descamps D, Collin G, Letourneur F, et al. Susceptibility of human immunodeficiency virus type 1 group O isolates to

antiretroviral agents: in vitro phenotypic and genotypic analyses. J Virol 1997;71 (11):8893–8.

[82] Tantillo C, Ding J, Jacobo-Molina A, et al. Locations of anti-AIDS drug binding sites and resistance mutations in the three-dimensional structure of HIV-1 reverse transcriptase. Implications for mechanisms of drug inhibition and resistance. J Mol Biol 1994;243 (3):369–87.

[83] Apetrei C, Descamps D, Collin G, et al. Human immunodeficiency virus type 1 subtype F reverse transcriptase sequence and drug susceptibility. J Virol 1998; 79:3534–8.

[84] Shafer RW, Eisen JA, Merigan TC, Katzenstein DA. Sequence and drug susceptibility of subtype C reverse transcriptase from human immunodeficiency virus type 1 seroconverters in Zimbabwe. J Virol 1997;71(7):5441–8.

[85] Birk M, Sönnerborg A. Variations in HIV-1 pol gene associated with reduced sensitivity to antiretroviral drugs in treatment-naive patients. AIDS 1998;12(18):2369–75.

[86] Loemba H, Brenner B, Parniak MA, et al. Genetic divergence of human immunodeficiency virus type 1 Ethiopian clade C reverse transcriptase (RT) and rapid development of resistance against nonnucleoside inhibitors of RT. Antimicrob Agents Chemother 2002;46(7):2087–94.

[87] Palmer S, Alaeus A, Albert J, Cox S. Drug susceptibility of subtypes A, B, C, D, and E human immunodeficiency virus type 1 primary isolates. AIDS Res Hum Retroviruses 1998;14(2):157–62.

[88] Brenner B, Turner D, Oliveira M, et al. A V106M mutation in HIV-1 clade C viruses exposed to efavirenz confers cross-resistance to non-nucleoside reverse transcriptase inhibitors. AIDS 2003;17(1):F1–F5.

[89] Petrella M, Brenner B, Loemba H, Wainberg MA. HIV drug resistance and implications for the introduction of antiretroviral therapy in resource-poor countries. Drug Resist Updat 2001; 4(6):339–46.

[90] Palella FJ, Jr., Delaney KM, Moorman AC, et al. Declining morbidity and mortality among patients with advanced human immunodeficiency virus infection. HIV Outpatient Study Investigators. N Engl J Med 1998;338(13):853–60.

[91] Wainberg MA, Friedland G. Public health implications of antiretroviral therapy and HIV drug resistance. JAMA 1998;279 (24):1977–83.

[92] Hirsch MS, Brun-Vézinet F, Clotet B, et al. Antiretroviral drug resistance testing in adults infected with human immunodeficiency virus type 1: 2003 recommendations of an International AIDS Society-USA Panel. Clin Infect Dis 2003;37 (1):113–28.

[93] Johnson VA, Brun-Vézinet F, Clotet B, et al. Drug resistance mutations in HIV-1. Top HIV Med 2003;11(6):215–21.

[94] Salomon H, Wainberg MA, Brenner B, et al. Prevalence of HIV-1 resistant to antiretroviral drugs in 81 individuals newly infected by sexual contact or injecting drug use. Investigators of the Quebec Primary Infection Study. AIDS 2000;14(2):F17–23.

[95] Yerly S, Kaiser L, Race E, et al. Transmission of antiretroviral-drug-resistant HIV-1 variants. Lancet 1999;354:729–33.

[96] Boden D, Hurley A, Zhang L, et al. HIV-1 drug resistance in newly infected individuals. JAMA 1999;282:1135–41.

[97] Little SJ, Holte S, Routy JP, et al. Antiretroviral-drug resistance among patients recently infected with HIV. N Engl J Med 2002;347:385–94.

[98] Hecht GM, Grant RM, Petropoulos CJ, et al. Sexual transmission of an HIV-1 variant resistant to multiple reverse-transcriptase and protease inhibitors. N Engl J Med 1998;339:307–11.

[99] Gandhi RT, Wurcel A, Rosenberg ES, et al. Progressive reversion of human immunodeficiency virus type 1 resistance mutations in vivo after transmission of a multiply drug-

resistant virus. Clin Infect Dis 2003;37:1693–8.

[100] Brenner BG, Routy JP, Petrella M, et al. Persistence and fitness of multidrug-resistant of human immunodeficiency virus type 1 acquired in primary HIV infection. J Virol 2002;76:1753–61.

[101] Verhofstede C, Wanzeele FV, Van der Gucht B, et al. Interruption of reverse transcriptase inhibitors or a switch from reverse transcriptase transcriptase to protease inhibitors resulted in a fast reappearance of virus strains with a reverse transcriptase inhibitor-sensitive genotype. AIDS 1999;13:2541–6.

[102] Devereux HL, Youle M, Johnson MA, Loveday C. Rapid decline in detectability of HIV-1 drug resistance mutations after stopping therapy. AIDS 1999;13: F123–F127.

[103] Jost S, Bernard MC, Kaiser L, et al. A patient with HIV-1 superinfection. N Engl J Med 2002;347:731–6.

[104] Ramos A, Hu DJ, Nguyen L, et al. Intersubtype human immunodeficiency virus type 1 superinfection following seroconversion to primary infection in two injecting intravenous drug users. J Virol 2002;76:7444–52.

[105] Gonzales MJ, Delwart E, Rhee SY, et al. Lack of detectable human immunodeficiency virus type 1 superinfection during 1072 person-years of observation. J Infect Dis 2003;188:397–405.

[106] Tsui R, Herring BL, Barbour JD, et al. Human immunodeficiency virus type 1 superinfection was not detected following 215 years of injection drug user exposure. J Virol 2004;78:94–103.

[107] Altfeld M, Allen TM, Yu XG, et al. HIV-1 superinfection despite broad CD8+ T-cell responses containing replication of the primary infection. Nature 2002;420:434–9.

[108] Koelsch KK, Smith DM, Little SJ, et al. Clade B HIV-1 superinfection with wild-type virus after primary infection with drug-resistant clade B virus. AIDS 2003;17:F11–F16.

[109] Brenner B, Routy JP, Quan Y, et al. and Co-Investigators of the

Quebec Primary Infection Study. Persistence of multidrug resistant HIV-1 in primary infection leading to superinfection. AIDS 2004;18:1653–60.

[110] Allen T, Altfeld M. HIV-1 superinfection. J Allergy Clin Immunol 2003;112(5):829–35.

[111] Smith D, Wong J, Hightower, et al. Incidence of HIV superinfection following primary infection. In: 11th Conference on Retroviruses and Opportunistic Infections; February 8–11, 2004.

[112] Petrella M, Oliveira M, Moisi D, et al. Differential maintenance of the M184V substitution in the reverse transcriptase of human immunodeficiency virus type 1 by various nucleoside antiretroviral agents in tissue culture. Antimicrob Agents Chemother 2004;48(11):4189–94.

[113] Turner D, Brenner B, Routy JP, et al. Diminished representation of HIV-1 variants containing select drug resistance-conferring mutations in primary HIV-1 infection. J AIDS 2004;37 (5):1627–31.

[114] Wainberg MA, Hsu M, Gu Z, et al. Effectiveness of 3TC in HIV clinical trials may be due in part to the M184V substitution in 3TC-resistant HIV-1 reverse transcriptase. AIDS 1996;10(Suppl 5):S3–S10.

[115] Baxter JD, Mayers DL, Wentworth DN, et al. A randomized study of antiretroviral management based on plasma genotypic antiretroviral resistance testing in patients failing therapy. CPCRA 046 Study Team for the Terry Beirn Community Programs for Clinical Research on AIDS. AIDS 2000;14:F83–F93.

[116] Colgrove RC, Pitt J, Chung PH, et al. Selective vertical transmission of HIV-1 antiretroviral resistance mutations. AIDS 1998;12:2281–8.

[117] Dickover RE, Garratty EM, Plaeger S, et al. Perinatal transmission of major, minor, and multiple maternal human immunodeficiency virus type 1 variants in utero and intrapartum. J Virol 2001;75:2194–203.

[118] Verhofstede C, Wanzeele FV, Van Der Gucht B, et al. Interruption of reverse transcriptase inhibitors or a switch from reverse transcriptase to protease inhibitors resulted in a fast reappearance of virus strains with a reverse transcriptase inhibitor-sensitive genotype. AIDS 1999;13:2541–6.

[119] Quinn TC, Wawer MJ, Sewankambo N, et al. Viral load and heterosexual transmission of human immunodeficiency virus type 1. Rakai Project Study Group. N Engl J Med 2000;342 (13):921–9.

[120] Yerly S, Vora S, Rizzardi P, et al. Acute HIV infection: impact on the spread of HIV and transmission of drug resistance. AIDS 2001;15 (17):2287–92.

[121] Wainberg MA, Friedland G. Public health implications of antiretroviral therapy and HIV drug resistance. JAMA 1998;279:1977–83.

[122] Yerly S, Kaiser L, Race E, et al. Transmission of antiretroviral-drug-resistant HIV-1 variants. Lancet 1999;354(9180):729–33.

[123] Phillips A. Will the drugs still work? Transmission of resistant HIV. Nat Med 2001;7 (9):993–4.

[124] Chaix ML, Descamps D, Harzic M, et al. Stable prevalence of genotypic drug resistance mutations but increase in non-B virus among patients with primary HIV-1 infection in France. AIDS 2003;17 (18):2635–43.

[125] Ammaranond P, Cunningham P, Oelrichs R, et al. No increase in protease resistance and a decrease in reverse transcriptase resistance mutations in primary HIV-1 infection: 1992-2001. AIDS 2003;17(2):264–7.

[126] Kuritzkes D. Drug resistance. Navigating resistance pathways. AIDS Read 2002;12:395–400.

[127] Nijhuis M, Deeks S, Boucher C. Implications of antiretroviral resistance on viral fitness.

Curr Opin Infect Dis 2001;14:23–8.

[128] Brenner B, Turner D, Wainberg M. HIV-1 drug resistance: can we overcome? Expert Opin Biol Ther 2002;2:751–61.

[129] Ait-Khaled M, Rakik A, Griffin P, et al. Mutations in HIV-1 reverse transcriptase during therapy with abacavir, lamivudine and zidovudine in HIV-1-infected adults with no prior antiretroviral therapy. Antivir Ther 2002;7:43–51.

[130] Ait-Khaled M, Stone C, Amphlett G, et al. M184V is associated with a low incidence of thymidine analogue mutations and low phenotypic resistance to zidovudine and stavudine. AIDS 2002;16:1686–9.

[131] Daar ES, Richman DD. Confronting the emergence of drug-resistant HIV type 1: impact of antiretroviral therapy on individual and population resistance. AIDS Res Hum Retroviruses 2005;21:343–57.

Chapter | 13 |

Pharmacology of antiretroviral drugs

Concepta Merry, Charles W. Flexner

INTRODUCTION

There may be no discipline in modern medicine in which clinical pharmacology is more relevant than in the care of the HIV-infected patient. In the developed world many patients currently take at least three antiretroviral (ARV) drugs plus medications for the prophylaxis and treatment of opportunistic infections in addition sometimes to medication for co-infections such as hepatitis B or C virus and/or a variety of medications for the management of chronic diseases such as hypertension and diabetes mellitus. In the developing world patients also take at least three ARV drugs plus medications for the prophylaxis and treatment of opportunistic infections in addition sometimes to medication for co-endemic diseases such as tuberculosis (TB), malaria, worm infestations or neglected tropical diseases and/or a variety of medications for the management of chronic diseases such as hypertension and diabetes mellitus [1]. Hence the potential for complex drug–drug interactions [2]. Selecting appropriate medications and constructing an effective ARV regimen can be difficult in this era of chronic polypharmacy. In addition to contending with drug resistance, the clinician is faced with drug–food effects, proper spacing of medications, drug–drug interactions, overlapping toxicities, and patient adherence with the regimen.

It is essential to ensure optimal dosing for patients, as high drug concentrations may be associated with more frequent adverse effects and low drug concentrations may be associated with the development of treatment failure [3, 4]. Sub-therapeutic drug concentrations can promote the emergence of resistant forms of HIV, and thus result in treatment failure [5]. Development of resistance compromises the response of the patient to future therapeutic interventions and may result in the transmission of resistant virus, which is more expensive and difficult to treat.

The main role of clinical pharmacology is to describe, quantify, and predict drug concentrations and response in order to design safe and effective regimens. The application of clinical pharmacology to HIV treatment is intended to optimize outcomes for individual patients and to prevent the emergence of drug-resistant virus. While an individualized approach to HIV treatment including therapeutic drug monitoring in selected patients may be the aim of treatment in the developed world and can be supported by clinical pharmacology, the combination of a public health approach to prescribing and shifting of tasks from highly skilled to less skilled health cadres in the developing world in reality limits the impact of clinical pharmacology to informing policy and generating recommendations.

Antiretroviral treatment guidelines are continuously updated and improved to reflect new data and novel drugs but the pharmacological principles underlying these guidelines tend to remain unchanged (http://www.aidsinfo.nih.gov/guidelines; http://www.who.int/hiv/pub/guidelines). The following sections review the clinical pharmacology of relevance to the optimal prescribing of ARV drugs.

ANTIRETROVIRAL DRUGS

There are currently five classes of drugs available for the treatment of HIV infection:

1. Nucleoside (NRTI) and nucleotide (NtRTI) reverse transcriptase inhibitors;
2. Non-nucleoside reverse transcriptase inhibitors (NNRTI);
3. Protease inhibitors (PI);

Table 13.1 Licensed antiretroviral drugs

NRTI and NtRTI[a]	NNRTI[a]	PI[a]	INSTI	EI
AZT	EFV	SQV	RAL	T-20
d4T	NVP	RTV		MVC
3TC	DLV	IDV		
ddC	ETR	APV		
ddI		FPV		
FTC		ATV		
ABC		NFV		
TDF		TPV		
		LPV/r		
		DRV		

[a]NRTI, nucleoside reverse transcriptase inhibitor; NtRTI, nucleotide reverse transcriptase inhibitor; NNRTI, non-nucleoside reverse transcriptase inhibitor; PI, protease inhibitor; INSTI. integrase strand transfer inhibitor; EI, entry inhibitor; AZT, zidovudine; EFV, efavirenz; SQV, saquinavir; RAL, raltegravir; T-20, enfuvirtide; d4T, stavudine; NVP, nevirapine; RTV, ritonavir; MVC, maraviroc; 3TC, lamivudine; DLV, delavirdine; IDV, indinavir; ddC, dideoxycytidine; ETR, etravirine; APV, amprenavir; ddI, didanosine; FPV, fosamprenavir; FTC, emtricitabine; ATV, atazanavir; ABC, abacavir; NFV, nelfinavir; TDF, tenofovir; TPV, tipranavir; LPV/r, lopinavir/ritonavir co-formulation; DRV, darunavir.

4. Entry inhibitors; and
5. Integrase inhibitors.

There are over 20 different original licensed ARV preparations (Table 13.1). There are also a growing number of fixed-dose co-formulations, pediatric formulations, and generically manufactured drugs. In practice the patient can only benefit from a smaller number of drugs used in combination. For example:

- Emtricitabine (FTC) is an analog of lamivudine (3TC), and therefore these drugs should not be co-prescribed;
- Fosamprenavir is a prodrug of amprenavir;
- Ritonavir is a potent PI with intrinsic ARV activity; it is poorly tolerated and is now prescribed mainly to boost the concentrations of other PIs; and
- Resistance to any single ARV may confer cross-resistance to other drugs in the same class, e.g. patients who develop resistance to nevirapine may also be resistant to efavirenz [6].

PHARMACOKINETIC DEFINITIONS

Figure 13.1 summarizes the key pharmacokinetic parameters that characterize orally administered drugs. There are limited data on the correlation between different pharmacokinetic parameters and clinical outcome for HIV-infected patients.

- Trough concentration: the concentration of drug in the blood immediately before the next dose is administered, although this does not necessarily represent the lowest concentration during a dosing interval.
- Minimum concentration (C_{min}): the lowest concentration of drug in the blood following the administered dose. The lowest drug concentration frequently occurs immediately before the next dose is administered; for these drugs, the minimum concentration and the trough concentration are identical. However, some drugs such as nelfinavir (NFV) have delayed absorption and the drug concentration falls even lower following the administered dose until the next dose is absorbed. Low minimum drug concentrations may be associated with increased risk of virologic failure for some ARVs [3].

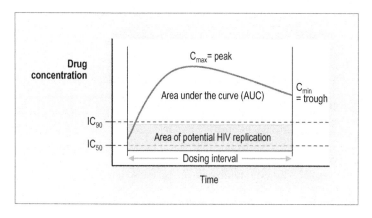

Figure 13.1 A summary of the key pharmacokinetic parameters that characterize orally administered drugs.

Low C_{min} may also occur due to drug–drug interactions or non-adherence.

- Peak concentration (C_{max}): the maximum concentration of drug measured in the blood following the administered dose. High peak concentrations correlate with drug toxicity for indinavir and possibly ritonavir [3, 7].
- Area under the curve (AUC): measure of the total net exposure of a patient to a drug over the dosing interval, usually based on plasma concentrations.
- Steady state: point at which the input mass of drug is equivalent to the mass eliminated from the body by clearance during any unit of time. For a drug administered every half-life, this takes approximately five half-lives to achieve.
- Half-life: the length of time it takes for the concentration of drug in the plasma to fall by 50%. This is important clinically, as different constituents of a triple-drug regimen may have different half-lives. Therefore, if the clinician stops all drugs at the same time, the drug with the shortest half-life is eliminated first, followed by the drug with the second shortest half-life, followed by the drug with the longest half-life. This exposes the patient's virus sequentially to triple therapy, dual therapy, and ultimately monotherapy. Drugs such as efavirenz and nevirapine have long half-lives and may pose a significant risk for the development of resistance in these circumstances. Therefore it is prudent to stop the individual components of a triple regimen at different times depending on the respective half-lives of the constituent drugs: e.g. a patient receiving a combination of stavudine (d4T), 3TC plus nevirapine could stop the nevirapine on day 1 and continue the d4T plus 3TC for at least 2 weeks to provide effective triple therapy as the nevirapine is eliminated from the body. Alternatively a PI could be introduced to provide cover during this elimination phase. The optimal interval between stopping NNRTIs and the other ARV drugs in the regimen is not known. This raises logistical issues in resource-limited settings where patients may receive a generic formulation of a fixed-dose combination of, for example, d4T plus 3TC plus nevirapine. For such patients, it may be preferable to stop the fixed-dose combination and continue the patient on either a fixed-dose dual combination of d4T plus 3TC or individually manufactured d4T plus 3TC during the elimination phase of nevirapine. However, either approach may be unpopular locally as prescribing the individual component drugs or a PI increases the drug acquisition costs and increases the complexity of care in a public health setting where task shifting is increasing. This clinical issue is even further complicated by the fact that certain ethnic groups, such as African-Americans, have an increased prevalence of genetic polymorphisms that result in a slower rate of clearance of NNRTIs such as efavirenz [8, 9].

DRUG METABOLISM

Intracellular phosphorylation

The NRTIs are prodrugs which are converted by host cellular enzymes in the cytoplasm to an active triphosphate. Occasionally, there may be competition for intracellular phosphorylation pathways by similar NRTIs; this can result in clinically relevant drug interactions. For example, zidovudine (azidothymidine; AZT) has been shown to impair the intracellular phosphorylation of d4T *in vitro*; when these two drugs were combined in clinical trials, this combination was associated with unfavorable outcomes as compared to using either drug without the other, or with other regimens containing two NRTIs [10].

Tenofovir is also a prodrug that is converted intracellularly to the active diphosphate. Since tenofovir starts with a single phosphate group, the diphosphate of this drug is analogous to an NRTI triphosphate. Purine nucleoside phosphorylase (PNP) is an enzyme responsible in part for the catabolic metabolism of didanosine (ddI). The activity of PNP is inhibited by tenofovir and tenofovir monophosphate, resulting in increased plasma concentrations of ddI [11]. Use of a reduced dose of enteric coated ddI (250 mg/day), with or without food, produces plasma ddI concentrations similar to that achieved with standard ddI dosing of 400 mg/day in the absence of tenofovir [12]. Hence it is recommended to either avoid the combination of tenofovir plus ddI or to reduce the dose of ddI if co-prescribed tenofovir with (http://www.aidsinfo.nih.gov/guidelines).

The combination of d4T with ddI is also no longer recommended as it is associated with unacceptably high levels of clinical toxicity, especially peripheral neuropathy and pancreatitis.

DRUG TRANSPORT PROTEINS

In addition to metabolism, which refers to chemical biotransformation usually mediated by enzymes in the liver, many drugs are subject to cellular influx or efflux mediated by drug transport proteins [13, 14]. The best known of these, P-glycoprotein (P-gp), is the product of the *mdr1* (multidrug resistance) gene first described as producing broad cross-resistance to certain kinds of cancer chemotherapy. P-gp is expressed in epithelial cells lining the intestinal mucosa, contributing to efflux of drugs back into the intestinal lumen. P-glycoprotein therefore contributes to the low bioavailability of certain drugs, for example some

HIV PIs. P-gp is also present in cells making up the blood–brain barrier, and can limit central nervous system penetration of drugs via efflux back into the systemic circulation. Several HIV PIs are substrates for and inhibitors of P-gp.

Cytochrome P450 enzymes

Cytochrome P-450 (CYP) enzymes are ubiquitous in higher vertebrates and are the major protective mechanism for chemical detoxification of xenobiotics, and drugs. This system consists of more than 12 families of enzymes common to all mammals [15]. In humans, the CYP1, CYP2, and CYP3 families are primarily responsible for drug metabolism, with the CYP3A subfamily accounting for metabolism of the largest number of drugs, including most HIV PIs and NNRTIs. CYP450-mediated drug metabolism largely takes place in the liver, although CYP enzymes are also present in other sites, including the intestinal wall. Intestinal drug metabolism contributes to the first-pass metabolism of many orally administered drugs, including saquinavir (SQV). Drugs may interact with CYP450 enzymes in one of three ways: (1) as a substrate, (2) as an inducer, and/or (3) as an inhibitor. Inhibitors of CYP3A4 can reduce drug metabolism in the intestinal tract and slow hepatic clearance, thus increasing systemic concentrations. Inducers of CYP metabolism accelerate clearance and decrease absorption and/or systemic concentrations.

Enzyme inhibition and boosted protease inhibitor therapy

Inhibitors of CYP-mediated biotransformation can be used to decrease the rate of hepatic clearance and increase concentrations of drugs subject to metabolism by the same pathway. HIV PIs can be CYP inducers, inhibitors, and substrates. As a consequence, these drugs can increase the concentrations of co-administered metabolized drugs, and are subject to having their own concentrations increased by other CYP inhibitors. Most of the currently approved HIV PIs are metabolized primarily by CYP3A4. The number and magnitude of potential drug interactions associated with these agents varies widely as a function of the relative potency of enzyme inhibition and induction.

Saquinavir was the first PI licensed for use in HIV-infection in the USA. The original formulation of this drug, a hard gel capsule, had low oral bioavailability. Ritonavir, the second HIV PI licensed for use in the USA, was poorly tolerated at the initially recommended dose of 600 mg twice daily, producing frequent nausea and vomiting. Ritonavir is a very potent inhibitor of CYP3A4, and as a result combined administration of SQV and ritonavir produced a mean 20-fold increase in steady-state SQV concentrations. Ritonavir affects SQV concentrations in two ways: first, by improving oral bioavailability through inhibition of intestinal CYP3A4 and possibly P-gp, and second, by

inhibiting hepatic CYP 3A4 and thus decreasing systemic clearance [16].

Fortunately, ritonavir is much better tolerated at lower doses, which retain most of the CYP 3A4 inhibition of higher-dose ritonavir. Today, ritonavir is used as a pharmacokinetic booster of other HIV PIs, and not for its own intrinsic ARV properties. With the exception of NFV, combining a low dose of ritonavir with most available HIV PIs improves the concentrations of the active PI, and may also allow a reduced dosing and dosing frequency of the co-administered drug. Aluvia/Kaletra is a fixed-dose combination of the PI lopinavir with a low dose of ritonavir 400/100 mg twice daily, abbreviated LPV/r. (It is customary to use a lower case "r" when abbreviating. The low doses of ritonavir used as a PK enhancer, e.g. ritonavir-boosted SQV, would be written SQV/r 1000/200 mg twice daily.) For dosing recommendations for ritonavir-boosted PI regimens, please consult the websites recommended at the end of this chapter.

Cobicistat is a promising new pharmacoenhancer alternative to ritonavir under development, although its toxicity profile is still unclear [17].

Patients who have failed multiple prior ARV regimens may be treated with a combination of two different PIs plus ritonavir in order to take advantage of the lack of cross-resistance between certain PIs, and the chance to treat with two active agents instead of one. So-called double-boosted or dual-boosted PI regimens utilize ritonavir to increase the concentrations of two ARV drugs at the same time. The pharmacokinetics of such regimens may be complex and difficult to predict, since there is the potential for both PIs to interact with ritonavir and with each other and referral to drug interaction websites is recommended (http://www.hiv-drug interactions.org and http://www.hivpharmacology.com).

Enzyme inhibition and drug interactions

Ritonavir not only boosts the concentrations of PIs but also the combination itself can inhibit the metabolism of other drugs metabolized by the CYP system. Therefore when initiating a ritonavir-boosted PI regimen it is important to check all other concomitant medications to check for potential drug interactions. It is equally important to check for potential drug interactions when withdrawing ritonavir-boosted PI therapy as previously efficacious concomitant medications may be less effective in the absence of the inhibitory effect. Broadly speaking, guidance on drug interactions resulting from inhibition of the CYP system falls into three categories:

- Contraindicated—Lovastatin plus lopinavir/ritonavir as the inhibitory effects of the boosted protease inhibitor results in unacceptable rates of myopathy and rhabdomyolysis [18].

- Dose adjustment recommended—Amprenavir, NFV, and indinavir are less potent inhibitors of CYP3A4 than ritonavir. All of these drugs increase the mean rifabutin AUC approximately twofold, but can be co-administered if the rifabutin dose is decreased by 50%.
- Careful co-prescribing and clinical monitoring—This is recommended when the magnitude of the interaction is small or when the co-prescribed drug has a wide therapeutic index, e.g. co-administration of fosamprenavir with diltiazem may increase the concentration of the calcium channel blocker and close clinical monitoring of the patient is recommended.

Enzyme induction and drug interactions

Enzyme induction refers to an increase in the rate of hepatic metabolism, mediated by increased transcription of mRNA encoding the genes for drug-metabolizing enzymes. This leads to a decrease in the concentrations of drugs metabolized by the same enzyme. Rifampicin is a potent inducer of CYP3A4 and can result in clinically significant decreases in plasma concentrations of many concomitant medications including PIs, non-nucleoside reverse transcriptase inhibitors, integrase inhibitors, and entry inhibitors. It is important to keep in mind that the doses of many concomitant medications will need to be adjusted when starting or stopping enzyme inducers. Similar to the clinical recommendations for enzyme inhibitors, the dosing guidelines for enzyme inducers fall into three broad categories:

- Contraindicated—e.g. rifampicin plus etravirine as co-administration may cause significant decreases in etravirine concentrations and lack of clinical efficacy.
- Dose adjustment recommended—e.g. Current guidelines recommend increasing the dose of efavirenz from 600 to 800 mg daily when co-administered with rifampicin to overcome the inducing effects of rifampicin.
- Careful co-prescribing and clinical monitoring—Co-administration of diltiazem (240 mg once daily) and efavirenz (600 mg for 14 days) results in a two-way drug interaction with decreases in diltiazem and increases in efavirenz levels, and current guidelines recommend that diltiazem dose adjustments should be guided by clinical response but no dose adjustment of efavirenz is necessary.

Many drugs exhibit complex effects on multiple CYP isoforms and drug transporters. For example, in addition to being inhibitors of CYP3A4, ritonavir and NFV are moderate hepatic enzyme inducers. They can increase activity of so-called phase 2 enzymes such as hepatic glucuronosyl transferase, as well as CYP. Both PIs decrease the AUC of the oral contraceptive ethinyl estradiol by about 40%. Patients taking ritonavir or NFV are advised to use alternative forms of birth control [19].

Endemic diseases and drug interactions

While these principles of pharmacology apply to drug interactions for any co-infection or co-morbidity, it is worth mentioning that at the time of writing there are very limited data on drug interactions between ARVs and drugs used to treat co-endemic diseases such as malaria. While there are limited data on co-treatment of HIV-TB-infected individuals there are few treatment options in resource-limited settings for patients on second-line ARV therapy.

Drug–food interactions

A number of environmental influences, besides concomitant medications, can influence pharmacokinetics. An especially important influence is food. Food can either increase or decrease the bioavailability of several drugs commonly used in HIV-infected patients. Furthermore, drug–food interactions may require a modification of the scheduling of administration of drugs during the day, and this can have a major effect on the quality of life of patients. Didanosine enteric-coated capsules must also be given on an empty stomach because administration with food decreases bioavailability [20]. The neuropsychiatric effects of efavirenz are exacerbated by taking the drug with food; hence the recommendation to take following a meal.

Specific food restrictions of ARVs are summarized in Table 13.2. This information must be incorporated into

Table 13.2 Recommendations for food for approved antiretroviral drugs		
TAKE WITH FOOD	TAKE ON EMPTY STOMACH	TAKE FOLLOWING A MEAL/AVOID HIGH FAT MEAL
TDF[a]	IDV[b]	EFV[a]
SQV	ddI	ETR
RTV		
NFV		
LPV/r		
ATV		
DRV		
FPV/r		
TPV		
[a]TDF and EFV can be taken with or without food. [b]IDV can also be taken with a light, low-fat snack.		

the counseling required for patients starting or modifying many ARV regimens. This can be particularly difficult for patients in the resource-limited setting who may only have one meal per day, or for patients who observe religious periods of fasting. It is important to consider these factors when prescribing ARVs.

Drug–traditional medicines interactions

Herbal remedies and nutritional supplements are widely used in HIV-infected patients, although the potential pharmacokinetic effects of these compounds are often ignored. Some herbal therapies contain ingredients capable of CYP inhibition or induction and have been implicated in drug interactions. For example, St John's wort contains a potent inducer of CYP3A4, and decreases the AUC of indinavir by over 50% [21]. There is also evidence that St John's wort decreases nevirapine concentrations by a similar magnitude [22]. The mechanism of this interaction appears to involve induction of both CYP3A4 and P-gp [23]. Patients taking HIV PIs and non-nucleoside reverse transcriptase inhibitors should be instructed to avoid St John's wort or any dietary supplement containing this herb.

Some nutritional supplements may also contain ingredients capable of affecting the concentrations of co-administered ARVs. Raw garlic inhibits the activity of CYP3A4 *in vitro* and in animals [24]. One study conducted in healthy volunteers found that garlic capsules taken b.i.d. for 3 weeks led to a mean decrease in the SQV AUC of approximately 50%, probably as a consequence of reduced bioavailability [25]. Other herbs with reported *in vitro* effects on CYP450-mediated metabolism include silymarin (milk thistle), ginseng, and skullcap, although clinical pharmacokinetic interaction data with these agents are contradictory or lacking [26]. Traditional and herbal medicines could be added to the list of agents capable of causing significant drug interactions. Clinicians could record information about use of these agents when taking medical histories, and consider them when adverse events or treatment failure appears with no other identifiable cause.

This is particularly important in resource-limited settings, where the majority of patients consult traditional healers prior to or in addition to medical doctors. It is important to include traditional healers in efforts to expand access to ARV in resource-limited settings, as they are key opinion leaders in the communities and have a significant impact on the health belief model for patients. Furthermore, the metabolism of many components of the traditional herbal medicines may be inhibited by drugs such as ritonavir. It is possible therefore, that Western medicines may be responsible for reduced clearance and heretofore unseen side effects of traditional medicines.

SPECIAL POPULATIONS

Renal and hepatic impairment

Since the majority of drugs are eliminated by renal or hepatic clearance, diseases altering the function of these organs can affect the concentrations of drugs. Table 13.3 lists ARVs for which the prescribing information recommends dose modification in the setting of renal or hepatic impairment. It is important to continuously monitor patients and adjust the drug doses accordingly to any identified changes in renal and hepatic function.

In particular, patients with HIV-related renal dysfunction may have marked improvements in renal function once started on effective ARV therapy. For further guidelines on dosing, please consult websites at the end of this chapter.

Low-weight individuals

There are limited data on the optimal dosing of ARV drugs in low-weight adults. This is particularly important in malnourished patients with advanced HIV disease in Africa, who may have a low body mass index, and also in many Asian patients who naturally tend to have lower body weights. It is currently recommended that the doses of d4T (Zerit) and ddI (Videx) be reduced in patients who weigh <60 kg [20, 27]. It is unclear whether the dose of ddI should be reduced to 200 mg/day in patients

Table 13.3 Antiretroviral drugs whose clearance is altered in patients with renal or hepatic insufficiency

RENAL INSUFFICIENCY	HEPATIC INSUFFICIENCY
ddi	ABC
3TC/FTC	NVP
TDF	ETR
D4T	SQV
NVP	IDV
ATV	APV/FPV
MVC	RTV
	TPV
	DRV
	ATV
	RAL

weighing <60 kg who are also receiving tenofovir, and it may be prudent to avoid this combination in such patients. It is important to continuously monitor weight, as patients who have been very ill may gain significant weight once they respond to ARV therapy.

Pediatrics

Growth and development may result in rapid changes in the activity of some drug-metabolizing enzymes. In addition, changes in body surface area and liver blood flow can alter the elimination of metabolized drugs. Other developmental changes that can effect drug concentrations include changes in gastric function, intestinal motility, percentage body fat, concentrations of plasma proteins, and renal function.

Unlike the developed world, children represent a significant proportion of HIV-infected individuals in the developing world. Frequently encountered problems include inaccurate dosing, unpalatable formulations, and formulations that are cumbersome to administer. There are an increasing number of pediatric formulations available for HIV-infected children for facilitating ease of administration for the caregivers.

Pregnancy

The current guidelines for the care of a HIV-infected woman during pregnancy and after delivery for both mother and newborn child vary from country to country, largely dictated by the local finances and healthcare delivery capacity. However, there are common basic pharmacological principles regardless of geography. Avoidance of teratogenic drugs like efavirenz during the first trimester of pregnancy, in women who wish to become pregnant or in women who do not use a reliable form of contraception is recommended. In addition, the concentrations of some medications may be altered during pregnancy. Available data suggest that the concentrations of some ARVs measured at various time points during pregnancy are on aver-

age lower than those in the non-pregnant woman [28–31]. The mechanism for the difference in pharmacokinetic profiles during pregnancy is multifactorial. Possible contributors include induction of hepatic drug metabolizing enzymes, changes in gastrointestinal transit times, increases in body water and fat, and changes in expression of drug transporters such as P-gp [32].

There is no evidence that pregnancy increases the risk of nevirapine toxicity over that of non-pregnant women but it is not recommended that nevirapine-based regimens be initiated in pregnant women with CD4 counts of >250 cells/mm^3.

Ethnic variations in pharmacokinetics

The influence of genetic factors on drug metabolism and drug concentrations is an important area of clinical research, particularly as ARVs are being initiated in different geographic regions. The field of pharmacogenetics identifies specific genetic polymorphisms that might explain inter-individual differences in drug concentrations. As discussed above, emerging data suggest differences in drug concentrations of ARVs in certain ethnic groups.

CONCLUSION

Clinical pharmacology is an integral part of the management of patients with HIV infection. The increasing number of ARVs and the increasing availability of ARVs in resource-limited settings raises new logistical and prescribing issues that need to be addressed in order to ensure optimal outcomes for patients in diverse regions.

ACKNOWLEDGMENTS

Thank you to David Burger for providing the HIV drug-interactions websites.

REFERENCES

[1] Lamorde M, Byakika-Kibwika P, Merry C. Antiretroviral therapy in developing countries—pharmacologic considerations. Curr Opin HIV AIDS 2008;3(3):252–7.

[2] Barry M, Mulcahy F, Merry C. Pharmacokinetics and potential interactions amongst antiretroviral agents used to treat patients with HIV infection. Clin Pharm 1999;36:289–304.

[3] Burger D, Hugen P, Reiss P, et al. ATHENA Cohort Study Group. Therapeutic drug monitoring of nelfinavir and indinavir in treatment-naive HIV-1-infected individuals. AIDS 2003;17:1157–65.

[4] Li RC, Zhu M, Schentag JJ. Achieving an optimal outcome in the treatment of infections. The role of clinical pharmacokinetics and

pharmacodynamics of antimicrobials. Clin Pharm 1999;37:1–16.

[5] Molla A, Korneyeva M, Gao Q, et al. Ordered accumulation of mutations in HIV protease confers resistance to ritonavir. Nat Med 1996;2:760–6.

[6] Antinori A, Zaccarelli M, Cingolani A, et al. Cross-resistance among nonnucleoside reverse transcriptase inhibitors limits

recycling efavirenz after nevirapine failure. AIDS Res Hum Retroviruses 2002;18:835–8.

[7] Gatti G, Di Biagio A, Casazza R, et al. The relationship between ritonavir plasma levels and side-effects: implications for therapeutic drug monitoring. AIDS 1999;13:2083–9.

[8] Haas DW, Ribaudo HJ, Kim RB, et al. Pharmacogenetics of efavirenz and central nervous system side effects: an Adult AIDS Clinical Trials Group study. AIDS 2004;18 (18):2391–400.

[9] Ramachandran G, Hemanth Kumar AK, Rajasekaran S, et al. CYP2B6 G516T polymorphism but not rifampin coadministration influences steady-state pharmacokinetics of efavirenz in human immunodeficiency virus-infected patients in South India. Antimicrob Agents Chemother 2009;53(3):863–8.

[10] Hoggard PG, Kewn S, Barry MG, et al. Effects of drugs on 2′,3′-dideoxy-2′,3′-didehydrothymidine phosphorylation in vitro. Antimicrob Agents Chemother 1997;41(6):1231–6.

[11] Ray AS, Olson L, Fridland A. Role of purine nucleoside phosphorylase in interactions between 2′,3′-dideoxyinosine and allopurinol, ganciclovir, or tenofovir. Antimicrob Agents Chemother 2004;48(4):1089–95.

[12] Kearney BP, Sayre JR, Flaherty JF, et al. Drug–drug and drug–food interactions between tenofovir disoproxil fumarate and didanosine. J Clin Pharmacol 2005;45(12):1360–7.

[13] Kim RB. Drug transporters in HIV therapy. Top HIV Med 2003;11 (4):136–9.

[14] Speck RR, Yu XF, Hildreth J, Flexner C. Differential effects of p-glycoprotein and multidrug resistance protein-1 on productive human immunodeficiency virus infection. J Infect Dis 2002;186 (3):332–40.

[15] Benet LZ, Kroetz DL, Sheiner LB. Pharmacokinetics: dynamics of drug absorption, distribution, and elimination. In: Hardman JG, Limbird LE, editors. The Pharmacological Basis of

Therapeutics. 9th ed. New York: McGraw-Hill; 1996.

[16] Drewe J, Gutmann H, Fricker G, et al. HIV protease inhibitor ritonavir: a more potent inhibitor of P-glycoprotein than the cyclosporine analog SDZ PSC 833. Biochem Pharmacol 1999;57:1147–52.

[17] Cohen C, Shamblaw D, Ruane P. The single-tablet, fixed-dose regimen of elvitegravir/GS-9350/emtricitabine/tenofovir DF (Quad) achieves a high rate of virologic suppression and GS-9350 is an effective booster. In: 17th Conference on Retroviruses and Opportunistic Infections (CROI 2010). 2010. San Francisco; February 16–19, Abstract 58LB.

[18] Abbott Laboratories. Kaletrar (lopinavir/ritonavir) tablets, oral solution. Full prescribing information, 2010. North Chicago, IL 60064.

[19] Ouellet D, Hsu A, Qian J, et al. Effect of ritonavir on the pharmacokinetics of ethinyl estradiol in healthy female volunteers, In: XIth International Conference on AIDS. Vancouver, BC; 7–12 July, 1996.

[20] Videx EC. (Didanosine) product monograph. Princeton, NJ: Bristol Myers-Squibb; 2001.

[21] Piscitelli SC, Burstein AH, Chaitt D, et al. St. John's wort and indinavir concentrations. Lancet 2000;355:547–8.

[22] M.M.R. de Maat, Hoetelmans RMW, Mathot RAA, et al. Drug interaction between St. John's wort and nevirapine. AIDS 2001;15:420–1.

[23] Roby CA, Anderson GD, Kantor E, et al. St. John's wort: effect on CYP3A4 activity. Clin Pharmacol Ther 2000;67:451–7.

[24] Laroche M, Choudhri S, Gallicano K, Foster B. Severe gastrointestinal toxicity with concomitant ingestion of ritonavir and garlic. Can J Infect Dis 1998;9 (Suppl A):471.

[25] Piscitelli SC, Burstein AH, Welden N, et al. The effect of garlic supplements on the pharmacokinetics of saquinavir. Clin Infect Dis 2002;34:234–8.

[26] Lee LS, Andrade ASA, Flexner C. Natural health product–antiretroviral

drug interactions: pharmacokinetic and pharmacodynamic effects. Clin Infect Dis 2006;43:1052–9.

[27] Zerit→(Stavudine) product monograph. Princeton, NJ: Bristol Myers-Squibb; 2002.

[28] Mirochnick M, Best BM, Stek AM, et al, for the IMPAACT 1026s study team. Atazanavir pharmacokinetics with and without tenofovir during pregnancy. J Acquir Immune Defic Syndr 2011 Jan 28.

[29] Best BM, Stek AM, Mirochnick M, et al, International Maternal Pediatric Adolescent AIDS Clinical Trials Group 1026s Study Team. Lopinavir tablet pharmacokinetics with an increased dose during pregnancy. J Acquir Immune Defic Syndr 2010;54(4):381–8.

[30] van Heeswijk RP, Khaliq Y, Gallicano KD, et al. The pharmacokinetics of nelfinavir and M8 during pregnancy and post partum. Clin Pharmacol Ther 2004;76:588–97.

[31] Lamorde M, Byakika-Kibwika P, Okaba-Kayom V, et al. Suboptimal nevirapine steady-state pharmacokinetics during intrapartum compared with postpartum in HIV-1-seropositive Ugandan women. J Acquir Immune Defic Syndr 2010;55 (3):345–50.

[32] Kosel BW, Beckerman KP, Hayashi S, et al. Pharmacokinetics of nelfinavir and indinavir in HIV-1-infected pregnant women. AIDS 2003;17:1195–9.

Useful HIV drug-interactions websites

NIH. Online. Available: http://www.aidsinfo.nih.gov/guidelines.

WHO. Online. Available: http://www.who.int/hiv/pub/guidelines.

http://www.hivpharmacology.com.

http://www.hiv-druginteractions.org.

http://www.thebody.com/index/treat/interactions.html#overview.

http://www.hivguidelines.org/clinical-guidelines/adults/hiv-drug-drug-interactions/.

http://hivinsite.ucsf.edu/insite?page=ar-00-02.

http://www.hivclinic.ca/main/drugs_interact.html.

Chapter | 14 |

Complications resulting from antiretroviral therapy for HIV infection

David Nolan, Simon Mallal, Peter Reiss

INTRODUCTION

The treatment of HIV infection has passed through a number of distinct phases over the three decades of the HIV/AIDS pandemic, accompanied by significant shifts in both patients' and clinicians' perceptions of antiretroviral drug toxicity (Fig. 14.1). Prior to the introduction of 'highly active antiretroviral therapy' (HAART) regimens around 1996, any concerns regarding long-term drug toxicities were dramatically outweighed by the obvious short-term benefits and improved survival associated with these combination drug regimens. These benefits were soon realized, and the dramatic reduction in AIDS-related deaths following the introduction of HAART regimens marks a turning point in the progression of the HIV pandemic. At the same time, however, the 'early HAART era' from 1996 to around 2002 was characterized by the emergence of antiretroviral therapy (ART)-associated adverse events, which became an important source of morbidity and even mortality, threatening to outweigh AIDS-related events in frequency and overall detrimental effects on quality of life even in advanced HIV disease [1]. With evidence that numerous ART regimens have comparable efficacy in the treatment of HIV infection, the choice of therapy is now largely determined by the differential tolerability and risk of drug toxicity associated with individual HIV drugs.

We have now moved into a 'late HAART era', characterized by the availability of newer-generation antiretroviral drugs that combine durable potency with improved safety profiles (Fig. 14.2), in which the realistic prospect of survival with HIV infection into old age has increasingly focused our attention on the prevention and management of prevalent diseases among those who have survived with HIV infection for many years. This new era has also seen the introduction of new classes of antiretroviral drugs, most notably integrase

inhibitors (e.g. raltegravir) and CCR5 inhibitors (e.g. maraviroc), which thus far have proven to be safe and effective additions to the already wide range of available treatment options. Clinical experience with these newer agents is still relatively limited, however, and vigilance will need to be maintained to ensure that adverse events (for example, isolated case reports of rhabdomyolysis [2] and CNS toxicity [3] associated with raltegravir treatment) are reported and further characterized where possible. It is also apparent that while the incidence of adverse HIV drug reactions has decreased [4], previous drug toxicities involving end-organ damage (for example, neuropathy and lipoatrophy) can provide an ongoing burden of disease that may in turn contribute to an increased risk of diseases associated with aging. In this context, there is an ongoing need not only to prevent these complications whenever possible but also to develop effective treatment strategies for those affected by these complications of HIV therapy.

Antiretroviral drug toxicities cover a broad spectrum, due in part to the large number of drugs used for HIV treatment. These drug side effects will be considered in turn, with an emphasis on clinical management based on an understanding of individual drug toxicity profiles. The influence of host and disease-related factors in determining the risk of these adverse effects will also be considered.

ADVERSE EFFECTS OF ANTIRETROVIRAL TREATMENT IN THE EARLY PHASE OF THERAPY

Antiretroviral therapy complications that can occur in the early weeks of HIV treatment (i.e. within 12 weeks of treatment initiation) are of particular concern to

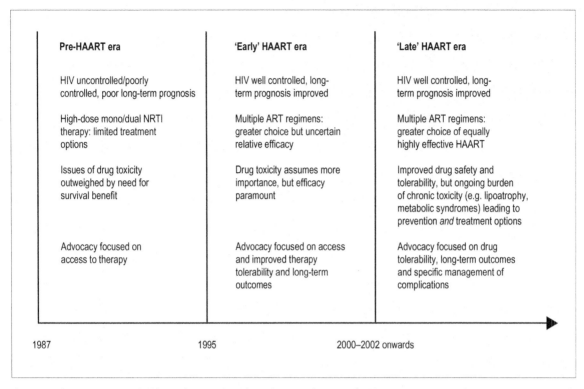

Pre-HAART era	'Early' HAART era	'Late' HAART era
HIV uncontrolled/poorly controlled, poor long-term prognosis	HIV well controlled, long-term prognosis improved	HIV well controlled, long-term prognosis improved
High-dose mono/dual NRTI therapy: limited treatment options	Multiple ART regimens: greater choice but uncertain relative efficacy	Multiple ART regimens: greater choice of equally highly effective HAART
Issues of drug toxicity outweighed by need for survival benefit	Drug toxicity assumes more importance, but efficacy paramount	Improved drug safety and tolerability, but ongoing burden of chronic toxicity (e.g. lipoatrophy, metabolic syndromes) leading to prevention *and* treatment options
Advocacy focused on access to therapy	Advocacy focused on access and improved therapy tolerability and long-term outcomes	Advocacy focused on drug tolerability, long-term outcomes and specific management of complications
1987	1995	2000–2002 onwards

Figure 14.1 Management priorities and perceptions through successive eras of HIV treatment.

patients and clinicians, as adverse events in the early phase of treatment can affect patients' perceptions of HIV treatment and can result in non-adherence or treatment discontinuation.

Mild cutaneous drug reactions can occur during the initial weeks of treatment, most notably associated with non-nucleoside reverse transcriptase inhibitors (NNRTIs; nevirapine, efavirenz, etravirine), protease inhibitors (PIs, especially fosamprenavir and darunavir), and less commonly with nucleoside analog reverse transcriptase inhibitors (NRTIs; tenofovir, or abacavir in the setting of the abacavir hypersensitivity reaction). These reactions are usually maculopapular in appearance, are generally non-progressive, and may not require cessation of therapy. However, assessment for the presence of mucosal involvement, fever, or signs of systemic involvement should be undertaken in order to exclude less common cases of more severe cutaneous drug reactions or systemic drug hypersensitivity reactions [5]. These more severe drug hypersensitivity reactions occur most commonly with abacavir or nevirapine therapy, although in both cases there have been significant advances in understanding the pathogenesis of these syndromes, which in turn have had a dramatic impact on clinical management.

Abacavir hypersensitivity reactions

Abacavir hypersensitivity reaction (HSR) was the most frequent adverse event associated with use of this drug, consistently reported in ~8% of predominantly Caucasian abacavir-exposed individuals in the pre-marketing phase of development. Fortunately, more recent, widespread genetic screening for *HLA-B*5701*, an allele strongly associated with abacavir hypersensitivity, has led to elimination of immunologically confirmed hypersensitivity. Abacavir HSR is commonly characterized by constitutional and gastrointestinal symptoms (fever, malaise, lethargy, vomiting, abdominal pain, diarrhea), with possible respiratory involvement and skin exanthema as a possible late manifestation. Symptoms associated with abacavir HSR overlap with many other clinical syndromes associated with HIV and ART, such as immune restoration inflammatory syndromes (IRIS), opportunistic diseases, and other drug hypersensitivity reactions (e.g. associated with NNRTIs or trimethoprim-sulfamethoxazole), which led to overdiagnosis and false-positive clinical diagnosis of abacavir hypersensitivity. Abacavir patch testing has been used as a research tool in clinical studies to overcome this problem and by identifying true immunologically mediated abacavir HSR (Fig. 14.3) [6].

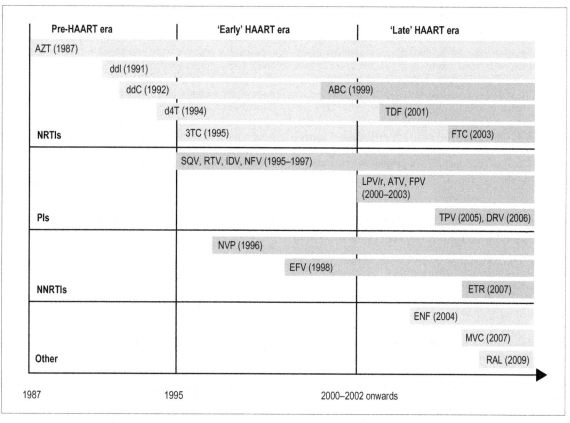

	Pre-HAART era	'Early' HAART era	'Late' HAART era
	AZT (1987)		
	ddI (1991)		
	ddC (1992)		ABC (1999)
	d4T (1994)		TDF (2001)
NRTIs		3TC (1995)	FTC (2003)
		SQV, RTV, IDV, NFV (1995–1997)	
			LPV/r, ATV, FPV (2000–2003)
PIs			TPV (2005), DRV (2006)
		NVP (1996)	
		EFV (1998)	
NNRTIs			ETR (2007)
			ENF (2004)
			MVC (2007)
Other			RAL (2009)

| 1987 | 1995 | 2000–2002 onwards |

Figure 14.2 Timeline of antiretroviral treatment availability. Dates of FDA approval are indicated. Abbreviations: NRTIs, nucleoside and nucleotide reverse transcriptase inhibitors; AZT, zidovudine; ddI, didanosine, ddC, Zalcitabine, ABC, abacavir; d4T, stavudine; TDF, tenofovir; 3TC, lamivudine; FTC, emtricitabine; PIs, HIV protease inhibitors; SQV, saquinavir; RTV, ritonavir; IDV, indinavir: NFV, nelfinavir; LPVr, lopinavir; ATV, atazanavir; FPV, fosamprenavir; TPV, tipranavir; DRV, darunavir; NVP, nevirapine; EFV, efavirenz; NNRTIs, non-nucleoside reverse transcriptase inhibitors; ETR, etravirine; ENF, enfurvitide (fusion inhibitor); MVC, maraviroc (CCR5 antagonist); RAL, raltegravir (integrase inhibitor).

Figure 14.3 Abacavir hypersensitivity demonstrated by erythematous and vesicular skin changes in response to a range of abacavir concentrations (as shown) in a petrolatum vehicle.

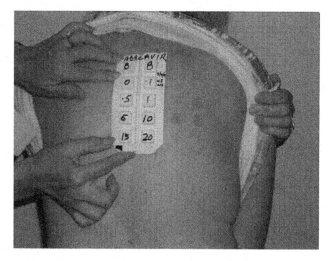

The large PREDICT-1 clinical trial, as well as numerous subsequent population-based studies, have demonstrated that *HLA-B*5701* screening eliminates abacavir HSR confirmed by patch testing [7], in keeping with studies of the immunological basis of this reaction [8]. The SHAPE study further demonstrated a 100% negative predictive value generalizes in both black and white patients [9]. Prospective genetic testing for *HLA-B*5701*, therefore, effectively prevents at-risk individuals being exposed to abacavir. It is an excellent example of cost-effective, personalized genetic medicine that has been incorporated into international HIV guidelines and widely implemented in primary practice [10].

Nevirapine hypersensitivity reactions

Adverse drug reactions associated with nevirapine lead to discontinuation of this treatment in ~6–7% of treated individuals, and unfortunately, rare fatal cases associated with fulminant liver injury and/or severe cutaneous eruptions such as toxic epidermal necrolysis continue to be reported [11]. Nevirapine safety data compiled prior to 2003 demonstrated that severe (grade 3–4) hepatotoxicity and rash occur during the early phase of treatment (within 12 weeks of treatment initiation) in ~5% of nevirapine recipients, and that low CD4 counts are relatively protective against the development of these severe toxicity syndromes [12]. These findings were subsequently reflected in the Federal Drug Administration (FDA) and European Medicines Agency (EMA) recommendations that nevirapine not be initiated in women with CD4 counts >250 cells/mm^3 or in men with CD4 counts >400 cells/mm^3 unless the benefit outweighs the risk. Subsequent studies have shown that the risk of nevirapine HSR among treatment-experienced patients with undetectable plasma HIV RNA levels (i.e. <400 copies/mL) prior to commencing nevirapine treatment is comparable to that of "low risk" treatment-naïve patients [11]. Conversely, studies in resource-limited settings where nevirapine is used as first-line therapy have not consistently confirmed an increased risk of adverse drug reactions (rash or hepatic injury) associated with baseline CD4 counts [13].

Nevirapine HSR appears to be relatively heterogeneous in nature, with variable expression of the component features of rash (Fig. 14.4), fever and constitutional illness, peripheral eosinophilia, and hepatotoxicity. It is particularly noteworthy that severe hepatic injury can occur in the absence of other clinical features. With regard to genetic risk factors, modest predictive values for nevirapine hypersensitivity have been associated with *HLA-DRB1*0101* (hepatotoxicity, fever, and/or rash in Caucasians with CD4 >25 percent) [14] and *HLA-B*3505* (rash alone in Asian (Thai) patients) [15].

Other potential pharmacogenetic strategies for preventing early treatment discontinuation

Many antiretroviral medications can cause symptoms that are prominent in the initial weeks of treatment and then generally abate with time (for example, vivid dreams, sleep disturbance, dizziness, and concentration difficulties with

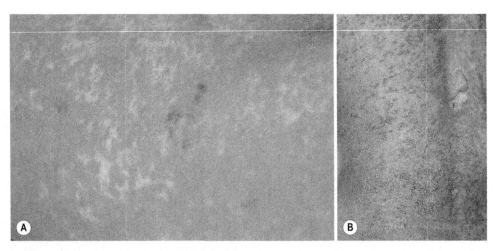

Figure 14.4 (A) Maculopapular rash in a patient with light skin receiving nevirapine. (B) Maculopapular rash in a patient with dark skin receiving nevirapine.

efavirenz; diarrhea associated with lopinavir/ritonavir; myalgias and nausea with zidovudine), and in these instances it is often useful to educate patients that these symptoms can be expected but are unlikely to persist. Other symptoms, such as the benign unconjugated hyperbilirubinemia associated with atazanavir, can become evident in the early weeks of treatment, but do not require a change in therapy unless associated with clinically apparent jaundice or scleral icterus.

Nevertheless, these side effects can persist in some patients, and although these symptoms are not generally severe, they are a relatively frequent cause for treatment modification. This has in fact become a fruitful area of pharmacogenetic investigation in recent times, with several robust genetic associations suggesting that the tolerability of several HIV medications may have a strong genetic component [16]. For example, relatively frequent (>10%) genetic variants associated with Gilbert syndrome (especially UDP-glucuronosyltransferase (UGT)1A1 polymorphism) are associated with high rates of early atazanavir discontinuation (62 versus 15%); while genetic variants that influence efavirenz metabolism are also associated with early discontinuation (71 versus 20%) [16]. No genetic risk factors for tenofovir or lopinavir discontinuation were identified in this study.

ADVERSE EFFECTS OF ANTIRETROVIRAL TREATMENT DURING LONG-TERM THERAPY

Here we will consider complications of ART that generally occur after the initial phase of treatment (i.e. beyond 3 months). Clinical syndromes that appear to have a clear association with antiretroviral medications will be considered first, with an emphasis on those conditions that are relatively rare in the general population (or confined to specific at-risk groups) but that are found more commonly in treated HIV-infected patients. A subsequent section will explore the more complex relationships between prevalent diseases of aging (e.g. cardiovascular disease) and the impact of HIV infection and treatment.

Complications of nucleoside and nucleotide reverse transcriptase inhibitor (NRTI) therapy

The spectrum of NRTI treatment complications has shifted significantly since the decline in the use of the thymidine analogue NRTIs, stavudine and zidovudine, as preferred NRTIs, in favor of the NRTI tenofovir and the non-thymidine NRTI abacavir (a guanosine analogue). These newer drugs have demonstrated an improved safety profile compared with their predecessors, but continue to require

vigilance when used in selected at-risk populations. In this section they will be considered first because of their more frequent use, rather than because of a greater propensity for complications.

Tenofovir renal safety

The renal safety of tenofovir has been a topic of interest since early reports (involving >30 cases) of significant renal toxicity with renal tubular damage and/or acute renal failure, with evidence of distinct renal pathological changes characterized by prominent proximal tubular injury [17]. In the large Gilead 903 study, in which participants had normal renal function at baseline, no evidence of significant renal toxicity could be identified over a 3-year treatment period using serum creatinine measures [18]. However, subsequent studies analyzed in a recent meta-analysis have demonstrated reproducible but modest reductions in glomerular filtration rate (of approximately 4 mL/min), with no discernible influence of tenofovir therapy on rates of acute or chronic renal injury or chronic renal failure, or of heavy proteinuria (>2 g/day), at the population level [19].

The overall prevalence of renal impairment or significant proteinuria in tenofovir-treated patients appears to have remained low at approximately 3% in both HIV-infected [20] and hepatitis B virus (HBV)-infected [21] populations, and attempts to identify useful clinical risk factors have not proved conclusive. Pre-existing renal impairment is known to be associated with risk of acute renal injury associated with tenofovir, and there is some evidence that alternative or additional explanations for renal impairment are frequent among tenofovir-treated patients with declining renal function [22]. However, current or previous renal impairment does not necessarily preclude the use of tenofovir in patients with limited treatment options [23], as long as renal function is appropriately monitored and proper dose adjustment is employed.

In this regard, simple measurements of serum creatinine levels have a limited capacity for capturing medication effects on renal function, so that the use of calculated methods such as the Cockcroft–Gault or CKD-EPI equation that adjust for body weight and gender are more useful for monitoring purposes. Assessment and monitoring of urinalysis for glycosuria and proteinuria, with quantification of urinary protein excretion (urinary protein/creatinine and microalbumin/creatinine ratio) in those with evidence of proteinuria, is also recommended, in light of the predilection for tenofovir to affect proximal tubular function. There have also been case reports of osteomalacia caused by phosphate wasting due to tenofovir-induced proximal renal tubular dysfunction. In addition to having proteinuria and/or glycosuria, patients with this problem may have hypophosphatemia and/or an elevated fractional excretion of phosphate.

Lactic acidosis, hyperlactatemia, and acute hepatic steatosis

Lactic acidosis is probably the most severe clinical manifestation of mitochondrial dysfunction, in which loss of mitochondrial oxidative function leads to increased reliance on "anaerobic" metabolism and the inevitable accumulation of lactate. In the setting of NRTI therapy, there is now an appreciation of a spectrum of clinical disease associated with elevated systemic lactate levels [24]. At one end of this spectrum is a relatively common syndrome of mild, asymptomatic, nonprogressive hyperlactatemia (generally >2.5 mmol/L), which appears to represent a "compensated" homeostatic system in which elevated lactate production is balanced by effective mechanisms of lactate clearance. While the degree of hyperlactatemia appears to be greater in the presence of stavudine or didanosine therapy than of zidovudine or abacavir, this syndrome appears to be benign irrespective of the choice of NRTI therapy.

An "intermediate" syndrome has also been described, characterized by symptomatic hyperlactatemia or hepatic steatosis without systemic acidosis, which is almost uniformly associated with stavudine therapy (incidence ~13/1,000 person-years). In this setting, lactate levels and symptoms can be controlled following modification of NRTI therapy.

The severe life-threatening hyperlactatemia syndromes, with lactic acidosis and hepatic steatosis, are relatively uncommon (1–2/1,000 person-years). A critical aspect of lactic acidosis is its unpredictability, as it typically occurs in patients who have been on stable NRTI regimens for months or even years, and is not heralded by increased lactate levels before the development of the fulminant syndrome. Host risk factors for NRTI-associated lactic acidosis include concurrent liver disease, female gender, and obesity, and while the majority of reported cases in recent years have involved stavudine-based ART, cases involving zidovudine therapy also occur. The cornerstone of management of this condition is early recognition of the clinical manifestations: abdominal symptoms including nausea, vomiting, anorexia, abdominal pain and distention, fatigue, with biochemical evidence of hepatocellular liver damage and lactate level generally >5 mmol/L. These clinical and laboratory abnormalities should lead to prompt cessation of NRTI therapy. A more recently identified clinical syndrome accompanying lactic acidosis is progressive, severe neuromuscular weakness mimicking the Guillain–Barré syndrome. Overall, the mortality associated with NRTI-associated lactic acidosis remains high (approximately 50%).

It is unfortunate to note that while this treatment complication has become exceedingly rare in developed countries with limited use of stavudine (or zidovudine), there are increasing reports of severe and fatal hyperlactatemia syndromes from resource-limited settings where stavudine is still frequently prescribed [25]. It is hoped that the implementation of updated treatment guidelines, along with increased recognition of the high costs associated with managing this and other drug toxicity syndromes associated with these thymidine analogue NRTI drugs [26], will soon change this situation.

Pancreatitis

The differential diagnosis for pancreatitis occurring in an HIV-infected individual includes direct didanosine and stavudine toxicity, severe PI-induced hypertriglyceridemia, and the effects of other drugs such as pentamidine. A diagnosis of pancreatitis includes clinical symptoms of abdominal pain combined with elevated serum amylase and/or lipase levels, thus excluding cases of isolated hyperamylasemia that have been associated with moderate to severe immune deficiency where the relationship between this biochemical abnormality and pancreatitis is uncertain.

The most comprehensive data concerning risk factors for NRTI-associated pancreatitis comes from the Johns Hopkins AIDS Service cohort ($n = 2,613$ cases) [27], with supporting data from the ACTG 5025 study. In these analyses, didanosine and stavudine were associated with roughly equivalent risk of pancreatitis, with estimated incidence rates of 0.8 and 1.1 cases per 100 person-years, respectively. Combining these drugs increased the risk approximately twofold, while concurrent didanosine and hydroxyurea use increased the relative risk approximately eightfold, including several fatal cases. More recently, cases of pancreatitis have been reported with concurrent use of didanosine and tenofovir, including with reduced doses of didanosine (250 mg/day), presumably due to the ability of tenofovir to "boost" didanosine effects *in vivo* [28].

Non-cirrhotic portal hypertension

A relatively rare syndrome (estimated prevalence ~8/10,000 patient-years) [29] of progressive portal hypertension associated with the development of ascites and varices has been noted among antiretroviral-treated patients. This syndrome is characterized by exuberant nodular regenerative hyperplasia and microvascular portal venopathy pathologically, and has been associated with didanosine exposure (odds ratio ~2), either alone or in combination with stavudine [29, 30], although cases have been described in the absence of exposure to these NRTIs [29]. Given the prominent role of venous thrombosis in the hepatic pathology, it is also proposed that additional factors such as enhanced microbial translocation from the gut and prothrombotic conditions may contribute to disease predisposition [31].

Neuropathy

The prevalence and long-term clinical impact of neuropathy is likely to be underestimated, as the symptoms are of gradual onset, and clinical signs of nerve damage are not always assessed in clinical practice. There is a definite contribution of HIV disease per se to the pathogenesis of a form of distal sensory neuropathy that is clinically and electrophysiologically indistinguishable from so-called "toxic neuropathy" from antiretroviral drugs [32]. It is therefore difficult to determine the relative contributions of disease- and drug-associated factors in the syndrome, as these effects are likely to be synergistic. The clinical syndrome common to both HIV-associated and toxic sensory polyneuropathy is dominated by peripheral pain and dysesthesia, with rare motor involvement.

In an international cohort study in which the overall prevalence of symptomatic peripheral neuropathy was approximately 50%, exposure to stavudine (odds ratio, OR 7.7) or didanosine (OR 3.2) were dominant risk factors, along with age >40 years (OR 2.9) [33].

Reversal of established neuropathy appears to be a slow process that is dependent on cessation of the offending NRTI, and there is limited evidence for treatment strategies other than topical capsaicin 8% [34], although several other agents such as gabapentin and tricyclic antidepressants have been used. As with any clinical neuropathy, a search for contributing factors such as diabetes, excessive alcohol consumption, and vitamin deficiencies (e.g. thiamine, B_{12}, and folate) should be undertaken in patients who have neuropathy.

Hematological complications of NRTI therapy

Zidovudine therapy has been associated with increased risk of anemia in ART recipients compared with other NRTIs (relative risk ~1.15), suggesting that this drug should be used with caution when hemoglobin levels are low prior to treatment. This may be particularly relevant when initiating ART in resource-poor countries where patients may be more prone to have reduced hemoglobin levels as a result of concomitant parasitic infection (malaria, hookworm), malnutrition, or genetically determined hemoglobinopathies. In this setting, monitoring for the presence of anemia appears to be a particularly cost-effective strategy when zidovudine therapy is being considered [35].

Recent studies have also suggested that combined full-dose didanosine and tenofovir treatment may contribute to a targeted toxicity against lymphocytes, resulting in reduced CD4 counts, despite the presence of undetectable viral loads [36], affecting approximately half of patients receiving this drug combination in one clinical trial. Hence, drug toxicity should be considered as a potential explanation when there is significant discordance between virological suppression and CD4 T cell responses in patients taking this non-recommended NRTI combination.

Lipoatrophy

The "lipodystrophy syndrome" represents a combination of complications first recognized among ART recipients in 1998. The clinical syndrome incorporates lipoatrophy (pathological loss of subcutaneous fat), as well as metabolic complications including dyslipidemia and insulin resistance that may be accompanied by abdominal or localized fat accumulation (Fig. 14.5). Examining the component features of the syndrome separately appears to be the best approach to clinical management. This is most apparent in the case of lipoatrophy, which is extremely uncommon in the general community, and is therefore strongly and specifically linked to ART [37]. Lipoatrophy is highly stigmatizing, as it has become a visible marker of HIV infection, causing the appearance of chronic illness and/or aging.

Thymidine analogue NRTI therapy alone is sufficient to cause lipoatrophy and is an independent risk factor for its occurrence in ART-treated individuals, with a 40–50% risk of clinically apparent lipoatrophy among stavudine recipients over a period of 3 years, compared with 10–20% in zidovudine-treated individuals [38]. Longitudinal studies have also demonstrated that body fat tends to remain stable or even increase in the first 6–12 months of therapy, and then to decline over the subsequent 12–24 months among patients receiving zidovudine- or stavudine-based treatment. Some degree of fat loss is common in patients receiving these drugs, so that lipoatrophy can be viewed as a pathological process of variable severity rather than a phenomenon that can be readily defined as "present" or "absent" [39]. In this context, the ability to recognize milder forms of lipoatrophy and to assess the rate of fat loss in the critical period from 6 to 24 months after initiating treatment with stavudine or zidovudine may allow for therapeutic intervention before fat loss becomes severe.

Substituting abacavir or tenofovir in patients with clinically apparent lipoatrophy has been associated with statistically significant but modest improvements in fat wasting [40], although increases in limb fat are often not apparent to either clinicians or patients. Therefore, it would seem prudent to focus on prevention of lipoatrophy, as fat restoration appears to be a slow and possibly incomplete process. Over 30 trials investigating HIV protease inhibitor discontinuation as a therapeutic strategy [40] have failed to demonstrate reversal of lipoatrophy, although metabolic abnormalities such as dyslipidemia and insulin resistance and occasionally intraabdominal visceral fat accumulation may improve.

The choice of NRTI therapy is therefore the primary management decision that affects the risk of lipoatrophy, irrespective of which additional drugs are included in the regimen (e.g. NNRTIs or PIs). Host factors are also important in determining the severity of lipoatrophy among patients receiving stavudine or zidovudine, with increased risk of lipoatrophy among those aged >40 years and among those with low pre-treatment CD4 count (<200 cells/mm^3), irrespective of the virological or immunological response to therapy. This argues against recommending delayed introduction of HIV treatment due to concerns regarding drug toxicities.

For those individuals affected by lipoatrophy, definitive treatments beyond NRTI switching are limited at present,

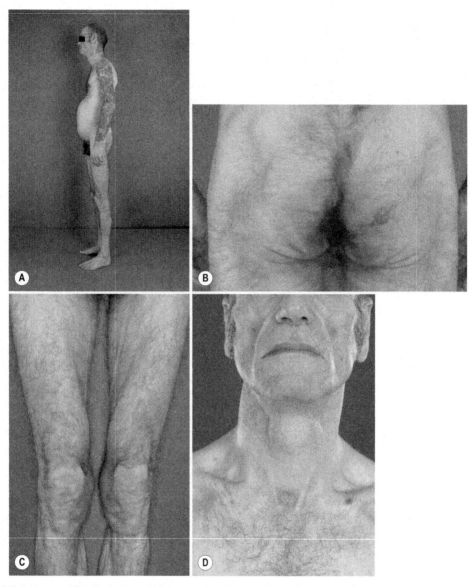

Figure 14.5 (A) Abnormal fat distribution with joint peripheral lipoatrophy and abdominal fat accumulation. (B) Subcutaneous fat atrophy of buttocks in the same patient. (C) Subcutaneous fat atrophy of the legs in the same patient. (D) Facial subcutaneous fat atrophy in the same patient.

and while there is some optimism regarding the potential role of pioglitazone treatment [41], consideration will need to be given to long-term safety data before this treatment strategy can be widely recommended. In the case of facial lipoatrophy, the dermal filler poly-L-lactic acid ("Newfill" or "Sculptra") has been approved by the US Food and Drug Administration (FDA) for this indication, and has proved safe and effective over extended follow-up. The use of high-fat or high-energy diets to promote fat gain in patients with lipoatrophy cannot be supported, even after the

causative NRTI drug has been removed, as the end-organ damage to subcutaneous adipose tissue depots means that this fat tissue is unable to effectively take up dietary fat, thereby increasing the risk of unwanted side effects such as visceral/abdominal fat accumulation and hypertriglyceridemia. In this respect, the presence of lipoatrophic damage to adipose tissue does appear to increase the long-term risk of "metabolic syndrome" complications, suggesting that vigilant monitoring for these complications needs to be maintained in patients with a history of lipoatrophy [42].

Complications of HIV protease inhibitor therapy

These adverse effects tend to be strongly associated with individual drugs within the PI class, rather than representing drug "class effects."

Abnormal liver function/liver enzyme abnormalities

Full-dose (but not low-dose) ritonavir has been associated with increased risk of hepatoxicity as defined by transaminase elevation (i.e. >five fold elevation of ALT and/or AST levels), with a relative risk of approximately four compared with other PI drugs. However, the presence of chronic viral hepatitis (i.e. hepatitis B or C) and/or alcohol abuse remain the most important risk factors for such hepatoxicity, which may reflect altered hepatic drug metabolism as well as the restoration of pathogenic inflammatory responses to hepatitis viruses following successful HIV therapy [43].

Gastrointestinal intolerance

Persistent diarrhea is a relatively frequent complication of nelfinavir therapy, affecting 20–50% of recipients. Of the other PI drugs, lopinavir and fosamprenavir have also been associated with diarrhea, particularly in the early weeks of treatment (incidence ~10%). Diarrhea seems to be much less common with the use of ritonavir-boosted atazanavir or darunavir.

Nephrolithiasis and renal dysfunction

Indinavir is associated with risk of renal calculus formation, affecting ~10% of recipients, and can also be associated with nephropathy in the absence of overt calculus formation. Indinavir-induced renal calculi (which are radiolucent) generally respond to hydration, diuresis, and urinary acidification. Indinavir is also associated with "retinoid" side effects, including dry lips and skin (~30%), and hair and nail changes including paronychia (~5%). There have now been >30 reports of renal calculi in atazanavir recipients, although clinical risk factors are not yet known. Atazanavir and lopinavir/ritonavir may also be associated with increased risk of chronic kidney disease [44].

Metabolic complications: dyslipidemia and insulin resistance

There is now definitive evidence that treatment with selected PIs can rapidly induce significant metabolic abnormalities, including but not limited to changes in plasma lipids and lipoproteins, in both HIV-infected and HIV-uninfected subjects, although it must also be acknowledged that metabolic effects of these drugs can no longer be considered "class effects." For example, indinavir has been shown to induce significant insulin resistance following short-term drug exposure in healthy control subjects [45], while lopinavir/ritonavir therapy under similar conditions is associated with elevated triglyceride levels but no significant impact on insulin sensitivity [46]. The newer PIs atazanavir [47] and darunavir [48] do not appear to have significant unfavorable effects on lipid or glucose metabolism, paving the way for *intra-class* PI switching strategies in response to treatment-induced dyslipidemia.

The effect of PI therapy on vascular disease risk is obviously strongly related to this issue, and will be discussed further below.

TOXICITY PROFILES OF NNRTIs

The NNRTIs efavirenz and nevirapine have proven to be highly effective HIV drugs that carry minimal risk of metabolic and gastrointestinal side effects, although differences in toxicity profiles attributable to "class effects" of NNRTI and PI drugs have become far less relevant with the development of more tolerable second-generation HIV protease inhibitors.

Efavirenz and central nervous system side effects

The efficacy of efavirenz-containing regimens and the much lower likelihood of severe hepatic and skin toxicities associated with nevirapine treatment have led to the adoption of efavirenz as a recommended first-line agent in various treatment guidelines. As mentioned earlier, the most frequent adverse effects associated with this drug are cognitive and neuropsychiatric, affecting approximately 15% of efavirenz recipients to at least a moderate extent within 1 month of initiating treatment. While these side effects generally resolve in the first 2–4 weeks of treatment, cohort studies have identified ongoing symptoms including dizziness, sadness, irritability, nervousness and mood changes, impaired concentration, and abnormal dreams [49]. Suicidal ideation has also been reported in a minority of patients, indicating that neuropsychiatric manifestations may be severe in some cases. While this list would appear to constitute a significant burden of toxicity, it is interesting to note that patients on efavirenz or nevirapine regimens consistently report equivalent improvements in quality of life. In cases where CNS side effects of efavirenz warrant treatment revision, substitution with an alternative medication, including etravirine, is associated with significant improvements in insomnia, abnormal dreams, and nervousness within weeks [50].

Rash

All NNRTI can cause rash during the initial weeks of therapy. Nevirapine is the most like to cause serious rash, which is discussed above under 'Nevirapine hypersensitivity reactions.' Rash due to efavirenz is often self-limited without the need for discontinuation. Etravirine may be associated with skin rash of varying severity, generally occurring within the first 4–6 weeks of treatment. In phase 3 trials approximately 2% of patients needed to discontinue etravirine because of rash.

IMPACT OF ANTIRETROVIRAL THERAPY ON PREVALENT DISEASES ASSOCIATED WITH AGING

The long-term success of ART has created new challenges relating to the management of HIV infection in aging patients, and in particular the potential effects of HIV infection and its treatment on the onset and severity of prevalent age-associated diseases (Fig. 14.6). It will soon be the case that the majority of HIV-infected individuals in developed settings will be older than 50 years of age, and while this proportion is lower in resource-limited settings (approaching 15%), it has been pointed out recently that the absolute number of older Africans living with HIV infection is already substantial at >3 million [51].

There is now some evidence of premature physiological aging with HIV infection, so that markers of physical frailty [52, 53], cerebral function [54], and atherosclerotic burden [55] are 10–15 years more advanced than expected. It is not known whether accelerated aging continues throughout the course of HIV infection and treatment, but proposed associations with persistent immune activation [56] appear to have a sound basis in recent research [57], with parallel examples in other branches of medicine [58]. One of the most profound insights in this area has come from the SMART study [57] and numerous substudies that have arisen from it, which have demonstrated increased adverse events, including all-cause mortality, among patients with untreated HIV infection. Importantly, CD4 counts and/or plasma HIV RNA levels did not deteriorate substantially in patients who interrupted treatment temporarily, and these standard markers of HIV disease progression did not predict the study's adverse outcomes. On the other hand, markers of immune activation and coagulation disturbance, which are generally not monitored in routine clinical practice, were more strongly associated with both infectious and non-infectious complications.

These findings place the effective treatment of HIV infection, with the maintenance of plasma aviremia, as the highest priority for clinical management during aging, and have also paved the way for consideration of earlier initiation of treatment in uncomplicated HIV infection [59]. While this question will soon be addressed formally in clinical trials, current treatment guidelines already recommend initiation of ART in asymptomatic patients with normal CD4 counts (>500 cells/mm^3) when the risk of co-morbid illness is elevated, as well as in older age groups [60], while treatment is recommended for all asymptomatic patients with CD4 counts below this threshold.

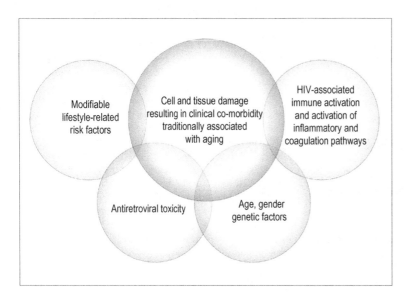

Figure 14.6 Multifactorial pathogenesis of aging-associated co-morbidities in the context of HIV infection.

CARDIOVASCULAR RISK AND HIV INFECTION

There is an increasing appreciation of the association between ART and metabolic complications such as dyslipidemia and insulin resistance, although considering specific "treatment phases" can help to clarify these issues. A central issue is that many of the metabolic endpoints are common in the general population and are therefore subject to many genetic (non-modifiable) and environmental (potentially modifiable) risk factors not specific to HIV infection nor its treatment. This is not to downplay the important role that antiretroviral agents have in the pathogenesis of metabolic complications, but to place these effects in a broader clinically relevant context.

Metabolic profile in the 'pre-treatment' phase: background risk and the influence of HIV infection

The "metabolic syndrome" incorporates lipid parameters (high triglyceride and low HDL-cholesterol values), abdominal obesity, and impaired glucose tolerance into a clinical entity that is present in more than 30% of adults (both male and female) in population studies [61]. This phenotype has a striking resemblance to the metabolic complications that have been incorporated into the "lipodystrophy syndrome," in that both are characterized by the presence of high levels of triglyceride-enriched lipoproteins, which manifests as an atherogenic lipid profile including high triglycerides, high apolipoprotein CIII, B and E, and elevated non-HDL-cholesterol levels [62]. Importantly, this syndrome is associated with a significantly increased risk of cardiovascular disease, even after adjustment for known cardiovascular risk factors, including LDL-cholesterol levels [61]. As may be expected, high saturated fat and calorie intake and low dietary fiber along with a sedentary lifestyle are significant risk factors.

Untreated HIV disease and immune deficiency are accompanied by changes in lipoprotein metabolism characterized by decreased levels of total, LDL-cholesterol, and HDL-cholesterol as well as decreased apolipoprotein B [63]. These metabolic parameters fall in parallel with CD4 counts, while progression to AIDS is associated with elevated triglyceride levels and an increase in more atherogenic small dense low-density lipoprotein particles [64].

Metabolic profile in the 'treatment' phase: metabolic complications of specific antiretroviral drugs

The use of any effective treatment regimen may counteract the lipid changes associated with HIV infection per se and to some extent restore plasma lipoprotein levels to those present prior to infection.

The role of selected PIs has been discussed above. With regard to NNRTI therapy, it is notable that treatment with nevirapine, and to a lesser extent efavirenz, has specific and potentially anti-atherogenic effects on HDL-cholesterol levels. For example, in the large 2NN trial, nevirapine therapy was associated with a 42.5% increase of HDL-cholesterol, while efavirenz had a more modest effect on HDL-cholesterol (33.7%) [65]. These differences remained, or even increased, after adjusting for changes in viral loads and CD4 counts indicating an independent effect of the drugs on lipids that could not be explained by suppression of HIV infection.

Monitoring and managing cardiovascular risk: incorporating multiple risk factors

Large-scale cohort studies have consistently shown that ART is associated with an increased risk of cardiovascular disease endpoints [66, 67], although traditional cardiovascular risk factors, particularly smoking [68], which is highly prevalent among HIV-infected patients, remain important independent predictors of cardiovascular events within HIV-infected patient populations [69]. It is therefore important to assess and manage global cardiovascular risk in HIV-infected patients, with particular attention to baseline (pre-treatment) values and metabolic responses to HIV treatment. Given that HDL-cholesterol levels as well as total and LDL-cholesterol levels are modulated by progressive HIV infection, and the importance of the non-HDL-cholesterol fraction in determining cardiovascular risk in the context of the metabolic syndrome, it may be useful to monitor the non-HDL-cholesterol fraction (total cholesterol minus HDL-cholesterol) in these individuals in order to capture the total burden of atherogenic triglyceride-rich lipoproteins.

With regard to the effects of HIV medications on cardiovascular risk, data from the large international D:A:D cohort have implicated three medications as potential risk factors [66, 67], and these effects have been incorporated into a cardiovascular risk calculator specific to HIV-infected populations [70]. Cumulative exposure to indinavir and lopinavir-ritonavir was associated with an increased risk of MI (relative rate per year, 1.1), with evidence that this effect was mediated at least in part by the effects of these medications on lipid levels. Current exposure to abacavir has also emerged as a possible risk factor, associated with a relative risk of ~1.9 in the D:A:D study [71], although this association has not been seen in clinical trials or some other cohort studies [72]. When considering the need to avoid these medications, it is important to consider the underlying absolute risk of cardiovascular disease attributable to traditional risk factors (including non-modifiable risk factors such as age and gender), in order to understand the benefit or harm that may result from this strategy. A useful approach to this issue has been provided by the Copenhagen HIV Programme [70], which has created a calculator that estimates the influence of ART based on the "number needed to harm." With respect to the true impact of abacavir treatment on cardiovascular risk, this remains an area of controversy [73, 74], and a pathogenic mechanism linked to myocardial events has been elusive thus far. Among those with existing cardiovascular disease or increased cardiovascular risk ($\geq$20% 10-year predicted risk), statins are recommended for their prognostic and survival benefit, irrespective of the baseline lipid values [75]. When choosing between particular statins, the potential for drug–drug interactions with particular antiretrovirals needs to be taken into account. Excellent and comprehensive guidelines have been established for the assessment and treatment of non-infectious co-morbidities, including cardiovascular risk and metabolic complications, in HIV-infected patients [76, 77], which recommend the use of standard treatment approaches based on global cardiovascular risk assessment.

BONE DENSITY AND HIV INFECTION

This topic has been the subject of a recent comprehensive review [78], which provides a practical approach for assessing and managing bone disease in the setting of HIV infection. The overall prevalence of osteoporosis in HIV-infected subjects is approximately 15%, more than three times greater than reported in HIV-uninfected controls, and there is strong evidence from the SMART study [79] and elsewhere that there is a decline in bone density during HIV treatment, particularly in the first year of therapy, of approximately 2–5%. With regard to specific antiretroviral agents, several studies have indicated an additional but non-progressive effect of tenofovir therapy on bone loss [80, 81] and increased bone turnover [81], which may relate to the effects of tenofovir on renal proximal tubular function. The clinical significance of this effect is uncertain [82] and needs to be considered in light of the overall risk factor profile for osteoporosis, a list that includes highly prevalent factors among HIV-infected patients, such as low body mass (especially lean body mass), smoking, drug and alcohol abuse, and hypogonadism.

There has also been considerable recent interest in the effects of vitamin D deficiency on bone health in HIV infection, given that vitamin D deficiency has been observed in the majority of HIV-infected individuals, that treatment with efavirenz appears to be associated with greater risk of this complication [83], and that of osteomalacia has been associated with tenofovir therapy.

Management guidelines have provided pathways for screening HIV-infected patients (particularly those over 50 years of age) for low bone density, as well as assessing serum vitamin D levels [78, 84]. These guidelines also establish criteria for treatment of established osteoporosis based on overall fracture risk, calculated using the FRAX tool [85], as well as the severity of bone loss and the presence of secondary factors.

CONCLUSION

- The toxicity profiles of antiretroviral drugs can to some extent be grouped based on drug classes, but important distinctions have also emerged among drugs within each class. Hence, the notion of "class effects" is not useful when considering the toxicity profiles of antiretroviral regimens.

- Antiretroviral medications that are now commonly used in resource-rich settings are characterized by favorable safety profiles as well as high levels of efficacy, so that severe treatment-associated toxicities have become an uncommon cause of morbidity and mortality.

- Adverse effects that occur during the early phase of treatment (i.e. <12 weeks) are now well characterized, and risk of some of these events appears to have a significant genetic component. This is most notable in the case of abacavir hypersensitivity reactions, where genetic screening for *HLA-B*5701* has dramatically increased medication safety.

- There is a range of adverse effects associated with long-term antiretroviral therapy, which are both medication- and organ-specific. Appropriate monitoring strategies are therefore determined by an understanding of the toxicity profiles of individual antiretroviral medications.

- Understanding the relationships between diseases associated with aging and HIV infection is becoming increasingly important in contemporary clinical practice, given that the majority of individuals living with HIV infection in the developed world will be >50 years of age within this decade.

- In this setting, establishing and sustaining effective virological suppression remains a high priority in HIV management, given evidence that viremic infection and associated inflammation is associated with an increased risk of serious infectious and non-infectious complications. The continued risk associated with residual inflammation in those with aviremic infection is an area of active research.

- Guidelines for the assessment and management of metabolic and other non-infectious complications of HIV treatment are evolving, which emphasizes the value of a holistic approach to risk management in order to prevent end-organ diseases such as cardiovascular events and bone fractures.

REFERENCES

[1] Reisler RB, Han C, Burman WJ, et al. Grade 4 events are as important as AIDS events in the era of HAART. J Acquir Immune Defic Syndr 2003;34:379–86.

[2] Croce F, Vitello P, Dalla Pria A, et al. Severe raltegravir-associated rhabdomyolysis: a case report and review of the literature. Int J STD AIDS 2010;21:783–5.

[3] Reiss KA, Bailey JR, Pham PA, Gallant JE. Raltegravir-induced cerebellar ataxia. AIDS 2010;24:2757.

[4] Rodger AJ, Curtis H, Sabin C, et al. British HIV Association (BHIVA) and BHIVA Clinical Audit and Standards Sub-Committee. Assessment of hospitalizations among HIV patients in the UK: a national cross-sectional survey. Int J STD AIDS 2010;21:752–64.

[5] Borrás-Blasco J, Navarro-Ruiz A, Borrás C, et al. Adverse cutaneous reactions associated with the newest antiretroviral drugs in patients with human immunodeficiency virus infection. J Antimicrob Chemother 2008;62:879–88.

[6] Phillips EJ, Sullivan JR, Knowles SR, et al. Utility of patch testing in patients with hypersensitivity syndromes associated with abacavir. AIDS 2002;16:2223–5.

[7] Mallal S, Phillips E, Carosi G, et al. PREDICT-1 Study Team. HLA-B*5701 screening for hypersensitivity to abacavir. N Engl J Med 2008;358:568–79.

[8] Chessman D, Kostenko L, Lethborg T, et al. Human leukocyte antigen class I-restricted activation of CD8+ T cells provides the immunogenetic basis of a systemic drug hypersensitivity. Immunity 2008;28:822–32.

[9] Saag M, Balu R, Phillips E, et al. Study of Hypersensitivity to Abacavir and Pharmacogenetic Evaluation Study Team. High sensitivity of human leukocyte antigen-B*5701 as a marker for immunologically confirmed abacavir hypersensitivity in white and black patients. Clin Infect Dis 2008;46:1111–8.

[10] Kauf TL, Farkouh RA, Earnshaw SR, et al. Economic efficiency of genetic screening to inform the use of abacavir sulfate in the treatment of HIV. Pharmacoeconomics 2010;28:1025–39.

[11] Kesselring AM, Wit FW, Sabin CA, et al. Nevirapine Toxicity Multicohort Collaboration. Risk factors for treatment-limiting toxicities in patients starting nevirapine-containing antiretroviral therapy. AIDS 2009;23:1689–99.

[12] Stern JO, Robinson PA, Love J, et al. A comprehensive hepatic safety analysis of nevirapine in different populations of HIV infected patients. J Acquir Immune Defic Syndr 2003;34(Suppl. 1):S21–S33.

[13] Peters PJ, Stringer J, McConnell MS, et al. Nevirapine-associated hepatotoxicity was not predicted by CD4 count ≥250 cells/μL among women in Zambia, Thailand and Kenya. HIV Med 2010;11:650–60.

[14] Martin AM, Nolan D, James I, et al. Predisposition to nevirapine hypersensitivity associated with HLA-DRB1*0101 and abrogated by low CD4 T-cell counts. AIDS 2005;19:97–9.

[15] Chantarangsu S, Mushiroda T, Mahasirimongkol S, et al. HLA-B*3505 allele is a strong predictor for nevirapine-induced skin adverse drug reactions in HIV-infected Thai patients. Pharmacogenet Genomics 2009;19:139–46.

[16] Lubomirov R, Colombo S, di Iulio J, et al. the Swiss HIV Cohort Study. Association of pharmacogenetic markers with premature discontinuation of first-line anti-HIV therapy: an observational cohort study. J Infect Dis 2011;203:246–57.

[17] Herlitz LC, Mohan S, Stokes MB, et al. Tenofovir nephrotoxicity: acute tubular necrosis with distinctive clinical, pathological, and mitochondrial abnormalities. Kidney Int 2010;78:1171–7.

[18] Mocroft A, Kirk O, Reiss P, et al. Estimated glomerular filtration rate, chronic kidney disease and antiretroviral drug use in HIV-positive patients. AIDS 2010;24:1667–78.

[19] Cooper RD, Wiebe N, Smith N, et al. Systematic review and meta-analysis: renal safety of tenofovir disoproxil fumarate in HIV-infected patients. Clin Infect Dis 2010;51(5):496–505.

[20] de Vries-Sluijs TE, Reijnders JG, et al. Long-term therapy with tenofovir is effective for patients co-infected with human immunodeficiency virus and hepatitis B virus. Gastroenterology 2010;139:1934–41.

[21] Horberg M, Tang B, Towner W, et al. Impact of tenofovir on renal function in HIV-infected, antiretroviral-naive patients. J Acquir Immune Defic Syndr 2010;53:62–9.

[22] Jones R, Stebbing J, Nelson M, et al. Renal dysfunction with tenofovir disoproxil fumarate-containing highly active antiretroviral therapy regimens is not observed more frequently: a cohort and case-control study. J Acquir Immune Defic Syndr 2004;37:1489–95.

[23] Young B, Buchacz K, Moorman A, et al. Renal function in patients with preexisting renal disease receiving tenofovir-containing highly active antiretroviral therapy in the HIV outpatient study. AIDS Patient Care STDS 2009;23:589–92.

[24] John M, Mallal S. Hyperlactatemia syndromes in people with HIV infection. Curr Opin Infect Dis 2002;15:23–9.

[25] Osler M, Stead D, Rebe K, et al. Risk factors for and clinical characteristics of severe hyperlactataemia in patients receiving antiretroviral therapy: a case-control study. HIV Med 2010;11:121–9.

[26] Bendavid E, Grant P, Talbot A, et al. Cost-effectiveness of antiretroviral regimens in the World Health Organization's treatment guidelines: a South African analysis. AIDS 2011;25:211–20.

[27] Moore RD, Keruly JC, Chaisson RE. Incidence of pancreatitis in HIV-

infected patients receiving nucleoside reverse transcriptase inhibitor drugs. AIDS 2001;15:617–20.

[28] Kirian MA, Higginson RT, Fulco PP. Acute onset of pancreatitis with concomitant use of tenofovir and didanosine. Ann Pharmacother 2004;38:1660–3.

[29] Cotte L, Bénet T, Billioud C, et al. The role of nucleoside and nucleotide analogues in nodular regenerative hyperplasia in HIV-infected patients: a case control study. J Hepatol 2011;54:489–96.

[30] Kovari H, Ledergerber B, Peter U, et al. Swiss HIV Cohort Study. Association of noncirrhotic portal hypertension in HIV-infected persons and antiretroviral therapy with didanosine: a nested case-control study. Clin Infect Dis 2009;49:626–35.

[31] Vispo E, Morello J, Rodriguez-Novoa S, Soriano V. Noncirrhotic portal hypertension in HIV infection. Curr Opin Infect Dis 2011;24:12–18.

[32] Keswani SC, Pardo CA, Cherry CL, et al. HIV-associated sensory neuropathies. AIDS 2002;16:2105–17.

[33] Cherry CL, Skolasky RL, Lal L, et al. Antiretroviral use and other risks for HIV-associated neuropathies in an international cohort. Neurology 2006;6:867–73.

[34] Phillips TJ, Cherry CL, Cox S, et al. Pharmacological treatment of painful HIV-associated sensory neuropathy: a systematic review and meta-analysis of randomised controlled trials. PLoS One 2010;5: e14433.

[35] Negredo E, Molto J, Burger D, et al. Unexpected CD4 cell count decline in patients receiving didanosine and tenofovir-based regimens despite undetectable viral load. AIDS 2004;18:459–63.

[36] Koenig SP, Schackman BR, Riviere C, et al. Clinical impact and cost of monitoring for asymptomatic laboratory abnormalities among patients receiving antiretroviral therapy in a resource-poor setting. Clin Infect Dis 2010;51:600–8.

[37] Palella Jr. FJ, Cole SR, Chmiel JS, et al. Anthropometrics and examiner-reported body habitus abnormalities in the multicenter AIDS cohort study. Clin Infect Dis 2004;38:903–7.

[38] Nolan D, Reiss P, Mallal S. Adverse effects of antiretroviral therapy for HIV infection: a review of selected topics. Expert Opin Drug Saf 2005;4:201–18.

[39] Podzamczer D, Ferrer E, Martínez E, et al. ABCDE Study Team. How much fat loss is needed for lipoatrophy to become clinically evident? AIDS Res Hum Retroviruses 2009;25:563–7.

[40] Barragan P, Fisac C, Podzamczer D. Switching strategies to improve lipid profile and morphologic changes. AIDS Rev 2006;8:191–203.

[41] Raboud JM, Diong C, Carr A, Grinspoon S, et al. A meta-analysis of six placebo-controlled trials of thiazolidinedione therapy for HIV lipoatrophy. HIV Clin Trials 2010;11:39–50.

[42] Hammond E, McKinnon E, Nolan D. Human immunodeficiency virus treatment-induced adipose tissue pathology and lipoatrophy: prevalence and metabolic consequences. Clin Infect Dis 2010;51:591–9.

[43] Núñez M. Clinical syndromes and consequences of antiretroviral-related hepatotoxicity. Hepatology 2010;52:1143–55.

[44] Mocroft A, Kirk O, Reiss P. EuroSIDA Study Group. Estimated glomerular filtration rate, chronic kidney disease and antiretroviral drug use in HIV-positive patients. AIDS 2010;24:1667–78.

[45] Noor MA, Lo JC, Mulligan K, et al. Metabolic effects of indinavir in healthy HIV-seronegative men. AIDS 2001;15:11–8.

[46] Lee GA, Seneviratne T, Noor MA, et al. The metabolic effects of lopinavir/ritonavir in HIV-negative men. AIDS 2004;18:641–9.

[47] Noor MA, Parker RA, O'Mara E, et al. The effects of HIV protease inhibitors atazanavir and lopinavir/ritonavir on insulin sensitivity in HIV-seronegative healthy adults. AIDS 2004;18:2137–44.

[48] Mills AM, Nelson M, Jayaweera D, et al. Once-daily darunavir/ritonavir vs. lopinavir/ritonavir in treatment-naive, HIV-1-infected patients: 96-week analysis. AIDS 2009;23 (13):1679–88.

[49] Lochet P, Peyriere H, Lotthe A, et al. Long-term assessment of neuropsychiatric adverse reactions associated with efavirenz. HIV Med 2003;4:62–6.

[50] Waters L, Fisher M, Winston A, et al. A phase IV, double-blind, multicentre, randomized, placebo-controlled, pilot study to assess the feasibility of switching individuals receiving efavirenz with continuing central nervous system adverse events to etravirine. AIDS 2011;25:65–71.

[51] Mills EJ, Rammohan A, Awofeso N. Ageing faster with AIDS in Africa. Lancet 2011;377:1131–3.

[52] Desquilbet L, Jacobson LP, Fried LP, et al. HIV-1 infection is associated with an earlier occurrence of a phenotype related to frailty. J Gerontol A Biol Sci Med Sci 2007; 62(11):1279–86.

[53] Oursler KK, Goulet JL, Crystal S, et al. Association of age and comorbidity with physical function in HIV-infected and uninfected patients: results from the Veterans Aging Cohort Study. AIDS Patient Care STDS 2011;25:13–20.

[54] Ances BM, Vaida F, Yeh MJ, et al. HIV infection and aging independently affect brain function as measured by functional magnetic resonance imaging. J Infect Dis 2010;201:336–40.

[55] Guaraldi G, Zona S, Alexopoulos N, et al. Coronary aging in HIV-infected patients. Clin Infect Dis 2009;49(11):1756–62.

[56] Deeks SG. HIV infection, inflammation, immunosenescence, and aging. Annu Rev Med 2011;62:141–55.

[57] Strategies for Management of Antiretroviral Therapy (SMART) Study Group. El-Sadr WM, Lundgren JD, Neaton JD, et al. CD4+ count-guided interruption of antiretroviral treatment. N Engl J Med 2006;355:2283–96.

[58] Yao X, Li H, Leng SX. Inflammation and immune system alterations in frailty. Clin Geriatr Med 2011;27:79–87.

[59] When To Start Consortium. Sterne JA, May M, Costagliola D, et al. Timing of initiation of

antiretroviral therapy in AIDS-free HIV-1-infected patients: a collaborative analysis of 18 HIV cohort studies. Lancet 2009;373:1352–63.

[60] Thompson MA, Aberg JA, Cahn P, et al. International AIDS Society-USA. Antiretroviral treatment of adult HIV infection: 2010 recommendations of the International AIDS Society-USA panel. JAMA 2010;304:321–33.

[61] Ford ES. The metabolic syndrome and mortality from cardiovascular disease and all-causes: findings from the National Health and Nutrition Examination Survey II Mortality Study. Atherosclerosis 2004;173:309–14.

[62] Sekhar RV, Jahoor F, White AC, et al. Metabolic basis of HIV-lipodystrophy syndrome. Am J Physiol Endocrinol Metab 2002;283:332–7.

[63] Grunfeld C, Pang M, Doerrler W, et al. Lipids, lipoproteins, triglyceride clearance, and cytokines in human immunodeficiency virus infection and the acquired immunodeficiency syndrome. J Clin Endocrinol Metab 1992;74:1045–52.

[64] Grunfeld C, Kotler DP, Hamadeh R, et al. Hypertriglyceridemia in the acquired immunodeficiency syndrome. Am J Med 1989;86:27–31.

[65] Van Leth F, Phanuphak P, Stroes E, et al. Nevirapine and efavirenz elicit different changes in lipid profiles in antiretroviral-therapy-naive patients infected with HIV-1. PLoS Med 2004;1:e19.

[66] Friis-Møller N, Thiébaut R, Reiss P, et al. Predicting the risk of cardiovascular disease in HIV-infected patients: the data collection on adverse effects of anti-HIV drugs study. Eur J Cardiovasc Prev Rehabil 2010;17(5):491–501.

[67] Worm SW, Sabin C, Weber R, et al. Risk of myocardial infarction in patients with HIV infection exposed to specific individual antiretroviral drugs from the 3 major drug classes: the data collection on adverse events of anti-HIV drugs (D:A:D) study. J Infect Dis 2010;201:318–30.

[68] Petoumenos K, Worm S, Reiss P, et al. Rates of cardiovascular disease following smoking cessation in patients with HIV infection: results from the D:A:D study. HIV Med 2011;12(7):412–21.

[69] Ford ES, Greenwald JH, Richterman AG, et al. Traditional risk factors and D-dimer predict incident cardiovascular disease events in chronic HIV infection. AIDS 2010;24:1509–17.

[70] D:A:D cardiovascular risk assessment tool and other risk calculators are located on the Copenhagen HIV Programme website: http://www.cphiv.dk/TOOLS/tabid/282/Default.aspx; [accessed February 9.02.11.].

[71] Kowalska JD, Kirk O, Mocroft A, et al. Implementing the number needed to harm in clinical practice: risk of myocardial infarction in HIV-1-infected patients treated with abacavir. HIV Med 2010;11:200–8.

[72] Ribaudo HJ, Benson CA, Zheng Y, et al. for the ACTG A5001/ALLRT Protocol Team. No risk of myocardial infarction associated with initial antiretroviral treatment containing abacavir: short and long-term results from ACTG A5001/ALLRT. Clin Infect Dis 2011;52:929–40.

[73] Reiss P. The art of managing human immunodeficiency virus infection: a balancing act. Clin Infect Dis 2009;49:1602–4.

[74] Costagliola D, Lang S, Mary-Krause M, et al. Abacavir and cardiovascular risk: reviewing the evidence. Curr HIV/AIDS Rep 2010;7:127–33.

[75] Heart Protection Study Collaborative Group. MRC/BHF Heart Protection Study of cholesterol lowering with simvastatin in 20,536 high-risk individuals: a randomised placebo-controlled trial. Lancet 2002;360:7–22.

[76] Lundgren JD, Battegay M, Behrens G, et al. EACS Executive Committee. European AIDS Clinical Society (EACS) guidelines on the prevention and management of metabolic diseases in HIV, HIV Med 2008;9:72–81. (available at: http://www.europeanaidsclinicalsociety.org/guidelinespdf/2_Non_Infectious_Co_Morbidities_in_HIV.pdf.

[77] Dube MP, Stein JH, Aberg JA, et al. Guidelines for the evaluation and management of dyslipidemia in human immunodeficiency virus (HIV)-infected adults receiving antiretroviral therapy: recommendations of the HIV Medical Association of the Infectious Disease Society of America and the Adult AIDS Clinical Trials Group. Clin Infect Dis 2003;37:613–27.

[78] McComsey GA, Tebas P, Shane E, et al. Bone disease in HIV infection: a practical review and recommendations for HIV care providers. Clin Infect Dis 2010;51:937–46.

[79] Grund B, Peng G, Gibert CL, et al. Continuous antiretroviral therapy decreases bone mineral density. AIDS 2009;23:1519–29.

[80] Cassetti I, Madruga JV, Suleiman JM, et al. The safety and efficacy of tenofovir DF in combination with lamivudine and efavirenz through 6 years in antiretroviral-naïve HIV-1-infected patients. HIV Clin Trials 2007;8(3):164–72.

[81] Stellbrink HJ, Orkin C, Arribas JR, et al. Comparison of changes in bone density and turnover with abacavir-lamivudine versus tenofovir-emtricitabine in HIV-infected adults: 48-week results from the ASSERT study. Clin Infect Dis 2010;51:963–72.

[82] Carr A, Hoy J. Low bone mineral density with tenofovir: does statistically significant mean clinically significant? Clin Infect Dis 2010;51:973–5.

[83] Brown TT, McComsey GA. Association between initiation of antiretroviral therapy with efavirenz and decreases in 25-hydroxyvitamin D. Antivir Ther 2010;15:425–9.

[84] European AIDS Clinical Society guidelines for the prevention and management of non-infectious co-morbidities in HIV are available at: http://www.europeanaidsclinicalsociety.org/guidelinespdf/2_Non_Infectious_Co_Morbidities_in_HIV.pdf..

[85] The FRAX tool is available at: http://www.sheffield.ac.uk/FRAX/.

Section | 3 |

Diseases associated with HIV infection

Chapter | 15 |

Oral complications of HIV infection

John S. Greenspan, Deborah Greenspan

INTRODUCTION

Oral lesions have been recognized as prominent features of the acquired immunodeficiency syndrome (AIDS) and human immunodeficiency virus (HIV) infection since the beginning of the epidemic, and continue to be important [1, 2]. Some of these changes are reflections of reduced immune function manifested as oral opportunistic conditions, which are often the earliest clinical features of HIV infection. Some, in the presence of known HIV infection, are highly predictive of the ultimate development of the full syndrome, whereas others represent the oral features of AIDS itself. The particular susceptibility of the mouth to HIV disease is a reflection of a wider phenomenon. Oral opportunistic infections occur in a variety of conditions in which the teeming and varied micro-flora of the mouth take advantage of local and systemic immunologic and metabolic imbalances. They include oral infections in patients with primary immunodeficiency, leukemia, and diabetes, and those resulting from radiation therapy, cancer chemotherapy, and bone marrow suppression. Oral lesions seen in association with HIV infection are classified in Table 15.1, and our general approach to the diagnosis and management of oral HIV disease is summarized in Table 15.2. Standardized definitions and diagnostic criteria for these lesions have been established and recently revised [3, 4].

In the prospective cohorts of HIV-infected homosexual and bisexual men in San Francisco, hairy leukoplakia was the most common oral lesion (20.4%), and pseudomembranous candidiasis the next most common (5.8%) [5]. The relationships between prevalence of oral lesions and CD4 count or HIV viral load shows fairly close correlations [6–10]. These lesions occur at an early stage after seroconversion and are predictors of progression [11]. Oral lesions are also common in HIV-infected women [9–13] and children [14, 15]. While their overall frequency has fallen with the introduction of antiretroviral therapy (ART), in both resource-rich and resource-poor countries among those who are treated for HIV infection, changes in their nature and relative frequency have been seen, with major decreases in Kaposi's sarcoma, lymphoma, oral candidiasis, and hairy leukoplakia, no changes in aphthous ulcers, and often increases in oral papillomavirus warts [16–18]. Some of the post-ART increases may represent oral aspects of the immune reconstitution inflammatory syndrome (IRIS) [19]. However, oral lesions are more common in people who smoke cigarettes [20].

CANDIDIASIS (ORAL CANDIDOSIS)

The pseudomembranous form of oral candidiasis/candidosis (thrush) was described in the first group of AIDS patients and is a harbinger of the full-blown syndrome in HIV-infected individuals [21, 22]. We have shown that both oral candidiasis and hairy leukoplakia predict the development of AIDS in HIV-infected patients independently of CD4 counts [23]. However, it is not well recognized that oral candidiasis can take several forms, some of them with subtle clinical appearances [24]. The most common form, pseudomembranous candidiasis, appears as removable white plaques on any oral mucosal surface (Fig. 15.1). These plaques may be as small as 1–2 mm or may be extensive and widespread. They can be wiped off, leaving an erythematous or even bleeding mucosal surface.

The erythematous form (Fig. 15.2) is seen as smooth red patches on the hard or soft palate, buccal mucosa, or dorsal surface of the tongue. These lesions may seem insignificant

Table 15.1 Oral lesions in HIV infection

FUNGAL	BACTERIAL	VIRAL	NEOPLASTIC	AUTOIMMUNE/ IDIOPATHIC
Candidiasis: pseudomembranous erythematous, angular cheilitis Histoplasmosis Cryptococcosis Penicillinosis	Periodontal disease Necrotizing stomatitis Tuberculosis MAC Bacillary angiomatosis Other	Herpes simplex Chickenpox Herpes zoster Cytomegalovirus lesions Hairy leukoplakia HPV lesions	Kaposi's sarcoma Non-Hodgkin's lymphoma Hodgkin's lymphoma Lip cancer	Salivary gland disease Aphthous ulcers ITP Other

Table 15.2 Diagnosis and management of oral HIV disease

CONDITION	DIAGNOSIS	MANAGEMENT
Fungal		
Candidiasis	Clinical appearance KOH preparation Culture	Antifungals Treatment for 2 weeks with systemic or topical agents Topical creams for angular cheilitis
Histoplasmosis	Biopsy	Systemic therapy
Geotrichosis	KOH preparation Culture	Polyene antifungals
Cryptococcosis	Culture Biopsy	Systemic therapy
Aspergillosis	Culture Biopsy	Systemic therapy
Bacterial		
Linear gingival erythema	Clinical appearance	Plaque removal, chlorhexidine
Necrotizing ulcerative periodontitis	Clinical appearance	Plaque removal, debridement, povidone-iodine, metronidazole, chlorhexidine
Necrotizing stomatitis	Clinical appearance Culture and biopsy (to exclude other causes)	Debridement, povidone-iodine, metronidazole, chlorhexidine
Mycobacterium avium complex	Culture Biopsy	Systemic therapy
Klebsiella stomatitis	Culture	Systemic therapy (based on antibiotic sensitivity testing)
Viral		
Herpes simplex	Clinical appearance Immunofluorescence on smears	Most cases are self-limiting Oral acyclovir or valacyclovir
Herpes zoster	Clinical appearance	Oral or intravenous acyclovir

Table 15.2 Diagnosis and management of oral HIV disease—cont'd

CONDITION	DIAGNOSIS	MANAGEMENT
Viral—cont'd		
Cytomegalovirus ulcers	Biopsy, immunohistochemistry for CMV	Ganciclovir
Hairy leukoplakia	Clinical appearance Biopsy; *in situ* hybridization for Epstein–Barr virus	Not routinely treated Oral acyclovir or valacyclovir for severe cases
Warts	Clinical appearance Biopsy	Excision
Neoplastic		
Kaposi's sarcoma	Clinical appearance	Palliative surgical or laser excision for some bulky or unsightly lesions; intralesional chemotherapy or sclerosing agents; radiation therapy; chemotherapy
Non-Hodgkin's lymphoma	Biopsy	Chemotherapy
Squamous cell carcinoma	Biopsy	Excision or radiation therapy or both
Other		
Recurrent aphthous ulcers	History Clinical appearance Biopsy (to exclude other causes)	Topical steroids, such as fluocinonide mixed 50/50 with orabase, applied to lesions 4 times a day Thalidomide for most severe cases
Immune thrombocytopenic purpura	Clinical appearance Hematological work-up	
Salivary gland disease	History Clinical appearance, Salivary flow measurements Biopsy (to exclude other causes); needle or labial salivary gland biopsy)	Salivary stimulants or change in systemic medication or both Consider use of Salagen or Evoxac Topical fluorides, toothpastes and rinses

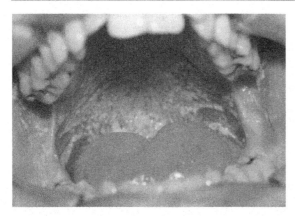

Figure 15.1 Pseudomembranous candidiasis.

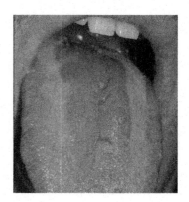

Figure 15.2 Erythematous candidiasis.

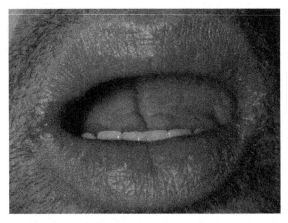

Figure 15.3 Angular cheilitis.

and may be missed unless a thorough oral mucosal examination is performed in good light.

Angular cheilitis (Fig. 15.3), due to *Candida* infection, presents as erythema, cracks, and fissures at the corner of the mouth. We have found that erythematous candidiasis is as serious a prognostic indicator of the development of AIDS as pseudomembranous candidiasis [24].

Denture stomatitis is frequently a form of erythematous candidiasis that occurs in association with the fitting surface of dentures. Clinically it appears as a smooth red area, often demarcating the outline of the denture on the palate. *Candida* also colonizes/inhabits the fitting surface of a plastic denture, and if the fitting surface of the denture is pressed into a *Candida* culture plate, prolific growth of colonies of the fungus will subsequently be seen.

Diagnosis of oral candidiasis involves potassium hydroxide preparation of a smear from the lesion (Fig. 15.4). Culture provides information about the species involved. However, because a positive candidal culture can be obtained from over 50% of the normal population, culture

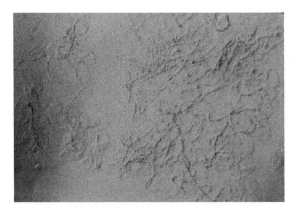

Figure 15.4 Potassium hydroxide preparation. Fungal hyphae and blastospores.

is usually not useful for diagnosis. It may be helpful in cases of oral candidiasis unresponsive to antifungal therapy to determine *Candida* spp. and/or possible azole-resistant candidiasis.

Treatment

Oral candidiasis in patients with HIV infection can be treated with oral or systemic therapy and sometimes a combination of both [25]. Our approach is as follows.

Oral topical agents include troches, tablets, creams, and suspensions. For an oral topical agent to be effective, adequate contact time is crucial. Suspensions are therefore probably not the best first choice. It is also important that sucrose is not used as a flavoring agent for several reasons, most particularly because of the risk of development of caries and the possibility of increased dental plaque production. For intraoral candidal lesions, effective agents include topical and systemic antifungal agents. Topical agents are effective if used consistently. They include nystatin vaginal tablets (Mycostatin), 100,000 units t.i.d., dissolved slowly in the mouth; or clotrimazole oral tablets (Mycelex), 10 mg, one tablet five times daily. Nystatin oral suspension, used as a mouthrinse and expectorated, is generally a less effective topical agent because of short contact time. Miconazole has recently become available in the USA as a 50-mg buccal tablet, to be placed by the patient at the mucogingival junction and left in place, where it dissolves slowly over several hours. The effectiveness of topical medications depends on adherence to recommended dosing regimens. Topical tablets and troches need adequate saliva to be effective. For those people with dry mouth, sipping a little water before use and occasionally during use of the medication can be helpful. When topical medications containing sucrose or dextrose that have the potential to cause caries are used, daily topical fluoride rinses should be used by those taking these medications frequently.

For those individuals who find it difficult to use these medications 4–5 times a day, systemic therapy can be considered. The azoles are frequently used for systemic therapy. There are many drug interactions, so care must be taken before these drugs are prescribed.

Fluconazole (Diflucan) is a systemic antifungal agent. The recommended dose is a 100-mg tablet, once daily for 14 days. Oral fluconazole is an effective antifungal agent that does not depend on gastric pH for absorption. Side effects include nausea and skin rash. Two 100-mg tablets are used on the first day, followed by one 100-mg tablet daily until the lesions disappear. Fluconazole is also available as an oral suspension, 10 mg/mL, and 10 mL used as a swish and swallow once per day [26]. Itraconazole is a systemic, triazole antifungal agent and is available as a capsule and suspension. Itraconazole oral solution has been evaluated in clinical trials as being an effective agent in the treatment of oral candidiasis, and salivary levels of itraconazole persist up to 8 h after dosing. Itraconazole capsules are now available as 100-mg caps, 2 to be taken once or twice/day for 2 weeks. This may be useful in cases that do not respond to fluconazole or clotrimazole. Antifungal therapy should be maintained for 2 weeks, and some patients may need maintenance therapy because of frequent relapse.

In the years before ART was widely used, many cases of oral candidiasis resistant to fluconazole were reported. Such complications are now rarely seen in countries where ART is widely available. Factors associated with the development of resistance include CD4 count < 100 cells/mm^3, previous use of fluconazole, and the emergence of new resistant strains of *Candida albicans* or the emergence of strains such as *Candida glabrata*, *Candida tropicalis*, and *Candida krusei*, which are inherently less sensitive to fluconazole [27]. However, in most cases, fluconazole is an extremely well-tolerated and effective antifungal agent.

For patients who develop oral candidiasis that appears unresponsive to therapy, voriconazole, a newer antifungal agent, may be useful, rather than as first-line therapy, as it is associated with more side effects than fluconazole.

Angular cheilitis usually responds to topical antifungal creams, such as nystatin-triamcinolone (Mycolog), clotrimazole (Mycelex), or ketoconazole (Nizoral). Patients with both intraoral candidiasis and angular cheilitis benefit from treatment with topical creams for the corners of the mouth as well as treatment for their intraoral lesions. Patients with denture stomatitis should be asked to remove their dentures before using intraoral topical medications and the dentures should be left out at night and left in a solution of three or four drops of bleach in a denture bowl. The dentures should be thoroughly rinsed and cleaned before placing them in the mouth.

Occasionally, other and unusual oral fungal lesions have been seen. They include histoplasmosis [28], geotrichosis [29], aspergillosis [30], *Penicillium marneffei* lesions, and cryptococcosis [31].

GINGIVITIS AND PERIODONTITIS

Unusual forms of gingivitis and periodontal disease [32] are seen in association with HIV infection, notably in groups where ART is not available such as in many geographic areas with high HIV prevalences. The gingivae may show a fiery red marginal line, known as linear gingival erythema, even in mouths showing absence of significant accumulations of plaque [33]. In early reports in the USA and Europe, the periodontal disease necrotizing ulcerative periodontitis occurred in approximately 30–50% of AIDS clinic patients [34] but was rarely seen in asymptomatic HIV-infected individuals [35]. It resembles, in some respects, acute necrotizing ulcerative gingivitis (ANUG) superimposed on rapidly progressive

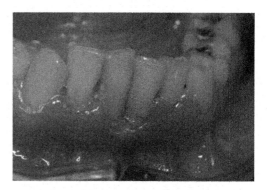

Figure 15.5 Necrotizing ulcerative periodontitis in HIV infection.

periodontitis (Fig. 15.5) and is frequently seen in African AIDS patients. Thus, there may be halitosis and a history of rapid onset. There is necrosis of the tips of interdental papillae, with the formation of cratered ulcers. However, in contrast to patients with ANUG, these patients complain of spontaneous bleeding and severe, deep-seated pain that is not readily relieved by analgesics. There may be rapid progressive loss of gingival and periodontal soft tissues and extraordinarily rapid destruction of supporting bone. Teeth may, therefore, loosen and even exfoliate. The periodontal disease often demonstrates alarming severity and a rapid rate of progression not seen by the majority of practicing dentists and periodontists prior to the AIDS epidemic. Exposure and even sequestration of bone may occur, producing necrotizing stomatitis lesions [36] similar to the noma seen in severely malnourished people in the Second World War, and more recently in developing countries in association with malnutrition and chronic infection, such as malaria. The pathologic and microbiologic features of these remarkable periodontal lesions are well documented [37]. Standard therapy for gingivitis and periodontitis is ineffectual. Instead, the therapeutic regimen that is effective [38] involves thorough debridement and curettage, followed by application of a combination of topical antiseptics, notably povidone-iodine (Betadine) irrigation followed with chlorhexidine (Peridex or PerioGard) mouthwashes, sometimes supplemented with a 4- to 5-day course of antibiotics, such as metronidazole (Flagyl) 250 mg q.i.d., Augmentin 250 mg (1 tab t.i.d.), or clindamycin 300 mg t.i.d. Treatment will fail if thorough local removal of bacteria and diseased hard and soft tissue is not achieved during the initial treatment phase and maintained long term. Our impression has been that the diagnosis and management of the periodontal complications of HIV/AIDS are challenging and are less likely to be successful unless carried out by, or under the supervision of, experienced dental health professionals.

OTHER BACTERIAL LESIONS

Cases have been described of oral mucosal lesions of tuberculosis and of lesions associated with unusual bacteria, including *Klebsiella pneumoniae* and *Enterobacter cloacae* [39]. These have been diagnosed using aerobic and anaerobic cultures and have responded to antibiotic therapy based on *in vitro* sensitivity assays. Oral ulcers caused by *Mycobacterium avium* have also been described [40], as have the lesions of bacillary angiomatosis [41].

VIRAL LESIONS

Herpes simplex

Oral lesions due to herpes simplex virus (HSV; see Chapter 34) were a common feature of HIV infection and are still occasionally seen. Diagnosis is usually made from the clinical appearance. The condition usually occurs as recurrent intraoral lesions with crops of small, painful vesicles that ulcerate. These lesions commonly appear on the hard palate or gingiva. Intraoral recurrent herpes simplex rarely occurs on keratinized mucosa. Smears from the lesions may reveal giant cells, and HSV can be identified using monoclonal antibodies and immunofluorescence. The lesions usually heal within 5–7 days, although they may recur in patients with lesions that have been present for 1–2 days treatment with acyclovir or valacyclovir. For those with frequent recurrence, it may be considered appropriate to treat them with oral acyclovir as soon as symptoms are reported. Usually, one 200-mg capsule of acyclovir taken five times a day is effective. Acyclovir 5% ointment may be useful for early labial HSV lesions. Acyclovir-resistant herpes of the lips and perioral structures have been described [42]. For herpes labialis, treatment with penciclovir topical cream applied to the lesions every 2 h for 4 days or the OTC preparation Abreva may be effective. For multiple lip lesions, systemic therapy may result in quicker resolution of the lesions.

Herpes zoster

Both chickenpox and herpes zoster (shingles; see Chapter 34) have occurred in association with HIV infection [43]. In orofacial zoster, the vesicles and ulcers follow the distribution of one or more branches of the trigeminal nerve on one side. Facial nerve involvement with facial palsy (Ramsay Hunt syndrome) may also occur. Prodromal symptoms may include pain referred to one or more teeth, which often prove to be vital and non-carious. The ulcers usually heal in 2–3 weeks, but pain may persist. Oral acyclovir in doses up to 4 g/day for 7–10 days or valacyclovir 1 g t.i.d. for 7 days may be used in severe cases, but occasionally patients must be hospitalized to receive intravenous acyclovir therapy.

Cytomegalovirus ulcers

Oral ulcers caused by cytomegalovirus (CMV; see Chapter 34) occasionally occur [44]. These ulcers can occur on any oral mucosal surface, and diagnosis is made by biopsy and immunohistochemistry. Oral ulcers due to CMV are usually seen in the presence of disseminated disease, but cases have occurred in which the oral ulcer was the first presentation. Whether to treat with ganciclovir or foscarnet depends on the severity of the viral infection, and a full work-up is indicated. Ulcers simultaneously infected by both HSV and CMV also occur [44].

Hairy leukoplakia

First seen on the tongue in men who have sex with men [45, 46], hairy leukoplakia has since been described in several oral mucosal locations, including the buccal mucosa, soft palate, and floor of mouth, and in all risk groups for AIDS. Hairy leukoplakia produces white thickening of the oral mucosa, often with vertical folds or corrugations (Fig. 15.6). The lesions range in size from a few millimeters to involvement of the entire dorsal surface of the tongue. The differential diagnosis includes pseudomembranous candidiasis, idiopathic leukoplakia, smoker's leukoplakia, epithelial dysplasia or oral cancer, white sponge nevus, and the plaque form of lichen planus. Biopsy reveals epithelial hyperplasia with a thickened parakeratin layer, showing surface irregularities, projections resembling 'hairs,' vacuolated prickle cells, and very little inflammation [47]. Epstein–Barr virus (EBV) can be identified in vacuolated and other prickle cells and in the cells of the superficial layers of the epithelium using cytochemistry, electron microscopy, Southern blotting, and *in situ* hybridization [47, 48]. For cases in which biopsy is not considered appropriate (e.g. hemophiliacs, children, large-scale epidemiologic studies), we and others have used cytospin and filter *in situ* hybridization techniques [49]. Langerhans' cells are sparse or absent from the lesion [50]. Hairy

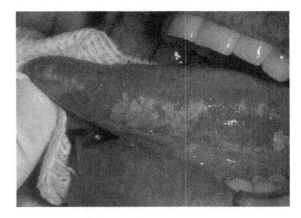

Figure 15.6 Hairy leukoplakia.

leukoplakia is not premalignant [51]. Indeed, the keratin profile of the lesion suggests reduced, rather than increased, cell turnover [52].

Almost all patients with hairy leukoplakia are HIV-infected and in the absence of modern ART, many would subsequently develop AIDS (median time 24 months) and die (median time 44 months) [23, 53, 54]. Rare cases have been described in HIV-uninfected individuals, usually in association with immunosuppression associated with organ transplantation [55]. Hairy leukoplakia has not been seen at sites other than the mucosal surfaces of the mouth [56].

Hairy leukoplakia apparently is an EBV-induced benign epithelial thickening. High doses of oral acyclovir appear to reduce the lesion clinically [57]; however, these effects are soon reversed after cessation of acyclovir therapy. Hairy leukoplakia occasionally may regress spontaneously [58].

It is not clear whether hairy leukoplakia is caused by direct infection or reinfection of maturing epithelial cells by EBV from the saliva, by EBV-infected B cells or pre-Langerhan's cells infiltrating the epithelium, or by latent infection of the basal cell layer [59]. EBV variants, unusual EBV types, and even multiple strains of EBV have been found in the lesion [60]. Hairy leukoplakia is a fertile model for studies of *EBV* gene expression [61, 62].

Warts

Oral lesions caused by human papillomavirus (HPV) [63] can occur as single or multiple papilliferous warts with multiple white and spike-like projections, as pink cauliflower-like masses (Fig. 15.7), as single projections, or as flat lesions resembling focal epithelial hyperplasia. In patients with HIV infection, we have seen numerous examples of each type. Southern blot hybridization has rarely revealed (as might be expected) HPV types 6, 11, 16, and 18, which usually are associated with anogenital warts, but sometimes shows HPV type 7, which is usually found in butcher's warts of the skin, or HPV types 13 and 32, previously associated with focal epithelial hyperplasia [64]. Novel HPV types are also found [65].

Sexual transmission thus seems to be rarely involved in these warts. Instead, they may be attributable to activation of latent HPV infection or perhaps autoinfection from skin and face lesions. Histologically, dysplastic warts due to novel HPV types have also been described [66] but are not associated with malignant transformation. Informed histopathological diagnosis is important because these benign lesions have sometimes been mistakenly diagnosed as premalignant dysplasia or even well-differentiated carcinoma.

If large, extensive, or otherwise troublesome, as is the case in significant numbers of patients who are on ART and present to specialized clinics with oral warts, these lesions can be removed using surgical or laser excision. In many cases, we have seen recurrence after therapy and even extensive spread throughout the mouth. Furthermore, our impression is that not only the frequency and severity but also the response to therapy of oral warts are worse in patients receiving ART. Topical agents such as podofilox (Condylox) and imiquimod (Aldara) have been tried, but there have been no published placebo-controlled studies showing efficacy with oral warts.

NEOPLASTIC DISEASE

Kaposi's sarcoma

Kaposi's sarcoma (KS; see Chapter 35) in patients with AIDS produces oral lesions in many cases [67, 68]. The lesions occur as red or purple macules, papules, or nodules (Fig. 15.8). Occasionally, the lesions are the same color as the adjoining normal mucosa. Although frequently they are asymptomatic, pain may occur because of traumatic ulceration with inflammation and infection. Bulky lesions may be visible or may interfere with speech and mastication. Diagnosis involves biopsy.

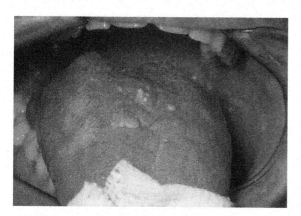

Figure 15.7 Papillomavirus warts.

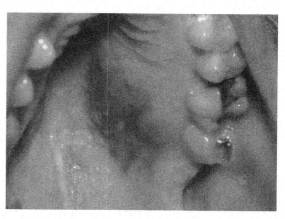

Figure 15.8 Kaposi's sarcoma.

Lesions at the gingival margin frequently become inflamed and painful because of plaque accumulation. Excision, by surgical means or by laser, is readily performed and can be repeated if the lesion again produces problems. Local radiation therapy has been used to reduce the size of such lesions. Oral lesions usually regress when patients receive chemotherapy for aggressive KS, and individual lesions may respond to local injection of vinblastine [69] or sclerosing agents. Unusual presentations of rapidly growing and sometimes solitary oral lesions of KS may follow initiation of ART. These may not respond well to local excision and may be an expression of the immune reconstitution inflammatory syndrome (IRIS) [70].

Lymphoma

Although not seen as frequently as with oral KS, oral lesions are a feature in patients with HIV-associated lymphoma, notably plasmablastic lymphoma (see Chapter 35) [71]. A biopsy may prove that poorly defined alveolar swellings, discrete oral masses, or non-healing ulcers in individuals who are HIV-infected are non-Hodgkin's lymphoma. No treatment is provided for the oral lesions separate from the systemic chemotherapy regimen that usually is used in such cases.

Carcinoma

On the issue of possible relationships between oral cancer and HIV infection, some studies indicate an increased risk of lip cancer, while one suggests an increase in several epithelial malignancies including tongue cancer. Frisch [72] examined cancer registry data from 11 US areas and found an association between HIV infection and lip cancer (relative risk 3.1 (1.9–4.8). Grulich and co-workers [73] in Australia found increases in lip cancer of 2.6 times the standard incidence rate. Demopoulos and co-workers [74] used cancer registry files at Bellevue Hospital in New York City and compared cancers in HIV-infected and HIV-uninfected individuals. HIV-infected patients with cancer were on average over a decade younger than HIV-uninfected patients (47.6 versus 60.3 years; $p = 0.04$). The cancers in HIV-infected people included lung, skin, penis, larynx, tongue, colon, and rectum. These findings indicate that we cannot exclude the possibility that these epithelial malignancies may be seen as HIV-infected people survive much longer under the influence of current and emerging ART.

OTHER LESIONS

Recurrent aphthous ulcers (RAU) are a common finding in the normal population. There is an impression [75], not substantiated by prospective studies of incidence, that RAU are more common among HIV-infected individuals.

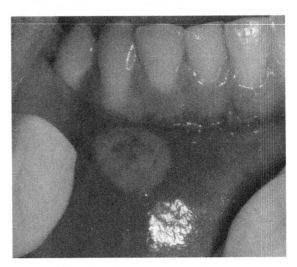

Figure 15.9 Recurrent aphthous ulcer.

These lesions occur as recurrent crops of small (1–2 mm) to large (1 cm) ulcers (Fig. 15.9) on the non-keratinized oral and oropharyngeal mucosa. They can interfere significantly with speech and swallowing and may present considerable problems in diagnosis. Location of RAU on the non-keratinized mucosa help in the differential diagnosis between RAU and HSV, as HSV lesions usually occur on keratinized mucosa. History may also be helpful, as typically those with RAU have experienced episodes of lesions occurring on areas such as the buccal mucosa, lateral margin of the tongue or floor of mouth, over many years, often starting in childhood. When they are large and persistent, biopsy may be indicated to exclude lymphoma. The histopathologic features of RAU are those of non-specific inflammation. Treatment with topical steroids is often effective in reducing pain and accelerating healing. Valuable agents include fluocinonide (Lidex), 0.05% ointment, mixed with equal parts of Orabase applied to the lesion up to six times daily, or clobetasol (Temovate), 0.05% mixed with equal parts of Orabase applied three times daily. These are particularly effective treatments for early lesions. Dexamethasone (Decadron) elixir, 0.5 mg/mL used as a rinse and expectorated, is also helpful, particularly when the location of the lesion makes it difficult for the patient to apply fluocinonide. Thalidomide, in defined protocols, has been found to be useful in very severe cases of steroid-resistant ulcers [76], but lower continuing doses do not prevent recurrences [77].

Immune thrombocytopenic purpura may produce oral mucosal ecchymoses or small blood-filled lesions. Spontaneous gingival bleeding may occur. Diagnosis by hematological evaluation is usually straightforward, but, as with any systemic condition presenting as oral lesions, full work-up is indicated.

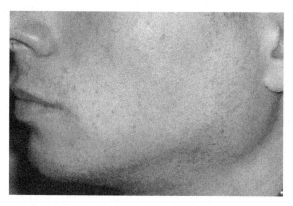

Figure 15.10 Parotid enlargement as part of diffuse infiltrative lymphocytosis syndrome (DILS).

Salivary gland enlargement, predominantly involving the parotids, is seen in pediatric AIDS patients [14] and among adults (Fig. 15.10) who are HIV-infected. This is one feature of the diffuse infiltrative lymphocytosis syndrome (DILS) [50, 78, 79]. HIV-infected children with parotid enlargement progress less rapidly than those without that condition [80]. No specific cause for HIV-associated salivary gland disease has been determined, although viral causes are suspected. The salivary gland enlargement of DILS in adults may be accompanied by elevated CD8 counts and labial salivary gland biopsy shows a CD8 lymphocytic infiltrate, reminiscent of the focal lymphocytic sialadenitis of Sjögren's syndrome, where, however, the infiltrate is predominantly of CD4 cells. Diagnosis to exclude lymphoma, leukemia, and other causes of salivary gland enlargement may involve labial salivary gland biopsy and major salivary gland needle biopsy. Some of these cases show xerostomia. Furthermore, the latter condition may be seen in association with HIV infection in the absence of salivary gland enlargement. The patient may complain of oral dryness, and there may be signs of xerostomia, such as lack of pooled saliva, failure to elicit salivary expression from Stensen's or Wharton's ducts, and obvious mucosal dryness. Tests of salivary function, notably stimulated parotid flow-rate determination, show reduced salivary flow. Some of these cases are attributable to side effects of the many medications that reduce salivation. Stimulation of salivary flow by use of sugar-free candy or sugar-free chewing gum or the use of Salagen or Evoxac may alleviate some of the discomfort. Topical fluorides and other preventive dentistry approaches are used to reduce the frequency of caries.

CONCLUSION

The oral manifestations of HIV infection occur as a variety of opportunistic infections, neoplasms, and other lesions. Some of them are common, perhaps the most common, features of HIV disease and are highly predictive of the development of AIDS. Their pattern, nature, and relative frequency appear to change in those on retroviral therapy. Clinicians caring for HIV-infected persons should become familiar with the diagnosis and management of this group of conditions.

The oral lesions of HIV infection present challenges of diagnosis and therapy. They also offer unrivaled opportunities to investigate the epidemiology, cause, pathogenesis, and treatment of mucosal diseases. As the epidemic progresses, it can be expected that further lesions will be observed and that additional rational and effective therapeutic approaches will be developed.

REFERENCES

[1] Gottlieb MS, Schroff R, Schantez HM. Pneumocystis carinii pneumonia and mucosal candidiasis in previously healthy homosexual men: evidence of a new acquired cellular immunodeficiency. N Engl J Med 1981;305:1425–31.

[2] Shiboski CH, Hodgson T, Challacombe SJ. Overview and research agenda arising from the 6th World Workshop on Oral Health and Disease in AIDS. Adv Dent Res 2011;23(1):7–9.

[3] EC-Clearinghouse on Oral Problems Related to HIV Infection and WHO Collaborating Centre on Oral Manifestations of the Human Immunodeficiency Virus. Classification and diagnostic criteria for oral lesions in HIV infection. J Oral Pathol Med 1993;22:289–91.

[4] Shiboski CH, Patton LL, Webster-Cyriaque JY, et al. The Oral HIV/ AIDS Research Alliance: updated case definitions of oral disease endpoints. J Oral Pathol Med 2009;38:481–8.

[5] Feigal DW, Katz MH, Greenspan D, et al. The prevalence of oral lesions in HIV-infected homosexual and bisexual men: three San Francisco epidemiological cohorts. AIDS 1991;5:519–25.

[6] Patton LL. Sensitivity, specificity, and positive predictive value of oral opportunistic infections in adults with HIV/AIDS as markers of immune suppression and viral burden. Oral Surg Oral Med Oral Pathol Oral Radiol Endod 2000;90:182–8.

[7] Chattopadhyay A, Caplan DJ, Slade GD, et al. Incidence of oral candidiasis and oral hairy leukoplakia in HIV-infected adults in North Carolina. Oral Surg Oral Med Oral Pathol Oral Radiol Endod 2005;99:39–47.

[8] Chattopadhyay A, Caplan DJ, Slade GD, et al. Risk indicators for

oral candidiasis and oral hairy leukoplakia in HIV-infected adults. Community Dent Oral Epidemiol 2005;33:35–44.

[9] Greenspan D, Komaroff E, Redford M, et al. Oral mucosal lesions and HIV viral load in the Women's Interagency HIV Study (WIHS). J Acquir Immune Defic Syndr 2000;25:44–50.

[10] Greenspan D, Gange S, Phelan JA, et al. Reduced incidence of oral lesions in HIV-1 infected women: changes with highly active antiretroviral therapy. J Dent Res 2004;83:145–50.

[11] Hilton JF, Donegan E, Katz MH, et al. Development of oral lesions in human immunodeficiency virus-infected transfusion recipients and hemophiliacs. Am J Epidemiol 1997;145:164–74.

[12] Shiboski CH, Hilton JF, Neuhaus JM, et al. Human immunodeficiency virus-related oral manifestations and gender. A longitudinal analysis. University of California, San Francisco Oral AIDS Center Epidemiology Collaborative Group. Arch Intern Med 1996;156:2249–54.

[13] Tappuni AR, Fleming GJ. The effect of antiretroviral therapy on the prevalence of oral manifestations in HIV-infected patients: a UK study. Oral Surg Oral Med Oral Pathol Oral Radiol Endod 2001;92:623–8.

[14] Flanagan MA, Barasch A, Koenigsberg SR, et al. Prevalence of oral soft tissue lesions in HIV-infected minority children treated with highly active antiretroviral therapies. Pediatr Dent 2001;22:287–91.

[15] Exposito-Delgado AJ, Vallejo-Bolanos E, Martos-Cobo EG. Oral manifestations of HIV infection in infants: a review article. Med Oral Patol Oral Cir Bucal 2004;9:410–20.

[16] Patton LL, McKaig R, Strauss R, et al. Changing prevalence of oral manifestations of human immuno-deficiency virus in the era of protease inhibitor therapy. Oral Surg Oral Med Oral Pathol Oral Radiol Endod 2000;89:299–304.

[17] Greenspan D, Canchola AJ, MacPhail LA, et al. Effect of highly active antiretroviral therapy on

frequency of oral warts. Lancet 1991;357:1411–12.

[18] Leao JC, Ribeiro MB, Carvalho AAT, et al. Oral complications of HIV disease. Clinics 2009;64:459–70.

[19] Tappuni A. Immune reconstitution inflammatory syndrome. Adv Dent Res 2011;23(1):90–6.

[20] Palacio H, Hilton JF, Canchola AJ, et al. Effect of cigarette smoking on HIV-related oral lesions. J Acquir Immune Defic Syndr Hum Retrovirol 1997;14:338–42.

[21] Klein RS, Harris CA, Small CR, et al. Oral candidiasis in high-risk patients as the initial manifestation of the acquired immunodeficiency syndrome. N Engl J Med 1984;311:354–8.

[22] Chidzonga MM, Mwale M, Malvin K, et al. Oral candidiasis as a marker of HIV disease progression among Zimbabwean women. J Acquir Immune Defic Syndr 2008;579–84.

[23] Katz MH, Greenspan D, Westenhouse J, et al. Progression to AIDS in HIV-infected homosexual and bisexual men with hairy leukoplakia and oral candidiasis. AIDS 1992;6:95–100.

[24] Dodd CL, Greenspan D, Katz MH, et al. Oral candidiasis in HIV infection: pseudomembranous and erythematous candidiasis show similar rates of progression to AIDS. AIDS 1991;5:1339–43.

[25] Pienaar ED, Young T, Holmes H. Interventions for the prevention and management of oropharyngeal candidiasis associated with HIV infection in adults and children. Cochrane Database Syst Rev 2010;11:CD003940.

[26] Pons V, Greenspan D, Debruin M. Therapy for oropharyngeal candidiasis in HIV-infected patients: a randomized, prospective multicenter study of oral fluconazole versus clotrimazole troches. Multicenter Study Group. J Acquir Immune Defic Syndr 1993;6:1311–16.

[27] Heald AE, Cox GM, Schell WA, et al. Oropharyngeal yeast flora and fluconazole resistance in HIV-infected patients receiving long-term continuous versus intermittent fluconazole therapy. AIDS 1996;10:263–8.

[28] Heinic G, Greenspan D, MacPhail LA, et al. Oral Histoplasma capsulatum in association with HIV infection: a case report. J Oral Pathol Med 1992;21:85–9.

[29] Heinic GS, Greenspan D, MacPhail LA, et al. Oral Geotrichum candidum infection in association with HIV infection. Oral Surg Oral Med Oral Pathol 1992;73:726–8.

[30] Shannon MT, Sclaroff A, Colm SJ. Invasive aspergillosis of the maxilla in an immunocompromised patient. Oral Surg Oral Med Oral Pathol 1990;70:425–7.

[31] Glick M, Cohen SG, Cheney RT, et al. Oral manifestations of disseminated Cryptococcus neoformans in a patient with acquired immunodeficiency syndrome. Oral Surg Oral Med Oral Pathol 1987;64:454–9.

[32] Robinson PG. The significance and management of periodontal lesions in HIV infection. Oral Dis 2002;8 (Suppl):91–7.

[33] Lamster I, Grbic J, Fine J, et al. A critical review of periodontal disease as a manifestation of HIV infection. In: Proceedings of the Second International Workshop on Oral Manifestations of HIV Infection, Chicago. Chicago: Quintessence Publishing Co; 1994.

[34] Masouredis CM, Katz MH, Greenspan D, et al. Prevalence of HIV-associated periodontitis and gingivitis in HIV-infected patients attending an AIDS clinic. J Acquir Immune Defic Syndr 1992;5:479–83.

[35] Winkler JR, Herrera C, Westenhouse J, et al. Periodontal disease in HIV-infected and uninfected homosexual and bisexual men [letter]. AIDS 1992;6:1041–3.

[36] Williams CA, Winkler JR, Grassi M, Murray PA. HIV-associated periodontitis complicated by necrotizing stomatitis. Oral Surg Oral Med Oral Pathol 1990;69:351–5.

[37] Zambon JJ, Reynolds H, Smutko J, et al. Are unique bacterial pathogens involved in HIV-associated periododontal diseases? In: Proceedings of the Second International Workshop on Oral

Manifestations of HIV Infection, Chicago. Chicago: Quintessence; 1994.

[38] Palmer GD. Periodontal therapy for patients with HIV infection. In: Proceedings of the Second International Workshop on Oral Manifestations of HIV Infection, Chicago. Chicago: Quintessence; 1994.

[39] Schmidt-Westhausen A, Fehrenbach FJ, Reichart PA. Oral Enterobacteriaceae in patients with HIV infection. J Oral Pathol 1990;19:229–31.

[40] Volpe F, Schimmer A, Barr C. Oral manifestations of disseminated *Mycobacterium avium*-intracellulare in a patient with AIDS. Oral Surg 1985;60:567–70.

[41] Speight PM. Epithelioid angiomatosis affecting the oral cavity as a first sign of HIV infection. Br Dent J 1991;171:367–70.

[42] Erlich KS, Mills J, Chatis P, et al. Acyclovir-resistant herpes simplex virus infections in patients with the acquired immunodeficiency syndrome. N Engl J Med 1989;320:293–6.

[43] Schiodt M, Rindum J, Bygbert I. Chickenpox with oral manifestations in an AIDS patient. Dan Dent J 1987;91:316–19.

[44] Heinic GS, Northfelt DW, Greenspan JS, et al. Concurrent oral cytomegalovirus and herpes simplex virus infection in association with HIV infection: a case report. Oral Surg Oral Med Oral Pathol 1993;75:488–94.

[45] Greenspan D, Greenspan JS, Conant M, et al. Oral "hairy" leucoplakia in male homosexuals: evidence of association with both papillomavirus and a herpes-group virus. Lancet 1984;2:831–4.

[46] Greenspan JS, Greenspan D, Palefsky JM. Oral hairy leukoplakia after a decade. Epstein-Barr Virus Report 1995;2:123–8.

[47] Greenspan JS, Greenspan D, Lennette ET, et al. Replication of Epstein–Barr virus within the epithelial cells of hairy leukoplakia, an AIDS-associated lesion. N Engl J Med 1985;313:1564–71.

[48] DeSouza YG, Greenspan D, Felton JR, et al. Localization of Epstein–Barr virus DNA in the epithelial cells of oral hairy leukoplakia using in-situ hybridization on tissue sections [Letter]. N Engl J Med 1989;320:1559–60.

[49] DeSouza YG, Freese UK, Greenspan D, et al. Diagnosis of Epstein–Barr virus infection in hairy leukoplakia by using nucleic acid hybridization and noninvasive techniques. J Clin Microbiol 1990;28:2775–8.

[50] Schiodt M, Dodd CL, Greenspan D, et al. Natural history of HIV-associated salivary gland disease. Oral Surg Oral Med Oral Pathol 1992;74:326–31.

[51] Daniels TE, Greenspan D, Greenspan JS, et al. Absence of Langerhans cells in oral hairy leukoplakia, an AIDS-associated lesion. J Invest Dermatol 1987;89:178–82.

[52] Williams DM, Leigh IM, Greenspan D, et al. Altered patterns of keratin expression in oral hairy leukoplakia: prognostic implications. J Oral Pathol Med 1991;20:167–71.

[53] Greenspan D, Greenspan JS, Hearst NG, et al. Oral hairy leukoplakia; human immunodeficiency virus status and risk for development of AIDS. J Infect Dis 1987;155:475–8.

[54] Greenspan D, Greenspan JS, Overby G, et al. Risk factors for rapid progression from hairy leukoplakia to AIDS: a nested case control study. J Acquir Immune Defic Syndr 1991;4:652–8.

[55] Itin P, Rufli I, Rudlinser R, et al. Oral hairy leukoplakia in a HIV-negative renal transplant patient: a marker for immunosuppression. Dermatologica 1988;17:126–8.

[56] Hollander H, Greenspan D, Stringari S, et al. Hairy leukoplakia and the acquired immunodeficiency syndrome. Ann Intern Med 1986;104:892.

[57] Resnick L, Herbst JHS, Ablashi DV, et al. Regression of oral hairy leukoplakia after orally administered acyclovir therapy. JAMA 1988;259:384–8.

[58] Katz MH, Greenspan D, Heinic GS, et al. Resolution of hairy leukoplakia: an observational trial of zidovudine versus no treatment [Letter]. J Infect Dis 1991;164:1240–1.

[59] Walling DW, Ray AJ, Nichols JE, et al. Epstein-Barr virus infection of Langerhans cell precursors as a mechanism of oral epithelial entry, persistence, and reactivation. J Virol 2007;81:7249–68.

[60] Walling DM, Edmiston SN, Sixbey JW, et al. Coinfection with multiple strains of the Epstein-Barr virus in human immunodeficiency virus-associated hairy leukoplakia. Proc Natl Acad Sci U S A 1992;89:6560–4.

[61] Palefsky JM, Penaranda ME, Pierik LT, et al. Epstein–Barr virus BMRF-2 and BDLF-3 expression in hairy leukoplakia. Oral Dis 1997;3 (Suppl.):171–6.

[62] Penaranda ME, Lagenaur LA, Pierik LT, et al. Expression of Epstein–Barr virus BMRF-2 and BDLF-3 genes in hairy leukoplakia. J Gen Virol 1997;78:3361–70.

[63] Syrjanen S. Human papillomavirus infection and its association with HIV. Adv Dent Res 2011;23 (1):84–9.

[64] Greenspan D, de Villiers EM, Greenspan JS, et al. Unusual HPV types in the oral warts in association with HIV infection. J Oral Pathol 1988;17:482–7.

[65] Volter C, He Y, Delius H, et al. Novel HPV types in oral papillomatous lesions from patients with HIV infection. Int J Cancer 1996;66:453–6.

[66] Regezi JA, Greenspan D, Greenspan JS, et al. HPV-associated epithelial atypia in oral warts in HIV+ patients. J Cutan Pathol 1994;21:217–23.

[67] Regezi JA, MacPhail LA, Daniels TE. Oral Kaposi's sarcoma: a 10-year retrospective histopathologic study. J Oral Pathol Med 1993;22:292–7.

[68] Ficarra G, Berson AM, Silverman S, et al. Kaposi's sarcoma of the oral cavity: a study of 134 patients with a review of the pathogenesis, epidemiology, clinical aspects, and treatment. Oral Surg Oral Med Oral Pathol 1988;66:543–50.

[69] Epstein JB, Scully C. Intralesional vinblastine for oral Kaposi's sarcoma in HIV infection. Lancet 1989;2:1100–1.

[70] Martin JN, Laker M, Kambugu A, et al. Kaposi's sarcoma-associated immune reconstitution inflammatory syndrome (KS-IRIS) in Africa: initial findings from a prospective evaluation. Infect Agents Cancer 2009;4(Suppl. 2): O17; 1–2.

[71] Sarode SS, Sarode GS, Patil A. Plasmablastic lymphoma of the oral cavity: a review. Oral Oncol 2010;46:146–53.

[72] Frisch M, Biggar RJ, Engels EA, et al. AIDS-Cancer Match Registry Study Group. Association of cancer with AIDS-related immunosuppression in adults. JAMA 2001;285:1736–45.

[73] Grulich AE, Li Y, McDonald A, et al. Rates of non-AIDS-defining cancers in people with HIV infection before and after AIDS diagnosis. AIDS 2002;16:1155–61.

[74] Demopoulos BP, Vamvakas E, Ehrlich JE, et al. Non-acquired immunodeficiency syndrome-defining malignancies in patients infected with human immunodeficiency virus. Arch Pathol Lab Med 2003;127:589–92.

[75] MacPhail LA, Greenspan JS. Oral ulceration in HIV infection: investigation and pathogenesis. Oral Dis 1997;3(Suppl):190–3.

[76] Jacobson JM, Greenspan JS, Spritzler J, et al. Thalidomide for the treatment of oral aphthous ulcers in patients with human immunodeficiency virus infection. National Institute of Allergy and Infectious Diseases AIDS Clinical Trials Group. N Engl J Med 1997;336:1487–93.

[77] Jacobson JM, Greenspan JS, Spritzler J, et al. Thalidomide in low intermittent doses does not prevent recurrence of human immunodeficiency virus-associated aphthous ulcers. J Infect Dis 2001;183:343–6.

[78] Itescu S, Dalton J, Zhang HZ, et al. Tissue infiltration in a CD8 lymphocytosis syndrome associated with human immunodeficiency virus-1 infection has the phenotypic appearance of an antigenically driven response. J Clin Invest 1993;91:2216–25.

[79] Itescu S, Brancato LJ, Winchester R. A sicca syndrome in HIV infection: association with HLA-DR5 and CD8 lymphocytosis [Letter]. Lancet 1989;2:466–8.

[80] Leggott PJ. Oral manifestations of HIV infection in children. Oral Surg Oral Med Oral Pathol 1992;73:187–92.

Chapter 16

Ocular manifestations of AIDS

James P. Dunn

INTRODUCTION

Ocular complications include both infectious and non-infectious disorders, and can affect virtually any part of the eye. Not only is prompt diagnosis and treatment of the more serious of these disorders essential in order to preserve vision and to help maintain quality of life, but simply recognizing HIV/AIDS-related eye disease can in many cases impact the systemic management of affected patients. This chapter will focus on the ocular manifestations of HIV/AIDS and the enormous impact over the past 15 years of potent antiretroviral therapy (ART).

EPIDEMIOLOGY

Although several of these conditions constitute AIDS-defining illnesses, most are not reportable diseases and the overall incidence of ocular complications is not precisely known. In general, however, ocular involvement in a person with AIDS is much more common in advanced disease—that is, patients with a CD4 count <200 cells/mm^3. In the pre-ART era, up to 49.1 events of vision loss to 20/200 or worse occurred per 100 eye-years, with the incidence of legal blindness as high as 14.8 per patient-year. The cost of treatment for, and loss of economic productivity from, ocular diseases is substantial [1].

The benefits of ART are numerous as regards to ocular manifestations. Not only is the incidence of ocular opportunistic infections such as cytomegalovirus (CMV) retinitis dramatically lower in the ART era but also many ophthalmic conditions may resolve with immune recovery alone, which allows for discontinuation of expensive and potentially toxic therapy for that specific condition. Consequently, the annual cost of treating patients with conditions such as CMV retinitis or progressive multifocal leukoencephalopathy (PML) can be significantly reduced.

It is important that persons with HIV/AIDS undergo regular eye examinations. While there is no standard frequency recommended, it should be remembered that these individuals often have limited access to healthcare, and may be at risk for many of the ocular complications of aging, including cataract, diabetic retinopathy, glaucoma, and refractive errors. Simply providing a proper pair of glasses to correct presbyopia in a patient over the age of 40 can have a huge benefit on that person's quality of life.

NON-INFECTIOUS RETINAL VASCULOPATHY

The most common ocular manifestation of HIV infection is a non-infectious retinal microvasculopathy (Fig. 16.1) [2]. The cause is unknown but is probably multifactorial; vascular sludging likely plays an important role. Clinical features include cotton-wool spots and, less commonly, intraretinal hemorrhages, Roth spots, and capillary non-perfusion. Vision is usually unaffected, and patients are otherwise asymptomatic. The cotton-wool spots are evanescent and appear clinically and histologically similar to cotton-wool spots found in other diseases such as diabetes. The significance of the non-infectious retinopathy is the correlation with the degree of immunosuppression. In one study, the retinopathy was found in 45% of patients with a CD4 count <50 cells/mm^3 compared with only 16% of patients with CD4 counts >50 cells/mm^3 [3]. Furthermore, the finding of a cotton-wool spot in a patient on routine examination with no other evident explanation (diabetes,

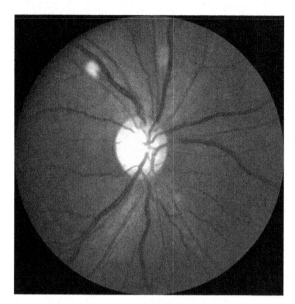

Figure 16.1 Cotton-wool spots (non-infectious retinal microvasculopathy).

hypertension, etc.) should prompt consideration for HIV testing.

There appears to be a cumulative dysfunction of the inner retina in patients with HIV disease, even in those taking ART, who have not had ocular opportunistic infections [4]. It is not clear whether this phenomenon represents an AIDS-associated primary neuropathy or secondary damage from non-infectious microvasculopathy. The retinopathy may be an indicator of vascular disease elsewhere in the body, in that the presence of non-infectious retinal microangiopathy has been significantly associated with mortality [5].

Retinal macrovasculopathy, including retinal artery and vein occlusions, occurred in 1.3% of nearly 2,500 consecutive HIV-infected patients [6]. There was a strong association between non-infectious retinal microvasculopathy and retinal vein occlusions (odds ratio 5.76). Complications, including severe vision loss, were common, with vision of 20/200 or worse in 40% of eyes. Hypertension or thrombotic disease was common in affected patients.

DISEASES OF THE ANTERIOR SEGMENT

While there are no AIDS-defining corneal infections, and with the exception of herpes zoster ophthalmicus their incidence does not appear to be significantly greater than in immunocompetent individuals, the presence of certain conditions should prompt consideration of possible immunosuppression. These include multiple molluscum contagiosum lesions, herpes zoster ophthalmicus in young

patients [7], multiple or bilateral herpes simplex virus lesions, and microsporidiosis. Jeng et al. have more extensively discussed anterior segment complications of AIDS [8].

Molluscum contagiosum virus (MCV) causes a severe, typically unilateral follicular conjunctivitis in otherwise healthy individuals. In contrast, MCV infection in patients with HIV infection tends to produce much more numerous and larger, often confluent lesions, but without itching or conjunctivitis, even when lesions are found on the ocular surface [9]. The lesions usually fade away with immune recovery, although patients with elevated CD4 counts can develop immune recovery inflammatory syndrome [10]. The differential diagnosis of cutaneous MCV includes bacillary angiomatosis and disseminated histoplasmosis or cryptococcosis. Treatment for cosmetically bothersome lesions includes surgical excision, chemocautery, or cryoablation.

Herpes simplex virus (HSV) can cause periocular, conjunctival, or corneal lesions. The disease is usually unilateral. Cutaneous vesicles can cross dermatomal distributions and the corneal epithelial lesions often have prominent dendrites, two features that help distinguish HSV from zoster keratitis. One large retrospective study that compared the incidence and clinical course of HSV keratitis in HIV-infected and HIV-uninfected patients found no difference in the incidence or type (epithelial or stromal) of keratitis, peripheral versus central location, or time needed for treatment response. However, recurrences were nearly 2.5 times more frequent in the HIV-infected patients [11]. Therapy includes topical trifluridine or ganciclovir or systemic acyclovir or similar drugs. Many ophthalmologists recommend secondary prophylaxis with oral antiviral therapy to reduce the risk of recurrence.

Varicella zoster virus (VZV) can cause cutaneous, conjunctival, or corneal disease in addition to intraocular disease (discussed below). The V1 dermatome is affected in herpes zoster ophthalmicus (HZO) and is the single most commonly affected dermatome in patients with shingles, but multidermatomal distribution is not uncommon. Keratitis, uveitis, and post-herpetic neuralgia are all more common in HZO in HIV-infected patients. These patients should be monitored closely after the development of HZO because of an increased risk of developing acute retinal necrosis [7]. Therapy includes intravenous acyclovir or high-dose oral valacyclovir; topical antivirals are ineffective for zoster keratitis, but topical corticosteroids may be necessary to control uveitis or stromal keratitis.

Microsporidiosis due to *Encephalitozoon* species can cause a chronic keratoconjunctivitis in HIV-infected patients with low CD4 counts. Symptoms include tearing and foreign body sensation. Clinical features include a bilateral papillary conjunctivitis with prominent hyperemia and diffuse punctate corneal epithelial erosions with intraepithelial infiltrates. In contrast to HIV-uninfected patients with microsporidiosis, the corneal stroma is not affected. The chronicity of the disease may be due to concurrent upper respiratory colonization. The diagnosis requires corneal scraping for Gram stain or electron microscopy. Therapy includes ART to improve host immunity, topical fumagillin, and systemic itraconazole or albendazole to control nasopharyngeal colonization [12].

Numerous other bacterial and fungal pathogens may cause ocular surface disease. Use of appropriate cultures, stains, fluorescent microscopy, electron microscopy, and/or PCR to identify the causative organism and allow specific therapy is essential.

A variety of miscellaneous anterior segment disorders have been reported. Dry eye is more common in HIV-infected patients, with nearly 18% of patients affected in one study [13]. As dry eye of any cause can increase the risk of contact lens-related problems, HIV-infected patients should be monitored closely for keratopathy and treated with supplemental ocular lubricants as needed. Whether HIV-infected patients are at increased risk for complications of keratorefractive surgery, or if such surgery poses a risk of HIV transmission due to viral particles released in the laser plume, is unclear.

Use of both inhaled crack cocaine and methamphetamine has been associated with infectious and non-infectious corneal ulceration. Putative mechanisms include direct toxic epitheliopathy, neurotrophic keratopathy, alkaline chemical keratopathy, and/or eye rubbing. Atypical pathogens are common [14], even though the conjunctival flora in patients with AIDS appears to be similar to that in HIV-uninfected individuals.

Atopic dermatitis and blepharitis may be more common or more severe in HIV-infected patients than in the general population, although definitive studies are lacking. Treatment for these conditions is similar to that for patients without HIV infection, although topical tacrolimus or other T-cell inhibitors should be avoided if possible because of the possible increased risk of Kaposi's sarcomas [8].

Pathanapitoon et al. examined 40 HIV-infected patients with uveitis and found 13/40 patients (32%) had detectable HIV-1 RNA [15]. The intraocular HIV load was greater than that found in plasma in three patients undergoing intraocular surgery, all of whom had bilateral anterior uveitis and/or vitritis without retinal lesions, with no identifiable cause of the uveitis otherwise noted. The uveitis in all three patients resolved after initiation of ART.

DISORDERS OF THE POSTERIOR SEGMENT

Cytomegalovirus retinitis is the most common ocular opportunistic infection in patients with AIDS. In the pre-ART era, more than 30% of patients with AIDS and advanced immunosuppression developed CMV retinitis, and median survival after the diagnosis was on the order of one year [2]. The infection spreads in a "brushfire"

pattern throughout the retina, causing full-thickness necrosis and blindness. Lesions may be single or multiple and unilateral or bilateral, affecting any part of the retina. Symptoms include visual field loss, decreased visual acuity, floaters, and photopsias, but pain, redness, and photophobia are not features, and it is not uncommon for patients to be completely asymptomatic. The presence of subjective scotomata varies with the location of the lesions. CMV retinitis may appear as intraretinal yellow necrotic lesions with retinal hemorrhages (fulminant/edematous retinitis), as less densely necrotic without hemorrhage (indolent/granular retinitis), or some combination of the two (Fig. 16.2). Both types, however, are characterized by a dry-appearing, granular border. There is often a mild vitritis and anterior chamber inflammation. The disease is described according to the location within the retina—zone 1 is within 3000 μm of the center of the fovea or 1500 μm of the optic nerve; zone 2 is located from the periphery of zone 1 to the ampulla of the vortex veins; and zone 3 from the periphery of zone 2 to the ora serrata. Zone 1 lesions are generally considered immediately sight-threatening and usually require more urgent therapy than do more peripheral lesions. Causes of vision loss include central retinal necrosis, rhegmatogenous retinal detachment, secondary optic nerve involvement, or exudative swelling along an active border adjacent to the fovea.

CMV retinitis is usually diagnosed clinically. Serologic testing is usually not helpful, since most adults are seropositive for CMV. In indeterminate cases, polymerase chain reaction (PCR) testing of aqueous or vitreous samples can help distinguish CMV retinitis from herpes simplex virus or varicella zoster retinitis. An elevated CMV viral load in blood samples may be the most predictive risk factor for

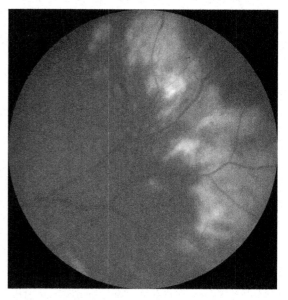

Figure 16.2 CMV retinitis. Note the granular border.

end-organ disease. In rare cases, endoretinal biopsy taken at the junction of necrotic and actively infected tissue may be necessary.

There are five drugs currently FDA-approved for treating CMV retinitis: intravenous ganciclovir, an intravitreal ganciclovir implant, oral valganciclovir, intravenous foscarnet, and intravenous cidofovir. In addition, intravitreal injections of ganciclovir and foscarnet are commonly used off-label to provide rapid intraocular drug levels in zone 1 lesions (i.e. most immediately vision-threatening). Most patients do not require intravitreous therapy, although it may be necessary in patients unable to undergo implant surgery and intolerant of the hematopoietic side effects of systemic ganciclovir. The ganciclovir implant provides intraocular drug levels roughly fourfold higher than those obtained with intravenous ganciclovir and controlled clinical trials have demonstrated its superiority over systemic therapy for control of retinitis. However, the implant does not reduce the risk of retinitis in the fellow eye or of extraocular CMV disease. Controlled studies have shown that a combination of the implant plus systemic therapy is the most effective, as it effectively controls retinitis while reducing the incidence of other end-organ CMV disease. Furthermore, presumably because of the reduction in the cross-activation of CMV and HIV, systemic anti-CMV therapy reduces mortality. Therefore, oral valganciclovir should always be used in the absence of specific contraindications.

As with other HIV-related infections, however, the most important treatment for CMV retinitis is immune recovery; all patients with CMV retinitis should be treated with ART unless there are medical contraindications or nonadherence to therapy is anticipated. All currently available therapy is virostatic, not virocidal, so patients who remain immunosuppressed require lifelong suppressive therapy, adding substantially to the cost and potential morbidity of treatment. Patients without immune recovery will on average get progression or breakthrough of retinitis, manifesting as new lesions or reactivation of a previously inactive lesion, within 2–3 months, even while continuing therapy. Development of ganciclovir resistance through UL97 or UL54 mutations is common within 6 months of therapy, but limited intraocular penetration across the blood–retina barrier with systemic therapy likely accounts for the initial episodes of recurrence. Antiviral resistance and breakthrough retinitis is much less common in ART-treated patients, but the increased mortality associated with the development of resistant CMV is of comparable magnitude in patients in the pre- and post-ART eras [16].

The widespread use of ART has had an enormous impact on the incidence, complications, and treatment of CMV retinitis, as summarized below, when compared to the pre-ART era:

1. The incidence of CMV retinitis has fallen 80–90% [17].
2. Visual field loss is decreased six- to sevenfold in patients with immune recovery (CD4 count > 100 cells/mm^3) [18].

3. Cessation of anti-CMV therapy is routinely possible in ART-treated patients who have maintained a CD4 count > 100 cells/mm^3 for at least 3 months [17].
4. The risk of retinal detachment in eyes with CMV retinitis is decreased in patients taking ART [17].
5. Mortality is decreased in patients with CMV retinitis taking ART compared to those patients not on ART.
6. ART-experienced patients who develop CMV retinitis have more asymptomatic disease, better visual acuity in the better eye, more bilateral disease, and less zone 1 involvement compared to ART-naïve patients [19].

ART is not a cure for CMV retinitis, and patients with CMV retinitis and immune recovery remain at increased risk of mortality and for progression of retinitis, retinal detachment, and vision loss [20]. Nonetheless, the risk of each of these complications is greater for patients with newly diagnosed retinitis than for patients with previously diagnosed, inactive retinitis and immune recovery.

The use of ART has resulted in the phenomenon known as immune recovery uveitis (IRU) [17], a term for a spectrum of inflammatory processes that include vitreous haze, optic disc edema, cystoid macular edema, epiretinal membrane formation, and vitreomacular traction (Fig. 16.3). In most, but not all, cases of IRU, the CMV retinitis is inactive; IRU does not occur in eyes without CMV retinitis or in patients without immune recovery. Affected patients usually complain of decreased vision and floaters but not of pain. Posterior synechiae are uncommon. IRU must be distinguished from other causes of intraocular inflammation in patients with CMV retinitis, including cidofovir-associated uveitis or ganciclovir implant-associated endophthalmitis, as well as non-CMV-associated uveitis, such as syphilis. Treatment for topical or periocular injections of corticosteroids is usually initiated, but the results are variable [21]. Vision loss is usually moderate but not severe [21] and can be due to cataract, vitreous haze, cystoid macular edema, and epiretinal membrane formation. IRU is now a leading cause of visual loss in patients with CMV retinitis.

Necrotizing herpetic retinopathy encompasses a spectrum of infectious retinitides caused by herpes simplex virus and varicella zoster virus. At one end of the spectrum is progressive outer retinal necrosis (PORN), which is almost always caused by VZV and occurs in patients with profound immunosuppression [22]. The retinitis can start in the macula or in the periphery with patchy, multifocal outer retinal lesions coalescing rapidly over several days throughout the retina in the absence of retinal vasculitis, vitreitis, or anterior uveitis. Retrolaminar optic nerve involvement may precede the retinitis, causing significant pain and decreased vision with an otherwise unremarkable examination, delaying the diagnosis for several days. Severe visual loss from the diffuse retinal necrosis, optic atrophy, and retinal detachment occur in the majority of patients. Treatment with intravenous acyclovir is usually ineffective [22]. Combination therapy with systemic foscarnet and

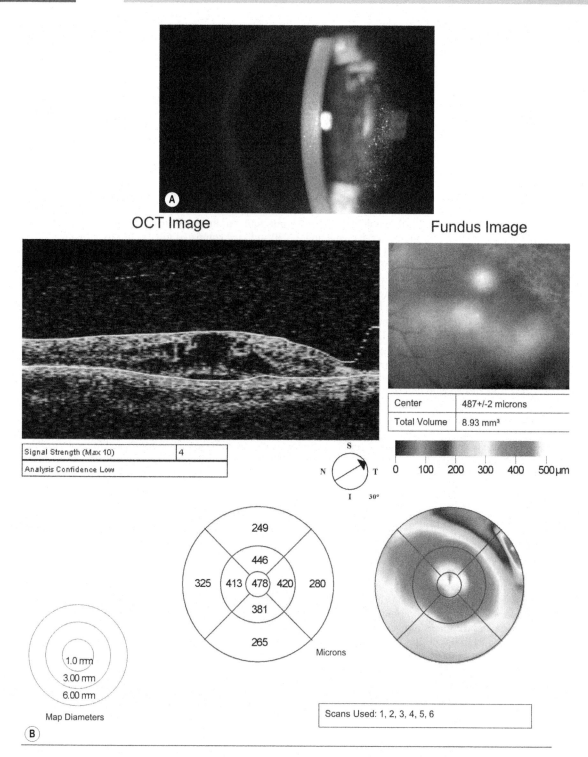

Figure 16.3 Immune recovery uveitis. (A) Keratic precipitates. (B) Optical coherence tomography showing macular edema.

intravitreal foscarnet or the ganciclovir implant may result in better visual outcomes by halting progression of retinitis and reducing the risk of retinal detachment [23]. It is essential to start patients on ART as soon as possible, as immune recovery offers the best chance of long-term control of PORN.

At the other end of the spectrum is acute retinal necrosis (ARN), which is characterized by a fulminant panuveitis with well-demarcated confluent areas of full-thickness retinitis, choroiditis, and papillitis. Unlike in PORN, the CD4 count is usually > 60 cells/mm^3 in patients with ARN. Varicella zoster virus and herpes simplex virus have both been associated with this disease. The retinitis is marked by deep retinal whitening, limited hemorrhage, and a rapid progression over days to weeks (that is, somewhat slower than in PORN but more rapid than in CMV retinitis). Traction retinal detachments occur in up to 75% of patients and blindness in 64% of patients within 2–3 months if treatment is not initiated. Late in the course of the disease, retinal breaks and detachments in the area of necrosis are common. Proliferative vitreoretinopathy often accompanies the retinal atrophy in the end stages of the disease. The treatment for ARN in AIDS patients is similar to that advocated in non-HIV patients. Therapy includes intravenous acyclovir or high-dose valacyclovir followed by indefinite oral therapy with acyclovir, valacyclovir, or famciclovir. While those immunocompetent patients with ARN are sometimes treated with oral corticosteroids to reduce vitreous inflammation, this approach is controversial in HIV patients because of concerns about additional immunosuppression; short-term prednisone therapy probably does not put the patient at significant risk. Laser demarcation along the posterior border of the retinitis is indicated to reduce the risk of retinal detachment. Some patients have necrotizing retinitis with features of both ARN and PORN; in such cases, it seems wise to err on the side of the more aggressive therapy used for the latter.

Ocular toxoplasmosis in HIV-infected patients is more likely to be bilateral and multifocal and to occur in the absence of pre-existing retinal scars (suggesting a higher incidence of acquired disease) compared to infection in HIV-uninfected patients [24]. A necrotizing retinopathy mimicking CMV retinitis may occur, but the borders of the lesion in toxoplasmosis are usually smooth without granularity, retinal hemorrhage is less common, and vitreous and anterior chamber inflammation is usually much greater in toxoplasmosis. A wide variety of treatments are used, with some variation of sulfa drugs and pyrimethamine the most commonly used. Intravitreal clindamycin may be helpful in patients who cannot tolerate systemic therapy. Secondary prophylaxis to prevent recurrence of disease was necessary in the pre-ART era. The incidence of both ocular toxoplasmosis and toxoplasmic encephalitis has decreased in the era of ART, and discontinuation of secondary prophylaxis is possible in patients with immune recovery [17].

Ocular syphilis in HIV-infected patients can cause optic neuritis, neuroretinitis, uveitis, and necrotizing retinitis.

The presence of a placoid choroidopathy or retinal arteriolitis with punctate inner retinitis may be pathognomonic. Conventional staging of syphilis may be difficult to apply to ocular disease, and it is recommended that all patients with ocular syphilis undergo neurosyphilis-type treatment regimens with intravenous penicillin to avoid the risk of inadequate therapy [25]. Rapid resolution of fundus abnormalities with intravenous penicillin is characteristic. The diagnosis should be based on clinical features and both reagin and specific (fluorescent treponemal antibody absorption test [FT-ABS] or microhemagglutination assay for *Treponema pallidum* [MHA-TP]) testing because of the risk of false-negative reagin tests. Despite the common association of HIV and syphilis, however, one large study did not find an increased incidence of ocular syphilis in HIV-infected compared to HIV-uninfected patients [26].

Tuberculosis (TB), like syphilis, is one of the "great mimickers" among ocular infections, and should always be considered in the differential of panuveitis. The presence of a choroidal nodule in patients at high risk of TB is highly suggestive of a tuberculoma. Findings that suggest a possible tuberculous cause of uveitis include broad-based posterior synechiae, retinal vasculitis, and a serpiginous-like choroiditis. The diagnosis can be difficult to make because chest films are often normal in extrapulmonary TB, organisms may be sparse in histopathologic specimens, and tuberculin skin tests have limited sensitivity [27]. Treatment with a four-drug regimen and oral corticosteroids is recommended for patients with tuberculous uveitis.

Pneumocystis carinii choroidopathy (PCC), or choroidal pneumocystosis, is a rare disseminated form of *P. carinii* infection that occurs only in patients treated with aerosolized pentamidine for *P. carinii* pneumonia (PCP) prophylaxis. The aerosolized treatment is effective for prevention of pulmonary disease but does not achieve adequate serum levels to prevent extrapulmonary infection. Affected patients typically show severe wasting but have normal chest X-rays. Ocular findings include multiple cream- or orange-colored choroidal infiltrates ranging from 300 to 3000 (two optic disc diameters) in size, which can become confluent. The overlying retinal vasculature is completely normal and there is no vitreitis. Vision is usually unaffected. Treatment with intravenous pentamidine or trimethoprim-sulfamethoxazole (TMP-SMX) is effective. Widespread use of prophylaxis against PCP with TMP-SMX or other systemic agents has virtually eliminated PCC.

NEURO-OPHTHALMOLOGIC DISORDERS

There are numerous causes of neuro-ophthalmic complications of AIDS, including infections, neoplasms, and degenerative disorders. Manifestations include optic neuropathy, cranial nerve palsies, loss of vision, diplopia, papilledema, visual field deficits, and abnormal eye movements. Cryptococcosis and toxoplasmosis are the most common central nervous system (CNS) infections in patients with AIDS [28]. Diseases caused by these organisms have become less frequent in the ART era but remain significant causes of morbidity and mortality, especially in patients with limited access to care [29]. The diagnosis is usually based on clinical findings, serology, spinal fluid analysis (including PCR), and imaging studies; brain biopsy is occasionally necessary, particularly when distinguishing intracranial toxoplasmosis from CNS lymphoma.

In contrast to immunocompetent patients with ocular toxoplasmosis, patients with AIDS are more likely to have acquired disease (as opposed to reactivation of congenitally acquired disease) and intracranial involvement. Jabs reported a relative risk of 19.9% for the development of CNS disease in patients with ocular toxoplasmosis, whereas only 12% of patients with CNS involvement had ocular disease [2]. Ocular manifestations are usually due to the mass effect of the infection within the brain, causing cranial nerve palsies and visual field defects. The manifestations of retinal involvement are discussed elsewhere in this chapter. Lifelong maintenance therapy is indicated to prevent recurrence in patients who remain immunosuppressed, but most ophthalmologists discontinue therapy in ART-treated patients if the CD4 count increases above 200 cells/mm^3 [30].

Over 75% of those affected with cryptococcal disease have a CD4 count of < 50 cells/mm^3. The most common presentation is chronic meningitis, with headache, nausea, and photophobia. Mass lesions (cryptococcomas) can cause focal neurologic deficits. Cryptococcal meningitis is the most common cause of papilledema in patients with AIDS, although it is seen in less than 10% of affected patients [31]. Ocular manifestations include sixth nerve palsies, decreased peripheral vision, and loss of central vision. A small subset of patients can develop sudden, severe, bilateral vision loss, with or without papilledema, presumably due to perineuritic adhesive arachnoiditis [32]. Metastatic choroidal lesions, similar to those seen in TB, may be present (Fig. 16.4).

Progressive multifocal leukoencephalopathy (PML) is a demyelinating disease caused by the polyoma JC virus and occurs in patients with profound immunosuppression from AIDS or iatrogenic immunosuppression [33]. In the pre-ART era, PML was a terminal diagnosis [34], but immune recovery from ART can result in substantial improvement. Ocular manifestations include retrochiasmal visual field defects, occipital blindness, and nuclear and supranuclear palsies. A high index of suspicion is necessary to make the diagnosis, as the remainder of the ocular examination may be unremarkable.

Other causes of neuro-ophthalmic disorders include tuberculous meningitis, AIDS-related dementia complex, intracranial zoster, and CNS lymphoma. The incidence is greater in developing countries [35]. Ocular non-Hodgkins's lymphoma (NHL) is much less common than CNS disease but can occur within the retina, choroid, or orbit.

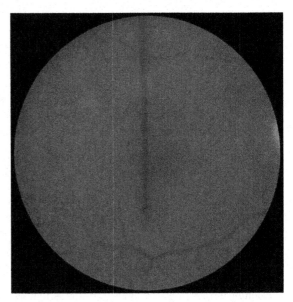

Figure 16.4 Cryptococcal choroiditis. The patient had concurrent meningitis.

Choroidal involvement is associated with systemic NHL, whereas retinal involvement is more commonly associated with CNS lymphoma and may mimic the necrotizing retinitis caused by CMV, toxoplasmosis, or syphilis.

The effect of direct HIV infection in neuro-ophthalmic disease is less well established. Although primary HIV infection can cause neurologic disease, optic neuropathy directly attributed to HIV is uncommon [36]. Patients with AIDS show a decrease in optic nerve axons, even in the absence of visual signs or symptoms. Reversal of optic neuropathy has been successful in some patients after initiation of ART. Furthermore, 10–15% of patients with AIDS but without ocular opportunistic infections will have a presumed neuroretinal disorder (HIV-NRD), manifested by reduced contrast sensitivity and abnormal visual fields [37]. Proposed mechanisms include direct infection of neural tissue, indirect damage due to immune reaction against HIV infection, and HIV microangiopathy-related cumulative damage to the optic nerve and retina.

CNS disease may paradoxically worsen after initiation of ART due to the immune recovery inflammatory syndrome in virtually all of these conditions. The exact pathophysiology, primary risk factors, and appropriate treatment remain uncertain, although systemic corticosteroids are often used [10].

NEOPLASTIC DISORDERS

Guech-Ongey et al. have identified three eye cancers that are significantly more common in patients with HIV/AIDS in the United States: conjunctival squamous cell carcinoma (SCC), primary ocular lymphoma, and Kaposi's sarcoma [38]. While the overall incidence is low (73 eye cancers among nearly half a million patients with HIV/AIDS in the US Cancer Match Registry Study from 1980 to 2004), the standardized incidence ratios per 100,000 population for the three cancers were 12.2, 21.7, and 109, respectively.

Kaposis sarcoma is the most common ocular neoplasm in patients with HIV/AIDS; however, the incidence has decreased markedly in the era of ART [39]. The causative agent is human herpesvirus type 8, which is sensitive to ganciclovir [40]. Lesions are usually found in the inferior conjunctival fornix, mimicking a subconjunctival hemorrhage, or less often on the eyelid, where they appear as raised, purple nodules. There is no intraocular spread and vision is not affected. As with many viral eye diseases, ART is the most effective definitive therapy. Lid lesions requiring more acute intervention because of entropion or trichiasis may respond to intralesional or systemic chemotherapy, cryotherapy, surgical debulking, or radiation, but this is not usually necessary.

Traditional risk factors for conjunctival SCC include age >50 years, Hispanic race, and residence in regions with high-solar ultraviolet radiation, but AIDS patients tend to be younger and more commonly female [41]. There is a strong association of SCC with human papillomavirus, but not all conjunctival tumors demonstrate presence of HPV [42]. Clinical features include a gelatinous or scaly lesion overlapping the limbus with extension onto the cornea of one eye only; leukoplakia is common. Treatment involves wide excision with freeze–thaw cryotherapy to the adjacent margins. The resulting epithelial defect may be left to heal by secondary intention, or more commonly is covered by an amniotic membrane graft or conjunctival autograft. Topical antimetabolites such as mitomycin-C, cidofovir, interferon-α, or 5-flurouracil are usually given postoperatively, but the recurrence rate is high. The disease can be fatal if it metastasizes to regional or distant lymph nodes or spreads intracranially.

DRUG-INDUCED OCULAR COMPLICATIONS

Several drugs used in the treatment of HIV-related eye disease can cause ocular side effects. The most well known is ethambutol, which can cause a dose-related optic neuropathy with decreased color vision and central or centrocecal scotomata. Patients with renal failure or taking doses of more than 15 mg/kg/day are at greatest risk.

Rifabutin can cause acute anterior uveitis, particularly when taken in high doses (600 mg per day) or concurrently with other drugs such as clarithromycin or ethambutol that may affect metabolic clearance of rifabutin [43]. The pathophysiology remains unclear. Manifestations include unilateral or bilateral acute uveitis with or without hypopyon, mimicking HLA-B27-associated uveitis or endophthalmitis. Treatment is aggressive topical corticosteroid therapy and cessation of rifabutin therapy. Retinal vasculitis has also been reported [44]. Less commonly, asymptomatic peripheral corneal endothelial deposits may occur, for which treatment is not necessary.

Cidofovir, now used most commonly to treat ganciclovir- and foscarnet-resistant CMV retinitis, can cause acute anterior uveitis, often with hypotony and extensive posterior synechiae formation [45]. Onset usually occurs after the patient has received 3–5 doses of the medication. The risk is increased in patients taking other nephrotoxic medications and irreversible hypotony may develop if cidofovir therapy is continued. Cessation of the drug and treatment with topical corticosteroids is usually effective. Subsequent resumption of cidofovir should be undertaken with great caution and only if no other treatment options for CMV retinitis are available.

Ritonavir was recently linked with a developed retinal pigment epitheliopathy, macular telangiectasis, and intra-retinal crystalline deposits [46]. The three patients reported all had CD4 counts >100 cells/mm^3.

Interferon-α can cause an ischemic retinopathy with cotton-wool spots, retinal hemorrhages, arteriolar hemorrhages, and capillary non-perfusion. Cystoid macular edema has also been reported. In one study, 35% of patients co-infected with HCV and HIV developed intraocular pathology [47].

FUTURE DIRECTIONS

Clearly, the most important intervention that can be undertaken both to prevent and to treat the ocular complications of HIV/AIDS is the initiation and maintenance of ART. Immune recovery inflammatory syndrome (IRIS) is a broad term for the paradoxical exacerbation of inflammation in immunosuppressed patients with a variety of pathogens and who are treated with ART. The most well-known ocular manifestation is immune recovery uveitis in patients with CMV retinitis [17]. Identification of patients at risk for IRU and improvement in the treatment of this disorder remain a high priority for ophthalmologists managing patients with AIDS. Nonetheless, the overwhelming benefits in terms of reduced incidence of disease, better outcomes in patients with ocular manifestations, enhanced quality of life, and reduced cost would appear to far outweigh the risks of IRU.

Rapid diagnosis of intraocular infections is critical for initiation of the most directed therapy. The utility of PCR testing appears greatest for viral infections, but is less useful for bacterial and protozoal infections, in which the more cumbersome intraocular antibody analysis may be more sensitive [48]. Development of multiplex PCR testing for all common ocular pathogens will enhance diagnostic speed and accuracy.

Among the promising new areas of research is the field of genomics. In recent years, host genetic factors have been identified that indicate different haplotypes can either increase or decrease the risk of CMV retinitis as a result of how they modulate host immune reactions through an IL-10 receptor mediated immune-suppression pathway [49]. Similarly, variants in the IL-10-related pathway and chemokine receptor ligand polymorphisms in RANTES may alter the risk of developing a neuroretinal dysfunction that results in reduced contrast sensitivity, abnormal visual fields, and impaired reading speed [37]. Another study by Hendrickson et al. found that, among HIV-infected patients of western European descent who carried the mitochondrial haplogroup J, there was an 80% decrease in this neuroretinal disorder compared to matched patients without haplogroup J [50].

Finally, ongoing epidemiological studies such as the Longitudinal Studies of the Ocular Complications of AIDS (LSOCA) hope to determine whether disorders such as cataracts are more common in patients with AIDS independent of CMV retinitis and whether careful evaluation of the retinal vasculature may help clinicians identify those patients at greatest risk for development of dyslipidemia syndromes associated with ART.

CONCLUSION

The incidence of ocular complications in patients with HIV/AIDS has declined significantly since the widespread usage of ART. Non-infectious retinal microvasculopathy remains the most common ocular manifestation and CMV retinitis the most common ocular opportunistic infection. Many virally mediated ocular diseases are responsive to ART alone. Although initial specific therapy (e.g. in CMV retinitis) is still indicated because of enhanced ocular and systemic outcomes, ongoing immune recovery frequently allows discontinuation of these specific therapies, resulting in decreased morbidity and medical care costs. Identifying and treating patients who develop ocular complications as a result of intolerance, poor adherence, or lack of access to ART remains a priority. For patients who experience immune recovery, emphasis by ophthalmologists is gradually shifting toward surveillance of treated disorders and monitoring for other chronic eye diseases such as cataracts and diabetic retinopathy.

REFERENCES

[1] Mahadevia PJ, Gebo KA, Pettit K, et al. The epidemiology, treatment patterns, and costs of cytomegalovirus retinitis in the post-HAART era among a national managed-care population. J Acquir Immune Defic Syndr 2004;36:972–7.

[2] Jabs DA. Ocular manifestations of HIV infection. Trans Am Ophthalmol Soc 1995;93:623–83.

[3] Kuppermann BD, Petty JG, Richman DD, et al. Correlation between CD4+ counts and prevalence of cytomegalovirus retinitis and human immunodeficiency virus-related noninfectious retinal vasculopathy. Am J Ophthalmol 1993;115:575–82.

[4] Falkenstein IA, Bartsch DU, Azen SP, et al. Multifocal electroretinography in HIV-positive patients without infectious retinitis. Am J Ophthalmol 2008;146:579–88.

[5] Lai TY, Wong RL, Luk FO, et al. Ophthalmic manifestations and risk factors for mortality of HIV patients in the post-highly active anti-retroviral therapy era. Clin Experiment Ophthalmol 2011;39:99–104.

[6] Dunn JP, Yamashita A, Kempen JH, Jabs DA. Retinal vascular occlusion in patients infected with human immunodeficiency virus. Retina 2005;25:759–66.

[7] Sellitti TP, Huang AJ, Schiffman J, Davis JL. Association of herpes zoster ophthalmicus with acquired immunodeficiency syndrome and acute retinal necrosis. Am J Ophthalmol 1993;116:297–301.

[8] Jeng BH, Holland GN, Lowder CY, et al. Anterior segment and external ocular diseases associated with human immunodeficiency virus disease. Surv Ophthalmol 2007;52:329–68.

[9] Charles NC, Friedberg DN. Epibulbar molluscum contagiosum in acquired immune deficiency syndrome. Case report and review of the literature. Ophthalmology 1992;99:1123–6.

[10] Dhasmana DJ, Dheda K, Ravn P, et al. Immune reconstitution inflammatory syndrome in HIV-infected patients receiving antiretroviral therapy: pathogenesis, clinical manifestations and management. Drugs 2008;68:191–208.

[11] Hodge WG, Margolis TP. Herpes simplex virus keratitis among patients who are positive or negative for human immunodeficiency virus: an epidemiologic study. Ophthalmology 1997;104:120–4.

[12] Rossi P, Urbani C, Donelli G, Pozio E. Resolution of microsporidial sinusitis and keratoconjunctivitis by intraconazole treatment. Am J Ophthalmol 1999; 127:210–2.

[13] Kahraman G, Krepler K, Franz C, et al. Seven years of HAART impact on ophthalmic management of HIV-infected patients. Ocul Immunol Inflamm 2005;13:213–18.

[14] Ghosheh FR, Ehlers JP, Ayres BD, et al. Corneal ulcers associated with aerosolized crack cocaine use. Cornea 2007;26:966–99.

[15] Pathanapitoon K, Riemens A, Kongyai N, et al. Intraocular and plasma HIV-1 RNA loads and HIV uveitis. AIDS 2011;25:81–6.

[16] Jabs DA, Martin BK, Forman MS. Cytomegalovirus Retinitis and Viral Resistance Study. Mortality associated with resistant cytomegalovirus among patients with cytomegalovirus retinitis and AIDS. Ophthalmology 2010;117:128–32.

[17] Goldberg DE, Smithen LM, Angelilli A, Freeman WR. HIV-associated retinopathy in the HAART era. Retina 2005;25:633–49.

[18] Thorne JE, Van Natta ML, Jabs DA, et al. Visual field loss in patients with cytomegalovirus retinitis. Ophthalmology 2011;118:895–901.

[19] Holland GN, Vaudaux JD, Shiramizu KM, et al. Characteristics of untreated AIDS-related cytomegalovirus retinitis. II. Findings in the era of highly active antiretroviral therapy (1997–2000). Am J Ophthalmol 2008;145:12–22.

[20] Jabs DA, Ahuja A, Van Natta M, et al. Course of cytomegalovirus retinitis in the era of highly active antiretroviral therapy: five-year outcomes. Ophthalmology 2010;117:2152–61.

[21] Thorne JE, Jabs DA, Kempen JH, et al. Incidence of and risk factor for visual acuity loss among patients with AIDS and cytomegaloviral retinitis in the era of highly active antiretroviral therapy. Ophthalmology 2006;113:1432–40.

[22] Engstrom RJ, Holland GN, Margolis TP, et al. The progressive outer retinal necrosis syndrome. A variant of necrotizing herpetic retinopathy in patients with AIDS. Ophthalmology 1994;101:1488–502.

[23] Scott IU, Luu KM, Davis JL. Intravitreal antivirals in the management of patients with acquired immunodeficiency syndrome with progressive outer retinal necrosis. Arch Ophthalmol 2002;120:1219–22.

[24] Holland GN, Engstrom RJ, Glasgow BJ, et al. Ocular toxoplasmosis in patients with the acquired immunodeficiency syndrome. Am J Ophthalmol 1988;106:653–7.

[25] Browning DJ. Posterior segment manifestations of active ocular syphilis, their response to a neurosyphilis regimen of penicillin therapy, and the influence of human immunodeficiency virus status on response. Ophthalmology 2000;107:2015–23.

[26] Hodge WG, Seiff SR, Margolis TP. Ocular opportunistic infection incidences among patients who are HIV positive compared to patients who are HIV negative. Ophthalmology 1998;105:895–900.

[27] Wroblewski KJ, Hidayat AA, et al. Ocular tuberculosis: a clinicopathologic and molecular study. Ophthalmology 2011;118:772–7.

[28] Sacktor N, Lyles RH, Skolasky R, et al. HIV-associated neurologic diseases incidence changes: Multicenter AIDS Cohort Study, 1990–1998. Neurology 2001;56:257–60.

[29] Dromer F, Mathoulin-Pelissier S, Fontanet A, et al. Epidemiology of HIV-associated cryptococcosis in France (1985–2001): comparison of the pre- and post-HAART era. AIDS 2004;18:555–62.

[30] Holland GN, Lewis KG. An update on current practices in the management of ocular toxoplasmosis. Am J Ophthalmol 2002;134:102–14.

[31] Chuck SL, Sande MA. Infections with Cryptococcus neoformans in the acquired immunodeficiency syndrome. N Engl J Med 1989;321:794–9.

[32] Lipson BK, Freeman WR, Beniz J, et al. Optic neuropathy associated with cryptococcal arachnoiditis in AIDS patients. Am J Ophthalmol 1989;107:523–7.

[33] White MK, Khalili K. Pathogenesis of progressive multifocal leukoencephalopathy—revisited. J Infect Dis 2011;203:578–86.

[34] Ormerod LD, Rhodes RH, Gross SA, et al. Ophthalmologic manifestations of acquired immune deficiency-associated progressive multifocal leukoencephalopathy. Ophthalmology 1996;103:899–906.

[35] Mwanza J-C, Nyambo LK, Tylleskar T, Plant GT.

[   ] Neuro-ophthalmological disorders in HIV infected subjects with neurological manifesations. Br J Ophthalmol 2004;88:1455–9.

[36] Goldsmith P, Jones RE, Ozuzu GE, et al. Optic neuropathy as the presenting feature of HIV infection: recovery of vision with highly active antiretroviral therapy. Br J Ophthalmol 2000;84:551–3.

[37] Sezgin E, Hendrickson SL, Jabs DA, et al. Effect of host genetics on incidence of HIV neuroretinal disorder in patients with AIDS. J Acquir Immune Defic Syndr 2010;54:343–51.

[38] Guech-Ongey M, Engels EA, Goedert JJ, et al. Elevated risk for squamous cell carcinoma of the conjunctiva among adults with AIDS in the United States. Int J Cancer 2008;122:2590–3.

[39] Goedert JJ. The epidemiology of acquired immunodeficiency syndrome malignancies. Semin Oncol 2000;27:390–401.

[40] Martin DG, Kuppermann BD, Wolitz RA, et al. Oral ganciclovir for patients with cytomegalovirus retinitis treated with a ganciclovir implant. Roche Ganciclovir Study Group. N Engl J Med 1999;340:1063–70.

[41] Gichuhi S, Irlam JH. Intervention for squamous cell carcinoma of the conjunctiva in HIV-infected individuals (Review). Cochrane Database Syst Rev 2007;(2): CD005643.

[42] Lewallen S, Shroyer DR, Keyser RB, et al. Aggressive conjunctival squamous cell carcinoma in three young Africans. Arch Ophthalmol 1996;114:215–18.

[43] Shafran SD, Singer J, Zarowny DP, et al. Determinants of rifabutin-associated uveitis in patients treated with rifabutin, clarithromycin, and ethambutol for Mycobacterium avium complex bacteremia: a multivariate analysis. Canadian HIV Trials Network Protocol 010 Study Group. J Infect Dis 1998;177:252–5.

[44] Skolik S, Willermain F, Caspers LE. Rifabutin-associated panuveitis with retinal vasculitis in pulmonary tuberculosis. Ocul Immunol Inflamm 2005;13: 483–5.

[45] Aker ME, Johnson DW, Burman WJ, et al. Anterior uveitis and hypotony after intravenous cidofovir for the treatment of cytomegalovirus retinitis. Ophthalmology 1998;105:651–7.

[46] Roe RH, Jumper JM, Gualino V, et al. Retinal pigment epitheliopathy, macular telangiectasis, and intraretinal crystalline deposits in HIV-positive patients receiving ritonavir. Retina 2011;31:559–65.

[47] Farel C, Suzman DL, McLaughlin M, et al. Serious ophthalmic pathology compromising vision in HCV/HIV co-infected patients treated with peginterferon alpha-2b and ribavirin. AIDS 2004;18: 1805–9.

[48] Westeneng AC, Rothova A, de Boer JH, de Groot-Mijnes JD. Infectious uveitis in immunocompromised patients and the diagnostic value of polymerase chain reaction and Goldmann-Witmer coefficient in aqueous

analysis. Am J Ophthalmol 2007;144:781–5.

[49] Sezgin E, Jabs DA, Hendrickson SL, et al. Effect of host genetics on the development of cytomegalovirus retinitis in patients with AIDS. J Infect Dis 2010;202:606–13.

[50] Hendrickson SL, Jabs DA, Van Natta M, et al. Mitochondrial haplogroups are associated with risk of neuroretinal disorder in HIV-positive patients. J Acquir Immune Defic Syndr 2010;53:451–5.

Chapter 17

Global HIV and dermatology

Toby Maurer, Robert Michelleti

SKIN DISEASE IN HIV

HIV-infected patients carry a heavy burden of cutaneous illness. As many as 90% have at least one skin disease; most have several [1, 2]. Mucocutaneous diseases in HIV patients are a significant source of morbidity. They can cause chronic itching or pain, lead to secondary superinfection, or reflect the presence of a life-threatening malignancy or invasive infection.

Importantly, skin disease is also a clinical marker of immunosuppression. Many conditions are seen preferentially in those with low CD4 counts, while a high number of skin diseases correlate with low CD4 and worse prognosis [3, 4]. Skin conditions in HIV-infected patients may occur as a manifestation of HIV itself, an opportunistic infection, a neoplastic process, a primary dermatologic condition, a drug reaction, or as part of the immune reconstitution inflammatory syndrome. Appropriate recognition and treatment of these conditions is vital to the care of patients with HIV.

PRIMARY HIV

Acute retroviral syndrome (ARS) or primary HIV infection may be the presenting sign in 40–90% of patients. It is often asymptomatic and non-specific. ARS consists of a mononucleosis-like illness with fever, lymphadenopathy, pharyngitis, and neurologic symptoms. The skin rash may be recognized in about half of symptomatic patients and typically is a non-specific maculopapular exanthem [5, 6]. Oral and genital ulcers may also occur, as may infiltrated plaques on the chest and back [7, 8]. There should be a high index of suspicion for HIV infection in patients

presenting with these symptoms [9]. Patients with primary HIV infection may be highly infectious because of the presence of a high viral burden in blood and genital secretions [10]. Confirmation of ARS can be made by finding positive plasma HIV RNA and negative HIV antibody [11]. Treatment with ART early in this phase may decrease the severity of the disease, alter the initial viral set point, and reduce the rate of viral replication. However, therapy may cause drug toxicities and potential resistance if it fails [8]. Studies to determine the optimal time to start therapy are ongoing.

PIGMENTATION

HIV infection is associated with pigment disorders, both hyperpigmentation and hypopigmentation. Hyperpigmentation has been reported in HIV-infected persons with background pigment. Advanced HIV infection and immunosuppression has also been associated with more diffuse hyperpigmentation. In a Chinese HIV-infected population in Malaysia, hyperpigmentation was the most common skin disorder, representing 36% of the whole group studied, while 47% of an Indian population in a separate study were affected [4, 12]. Pigmentation is most commonly seen in sun-exposed areas but becomes more diffuse over the body. Photodistributed hyperpigmentation has been noted with CD4 counts < 100 cells/mm^3 and may be the presenting sign of HIV infection [13]. Gray coloration of the nails and pigmented oral mucosa may be other markers of more advanced stages of immunosuppression with CD4 counts < 200 cells/mm^3 [14, 15]. Cutaneous hyperpigmentation has also been linked with eczematous features, in both the acute and chronic forms [16].

Several reasons for hyperpigmentation have been postulated [17]. Medications used for the treatment and prophylaxis of AIDS-related conditions can cause photosensitivity [18]. These drugs include trimethoprim-sulfamethoxazole, azithromycin, dapsone, ketoconazole, and anti-tuberculosis drugs. Antiretroviral medications like indinavir, saquinavir, and efavirenz have been associated with photosensitivity [19]. Zidovudine (AZT) may result in the hyperpigmentation of the nails, oral mucosa, and skin and appears to be related to increased melanogenesis and not to drug deposition or photosensitivity [20]. Concomitant diseases in HIV-infected individuals, such as *Porphyria cutanea tarda*, which causes photosensitivity, and *Mycobacteria avium intracellulare*, which can affect the adrenal glands and cause adrenal suppression, can eventuate in hyperpigmentation [21]. Sunscreen (SPF15 or higher) and avoidance of sun exposure can improve symptoms.

Pigmented oral lesions are not uncommon, particularly in India and Africa [22]. Similar oral lesions are noted in Caucasians with HIV infection who have not been on any medications.

Hypopigmentation in HIV infection in the form of vitiligo has been reported. Vitiligo has been considered to be an autoimmune disorder like alopecia areata, possibly reflecting concomitant B-cell dysfunction in HIV infection, though the mechanism is poorly understood. Both the onset and resolution of vitiligo have been reported in persons with increasing CD4 cell counts on antiretroviral therapy (ART) [23, 24].

ITCHING

Itching is a common complaint among HIV-infected patients. Pruritus without a rash is less common than originally thought and can be associated with concomitant systemic diseases like hepatitis C, chronic renal failure, lymphomas, and methamphetamine use. When a pruritic dermatitis is noted, a careful history and physical examination usually reveals a primary dermatologic condition for which standard treatment for the underlying condition can proceed. Included in this heterogeneous group of diseases are xerosis, eczema, seborrheic dermatitis, psoriasis, *Staphylococcal aureus* folliculitis, eosinophilic folliculitis, prurigo nodularis, pruritic papular eruption (PPE) of HIV, arthropod assaults, scabies, and drug rashes. Biopsy and cultures of lesions can be helpful in distinguishing these conditions [16].

As early as 1983, reports from sub-Saharan Africa, Haiti, Brazil, and Thailand described an eruption of intensely pruritic papules and nodules that begins on the extensor surfaces of the extremities and subsequently involves the trunk and face [25–28]. Called the pruritic papular eruption of HIV, these lesions have not been reported in Europe or America but are exceedingly common in the tropics, affecting 11–46% of HIV-infected patients in those regions. When present, PPE is highly predictive of HIV infection

and in fact is often the presenting sign [29, 30]. A marker of more advanced immunosuppression, it may improve dramatically with effective ART [31]. Biopsy findings include a mild to moderate dermal perivascular and periadnexal infiltrate. Early lesions biopsied in Uganda have revealed histology consistent with arthropod bites [32]. It has been hypothesized that this condition represents an altered and hyperactive immune response to arthropod bites [33, 34]. Cytokine profiles of individuals with PPE show lower levels of interleukin-2 and γ-interferon, arguing for a dysregulated immune system [35]. In addition to immune reconstitution, potent topical steroids, antihistamines, and ultraviolet light may bring symptomatic relief [36–39]. Eosinophilic folliculitis (EF) has been reported in Southeast Asia, Africa, India, Europe, and North America [16, 22, 40, 41]. This disease presents with pruritic urticarial papules and nodules on the scalp, neck, face, upper chest, and back and is therefore differentiated clinically from PPE. It is usually associated with a nadir CD4 count < 100 cells/mm^3 and a current CD4 count < 200 cells/mm^3. This condition can also be seen in individuals starting ART as part of an immune reconstitution syndrome [42]. Clinicians should be aware of this possibility and should not confuse the eruption with a medication reaction or stop therapy. The pathogenesis of EF remains elusive [43]; however, it presumably involves an enhanced Th2 response with elevated interleukin-4, interleukin-5, and chemokine recruitment of eosinophils [44]. Histologically, there is a predominant perifollicular infiltrate of eosinophils [38, 45]. Biopsy of lesions can differentiate this condition from other pruritic disorders. Treatment [46] options include waiting out the immune reconstitution period (the first 12 weeks of ART), potent topical steroids and antihistamines, itraconazole, UVB therapy, and isotretinoin [47].

Prurigo nodularis has been reported globally and is characterized by pruritic dome-shaped nodules initially presenting on the photoexposed areas of the extremities and eventually involving the trunk [16]. These nodules are bilateral and symmetric and appear in persons with background pigment, usually with CD4 counts < 100 cells/mm^3. The incessant rubbing and scratching of these lesions can lead to lichenification of the skin as well as pigment change, both hyper- and hypopigmentation. A search for an underlying, treatable condition like scabies or eczema is warranted [48, 49]. Immune reconstitution and reduction of viremia with ART are helpful. Regimens that include raltegravir may be particularly useful in refractory cases [50]. Potent topical steroids and antihistamines are of benefit. Ultraviolet light and thalidomide have been somewhat helpful when other therapies have failed [51].

Scabies is noted globally and usually presents with pruritic papules with accentuation in the intertriginous areas, genitalia, and fingerwebs [48, 49]. With advancing immunosuppression, the infestation may become more widespread and refractory to treatment [52]. Crusted scabies may also occur with advanced HIV and presents with thick crusts that are non-pruritic and teeming with mites [53]. Outbreaks of scabies in institutional settings like orphanages, hospitals, and hospices are particularly challenging [54]. Topical treatment of scabies is with benzyl benzoate 10%, sulfiram 2% (in Europe), or permethrin 5% cream (available in the USA and UK). Gamma-benzene hexachloride (lindane) is contraindicated in HIV, as it has been associated with the development of peripheral neuropathies. Oral ivermectin can also be used for treatment of scabies in an institution or for crusted scabies. Treatment of contacts and proper cleaning of garments and linens is essential in treatment and infection control, particularly in institutional settings [55, 56]. The risk of secondary staphylococcal and streptococcal infection of scabietic lesions is high in tropical environments, so antibacterial therapy should also be used when necessary [57–59].

STAPHYLOCOCCAL AUREUS SKIN INFECTIONS

Staphylococcus aureus is the most common cutaneous bacterial infection in patients with HIV disease [60]. Community-acquired infections of subcutaneous and deep tissues are common throughout the world [61]. In the Caribbean Islands and Africa, bacterial infection in HIV represent up to 40% of all skin diseases as either primary infection or secondary superinfection of eczema or scabies [62].

Rates of *S. aureus* carriage are high, and persistent colonization among HIV-infected patients is common. These factors increase the risk of soft tissue infections [63–65]. *Staphylococcus aureus* in the skin can manifest in many ways, including bullous impetigo, ecthyma, folliculitis, abscesses, and furuncles. Occasionally, infected follicles coalesce to form violaceous plaques that may be studded with pustules. Rarely, abscesses of the muscle (pyomyositis) as well as deep tissue involvement in the form of necrotizing fasciitis may occur.

Over the past decade, HIV-infected patients have shown a high and growing rate of soft tissue infection with methicillin-resistant *S. aureus* (MRSA). In Cook County, Illinois, the incidence of MRSA infection among HIV-infected patients was six times higher than among HIV-uninfected patients, while between 2000–2003 and 2004–2007, the incidence of MRSA among HIV patients increased 3.6-fold [66]. Risk factors for the development of MRSA in HIV include low CD4 counts, recent hospitalization or antibiotic exposure, high-risk sexual practices, intravenous drug use, and environmental exposures [67, 68]. Some studies suggest the widespread use of trimethoprim-sulfamethoxazole prophylaxis may increase rates of *S. aureus* resistance to that medication [69]; however, this does not always appear to be the case [70].

Knowing the organism and its sensitivities is imperative where at all possible. Otherwise, local resistance patterns should guide empiric therapy. Increasing resistance to β-lactam drugs and fluoroquinolones has been reported. Erythromycin, clindamycin, sulfamethoxazole, gentamicin, and intravenous vancomycin are still used. Tetracycline drugs are being used with more frequency [71]. Linezolid is an expensive alternative and should be reserved for cases in which there is documented resistance to the abovementioned antibiotics [72]. Incision and drainage of abscesses is critical. Hibiclens and Betadine washes may have a role but can often dry out the skin, leading to eczematous eruptions prone to secondary bacterial infections. Mupirocin ointment reduces carriage rates in HIV but does not decrease infection rates and there is concern for emerging mupirocin resistance [73, 74]. Rifampin can be used in combination with other antibiotics to reduce carriage rates of *S. aureus*. It acts synergistically with other antibiotics but cannot be used with many of the antiretroviral medications, particularly the protease inhibitors, because of drug–drug interactions [75]. In Mali, an algorithm for treatment of skin diseases was developed. Patients were first evaluated for signs of pyoderma by looking for presence of yellow crusts, pus, sores, or blisters. Depending on the degree of pyoderma, patients were treated with topical antiseptics or oral antibiotics and returned for a follow-up visit. Abscesses were incised and drained and not treated with antibiotics. The use of this algorithm correctly identified pyodermas and secondarily infected eczemas 96–98% of the time and decreased the use of steroids and antifungals [48].

BACILLARY ANGIOMATOSIS

Bacillary angiomatosis (BA), a treatable opportunistic infection, can present with vascular, easily friable papules or subcutaneous nodules in patients with advanced HIV disease. The agents causing this infection have been classified as *Bartonella*, and at least 15 species have been identified worldwide in association with various vectors [22, 76]. Cutaneous manifestations of BA in the HIV-infected population are primarily caused by two species, *Bartonella henselae* and *Bartonella quintana* [77, 78]. Epidemiologically, *B. henselae* has been associated with cat and flea exposure. *B. quintana* has been associated with low income, homelessness, and exposure to lice [79]. BA has been reported in North and South America, Europe, India, and Africa [76, 80–84]. Studies from multiple regions have shown that the seroprevalence among HIV-infected patients is high [85–87]. In countries where Kaposi's sarcoma (KS) is prevalent, BA may be under-recognized, as it can mimic the vascular lesions typically associated with KS. Diagnostic accuracy is important because the response of BA to prompt antibiotic therapy can be excellent, whereas the prognosis of untreated, disseminated BA or KS is more guarded. Lesions of BA may also be confused with pyogenic granuloma and lymphoma [88].

Bacillary angiomatosis initially was considered a disorder of the skin, but systemic involvement is common. Visceral disease may present as osseous lesions, hepatic and splenic tumors, lymph node disease, pulmonary lesions, brain lesions, bone marrow, and widespread fatal systemic involvement. Bacillary angiomatosis can present with unexplained fever, bacteremia, or endocarditis in HIV-infected patients [89]. Lesions should be biopsied and examined with hematoxylin and eosin staining and Warthin–Starry silver staining, which reveals the organisms. Culture, indirect fluorescent antibody testing, and polymerase chain reaction can be performed on lesions and serum. Immunohistochemical staining for anti-HHV8 can be used to differentiate KS from BA [90].

Treatment with erythromycin or doxycycline for at least 3 months is recommended even though cutaneous lesions resolve in 3–4 weeks. Relapses can occur if treatment is not continued appropriately. Severely ill patients should be treated with i.v. doxycycline with either gentamicin or rifampin for at least 4 months.

CANCRUM ORIS

Noma, or cancrum oris, is an infectious disease that starts as necrotizing ulcerative gingivitis, progresses with tumefaction, and destroys adjacent structures around and deep to the area [91]. It occurs in countries where there is extreme poverty, malnutrition, and HIV, particularly in sub-Saharan Africa [92]. It tends to occur in children and young adults (2–16) [93]. Local debridement and antibiotics are established treatments, but in the absence of timely therapy, mortality is high [94].

SYPHILIS

Worldwide, there has been a dramatic increase in the reported number of cases of syphilis in recent years [95–99]. The majority of cases in large urban settings have been in men, particularly men having sex with men [100, 101]. In Europe and the USA, the overall proportion of syphilis patients co-infected with HIV is 50% [102]. Over 70% of these co-infected patients were already aware of their HIV infection at the time that they were diagnosed with syphilis [98, 103–106]. Methamphetamine use has been implicated in the rising incidence of syphilis in the USA and Europe, particularly with cases of re-infection of syphilis [107, 108]. Among women with syphilis and HIV, sex work, limited or no use of condoms, and alcohol and drug use were found to be risk factors [95, 98]. Screening of syphilis, even in asymptomatic HIV-infected patients, is recommended [109, 110].

Primary and secondary cutaneous presentations of syphilis are similar in HIV- and non-HIV-infected individuals [111]. Lesions include chancres, sometimes with rapid evolution to secondary stages, papulosquamous lesions on the trunk and palmar/plantar regions, patchy alopecia, and osteochondritis of the sternal region [112–114]. Uveitis with or without rash is another common manifestation [115]. Oral lesions are also common [22]. Tertiary cutaneous lesions are characterized by verrucous or hyperkeratotic nodules. Lues maligna has been reported in HIV infection [116]. Skin biopsies or dark field microscopy of cutaneous lesions demonstrates spirochetes and establishes the diagnosis [110]. Negative serologic tests may not be adequate for ruling out secondary syphilis, as HIV infection may delay development of serologic evidence of *Treponema pallidum*. However, for the majority of patients, serologic testing is adequate [117].

Central nervous system (CNS) involvement may manifest early in HIV, and relapse in the CNS may be more common even after standard treatment. Clinicians should carefully follow HIV-infected patients who have been treated with standard therapies for early syphilis. If CNS signs or symptoms develop, clinicians should perform appropriate evaluation for early CNS relapse, including lumbar puncture and VDRL of the cerebrospinal fluid [118]. Lumbar puncture of patients with CD4 < 350 cells/mm^3 and/or rapid plasma reagin (RPR) titer $\geq 1{:}32$ without regard to stage may improve the ability to diagnosis neurosyphilis [119] in asymptomatic patients.

The CDC recommends treating primary and secondary syphilis with 2.4 million units of benzathine penicillin given intramuscularly at a single session. Some specialists recommend benzathine penicillin 2.4 million units intramuscularly, once per week for 2 or 3 weeks. In late latent disease, three doses of benzathine penicillin are recommended 1 week apart. For penicillin-allergic patients, doxycycline and tetracycline are recommended. Erythromycin is not recommended because treatment failures have been noted with azithromycin [120]. Since the relapse rate of neurosyphilis is approximately 17% in patients treated with standard regimens, HIV-infected patients should be evaluated clinically and serologically for treatment failure at 3, 6, 9, 12, and 24 months after therapy. Although of unproven benefit, some specialists recommend a CSF examination 6 months after therapy [117].

Serologic clearance of syphilis appears largely unaffected by HIV status in the "highly active" ART era (91.8% in HIV-infected versus 98.3% in HIV-uninfected, $p = 0.14$) [121]. HIV-infected patients who meet the criteria for treatment failure should be managed in the same manner as HIV-uninfected patients (i.e. a CSF examination and re-treatment). CSF examination and re-treatment also should be strongly considered for patients whose nontreponemal test titers do not decrease fourfold within 6–12 months of therapy. Most specialists would re-treat patients with benzathine penicillin G administered as three doses of 2.4 million units i.m. each at weekly intervals, if CSF examinations are normal [117].

Patients with neurosyphilis should be treated with crystalline penicillin G, 2.4 million units i.v. every 4 hours for at least 10 days [117].

CUTANEOUS TUBERCULOSIS

Cutaneous and intraoral tuberculosis (TB), like pulmonary TB, appear to be more common among HIV-infected patients [122] than in the general population. Lesions have been described most frequently in India, Brazil, Thailand, and Africa [22, 123–127]. Many such cases have been associated with pulmonary disease, but this need not be the case [123]. In several instances, unsuspected pulmonary disease was discovered on chest X-ray and sputum samples after the diagnosis of cutaneous disease was made. This is particularly true of TB in the oral cavity [124]. Lesions present most often as scrofuloderma [125] or the infiltrated plaques of lupus vulgaris. Single or multiple lesions, nodules, or papillomas are also seen such that cutaneous TB can mimic fungal or bacterial infections, KS, neoplastic processes, and herpetic infections and should be considered in the differential diagnosis of those diseases [126]. Disseminated military TB may also mimic the papular pruritic eruption of HIV and should be considered if the eruption fails to improve with antiretrovirals alone. Biopsy and tissue culture confirm the diagnosis [123, 127]. An id reaction in the form of papulonecrotic id has also been described in a patient with immune reconstitution [128, 129].

Mycobacterium avium-intracellulare (MAI) infrequently presents with skin manifestations, although it has been reported to form single or multiple nodules and cervical lymphadenitis in persons whose CD4 counts are < 200 cells/mm^3 [130]. A search for systemic disease should be undertaken with blood cultures and bone marrow aspirates for culture [131]. MAI is seen more frequently in the developed world and has been infrequently reported in Trinidad, Kenya, and other places [132].

LEPROSY

Studies have indicated that HIV infection does not affect the clinical presentation or incidence of leprosy [133]. However, immunosuppression due to HIV infection may cause a relapse of leprosy in persons already treated [134]. Several reports document inflammatory and vasculo-ulcerative reactions of leprosy within 2–6 months after starting ART [135–137]. This is thought to be part of the immune reconstitution syndrome and has been documented particularly in patients whose CD4 counts were < 100 cells/mm^3 when initiating ART. Occasionally, anti-inflammatory medications such as prednisone and thalidomide have been used in addition to leprosy and HIV medications with varying success. While leprosy may worsen during the first few weeks of ART when there is immune reconstitution, lesions improve with appropriate multidrug therapy for leprosy [138].

NOCARDIOSIS

Nocardiosis is a localized infection or disseminated infection caused by an aerobic actinomyces that is geographically distributed worldwide. It has been reported in HIV-infected patients in the USA, Africa, and Thailand [139, 140]. There are fewer reports of *Nocardia* and HIV infection from Europe, although there have been recent reports from Spain and France. *Nocardia* predominantly affects the pulmonary system. Skin is the second most common site of infection and presents as cutaneous or subcutaneous abscesses [141]. Intravenous drug use has been identified as a risk factor in HIV-infected patients. Most HIV-infected patients with *Nocardia* have CD4 cell counts < 200 cells/mm^3, with the majority having a known diagnosis of AIDS at the time of infection [142]. Diagnosis can be made by using a modified acid fast stain on tissue or by culturing tissue, fluid, or blood [142]. The treatment of choice is trimethoprim-sulfamethoxazole, though dual therapy is often used [143]. Sensitivities to cultured material can be done. In a study from Thailand, patients who were resistant to trimethoprim-sulfamethoxazole succumbed to death [139]. Imipenem, amikacin, minocycline, amoxicillin-clavulanic acid, and third-generation cephalosporins have been proposed with unclear outcomes. Where possible, debridement of skin lesions is indicated as adjunctive therapy to antibiotics. Previous studies have reported that most patients respond to therapy in an average of 4 months. Cessation of therapy can be followed by recurrence and progression of disease despite reinitiation of therapy. Some authors have suggested that lifelong therapy should be instituted in the treatment of nocardiosis in HIV co-infected patients, particularly those who have evidence of advanced HIV disease. It is unclear what role ART has in this group of patients.

LEISHMANIA

Leishmania—cutaneous, mucocutaneous, and visceral—has been reported in HIV co-infected persons [144, 145]. This is a protozoan disease transmitted by the sandfly and occurs in HIV-infected patients who live in or have traveled to endemic areas. In Spain and southwest Europe, there is a high prevalence of visceral leishmaniasis (kala-azar) among HIV-infected patients [146, 147]. The absence of an effective TH1 immune response, as seen in HIV infection, increases the risk of progression from asymptomatic disease to visceral leishmaniasis. It may also lead to poor treatment response and frequent relapses [148]. Conversely, leishmania induces more robust HIV replication [149]. Co-infected patients with cutaneous leishmaniasis can present with a few spontaneously healing lesions, diffuse non-healing lesions, mucocutaneous lesions, or localized or diffuse hyperpigmentation. Diagnosis is made by biopsy demonstrating amastigotes in the tissue [145]. Bone marrow can be biopsied in cases of suspected visceral involvement [144]. However, it should be noted that in persons with visceral leishmaniasis, any skin lesion (not only those of leishmania) can harbor amastigotes due to generalized involvement of macrophages [150]. Culture of tissue is standard so that the species of leishmania can be identified and correct therapy can proceed, particularly for *Leishmania braziliensis* and *L. panamensis*, so that the risk of mucocutaneous disease can be reduced [145]. Local therapy can be used for localized lesions and includes cryotherapy and paromycin ointment. Proven therapies include antimonials, pentamidine, amphotericin B, interferon with antimony, and miltefosine [151]. All HIV-infected patients should be carefully monitored after treatment to ensure that treatment was successful and that relapses do not occur.

SUPERFICIAL FUNGAL (DERMATOPHYTE) INFECTIONS

Superficial mycoses are particularly prevalent in developing countries and account for up to 50% of dermatologic disease in HIV-infected patients [152]. It is not clear whether the prevalence among HIV patients is increased compared to the general population, but cutaneous involvement may be more widespread, severe, or atypical [153, 154].

TINEA OF THE SKIN, HAIR, AND NAILS

Clinically, tinea corporis is characterized by well-demarcated, annular, erythematous, scaling plaques with central clearing. The hands, feet, lower trunk, groin, and buttocks are commonly involved. Onychomycosis is characterized by opacification and thickening of the nails. It is quite common among HIV-infected patients despite the use of ART [155]. Tinea can spread to hair-bearing areas, especially on the face and lower legs, presenting like plaques of folliculitis known as Majocchi's granuloma. Direct examination of skin scrapings and culture for identification of species is helpful. The most common causal organism is *Trichophyton rubrum* [156].

Tinea of the palms, soles, and other localized areas of the body can be treated with topical imidazoles or terbinafine. If extensive areas are involved, oral antifungals may be a more effective alternative that can be used for shorter periods of time [157]. For tinea involving hair follicles, oral antifungals are required for approximately one month. For nail infections, oral antifungals are required but should

be used selectively for patients in whom potential benefits outweigh risks. Relapse rates for onychomycosis are high, while transaminitis and drug–drug interactions through the cytochrome P450 system can complicate treatment. Oral terbinafine can be taken daily for 3 months at a dose of 250 mg. Itraconazole can be taken 7 days per month for 3 months at a dose of 400 mg. Griseofulvin requires a 12- to 18-month course; the success rate is lower, but it is the least hepatotoxic. The efficacy and relapse rates of onychomycosis in the HIV-infected population bear further study.

DEEP (SYSTEMIC) FUNGAL INFECTIONS

Invasive or systemic fungal infections reported in HIV include cryptococcosis, histoplasmosis, sporotrichosis, aspergillosis, coccidiomycosis, actinomycosis, phaeohyphomycosis, and chromoblastomycosis.

Cryptococcosis

Approximately 10–15% of patients with HIV disease and cryptococcosis have skin lesions [158]. By definition, these patients have disseminated disease, for which skin lesions may be the only clue. While the prognosis is poor, early disease recognition may be advantageous. Patients presenting with cryptococcosis have CD4 counts under 200. Skin lesions can occur anywhere on the body and present as pearly 2- to 5-mm translucent papules that resemble molluscum. However, unlike molluscum, they present over a short period of time [159]. Large gelatinous plaques with umbilicated areas may also occur. Diagnosis is established by skin biopsy and culture. A systemic work-up should be performed with particular attention to possible CNS disease. Treatment is with systemic antifungals that include amphotericin B, flucytosine, fluconazole, and itraconazole. Maintenance therapy should be continued for life. The role of successful ART therapy is unknown with regard to maintenance therapy.

Histoplasmosis

The incidence of disseminated histoplasmosis is between 5 and 20% in patients with AIDS living in endemic areas [160]. *Histoplasma capsulatum* is endemic to Texas and the Ohio and Mississippi River Valleys in the USA, Mexico, Panama, and South America [161–163]. Histoplasmosis has also been described in Europe and is probably underdiagnosed in Africa. Skin involvement occurs in 10–17% of patients with advanced HIV disease (CD4 <100 cells/mm^3). The cutaneous lesions are not specific and present as erythematous macules, papules, pustules, acneiform lesions, ulcerations, and crusting plaques, mostly on the face and chest [164]. The diagnosis should be suspected in persons living in or coming from endemic areas who present with fever, respiratory symptoms, weight loss, and diarrhea. Most patients have concomitant pulmonary disease [165]. Sepsis, disseminated intravascular coagulopathy, and renal failure can be seen [166]. Histologic analysis of the skin may demonstrate granulomas. Organisms are seen with methamine silver stain. Bone marrow is positive in 75% of cases, and blood culture is positive in 50–70% of cases. Treatment consists of amphotericin B and itraconazole. In those who survive, relapse is common, so lifelong maintenance treatment is required. *Histoplasma duboisii* has been identified on the African continent, both West and Central African countries, and presents most commonly with mucocutaneous lesions in 38–82% of cases. Ulcerated and crusted papules are seen. Cutaneous lesions tend to be papules with ulceration and crusting.

Sporotrichosis

Sporotrichosis has been reported worldwide and is seen with increased incidence among immunosuppressed patients [167]. Sporotrichosis in HIV can disseminate either from local lesions or from asymptomatic pulmonary infections that spread hematogenously to the skin and joints. It can present with widespread cutaneous ulcers and subcutaneous nodules. Disseminated sporotrichosis occurs in patients with CD4 counts < 200 cells/mm³ and in alcoholics. Skin biopsies and cultures establish the diagnosis. Amphotericin B and itraconazole are used for treatment. Potassium iodide solution (SSKI) should not be used in patients with HIV and sporotrichosis because of a lack of efficacy. Lesions may initially worsen when starting ART because of immune reconstitution [168]. Like the other systemic fungal diseases, lifelong therapy is needed to prevent relapses [169].

Aspergillosis

Cutaneous aspergillosis can occur as a primary or secondary infection. The latter is from hematogenous spread or extension from underlying structures. Primary cutaneous aspergillosis is associated with local skin injury (from tape and intravenous catheter sites) and neutropenia [170]. Lesions can appear as erythematous or violaceous indurated papules or plaques with overlying pustules, ulcers, or eschar. Treatment includes local debridement and systemic antifungal therapy with amphotericin B, voriconazole, itraconazole, or caspofungin [171].

PENICILLIUM

Penicillium marneffei is a common fungal infection presenting in HIV co-infected persons in Southeast Asia, particularly Thailand and the Southern part of China. [12, 172, 173] Most common during the rainy season

[174], presenting symptoms include molluscum-like skin lesions, acneiform, and folliculocentric lesions with fever, anemia, and weight loss. Diagnosis can be established by analysis of blood and bone marrow aspirates with Wright stain. Touch smears of tissue as well as biopsies of lymph node and skin can be used to establish a diagnosis. Tissue culture is definitive and reveals a dimorphic fungus. CD4 counts are usually well below 100 in patients presenting with this diagnosis. Mortality is very high for untreated patients. Treatment consists of amphotericin B or itraconazole [172]. An immune reconstitution syndrome has been described in patients with penicilliosis initiation ART [175].

HERPES SIMPLEX VIRUS (HSV) AND VARICELLA-ZOSTER VIRUS (VZV)

Herpes simplex virus and varicella-zoster virus infection are commonly seen in HIV patients worldwide. The presentation is generally typical, with multiple tiny vesicles, punched-out erosions, or crusts. Atypical or extensive ulcerative, vegetative, or tumor-like lesions may also occur [176]. HSV infection leads to increased transmission of HIV, but randomized, controlled trials have failed to show lower HIV transmission among those treated with daily suppressive therapy for HSV [177]. VZV re-activation is 10 times more common in HIV than the general population [178]. Complications such as blindness (when the V1 distribution is affected) and post-herpetic neuralgia can cause significant morbidity.

HUMAN PAPILLOMAVIRUS (HPV)

Cutaneous warts occur more frequently in HIV-infected men and women. They are more extensive and more difficult to treat than warts in immunocompetent patients. Unusual wart types and an epidermodysplasia verruciformis-like syndrome called acquired epidermodysplasia verruciformis have been reported in HIV-infected individuals [179, 180]. The warts themselves rarely cause symptoms unless they are on the soles of the feet and around the fingernails, where they may cause excruciating pain. Due to the frequent presence of high-risk HPV types, there is a risk of malignant transformation. Unfortunately, the advent of ART has not reduced the number or severity of warts, while the incidence of intraoral warts has actually increased [181].

Treatment of warts in HIV patients is the same as for those without HIV and has an approximately 50% success rate. Relapse of warts is especially common. Destructive modes of therapy include liquid nitrogen every 3–6 weeks, salicylic acid, laser, and excision. Immunomodulatory therapy in the form of imiquimod has had less promising results on cutaneous warts. Topical cidofovir has been used but is very expensive to formulate [182].

MALIGNANCIES OF THE SKIN

The incidence of cutaneous malignancies, including basal cell carcinoma, squamous cell cancer, and melanoma, is increased in HIV-infected patients compared to the general population [60, 183–185]. Risk factors for development of these cancers include Caucasian/non-Hispanic race, increasing age, and longer duration of HIV infection, independent of age and history of opportunistic infections. Tumors may develop throughout the range of CD4 counts. This risk remains elevated and unchanged despite ART [186]. The diagnosis of cutaneous malignancies is the same in the HIV-infected patient as in the uninfected patient [187, 188]. Basal cell and squamous cell cancers should be treated in the same manner as non-melanoma skin cancers in the general population. Close follow-up for metastatic squamous cell cancer is recommended because tumor surveillance may be altered in the HIV-infected patient. Similarly, in HIV-infected patients with melanoma, tumors may be more aggressive, independent of CD4 count. ART may maintain the immune and tumor surveillance systems, so ART is suggested for patients with HIV and malignancy, regardless of CD4 count. Close follow-up for recurrent or metastatic tumors is recommended in persons with melanoma and HIV, as there is a higher incidence of metastasis and recurrence.

Kaposi's sarcoma (KS) is frequently seen in patients with AIDS, particularly in Africa. A low-grade vascular tumor associated with human herpesvirus 8, KS typically presents as asymptomatic, flat, violaceous or reddish-brown patches, papules, or plaques favoring the head and neck, palate, upper chest, genitals, thighs, legs, and plantar surfaces. Skin biopsy is necessary to differentiate KS from clinically similar cutaneous conditions such as bacillary angiomatosis, lymphoma, pyogenic granuloma, lichen planus, warts, sarcoid, or even postinflammatory hyperpigmentation. Immune reconstitution with ART is the treatment of choice in early disease. Chemotherapeutic agents for advanced disease are less often available in the developing world. Thus, recognition and confirmation of KS at its earliest stages when ART can be started may be the best hope of controlling disease.

PSORIASIS

Psoriasis in HIV has been reported since the early days of the epidemic [16, 27]. It presents in HIV as in non-HIV-infected persons with large, marginated silvery-scaled plaques. Often, there is nail pitting. Arthritis may be a component of psoriasis, particularly in HIV disease, presenting as a Reiter's-like syndrome [189]. All clinical manifestations of psoriasis occur in HIV patients, but the inverse (flexural), guttate, and erythrodermic forms are seen most often.

Pruritus can be a frequent problem with psoriasis and can lead to significant discomfort and secondary *S. aureus* infections. In KwaZulu-Natal, South Africa, psoriasis affected young black patients and was the most frequent reason for admission to dermatology wards [190].

Psoriasis may appear early in HIV infection and can be exacerbated by declining CD4 count and increasing viral load. Thus, the severity of psoriasis can be a marker for worsening immunosuppression [191]. ART is considered a first-line treatment for moderate-to-severe psoriasis in HIV patients [192]. It has shown efficacy in case reports [193] and in an open-label study of zidovudine [194]. Effective treatment of HIV decreases the inflammatory mediator TNF-α, which is elevated in HIV infection and plays a key role in the pathogenesis of psoriasis. Other first-line treatments of mild-to-moderate psoriasis include topical medications, such as corticosteroids and vitamin D analogs (calcipotriene). Ultraviolet light therapy has shown efficacy without evidence of adverse immunologic effects. Oral retinoids can be used as second-line agents [195]. Immunosuppressants such as cyclosporine, methotrexate, and TNF-α inhibitors have been used to treat psoriasis in HIV patients. There are precautions that need to be taken in the HIV population when considering TNF blockers like underlying TB, hepatitis B, and propensity to leukoencephalitis [192, 196]. To date, there are few long-term data, so these agents should be used cautiously and reserved for severe, refractory cases [197, 198].

SEBORRHEIC DERMATITIS

Seborrheic dermatitis is an inflammatory eruption usually affecting the scalp and central areas of the face, particularly around the eyebrows and nasolabial folds. Early in the AIDS epidemic, the prevalence of this disease ranged from 40 to 80%, whereas in the general population, the prevalence approximated 5% [16, 199]. More recent studies show that the burden of disease in HIV-infected patients remains high [4, 200]. A larger percentage of patients with advanced disease present with seborrheic dermatitis compared to those with early-stage disease. However, seborrheic dermatitis can be seen throughout the disease spectrum. Seborrheic dermatitis has been noted worldwide [201–203]. One study noted that persons on ART had less seborrheic dermatitis than those who were not on ART. As CD4 counts increased on ART, seborrheic dermatitis was reduced by half compared with those not treated with ART [204, 205]. With HIV infection, occasionally seborrheic dermatitis will occur on the center of the chest, axilla, and groin. The scale is usually fine, loose, or waxy on red or pink poorly defined patches. Pruritus is generally mild. In individuals with background pigmentation, seborrheic dermatitis can appear as hypopigmented areas. When seborrheic dermatitis presents in the groin or axilla, it can be intensely red and can present like inverse psoriasis.

This morphology has been termed sebopsoriasis. The etiology of seborrheic dermatitis remains unclear, but it appears that *Malassezia* species (*Pityrosporum ovale*) may play a role [206].

Treatment consists of mild topical steroids (e.g. 1% hydrocortisone ointment) and topical imidazole creams (clotrimazole or ketoconazole) applied together twice daily, which reduce both the inflammatory response and the amount of *P. ovale*. For the scalp, tar, zinc, ketoconazole, or selenium sulfide shampoos can be used. Because seborrheic dermatitis is a chronic condition, maintenance therapy is required, usually consisting of therapy with these agents twice weekly [207].

XEROSIS AND ATOPIC DERMATITIS

Xerosis affects 20–30% of patients with HIV, while a substantial subset are affected by atopic dermatitis or xerotic eczema [208, 209]. These conditions are more commonly seen in those with lower CD4 counts, reflecting a possible immunologic role. HIV infection, particularly advanced disease, is characterized by a TH1/TH2 imbalance [210] that likely exacerbates or predisposes to atopic dermatitis, a Th2-mediated condition [211]. Epidermal barrier dysfunction, a key pathogenetic feature of atopic dermatitis [212], has been demonstrated in HIV-infected patients, even those without clinical xerosis or background atopy. Data suggest Th2 cytokines provoke barrier dysfunction, thereby enabling a cycle of antigen penetration and cutaneous inflammation in Th2-predominant HIV patients [213].

Clinically, atopic dermatitis is characterized by pruritic scaly plaques, particularly in flexural areas. The distribution of atopic dermatitis may differ with ethnicity. In Black Africans, atopic dermatitis involves the extensor surfaces, affecting the elbow and wrist joints. The face is predominantly involved. Treatment for xerosis and atopic dermatitis is the same as in the non-HIV-infected population. Bathing should be minimized, and gentle soaps should be used. Frequent application of emollients is essential. Topical steroids and sedating antihistamines are useful for flares. Initiation of ART leads to resolution of xerosis and atopic dermatitis in some patients [214].

RECURRENT APHTHOUS STOMATITIS

Aphthoses in HIV-infected patients can be larger and more difficult to treat. They can occur intraorally or in the anogenital region. They can be extremely painful, and the diagnosis should be established by biopsy to rule out other infectious causes or neoplasms. The worst of these has been seen in patients who present with profound neutropenia as well as HIV disease with CD4 counts < 200 cells/mm^3. Local injection with steroids, application of high-potency steroids, and thalidomide can be useful in the treatment of these ulcers [215].

DRUG ERUPTIONS

Many drugs used in the treatment of HIV and AIDS-associated opportunistic infections can cause hypersensitivity reactions. Though the pathophysiology of these reactions is poorly understood, both immunologic and genetic factors (through the major histocompatibility complex) play a role [216]. Whatever the cause, drug eruptions are many times more common among HIV patients than in the general population [217] and should be recognized promptly to minimize morbidity and mortality [218]. Abacavir hypersensitivity, a serious drug reaction characterized by at least two of the following symptoms—morbilliform dermatitis, lymphadenopathy, fever, gastrointestinal symptoms, respiratory symptoms, myalgia, and malaise—occurs in about 5% of patients within the first 8 weeks of therapy and can be fatal on rechallenge [219]. HLA-B*5701 positivity represents a strong genetic predisposition to abacavir hypersensitivity. It is much less common among those of African descent than among those of other ethnicities. A history of allergy to nevirapine and naivety to ART also increase the risk of developing abacavir hypersensitivity [219].

Cutaneous side effects to protease inhibitors are few and occur within the first 4 months of treatment, with the majority of reactions occurring within the first 4 weeks [220]. Hypersensitivity reactions have been reported frequently with the non-nucleoside reverse transcriptase inhibitors (NNRTIs) nevirapine and efavirenz, usually presenting as a morbilliform rash, with or without fever, developing 1–3 weeks after initiation of the drug. Drug photosensitivity has been reported with efavirenz. Amprenavir has a cutaneous hypersensitivity profile similar to that of the NNRTIs [221]. Nevirapine rash is seen in about 17% of patients and may be related to HLA type and depletion of CD4 cells. Antihistamine or prednisone pretreatments do not appear to decrease the development of NNRTI drug eruptions [222, 223]. Nevirapine has been associated with serious reactions, including DRESS (drug rash with eosinophilia and systemic symptoms), Stevens–Johnson syndrome, and toxic epidermal necrolysis. Thus, this drug and others in its class should be discontinued at the first sign of rash [224].

Sulfonamide rashes and drug hypersensitivity are common among HIV-infected patients, presenting with a wide variety of cutaneous reactions [225]. Clindamycin has also been implicated as a common antibiotic cause of cutaneous reactions [226]. The mechanism of hypersensitivity reactions to antibiotics in HIV has been explored and includes the inability of HIV-infected cells to deal with reactive metabolites of these drugs. Desensitization protocols for sulfonamides may allow for continued use of the drug.

TB drugs can also play a role in drug eruptions. In many countries, multiple TB medications are combined into one drug and it can be impossible to sort out the culprit [227].

REFERENCES

[1] Uthayakumar S, Nandwani R, Drinkwater T. The prevalence of skin disease in HIV infection and its relationship to the degree of immunosuppression. Br J Dermatol 1997;137(4):595–8.

[2] Jensen B, Weismann K, Sindrup J, et al. Incidence and prognostic significance of skin disease in patients with HIV/AIDS: a 5-year observational study. Acta Derm Venereol 2000;80(2):140–3.

[3] Goh B, Chan R, Sen P, et al. Spectrum of skin disorders in human immunodeficiency virus-infected patients in Singapore and the relationship to CD4 lymphocyte counts. Int J Dermatol 2007;46(7):695–9.

[4] Singh H, Singh P, Tiwari P, et al. Dermatological manifestations in HIV-infected patients at a tertiary care hospital in a tribal (Bastar) region of Chhattisgarh, India. Indian J Dermatol 2009;54 (4):338–41.

[5] Sued O, Miró J, Alquezar A, et al. Primary human immunodeficiency virus type 1 infection: clinical, virological and immunological characteristics of 75 patients (1997–2003). Enferm Infecc Microbiol Clin 2006;4:238–44.

[6] Chu C, Selwyn P. Diagnosis and initial management of acute HIV infection. Am Fam Physician 2010;81(10):1239–44.

[7] Porras-Luque JI, Valks R, Casal EC, et al. Generalized exanthem with palmoplantar involvement and genital ulcerations. Acute primary HIV infection. Arch Dermatol 1998;134:1279–82.

[8] Sun HY, Chen MJ, Hung CC, et al. Clinical presentations and virologic characteristics of primary human immunodeficiency virus type-1 infection in a university hospital in Taiwan. J Microbiol Immunol Infect 2004;37:271–5.

[9] Kobayashi S, Segawa S, Kawashima M, et al. A case of symptomatic primary HIV infection. J Dermatol 2005;32:137–42.

[10] Daar ES, Moudgil T, Meyer RD, et al. Transient high levels of viremia in patients with primary human immunodeficiency virus type 1 infection. N Engl J Med 1991;324:961–4.

[11] Taiwo BO, Hicks CB. Primary human immunodeficiency virus. South Med J 2002;95:1312–7.

[12] Jing W, Ismail R. Mucocutaneous manifestations of HIV infection: a retrospective analysis of 145 cases in a Chinese population in Malaysia. Int J Dermatol 1999;38:457–63.

[13] Wong SN, Khoo LS. Chronic actinic dermatitis as the presenting feature of HIV infection in three Chinese males. Clin Exp Dermatol 2003;28:265–8.

[14] Namakoola I, Wakeham K, Parkes-Ratanshi R, et al. Use of nail and oral pigmentation to determine ART eligibility among HIV-infected Ugandan adults. Trop Med Int Health 2010;15(2):259–62.

[15] Scarborough M, Gordon S, French N, et al. Grey nails predict low CD4 cell count among untreated patients with HIV infection in Malawi. AIDS 2006;20 (10):1425–7.

[16] Gelfand JM, Rudikoff D. Evaluation and treatment of itching in HIV-infected patients. Mt Sinai J Med 2001;68:298–308.

[17] Bilu D, Mamelak AJ, Nguyen RH, et al. Clinical and epidemiologic characterization of photosensitivity in HIV-positive individuals. Photodermatol Photoimmunol Photomed 2004;20:175–83.

[18] Joyner S, Lee D, Hay P, et al. Hydroxyurea-induced nail pigmentation in HIV patients. HIV Med 1999;1:40–2.

[19] Terheggen F, Frissen J, Weigel H, et al. Nail, hair and skin hyperpigmentation associated with indinavir therapy. AIDS 2004;18:1612.

[20] Rahav G, Maayan S. Nail pigmentation associated with zidovudine: a review and report of a case. Scand J Infect Dis 1992;24:557–61.

[21] Grover C, Kubba S, Bansal S, et al. Pigmentation: a potential cutaneous marker for AIDS. J Dermatol 2004;31:756–60.

[22] Lanjewar DN, Bhosale A, Iyer A. Spectrum of dermatopathologic lesions associated with HIV/AIDS in India. Indian J Pathol Microbiol 2002;45:293–8.

[23] Antony FC, Marsden RA. Vitiligo in association with human immunodeficiency virus infection. J Eur Acad Dermatol Venereol 2003;17:456–8.

[24] Seyedalinaghi S, Karami N, Hajiabdolbaghi M, et al. Vitiligo in a patient associated with human immunodeficiency virus infection and repigmentation under antiretroviral therapy. J Eur Acad Dermatol Venereol 2009;23 (7):840–1.

[25] Colebunders R, Mann JM, Francis H, et al. Generalized papular pruritic eruption in African patients with human immunodeficiency virus infection. AIDS 1987;1:117–21.

[26] Bason MM, Berger TG, Nesbitt Jr. LT. Pruritic papular eruption of HIV-disease. Int J Dermatol 1993;32:784–9.

[27] Sivayathorn A, Srihra B, Leesanguankul W. Prevalence of skin disease in patients infected with human immunodeficiency virus in Bangkok, Thailand. Ann Acad Med Singapore 1995;24:528–33.

[28] Ishii N, Nishiyama T, Sugita Y, et al. Pruritic papular eruption of the acquired immunodeficiency syndrome. Acta Derm Venereol 1994;74:219–20.

[29] Liautaud B, Pape J, DeHovitz J, et al. Pruritic skin lesions: a common presentation of acquired immunodeficiency syndrome. Arch Dermatol 1989;125:629–32.

[30] Boonchai W, Laohasrisakul R, Manonukul J, et al. Pruritic papular eruption in HIV seropositive patients: a cutaneous marker for immunosuppression. Int J Dermatol 1999;38:348–50.

[31] Castelnuovo B, Byakwaga H, Menten J, et al. Can response of a pruritic papular eruption to antiretroviral therapy be used as a clinical parameter to monitor virological outcome? AIDS 2008;22:269–73.

[32] Resneck Jr JS, van Beek M, Furmanski L, et al. Etiology of pruritic papular eruption with HIV infection in Uganda. JAMA 2004;292:2614–21.

[33] Penneys NS, Nayar JK, Bernstein H, et al. Chronic pruritic eruption in patients with acquired immunodeficiency syndrome associated with increased antibody titers to mosquito salivary gland antigens. J Am Acad Dermatol 1989;21:421–5.

[34] Rosatelli JB, Roselino AM. Hyper-IgE, eosinophilia, and immediate cutaneous hypersensitivity to insect antigens in the pruritic papular eruption of human immunodeficiency virus. Arch Dermatol 2001;137:672–3.

[35] Aires JM, Rosatelli JB, de Castro Figueiredo JF, et al. Cytokines in the pruritic papular eruption of HIV. Int J Dermatol 2000;39:903–6.

[36] Pardo RJ, Bogaert MA, Penneys NS, et al. UVB phototherapy of the pruritic papular eruption of the acquired immunodeficiency syndrome. J Am Acad Dermatol 1992;26:423–8.

[37] Resneck Jr JS, van Beek M, Furmanski L, et al. Etiology of pruritic papular eruption with HIV infection in Uganda. JAMA 2004;292:2614–21.

[38] McCalmont TH, Altemus D, Maurer T, et al. Eosinophilic folliculitis. The histologic spectrum. Am J Dermatopathol 1995;17:439–46.

[39] Navarini A, Stoeckle M, Navarini S, et al. Antihistamines are superior to topical steroids in managing human immunodeficiency virus (HIV)-associated papular pruritic eruption. Int J Dermatol 2010;49:83–6.

[40] Ho MH, Chong LY, Ho TT. HIV-associated eosinophilic folliculitis in a Chinese woman: a case report and a survey in Hong Kong. Int J STD AIDS 1998;9:489–93.

[41] Hayes BB, Hille RC, Goldberg LJ. Eosinophilic folliculitis in 2 HIV-positive women. Arch Dermatol 2004;140:463–5.

[42] Rajendran P, Doley J, Heaphy M, et al. Eosinophilic folliculitis: before and after the introduction of antiretroviral therapy. Arch Dermatol 2005;141(10):1227–31.

[43] Teofoli P, Barbieri C, Pallotta S, et al. Pruritic eosinophilic papular eruption revealing HIV infection. Eur J Dermatol 2002;12:600–602.

[44] Cedeno-Laurent F, Gomez-Flores M, Mendez N, et al. New insights into HIV-1-primary skin disorders. J Int AIDS Soc 2011;14:5.

[45] Holmes RB, Martins C, Horn T. The histopathology of folliculitis in HIV-infected patients. J Cutan Pathol 2002;29:93–5.

[46] Annam V, Yelikar BR, Inamadar AC, et al. Clinicopathological study of itchy folliculitis in HIV-infected patients. Indian J Dermatol Venereol Leprol 2010;76(3):259–62.

[47] Ellis E, Scheinfeld N. Eosinophilic pustular folliculitis: a comprehensive review of treatment options. Am J Clin Dermatol 2004;5:189–97.

[48] Mahe A, Faye O, N'Diaye HT, et al. Definition of an algorithm for the management of common skin diseases at primary health care level in sub-Saharan Africa. Trans R Soc Trop Med Hyg 2005;99:39–47.

[49] Nnoruka EN. Current epidemiology of atopic dermatitis in south-eastern Nigeria. Int J Dermatol 2004;43:739–44.

[50] Unemori P, Leslie K, Maurer T. Persistent prurigo nodularis responsive to initiation of combination therapy with raltegravir. Arch Dermatol 2010;146(6):682–3.

[51] Maurer T, Poncelet A, Berger T. Thalidomide treatment for prurigo nodularis in human immunodeficiency virus-infected subjects: efficacy and risk of neuropathy. Arch Dermatol 2004;140:845–9.

[52] Thappa DM, Karthikeyan K. Exaggerated scabies: a marker of HIV infection. Indian Pediatr 2002;39:875–6.

[53] Brites C, Weyll M, Pedroso C, et al. Severe and Norwegian scabies are strongly associated with retroviral (HIV-1/HTLV-1) infection in Bahia, Brazil. AIDS 2002;16:1292–3.

[54] Geoghagen M, Pierre R, Evans-Gilbert T, et al. Tuberculosis, chickenpox and scabies outbreaks in an orphanage for children with HIV/AIDS in Jamaica. West Indian Med J 2004;53:346–51.

[55] Buffet M, Dupin N. Current treatments for scabies. Fundam Clin Pharmacol 2003;17:217–25.

[56] Osborne GE, Taylor C, Fuller LC. The management of HIV-related skin disease. Part I: infections. Int J STD AIDS 2003;14:78–88.

[57] Reid H, Birju B, Holder Y, et al. Epidemic scabies in four Caribbean islands, 1981–1988. Trans R Soc Trop Med Hyg 1990;84:298–300.

[58] Currie B, Carapetis J. Skin infections and infestations in Aboriginal communities in northern Australia. Aust J Dermatol 2001;41:139–41.

[59] Hay R. Scabies and pyodermas—diagnosis and treatment. Dermatol Ther 2009;22(6):466–74.

[60] Castano-Molina C, Cockerell CJ. Diagnosis and treatment of infectious diseases in HIV-infected hosts. Dermatol Clin 1997;15:267–83.

[61] Barro-Traore F, Traore A, Konate I, et al. Epidemiological features of tumors of the skin and mucosal membranes in the department of dermatology at the Yalgado Ouedraogo National Hospital, Ouagadougou, Burkina Faso. Sante 2003;13:101–4.

[62] Geoghagen M, Pierre R, Evans-Gilbert T, et al. Tuberculosis, chickenpox and scabies outbreaks in an orphanage for children with HIV/AIDS in Jamaica. West Indian Med J 2004;53:346–51.

[63] Shapiro M, Smith KJ, James WD, et al. Cutaneous microenvironment of human immunodeficiency virus (HIV)-seropositive and HIV-seronegative individuals, with special reference to Staphylococcus aureus

colonization. J Clin Microbiol 2000;38:3174–8.

[64] Alexander E, Morgan D, Kesh S, et al. Prevalence, persistence, and microbiology of *Staphylococcus aureus* nasal carriage among hemodialysis outpatients at a major New York hospital. Diagn Microbiol Infect Dis 2011;70 (1):37–44.

[65] Shet A, Mathema B, Mediavilla JR, et al. Colonization and subsequent skin and soft tissue infection due to methicillin-resistant *Staphylococcus aureus* in a cohort of otherwise healthy adults infected with HIV Type 1. J Infect Dis 2009;200:88–93.

[66] Popovich K, Weintsein R, Aroutcheva A, et al. Community-associated methicillin-resistant *Staphylococcus aureus* and HIV: intersecting epidemics. Clin Infect Dis 2010;50:979–87.

[67] Lee NE, Taylor MM, Bancroft E, et al. Risk factors for community-associated methicillin-resistant *Staphylococcus aureus* skin infections among HIV-positive men who have sex with men. Clin Infect Dis 2005;40:1529–34.

[68] Imaz Am Pujol M, Barragan P. Community associated methicillin-resistant *Staphylococcus aureus* in HIV-infected patients. AIDS Rev 2010;12(3):153–63.

[69] Martin J, Rose D, Hadley W, et al. Emergence of trimethoprim-sulfamethoxazole resistance in the AIDS era. J Infect Dis 1999;180 (6):1809–18.

[70] Krucke GW, Grimes DE, Grimes RM, Dang TD. Antibiotic resistance in *Staphylococcus aureus*-containing cutaneous abscesses of patients with HIV. Am J Emerg Med 2009;27:344–7.

[71] Ruhe JJ, Monson T, Bradsher RW, et al. Use of long-acting tetracyclines for methicillin-resistant *Staphylococcus aureus* infections: case series and review of the literature. Clin Infect Dis 2005;40:1429–34.

[72] Ellis MW, Lewis JS 2nd. Treatment approaches for community-acquired methicillin-resistant *Staphylococcus aureus* infections. Curr Opin Infect Dis 2005;18:496–501.

[73] Kluytmans JA, Wertheim HF. Nasal carriage of *Staphylococcus aureus* and prevention of nosocomial infections. Infection 2005;33:3–8.

[74] Gordon RJ, Chez N, Jia H, et al. The NOSE study (nasal ointment for *Staphylococcus aureus* eradication): a randomized controlled trial of monthly mupirocin in HIV-infected individuals. J Acquir Immune Defic Syndr 2010;55 (4):466–72.

[75] Niemi M, Backman JT, Fromm MF, et al. Pharmacokinetic interactions with rifampicin: clinical relevance. Clin Pharmacokinet 2003;4:819–50.

[76] Frean J, Arndt S, Spencer D. High rate of *Bartonella henselae* infection in HIV-positive outpatients in Johannesburg, South Africa. Trans R Soc Trop Med Hyg 2002;96:549–50.

[77] Koehler JE. *Bartonella*-associated infections in HIV-infected patients. AIDS Clin Care 1995;7:97–102.

[78] Koehler JE, Sanchez MA, Tye S, et al. Prevalence of *Bartonella* infection among human immunodeficiency virus-infected patients with fever. Clin Infect Dis 2003;37:559–66.

[79] Plettenberg A, Lorenzen T, Burtsche BT, et al. Bacillary angiomatosis in HIV-infected patients—an epidemiological and clinical study. Dermatology 2000;201:326–31.

[80] Lanjewar DN, Bhosale A, Iyer A. Spectrum of dermatopathologic lesions associated with HIV/AIDS in India. Indian M Pathol Microbiol 2002;45:293–8.

[81] Minga KA, Gberi I, Boka MB, et al. Bacillary angiomatosis in an adult infected with HIV-1 at an early stage of immunodepression in Abidjan, Cote d'Ivoire. Bull Soc Pathol Exot 2002;95:34–6.

[82] Ciervo A, Petrucca A, Ciarrocchi S, et al. Molecular characterization of first human *Bartonella* strain isolated in Italy. J Clin Microbiol 2001;39:4554–7.

[83] Gazineo JL, Trope BM, Maceira JP, et al. Bacillary angiomatosis: description of 13 cases reported in five reference centers for AIDS treatment in Rio de Janeiro, Brazil.

Rev Inst Med Trop Sao Paulo 2001;43:1–6.

[84] Mateen F, Newstead J, McClean K. Bacillary angiomatosis in an HIV-positive man with multiple risk factors: a clinical and epidemiological puzzle. Can J Infect Dis Med Microbiol 2005;16 (4):249–52.

[85] Lamas C, Mares-Guia M, Rozental T, et al. *Bartonella* spp. infection in HIV positive individuals, their pets and ectoparasites in Rio de Janeiro, Brazil: serological and molecular study. Acta Trop 2010;115 (1–2):137–41.

[86] Pons I, Sanfeliu I, Noqueras M, et al. Seroprevalence of *Bartonella* spp. infection in HIV patients in Catalonia, Spain. BMC Infect Dis 2008;8:58.

[87] Pape M, Kollaras P, Mandraveli K. Occurrence of *Bartonella henselae* and *Bartonella quintana* among human immunodeficiency virus-infected patients. Ann N Y Acad Sci 2005;1063:299–301.

[88] Rosales CM, McLaughlin MD, Sata T, et al. AIDS presenting with cutaneous Kaposi's sarcoma and bacillary angiomatosis in the bone marrow mimicking Kaposi's sarcoma. AIDS Patient Care STDS 2002;16:573–7.

[89] Koehler JE, Sanchez MA, Tye S, et al. Prevalence of *Bartonella* infection among human immunodeficiency virus-infected patients with fever. Clin Infect Dis 2003;37:559–66.

[90] Cheuk W, Wong KO, Wong CS, et al. Immunostaining for human herpesvirus 8 latent nuclear antigen-1 helps distinguish Kaposi sarcoma from its mimickers. Am J Clin Pathol 2004;121:335–42.

[91] Ibeziako SN, Nwolisa CE, Nwaiwu O. Cancrum oris and acute necrotising gingivitis complicating HIV infection in children. Ann Trop Paediatr 2003;23:225–6.

[92] Chidzonga MM. HIV/AIDS orofacial lesions in 156 Zimbabwean patients at referral oral and maxillofacial surgical clinics. Oral Dis 2003;9:317–22.

[93] Faye O, Keita M, N'diaye HT, et al. Noma in HIV-infected adults.

Ann Dermatol Venereol 2003;130:199–201.

[94] Bratthall D, Petersen P, Stjernsward J, et al. Oral and craniofacial diseases and disorders. In: Disease Control Priorities in Developing Countries. 2nd ed. Washington, DC: World Bank; 2006.

[95] Gutierrez-Galhardo MC, Valle G. F. do, Sa FC, et al. Clinical characteristics and evolution of syphilis in 24 HIV+ individuals in Rio de Janeiro, Brazil. Rev Inst Med Trop Sao Paulo 2005;47:153–7.

[96] Gare J, Lupiwa T, Suarkia DL, et al. High prevalence of sexually transmitted infections among female sex workers in the eastern highlands province of Papua New Guinea: correlates and recommendations. Sex Transm Dis 2005;32:466–73.

[97] Hesketh T, Tang F, Wang ZB, et al. HIV and syphilis in young Chinese adults: implications for spread. Int J STD AIDS 2005;16:262–6.

[98] Amo J del, Gonzalez C, Losana J, et al. Influence of age and geographical origin in the prevalence of high risk human papillomavirus in migrant female sex workers in Spain. Sex Transm Infect 2005;81:79–84.

[99] Nnoruka EN, Ezeoke AC. Evaluation of syphilis in patients with HIV infection in Nigeria. Trop Med Int Health 2005;10:58–64.

[100] Ryder N, Bourne C, Rohrsheim R. Clinical audit: adherence to sexually transmitted infection screening guidelines for men who have sex with men. Int J STD AIDS 2005;16:446–9.

[101] Dougan S, Elford J, Rice B, et al. Epidemiology of HIV among black and minority ethnic men who have sex with men in England and Wales. Sex Transm Infect 2005;81:345–50.

[102] Lautenschlager S. Sexually transmitted infections in Switzerland: return of the classics. Dermatology 2005;210:134–42.

[103] Bij AK van der, Stolte IG, Coutinho RA, et al. Increase of sexually transmitted infections, not HIV, among young homosexual men in Amsterdam:

are STIs still reliable markers for HIV transmission? Sex Transm Infect 2005;81:34–7.

[104] Sasse A, Defraye A, Ducoffre G. Recent syphilis trends in Belgium and enhancement of STI surveillance systems. Euro Surveill 2004;9:6–8.

[105] Cowan S. Syphilis in Denmark—outbreak among MSM in Copenhagen, 2003–2004. Euro Surveill 2004;9:25–7.

[106] Marcus U, Bremer V, Hamouda O. Syphilis surveillance and trends of the syphilis epidemic in Germany since the mid-90s. Euro Surveill 2004;9:11–4.

[107] Wong W, Chaw JK, Kent CK, et al. Risk factors for early syphilis among gay and bisexual men seen in an STD clinic: San Francisco, 2002–2003. Sex Transm Dis 2005;32:458–63.

[108] Fenton KA, Imrie J. Increasing rates of sexually transmitted diseases in homosexual men in Western Europe and the United States: why? Infect Dis Clin North Am 2005;19:311–31.

[109] Cohen CE, Winston A, Asboe D, et al. Increasing detection of asymptomatic syphilis in HIV patients. Sex Transm Infect 2005;81:217–19.

[110] Gilleece Y, Sullivan A. Management of sexually transmitted infections in HIV positive individuals. Curr Opin Infect Dis 2005;18:43–7.

[111] Sanchez MR. Infectious syphilis. Semin Dermatol 1994;13:234–42.

[112] Ortega KL, Rezende NP, Watanuki F, et al. Secondary syphilis in an HIV positive patient. Med Oral 2004;9:33–8.

[113] Baniandres Rodriguez O, Nieto Perea O, Moya Alonso L, et al. Nodular secondary syphilis in a HIV patient mimicking cutaneous lymphoma. Med Interna 2004;21:241–3.

[114] Dave S, Gopinath DV, Thappa DM. Nodular secondary syphilis. Dermatol Online J 2003;9:9.

[115] Doris JP, Saha K, Jones NP, et al. Ocular syphilis: the new epidemic. Eye 2006;20:703–5.

[116] Passoni LF, Menezes JA de, Ribeiro SR, et al. Lues maligna in

an HIV-infected patient. Rev Soc Bras Med Trop 2005;38:181–4.

[117] Centers for Disease Control and Prevention. Sexually transmitted diseases treatment guidelines 2002. MMWR 2002;51:1–98.

[118] Chan DJ. Syphilis and HIV co-infection: when is lumbar puncture indicated? Curr HIV Res 2005;3:95–8.

[119] Ghanem K, Moore R, Rompalo A, et al. Lumbar puncture in HIV-infected patients with syphilis and no neurologic symptoms. Clin Infect Dis 2009;48(6):816–21.

[120] Centers for Disease Control and Prevention (CDC). Azithromycin treatment failures in syphilis infections—San Francisco, California, 2002–2003. MMWR 2004;53:197–8.

[121] Thurnheer M, Weber R, Toutous-Trellu L, et al. Occurrence, risk factors, diagnosis and treatment of syphilis in the prospective observational Swiss HIV Cohort Study. AIDS 2010;24 (12):1907–16.

[122] Varshney A, Goyal T. Incidence of various clinic-morphological variants of cutaneous tuberculosis and HIV concurrence: a study from the Indian subcontinent. Ann Saudi Med 2011;31(2):134–9.

[123] Regnier S, Ouagari Z, Perez Z, et al. Cutaneous military resistant tuberculosis in a patient infected with human immunodeficiency virus: case report and literature review. Clin Exp Dermatol 34(8): e690–2.

[124] Miziara ID. Tuberculosis affecting the oral cavity in Brazilian HIV-infected patients. Oral Surg Oral Med Oral Pathol Oral Radiol Endod 2005;100:179–82.

[125] High WA, Evans CC, Hoang MP. Cutaneous miliary tuberculosis in two patients with HIV infection. J Am Acad Dermatol 2004;50: S110–13.

[126] Ramdial PK, Sing Y, Subrayan S, et al. Granulomas in acquired immunodeficiency syndrome-associated cutaneous Kaposi sarcoma: evidence for a role for *Mycobacterium tuberculosis*. J Cutan Pathol 2010;37(8):827–34.

[127] Chapman AL, Munkanta M, Wilkinson KA, et al. Rapid

detection of active and latent tuberculosis infection in HIV-positive individuals by enumeration of *Mycobacterium tuberculosis*-specific T cells. AIDS 2002;16:2285–93.

[128] Alsina M, Campo P, Toll A, et al. Papulonecrotic tuberculide in a human immunodeficiency virus type 1-seropositive patient. Br J Dermatol 2000;143:232–3.

[129] Jevtovic DJ, Salemovic D, Ranin J, et al. The prevalence and risk of immune restoration disease in HIV-infected patients treated with highly active antiretroviral therapy. HIV Med 2005;6:140–3.

[130] Boyd AS, Robbins J. Cutaneous *Mycobacterium avium intracellulare* infection in an HIV+ patient mimicking histoid leprosy. Am J Dermatol 2005;27:39–41.

[131] Tandon R, Kim K, Serrao R. Disseminated *Mycobacterium avium-intracellulare* infection in a person with AIDS with cutaneous and CNS lesions. AIDS Read 2007;17(11):555–60.

[132] Mahaisavariya P, Chaiprasert A, Khemngern S, et al. Nontuberculous mycobacterial skin infections: clinical and bacteriological studies. J Med Assoc Thai 2003;86:52–60.

[133] Pereira GA, Stefani MM, Araujo Filho JA, et al. Human immunodeficiency virus type 1 (HIV-1) and *Mycobacterium leprae* co-infection: HIV-1 subtypes and clinical, immunologic, and histopathologic profiles in a Brazilian cohort. Am J Trop Med Hyg 2004;71:679–84.

[134] Rath N, Kar HK. Leprosy in HIV infection: a study of three cases. Indian J Lepr 2003;75:355–9.

[135] Pignataro P, Rocha Ada S, Nery JA, et al. Leprosy and AIDS: two cases of increasing inflammatory reactions at the start of highly active antiretroviral therapy. Eur J Clin Microbiol Infect Dis 2004;23:408–11.

[136] Couppie P, Abel S, Voinchet H, et al. Immune reconstitution inflammatory syndrome associated with HIV and leprosy. Arch Dermatol 2004;140:997–1000.

[137] Visco-Comandini U, Longo B, Cuzzi T, et al. Tuberculoid leprosy in a patient with AIDS: a manifestation of immune restoration syndrome. Scand J Infect Dis 2004;36:881–3.

[138] Lockwood D, Lambert S. Human immunodeficiency virus and leprosy: an update. Dermatol Clin 2011;29(1):125–8.

[139] Mootsikapun P, Intarapoka B, Liawnoraset W. Nocardiosis in Srinagarind Hospital, Thailand: review of 70 cases from 1996–2001. Int J Infect Dis 2005;9:154–8.

[140] Jones N, Khoosal M, Louw M, et al. Nocardial infection as a complication of HIV in South Africa. J Infect 2000;41:232–9.

[141] Uttamchandani RB, Daikos GL, Reyes RR, et al. Nocardiosis in 30 patients with advanced human immunodeficiency virus infection: clinical features and outcome. Clin Infect Dis 1994;18:348–53.

[142] Javaly K, Horowitz HW, Wormser GP. Nocardiosis in patients with human immunodeficiency virus infection. Report of 2 cases and review of the literature. Medicine (Baltimore) 1992;71:128–38.

[143] Biscione F, Cecchini D, Ambrosioni J. Nocardiosis in patients with human immunodeficiency virus infection. Enferm Infecc Microbiol Clin 2005;23(7):419–23.

[144] Bosch RJ, Rodrigo AB, Sanchez P, et al. Presence of *Leishmania* organisms in specific and non-specific skin lesions in HIV-infected individuals with visceral leishmaniasis. Int J Dermatol 2002;41:670–5.

[145] Bittencourt A, Silva N, Straatmann A, et al. Post-kala-azar dermal leishmaniasis associated with AIDS. Braz J Infect Dis 2002;6:313–6.

[146] Agostoni C, Dorigoni N, Malfitano A, et al. Mediterranean leishmaniasis in HIV-infected patients: epidemiological, clinical, and diagnostic features of 22 cases. Infection 1998;26:93–9.

[147] Barrio J, Lecona M, Cosin J, et al. *Leishmania* infection occurring in herpes zoster lesions in an HIV-positive patient. Br J Dermatol 1996;134:164–6.

[148] Soni P, Prasad N, Khandelwal K. Unresponsive cutaneous leishmaniasis and HIV co-infection: report of three cases. Indian J Dermatol Venereol Leprol 2011;77(2):251.

[149] Ezra N, Ochoa M, Craft N. Human immunodeficiency virus and leishmaniasis. J Glob Infect Dis 2010;2(3):248–57.

[150] Gallego MA, Aguilar A, Plaza S, et al. Kaposi's sarcoma with an intense parasitization by *Leishmania*. Cutis 1996;57:103–5.

[151] Schraner C, Hasse B, Hasse U, et al. Successful treatment with miltefosine of disseminated cutaneous leishmaniasis in a severely immunocompromised patient infected with HIV-1. Clin Infect Dis 2005;40:e120–4.

[152] Johnson R. Dermatophyte infections in human immune deficiency virus (HIV) disease. J Am Acad Dermatol 2000;43(Suppl. 5):S135–42.

[153] Graham E, Rodwell J, Bayles C, et al. The prevalence of dermatophyte infection in patients infected with human immunodeficiency virus. Int J Dermatol 2008;47(4):339–43.

[154] Venkatesan P, Perfect J, Myers S. Evaluation and management of fungal infections in immunocompromised patients. Dermatol Ther 2005;18(1):44–57.

[155] Maurer T, Rodrigues LK, Ameli N, et al. The effect of highly active antiretroviral therapy on dermatologic disease in a longitudinal study of HIV type 1-infected women. Clin Infect Dis 2004;38:579–84.

[156] Rinaldi MG. Dermatophytosis: epidemiological and microbiological update. J Am Acad Dermatol 2000;43(5 Suppl. 1):S120–S124.

[157] Millikan LE. Role of oral antifungal agents for the treatment of superficial fungal infections in immunocompromised patients. Cutis 2001;68:6–14.

[158] Dharmshale S, Patil S, Gohil A, et al. Disseminated cryptococcosis with extensive cutaneous

involvement in AIDS. Indian J Med Microbiol 2006;24(3):228–30.

[159] Manfredi R, Mazzoni A, Nanetti A, et al. Morphologic features and clinical significance of skin involvement in patients with AIDS-related cryptococcosis. Acta Derm Venereol 1996;76:72–4.

[160] Ramdial P, Mosam A, Dlova NC, et al. Disseminated cutaneous histoplasmosis in patients infected with human immunodeficiency virus. J Cutan Pathol 2002;29:215–25.

[161] Calza L, Manfredi R, Donzelli C, et al. Disseminated histoplasmosis with atypical cutaneous lesions in an Italian HIV-infected patient: another autochthonous case. HIV Med 2003;4:145–8.

[162] Lo Cascio G, Ligozzi M, Maccacaro L, et al. Diagnostic aspects of cutaneous lesions due to *Histoplasma capsulatum* in African AIDS patients in nonendemic areas. Eur J Clin Microbiol Infect Dis 2003;22:637–8.

[163] Gutierrez ME, Canton A, Sosa N, et al. Disseminated histoplasmosis in patients with AIDS in Panama: a review of 104 cases. Clin Infect Dis 2005;40:1199–202.

[164] Couppie P, Roussel M, Thual N, et al. Disseminated histoplasmosis: an atypical ulcerous form in an HIV-infected patient. Ann Dermatol Venereol 2005;132:133–5.

[165] Bonifaz A, Chang P, Moreno K. Disseminated cutaneous histoplasmosis in acquired immunodeficiency syndrome: report of 23 cases. Clin Exp Dermatol 2009;34(4):481–6.

[166] Daher E, Silva G, Barros F. Clinical and laboratory features of disseminated histoplasmosis in HIV patients from Brazil. Trop Med Int Health 2007;12 (9):1108–15.

[167] Lopez-Romero E, Reyes-Montes M, Perez-Torres A, et al. *Sporothrix schenckii* complex and sporotrichosis, an emerging health problem. Future Microbiol 2011;6 (1):85–102.

[168] Gutierrez-Galhardo M, Francesconi do Valle A, Barros Fraga B, et al. Disseminated

sporotrichosis as a manifestation of immune reconstitution inflammatory syndrome. Mycoses 2008;53:78–80.

[169] Rocha MM, Dassin T, Lira R, et al. Sporotrichosis in patient with AIDS: report of a case and review. Rev Iberoam Micol 2001;18:133–6.

[170] Shetty D, Giri N, Gonzalez CE, et al. Invasive aspergillosis in human immunodeficiency virus-infected children. Pediatr Infect Dis J 1997;16:216–21.

[171] Stanford D, Boyle M, Gillespie R. Human immunodeficiency virus-related primary cutaneous aspergillosis. Australas J Dermatol 2000;41:112–6.

[172] Supparatpinyo K, Khamwan C, Baosoung V, et al. Disseminated *Penicillium marneffei* infection in southeast Asia. Lancet 1994;344:110–13.

[173] Duong TA. Infection due to *Penicillium marneffei*, an emerging pathogen: review of 155 reported cases. Clin Infect Dis 1996;23:125–30.

[174] Le T, Wolbers M, Chi N. Epidemiology, seasonality, and predictors of outcome of AIDS-associated *Penicillium marneffei* infection in Ho Chi Minh City, Vietnam. Clin Infect Dis 2011;52 (7):945–52.

[175] Amerson E, Maurer T. Immune reconstitution inflammatory syndrome and tropical dermatosis. Dermatol Clin 2011;29(1): 39–43.

[176] Cury K, Valin N, Gozlan J, et al. Bipolar hypertrophic herpes: an unusual presentation of acyclovir-resistant herpes simplex type 2 in an HIV-infected patient. Sex Transm Dis 2010;37:126–8.

[177] Celum C, Wald A, Lingappa JR, et al. Acyclovir and transmission of HIV-1 from persons infected with HIV-1 and HSV-2. N Engl J Med 2010;362:427–39.

[178] Gebo KA, Kalyani R, Moore RD, Polydefkis MJ. The incidence of, risk factors for, and sequelae of herpes zoster among HIV patients in the highly active antiretroviral therapy era. J Acquir Immune Defic Syndr 2005;40: 169–74.

[179] Palefsky JM. Cutaneous and genital HPV-associated lesions in HIV-infected patients. Clin Dermatol 1997;15:439–47.

[180] Degener AM, Laino L, Pierangeli A, et al. Human papillomavirus-32-positive extragenital Bowenoid papulosis (BP) in a HIV patient with typical genital BP localization. Sex Transm Dis 2004;31:619–22.

[181] Rodrigues LK, Maurert BT. Cutaneous warts in HIV-positive patients undergoing highly active antiretroviral therapy. Arch Dermatol 2001;137:1103–4.

[182] Toutous-Trellu L, Hirschel B, Piguet V, et al. Treatment of cutaneous human papilloma virus, poxvirus and herpes simplex virus infections with topical cidofovir in HIV positive patients. Ann Dermatol Venereol 2004;131:445–9.

[183] Cooley TP. Non-AIDS-defining cancer in HIV-infected people. Hematol Oncol Clin North Am 2003;17:889–99.

[184] Allardice GM, Hole DJ, Brewster DH, et al. Incidence of malignant neoplasms among HIV-infected persons in Scotland. Br J Cancer 2003;89:505–7.

[185] Rabkin CS, Biggar RJ, Horm JW. Increasing incidence of cancers associated with the human immunodeficiency virus epidemic. Int J Cancer 1991;47:692–6.

[186] Franceschi S, Lise M, Clifford G. Changing patterns of cancer incidence in the early-and late-HAART periods: the Swiss HIV Cohort Study. Br J Cancer 2010;103(3):416–22.

[187] Wilkins K, Dolev JC, Turner R, et al. Approach to the treatment of cutaneous malignancy in HIV-infected patients. Dermatol Ther 2005;18:77–86.

[188] Calista D. Five cases of melanoma in HIV positive patients. Eur J Dermatol 2001;11:446–9.

[189] Utikal J, et al. Reiter's syndrome-like pattern in AIDS-associated psoriasiform dermatitis. J Eur Acad Dermatol Venereol 2003;17:114–16.

[190] Mosam A, et al. The impact of human immunodeficiency virus/ acquired immunodeficiency

syndrome (HIV/AIDS) on skin disease in KwaZulu-Natal, South Africa. Int J Dermatol 2004;43:782–3.

[191] Mallon E, Bunker CB. HIV-associated psoriasis. AIDS Patient Care STDS 2000;14:239–46.

[192] Menon K, Van Voorhees A, Bebo B, et al. National Psoriasis Foundation. Psoriasis in patients with HIV infection: from the medical board of the National Psoriasis Foundation. J Am Acad Dermatol 2010;62(2):291–9.

[193] Fischer T, Schworer H, Vente C, et al. Clinical improvement of HIV-associated psoriasis parallels a reduction of HIV viral load induced by effective antiretroviral therapy. AIDS 1999;13:628–9.

[194] Duvic M, Crane MM, Conant M, et al. Ziduvudine improves psoriasis in human immunodeficiency virus-positive males. Arch Dermatol 1994;130:447–51.

[195] Buccheri L, Katchen BR, Karter AJ, Cohen SR. Acitretin therapy is effective for psoriasis associated with human immunodeficiency virus infection. Arch Dermatol 1997;133:711–15.

[196] Mikhail M, Weinberg JM, Smith BL. Successful treatment with etanercept of von Zumbusch pustular psoriasis in a patient with human immunodeficiency virus. Arch Dermatol 2008;144(4):453–6.

[197] Ting PT, Koo JY. Use of etanercept in human immunodeficiency virus (HIV) and acquired immunodeficiency syndrome (AIDS) patients. Int J Dermatol 2006;45:689–92.

[198] Morar N, Willis-Owen SA, Maurer T, Bunker CB. HIV-associated psoriasis: pathogenesis, clinical features, and management. Lancet Infect Dis 2010;10(7):470–8.

[199] Hira SK, Wadhawan D, Kamanga J, et al. Cutaneous manifestations of human immunodeficiency virus in Lusaka, Zambia. J Am Acad Dermatol 1988;19:451–7.

[200] Kim T, Lee K, Oh S. Skin disorders in Korean patients infected with human immunodeficiency virus and their association with a CD4 lymphocyte count: a preliminary study. J Eur Acad Dermatol Venereol 2010;24(12):1476–80.

[201] Tzung TY, Yang CY, Chao SC, et al. Cutaneous manifestations of human immunodeficiency virus infection in Taiwan. Kaohsiung J Med Sci 2004;20:216–24.

[202] Pitche P, Tchangai-Walla K, Napo-Koura G, et al. Prevalence of skin manifestations in AIDS patients in the Lome-Tokoin University Hospital (Togo). Sante 1995;5:349–52.

[203] Wiwanitkit V. Prevalence of dermatological disorders in Thai HIV-infected patients correlated with different CD4 lymphocyte count statuses: a note on 120 cases. Int J Dermatol 2004;43:265–8.

[204] Dunic I, Vesic S, Jevtovic DJ. Oral candidiasis and seborrheic dermatitis in HIV-infected patients on highly active antiretroviral therapy. HIV Med 2004;5:50–4.

[205] Muhammad B, Eligius L, Mugusi F, et al. The prevalence and pattern of skin diseases in relation to CD4 counts among HIV-infected police officers in Dar es Salaam. Trop Doct 2003;33:44–8.

[206] Pechere M, Krischer J, Remondat C, et al. Malassezia spp carriage in patients with seborrheic dermatitis. J Dermatol 1999;26:558–61.

[207] Gupta AK, Bluhm R. Seborrheic dermatitis. J Eur Acad Dermatol Venereol 2004;18:13–26.

[208] Lee D, Benson CA, Lewis CE, et al. Prevalence and factors associated with dry skin in HIV infection: the FRAM study. AIDS 2007;21:2051–7.

[209] Rudikoff D. The relationship between HIV infection and atopic dermatitis. Curr Allergy Asthma Rep 2002;2:275–81.

[210] Klein SA, Dobmeyer JM, Dobmeyer TS, et al. Demonstration of the Th1 to Th2 cytokine shift during the course of HIV-1 infection using cytoplasmic cytokine detection on single cell level by flow cytometry. AIDS 1997;11:1111–18.

[211] Lee GR, Flavell RA. Transgenic mice which overproduce Th2 cytokines develop spontaneous atopic dermatitis and asthma. Int Immunol 2004;16:1155–60.

[212] Palmer CN, Irvine AD, Terron-Kwiatkowski A, et al. Common loss-of-function variants of the epidermal barrier protein filaggrin are a major predisposing factor for atopic dermatitis. Nat Genet 2006;38:441–6.

[213] Gunathilake R, Schmuth M, Scharschmidt T, et al. Epidermal barrier dysfunction in non-atopic HIV: evidence for an "inside-to-outside" pathogenesis. J Invest Dermatol 2010;130:1185–8.

[214] Maurer T, Rodrigues LK, Ameli N, et al. The effect of highly active antiretroviral therapy on dermatologic disease in a longitudinal study of HIV type 1-infected women. Clin Infect Dis 2004;38:579–84.

[215] Gileva OS, Sazhina MV, Gileva ES, et al. Spectrum of oral manifestations of HIV/AIDS in the Perm region (Russia) and identification of self-induced ulceronecrotic lingual lesions. Med Oral 2004;9:212–15.

[216] Chaponda M, Pirmohamed M. Hypersensitivity reactions to HIV therapy. Br J Clin Pharmacol 2011;71(5):659–71.

[217] Pirmohamed M, Park B. HIV and drug allergy. Curr Opin Allergy Clin Immunol 2001;1(4):311–16.

[218] Introcaso CE, Hines JM, Kovarik CL. Cutaneous toxicities of antiretroviral therapy for HIV: part I. Lipodystrophy syndrome, nucleoside reverse transcriptase inhibitors, and protease inhibitors. J Am Acad Dermatol 2010;63(4):549–61.

[219] Chirouze C, Hustache-Mathieu L, Rougeot C, et al. Risk factors for Abacavir-induced hypersensitivity syndrome in the "real world" Pathol Biol (Paris) 2004;52:529–33.

[220] Rotunda A, Hirsch RJ, Scheinfeld N, et al. Severe cutaneous reactions associated with the use of human immunodeficiency virus medications. Acta Derm Venereol 2003;83:1–9.

[221] Phillips EJ, Kuriakose B, Knowles SR. Efavirenz-induced skin eruption and successful desensitization. Ann Pharmacother 2002;36:430–2.

[222] Wit FW, Wood R, Horban A, et al. Prednisolone does not prevent hypersensitivity reactions in antiretroviral drug regimens containing abacavir with or without nevirapine. AIDS 2001;15:2423–9.

[223] Launay O, Roudière L, Boukli N, et al. Assessment of cetirizine, an antihistamine, to prevent cutaneous reactions to nevirapine therapy: results of the viramune-zyrtec double-blind, placebo-controlled trial. Clin Infect Dis 2004;38:66–72.

[224] Fagot JP, Mockenhaupt M, Bouwes-Bavinck JN, et al. EuroSCAR Study Group. Nevirapine and the risk of Stevens–Johnson syndrome or toxic epidermal necrolysis. AIDS 2001;15:1843–8.

[225] Slatore CG, Tilles SA. Sulfonamide hypersensitivity. Immunol Allergy Clin North Am 2004;24:477–90.

[226] Wijsman JA, Dekaban GA, Rieder MJ. Differential toxicity of reactive metabolites of clindamycin and sulfonamides in HIV-infected cells: influence of HIV infection on clindamycin toxicity in vitro. J Clin Pharmacol 2005;45:346–51.

[227] Kouassi B, Horo K, Vilasco B, et al. Lyell's syndrome occurring in three HIV-positive patients undergoing anti-tuberculous therapy. Rev Mal Respir 2010;27(3):247–50.

Chapter | 18 |

Gastrointestinal disorders in HIV including diarrhea

Marie-Louise C. Vachon, Douglas T. Dieterich

INTRODUCTION

Gastrointestinal complaints are common among patients infected with human immunodeficiency virus (HIV). In the early days of the HIV epidemic, gastrointestinal (GI) illnesses, mostly diarrhea caused by opportunistic pathogens, were a major cause of death. Often, odynophagia caused by *Candida* esophagitis prevented patients from eating, and cryptosporidiosis and cytomegalovirus (CMV) infections prevented them from absorbing nutrients. The treatment of opportunistic pathogens has progressed only slightly in the almost 30-year history of HIV, but the successful treatment of HIV itself has caused mortality due to GI illnesses (excluding liver disease) to fade into the background. While many patients with HIV continue to have GI issues, the major cause of death in most cohorts is shifting from acquired immunodeficiency syndrome (AIDS) to liver disease. Understanding the importance of the gut-associated lymphoid tissue (GALT), commencing with the acute HIV infection, has highlighted the role the GI tract plays in the pathogenesis of HIV. Indeed the infection of the GALT by HIV may even contribute to liver disease. While the causes of GI illnesses have changed since the early days of the epidemic, there are numerous disorders of the GI tract that have a large impact on morbidity and mortality of HIV patients today: for example, drug-induced diarrhea and anorectal cancer.

GUT-ASSOCIATED LYMPHATIC TISSUE (GALT)

Recent research has emphasized the importance of the GALT in the pathogenesis of HIV in the gut, in the liver, and in the body overall. The primary target of HIV is the CD4 T cell compartment and the GALT contains the largest number of lymphocytes of any organ in the body, approximately 80% of the entire T cell population. The majority of gut and peripheral CD4 T cells are lost during the acute phase of HIV [1, 2]. This depletion of gut CD4 T cells and the resulting altered mucosal immunity persist into the chronic phase and despite effective antiretroviral therapy (ART) and peripheral CD4 T cell recovery [3–5]. This breach in the integrity of the gut mucosa allows bacteria and bacterial products, such as the endotoxins lipopolysaccharides (LPS) to cross over and reach the portal and systemic circulations. This process, referred to as microbial translocation, may contribute to the pro-inflammatory state characterizing chronic HIV infection [6]. Microbial translocation also occurs in inflammatory bowel disease (IBD) and is involved in its pathogenesis [7]. In a study of 26 patients with AIDS with a CD4 count < 300 cells/mm^3 and high plasma LPS levels, 65% of patients had at least one positive serological marker of IBD when tested for ASCA (anti-*Saccharomyces cerevisiae* antibody); pANCA (perinuclear anti-neutrophil antibody); anti-OmpC (antibody against outer membrane porin C of *E. coli*); and anti-CBir1 (antibody against bacterial flagellin) [8]. Forty-six percent of patients had an IBD-like serological pattern; 75% of them had a Crohn's disease-like pattern. This suggests that IBD markers may be useful for monitoring HIV-related inflammatory gut disease and requires further study. Massive depletion of the gut T cells may also make the gastrointestinal tract more susceptible to common pathogens.

ESOPHAGEAL DISORDERS

The epidemiology of esophageal disorders has changed in parallel with ART-induced immune reconstitution and consequent aging of the HIV-infected population.

Opportunistic GI disease has decreased significantly with combination ART (cART) [9]. In the developed world, HIV-infected patients presenting with esophageal symptoms often receive diagnoses similar to that of an immunocompetent host [10]. Dysphagia and odynophagia were common complaints of HIV-infected patients prior to cART [11]. Most of the time, the etiology was *Candida* esophagitis and, not infrequently, esophageal ulcers caused by either CMV or herpes simplex virus (HSV), or were idiopathic. Today, most patients have good control of their HIV infection with suppressed HIV RNA and CD4 T cell counts >200 cells/mm^3. Reflux symptoms are a major complaint and patients are found to have inflammatory gastropathy, gastroesophageal reflux disease (GERD), *Helicobacter pylori* infections, Barrett's esophagus, and gastric ulcers [11]. Since the HIV population is aging, these are all appropriate illnesses for these patient's age groups. In a given patient, the differential diagnosis depends on the degree of immunosuppression, reflected by the CD4 count, but also on other specific risk factors associated with each condition.

Although cART can help restore immunity and prevent opportunistic infections, those not taking ART, not adherent to ART, failing ART, or not optimally responding to ART may present with upper GI complaints and CD4 counts <200 cells/mm^3 [12]. Among these patients, upper endoscopy is diagnostic in about 75% of cases [13]. Opportunistic infections are likely involved and should be ruled out. *Candida* esophagitis caused by *Candida albicans* is the most common. (See Chapter 15 on oropharyngeal candidiasis.) At endoscopy, the typical appearance of the esophagus is hyperemic with yellow-white mucosal plaques that, when removed, uncover a friable mucosa. For *Candida* esophagitis, upper endoscopy with biopsy and culture is the diagnostic method of choice, although when presentation is highly suggestive of it, antifungal therapy can be attempted first [14]. Oral fluconazole is the drug of choice [15], but intravenous (IV) fluconazole can be used as needed. Other azoles (itraconazole, ketoconazole, posaconazole, voriconazole) and echinocandins (caspofungin, micafungin, anidulafungin) are also effective against *Candida* and can be used in certain cases [14]. Advanced immunosuppression, especially with CD4 counts <50 cells/mm^3, increases the risk of developing refractory candidiasis that has a poor prognosis [16]. Refractory candidiasis is usually defined as mucosal candidiasis that fails to resolve despite 7–14 days of daily fluconazole ($\geq$200 mg daily). Long-term exposure to azole antifungal agents also predisposes to selection of fluconazole-resistant *Candida* strains, such as *C. glabrata* and *C. krusei*, although most cases of refractory candidiasis are caused by *C. albicans* with high minimal inhibitory concentrations (MIC) to fluconazole [16]. Esophageal candidiasis should also be suspected when other risk factors are present whether the CD4 count is above or below 200 cells/mm^3. These risk factors include acute HIV infection, use of broad-spectrum antibiotics, corticosteroids, diabetes mellitus, and immunosuppression due to leukemia, lymphoma, transplantation, or antineoplastic agents. Primary and secondary (except when recurrences are frequent or severe) prophylaxis of mucosal candidiasis disease are not recommended because of the low mortality of the disease, effectiveness of therapy in the acute setting, and the risk for development of antifungal resistance [14].

When the CD4 count decreases <100 cells/mm^3, other pathogens are found alone or, most commonly, in association with candidiasis such as HSV and, as immunosuppression further increases, CMV, mycobacterial infections, and other opportunistic pathogens, at a lesser frequency (Fig. 18.1A). Symptoms from HSV and CMV esophagitis are similar to candidiasis. Dysphagia, odynophagia, nausea, fever, and epigastric pain are the most common presenting symptoms. The diagnosis of HSV esophagitis is made at upper endoscopy. Classically, multiple small superficial ulcers with or without vesicles are seen in the distal third of the esophagus (Fig. 18.1B) [17]. Recovery of the virus in culture is diagnostic, although typical herpetic lesions can be seen on biopsy as well. Although HSV-1 is found in the majority of cases, HSV-2 has been reported [17]. Acyclovir, oral, or IV is the usual treatment. CMV esophagitis is also diagnosed at upper endoscopy. Unique or multiple large, shallow ulcers in the middle or distal esophagus are seen (Fig. 18.1C) [18]. Culture is neither sensitive nor specific. Definitive diagnosis is made by (1) histopathology showing large intranuclear inclusions with an owl-eye appearance (Fig. 18.1D) and (2) positive immunohistochemical or direct fluorescent staining techniques for CMV. Treatment is oral valganciclovir or IV ganciclovir. Kaposi's sarcoma (KS), caused by human herpesvirus type 8 (HHV-8), is more common at CD4 counts <200 cells/mm^3, but can occur at any CD4 count. Treatment of esophagitis in the HIV immunosuppressed patient should also include timely instituted cART. Guidelines for prevention and treatment of specific opportunistic infections in HIV-infected patients are available [14]. Idiopathic (aphthous) ulcerations of the esophagus are found in approximately 5% of patients with AIDS and esophagitis [19]. Thalidomide and corticosteroids have been used to treat these [20]. HIV-infected patients without immunosuppression presenting with upper GI complaints can be evaluated the same way as immunocompetent hosts.

GASTRIC DISORDERS

The most common gastric disorders diagnosed in HIV patients are similar to those seen in non-HIV-infected patients although opportunistic infections must be considered, especially in those with lower CD4 counts. *Helicobacter pylori* infections are often identified in HIV-infected patients and can lead to gastritis and gastroduodenal ulcers in these patients, similar to the general population. *Helicobacter pylori*

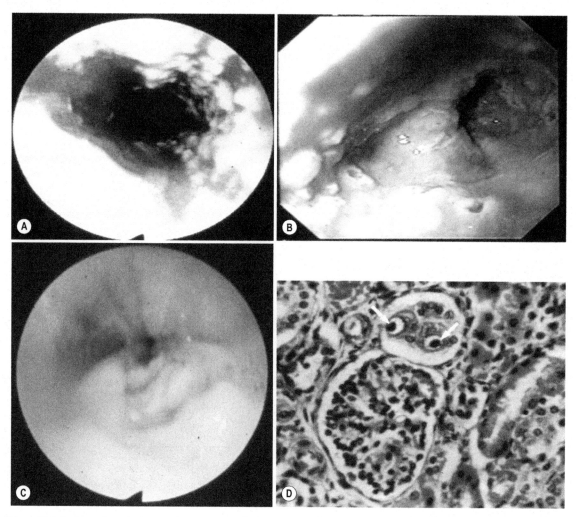

Figure 18.1 Endoscopic and microscopic appearance of opportunistic infections of the lower GI tract. (A) Cytomegalovirus (CMV) in association with *candida* esophagitis. (B) Herpes simplex virus (HSV) esophagitis with classic HSV vesicles. (C) CMV esophageal ulcer. (D) CMV inclusion bodies or owl's eye appearance of CMV ulcer biopsy demonstrated by arrows.

is a small, microaerophilic, curved rod that has the ability to live and multiply in the acid gastric milieu, establishing colonization or infection. Data on incidence of *H. pylori* infections among HIV-infected patients compared to the general population are conflicting, but it seems that patients with AIDS have a lower incidence than HIV-infected patients without AIDS or HIV-uninfected patients [21]. The cause for this is unknown. It may be explained by repetitive antibiotic treatments in AIDS patients and widespread use of antacids medications for upper GI symptoms [22]. *Helicobacter pylori* is usually diagnosed by serology, urea breath testing, stool antigen detection, or endoscopy with biopsy specimens that allows for microscopic examination, urease

detection, and culture. In a recent report of upper GI endoscopic findings in the cART era, *H. pylori* infections were identified in 40% of endoscopic biopsies and were more frequent than during the pre-ART era (11%) [11]. The two main indications for performing an endoscopy were abdominal discomfort (31%), and reflux symptoms (16%). The clinical presentation and treatment options for *H. pylori* infection do not differ from those for HIV-uninfected patients [21]. However, careful attention must be paid when choosing treatment regimens because of potential drug–drug interactions (DDIs) between proton pump inhibitors (PPIs) and certain antiretrovirals, mostly the protease inhibitor (PI) atazanavir (see Table 18.1).

Table 18.1 Preferred and alternative initial therapies of *Helicobacter pylori* infection,[a] treatment duration, eradication rate, and potential for drug–drug interactions (DDIs) with ART

REGIMEN [23]	DURATION	ERADICATION RATE	POTENTIAL FOR DDIs [24]
Preferred initial therapy[b]			
Not penicillin-allergic			
(1) Proton pump inhibitor (PPI)[c] + (2) Clarithromycin 500 mg twice daily + (3) Amoxicillin 1 g twice daily	7–14 days	70–85%	Atazanavir (ATZ) has pH-dependent absorption and is both a substrate + inhibitor of CYP3A. Co-administration with a PPI may result in loss of therapeutic effect of ATZ and emergence of ATZ resistance. *Co-administration is not recommended*
Penicillin-allergic			
(1) PPI[c] + (2) Clarithromycin 500 mg twice daily + (3) Metronidazole 500 mg twice daily	7–14 days	70–85%	Clarithromycin can increase plasma levels of delavirdine
Alternative initial therapy[d]			
(1) PPI[c] + (2) Bismuth sub-salicylate 525 mg 4 times daily + (3) Metronidazole 250 mg 4 times daily + (4) Tetracycline 500 mg 4 times daily	10–14 days	75–90%	Indinavir, saquinavir, and delavirdine have acidic pH-dependent absorption and can raise gastric pH. Spacing of PPIs with these medications and ritonavir boosting are recommended to overcome the potential interaction
OR			
(1) PPI[c] + (2) Bismuth sub-citrate 420 mg 4 times daily + (3) Metronidazole 375 mg 4 times daily + (4) Tetracycline 375 mg 4 times daily	10–14 days	75–90%	

[a]Recommendations for HIV-infected patients do not differ from HIV-uninfected patients [23].
[b]For patients who have not recently or repeatedly received macrolide and/or metronidazole treatment.
[c]Lanzoprazole 30 mg twice daily, omeprazole 20 mg twice daily, pantoprazole 40 mg twice daily, rabeprazole 20 mg twice daily, or esomeprazole 40 mg daily.
[d]For patients from areas of high prevalence (>20%) of resistance to clarithromycin or metronidazole, or with recent exposure to clarithromycin or metronidazole.

Upper GI illnesses in patients with HIV-related immunodeficiency may be caused by opportunistic infections or neoplasms. CMV may cause erosive gastritis with or without aphthous ulcerations, and solitary superficial and deep ulcerations that may be associated with esophageal involvement [25]. Since CMV usually arises in deeply immunosuppressed patients (CD4 T cell count <50 cells/mm^3), concomitant opportunistic pathogens such as *Candida* species and HSV may be present. Other rare gastric infections that have been reported in HIV-infected patients include cryptosporidiosis, histoplasmosis, cryptococcosis, leishmaniasis, toxoplasmosis, syphilis, bacillary angiomatosis, schistosomiasis, and strongyloidosis. The incidence of KS and non-Hodgkin lymphoma (NHL), two of the three AIDS-defining malignancies, has declined significantly in the post-cART era [26]. KS, caused by HHV-8, may affect any part of the GI tract with or without concurrent mucocutaneous involvement.

Gastric KS is rarely symptomatic but can present with abdominal discomfort, nausea, vomiting, and dyspepsia. Rare severe complications such as bleeding and perforation can occur [27]. At endoscopy, KS typically appears as red or purple, small submucosal vascular nodules without ulceration. The mainstay of treatment in patients with HIV is cART for restoring immunity. Additional treatment options include local treatment for bleeding lesions and systemic chemotherapy. The stomach is the more common site of gastrointestinal NHL. Diagnosis and treatment are similar to those for HIV-uninfected patients.

DIARRHEA

Since the beginning of the HIV epidemic, chronic diarrhea has been one of the signature manifestations of advanced HIV infection and AIDS. In developing countries, diarrhea is often due to opportunistic infections in patients with decreased immunity and remains a major cause of malnutrition, wasting syndrome, and mortality [28, 29]. In developed countries in which patients have wide access to cART and therefore live longer, the incidence of opportunistic infections is less, although the incidence of chronic diarrhea has remained stable, reflecting a change in underlying causes [30]. In these patients with a partially reconstituted immune system due to cART, diarrhea is still a common complaint and can lead to significant discomfort. ART (mostly PI)-associated diarrhea, and causes of diarrhea seen in HIV-uninfected patients, including *Clostridium difficile*-associated diarrhea, are predominant in this patient population [31, 32].

Diarrhea can be acute or chronic. Acute diarrhea is defined as the occurrence of at least three loose or watery stools daily for 3 days and up to 2 weeks. Chronic diarrhea is diagnosed when symptoms have been present for more than 4 weeks [33]. When evaluating a patient with acute or chronic diarrhea, a careful history is essential to help prioritize the differential diagnosis and decide on pertinent diagnostic studies to request. Key elements of the history of diarrhea in HIV-infected patients include the most recent CD4 T cell count, past history of opportunistic infections, past history of diarrheal illnesses, practice of unsafe sex, recent and present antibiotic use, HIV regimen, and adherence to treatment. All other pertinent elements of the questionnaire of patients with diarrhea should also be obtained. Characterization of the diarrhea (volume, duration, frequency) and associated symptoms (nausea, abdominal cramps, bleeding, weight loss, fever, and others) can be helpful for attempting to differentiate small- versus large-bowel disease, but symptoms can easily overlap. Upper abdominal cramping and bloating suggest small-bowel involvement or enteritis; hematochezia, tenesmus, and lower abdominal cramping suggest colonic involvement

(see below). Patients with CD4 T cell counts >200 cells/mm^3 are likely to be diagnosed with diseases similar to those of HIV-uninfected patients unless ART-induced diarrhea is the likely diagnosis. PIs are the ART class most likely to cause diarrhea. The inevitable use of ritonavir for PI boosting contributes to this risk. The two preferred PIs as initial HIV therapy in 2011 according to the DHHS guidelines [34], atazanavir/ritonavir and darunavir/ritonavir, have been reported to cause diarrhea in 3 and 4%, respectively, compared to 10–11% for lopinavir/ritonavir and 13% for fosamprenavir/ritonavir after 1 year of treatment in previously naïve-to-ART patients [35–37]. Causes of diarrhea other than opportunistic infections should also be considered in HIV-infected patients and diagnosed with conventional tests. The most frequent pathogens causing non-opportunistic infectious diarrhea in HIV-infected patients are the bacteria *Salmonella*, *Shigella*, *Campylobacter*, *Yersinia*, *Vibrio*, *E. coli*, *C. difficile*, and others; the viruses rotavirus, Norwalk, and adenovirus; and the parasites *Giardia*, *Entamoeba*, and *Blastocystis*. Antibiograms of isolated bacteria are helpful since resistance to commonly used antibiotics has been described [38]. Salmonellosis, although not considered an opportunistic infection, is about 100 times more frequent in HIV patients than in immunocompetent hosts [39]. Recurrent *Salmonella* bacteremia in an HIV patient establishes a diagnosis of AIDS. Celiac disease, inflammatory bowel disease, diverticulitis, ischemic colitis, appendicitis, and others must also be considered, depending on the clinical presentation.

The degree of immunosuppression, represented by the CD4 T cell count, is one of—if not—the most useful pieces of information when evaluating such patients. Those with CD4 T cell counts <200 cells/mm^3, but mostly those with CD4 T cell counts <100 cells/mm^3, are more likely to be diagnosed with opportunistic infections and special diagnostic studies should be undertaken. See Figure 18.2 for a suggested approach to the HIV-infected patient with diarrhea. In patients with severe immunodeficiency (CD4 T cell <100 cells/mm^3), opportunistic pathogens, such as cryptosporidia (*Cryptosporidium parvum*, *C. hominis*, and others), microsporidia (*Enterocytozoon bieneusi*, *Encephalitozoon intestinalis*, and others), CMV, and mycobacteria (*Mycobacterium avium* complex [MAC] and *M. tuberculosis*) are expected, alone or in combination, and should be ruled out carefully [40, 41]. Studies performed in men who have sex with men (MSM) with AIDS and diarrhea before cART became available identified one or more enteric pathogens in 68–85% of patients [42, 43]. Cryptosporidiosis is diagnosed by microscopic examination of stool samples. It should be specifically requested when stool samples are sent to the laboratory since they can easily be missed during routine stool examinations. Acid-fast staining methods (usually the modified Ziehl–Neelsen stain) can be used. They allow differentiation of the small *Cryptosporidium* oocysts (which stain pink or red) from yeasts and stool debris (which stain green or blue). Immunofluorescent

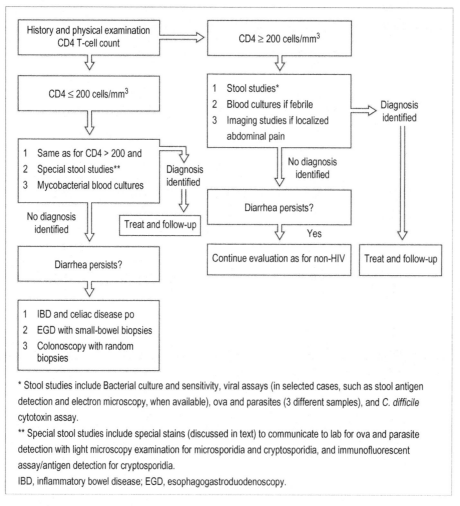

Figure 18.2 Suggested approach to the HIV-infected patient with diarrhea. IBD, Inflammatory bowel disease; EGD, Esophagogastroduodenoscopy; po, by mouth.

assays and antigen-detection assays are also available. *Cryptosporidium* can also be detected with hematoxylin and eosin staining of small intestinal biopsies. Microsporidia can be found in stool samples when special staining methods such as modified trichrome stain (chromotrope 2R) and calcofluor white are used. Small intestinal biopsies stained with these two techniques, Giemsa, hematoxylin and eosin, and other methods can make the diagnosis. Electron microscopy is used to identify microsporidia at the species level. The two other protozoa, *Isospora belli* and *Cyclospora cayetanensis*, can be detected with the modified Ziehl–Neelsen stain (which appears red) and both are autofluorescent blue under ultraviolet fluorescence microscopy. When stool samples are repeatedly negative and diarrhea persists, upper endoscopy and colonoscopy with random biopsies of small intestine and colon are recommended.

The yield of upper endoscopy in HIV patients with chronic diarrhea is between 11 and 36%, with cryptosporidia and microsporidia being the most frequently identified pathogens [44]. For colonoscopy, the yield is 27–42%, with CMV being the most common diagnosis [44]. MAC can infect the small bowel of severely immunosuppressed patients (usually with CD4 count < 50 cells/mm^3) and results in disseminated disease. Patients can present with malabsorptive diarrhea, abdominal pain, fever, night sweats, and weight loss. Mycobacterial blood cultures are helpful for diagnosing disseminated disease. Blood cultures are positive in approximately 90% of patients with disseminated disease and were as high as 99% when two specimens were taken in one study [45]. Endoscopy with small-bowel biopsy and acid-fast staining can identify MAC, which can also grow in appropriate media.

Acute and chronic diarrhea can come from the small intestine, large intestine, or both, respectively referred to as enteritis, colitis, and enterocolitis. The main symptoms of enteritis are bloating, abdominal cramps, and profuse diarrhea (>2 L/day) associated with dehydration and malabsorption, leading to weight loss. Protozoa are the most common pathogens causing enteritis in these patients. Cryptosporidia (mostly *C. parvum*) and microsporidia (mostly *Enterocytozoon bieneusi* and *Encephalitozoon intestinalis*) are most frequently isolated in immunosuppressed patients. Other common infectious pathogens of the small intestine are the bacteria *Shigella*, *Salmonella*, *Campylobacter*, *E. coli*, *Yersinia*, and *Vibrio*; the parasites *Giardia lamblia*, *Entamoeba histolytica*, *Isospora belli*, and *Cyclospora cayetanensis*; the mycobacteria MAC and *M. tuberculosis*; and the viruses CMV, herpes simplex, and HHV-8 presenting as KS. Rare agents of enteritis include, but are not limited to, *Pneumocystis jiroveci*, *Candida* sp., *Paracoccidiodes braziliense*, *Mucor* sp., *Histoplasma capsulatum*, *Treponema pallidum*, and *Schistosoma* sp. Noninfectious causes of enteritis, such as diverticulitis, ischemic enteritis, appendicitis, sarcoidosis, lymphoma, and carcinoma, should be included in the differential diagnosis. In addition, idiopathic AIDS enteropathy, profuse diarrhea associated with malnutrition and wasting without an infectious pathogen identified, has been recognized in HIV/AIDS patients, and is a diagnosis of exclusion. Viral pathogens, including HIV itself, and associated inflammatory and immunological responses, are potentially involved in the pathogenesis [46].

Symptoms suggestive of colitis are lower abdominal cramps, frequent small loose stools, rectal bleeding, and tenesmus. CMV colitis in patients with AIDS may lead to profuse watery diarrhea, abdominal pain, fever, and bloody diarrhea. Before effective cART was available, CMV colitis was a frequent cause of diarrhea. In immunosuppressed patients in whom a cause for diarrhea is identified on colonic biopsies, CMV is still one of the most frequently encountered pathogens [47, 48]. The typical colonoscopic finding in patients with CMV colitis is distal patchy colitis with ulcerations (Figs 18.3A and 18.3B) [49]. In a study of 56 HIV/AIDS patients with CMV colitis, colonoscopy showed colitis associated with ulcers in 39% of patients, ulceration alone in 38%, and colitis alone in 21%. Subepithelial hemorrhage was frequent [49]. Ulcerations at colonoscopy combined with the typical CMV inclusion bodies or owl-eye appearance at microscopic examination of colonic biopsies signal the diagnosis of CMV colitis. CMV can also be cultured, but a positive culture alone is not diagnostic. Treatment is usually with IV ganciclovir or IV foscarnet, although oral valganciclovir can be administered [14, 50, 51]. *Clostridium difficile* is associated with antibiotic use, although it can present in the absence of such history. The absence of recent antibiotic use in the history of a patient with HIV and diarrhea should not be a reason for excluding *C. difficile*-associated diarrhea. In one study, *C. difficile*

was the most commonly recognized cause of bacterial diarrhea in HIV patients, accounting for 4.1 cases per 1000 persons-years [31]. Diagnosis is typically made, similarly to HIV-uninfected patients, by the detection of *C. difficile* cytotoxins in stools or at colonoscopy by demonstration of colitis with pseudomembranes (Fig. 18.3C). Treatment is similar to that of HIV-uninfected patients; however, the incidence of metronidazole-resistant *C. difficile* seems anecdotally to be increasing and, often, treatment will require combination treatment with both metronidazole and oral vancomycin. Non-infectious colon diseases such as diverticulitis, inflammatory bowel disease, and cancer must also be part of the differential diagnosis, as appropriate.

Treatment of diarrhea in HIV-infected patients depends on the underlying cause. Adequate fluid and electrolyte support is given to dehydrated patients; nutritional supplements and symptomatic treatment of diarrhea with antimotility agents are often needed. Restoration of the immune system with effective cART is the mainstay of treatment in patients with diarrhea due to opportunistic infections, especially in patients with cryptosporidia and microsporidia for which truly effective targeted therapies are not available. For cryptosporidia, nitazoxanide in conjunction with cART has shown some benefit [52]. No effective targeted therapy is available for *E. bieneusi*; *E. intestinalis* may respond to albendazole [53, 54]. TMP-SMX is effective against *Isospora belli* and *Cyclospora cayetanensis*. A lifelong suppressive therapy is usually recommended in patients with AIDS due to the high recurrence rates. Comprehensive reviews of treatment of opportunistic infections, including treatment of CMV and mycobacterial infections, have been published recently [14, 46].

ANORECTAL DISORDERS

Anorectal disorders are an important component of HIV GI care, especially in HIV MSM. The incidence of anorectal pathologies has been affected by cART [55]. Anorectal pathologies seen in HIV patients are diverse and include anal fissures, fistulae, perirectal abscesses, ulcerations, proctitis, and cancer. Human papillomavirus (HPV) infects anal epithelia in men and women similarly to cervical epithelia in women. Infections with oncogenic HPV genotypes (mostly HPV-16 and HPV-18) can lead to anal condyloma, anal squamous intraepithelial lesions (SIL), and anal squamous carcinoma [56]. Abnormal anal Papanicolaou smears are a common finding in men with AIDS (39% in one study) and are significantly associated with lower CD4 T cell counts [57]. Indeed, the incidence of high-grade anal intraepithelial neoplasia (AIN), the likely anal cancer precursor lesion, and the incidence of anal cancer are higher in patients with HIV/AIDS than in HIV-uninfected patients

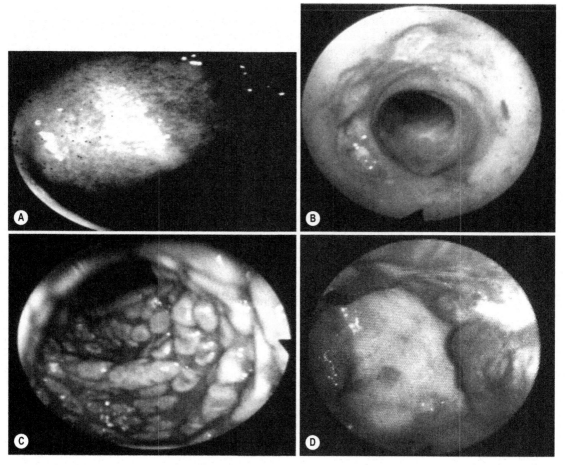

Figure 18.3 Endoscopic appearance of opportunistic infections of the lower GI tract. (A) Cytomegalovirus (CMV) patchy colitis. (B) CMV ulcers of colon mucosa. (C) *Clostridium difficile* colitis with pseudomembranes. (D) Raised red, confluent lesions of Kaposi's sarcoma (KS) of the rectum.

[58]. Although no recommendations exist for routine anal cytology screening of HIV-infected patients in 2011, some experts recommend routine anal cytology in HIV-infected MSM [14]. The quadrivalent HPV vaccine Gardasil is now approved by the FDA for use in both women and men aged 9 to 26 years, but data on safety and efficacy in HIV-infected patients, especially HIV-infected MSM, are not yet available. Proctitis is one of the possible clinical presentations of sexually transmitted infections, usually associated with unprotected anal intercourse. Purulent anal discharge, tenesmus, and rectal pain are the classical symptoms. The pathogens usually involved are *Neisseria gonorrhoeae*, *Chlamydia trachomatis*, herpes simplex, *Treponema pallidum*, and CMV. *Chlamydia trachomatis* serovars L1, L2, or L3, causing lymphogranuloma venereum (LGV), can lead to severe proctitis [59]. Diagnosis and treatments are similar to those for HIV-uninfected patients. The rectum can also be the site of opportunistic infections. HSV and

CMV infections, as described with esophagitis and colitis, can cause perianal and rectal ulcerations, with associated pain, tenesmus, and bleeding. Endoscopy can also reveal KS that typically appears as red or purple submucosal vascular nodules, similar to its appearance in the upper GI tract (Fig. 18.3D).

CONCLUSION

The role of the GI tract in HIV has changed dramatically over the 30+ years of the HIV epidemic. In the early days it served as the portal of entry, and the major infected organ system. The huge advances in ART of the past three decades have changed our perspective on the GI tract in HIV patients. In developed countries, we rarely see patients with low CD4 counts and opportunistic infections, except in liver and kidney transplant recipients with HIV. That prospect was totally inconceivable at the beginning of the epidemic. We see the diseases of the aging GI tract in our aging HIV population, like Barrett's esophagus and *C. difficile* infections, either with or without prior antibiotic treatment, probably due to alterations in normal colonic flora. As new research sheds light on the GALT and the importance of the gut immune system, the GI tract is assuming a more important role in the pathogenesis of HIV again.

REFERENCES

[1] Mehandru S, Poles MA, Tenner-Racz K, et al. Primary HIV-1 infection is associated with preferential depletion of CD4$^+$ T lymphocytes from effector sites in the gastrointestinal tract. J Exp Med 2004;200 (6):761–70.

[2] Brenchley JM, Schacker TW, Ruff LE, et al. CD4+ T cell depletion during all stages of HIV disease occurs predominantly in the gastrointestinal tract. J Exp Med 2004;200(6):749–59.

[3] Poles MA, Boscardin WJ, Elliott J, et al. Lack of decay of HIV-1 in gut-associated lymphoid tissue reservoirs in maximally suppressed individuals. J Acquir Immune Defic Syndr 2006;43(1):65–8.

[4] Mehandru S, Poles MA, Tenner-Racz K, et al. Lack of mucosal immune reconstitution during prolonged treatment of acute and early HIV-1 infection. PLoS Med 2006;3(12):e484.

[5] Guadalupe M, Reay E, Sankaran S, et al. Severe CD4+ T cell depletion in gut lymphoid tissue during primary human immunodeficiency virus type 1 infection and substantial delay in restoration following highly active antiretroviral therapy. J Virol 2003;77(21):11708–17.

[6] Brenchley JM, Price DA, Schacker TW, et al. Microbial translocation is a cause of systemic immune activation in chronic HIV infection. Nat Med 2006;12 (12):1365–71.

[7] Gardiner KR, Halliday MI, Barclay GR, et al. Significance of systemic endotoxaemia in inflammatory bowel disease. Gut 1995;36(6):897–901.

[8] Kamat A, Ancuta P, Blumberg RS, Gabuzda D. Serological markers for inflammatory bowel disease in AIDS patients with evidence of microbial translocation. PLoS One 2010;5(11):e15533.

[9] Monkemuller KE, Call SA, Lazenby AJ, Wilcox CM. Declining prevalence of opportunistic gastrointestinal disease in the era of combination antiretroviral therapy. Am J Gastroenterol 2000;95 (2):457–62.

[10] Wilcox CM, Saag MS. Gastrointestinal complications of HIV infection: changing priorities in the HAART era. Gut 2008;57 (6):861–70.

[11] Nkuize M, De Wit S, Muls V, et al. Upper gastrointestinal endoscopic findings in the era of highly active antiretroviral therapy. HIV Med 2010;11(6):412–17.

[12] Monkemuller KE, Lazenby AJ, Lee DH, et al. Occurrence of gastrointestinal opportunistic disorders in AIDS despite the use of highly active antiretroviral therapy. Dig Dis Sci 2005;50(2):230–4.

[13] Bashir RM, Wilcox CM. Symptom-specific use of upper gastrointestinal endoscopy in human immunodeficiency virus-infected patients yields high dividends. J Clin Gastroenterol 1996;23(4):292–8.

[14] Centers for Disease Control and Prevention. Guidelines for prevention and treatment of opportunistic infections in HIV-infected adults and adolescents. MMWR 2009;58(No. RR-4):84–91.

[15] Pappas PG, Rex JH, Sobel JD, et al. Guidelines for treatment of candidiasis. Clin Infect Dis 2004;38 (2):161–89.

[16] Fichtenbaum CJ, Koletar S, Yiannoutsos C, et al. Refractory mucosal candidiasis in advanced human immunodeficiency virus infection. Clin Infect Dis 2000;30 (5):749–56.

[17] Genereau T, Lortholary O, Bouchaud O, et al. Herpes simplex esophagitis in patients with AIDS: report of 34 cases. The Cooperative Study Group on Herpetic Esophagitis in HIV Infection. Clin Infect Dis 1996;22(6):926–31.

[18] Wilcox CM, Diehl DL, Cello JP, et al. Cytomegalovirus esophagitis in patients with AIDS. A clinical, endoscopic, and pathologic correlation. Ann Intern Med 1990;113(8):589–93.

[19] Bonacini M, Young T, Laine L. The causes of esophageal symptoms in human immunodeficiency virus infection. A prospective study of 110 patients. Arch Intern Med 1991;151 (8):1567–72.

[20] Johnson L, Jarvis JN, Wilkins EG, Hay PE. Thalidomide treatment for refractory HIV-associated colitis: a case series. Clin Infect Dis 2008;47 (1):133–6.

[21] Romanelli F, Smith KM, Murphy BS. Does HIV infection alter the incidence or pathology of *Helicobacter pylori* infection? AIDS Patient Care STDS 2007;21(12):908–19.

[22] Logan RP, Polson RJ, Rao G, et al. *Helicobacter pylori* and HIV infection. Lancet 1990;335(8703):1456.

[23] Chey WD, Wong BC, Practice Parameters Committee of the American College of Gastroenterology. American College of Gastroenterology guideline on the management of *Helicobacter pylori* infection. Am J Gastroenterol 2007;102(8):1808–25.

[24] McCabe SM, Smith PF, Ma Q, Morse GD. Drug interactions between proton pump inhibitors and antiretroviral drugs. Expert Opin Drug Metab Toxicol 2007;3 (2):197–207.

[25] Farman J, Lerner ME, Ng C, et al. Cytomegalovirus gastritis: protean radiologic features. Gastrointest Radiol 1992;17(3):202–6.

[26] Engels EA, Biggar RJ, Hall HI, et al. Cancer risk in people infected with human immunodeficiency virus in

the United States. Int J Cancer 2008;123(1):187–94.

[27] Friedman SL. Gastrointestinal and hepatobiliary neoplasms in AIDS. Gastroenterol Clin North Am 1988;17(3):465–86.

[28] Lawn SD, Harries AD, Anglaret X, et al. Early mortality among adults accessing antiretroviral treatment programmes in sub-Saharan Africa. AIDS 2008;22(15):1897–908.

[29] Dillingham RA, Pinkerton R, Leger P, et al. High early mortality in patients with chronic acquired immunodeficiency syndrome diarrhea initiating antiretroviral therapy in Haiti: a case-control study. Am J Trop Med Hyg 2009;80(6):1060–4.

[30] Call SA, Heudebert G, Saag M, Wilcox CM. The changing etiology of chronic diarrhea in HIV-infected patients with CD4 cell counts less than 200 cells/mm³. Am J Gastroenterol 2000;95(11):3142–6.

[31] Sanchez TH, Brooks JT, Sullivan PS, et al. Bacterial diarrhea in persons with HIV infection, United States, 1992–2002. Clin Infect Dis 2005;41(11):1621–7.

[32] Guest JL, Ruffin C, Tschampa JM, et al. Differences in rates of diarrhea in patients with human immunodeficiency virus receiving lopinavir-ritonavir or nelfinavir. Pharmacotherapy 2004;24(6):727–35.

[33] Beatty GW. Diarrhea in patients infected with HIV presenting to the emergency department. Emerg Med Clin North Am 2010;28(2):299–310.

[34] Panel on Antiretroviral Guidelines for Adults and Adolescents. Guidelines for the use of antiretroviral agents in HIV-1-infected adults and adolescents. Department of Health and Human Services. January 10, 2011. pp. 1–166. Available at http://www.aidsinfo.nih.gov/ContentFiles/AdultandAdolescentGL.pdf.

[35] Molina JM, Andrade-Villanueva J, Echevarria J, et al. Once-daily atazanavir/ritonavir versus twice-daily lopinavir/ritonavir, each in combination with tenofovir and emtricitabine, for management of antiretroviral-naive HIV-1-infected patients: 48 week efficacy

and safety results of the CASTLE study. Lancet 2008;372(9639):646–55.

[36] Ortiz R, Dejesus E, Khanlou H, et al. Efficacy and safety of once-daily darunavir/ritonavir versus lopinavir/ritonavir in treatment-naive HIV-1-infected patients at week 48. AIDS 2008;22(12):1389–97.

[37] Eron Jr J, Yeni P, Gathe Jr J, et al. The KLEAN study of fosamprenavir-ritonavir versus lopinavir-ritonavir, each in combination with abacavir-lamivudine, for initial treatment of HIV infection over 48 weeks: a randomised non-inferiority trial. Lancet 2006;368(9534):476–82.

[38] Ko WC, Yan JJ, Yu WL, et al. A new therapeutic challenge for old pathogens: community-acquired invasive infections caused by ceftriaxone- and ciprofloxacin-resistant Salmonella enterica serotype Choleraesuis. Clin Infect Dis 2005;40(2):315–18.

[39] Hsu RB, Tsay YG, Chen RJ, Chu SH. Risk factors for primary bacteremia and endovascular infection in patients without acquired immunodeficiency syndrome who have nontyphoid salmonellosis. Clin Infect Dis 2003;36(7):829–34.

[40] Datta D, Gazzard B, Stebbing J. The diagnostic yield of stool analysis in 525 HIV-1-infected individuals. AIDS 2003;17(11):1711–13.

[41] Weber R, Ledergerber B, Zbinden R, et al. Enteric infections and diarrhea in human immunodeficiency virus-infected persons: prospective community-based cohort study. Swiss HIV Cohort Study. Arch Intern Med 1999;159(13):1473–80.

[42] Smith PD, Lane HC, Gill VJ, et al. Intestinal infections in patients with the acquired immunodeficiency syndrome (AIDS). Etiology and response to therapy. Ann Intern Med 1988;108(3):328–33.

[43] Laughon BE, Druckman DA, Vernon A, et al. Prevalence of enteric pathogens in homosexual men with and without acquired immunodeficiency syndrome. Gastroenterology 1988;94(4):984–93.

[44] Wilcox CM. Etiology and evaluation of diarrhea in AIDS: a global perspective at the millennium. World J Gastroenterol 2000;6(2):177–86.

[45] Stone BL, Cohn DL, Kane MS, et al. Utility of paired blood cultures and smears in diagnosis of disseminated Mycobacterium avium complex infections in AIDS patients. J Clin Microbiol 1994;32(3):841–2.

[46] Cello JP, Day LW. Idiopathic AIDS enteropathy and treatment of gastrointestinal opportunistic pathogens. Gastroenterology 2009;136(6):1952–65.

[47] Huppmann AR, Orenstein JM. Opportunistic disorders of the gastrointestinal tract in the age of highly active antiretroviral therapy. Hum Pathol 2010;41(12):1777–87.

[48] Orenstein JM, Dieterich DT. The histopathology of 103 consecutive colonoscopy biopsies from 82 symptomatic patients with acquired immunodeficiency syndrome: original and look-back diagnoses. Arch Pathol Lab Med 2001;125(8):1042–6.

[49] Wilcox CM, Chalasani N, Lazenby A, Schwartz DA. Cytomegalovirus colitis in acquired immunodeficiency syndrome: a clinical and endoscopic study. Gastrointest Endosc 1998;48(1):39–43.

[50] Dieterich DT, Kotler DP, Busch DF, et al. Ganciclovir treatment of cytomegalovirus colitis in AIDS: a randomized, double-blind, placebo-controlled multicenter study. J Infect Dis 1993;167(2):278–82.

[51] Dieterich DT, Poles MA, Dicker M, et al. Foscarnet treatment of cytomegalovirus gastrointestinal infections in acquired immunodeficiency syndrome patients who have failed ganciclovir induction. Am J Gastroenterol 1993;88(4):542–8.

[52] Rossignol JF, Hidalgo H, Feregrino M, et al. A double-'blind' placebo-controlled study of nitazoxanide in the treatment of cryptosporidial diarrhoea in AIDS patients in Mexico. Trans R

Soc Trop Med Hyg 1998;92 (6):663–6.

[53] Dieterich DT, Lew EA, Kotler DP, et al. Treatment with albendazole for intestinal disease due to *Enterocytozoon bieneusi* in patients with AIDS. J Infect Dis 1994;169 (1):178–83.

[54] Molina JM, Chastang C, Goguel J, et al. Albendazole for treatment and prophylaxis of microsporidiosis due to *Encephalitozoon intestinalis* in patients with AIDS: a randomized double-blind controlled trial. J Infect Dis 1998;177(5):1373–7.

[55] Gonzalez-Ruiz C, Heartfield W, Briggs B, et al. Anorectal pathology in HIV/AIDS-infected patients has not been impacted by highly active antiretroviral therapy. Dis Colon Rectum 2004;47 (9):1483–6.

[56] Zbar AP, Fenger C, Efron J, et al. The pathology and molecular biology of anal intraepithelial neoplasia: comparisons with cervical and vulvar intraepithelial carcinoma. Int J Colorectal Dis 2002;17(4):203–15.

[57] Palefsky JM, Gonzales J, Greenblatt RM, et al. Anal intraepithelial neoplasia and anal papillomavirus infection among homosexual males with group IV HIV disease. JAMA 1990;263 (21):2911–16.

[58] Chiao EY, Giordano TP, Palefsky JM, et al. Screening HIV-infected individuals for anal cancer precursor lesions: a systematic review. Clin Infect Dis 2006;43(2): 223–33.

[59] Quinn TC, Goodell SE, Mkrtichian E, et al. *Chlamydia trachomatis* proctitis. N Engl J Med 1981;305(4):195–200.

Chapter | 19 |

Primary neurological manifestation of HIV/AIDS

David B. Clifford, Mengesha A. Teshome

INTRODUCTION

In the past 30 years we have learned much about the biology and treatment of human immunodeficiency virus (HIV). Emphasis on prevention and a laudable global effort to increase access to treatment are encouraging developments. In 2010, UNAIDS reported declining new HIV infections in many countries most affected by the epidemic. Between 2001 and 2009, HIV incidence fell by more than 25% in 33 countries, 22 of which were in sub-Saharan Africa. Countries that were most affected in sub-Saharan Africa—Ethiopia, Nigeria, South Africa, Zambia, and Zimbabwe—have either stabilized or are showing signs of decline. Unfortunately, in 7 countries, 5 of them in Europe and Central Asia, HIV incidence increased by more than 25%. However, realizing that 33.3 million people live with HIV, HIV remains a major health challenge, particularly in sub-Saharan Africa where 22.5 million (68% of the global total) live.

Neurological complications of HIV infection continue to cause significant morbidity. Reports from a growing number of countries confirm tragic persistence of cognitive and neuropathic complications of HIV. Our descriptions in this chapter are often based on more detailed observations made in the Western world. However, reports from the developing world are increasingly replicating the experience from the West, suggesting that neurological conditions are important throughout the global epidemic. While no firm evidence contradicts this expectation, the importance of viral and host genetics in determining disease manifestations is undeniable, as is knowledge that these factors are different in various parts of the world. It is also certain that co-infections influence the course of HIV disease, and these are well known to differ in the developing world, again

providing factors that may well alter the natural history of HIV neurological disease.

NeuroAIDS issues may be considered as primary complications, including conditions that are in some way the direct consequence of the HIV infection, or secondary complications (Box 19.1). The primary complications include a spectrum of HIV-associated neurocognitive disorders (HAND), HIV-associated myelopathy, and HIV-associated peripheral neuropathy. Secondary complications result as a consequence of the immunodeficient state of the host (Box 19.1). Neurological infections that fall into this category include cryptococcal meningitis, toxoplasmic encephalitis, cytomegalovirus encephalitis and radiculomyelitis, progressive multifocal leukoencephalopathy, and varicella zoster complications. This chapter will focus on the primary neuroAIDS complications while many of the secondary complications are described elsewhere in the text.

The frequency of neurological complications has changed as the epidemic has evolved, being profoundly impacted by therapeutic practices and perhaps by varying underlying risks in various affected populations. Both the primary HIV-associated complications and the secondary complications occur more frequently in advanced stages of HIV, when the immune system is most impaired. HIV-associated dementia (HAD), HIV-associated myelopathy, and peripheral neuropathy all are seen most commonly after the CD4 count drops below 200 cells/mm^3. Often primary neurological manifestations are not noticed when early development of opportunistic illnesses supervene, masking the anticipated course of disease progression. As more subjects in developing countries are managed to prevent and treat secondary complications we anticipate a rapid emergence of clinical recognition of primary HIV-associated neurological complications. Furthermore, with more successful HIV therapy, most patients retain a higher level of immunity and live longer, resulting in an actual increase in the prevalence of HAND in populations of long-term survivors.

Diagnostic rules in the setting of HIV deserve some special cautions. While in most fields of medicine, a single disease should be sought to understand most patients' complaints. In AIDS, neurological complications often are superimposed on an ongoing process with a different etiology. Drug toxicity may add other facets to neurological conditions. Clinical features often reflect the sum of deficits from multiple pathophysiologic perturbations. In addition, AIDS patients are susceptible to the same neurological diseases as patients who do not have HIV infection and thus the clinician must not always leap to unusual diagnoses in the setting of HIV disease, considering as well conditions common in the immunocompetent population.

EPIDEMIOLOGY

Neurological complications of HIV infection are common manifestations of the AIDS illness [1]. Pre-combination antiretroviral therapy (cART) era investigations documented that two-thirds of patients with AIDS developed HAD. Although, after successful introduction of antiretroviral therapy, the incidence of frank dementia declined significantly, milder cognitive difficulties and HIV-associated peripheral neuropathies have persisted. The CNS HIV Antiretroviral Therapy Effects Research (CHARTER) study, a multicenter NIH study, evaluated over 1,500 HIV-infected individuals in the USA and found 53% had cognitive impairment [2].

The risk of impairment was higher in those with co-morbidities. The same study also found evidence of peripheral neuropathy in more than half of the subjects. Early studies in Uganda support the prevalence of neurologic impairment in less developed settings [3]. A recent report found HAND in 23.5% of HIV-infected patients seen at HIV care centers in South Africa [4].

PATHOPHYSIOLOGY, PATHOGENESIS, AND GENETICS

Primary HIV-associated complications result from infection in the nervous system, and respond to antiretroviral therapy. The mechanism by which HIV infection leads to HAD is likely multifactorial. HIV enters the brain and CSF almost immediately after systemic infection, probably via HIV-infected monocytes, which then differentiate into macrophages. The virus can be recovered from the nervous system throughout the illness. However, productive infection is almost exclusively localized in monocytes and macrophages and mainly occurs late in the disease. Neurons are rarely if ever infected, and astroglial cells, while they may be infected, do not seem to support replication. The consequences of astroglial infection remain uncertain. However, recent research supports an association of HAD with astrocyte infection, suggesting that these cells controlling the environment in the brain could be critical and require further study [5]. It seems likely that much of the pathological consequence of the HIV infection in the brain is driven by immune response to infection rather than directly correlated to the viral load in the CNS. Cytokine production is more closely linked with the degree of HAD than the viral load. However, replicative HIV infection in the CNS, reflected by increasing HIV RNA viral loads in the CSF, has been loosely associated with primary HAD prior to the cART era [6]. Pathologic changes are found in the deep gray matter of the brain, in white matter, and eventually in the cortex, resulting in loss of neurons and simplified dendritic structures [7].

While most people are susceptible to HIV, infection requires both CD4 receptors and chemokine receptors. Viral isolates may evolve in a host from CCR5 receptor dependent (R5) to viral tropism using the CXCR4 (X4) co-receptors. Generally, primary brain isolates are of the R5 class consistent with the fact that CCR5 is the predominant receptor on monocytes and macrophages, the primary cells with replicative infection in the brain. It is interesting that some people are protected from HIV infection by a genetic mutation in the CCR5 chemokine receptor that prevents it from participating as a co-receptor for cellular infection. A leukemia patient who received a bone marrow transplant from a donor with a non-binding CCR5 cell surface protein has been reported as showing evidence of a cure of HIV infection 3 years after receiving the transplant, including no evidence of the virus on brain biopsy [8].

Understanding factors predicting the subset of HIV-infected persons who develop neurological disease is a fundamental problem of great significance. There are likely to be both host and viral factors that predispose to development of the primary HIV complications. Understanding these should provide greater understanding of the diseases as well as opportunities to protect people from their consequences.

HIV-ASSOCIATED NEUROCOGNITIVE DISORDERS (HAND)

Clinical features

HIV-associated neurocognitive disorders (HAND) include a spectrum of cognitive impairments that range from asymptomatic neurocognitive impairment (ANI) to a severe form, HAD. Early on, it had been noted that HAND varied in severity and affected different domains of brain function, resulting in a variety of cognitive, motor, and behavioral manifestations. A consensus nomenclature for study of HAND was developed in 2007 by experts who presented a modified comprehensive classification of HAND [9]. In this classification, three HAND conditions are characterized: ANI, HIV-associated mild neurocognitive impairment (MND), and HAD. The work group emphasized the possibility of bidirectional temporal changes in diagnosis. These conditions should be classified using a variety of specific clinical and laboratory-based methods, depending upon the resources available where the patients are being evaluated. Ideally, baseline neuropsychological (NP) assessment should be part of the clinical evaluation. Where NP testing is not available, presence of cognitive impairment involving two or more ability domains may be suggested by quantitative neuropsychological testing using demographically appropriate normative cutoffs. Tools of value for screening include the HIV Dementia Scale, the International HIV Dementia Scale, Mattis Dementia Rating Scale, and the Montreal Cognitive Assessment (MoCA). Recent interest in use of the MoCA includes availability in multiple languages, balanced simple assessment of several domains, and low cost (free access at http://www.mocatest.org).

ANI and MND must both have documented neurocognitive impairment, but only in the case of MND does this impact on activities of daily living. The Frascati-proposed diagnostic criteria defines ANI and MND by performance at least 1 standard deviation (SD) below the mean of demographically adjusted normative scores in at least two cognitive areas (attention-information processing, language, abstraction-executive, complex perceptual motor skills, memory, including learning and recall, simple motor skills, or sensory perceptual abilities), with MND having evidence of functional impairment in daily living. HAD has a more profound impact on motor, cognitive, and

---

Box 19.2 Salient clinical features of HIV-associated dementia

Cognitive changes
- Reduced concentration, inability to focus thoughts or finish tasks
- Decreased reading, less interest in TV
- Decreased memory, making lists, needing reminders
- Speech changes, slowing, sometimes word-finding difficulty

Motor changes
- Slow initiation of movement
- Imbalance, clumsiness
- Weakness
- Sometime myoclonus
- Changes in bladder function, urgency, incontinence

Behavioral changes
- Personality changes, flat affect
- Depressed appearance
- Sleep disturbance, generally hypersomnia
- Rarely psychotic thought

---

behavioral problems that develop in advancing HIV infection (Box 19.2). Early signs and symptoms of HAND may be subtle, but evolution to HAD occurs mainly in untreated HIV. Before cART, patients often presented with insidious onset of reduced work productivity, poor concentration, mental slowing, and forgetfulness. The cognitive decline was often characterized by slowed thought and speech, which the patient as well as examiners may recognize. Habits of reading and recreation are impacted early, while productivity drops. Apathy and withdrawal from hobbies and social activities are common and must be differentiated from depression. Motor slowing is also typical, and has provided convenient means of documenting advancing neurological involvement. Imbalance, clumsiness, and weakness are common motor complaints. Behavioral changes are less common, but may be dramatic manifestations of the neurological involvement. Flattened affect is typical, and develops even without overt affective disorder. Other manifestations include sleep disturbance, psychosis, and seizures. Occasional frank psychotic episodes develop.

As the disease advances, global dementia with memory loss and language impairment develops, culminating in a virtual vegetative state. Neuropsychological evaluation reveals features suggestive of a subcortical dementia, such as is seen in Parkinson's disease. Early in the course of CNS disease, patients develop psychomotor slowing, memory loss, and word-finding difficulties. As the stage of the disease advances, severe psychomotor retardation and language impairment become obvious, leading to akinetic mutism. Clinicians sometimes comment on parallels with Parkinson's disease, and indeed the earliest regions of the brain affected in HIV include the basal ganglia. More recent studies reveal that loss of dopamine transporters in basal ganglia correlate with progressive cognitive disability. The greater dopamine transporter decrease in the putamen than in the caudate parallels that observed in Parkinson's disease [10].

While this description is important in untreated populations, it is almost never encountered in treated patients. HAND is most commonly seen today as either ANI or MND in early stages of the disease, or in treated patients, function may reveal subtle changes best documented by formalized neuropsychological testing. While progression to HAD on treatment is exceedingly rare, a new uncommon condition of an acute or subacute encephalitis occurring while patients are on therapy, potentially consistent with HIV cerebral immune reconstitution inflammatory syndrome (IRIS), has been described. This causes white matter changes in scans, and on brain biopsy is characterized by intense CD8 lymphocyte infiltration. Corticosteroid therapy as well as enhanced HIV therapy may be most effective in managing this serious encephalitic complication [11].

Diagnosis

Diagnosis of HAND is achieved by excluding alternative causes and recognizing patterns of illness associated with primary disease. While challenging in advanced patients, these conditions are even harder to fulfill in milder conditions, particularly when many co-morbid issues might also contribute to the findings. These conditions are generally clearest when the HIV disease is advanced, as defined by low CD4 counts (most often <250 cells/mm^3). While HAND is now often diagnosed in patients with a higher CD4 count, it remains problematic to ascribe neurologic problems to the viral disease in well-controlled patients with an intact immune system. Nevertheless, most investigators believe evidence supports HAND even in the presence of virologically successful antiretrovirals (ARV) and functional immune reconstitution.

Recommended investigations for HAND include assessing HIV control by current and nadir CD4 count and viral load measurements, including CSF viral loads. Brain MR and CT imaging studies are most important for ruling out alternative diagnoses, but may support a diagnosis of HAND when typical atrophy or white matter disease is demonstrated (Fig. 19.1). MR spectroscopy has been extensively used in the research setting seeking non-invasive means of monitoring CNS disease. Markers of gliosis or inflammation appear to occur early with late loss of neuronal markers. Some reports correlate these measures with treatment as well as disease progression, but to date MR spectroscopy has been of little practical use in tracking the CNS disease in the clinic. Functional MRI is not yet widely applied, but early studies suggest that before performance

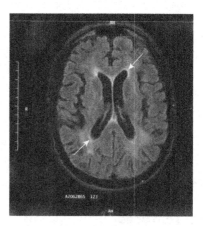

Figure 19.1 MR scan of a patient with HIV-associated dementia. Note the marked, widespread cortical atrophy, ventricular enlargement and diffuse changes in the subcortical white matter (arrows).

deteriorates, recruitment patterns change, engaging larger brain regions to perform tasks in affected individuals. Brain perfusion measured with MR by arterial spin labeling studies has suggested that HIV infection results in decreased perfusion to the brain which is only partially corrected by ARV [12]. Positron emission tomography (PET) has revealed abnormalities in subcortical metabolism early, with advancing hypometabolism globally in later stages; however, use of PET is limited due to costs and complexity.

CSF is rarely completely normal in HAND but the mild lymphocytic cellular response and mild elevation of protein most often encountered are not diagnostic. Elevated immunoglobulins, not rarely with oligoclonal banding, may be detected. Even after complete viral suppression with cART, there is the suggestion that there remains at least somewhat elevated inflammatory response in the CSF [13]. Careful analysis of CSF helps to exclude other etiologic causes of altered neurologic status. In untreated patients more elevated HIV viral loads in CSF are typical but not diagnostic of primary HIV neurological disease, but the association of cognitive impairment with viral load appears even less reliable in the era of cART. CSF cytokine elevations have correlated with HAD, but the more common mild HAND manifestations do not have substantial elevations.

There is a critical need for better-validated, quantitative biomarkers of early neuroAIDS disease, particularly means of determining which subjects may suffer progressive deterioration and thus be candidates for interventions and clinical trials.

Treatment

There is no specific therapy available for cognitive decline in AIDS. Optimal therapy of HIV is a uniform goal once the diagnosis is established. Because lower nadir CD4 has been suggested to increase the risk of HAND, neurological manifestations are a good rationale driving expert recommendations for earlier and more aggressive use of ARV in HIV infection. The central importance of antiretroviral therapy with relation to CNS manifestations is undeniable. Prior to introduction of ARV, the prevalence of HAD was typically at least 60–70% in advanced disease. Introduction of zidovudine was associated with improvement in cognitive performance and in a small placebo-controlled trial of high doses of zidovudine in subjects with active dementia [14]. In the early years of HIV therapy, incidence of HAD dropped to ∼7% per year, with roughly 20% prevalence in the population. HAD has become rare in patients responding well to ARV with controlled viral loads, with estimated incidence now much less than 5%. Thus, amelioration of marked cognitive impairment can be added to the other major benefits of cART. However, even the lower incidence of dementia when coupled with much longer survival has resulted in stable or even increasing numbers of cognitively impaired patients in some clinics [1].

Antiretroviral drugs may vary in their effectiveness in the CNS compartment with several, particularly highly protein-bound protease inhibitors, probably having limited access to the brain. Determining whether designing therapy for CNS penetration could improve cognitive outcomes is an active topic for investigation [15]. The CNS penetration effectiveness (CPE) ranking of different ARV agents derived from information about the properties of individual ARV is used to study this issue. At present observations are not conclusive regarding the value of CPE for managing therapy. Some reports show correlation between poor penetration score and higher CSF viral loads [16]. However, other studies do not uniformly support the importance of CPE since mild HAND may be seen unrelated to CPE scores [17]. Neuroprotective strategies distinct from ARV continue to be investigated but none have been demonstrated to be effective beyond HIV therapy.

The latest expert recommendations for HIV therapy continue a trend toward earlier initiation of ARV at higher CD4 counts, often in patients < 500 cells/mm^3 (http://aidsinfo.nih.gov). There is general support for aggressive and consistent use of cART once symptomatic disease, including neurological disease, is identified. Data analysis from the CHARTER study showed an association of HAND with lower nadir CD4 rather than current CD4 status. A challenge for therapeutic development resides in balancing the degree and durability of viral response with the cost and complications of the therapy, including side effects and secondary toxicities. With declining toxicity, earlier therapy has become more attractive and now dominates treatment recommendations. Treatment of HIV within the CNS may be even more difficult than systemic infection, since the virus is harbored in longer-lived cells and may be exposed to lower and less effective levels of ARV due to the blood–brain barrier. The quantity and quality of information on CNS efficacy of HIV therapy is suboptimal. CNS penetration of ARV may contribute to efficacy, while active transport of other drugs out of the central compartment could drive outcomes [18]. Despite these theoretical concerns, decline in the incidence of neurological complications has closely followed improvement in systemic HIV therapy, and concerns about CPE of therapies remain to be validated. Thus, the clinician's first task is to construct the most effective and best-tolerated HIV therapy overall. If HAND is present, it is reasonable to consider CPE in the choice of therapies, but this should not yet be considered an overriding consideration, pending more information about this approach to therapy. Based primarily on CSF penetration (which is not necessarily the same as brain penetration), optimal nucleoside reverse transcriptase inhibitors (NRTIs) include zidovudine, stavudine, and abacavir. Nevirapine appears to cross the blood–brain barrier well and is theoretically a favorable drug from the non-nucleoside reverse transcriptase inhibitors (NNRTIs) class, but there is also documentation of therapeutic efficacy with efavirenz [19]. From the protease inhibitors (PIs) class of ARV, indinavir is the least protein bound and has best evidence of efficacy in the CNS, but is rarely prescribed due to side effects and frequent dosing. Relatively better PI drugs for CPE include ritonavir-boosted lopinavir or darunavir. The newer CCR5 antagonist maraviroc and the integrase inhibitor raltegravir both seem to have moderately good CPE scores, making them reasonable additions to salvage regimens with drug-resistant virus.

Measuring the efficacy of primary neuroAIDS therapy remains more challenging than systemic therapy. In cases of clear-cut neurological impairment, a rather dramatic clinical improvement may at times be noted, and the benefits of therapy are easily appreciated. However, with more subtle disabilities, it is much harder to document a response to therapy. For clinical trial development of treatment, repeated well-validated neuropsychometric measures to reflect the clinical response to therapy are generally employed. Viral load in CNS, which generally is lower than systemic values, has poor correlation with severity of neurological disease and often provides little guidance for therapy. However, occasional cases of CSF viral replication even when viremia is controlled are reported, and neurological improvement may be directed by the characteristics of the CSF virus [20].

Driven by the concern that viral infection is not eliminated from the brain by antiviral therapy, considerable effort has been placed in protective strategies to block presumed neurotoxic brain damage [21]. To date, small controlled studies have evaluated the toxicity, safety, and tolerability of different presumed protective drugs and failed to demonstrate neuroprotective properties. Recent trials of minocycline have also failed to reverse cognitive deficits during controlled trials [22]. At present no adjuvant therapy can be recommended outside of the clinical trial setting.

HIV NEUROPATHY

Clinical features

HIV-associated sensory neuropathy (HIV-SN) is a major source of morbidity among AIDS patients, affecting approximately 30% of AIDS patients. Other potentially treatable peripheral nerve diseases occur in HIV related to other infectious agents and immune-mediated mechanisms. However, the most common forms of distal sensory polyneuropathy (DSN) are HIV-SN and antiretroviral toxic neuropathy (ATN). These two forms are phenotypically identical. They present as a length-dependent neuropathy with distal to proximal development of symptoms. A mixture of negative symptoms including numbness and sensory loss along with positive dysesthetic and painful aching or burning is typical. Symptoms are generally worse at night and can be aggravated by innocuous stimuli, such as bed sheets or wearing shoes. Abnormalities on neurological examination are limited to sensory nerve function and include reduced or absent ankle reflexes and increased vibratory and pin sensation thresholds. International studies in Southeast Asia have confirmed that taller patients are more likely to suffer neurotoxic neuropathy, and thus an algorithm making greater effort to avoid stavudine in tall patients would make sense [23]. In the USA and Europe, the decline in use of stavudine and didanosine has been accompanied by a reduction in toxic neuropathies, but the overall burden of neuropathies remains high in most HIV clinics, and is particularly troublesome in international sites where frequent use of stavudine continues. A study from South Africa revealed a 57% prevalence of symptomatic neuropathy among stavudine-exposed South Africans [24].

Diagnosis

Without a definitive test, diagnosis of HIV-associated neuropathy requires typical presentation and exclusion of alternative diagnoses. The typical pattern of symmetric distal sensory loss is characteristic. Asymmetric neuropathies, or those with substantial motor involvement, suggest an alternate diagnosis. Physiologic testing may be of limited value in HIV-SN. Affected patients can often test normally on routine nerve conduction study. This reflects the prominent small-caliber sensory nerve involvement in HIV-SN while nerve conduction tests preferentially evaluate larger nerve fibers. Skin biopsy and visualization of epidermal nerve fibers is a useful diagnostic tool in research settings and theoretically could allow monitoring treatment aimed at nerve regeneration [25]. Reduced fiber density, increased frequency of fiber varicosities, and fiber fragmentation are prominent features of skin biopsy from patients with HIV-SN. A clinically similar syndrome is often caused by dideoxynucleoside drugs used to treat HIV, including didanosine (DDI), stavudine (D4T), and in the past by zalcitabine (DDC). While both DSN and ATN can coexist in a single patient, temporal profile of symptoms in relation to introduction and termination of neurotoxic medications can help in distinguishing the active pathophysiologic process. PIs have also been associated with neuropathy, although this association has not been consistent, or strong [26].

Predisposing conditions for neuropathy, including diabetes, nutritional deficiency, alcohol abuse, or prior chemotherapy, may contribute to development of symptomatic neuropathy. Prior to cART, DSN was associated with advanced HIV disease, with lower CD4 count and higher viral load. Advancing age remains a consistent and significant risk factor of increasing importance with the aging of HIV patients [27]. In the developing world, ATN is still important. Symptoms typically begin from a few weeks to 6 months after introduction of toxic medications. Symptoms may worsen at least for a few weeks after discontinuation of the offending agent, followed by at least partial improvement in most, but not all, patients.

The main pathologic features that characterize DSN and ATN include "dying back" axonal degeneration of long axons in distal regions, loss of unmyelinated fibers, and variable degree of macrophage infiltration in peripheral nerve and dorsal root ganglia. Marked activation of macrophages as well as the effect of proinflammatory cytokines appears to be the main immunopathogenic factor in DSN [28]. Interference with DNA synthesis and mitochondrial abnormalities produced by nucleoside antiretroviral drugs have been postulated as pathologic factors involved in ATN.

Treatment

Treatment for HIV-SN includes optimizing the environment for the nerves by assuring excellent nutritional status and minimal toxic insults. In case of ATN, the suspected agent should be discontinued or at least the dose should be reduced. In the current era, it is rarely necessary to continue toxic nucleosides when there is access to the full selections of ARV. Symptomatic therapy is often needed for pain. Several drugs often used for neuropathic pain are apparently less effective in HIV-SN. Currently, the only therapies shown to be effective against pain by randomized, placebo-controlled clinical trials are smoked tetrahydrocannabinol [29] and lamotrigine [30]. Gabapentin in doses of 1,800 to 3,600 mg/day has provided helpful amelioration for chronic pain, but it is often necessary to employ long-acting narcotic drugs to provide reasonable quality of life in the face of troubling pain. A randomized clinical trial testing pregabalin, a related anticonvulsant used for neuropathic pain syndromes, failed to confirm activity in the face of a very potent placebo response [31].

A sometime lethal neuromuscular syndrome seen after lactic acidosis remains important in developing countries where stavudine is used extensively [32]. It typically occurs several weeks after lactic acidosis associated with d-drug toxicity [33]. Patients develop severe weakness and subacute painful neuropathic symptoms. Reflexes are depressed, and muscle biopsies suggest mitochondrial myopathy as well as neuropathic changes. It occurs more commonly in women than men. Eye movements may be restricted. Supportive therapy, and avoidance of mitochondrial toxins allow recovery of many of these patients, but notable mortality has been associated with this condition.

HIV-1-ASSOCIATED VACUOLAR MYELOPATHY

Clinical features

Vacuolar myelopathy is the most common chronic myelopathy associated with HIV infection. It occurs during the late stage of HIV infection, when CD4 counts are very low. It is often seen in conjunction with HAD, peripheral neuropathies, opportunistic CNS, and peripheral nervous system infections. In the early years of HIV when therapy was quite limited, myelopathy was clinically noted in up to 20% of adult HIV patients, while pathologic study of the spinal cord indicated involvement in over half of AIDS autopsies. Pathophysiologic data are limited but it has been suggested that infiltration of the cord with HIV-infected cells secreting neurotoxic factors, neurotoxic HIV proteins, or underutilization of vitamin B_{12} could underlie this devastating disorder. The vacuolar degeneration of heavily myelinated tracts including the corticospinal tract results in progressive spastic diplegia (paraplegia), often with urinary bladder involvement and sensory ataxia. Both dorsal column and spinothalamic sensory deficits are often observed in these patients.

Diagnosis

Laboratory studies focus on exclusion of treatable causes like vitamin B_{12} deficiency and compressive myelopathy. It is critical not to ascribe myelopathy to HIV without imaging the spinal cord for treatable compressive lesions. A negative imaging study with MRI, normal level for vitamin B_{12}, and negative HTLV-1 status are important exclusions before HIV-associated vacuolar myelopathy is accepted as a diagnosis.

Treatment

Treatment for myelopathy is best addressed by optimized ARV. The high prevalence of this disorder in untreated HIV disease is substantially different from the experience in the era of cART where myelopathy is very rarely encountered in treated subjects. When treatment is started in patients beginning to demonstrate signs of myelopathy, it is arrested and partially reversed in many cases. In addition to ARV treatment, care in nutrition is likely to contribute to better outcomes.

CONCLUSION

Primary neurological complications at every level of the nervous system have been a significant part of the impact of HIV infection throughout the world. While these manifestations may be veiled by the acute illnesses complicating untreated disease, they are present in the much larger group of people suffering HIV in developing countries, and are likely to be noted more prominently as therapy is introduced. Because the actual manifestations of these diseases are likely to be dependent on both viral and host genetics, each having significant differences in various parts of the world, it will be critical to study the presentation and course of these complications in the different settings where HIV is prevalent, as unique features that could influence outcomes are likely to emerge.

REFERENCES

[1] McArthur JC, Steiner J, Sacktor N, Nath A. Human immunodeficiency virus-associated neurocognitive disorders mind the gap. Ann Neurol 2010;67:699–714.

[2] Heaton RK, Clifford DB, Franklin Jr DR, et al. HIV-associated neurocognitive disorders persist in the era of potent antiretroviral therapy. CHARTER study. Neurology 2010;75:2087–96.

[3] Sacktor NC, Wong M, Nakasujja N, et al. The International HIV Dementia Scale: a new rapid screening test for HIV dementia. AIDS 2005;19:1367–74.

[4] Joska JA, Gouse H, Paul RH, et al. Does highly active antiretroviral therapy improve neurocognitive function? A systematic review. J Neurovirol 2010;16:101–14.

[5] Churchill MJ, Wesselingh SL, Cowley D, et al. Extensive astrocyte infection is prominent in human immunodeficiency virus—associated dementia. Ann Neurol 2009;66:253–8.

[6] Ellis RJ, Hsia K, Spector SA, et al. Cerebrospinal fluid human immunodeficiency virus Type 1 RNA levels are elevated in neurocognitively impaired individuals with acquired immunodeficiency syndrome. Ann Neurol 1997;42:679–88.

[7] Sá MJ, Madeira MD, Ruela C, et al. AIDS does not alter the total number of neurons in the hippocampal formation but induces cell atrophy: a stereological study. Acta Neuropathol 2000;99:643–53.

[8] Allers K, Hutter G, Hofmann J, et al. Evidence for the cure of HIV infection by CCR5D32/D32 stem cell transplantation. Blood 2011;117(10):2791–9.

[9] Antinori A, Arendt G, Becker JT, et al. Updated research nosology for HIV-associated neurocognitive disorders. Neurology 2007;69(18):1789–99.

[10] Wang GJ, Chang L, Volkow ND, et al. Decreased brain dopaminergic transports in HIV-associated dementia patients. Brain 2004;127:2452–8.

[11] Lescure FX, Gray F, Savatovsky J, et al. Lymphocytes T8 infiltrative encephalitis: a new form of neurological complication in HIV infection. In: XVIII International AIDS Conference; 2010.

[12] Ances BM, Liang CL, Leontiev O, et al. Effects of aging on cerebral blood flow, oxygen metabolism, and blood oxygenation level dependent responses to visual stimulation. Hum Brain Mapp 2009;30:1120–32.

[13] Eden A, Price RW, Spudich S, et al. Immune activation of the central nervous system is still present after > 4 years of effective highly active antiretroviral therapy. J Infect Dis 2007;196(12): 1779–83.

[14] Sidtis JJ, Gatsonis C, Price RW, et al. Zidovudine treatment of the AIDS dementia complex: results of a placebo-controlled trial. Ann Neurol 1993;33:343–9.

[15] Letendre SL, McCutchan JA, Childers ME, et al. Enhancing antiretroviral therapy for human immunodeficiency virus cognitive disorders. Ann Neurol 2004;56:416–23.

[16] Letendre S, Marquie-Beck J, Capparelli E, et al. Validation of the CNS penetration-effectiveness rank for quantifying antiretroviral penetration into the central nervous system. Arch Neurol 2008;65 (1):65–70.

[17] Simioni S, Cavassini M, Annoni JM, et al. Cognitive dysfunction in HIV patients despite long-standing suppression of viremia. AIDS 2010;24:1243–50.

[18] Choo EF, Leake B, Wandel C, et al. Pharmacological inhibition of P-glycoprotein transport enhances the distribution of HIV-1 protease inhibitors into brain and testes. Drug Metab Dispos 2000;28:655–60.

[19] Tashima K, Caliendo AM, Ahmad M, et al. Cerebrospinal fluid human immunodeficiency virus type 1 (HIV-1) suppression and efavirenz drug concentrations in HIV-1-infected patients receiving combination therapy. J Infect Dis 1999;180:862–4.

[20] Canestri A, Lescure FX, Jaureguiberry S, et al. Discordance between cerebral spinal fluid and plasma HIV replication in patients with neurological symptoms who are receiving suppressive antiretroviral therapy. Clin Infect Dis 2010;50:773–8.

[21] Clifford DB. Human immunodeficiency virus-associated dementia. Arch Neurol 2000;57:321–4.

[22] Zink MC, Uhrlaub J, DeWitt J, et al. Neuroprotective and anti-human immunodeficiency virus activity of minocycline. JAMA 2005;293:2003–11.

[23] Cherry CL, Affandi JS, Imran D, et al. Age and height predict neuropathy risk in patients with HIV prescribed stavudine. Neurology 2009;73:315–20.

[24] Wadley AL, Cherry CL, Price P, Kamerman PR. HIV neuropathy risk factors and symptom characterization in stavudine-exposed South Africans. J Pain Symptom Manage 2011;41 (4):700–6.

[25] Polydefkis M, Yiannoutsos CT, Cohen BA, et al. Reduced intraepidermal nerve fiber density in HIV-associated sensory neuropathy. Neurology 2002;58:115–19.

[26] Ellis RJ, Marquie-Beck J, Delaney P, et al. Human immunodeficiency virus protease inhibitors and risk for peripheral neuropathy. Ann Neurol 2008;64:566–72.

[27] Watters MR, Poff PW, Shiramizu BT, et al. Symptomatic distal sensory polyneuropathy in HIV after age 50. Neurology 2004;62:1378–83.

[28] Keswani SC, Pardo CA, Cherry CL, et al. HIV-associated sensory neuropathies. AIDS 2002;16:2105–17.

[29] Abrams DI, Jay CA, Shade SB, et al. Cannabis in painful HIV-associated sensory neuropathy. A randomized placebo-controlled trial. Neurology 2007;68:515–21.

[30] Simpson DM, McArthur JC, Olney R, et al. Lamotrigine for HIV-associated painful sensory neuropathies. Neurology 2003;60:1508–14.

[31] Simpson DM, Schifitto G, Clifford DB, et al. Pregabalin for painful HIV neuropathy. A randomized, double-blind, placebo-controlled trial. Neurology 2010;74:413–20.

[32] Vidal JE, Clifford D, Ferreira CM, Penalva de Oliveira AC. HIV-associated neuromuscular weakness syndrome in Brazil. Report of the two first cases. Arq Neuropsiquiatr 2007;65:848–51.

[33] Simpson D, Estanislao L, Evans S, et al. HIV associated neuromuscular weakness syndrome. AIDS 2004;18:1403–12.

Chapter | 20 |

Psychiatric barriers and the international AIDS epidemic

Chiadi U. Onyike, Andrew F. Angelino, Glenn J. Treisman

INTRODUCTION

The analysis of causation and intervention in the HIV/AIDS epidemic has relied on the classic epidemiologic triad of host, agent, and environmental factors. Yet the HIV/AIDS epidemic differs from earlier pandemics in the sense that behavior is the principal vector of its spread. HIV infection is propagated by behaviors that involve intimate physical contact or exposure to blood or body secretions. In the early years of the epidemic the identified vulnerable host groups were *h*omosexuals, *h*eroin addicts, *H*aitians, and *h*emophiliacs (the 4-H group), which pointed to the specific behaviors that served as vectors for the viral agent. It is now recognized, especially in high-income countries, that psychiatric disability has facilitated the spread of this virus [1]. Nearly 30 years later health promotional efforts in high-income countries has slowed the epidemic considerably, in terms of overall prevalence, but transmission has continued apace among subgroups who are unable to modify their behavior without active assistance. It has become clear that psychiatric disorders, besides their role in the spread of the virus through the risk behaviors that they provoke or promote, also impact outcomes adversely by undermining help seeking and treatment adherence (Fig. 20.1). HIV/AIDS is also associated with secondary psychiatric states, such as depression, anxiety, mania, delirium, cognitive impairment, and dementia [2]. Therefore the intersections of HIV/AIDS and psychiatric disorder require examination in any discussion of HIV/AIDS prevention, treatment, and prognosis.

It is well established that psychiatric disorders generally have adverse impacts on health awareness, health-seeking behavior, and treatment adherence. The World Health Organization (WHO) estimates [3] show that neuropsychiatric disorder is highly prevalent worldwide—the 12-month prevalence (interquartile range, IQR) is 18.1–36.1% for DSM-IV disorders and 0.8–6.8% for Serious Mental Illness (i.e., a DSM-IV disorder, other than substance abuse, that causes serious disability). Furthermore, neuropsychiatric disorders are also major contributors to disability; Serious Mental Illness results in 49–184 days/year out of role, Moderate Mental Illness in 21–109, and Mild Mental Illness in 12–67 [3]. The WHO Mental Health Gap Action Programme [4] has reported that depression, with lifetime prevalence of major depression or dysthymia estimated at 12.1%, is the single largest contributor to non-fatal burden of disease and is responsible for a high number of lost disability adjusted life years (DALYs) worldwide. It is the fourth leading cause of disease burden (in terms of DALYs) globally and is projected to increase to the second leading cause in 2030. Suicide, an important complication of depression, is the third leading cause of death worldwide in people aged between 15 and 34 years, and the thirteenth leading cause of death for all ages combined. It also represents 1.4% of the global disease burden (in DALYs). Alcohol use disorders, schizophrenia, and dementia are also important contributors to disease burden. An estimated 24.3 million people have dementia worldwide, a figure predicted to double every 20 years, and 60% of those with dementia live in middle- or low-income countries.

Global disparities in the global HIV/AIDS situation are also substantial, despite notable progress in the prevention of new infections and expansion of treatment in the past decade. According to the latest Global Summary of the HIV and AIDS Epidemic published in 2010 [5], there has been a 19% decline in HIV-related deaths since 1999, a 25% drop in the incidence of new infections in 33 countries (22 of these in Africa), and a 26% reduction worldwide in the frequency of mother-to-child transmission. In 2009

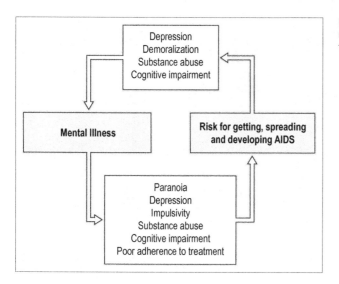

Figure 20.1 Psychiatric disorders play an important role in both the spread of the virus through behavior and the impact on treatment response.

alone, 1.2 million patients received treatment for the first time, representing an increase in the number of people receiving treatment of 30% in a single year! Still there is much work to be done. The majority of new infections (69%) still occur in sub-Saharan Africa, and also seven middle- and low-income countries in Eastern Europe and Central Asia experienced a 25% increase in HIV incidence in the past decade. Today almost 50% of the 33.3 million adults and children living with HIV reside in middle- and low-income countries [5], and the reduction in mother-to-child transmission still translates to 370,000 new children with the infection who mostly reside in low-income countries. Also 35% (5.3 million) of the 15 million in need living in these countries are receiving anti-retroviral treatment.

Economically disadvantaged people have limited access to psychiatric treatment and chronic psychiatric illness contributes to this problem through the tendency to restrict and deplete economic resources and cause economic "downward drift" into poverty. Generally, psychiatric care is least available to those who will need it the most (i.e., individuals suffering severe mental illness). This applies in high- and low-income countries [6], but is probably more acute in low-income countries where public mental health services may be deficient or practically absent. Generally, the countries most severely affected by HIV have the least developed resources for HIV treatment and for mental health. The 15 million living with HIV in low- and middle-income countries have very limited access to psychiatric services. The unmet need for mental disorders and serious mental illness is high in these countries: a survey in Nigeria found that only 1.2% of individuals received any treatment in the 12 months preceding the study [7]. This problem reflects a scarcity of treatment resources: 52% of low-income countries provide community-based care, compared with 97% of high-income countries. The median number of

psychiatric hospital beds reaches as low as 0.33 per 10,000 in Africa and Southeast Asia [8]. Ultimately the principal factor limiting psychiatric care in middle- and low-income countries is the scarcity of professionals. Low-income countries have a median of 0.05 psychiatrists and 0.16 psychiatric nurses per 100,000 population, whereas high-income countries have a 200-fold higher ratio of psychiatric mental health-workers to population [8]. Treatment of psychiatric disorders is further constrained by the unavailability of essential medicines in low-income countries; about a quarter of these countries do not provide any psychotropic medicines in primary-care settings and in many others supplies are insufficient or irregular [8]. Therefore, patients and families are often forced to pay for medicines. Since these costs are relatively high in low-income countries, the result is that treatment, where it exists, is unaffordable for many. It is also worth noting that over 85% of controlled trials for cost-effective treatments are conducted in high-income countries [9]. Another key factor, and one that limits prospects for progress in the development of psychiatric services, is the lack of prioritization of mental health in national health policies and of advocacy for it at the community level [10]—a problem exacerbated by misperceptions about the cost–benefits of providing these services.

Cultural values and beliefs play a substantial role in mental health care in middle- and low-income countries [7, 11, 12]. Mental illness carries a high stigma and is often attributed to religio-magical phenomena, in which the illness represents retribution meted out by ancestors or possession by evil spirits. In some countries, such as in Uganda, those who are mentally ill are excluded from employment or voting. In many others, they are excluded from full social participation in a variety of ways that limit schooling, marriage opportunities, and forming of social networks. On the other hand, there is reliance in some areas on traditional healers who are frequently included in policy initiatives and form a substantial component of the community mental health resource. In East Africa, 70–100% of individuals consult a traditional healer as first line of care [13–15]. However, utilization of traditional methods for psychiatric care is low in many places. In Nigeria, for example, less than 5% of individuals with a psychiatric illness consult a traditional healer and about the same number seek formal psychiatric care. Cultural factors are also critical in the expression of psychological distress and psychiatric disorders and to their detection during screening programs and clinical care—lack of sophistication regarding local expressions and/or reliance on standard screening instruments that have not been culturally adapted may result in failure to detect cases.

As a consequence of the low coverage of both antiretroviral and psychiatric treatment in middle- and low-income countries, many patients who have psychological distress and/or psychiatric disorders go without antiretroviral treatment— from either not having sought it or not being able to maintain adherence. Generally, psychological distress and social isolation are factors in seeking antiretroviral treatment and yet often go unnoticed, especially when there is no overt symptomatology [16–18]. Longitudinal studies also confirm what had already been demonstrated in high-income countries, that psychological distress and psychiatric disorders contribute to low initiation and non-adherence in young [16, 19] and older [20] individuals suffering HIV and AIDS. A newly emerged issue is the nature of relationships between aging, cognitive dysfunction (discussed below) and adherence to antiretroviral therapy. Cognitive dysfunction and dementia have been associated with higher rates of non-adherence [20, 21], and reciprocity in the adverse relationship between cognition and adherence has also been demonstrated [22].

Thus far we have covered two aspects to the relationship between psychiatric disorders and the HIV epidemic. One aspect involves the effects of psychiatric disorders on self-management of exposure risk, and the other had to do with effects on access and utilization of treatment services. There is yet another dimension to the psychiatric aspects of the HIV/AIDS infection, having to do with secondary psychiatric disorders developing as a consequence of the infection. We now address this issue.

Psychiatric disorders differ in their etiology, causal pathways, and correlates, and also in their treatments. While in the USA there has been a great focus on "disease" psychiatry and the use of disease-based criteria for conditions (such as those used in the DSM-IV), many psychiatric conditions are not diseases and do not fit well into this model but still have a huge impact on HIV infection. We will discuss psychiatric diseases, which are (or are presumed to involve) brain lesions first, and then discuss problems of addictions and problems of temperament and endowment. We also acknowledge that problems originating in a person's

experience have a profound influence on their ability to accept treatment as well. For instance, those persons who have experienced misuse at the hands of trusted paternal figures will manifest their distrust when accessing medical care, as they do in other areas of their lives. Likewise, those who experienced abnormal sexual experiences at vulnerable developmental stages are at high risk for manifesting promiscuity and prostitution. The treatment of these issues here is intended to deliver on breadth, rather than depth; a detailed review of these subjects is beyond the scope and space of this chapter.

CHRONIC MENTAL ILLNESS AND HIV INFECTION

A subset of patients with chronic mental illnesses such as recurrent severe major depression, schizophrenia, and bipolar affective disorder have been identified as constituting a high-risk population that manifests HIV risk behaviors at higher-than-average rates, but these observations have been made in high-income countries. The prevalence rate of HIV among the chronically mentally ill in the USA has been estimated to be between 4 and 20% [23–28]. Risk behaviors associated with HIV infection are also frequently observed in this population; early studies of chronically hospitalized patients in New York City [29] and patients attending community mental health clinics in Melbourne, Australia [30] showed that patients with mental illness were more likely to participate in unprotected casual sex and injection drug use when compared with the general population. This observation has been replicated in other studies [31–34], cementing the observation that individuals who suffer chronic mental illness manifest higher rates of behaviors that put them at risk for HIV infection.

Besides increasing their exposure to the virus, patients with mental illnesses are impaired in their ability to adhere to the complicated medication regimens necessary to suppress viral replication and HIV disease (discussed earlier, see also Campos et al. [35] and Venkatesh et al. [36]). Successful treatment requires consistently taking at least 90% of prescribed antiretroviral medications, with faithfulness to the dosage and to the schedule. Unfortunately, adherence rates vary widely in individuals with chronic mental illness, ranging from 32 to over 80%, depending on the group and the duration over which adherence is being monitored. For example, an analysis of data from a sample of 115 patients attending a Los Angeles HIV clinic found three-day, one-week, and one-month adherence success rates (taking 95% of doses) of 58.3, 34.8, and 26.1%, respectively. Three-day adherence was strongly associated with mental health status, social support, patient–physician relationship, and experience of adverse effects [37]. Another study estimated sustained viral suppression in only 25–40%

of patients [38]. In both studies, mental illness was a factor in non-adherence to treatment. Psychosocial interventions geared toward improving autonomy, self-efficacy, and community support can improve adherence and may, therefore, be useful adjuncts to psychiatric regimens in optimizing adherence. For example, a study evaluated predictors of high ART adherence ($\geq 90\%$), measured by electronic drug monitors, after enrollment in a randomized controlled trial testing behavioral interventions to improve ART adherence [39]. High motivation, positive coping styles, and high levels of interpersonal support were positively associated with adherence, whereas passive belief in divine intervention was negatively associated with adherence.

MOOD DISORDERS IN HIV/AIDS

Affective disorders (mood disorders), particularly major depression, are the most common co-morbid psychiatric conditions in patients suffering from HIV disease. The prevalence of major depression in those with HIV in the USA has been estimated at 15–40%. The prevalence exceeds 50% in persons with HIV seeking psychiatric treatment [40]. Nevertheless, any evaluation for depression must also consider other states such as demoralization, dementia, and delirium, all of which are common in those with HIV and AIDS. While checklists can be useful for screening, a detailed history that explores the patient's mood, self-attitude, vital sense, hedonic capacity, and neurovegetative symptoms (i.e., appetite and sleep) will help in establishing the diagnosis. The importance of identifying and treating depression rests on the opportunity to improve quality of life, reduce high-risk behaviors, and improve treatment adherence.

While some cases appear to have developed as adverse reactions to anti-retroviral agents, it is also well established that advanced HIV can trigger a secondary mania. An early study in a large clinical cohort showed 8% of the patients with AIDS had mania, a tenfold higher 6-month prevalence than in the general population [41], also characterizing the phenotype of the mania showing its association with the late stage of HIV infection with an appearance similar to a delirium. Secondary mania has also been documented in Africa, with high prevalence and a phenotype showing marked euphoria, irritability, aggression, and combinations of auditory and visual hallucination [42, 43]. The predominant mood appears to be irritability and an involved work-up for delirium (Box 20.1) needs to be completed prior to making this diagnosis.

Diagnosis of mood disorders is complicated in the global community by different standards and beliefs regarding mental illness, and variation in the manner of presentation. As we noted earlier, depression inventories familiar to practitioners and researchers in high-income Anglophone countries can show low utility in the diagnosis or

---

---

understanding of mental illness in African, South American, or Central Asian contexts. An excellent example derives from a study conducted in Uganda that examined local perceptions of the impact HIV had on mental health. Interviewees described two local syndromes, *Yo'kwekyawa* (translated as "hating oneself") and *Okwekubaziga* (translated as "pitying oneself"), as resulting from HIV infection [44]. Both terms encompass many aspects of what we understand as major depression and give strength to the notion that those affected with HIV anywhere in the world are likely to have similar mental health manifestations (like depression), though they may not describe it in a manner familiar to the Western world.

HIV-ASSOCIATED NEUROCOGNITIVE DISORDERS

HIV-associated neurocognitive disorder (HAND), discussed more fully in Chapter 19, remains common in the era of *antiretroviral therapy* (ART) [45, 46]. HIV infection of the CNS occurs early in the illness. Studies show that ART treatment ameliorates HAND, but it appears that resolution is usually incomplete [47]. Thus, HAND prevalence rates still range from 30 to 50%. While the profile of cognitive impairment has changed little in the ART era, nosology has changed in tandem with new discoveries. The latest nosology defines three states according to formal criteria

[48], representing a continuum of HIV-associated cognitive disorder:

(1) *HIV-associated asymptomatic neurocognitive impairment* (ANI, a subclinical state demonstrated by testing in two or more cognitive domains);

(2) *HIV-associated mild neurocognitive disorder* (MND, manifesting cognitive impairment with mild functional disability); and

(3) *HIV-associated dementia* (HAD, characterized by marked cognitive impairment and marked functional disability).

Impairments of attention, abstraction, memory and learning, speech, and language, and abnormal psychomotor and fine motor functions are the most common features of the dementia. AIDS dementia also manifests apathy, irritability, hyperactivity, agitation, insomnia, euphoria, and psychosis. Given its features, HAD may mimic (or be mimicked by) HIV-associated delirium, depression, or mania). AIDS delirium presents with fluctuating levels of alertness, attention, and arousal, along with lapses in memory and perceptual abnormalities, and may co-occur with dementia in advanced cases of AIDS. Thus it may present a diagnostically frustrating picture that relies on interviews of close relatives and friends, careful observation, and diagnostic testing for clarity. Delirium in AIDS can reflect metabolic disturbances, electrolyte imbalance, encephalitis, sepsis, or the adverse effects of medications. Opportunistic CNS infections such as progressive multifocal leukoencephalopathy (PML), cytomegalovirus encephalitis, cryptococcal meningitis, toxoplasmosis, and varicella-zoster virus encephalitis may cause or contribute to delirium. Delirium in AIDS has an unfavorable prognosis [49], particularly when untreated. Therefore, aggressive evaluation and management is always warranted.

HIV AND SUBSTANCE ABUSE

Intravenous drug use holds a prime place in the discussion of substance abuse, as it is a direct route of infection and spread of HIV. It is a major player in the ongoing AIDS epidemic in Asia, Eastern Europe, Latin America, and developed countries. From India to China, HIV prevalence in communities of injection drug users (IDUs) has increased from 0 to 50% within 6 months; and the map of HIV spread throughout Southeast Asia by virus strain follows, not coincidentally, heroin trafficking patterns in the region [50]. Other substance use disorders play an important role in the transmission of HIV through the promotion of high-risk behaviors. Since behavior is the principal vector of HIV transmission everywhere, it is the main factor driving the epidemic.

Substance abuse, whether of alcohol, narcotics, stimulants, or other substances, is a problem of worldwide scope. The global burden of disease ranks substance use disorders among the top 10 causes of morbidity globally. The susceptibility to addiction is complex, involving cultural, social, psychological, genetic, and psychiatric factors. In the Western hemisphere addictions have been for sometime conceptualized as diseases, a useful approach for de-stigmatizing patients who suffer these chronic problems and for mobilizing family and community support for their care. While some data show that brain pathology can foster or perpetuate certain substance use disorders, descriptions of these behaviors in terms that emphasize or illustrate how they become self-perpetuating as a result of recruitment of the brain's normal reward systems (the reader is referred to McHugh and Slavney [51] for more discussion) has proved to be a profitable approach to their analysis and treatment.

To understand how this works, it is necessary to examine what behavior is and how it is perpetuated. In simple terms, behavior can be defined as self-directed actions; thus, something one does. In general, behaviors are elicited by stimuli (typically environmental but sometimes endogenous). The behavior reshapes, extinguishes, or modifies stimuli such as to elicit CNS-mediated reward responses such as pleasure or satiation. It is conditioning by this reward that "drives" behaviors such as the insertion of a needle into your arm, "chasing the dragon," visiting a brothel, or having high-risk sex. In other words a positive response elicited within the brain not only increases the likelihood the behavior will be repeated in the future but also that it will be the preferred behavioral response.

Behaviors stimulate the brain's internal reward circuitry. Neurotransmitters mediating the reward response are released, leading to a sense of pleasure. With the waning of the pleasure comes an urge, or craving, to accomplish the behavior that originated in the good feelings. Such a positive feedback loop can be very helpful when increasing the frequency of behaviors needed for survival such as sleeping, eating, and sex. However, such a loop, if not tightly regulated, can lead to an excessive focus on a particular behavior. If you eat enough or sleep enough, you lose interest in that activity temporarily. The loop is "off." Drugs and alcohol can activate this loop and drive it out of control. Genetics, environment, and circumstances all play a role in both the predisposition to drug use and the intensity of reward their use elicits. Psychiatric illnesses also play a role in determining the disposition to using drugs and the vulnerability of the reinforcement loop. Understanding and appreciation of the stimulus–behavior–reward cycle provides opportunity for intervention by removing the stimulus, proscribing (and stigmatizing) the behavior, or blunting the reward experience (see Treisman and Angelino [52] for further discussion).

PERSONALITY, TEMPERAMENT, AND HIV

Since ancient times, healers have recognized personality types and pointed to behaviors associated with those types. Today the four humors of Greek medicine—melancholic, choleric, sanguine, and phlegmatic—still carry heuristic value as personality descriptors. Today there are a great many approaches to characterizing personality, from Freudian and other psychodynamic theories proposing failure to complete stages of formative experience (e.g., oral, anal types), to others that describe personality in terms of their impact on others (antisocial, avoidant), and yet others that describe in terms of behavioral characteristics (risk-taking, pleasure-seeking). Regardless which set of descriptors, one can see that careful, anxious, and risk-avoidant people are at lower risk for HIV, while those who are risk-taking, emotion-driven, and relatively unconcerned with their future well-being are at higher risk for acquiring the infection. Likewise those who tend to be unconcerned about their responsibilities to others might knowingly continue to spread HIV, showing little regard for the impact they have on others. A small amount of research has examined the roles personality type plays in HIV infection and outcomes, mostly in Western and high-income cultures, and this issue continues to be of crucial importance to halting the HIV epidemic. People with certain personality types are "vulnerable" to situations that might expose them to HIV, and need adequate coaching in advance to help them avoid the trap their vulnerabilities might set for them.

Lastly, psychiatric disorders often compound each other in co-morbid situations. Major depression increases the likelihood of alcohol abuse, and alcohol abuse worsens major depression, clouds judgment and erodes self-discipline and self-attitude, and undermines relationships with others who might provide guidance and restraint. People who are risk-taking or those that are highly anxious are also more likely to overuse alcohol, or other substances, and thus are vulnerable to these complications, each of which compound the risk for acquiring HIV and related conditions, such as hepatitis C, gonorrhea and other STDs, and a host of other behaviorally transmitted infections.

PSYCHOPHARMACOLOGY IN HIV-INFECTED INDIVIDUALS

The core requirement of treatment is accurate diagnosis. For the last half of the 20th century, the international efforts in psychiatry focused on whether the same conditions exist across cultures and if they have similar courses and responses to treatment. With the exception of some culture-specific conditions, the common psychiatric disorders have similar prevalence around the world and appear to respond similarly to treatment. While there are differences in the approved drugs from one country to another, the majority of the pharmacological classes are available, although there are distinct cultural beliefs about the use of medications to treat psychiatric disorders.

Psychopharmacologic agents can be divided up into the classes in Table 20.1. We have given generic names for several of the common drugs in each class, but the list is not

Table 20.1 Commonly used psychotropic medications in HIV-infected patients

CLASS OF AGENT	GENERIC NAMES	ADVANTAGES	DISADVANTAGES
Antidepressant			
SSRI	Citalopram, Dapoxetine, Fluoxetine, Paroxetine, Sertraline, Vilazodone (others)	Easy to use, well tolerated, now mostly off patent and inexpensive, relatively few drug interactions	Serotonin syndrome, decreased sexual drive and anorgasmia, GI activation
SNRI	Duloxetine, Milnacipran, Venlafaxine (others)	Easy to use, well tolerated, helpful for chronic pain, relatively few drug interactions	Serotonin syndrome, decreased sexual drive and anorgasmia, GI activation
Tricyclic antidepressant	Desipramine, Doxepin, Nortriptyline (others)	Hypnotic (for sleep), increased appetite, useful for chronic pain, meaningful therapeutic blood levels	Need monitoring for narrow margin of safety, anticholinergic and alpha-blocking, cardiotoxic and can be fatal in overdose, lowers seizure threshold
Aminoketone	Bupropion (originally called Amfebutamone)	No sexual side effects, activating, no weight gain	Jittery feelings, lowers seizure threshold
Tetracyclic	Mianserin, Mirtazepine	Appetite stimulating, safer in overdose than tricyclic antidepressants, useful in pain, promotes sleep	Weight gain, sedation

Table 20.1 Commonly used psychotropic medications in HIV-infected patients—cont'd

CLASS OF AGENT	GENERIC NAMES	ADVANTAGES	DISADVANTAGES
Antipsychotic			
Typical (or first generation)	Chlorpromazine, Haloperidol (many others)	Inexpensive, sedating and tranquilizing	Dystonia, bradykinesia, tardive dyskinesia, anticholinergic, alpha-blocking, neuroleptic malignant syndrome
Atypical (or second generation)	Amisulpride, Aripiprazole, Asenapine, Blonanserin, Clotiapine, Clozapine, Iloperidone, Lurasidone, Mosapramine, Olanzapine, Paliperidone, Perospirone, Quetiapine, Remoxipride, Risperidone, Sertindole, Sulpiride, Ziprasidone, Zotepine	Much less dystonia, bradykinesia, tardive dyskinesia, anticholinergic, alpha-blocking, possibly less neuroleptic malignant syndrome	Many still on patent, weight gain, metabolic syndrome, QT prolongation (agrualocytosis with clozapine)
Sedative-hypnotic (anxiolytic)			
Benzodiazepine	Alprazolam, Bromazepam, Chlordiazepoxide, Cinolazepam, Clobazam, Clonazepam, Cloxazolam, Clorazepate, Diazepam, Estazolam, Flunitrazem, Flurazepam, Halazepam, Ketazolam, Loprazolam, Lorazepam, Lormetazepam, Medazepam, Midazolam, Nitrazepam, Nordazepam, Oxazepam, Phenazepam, Pinazepam, Prazepam, Quazepam, Temazepam, Tetrazepam, Triazolam	Pleasant sedation, effective anxiolytic, good panic attack abortive agents, most widely used psychopharmacologic agents	Numerous drug interactions with HIV medications, addictive, cognitive impairment, physical dependence with potentially life-threatening withdrawal, respiratory suppression
Non-benzodiazepine	Eszopiclone, Zaleplon, Zolpidem, Zopiclone	Possibly less addictive, less physical dependence, less respiratory suppression	Rapid sleep habituation with subsequent dependence for sleep in many patients, cognitive impairment

exhaustive. Studies in a variety of settings have shown that these agents are similarly effective in HIV-infected patients when compared with those at risk or in control groups. We have put in only the most major advantages and disadvantages by class, but there are numerous subtle issues within each class. The long lists of antipsychotics and benzodiazepines demonstrate the heterogeneity of the availability of the drugs in different countries.

Generally, as compared with non-HIV-infected patients, the following guidelines are useful in HIV settings:

- Psychotropic medications for every psychiatric condition have been shown to work as well in HIV-infected individuals as in non-infected individuals.

- Care should be taken in using psychotropic medications in debilitated patients—they should be started at low doses and titrated up slowly to effective doses (Start Low-Go Slow).

- In general, in contrast to sedative-hypnotic agents, antidepressant and antipsychotic medications have few clinically significant drug–drug interactions with antiretrovirals, but each individual patient should be monitored for onset of side effects and reduced efficacy to avoid poor outcomes.

- Benzodiazepines should be used with great caution, as some interact with certain antiretrovirals and can lead to serious adverse outcomes.

- Psychotherapy and education are essential to successful treatment. Patient adherence is driven mostly by patient attitudes toward taking psychotropic medication—if the patient does not take the medication it cannot work. On the positive side, adherence to psychiatric medications predicts adherence to ART.

- There are clinically significant drug–drug interactions between methadone and efavirenz and ritonavir for which dose adjustments of methadone are required. Buprenorphine (a partial agonist for the opioid receptor) may require less adjustment. Many patients on opiates will experience changes with the initiation of ART, and will require careful monitoring with treatment initiation and regimen changes.

CONCLUSION

Recognition and treatment of mental illness in the global fight against HIV/AIDS is paramount: mental and behavioral disorders are not only more likely to develop in the infected patient, but also they are important risk factors for HIV acquisition and transmission of the infection. Furthermore, these disorders deplete their victims economically and socially and undermine the potential for treatment success by impairing adherence. The complex interplay of HIV/AIDS and mental illness can be daunting,

in the sense of the challenges posed for designing and implementing public health interventions. Fortunately there is international consensus and action for HIV/AIDS treatment and prevention worldwide, and indications of progress. What is needed next is the scaling up of mental health services in middle- and low-income countries, to eliminate the mismatch between need and services. Scaling up of services will involve community education activities, consensus building, engagement of community resources, establishment of secure funding, training of psychiatrist and other psychiatric health workers, infrastructure development, and monitoring and evaluation activities [10, 53]. There is also evidence that simple pharmacologic regimens and community-based rehabilitation models can be implemented in low-income countries [9]. By addressing the psychiatric morbidity surrounding HIV, we can reduce the global burden of disease and reduce further spread of AIDS. Separately, programs might be implemented to increase the rates of ART compliance through programs that promote knowledge and self-efficacy, especially in those who suffer psychiatric disorders. While the HIV/AIDS situation in low-income countries remains urgent, the latest global reports show that we are making progress in the fight against this epidemic. WHO initiatives aimed at addressing mental health gaps in middle- and low-income countries promise additional means for increasing and extending successes against the HIV/AIDS epidemic.

REFERENCES

[1] Angelino AF, Treisman GJ. Issues in co-morbid severe mental illnesses in HIV infected individuals. Int Rev Psychiatry 2008;20(1):95–101.

[2] Treisman G, Angelino A. Interrelation between psychiatric disorders and the prevention and treatment of HIV infection. Clin Infect Dis 2007;45(Suppl. 4): S313–S317.

[3] Kessler RC, Aguilar-Gaxiola S, Alonso J, et al. The global burden of mental disorders: an update from the WHO World Mental Health (WMH) surveys. Epidemiol Psichiatr Soc 2009;18(1):23–33.

[4] World Health Organization. mhGAP: Mental Health Gap Action Programme: scaling up care for mental, neurological, and substance use disorders. 2008.

[5] Joint United Nations Programme on AIDS (UNAIDS). Global Report: UNAIDS Report on the Global AIDS Epidemic 2010 [Internet]. Available

from: http://www.unaids.org/globalreport/Global_report.htm.

[6] Wang PS, Aguilar-Gaxiola S, Alonso J, et al. Use of mental health services for anxiety, mood, and substance disorders in 17 countries in the WHO world mental health surveys. Lancet 2007;370 (9590):841–50.

[7] Gureje VO, Lasebikan O. Use of mental health services in a developing country. Results from the Nigerian survey of mental health and well-being. Soc Psychiatry Psychiatr Epidemiol 2006;41 (1):44–9.

[8] Saxena S, Thornicroft G, Knapp M, Whiteford H. Resources for mental health: scarcity, inequity, and inefficiency. Lancet 2007;370 (9590):878–89.

[9] Patel V, Aroya R, Chatterjee S, et al. Global Mental Health 3–Treatment and prevention of mental disorders in low-income and middle-income

countries. Lancet 2007;370:991–1005.

[10] Saraceno B, van Ommeren M, Batniji R, et al. Barriers to improvement of mental health services in low-income and middle-income countries. Lancet 2007;370 (9593):1164–74.

[11] Gureje O, Lasebikan VO, Ephraim-Oluwanuga O, et al. Community study of knowledge of and attitude to mental illness in Nigeria. Br J Psychiatry 2005;186:436–41.

[12] Corrigan PW, Watson AC, Warpinski AC, Gracia G. Stigmatizing attitudes about mental illness and allocation of resources to mental health services. Community Ment Health J 2004;40(4):297–307.

[13] Kiima DM, Njenga FG, Okonji MM, Kigamwa PA. Kenya mental health country profile. Int Rev Psychiatry 2004;16(1–2):48–53.

[14] Ndyanabangi S, Basangwa D, Lutakome J, Mubiru C. Uganda

mental health country profile. Int Rev Psychiatry 2004;16 (1–2):54–62.

[15] Mayeya J, Chazulwa R, Mayeya PN, et al. Zambia mental health country profile. Int Rev Psychiatry 2004;16 (1–2):63–72.

[16] Nakimuli-Mpungu E, Mutamba B, Othengo M, Musisi S. Psychological distress and adherence to highly active anti-retroviral therapy (HAART) in Uganda: a pilot study. Afr Health Sci 2009;9(Suppl. 1): S2–S7.

[17] Pence BW. The impact of mental health and traumatic life experiences on antiretroviral treatment outcomes for people living with HIV/AIDS. J Antimicrob Chemother 2009;63(4):636–40.

[18] Tessema B, Biadglegne F, Mulu A, et al. Magnitude and determinants of nonadherence and nonreadiness to highly active antiretroviral therapy among people living with HIV/AIDS in Northwest Ethiopia: a cross-sectional study. AIDS Res Ther 2010;7:2.

[19] Olisah VO, Baiyewu O, Sheikh TL. Adherence to highly active antiretroviral therapy in depressed patients with HIV/AIDS attending a Nigerian university teaching hospital clinic. Afr J Psychiatry (Johannesbg) 2010;13(4):275–9.

[20] Nakimuli-Mpungu N, Nakasujja N, Akena HD, et al. Effect of older age at initiation of antiretroviral therapy on patient retention in an urban ART program in Uganda. Neurobehav HIV Med 2011;31–8.

[21] Ettenhofer M, Hinkin C, Castellon S, et al. Aging, neurocognition, and medication adherence in HIV infection. Am J Geriatr Psychiatry 2009;17 (4):281–90.

[22] Ettenhofer ML, Foley J, Castellon SA, Hinkin CH. Reciprocal prediction of medication adherence and neurocognition in HIV/AIDS. Neurology 2010;74 (15):1217–22.

[23] Cournos F, McKinnon K. HIV seroprevalence among people with severe mental illness in the United States: a critical review. Clin Psychol Rev 1997;17(3):259–69.

[24] Rosenberg SD, Goodman LA, Osher FC, et al. Prevalence of HIV,

hepatitis B, and hepatitis C in people with severe mental illness. Am J Public Health 2001;91 (1):31–7.

[25] Rosenberg SD, Drake RE, Brunette MF, et al. Hepatitis C virus and HIV co-infection in people with severe mental illness and substance use disorders. AIDS 2005;19(Suppl. 3):S26–S33.

[26] Pirl WF, Greer JA, Weissgarber C, et al. Screening for infectious diseases among patients in a state psychiatric hospital. Psychiatr Serv 2005;56(12):1614–16.

[27] Joska JA, Kaliski SZ, Benatar SR. Patients with severe mental illness: a new approach to testing for HIV. S Afr Med J 2008;98 (3):213–17.

[28] Maling S, Todd J, Van der Paal L, et al. HIV-1 seroprevalence and risk factors for HIV infection among first-time psychiatric admissions in Uganda. AIDS Care 2011;23 (2):171–8.

[29] Volavka J, Convit A, Czobor P, et al. HIV seroprevalence and risk behaviors in psychiatric inpatients. Psychiatry Res 1991;39(2):109–14.

[30] Davidson S, Judd F, Jolley D, et al. Risk factors for HIV/AIDS and hepatitis C among the chronic mentally ill. Aust N Z J Psychiatry 2001;35(2):203–9.

[31] McKinnon K, Carey MP, Cournos F. Research on HIV, AIDS, and severe mental illness: recommendations from the NIMH National Conference. Clin Psychol Rev 1997;17(3):327–31.

[32] McKinnon K, Cournos F. HIV infection linked to substance use among hospitalized patients with severe mental illness. Psychiatr Serv 1998;49(10):1269.

[33] Cournos F, McKinnon K, Sullivan G. Schizophrenia and comorbid human immunodeficiency virus or hepatitis C virus. J Clin Psychiatry 2005;66(Suppl. 6):27–33.

[34] Newville H, Haller DL. Psychopathology and transmission risk behaviors in patients with HIV/ AIDS. AIDS Care 2010;22 (10):1259–68.

[35] Campos LN, Guimarães MD, Remien RH. Anxiety and depression symptoms as risk factors for non-adherence to antiretroviral therapy

in Brazil. AIDS Behav 2010;14 (2):289–99.

[36] Venkatesh KK, Srikrishnan AK, Mayer KH, et al. Predictors of nonadherence to highly active antiretroviral therapy among HIV-infected South Indians in clinical care: implications for developing adherence interventions in resource-limited settings. AIDS Patient Care STDS 2010;24(12):795–803.

[37] Murphy DA, Marelich WD, Hoffman D, Steers WN. Predictors of antiretroviral adherence. AIDS Care 2004;16 (4):471–84.

[38] Lucas GM, Chaisson RE, Moore RD. Highly active antiretroviral therapy in a large urban clinic: risk factors for virologic failure and adverse drug reactions. Ann Intern Med 1999;131(2):81–7.

[39] Finocchario-Kessler S, Catley D, Berkley-Patton J, et al. Baseline predictors of ninety percent or higher antiretroviral therapy adherence in a diverse urban sample: the role of patient autonomy and fatalistic religious beliefs. AIDS Patient Care STDS 2011;25(2):103–11.

[40] American Psychiatric Association . Practice guideline for the treatment of patients with HIV/AIDS. Work Group on HIV/AIDS. Am J Psychiatry 2000;157(Suppl. 11):1–62.

[41] Lyketsos CG, Hanson AL, Fishman M, et al. Manic syndrome early and late in the course of HIV. Am J Psychiatry 1993;150 (2):326–7.

[42] Nakimuli-Mpungu E, Musisi S, Mpungu S, Katabira E. Primary mania versus HIV-related secondary mania in Uganda. Am J Psychiatry 2006;163 (8):1349–54.

[43] Nakimuli-Mpungu E, Musisi S, Mpungu S, Katabira E. Early-onset versus late-onset HIV-related secondary mania in Uganda. Psychosomatics 2008;49(6):530–4.

[44] Wilk CM, Bolton P. Local perceptions of the mental health effects of the Uganda acquired immunodeficiency syndrome epidemic. J Nerv Ment Dis 2002;190 (6):394–7.

[45] Robertson K, Liner J, Hakim J, et al. NeuroAIDS in Africa. J Neurovirol 2010;16(3):189–202.

[46] Tozzi V, Balestra P, Libertone R, Antinori A. Cognitive function in treated HIV patients. Neurobehav HIV Med 2010;95–113.

[47] Joska JA, Gouse H, Paul RH, et al. Does highly active antiretroviral therapy improve neurocognitive function? A systematic review. J Neurovirol 2010;16(2):101–14.

[48] Antinori A, Arendt G, Becker JT, et al. Updated research nosology for HIV-associated neurocognitive disorders. Neurology 2007;69 (18):1789–99.

[49] Uldall KK, Ryan R, Berghuis JP, Harris VL. Association between delirium and death in AIDS patients. AIDS Patient Care STDS 2000;14(2):95–100.

[50] Cohen J. Asia and Africa: on different trajectories? Science 2004;304(5679):1932–8.

[51] McHugh PR, Slavney PR. The Perspectives of Psychiatry. 2nd ed. Baltimore, MD: Johns Hopkins University Press; 1998.

[52] Treisman GJ, Angelino AF. The Psychiatry of AIDS: A Guide to Diagnosis and Treatment. Baltimore, MD: Johns Hopkins University Press; 2004.

[53] Thornicroft G, Alem A, Antunes Dos Santos R, et al. WPA guidance on steps, obstacles and mistakes to avoid in the implementation of community mental health care. World Psychiatry 2010;9(2): 67–77.

Chapter | 21 |

Cardiovascular complications of HIV infection

Rakesh K. Mishra

INTRODUCTION

The landscape of cardiovascular disease in HIV-infected patients has changed significantly since the introduction of potent antiretroviral therapy (ART). In the early years of the epidemic, the principal cardiovascular manifestations of HIV were dilated cardiomyopathy, pericardial disease, pulmonary hypertension, and neoplastic involvement of the heart. ART has been revolutionary in the care of HIV, significantly reducing the incidence of opportunistic infections and, thereby, prolonging life [1]. However, ART, especially one of its components, the protease inhibitors, can be associated with significant metabolic abnormalities including insulin resistance, lipid abnormalities such as decreased high-density lipoproteins (HDL) and increased triglycerides, and fat redistribution with loss of peripheral fat and intra-abdominal fat accumulation [2]. Therefore, it is not surprising that, as the incidence of dilated cardiomyopathy, pericardial disease, and neoplastic involvement of the heart has decreased, the incidence of cardiovascular disease has increased since the introduction of ART. The prolongation of life with ART and the consequently longer exposure to this therapy and HIV itself may all be factors in the increasing incidence and prevalence of cardiovascular disease in HIV-infected patients.

This review will discuss the most common cardiovascular complications of HIV diseases (Box 21.1), including coronary artery disease, cardiomyopathy and congestive heart failure, pericardial disease, pulmonary hypertension, endocarditis, and neoplastic involvement of the heart. For each of these conditions, there will be a focus on trends in the incidence, prevalence, and disease course from the pre-ART to the current era.

CORONARY ARTERY DISEASE

With the advent of ART and improved survival with HIV infection, there is now increasing epidemiological overlap between patients with HIV infection and those at risk for coronary artery disease (CAD). In addition to traditional risk factors for CAD, HIV infection itself and certain antiretroviral combinations may also contribute to the increased risk of CAD. Many large cohort studies have found a higher prevalence of traditional CAD risk factors among HIV-infected patients, including higher rates of smoking, lower high-density lipoprotein cholesterol (HDL-C), and higher triglyceride levels [3, 4]. However, the increased risk of CAD events persists despite adjustment for these traditional risk factors [5]. This suggests a role for both the HIV infection itself and, perhaps, certain components of ART in cardiovascular risk. HIV accelerates atherosclerosis through direct effects on cholesterol processing and transport, attraction of monocytes to the intimal wall, and activation of monocytes to induce an inflammatory response and endothelial proliferation [6]. In a large study of patients enrolled in the Kaiser Permanente database, the overall CAD event rate among HIV-infected patients was significantly greater than that of HIV-uninfected controls [7]. Interestingly, the age-adjusted CAD and myocardial infarction (MI) hospitalization rates were not significantly different before and after the introduction of protease inhibitors (PI) or before and after the initiation of other antiretroviral agents. Carotid intimal medial thickness (IMT), a marker of subclinical CAD, is increased in HIV-infected patients compared with those without HIV [8]. The fat redistribution and metabolic change in HIV infection (FRAM) investigators found that the statistically significant increase in carotid IMT in HIV-infected patients persisted after adjustment for both demographics and traditional CAD risk factors [9]. In this study, the effect of HIV on carotid IMT was similar to the effects of male sex, current smoking, and diabetes. In a recent study of non-smoking HIV-infected male patients, duration of HIV infection, not ART use, was associated with increased carotid IMT [10]. Moreover, the rate of MI in HIV-infected patients, though still higher than in controls, has declined in recent years [11]. This reduction in risk is likely associated with increasing use of lipid-lowering therapy in these patients, along with the use of newer ART agents.

In addition to HIV itself, ART has been implicated in increasing the risk of CAD. The HIV Outpatient Study (HOPS), a large prospective observational study, found an increase in the incidence of MI after the introduction of PIs in 1996 [12]. The Data Collection on Adverse Events of Anti-HIV Drugs (D:A:D) Study Group, another large prospective observational study, found an increasing incidence of MI with increasing exposure to combination ART [13]. In a follow-up study from the same group, there was an increased risk of MI per year of exposure to PIs [14]. Adjustment for serum lipids attenuated, but did not obliterate, this effect. And, finally, there have been conflicting findings on the association between abacavir use and an increased risk of MI [15, 16]. A recent meta-analysis by the US Food and Drug Administration of 26 randomized control trials showed no increase in the risk of MI with abacavir use [17], whereas a large observational study has suggested a possible link [15]. The expert opinions in the field have concluded that the overall increase in risk of CVD events associated with ART is modest, is outweighed by their effectiveness in controlling HIV disease, and should be combated with modulation of traditional cardiovascular risk factors.

Both HIV and ART are associated with dyslipidemia. After seroconversion, there is a decrease in total cholesterol, low-density lipoprotein cholesterol (LDL-C), and HDL-C [18]. This is followed by increases in levels of triglycerides and very low-density lipoprotein cholesterol (VLDL-C) [19]. In fact, increasing plasma HIV RNA levels are associated with decreasing levels of HDL-C and LDL-C

and increasing levels of triglycerides and VLDL-C; decreasing CD4 counts are associated with lower levels of HDL-C [20]. After the initiation of ART, lipid levels return to either baseline levels or higher levels, except HDL-C, which remains low [18]. These changes may represent a general restoration to health or may be the result of direct medication effects. Most PIs raise lipid levels [6]. Non-nucleoside reverse transcriptase inhibitors (NNRTIs) are also associated with lipid abnormalities but to a lesser extent than PIs. However, the effects on lipids vary with each specific drug within a class. For example, within the class of PIs, lopinavir/ritonavir and tipranavir/ritonavir are associated with more significant increases in lipid levels, particularly triglycerides, while atazanavir/ritonavir and darunavir/ritonavir cause more modest lipid changes [6]. Several mechanisms by which ART could lead to dyslipidemia have been proposed (Box 21.2) [21].

The Infectious Disease Society of America (IDSA) and the Adult AIDS Clinical Trials Group (ACTG) have provided guidelines for the evaluation and management of dyslipidemia in HIV-infected adults receiving ART. These guidelines draw heavily upon the National Cholesterol Education Program Adult Treatment Panel III guidelines. A subsequent implications paper should be considered in conjunction with these guidelines [22]. These topics have been reviewed extensively elsewhere [23] and a summary of these guidelines is provided in Figure 21.1.

Figure 21.1 General approach to lipid disorders and cardiovascular risk in HIV-infected patients receiving ART per the guidelines of the Infectious Disease Society of America and the Adult AIDS Clinical Trials Group. CHD, coronary heart disease; HDL, high-density lipoprotein; LDL, low-density lipoprotein.

Adapted from Dubé MP, Stein JH, Aberg JA, et al. Guidelines for the evaluation and management of dyslipidemia in human immunodeficiency virus (HIV)-infected adults receiving antiretroviral therapy: recommendations of the HIV Medical Association of the Infectious Disease Society of America and the Adult AIDS Clinical Trials Group. Clin Infect Dis 2003; 37:613–27.

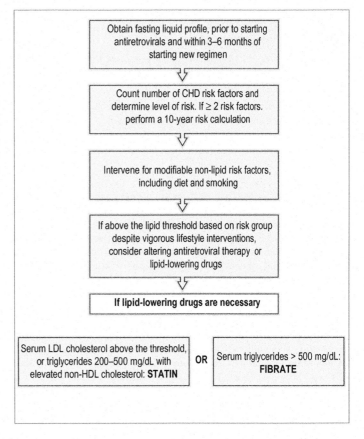

CARDIOMYOPATHY AND CONGESTIVE HEART FAILURE

Heart muscle disease is one of the most important cardiovascular manifestations of HIV infection. This may present as dilated cardiomyopathy (DCM), myocarditis, or isolated left or right ventricular dysfunction [24]. In the pre-ART era, clinical and pathological studies showed a nearly 30% prevalence of cardiomyopathy in patients with HIV, with an annual incidence of 15.9/1000 cases [25, 26]. DCM carries a poor prognosis in patients with HIV. In a 4-year prospective echocardiographic study survey of 296 patients with HIV infection, DCM was associated with a CD4 count of <100 cells/mm^3 and significantly reduced survival time [27]. DCM tends to occur late in the course of HIV infection. The exact prevalence of myocarditis in patients with HIV infection has been difficult to establish, with estimates ranging from 6 to 52% [26, 28]. It is likely that myocarditis and DCM represent a continuum of disease progression.

Since the introduction of ART, there has been a decline in the incidence and prevalence of DCM. In a single-center retrospective study comparing the prevalence of cardiovascular complications of HIV disease before and after ART, the prevalence of DCM decreased from 8.1 to 1.8% [29]. A more recent report from the Study to Understand the Natural History of HIV/AIDS in the Era of Effective Therapy (SUN Study) showed a persistently high prevalence of subclinical cardiac structural and functional abnormalities in outpatients with HIV on ART [30]. While nearly two-thirds of the patients had LV systolic or diastolic dysfunction, left ventricular hypertrophy, left atrial enlargement, or pulmonary hypertension, less that 2% had moderate or severe LV systolic dysfunction and 11% had moderate or severe diastolic dysfunction. However, DCM continues to be a significant cardiovascular complication of HIV where access to ART is limited. In a recent study of 416 HIV-infected patients in Rwanda, DCM was documented by echocardiography in 71 (17.7%) of them [31]. By both univariate and multivariate analysis, low socioeconomic status, estimated duration of HIV-1 infection, CD4 count, HIV-1 viral load, CDC stage B and C of HIV disease, and low plasma level of selenium were factors significantly associated with the development of cardiomyopathy.

The pathogenesis of DCM continues to be an area of intense study (Box 21.3). HIV may damage cardiac myocytes

> **Box 21.3 Common causes of HIV-associated dilated cardiomyopathy [24]**
>
> - Myocarditis: HIV, Coxsackie virus group B, Epstein–Barr virus, cytomegalovirus, echovirus, *Toxoplasma gondii*
> - Autoimmunity
> - Metabolic: selenium, vitamin B_{12}, carnitine deficiency
> - Endocrine: thyroid hormone, growth hormone, adrenal insufficiency, hyperinsulinemia

by a direct cytolytic effect or through an "innocent bystander" reaction [25, 28]. Infection of myocardial cells by HIV-1 has been demonstrated in a patchy distribution [28]. The mechanism by which HIV infection enters cardiac myocytes, which do not possess CD4 receptors, is not clear. It has been hypothesized that other cells in the myocardium—such as dendritic cells—play a role not only as a reservoir but also as antigen-presenting cells in the context of the major histocompatibility complex and as activators of cytokines that contribute to tissue damage [32]. In a more recent study comparing histopathological sections from HIV-infected patients with and without cardiomyopathy, the expression of HIV envelope protein glycoprotein 120 (gp120) and HIV replication were noted to be more prominent in T-cells and macrophages, which also produce higher levels of pro-inflammatory cytokines, than in cardiac myocytes, in which HIV does not replicate [33]. Although HIV has been detected in cardiac tissue, these findings suggest that an indirect mechanism initiated by inflammatory cells and cytokines or perhaps even a secondary viral infection such as cytomegalovirus, group B Coxsackie virus, Epstein–Barr virus, or adenovirus mediates the high incidence of myocarditis with potential progression to DCM among HIV-infected patients rather than an HIV-specific infection of cardiomyocytes [34].

There is a growing body of evidence that suggests that autoimmune mechanisms may also play an important role in the development of cardiomyopathy in HIV-infected patients [32, 35]. Uncontrolled hypergammaglobulinemia from T-helper cell dysfunction and increased concentrations of circulating immune complex have been associated with cardiac inflammation [36]. HIV protein transcription also may alter the surface of cardiac myocytes with induction of cell-surface immunogenic proteins leading to production of cardiac autoantibodies that, in turn, could trigger cardiomyocyte destruction. In patients with LV dysfunction and evidence of myocarditis, immunohistologic findings have revealed induced expression of major histocompatibility class I antigen on myocytes and increased numbers of infiltrating CD8$^+$ T lymphocytes [37]. In a study of 74 HIV-infected patients including 28 with echocardiographic evidence of heart muscle disease, cardiac autoantibodies detected by indirect immunofluorescence were more common in the HIV-infected patients (15%),

particularly the HIV heart muscle disease group (21%), than in HIV-uninfected controls (3.5%) [38]. In addition, abnormal anti-α myosin autoantibody concentrations were found more often in HIV patients with heart muscle disease (43%) than in HIV-infected patients with normal hearts (19%) or in HIV-uninfected controls (3%).

Nutritional abnormalities also may play a role in some patients, especially late in HIV infection and particularly in the resource-poor setting. Deficiencies of selenium, vitamin B_{12}, and carnitine have been reported and associated with left ventricular dysfunction [31, 39]. Other metabolic and endocrine abnormalities that have been associated with cardiac dysfunction include hypothyroidism, growth hormone deficiency, hypoadrenalism, and hyperinsulinism [34, 36].

The role of certain drugs used to treat HIV in the development of cardiomyopathy remains controversial. The nucleoside reverse transcriptase inhibitor (NRTI) zidovudine has been associated with diffuse destruction of ultra-structures and inhibition of mitochondrial DNA replication, resulting in lactic acidosis that contributes to myocardial dysfunction [40, 41]. However, zidovudine neither improved nor worsened the cardiac abnormalities in a prospective study of 24 children [42], and in adults, it does not seem to be associated with myocardial dysfunction [43].

Drugs used to treat complications of HIV infection also have been associated with dilated cardiomyopathy. Amphotericin B, used to treat disseminated fungal infections, is associated with a reversible dilated cardiomyopathy and may cause hypertension and bradycardia [44]. Doxorubicin, which is used to treat Kaposi's sarcoma, is associated with cardiomyopathy in a dose-related manner [45]. Foscarnet treatment of cytomegalovirus infection may cause cardiomyopathy as well [46]. Interferon-α, an immunomodulator that is used as an antineoplastic and antiviral for concomitant hepatitic C infection, can also cause cardiomyopathy, although arrhythmia and myocardial ischemia are more common [47]. Finally, as survival with HIV infection increases and risk factors for atherosclerosis develop due to aging and the use of ART, CAD and MI are increasingly common phenomena that may contribute to left ventricular systolic dysfunction, as discussed above.

PERICARDIAL DISEASE

In the pre-ART era, pericardial effusion was one of the most common clinically relevant cardiac complications in patients with HIV infection, with an annual incidence of 11% [48]. Pericardial effusion can have a wide range of manifestations including the asymptomatic effusion incidentally detected by echocardiography or routine chest imaging, cardiac tamponade, acute or chronic pericarditis, and, uncommonly, constrictive pericardial disease. A review of 15 autopsy and echocardiographic studies that included 1139 HIV-infected patients revealed that approximately 21%

had a pericardial effusion, most of which were without an identifiable cause and were asymptomatic [49]. A male predominance in the development of pericardial effusions has been reported [50]. Dyspnea and edema were common presenting symptoms, whereas chest pain was uncommon [50]. Most of the effusions were small, with a lower prevalence of moderate to large pericardial effusions [48, 50, 51]. Variables associated with moderate to large pericardial effusions were congestive heart failure, Kaposi's sarcoma, tuberculosis, and pulmonary infections of all etiologies [51]. Tamponade requiring emergent pericardiocentesis was rare, as was acute pericarditis [48, 51]. In the pre-ART era, the development of a pericardial effusion was a poor prognostic marker in patients with HIV [48]. HIV-infected patients with pericardial effusion had shorter survival (36% at 6 months) than individuals without effusions (93% at 6 months, relative risk 2.2, 95% CI, 1.2–4, $p < 0.01$). Pericardiocentesis is currently recommended only in large, symptomatic effusions, for diagnostic evaluation of systemic illness, or for the management of acute cardiac tamponade [39]. The prevalence of pericardial effusions has declined dramatically since the introduction of ART [29, 52]. However, in sub-Saharan Africa, pericardial disease continues to be a frequent initial manifestation of HIV-related cardiac disease [53].

In the developed world, most pericardial effusions in patients with HIV infection are idiopathic. However, in sub-Saharan Africa, *Mycobacterium tuberculosis* was the underlying cause in up to 70% of cases of pericardial effusion [53]. Culture of pericardial fluid usually is unrevealing (although pericardial biopsy has a higher yield), but other uncommon opportunistic infections and neoplasms can be diagnosed (Box 21.4).

PULMONARY HYPERTENSION

Pulmonary arterial hypertension (PAH) is a rare but serious cardiovascular complication of HIV infection. The most common presenting symptom is dyspnea (83%), followed by peripheral edema, syncope, and chest pain [54]. The prevalence of PAH in HIV-infected individuals (0.5%) is higher than in the general population and has not changed significantly since the introduction of ART [54–56]. However, the annual incidence of PAH has declined from 0.21% in the pre-ART era to 0.03% recently and this may be due to higher CD4 counts with a decrease in overall immune activation [54]. Though overall survival has improved in the ART era, patients with HIV-associated PAH continue to have a worse prognosis, with reduced median survival, than HIV-infected patients without PAH [54, 57]. About two-thirds of deaths in HIV-infected patients with PAH are due to the direct sequelae of PAH, such as right ventricular failure, cardiogenic shock, and sudden cardiac death [58, 59]. The histopathological findings in HIV-infected patients with PAH are similar to those seen in idiopathic PAH: the majority have pulmonary arteriopathy with medial hypertrophy, intimal thickening and/or plexiform lesions (89%), with veno-occlusive disease in 7% and thrombotic pulmonary arteriopathy in 4% [58]. Though HIV infection is regarded as a risk factor for the development of PAH, it is unlikely that direct infection of the pulmonary vascular endothelium is the mechanism. Even with the use of highly sensitive techniques such as polymerase chain reaction (PCR) and *in situ* hybridization, the virus has not been identified in the pulmonary endothelium of HIV-infected patients with PAH [60]. It is thus likely that HIV plays an indirect role in the pathogenesis of PAH, through mediators such as growth factors and cytokines. The HIV envelope glycoprotein (gp120) stimulates macrophage secretion of endothelin-1, a potent vasoconstrictor that is implicated in other forms of PAH [61]. Pro-inflammatory cytokines such as interleukin-1β, interleukin-6, and tumor necrosis factor-α are elevated in HIV-infected patients and are also implicated in the development of PAH [62]. Interleukin-1β is also linked to the production of platelet-derived growth factor, a growth factor implicated in vascular remodeling in PAH [63]. In addition to primary pulmonary hypertension, secondary causes due to talc exposure in injection drug users, chronic liver disease, interstitial lung disease, and coagulopathies also contribute to HIV-associated pulmonary hypertension.

> ### Box 21.4 **Common causes of HIV-associated pericardial effusion**
>
> - Idiopathic: capillary leak
> - Malignant: Kaposi's sarcoma, lymphoma
> - Infectious: bacterial—*Staphylococcus*, *Streptococcus*, *Proteus*, *Nocardia*, *Pseudomonas*, *Klebsiella*, *Enterococcus*, *Listeria*, *Mycobacteria*
> - Viral: HIV, herpes simplex virus, cytomegalovirus
> - Fungal/protozoan: *Cryptococcus*, *Histoplasma*, *Toxoplasma*
> - Hypothyroidism

ENDOCARDITIS

Before the introduction of ART, non-bacterial thrombotic endocarditis ("marantic" endocarditis) was relatively common, with a prevalence of 3 to 5% in AIDS patients, particularly in those with HIV-wasting syndrome [25]. Marantic endocarditis is characterized by the presence of fibrin-rich collections of platelets and erythrocytes that adhere to valves, forming a fibrin mesh with relatively little inflammatory reaction. Systemic embolism is common, but most episodes are clinically silent. The diagnosis of non-bacterial thrombotic endocarditis is usually made post mortem.

Infective endocarditis (IE) occurs at a similar rate among patients with HIV infection, as in other groups of individuals at increased risk such as intravenous drug users [39]. Recently the incidence of IE in HIV-infected patients who use intravenous drugs has decreased from 20.5 per 1,000 person-years in the pre-ART era to 6.6 per 1,000 person-years [64]. Those with advanced immunosuppression are more likely to develop IE. Intravenous drug users frequently have right-sided valvular infections due to *Staphylococcus aureus*, *Streptococcus pneumonia* and *Streptococcus virideans* [39, 65]. Although presentations of IE usually are similar among HIV-infected and non-infected patients, survival with endocarditis is worse in individuals with HIV infection, particularly in those with more advanced HIV disease [64, 65].

NEOPLASMS

The most common cardiac neoplasms in HIV-infected patients are Kaposi's sarcoma and non-Hodgkin's lymphoma. A recent autopsy study demonstrated a marked decline in the prevalence of Kaposi's sarcoma from 17 to 3% since the introduction of ART [66]. Although malignant lymphomas of the heart are rare, lymphomas were identified in 5 to 10% of patients with HIV infection in the pre-ART era, which is a 60–100 times higher prevalence than expected in the general population [36, 67]. A statistically significant reduction in the incidence of non-Hodgkin's lymphoma has been demonstrated since the widespread introduction of ART, although this reduction has not been as dramatic as that for Kaposi's sarcoma [68].

HIV-associated lymphomas are typically derived from B-lymphocytes and are high grade. Metastatic lymphomas of the heart are more common than primary cardiac lymphomas, which tend to be rare. Most patients have disseminated disease at the time of their initial presentation, although some patients may have primary lymphomas involving only the pericardium [69]. In general, AIDS-associated lymphomas are found in patients with low CD4 counts; however, non-Hodgkin's lymphoma may occur in patients with less

advanced immune suppression. The prognosis of patients with HIV-associated cardiac non-Hodgkin's lymphoma is poor, although remission has been observed in patients treated with combination chemotherapy.

Autopsy studies have demonstrated that cardiac involvement with Kaposi's sarcoma was usually due to disseminated disease with metastases involving the pericardium [70]. Metastases to subepicardial adipose tissue adjacent to major coronary arteries have also been described [70]. Though cardiac involvement with Kaposi's sarcomas has usually been discovered at autopsy, bloody pericardial effusions may be discovered by imaging or pericardiocentesis in patients with advanced disease.

CONCLUSION

HIV infection and AIDS have reached global epidemic proportions. Although ART is very effective at improving survival with HIV infection, it is not widely available in regions of the world that are most affected. In patients who are not on ART, end-stage complications of AIDS that affect the heart, including dilated cardiomyopathy, myocarditis, pericardial effusion, pulmonary hypertension, endocarditis, and involvement of the heart with neoplasms, are not uncommon. In parts of the world where ART is used frequently, complications related to aging, HIV replication itself with consequent immune activation, the use of ART and the high prevalence of risk factors such as diabetes mellitus, smoking, hyperlipidemia, and obesity all contribute to the overlapping epidemiology and disease manifestations of CAD in patients with HIV infection.

ACKNOWLEDGMENT

I acknowledge the use of content written by James H. Stein, author of this chapter in the previous edition.

REFERENCES

[1] Boccara F. Cardiovascular complications and atherosclerotic manifestations in the HIV-infected population: type, incidence and associated risk factors. AIDS 2008;22(Suppl. 3):S19–S26.

[2] Khunnawat C, Mukerji S, Havlichek Jr D, et al. Cardiovascular manifestations in human immunodeficiency virus-infected patients. Am J Cardiol 2008;102:635–42.

[3] Saves M, Chene G, Ducimetiere P, et al. Risk factors for coronary heart disease in patients treated for human immunodeficiency virus infection compared with the general population. Clin Infect Dis 2003;37:292–8.

[4] Kaplan RC, Kingsley LA, Sharrett AR, et al. Ten-year predicted coronary heart disease risk in HIV-infected men and women. Clin Infect Dis 2007;45:1074–81.

[5] Triant VA, Lee H, Hadigan C, Grinspoon SK. Increased acute myocardial infarction rates and cardiovascular risk factors among

patients with human immunodeficiency virus disease. J Clin Endocrinol Metab 2007;92:2506–12.

[6] Malvestutto CD, Aberg JA. Coronary heart disease in people infected with HIV. Cleve Clin J Med 2010;77:547–56.

[7] Klein D, Hurley LB, Quesenberry Jr CP, Sidney S. Do protease inhibitors increase the risk for coronary heart disease in patients with HIV-1 infection? J Acquir Immune Defic Syndr 2002;30:471–7.

[8] Hulten E, Mitchell J, Scally J, et al. HIV positivity, protease inhibitor exposure and subclinical atherosclerosis: a systematic review and meta-analysis of observational studies. Heart 2009;95:1826–35.

[9] Grunfeld C, Delaney JA, Wanke C, et al. Preclinical atherosclerosis due to HIV infection: carotid intima-medial thickness measurements from the FRAM study. AIDS 2009;23:1841–9.

[10] Desvarieux M, Meynard JL, Boccara F, et al. Carotid atherosclerosis is related to HIV duration and anti-inflammatory profile and not to ARV exposure: The CHIC controlled study. In: CROI. Boston, MA. 2011.

[11] Hurley LB, Leyden W, Xu L. Updated surveillance of cardiovascular event rates among HIV-infected and HIV-uninfected Californians, 1996 to 2008. In: CROI. Montreal, Canada. 2009.

[12] Holmberg SD, Moorman AC, Williamson JM, et al. Protease inhibitors and cardiovascular outcomes in patients with HIV-1. Lancet 2002;360:1747–8.

[13] Friis-Moller N, Sabin CA, Weber R, et al. Combination antiretroviral therapy and the risk of myocardial infarction. N Engl J Med 2003;349:1993–2003.

[14] Friis-Moller N, Reiss P, Sabin CA, et al. Class of antiretroviral drugs and the risk of myocardial infarction. N Engl J Med 2007;356:1723–35.

[15] Sabin CA, Worm SW, Weber R, et al. Use of nucleoside reverse transcriptase inhibitors and risk of myocardial infarction in HIV-infected patients enrolled in the D:A:D study: a multi-cohort collaboration. Lancet 2008;371:1417–26.

[16] Lichtenstein KA, Armon C, Buchacz K, et al. Low CD4+ T cell count is a risk factor for cardiovascular disease events in the HIV outpatient study. Clin Infect Dis 2010;51:435–47.

[17] Ding X, Andraca-Carrera E, Cooper C, et al. No association of myocardial infarction with ABC use: an FDA meta-analysis. In: CROI. Boston, MA. 2011.

[18] Riddler SA, Smit E, Cole SR, et al. Impact of HIV infection and HAART on serum lipids in men. JAMA 2003;289:2978–82.

[19] Grunfeld C, Pang M, Doerrler W, et al. Lipids, lipoproteins, triglyceride clearance, and cytokines in human immunodeficiency virus infection and the acquired immunodeficiency syndrome. J Clin Endocrinol Metab 1992;74:1045–52.

[20] El-Sadr WM, Mullin CM, Carr A, et al. Effects of HIV disease on lipid, glucose and insulin levels: results from a large antiretroviral-naive cohort. HIV Med 2005;6:114–21.

[21] Stein JH. Dyslipidemia in the era of HIV protease inhibitors. Prog Cardiovasc Dis 2003;45:293–304.

[22] Grundy SM, Cleeman JI, Merz CN, et al. Implications of recent clinical trials for the National Cholesterol Education Program Adult Treatment Panel III guidelines. Circulation 2004;110:227–39.

[23] Stein JH. Managing cardiovascular risk in patients with HIV infection. J Acquir Immune Defic Syndr 2005;38:115–23.

[24] Currie PF, Boon NA. Immunopathogenesis of HIV-related heart muscle disease: current perspectives. AIDS 2003;17(Suppl. 1):S21–S28.

[25] Barbaro G, Di Lorenzo G, Grisorio B, Barbarini G. Cardiac involvement in the acquired immunodeficiency syndrome: a multicenter clinical-pathological study. Gruppo Italiano per lo Studio Cardiologico dei pazienti affetti da AIDS Investigators. AIDS Res Hum Retroviruses 1998;14:1071–7.

[26] Levy WS, Simon GL, Rios JC, Ross AM. Prevalence of cardiac abnormalities in human immunodeficiency virus infection. Am J Cardiol 1989;63:86–9.

[27] Currie PF, Jacob AJ, Foreman AR, et al. Heart muscle disease related to HIV infection: prognostic implications. BMJ 1994;309:1605–7.

[28] Barbaro G, Di Lorenzo G, Grisorio B, Barbarini G. Incidence of dilated cardiomyopathy and detection of HIV in myocardial cells of HIV-positive patients. Gruppo Italiano per lo Studio Cardiologico dei Pazienti Affetti da AIDS. N Engl J Med 1998;339:1093–9.

[29] Pugliese A, Isnardi D, Saini A, et al. Impact of highly active antiretroviral therapy in HIV-positive patients with cardiac involvement. J Infect 2000;40:282–4.

[30] Mondy KE, Gottdiener J, Overton ET, et al. High prevalence of echocardiographic abnormalities among HIV-infected persons in the era of highly active antiretroviral therapy. Clin Infect Dis 2011;52:378–86.

[31] Twagirumukiza M, Nkeramihigo E, Seminega B, et al. Prevalence of dilated cardiomyopathy in HIV-infected African patients not receiving HAART: a multicenter, observational, prospective, cohort study in Rwanda. Curr HIV Res 2007;5:129–37.

[32] Barbaro G, Di Lorenzo G, Soldini M, et al. Intensity of myocardial expression of inducible nitric oxide synthase influences the clinical course of human immunodeficiency virus-associated cardiomyopathy. Gruppo Italiano per lo Studio Cardiologico dei pazienti affetti da AIDS (GISCA). Circulation 1999;100:933–9.

[33] Twu C, Liu NQ, Popik W, et al. Cardiomyocytes undergo apoptosis in human immunodeficiency virus cardiomyopathy through mitochondrion- and death receptor-controlled pathways. Proc Natl Acad Sci U S A 2002;99:14386–91.

[34] Barbaro G. Pathogenesis of HIV-associated heart disease. AIDS 2003;17(Suppl. 1):S12–S20.

[35] Chi D, Henry J, Kelley J, et al. The effects of HIV infection on endothelial function. Endothelium 2000;7:223–42.

[36] Rerkpattanapipat P, Wongpraparut N, Jacobs LE, Kotler MN. Cardiac manifestations of acquired immunodeficiency syndrome. Arch Intern Med 2000;160:602–8.

[37] Herskowitz A, Wu TC, Willoughby SB, et al. Myocarditis and cardiotropic viral infection associated with severe left ventricular dysfunction in late-stage infection with human immunodeficiency virus. J Am Coll Cardiol 1994;24:1025–32.

[38] Currie PF, Goldman JH, Caforio AL, et al. Cardiac autoimmunity in HIV related heart muscle disease. Heart 1998;79:599–604.

[39] Barbaro G. Cardiovascular manifestations of HIV infection. Circulation 2002;106:1420–5.

[40] Fantoni M, Autore C, Del Borgo C. Drugs and cardiotoxicity in HIV and AIDS. Ann N Y Acad Sci 2001;946:179–99.

[41] Herskowitz A, Willoughby SB, Baughman KL, et al. Cardiomyopathy associated with antiretroviral therapy in patients with HIV infection: a report of six cases. Ann Intern Med 1992;116:311–13.

[42] Lipshultz SE, Orav EJ, Sanders SP, et al. Cardiac structure and function in children with human immunodeficiency virus infection treated with zidovudine. N Engl J Med 1992;327:1260–5.

[43] Jacob AJ, Sutherland GR, Bird AG, et al. Myocardial dysfunction in patients infected with HIV: prevalence and risk factors. Br Heart J 1992;68:549–53.

[44] Arsura EL, Ismail Y, Freedman S, Karunakar AR. Amphotericin B-induced dilated cardiomyopathy. Am J Med 1994;97:560–2.

[45] Bristow MR, Mason JW, Billingham ME, Daniels JR. Doxorubicin cardiomyopathy: evaluation by phonocardiography, endomyocardial biopsy, and cardiac catheterization. Ann Intern Med 1978;88:168–75.

[46] Brown DL, Sather S, Cheitlin MD. Reversible cardiac dysfunction associated with foscarnet therapy for cytomegalovirus esophagitis in an AIDS patient. Am Heart J 1993;125:1439–41.

[47] Sonnenblick M, Rosin A. Cardiotoxicity of interferon. A review of 44 cases. Chest 1991;99:557–61.

[48] Heidenreich PA, Eisenberg MJ, Kee LL, et al. Pericardial effusion in AIDS. Incidence and survival. Circulation 1995;92:3229–34.

[49] Estok L, Wallach F. Cardiac tamponade in a patient with AIDS: a review of pericardial disease in patients with HIV infection. Mt Sinai J Med 1998;65:33–9.

[50] Hsia J, Ross AM. Pericardial effusion and pericardiocentesis in human immunodeficiency virus infection. Am J Cardiol 1994;74:94–6.

[51] Silva-Cardoso J, Moura B, Martins L, et al. Pericardial involvement in human immunodeficiency virus infection. Chest 1999;115:418–22.

[52] Bijl M, Dieleman JP, Simoons M, van der Ende ME. Low prevalence of cardiac abnormalities in an HIV-seropositive population on antiretroviral combination therapy. J Acquir Immune Defic Syndr 2001;27:318–20.

[53] Ntsekhe M, Mayosi BM. Cardiac manifestations of HIV infection: an African perspective. Nat Clin Pract Cardiovasc Med 2009;6:120–7.

[54] Zuber JP, Calmy A, Evison JM, et al. Pulmonary arterial hypertension related to HIV infection: improved hemodynamics and survival associated with antiretroviral therapy. Clin Infect Dis 2004;38:1178–85.

[55] Speich R, Jenni R, Opravil M, et al. Primary pulmonary hypertension in HIV infection. Chest 1991;100:1268–71.

[56] Sitbon O, Lascoux-Combe C, Delfraissy JF, et al. Prevalence of HIV-related pulmonary arterial hypertension in the current antiretroviral therapy era. Am J Respir Crit Care Med 2008;177:108–13.

[57] Opravil M, Pechere M, Speich R, et al. HIV-associated primary pulmonary hypertension. A case control study. Swiss HIV Cohort Study. Am J Respir Crit Care Med 1997;155:990–5.

[58] Mehta NJ, Khan IA, Mehta RN, Sepkowitz DA. HIV-related pulmonary hypertension: analytic review of 131 cases. Chest 2000;118:1133–41.

[59] Nunes H, Humbert M, Sitbon O, et al. Prognostic factors for survival in human immunodeficiency virus-associated pulmonary arterial hypertension. Am J Respir Crit Care Med 2003;167:1433–9.

[60] Mette SA, Palevsky HI, Pietra GG, et al. Primary pulmonary hypertension in association with human immunodeficiency virus infection. A possible viral etiology for some forms of hypertensive pulmonary arteriopathy. Am Rev Respir Dis 1992;145:1196–200.

[61] Ehrenreich H, Rieckmann P, Sinowatz F, et al. Potent stimulation of monocytic endothelin-1 production by HIV-1 glycoprotein 120. J Immunol 1993;150:4601–9.

[62] Humbert M, Monti G, Brenot F, et al. Increased interleukin-1 and interleukin-6 serum concentrations in severe primary pulmonary hypertension. Am J Respir Crit Care Med 1995;151:1628–31.

[63] Schermuly RT, Dony E, Ghofrani HA, et al. Reversal of experimental pulmonary hypertension by PDGF inhibition. J Clin Invest 2005;115: 2811–21.

[64] Gebo KA, Burkey MD, Lucas GM, et al. Incidence of, risk factors for, clinical presentation, and 1-year outcomes of infective endocarditis in an urban HIV cohort. J Acquir Immune Defic Syndr 2006;43:426–32.

[65] Nahass RG, Weinstein MP, Bartels J, Gocke DJ. Infective endocarditis in intravenous drug users: a comparison of human immunodeficiency virus type 1-negative and -positive patients. J Infect Dis 1990;162:967–70.

[66] Morgello S, Mahboob R, Yakoushina T, et al. Autopsy findings in a human immunodeficiency virus-infected population over 2 decades: influences of gender, ethnicity, risk factors, and time. Arch Pathol Lab Med 2002; 126:182–90.

[67] Aboulafia DM. Human immunodeficiency virus-associated neoplasms: epidemiology, pathogenesis, and review of current therapy. Cancer Pract 1994;2:297–306.

[68] Appleby P, Beral V, Newton R, Reeves G. Highly active antiretroviral therapy and incidence of cancer in human immunodeficiency virus-infected adults. J Natl Cancer Inst 2000;92:1823–30.

[69] Aboulafia DM, Bush R, Picozzi VJ. Cardiac tamponade due to primary pericardial lymphoma in a patient with AIDS. Chest 1994;106:1295–9.

[70] Silver MA, Macher AM, Reichert CM, et al. Cardiac involvement by Kaposi's sarcoma in acquired immune deficiency syndrome (AIDS). Am J Cardiol 1984;53:983–5.

Chapter | 22 |

Endocrine complications of HIV infection

Steven A. Taylor, Carl Grunfeld, Morris Schambelan

INTRODUCTION

A wide spectrum of endocrine complications is associated with HIV infection and AIDS. Although these disorders may reflect changes induced by HIV itself, more often they are a consequence of systemic illness, opportunistic infections (OIs), neoplasm, body composition changes, HIV-related therapies, and/or restoration of health. The use of highly active antiretroviral therapy (HAART) clearly altered the endocrinologic manifestations of HIV. As the incidence of glandular infiltration by OIs and neoplasm has declined, attention has focused on the metabolic complications of therapy. Studies performed in the pre-HAART era remain relevant, however, to the management of patients where there is limited access to HIV care and to those who become resistant to antiretroviral therapy (ART). Understanding these disorders is crucial to the ongoing care of HIV-infected patients. This chapter describes the endocrine complications of HIV disease and provides a general approach to management, primarily referencing high-quality review articles, rather than the primary references, due to space limitations.

THE THYROID

Thyroid pathology

Clinically significant OIs of the thyroid occur very rarely in patients with AIDS, and the advent of ART has further reduced the frequency. In an autopsy study, two-thirds of thyroids examined demonstrated pathologic changes, though no patients had pre-mortem clinical thyroid disease. Indeed, more than one OI was found in the majority of specimens [1]. Pathogens infecting the thyroid included *Pneumocystis jiroveci*, cytomegalovirus (CMV), *Cryptococcus neoformans*, *Aspergillus fumigatus*, *Rhodococcus equi*, *Haemophilus influenzae*, *Microsporidia*, *Histoplasma capsulatum*, *Paracoccidioides brasiliensis*, *Mycobacterium avium intracellulare*, and *Mycobacterium tuberculosis*. *Pneumocystis jiroveci* was the most common OI of the thyroid, occurring primarily among patients receiving aerosolized pentamidine [2]. Clinical manifestations of thyroiditis are variable and may include signs and symptoms of either hyper- or hypothyroidism. Palpation of the thyroid gland may reveal localized tenderness and/or fluctuance; systemic signs of infection may be present. Functional testing may reveal transient hyperthyroidism (that may not require treatment), euthyroidism, or hypothyroidism. HIV has also been isolated from thyroid tissue of infected patients with Graves' disease (GD), though it is unclear whether HIV is involved in the pathogenesis of this autoimmune thyroid disorder [3].

Neoplastic infiltration of the thyroid is uncommon in patients with AIDS. Only two cases of thyroid lymphoma, one case of thyroid carcinoma, and one case of acute myelogenous leukemia presenting as a thyroid mass [4] have been reported. There have been a few cases of Kaposi's sarcoma (KS) involving the thyroid gland in patients with pre-existing cutaneous lesions. Other frequent pathologic changes of the thyroid include non-specific focal chronic inflammation, colloid goiter, and lipomatosis [1].

Alterations in thyroid function

Although asymptomatic HIV-infected patients with stable body weight are usually clinically euthyroid, abnormal thyroid homeostasis is often present in patients with AIDS. In non-thyroidal illness (NTI), inhibition of peripheral T4 to

T3 conversion and reduced reverse T3 (rT3) clearance results in low T3 and elevated rT3, usually accompanied by normal thyroid-stimulating hormone (TSH) levels. The characteristic changes of NTI differ from those observed in AIDS patients, who often have higher T3 levels and lower rT3 levels than would generally be expected. The increased thyroid hormone-binding globulin (TBG) levels associated with HIV infection do not explain these findings [5]. The abnormalities of thyroid testing in HIV-infected individuals compared with seronegative patients with NTI are presented in Table 22.1. The maintenance of normal T3 levels among AIDS patients has led to concern that the protective effects that reduction of T3 provides in NTI, such as lowering metabolic rate, ameliorating weight loss, and decreasing protein catabolism, may be compromised. Lower T3 levels are observed, however, during secondary infection and anorexia. Patients with asymptomatic HIV infection have been reported to demonstrate characteristics of compensated hypothyroidism including high-normal range 24-h TSH profiles, lower free T4 levels, and a greater TSH response to TRH infusion [6]. These alterations in thyroid hormone physiology may be adaptive to chronic illness, decreased energy intake, or the increased metabolic demands of HIV infection. Still, there is little evidence to suggest those with asymptomatic HIV infection be routinely screened for thyroid dysfunction [7]. If hyper- or hypothyroidism are clinically suspected, a physical examination that includes an assessment of the thyroid gland should be performed followed by measurement of TSH level. HIV-infected patients with an acute illness, such as local or systemic infection, may have thyroid function test (TFT) results consistent with NTI. In this instance, TFTs should be repeated a few weeks after recovery from illness to document resolution of abnormalities. Use of exogenous thyroid hormone is not indicated in the setting of NTI.

Effects of antiretroviral and other therapies

Rifampin, ketoconazole, and ritonavir may alter thyroid function by accelerating the metabolic clearance of thyroid hormone and can precipitate hypothyroidism in patients with marginal thyroid reserve; thus, higher doses of thyroxine may be necessary in patients receiving concomitant replacement therapy [2].

Treatment of hepatitis C infection with interferon-α (INF-α) has been associated with the development of autoimmune thyroid diseases (AITD) such as GD, Hashimoto's thyroiditis, and subacute or destructive thyroiditis. Since individuals with pre-existing or recently detected thyroid autoantibodies (i.e. thyroid peroxidase [TPOAb] and thyroglobulin [TgAb] antibodies) are at higher risk for INF-α-induced AITD, practitioners should test TSH, free T4, and thyroid antibodies before initiation of INF-α treatment, followed by measurement of TSH every 8–12 weeks during treatment [8]. IFN-α treatment should be delayed until correction of pre-existing thyroid dysfunction. If thyroid dysfunction develops during treatment, IFN-α need not be discontinued unless destructive thyroiditis with severe symptoms refractory to β-blockers or GD requiring high doses of anti-thyroidal medications develops. Although most patients who develop thyroid dysfunction during treatment with INF-α normalize after it is discontinued, a minority continue to require treatment [8].

Since the introduction of HAART, AITD has been reported as a late complication of immune reconstitution, typically presenting as GD 1–2 years after initiation of therapy [9]. The onset of AITD is temporally consistent with thymic production of naïve CD4 T cells (the "late" phase of T cell repopulation), and immune dysregulation in those with genetic predisposition may result in thyroid-specific autoimmunity.

Treatment considerations

Subtle alterations in thyroid function in HIV-infected individuals must be interpreted in their clinical context. In patients with clinically significant and biochemically confirmed hypothyroidism, low doses of replacement therapy (levothyroxine 25–50 μg daily) should be prescribed initially, with gradual titration and monitoring of TSH levels. Clinical management for patients with hyperthyroidism and coexisting HIV infection is similar to that for immunocompetent individuals, except that a tender or nodular thyroid gland in a patient with advanced HIV disease should prompt further investigation for an OI or malignancy of the thyroid. Diagnostic evaluation includes

	SERONEGATIVE NTI	HIV-INFECTED, STABLE	HIV-INFECTED, SICK
T3	↓↓	Normal	↓
rT3	↑	↓	↓ or Normal
TBG	↑	↑	↑↑
T4	Normal or ↓	Normal	Normal
TSH	Normal, may be ↑ during recovery	Normal	Normal

Table 22.1 Alterations in thyroid function in HIV infection

NTI, non-thyroidal illness.
From Sellmeyer DE, Grunfeld C. Endocrine and metabolic disturbances in human immunodeficiency virus infection and the acquired immune deficiency syndrome. Endocr Rev 1996; 17:518–532.

fine needle aspiration (FNA) biopsy of the affected gland. *Pneumocystis jiroveci* organisms can be demonstrated with Gomori's methenamine silver stain. FNA should also be considered in patients with disseminated KS who present with a thyroid nodule to identify the rare case of KS of the thyroid.

THE ADRENAL

Adrenal pathology

Although pathologic involvement of the adrenal gland was frequently noted during autopsy in the pre-HAART era, clinical adrenal insufficiency (AI) was relatively rare. This is likely explained by the fact that greater than 90% of the adrenal cortices must be destroyed for AI to ensue. Cytomegalovirus adrenalitis was the most common finding. *Mycobacterium tuberculosis*, *M. avium intracellulare*, *C. neoformans*, and *Toxoplasma gondii* also infect the adrenal gland. Infiltration with KS or lymphoma, hemorrhage, fibrosis, infarction, and focal necrosis were also reported [2].

Alterations in adrenal function

HIV-infected individuals may demonstrate changes in steroid metabolism, including an elevation in basal cortisol levels that may be accompanied by decreased responsiveness to ACTH stimulation. Lower levels of ACTH and the weak adrenal androgen dehydroepiandrosterone (DHEA) are often observed, along with impaired adrenal reserve of the 17-deoxysteroids (corticosterone, deoxycorticosterone, and 18-OH-deoxycorticosterone) [10]. Factors such as cytokines, acting independently of the pituitary gland, may directly enhance cortisol biosynthesis in the absence of an increase in ACTH. In some HIV-infected patients, however, the combination of increased cortisol and ACTH levels suggests hypothalamic activation, although those with late-stage HIV disease often have an attenuated pituitary–adrenal response to corticotropin-releasing hormone (CRH). Compensatory rises in ACTH levels may also develop in those with subclinical AI due to physiologic hormonal feedback mechanisms. In AIDS patients who present with elevated levels of both cortisol and ACTH but manifest paradoxical Addisonian features, peripheral glucocorticoid resistance may be present [11]. Levels of DHEA decline with advancing age and chronic illness, in contrast to levels of cortisol, which remain relatively stable. Interest in DHEA therapy among the HIV community was motivated by studies showing that DHEA inhibits HIV-1 replication and activation *in vitro*. Cross-sectional studies have associated low DHEA levels and elevated cortisol/DHEA ratios with advanced HIV infection, and low serum concentrations of DHEA have been significantly correlated with CD4 T cell count, weight loss, and progression to AIDS. Small placebo-controlled trials of oral administration of DHEA showed improved quality of life in patients with AIDS without change in CD4 T cell count [12]. However, a recent 6-month randomized, double-blind, placebo-controlled study of 40 HIV-infected subjects with suppressed viral loads showed no changes in immune parameters, lean muscle mass, or bone density following treatment with oral DHEA [13]. DHEA cannot be recommended in the routine treatment of HIV-infected patients until its efficacy has been proven in larger, randomized clinical trials evaluating multiple outcomes.

Effects of antiretroviral and other therapies

Although the dorsocervical fat pad enlargement and visceral adiposity seen in some HIV-infected patients appears phenotypically similar to Cushing's syndrome, overt hypercortisolism has not been found in affected patients [14]. The demonstration of both normal diurnal cortisol excretion and normal response to exogenous CRH administration provides additional evidence that the development of central lipohypertrophy cannot be attributed to abnormal cortisol metabolism, though some have hypothesized that it may be related to the increased cortisol/DHEA ratio observed in these patients. Iatrogenic Cushing's syndrome, however, can occur in patients treated concomitantly with ritonavir and nasal or inhaled fluticasone (for allergic rhinitis or asthma). Ritonavir prolongs the half-life of fluticasone via effects on CYP3A4, leading to much higher plasma levels of fluticasone than pharmacologically intended and classic physical manifestations of glucocorticoid excess. When given in conjunction with ritonavir, intra-articular triamcinolone used in the treatment of osteoarthritis may also be associated with signs and symptoms of glucocorticoid excess, though the mechanism for this is unclear. Upon steroid withdrawal, secondary adrenal suppression may ensue. Associated conditions such as osteoporosis or diabetes may be induced or exacerbated. Practitioners should be aware of these potential interactions in order to avoid delays in diagnosis among patients who have pre-existing central lipohypertrophy that might mask the clinical features of Cushing's syndrome. These patients should be examined for cardinal signs of Cushing's syndrome, including violaceous striae, bruising, and proximal muscle weakness.

Multiple medications used to treat complications of HIV may affect adrenocortical function. AI may be induced in patients with impaired adrenal reserve by conazoles (keto-, flu- and itraconazole) through inhibition of cortisol biosynthesis. Rifampin may also induce AI by increasing the metabolic clearance of cortisol. A syndrome of mineralocorticoid excess has been reported in patients on high-dose itraconazole [15]. Megestrol acetate, a progestational agent used as an appetite stimulant in the treatment of AIDS-wasting, can suppress both the hypothalamic–pituitary–adrenal

(HPA) axis and the hypothalamic–pituitary–gonadal (HPG) axis due to its intrinsic glucocorticoid-like activity. Some patients receiving long-term therapy may develop iatrogenic Cushing's syndrome and/or diabetes mellitus, as well as adrenal failure when treatment is suddenly discontinued. Opiate use, often seen coexisting with HIV infection, can blunt cortisol secretion in response to ACTH stimulation [16].

Treatment considerations

The alterations in steroid metabolism observed in patients with HIV infection may be adaptive to chronic illness and may not require treatment. Estimates of the prevalence of AI vary considerably, depending on the population studied, whether patients manifest clinical signs and symptoms, and the method of diagnostic testing used. AI is clearly more common in HIV-infected patients than in the general population. The diagnosis should be considered in patients who present with malaise, orthostatic hypotension, nausea, abdominal pain, weight loss, hyponatremia, and hypoglycemia. The appropriate method of adrenal function testing, however, is controversial. Although the ACTH stimulation test (administration of 250 µg cosyntropin) is the most widely used, it may not identify all patients with impaired pituitary reserve. In several reported cases, insulin-induced hypoglycemia or the metyrapone test was used to diagnose AI in HIV-infected patients. Further, the sensitivity of the ACTH stimulation test falls with acute or chronic illness, which is associated with impaired cortisol protein binding and reduced cortisol binding protein levels. Total cortisol levels may be low due to these factors, though biologically active free cortisol levels may be normal or high. Several factors limit the reliability of free cortisol assays in the clinical assessment for AI. If AI is suspected in the setting of intercurrent illness, an assessment for typical risk factors—especially recent use or discontinuation of glucocorticoids—should ensue. If suspicion persists based on results of dynamic laboratory testing, treatment should be instituted.

Patients with documented AI should be treated with glucocorticoid replacement therapy and require increased doses during periods of stress. If primary adrenal failure is present with evidence of concomitant mineralocorticoid deficiency (hyperkalemia and metabolic acidosis), the addition of fludrocortisone should be considered. Controversy exists regarding whether patients with elevated basal cortisol levels, but a blunted response to standard single-dose ACTH stimulation, should be treated with glucocorticoid therapy. Some of these patients probably do not require chronic glucocorticoid replacement, as they show adequate cortisol response after receiving supraphysiologic ACTH stimulation for 3 consecutive days [10]. These challenging cases must be evaluated individually, with the goal of minimizing unnecessary glucocorticoid

exposure. Administration of short-term, supplementary glucocorticoids to symptomatic patients who demonstrate a subnormal rise in cortisol levels during periods of stress is reasonable.

THE PANCREAS

Pancreatic pathology

Morphologic abnormalities of the pancreas are common at autopsy in AIDS patients (up to 90%); however, most lesions are asymptomatic [17]. Pancreatic OIs such as mycobacteria, toxoplasmosis, CMV, and *P. jiroveci* have been documented, with presentation similar to that of pancreatitis due to other causes [18]. The most common pancreatic OI is tuberculosis, presenting with diverse manifestations, such as masses mimicking carcinoma, obstructive jaundice, pancreatitis, gastrointestinal bleeding, and generalized lymphadenopathy. It may be diagnosed by abdominal computed tomography followed by FNA biopsy. HIV-associated neoplasms rarely affect the pancreas, although primary pancreatic lymphoma [19] and KS have been reported, the latter successfully treated with intensive ART and paclitaxel [20].

Alterations in glucose homeostasis and effects of antiretroviral therapy

Prior to the advent of HAART, symptomatic HIV-infected men were found to have increased insulin sensitivity of peripheral tissues compared with non-infected controls. Recent studies found conflicting evidence as to whether insulin sensitivity is altered among asymptomatic HIV-infected individuals who are ARV-naïve. Following the introduction of HAART with protease inhibitors (PIs), abnormalities of glucose metabolism including insulin resistance, impaired insulin secretion, hyperglycemia, and frank diabetes were reported. However, it was unclear whether restoration of health, immune reconstitution, body composition changes, or other antiretrovirals contributed to these disturbances. Subsequent studies of individual PIs among healthy, HIV-seronegative volunteers minimized confounding by HIV-related factors and demonstrated a spectrum of effects of PIs on glucose metabolism [21–28]. For instance, although a single dose of indinavir and ritonavir-boosted lopinavir were found to acutely induce insulin resistance, amprenavir and boosting-dose ritonavir did not. After 4 weeks of treatment, insulin resistance and increased fasting glucose occurred with indinavir but not with ritonavir-boosted lopinavir. Endogenous glucose production (EGP) was increased following administration of indinavir compared to placebo. This finding, indicating an indinavir-induced reduction in the ability of insulin to blunt EGP that may lead to hyperglycemia and a predisposition to diabetes, was not shown with amprenavir. More recently, though it was initially reported that PIs as a class impair pancreatic β-cell insulin secretion in HIV-infected patients, there was no effect on insulin secretion after healthy HIV-seronegative volunteers were given ritonavir-boosted lopinavir for 4 weeks. Thus, PIs do not have a singular class effect on glucose metabolic pathways, and the distinct effects of individual PIs on glucose metabolism must be taken into account when tailoring antiretroviral regimens.

Non-nucleoside reverse transcriptase inhibitors (NNRTIs) have not been associated with derangements in glucose metabolism. Impaired glucose homeostasis occurs in PI-naïve patients treated with nucleoside reverse transcriptase inhibitors (NRTIs). The effects of NRTIs on glucose metabolism should, therefore, also be systematically studied.

Effects of other therapies

Pentamidine, used in the prevention and treatment of *P. jiroveci*, may cause pancreatic β-cell toxicity when administered either intravenously or aerosolized. Acute insulin secretion and resultant hypoglycemia may be followed by β-cell destruction and diabetes mellitus [2]. Acute pancreatitis rarely occurs with pentamidine, trimethoprim-sulfamethoxazole, the NRTIs ddI and ddC, ritonavir-induced hypertriglyceridemia and antifungal treatment with liposomal amphotericin B, micafungin, griseofulvin, fluconazole, itraconazole, and voriconazole [15].

The intrinsic glucocorticoid-like activity of megestrol acetate may exacerbate or cause hyperglycemia, although the incidence of this complication is low. Growth hormone (GH) can induce insulin resistance and predispose to hyperglycemia and diabetes. A small increase in hemoglobin A_{1c} accompanies tesamorelin treatment to reduce visceral adipose tissue. Ketoconazole, fluconazole, and voriconazole have been associated with hypoglycemia, though the underlying mechanisms are unknown [15]. Additionally, co-administration of fluconazole with the oral hypoglycemic medications tolbutamide, glimepiride, and nateglinide increase their peak plasma concentrations, increasing risk of hypoglycemia.

Treatment considerations

Recommendations for managing the metabolic complications of HIV infection, including abnormalities in glucose homeostasis, have been published [29]. If ART includes a PI associated with changes in glucose homeostasis, fasting glucose should be monitored before initiation, at the time of a change in therapy, 3 to 6 months after starting or switching therapy, and at least annually during therapy. For patients with risk factors for type 2 diabetes and those with lipoatrophy or lipohypertrophy, an oral glucose tolerance test may be considered. If possible, PIs most associated with insulin resistance should be avoided for

patients with pre-existing glucose intolerance or those with first-degree relatives with diabetes.

Treatment of diabetes in HIV-infected patients should emphasize healthy diet, regular exercise, and maintenance of normal body weight. Among the accepted first-line oral medications for diabetes, preference may be given to metformin. Metformin should be avoided in those with a history of renal disease or lactic acidemia, a recognized adverse effect of NRTIs. Agents from other oral hypoglycemic classes may be used in the management of HIV-infected type 2 diabetics, but results will likely not differ from the general population. The thiazolidinedione (TZD) pioglitazone may be used, but TZDs reduce bone mineral density (BMD) and increase fractures; pioglitazone should be used with care in a population already at risk of low BMD and fracture. If adequate glycemic control is not achieved with oral agents, an insulin-based regimen should be started. Metformin and pioglitazone do not necessarily need to be discontinued in this instance.

In addition, clinicians should be aware of potential interactions between PIs and hypoglycemic agents. Ritonavir and nelfinavir induce CYP2C9, which may reduce concentrations of selected sulfonylureas and TZDs [29].

ABNORMALITIES OF LIPID METABOLISM

High-density lipoprotein (HDL) levels decrease early in untreated HIV infection, often by as much as 50%, followed by smaller decreases in low-density lipoprotein (LDL) and then by increases in triglycerides. The circulating level of HIV RNA accounts for some of the change. Lower CD4 T cell counts are associated with lower HDL levels.

Effects of antiretroviral drugs and other therapies

In early studies of AZT therapy, triglycerides were reduced. Triglycerides increase with specific antiretroviral drugs, including efavirenz and ritonavir. The latter increases triglycerides in a dose-dependent manner in both HIV-infected patients and healthy volunteers.

LDL levels increase with most ART regimens, but not to high levels, which may reflect restoration to health. LDL levels are not increased by PIs in healthy volunteers.

NNRTIs raise HDL levels, though usually not back to normal. Nevirapine can induce a 50% increase in HDL, while efavirenz induces smaller increases. Nevirapine increases HDL in non-infected infants treated to prevent vertical transmission. Small changes in HDL may occur with other antiretroviral drugs, but results have varied. Tenofovir may improve the atherogenic lipid profile.

Anabolic steroids, especially oral preparations, increase LDL and decrease HDL levels. The combination of HIV and oxandrolone can induce extremely low HDL levels. Ketoconazole causes a dose-dependent reduction in LDL and total cholesterol and an increase in triglycerides without affecting VLDL or HDL levels [15]. Case reports describe hypercholesterolemia and hypertriglyceridemia with itraconazole and voriconazole, though the mechanism is unclear.

Treatment considerations

PIs, which inhibit CYP3A4, may cause up to a 32-fold increase in simvastatin and lovastatin levels; these statins should be avoided when PIs are used. Atorvastatin activity increases twofold with PIs, and high doses of atorvastatin should not be used. Conversely, pravastatin levels decrease with PI co-administration. Lopinavir/ritonavir and atazanavir/ritonavir increase rosuvastatin levels by an unknown pathway. Statins reduce cholesterol levels in HIV-infected subjects similar to those in the general population. Due to the many contributors to hypertriglyceridemia, triglyceride levels are less likely to reach goals in HIV-infected patients.

BONE

Bone pathology

Osteomyelitis is associated with mortality rates in excess of 20% in HIV-infected patients, underscoring the need to quickly recognize and treat this entity [30]. As in immunocompetent individuals, *Staphylococcus aureus* is the pathogen most commonly implicated in osteomyelitis in HIV-infected individuals. Osteomyelitis in HIV-infected patients has also been reported to be caused by *Salmonella* spp., *Nocardia asteroides*, *Streptococcus pneumoniae*, *Neisseria gonorrhoeae*, CMV, *Aspergillus* spp., *T. gondii*, *Torulopsis glabrata*, *C. neoformans*, Mycobacteria and *Coccidioides immitis* [30]. *Bartonella* infection particularly occurs with CD4 counts < 100 cells/mm^3. Systemic signs of infection and complaints of local bone pain should raise suspicion for osteomyelitis. Radiologic evaluation assists in the diagnosis, and bone biopsy isolates causative organisms to direct therapy.

Systemic non-Hodgkin's lymphoma (NHL) and KS may invade bone, typically with CD4 counts < 200 cells/mm^3. Twenty to thirty percent of patients with systemic NHL have bone involvement [31]. In contrast, widespread KS rarely involves the skeleton, but may result from direct invasion from a nearby soft tissue lesion. Bone biopsy is necessary to diagnose NHL and KS; both portend a poor response to treatment.

Osteonecrosis, death of bone resulting from circulatory insufficiency, is another complication of HIV infection that may present as either unilateral or bilateral bone or joint pain. Osteonecrosis of the hip was detected by MRI in 4.4% of 339 asymptomatic HIV-infected patients in a cross-sectional study compared to none of the seronegative controls [32]. The shoulder may also be affected. Osteonecrosis may be associated with prior glucocorticoid use. Unfortunately, surgical intervention remains the only available treatment for symptomatic osteonecrosis.

Alterations in bone and mineral metabolism

Reduced bone mineral density (BMD) is more common in HIV-infected individuals, though the reasons for this remain unclear. Histomorphometric analyses found altered bone remodeling prior to the introduction of HAART [33]. Multiple studies have shown increased prevalence of osteopenia and osteoporosis in treated HIV-infected patients. Reduced BMD in HIV infection is likely multifactorial, with possible contributions from weight loss, malnutrition, malabsorption (leading to vitamin D deficiency), hypogonadism, antiretrovirals, and traditional risk factors for osteoporosis (gender, low BMI, age, menopause, smoking, and injection drug use). Increased fracture rates have been reported.

Calcium and phosphate homeostasis, critical in bone remodeling, may be altered in HIV infection and have untoward skeletal consequences. Some patients with HIV disease and low BMD may have vitamin D insufficiency with secondary hyperparathyroidism. Vitamin D insufficiency may result in hypocalcemia, which may also be related to inadequate parathyroid hormone responses, compromised nutritional state, or medications used to treat opportunistic infections. Primary hypoparathyroidism resulting in hypocalcemia and hyperphosphatemia may rarely occur due to direct glandular infiltration by malignancy or infection, including *P. jiroveci*. Alternatively, hypercalcemia may occur from increased production of 1,25-dihydroxyvitamin D by NHL or granulomas from infectious pathogens, including *M. tuberculosis*, *M. avium intracellulare*, *P. jiroveci*, and *C. neoformans*. Treatment of *C. immitis* has been associated with hypercalcemia of unclear etiology. Immune reconstitution has been associated with hypercalcemia in the setting of CMV infection.

Effects of antiretroviral and other therapies

Following the introduction of PI-based ART, decreased BMD was reported among treated HIV-infected individuals. Most cross-sectional studies have since demonstrated that HIV-infected men and women treated with any ART regimen have lower BMD. Several studies have shown reduction of BMD after initiation of ART, with the greatest reductions seen in regimens using tenofovir. Medications used in the treatment of complications that may contribute to development of osteoporosis include corticosteroids, pentamidine, megestrol acetate, and ketoconazole. Heroin users have 11% lower lumbar BMD than controls. This effect may be partially attributed to opiate-associated hypogonadism. Renal electrolyte wasting leading to hypocalcemia and hypophosphatemia can occur with cidofovir for CMV treatment or with ART with tenofovir or adefovir. Amphotericin B and nystatin have been associated with renal magnesium wasting, leading to hypomagnesemia, resultant hypoparathyroidism, and hypocalcemia [15]. Foscarnet, used in the treatment of CMV retinitis, may cause hypocalcemia or hypomagnesemia. It binds circulating calcium and magnesium and can result in reductions in the ionized forms of both. Foscarnet-complexed calcium can precipitate in tissues, including the kidney. This may contribute to renal magnesium wasting, which also occurs with foscarnet administration. Pentamidine can also cause hypocalcemia and hypomagnesemia, while trimethoprim-sulfamethoxazole, ketoconazole, and aminoglycosides are associated with hypocalcemia. Hypercalcemia has been reported with caspofungin, though the mechanism by which it occurs is unclear [15]. Ketoconazole, rifampin, and rifabutin alter vitamin D metabolism but rarely change ionized calcium levels.

Treatment considerations

Screening for osteoporosis with bone densitometry among HIV-infected individuals remains controversial. However, if osteoporosis is present or a fragility fracture occurs in the setting of osteopenia, work-up for secondary causes of osteoporosis, including vitamin D insufficiency and hypogonadism, should be initiated. If present, these disorders should be treated. Patients should be encouraged to address modifiable risk factors (e.g. smoking), engage in weight-bearing exercise, and increase intake of calcium and vitamin D. Studies investigating the effects of switching antiretroviral regimen on BMD have been small and of short duration; therefore no clear recommendations can be made in this regard.

Once reversible causes of bone loss are addressed, the use of bisphosphonates should be considered in the treatment of HIV-related osteoporosis. Both alendronate and zoledronic acid, administered with or without supplementation with calcium and vitamin D, improve BMD at the lumbar spine and hip in HIV-infected individuals. Currently, data on other agents that increase BMD in the setting of HIV-associated bone loss are inadequate.

REPRODUCTIVE HEALTH IN MEN

Testicular pathology

Histopathologic changes in the testes were commonly found in autopsy studies among men with AIDS and included hypospermatogenesis, interstitial inflammation, and atrophy. Pathologic damage to the testes is associated with decreased testosterone and bioavailable testosterone, as well as increased serum gonadotropin levels [34]. Not surprisingly, testicular atrophy is more likely to be found in AIDS patients with lower BMI and may be caused by HIV infection itself, medication-related toxicity, or OIs including CMV, *T. gondii*, and *M. avium intracellulare*. AIDS patients are also at greater risk for the development of testicular malignancies, including KS, lymphoma, and germ cell tumors.

Alterations in sex hormones

Early in the course of HIV infection, hyperresponsiveness of luteinizing hormone (LH) to infusion of gonadotropin-releasing hormone (GnRH) may explain the normal or, in some cases, elevated, total and free testosterone levels [35]. As HIV disease progresses to AIDS, testosterone levels usually decrease. With the advent of HAART, the incidence of hypogonadism in HIV-infected men has declined from 40 to 20%. Hypogonadism may be accompanied by decreased muscle mass and strength, generalized fatigue, reduced libido and mood, gynecomastia, normocytic anemia, and reduced bone mineral density.

In the post-HAART era, direct testicular and pituitary pathology causing hypogonadism have become far less common. Hypogonadotropic hypogonadism is now more likely to be multifactorial in nature and may be due to chronic illness, altered cytokine profiles, OIs, medications, weight loss, or cachexia and associated malnutrition. The loss of lean body mass (LBM) and muscle strength in patients with the AIDS-wasting syndrome may be partially attributable to coexisting hypogonadism. In contrast to the decreased levels of testosterone, serum and urinary levels of estrogens may be elevated in HIV-infected men [36].

Increased sex hormone-binding globulin (SHBG) levels have been observed in this population. Increased SHBG can increase total testosterone levels; therefore, assessment of free or bioavailable testosterone in a special endocrine referral lab may be required to diagnose male hypogonadism in some cases. Primary hypogonadism is marked by elevated LH and follicle-stimulating hormone (FSH) levels, while LH and FSH levels are either low or inappropriately normal in secondary hypogonadism.

Sexual dysfunction is a common complaint among men with advanced HIV disease, with an estimated prevalence of nearly 60%. Although erectile and ejaculatory dysfunction, as well as loss of libido, are often attributed to low testosterone levels, other factors may also be contributory, including neurologic disease, systemic illness, drug effects, weakness, low energy, and psychosexual issues [35].

Gynecomastia in HIV-infected men may be due to hypoandrogenism and/or elevated estrogen levels, liver disease, or the use of commonly implicated medications. Gynecomastia is also common among healthy men as they age.

Effects of antiretroviral and other therapies

A number of medications used in the treatment of HIV and its related disorders affect the reproductive health of men. Systemic glucocorticoid therapy, megestrol acetate, and opiates can cause hypogonadotropic hypogonadism. Ketoconazole, particularly at higher doses, and chronic use of alcohol and marijuana impair testosterone production [16]. These drugs, as well as ART, may lead to gynecomastia in HIV-infected men. Though gynecomastia was initially attributed to PIs, other antiretroviral medications, such as the NNRTI efavirenz, have been associated with its development.

Sexual dysfunction has been associated with PI therapy in reports of affected men without any other apparent etiology. In some of these patients and in those with low libido, raised serum estradiol levels were found.

Treatment considerations

After both confirming hypogonadism with repeated morning measurements of testosterone utilizing a reliable laboratory assay and excluding reversible etiologies, symptomatic patients with primary or secondary hypogonadism should be offered therapy with replacement doses of testosterone. Testosterone is usually administered by intramuscular injection every 2–3 weeks using testosterone esters (e.g. enanthate and cypionate) or by transdermal delivery via patch or gel. Although the testosterone patch and gel avoid the large fluctuations in circulating testosterone levels seen with injections, transdermal therapy does not always produce therapeutic testosterone levels at recommended doses. Clinical assessment of the response and subsequent laboratory monitoring of testosterone concentration should be performed, along with periodic measurements of HDL cholesterol, hematocrit, and prostate-specific antigen. Hypogonadal men with HIV-associated weight loss treated with physiologic testosterone therapy with or without concurrent resistance training show improvement in LBM, muscle strength, bone mineral density, and quality of life [37]. Anemia associated with hypogonadism is ameliorated by testosterone. Caution should be used when treating sedentary obese men with hypogonadism, as testosterone increases cardiac events in this population. Given the potential risks, use of supraphysiologic testosterone therapy in eugonadal HIV-infected men with weight loss is not recommended.

Treatment options for reversing HIV-associated gynecomastia have not been systematically evaluated. Cosmetic surgery to debulk mammary tissue may be considered. A case report describes successful treatment of an HIV-infected man with the selective estrogen receptor modulator tamoxifen [38].

In managing erectile dysfunction in HIV-infected men on ART, clinicians should be aware that PIs increase levels of phosphodiesterase type 5 inhibitors (PDE5-Is) including sildenafil, tadalafil, and vardenafil. To reduce the risk of PDE5-I-associated toxicities, low doses of PDE5-Is should be used cautiously in PI-treated patients.

Fertility and reproduction

Analysis of semen among men with early HIV disease is usually normal and compatible with fertility. In contrast, men with advanced stages of HIV often have oligospermia and morphologically abnormal sperm [35]. ART with zidovudine does not adversely affect sperm production or quality. Treatment with testosterone or anabolic steroids is associated with azoospermia.

Sperm washing has been described as a safe and effective method of achieving pregnancy among HIV-discordant couples, though concern about the risk of infection transmission to seronegative women is not completely eradicated by this process [39].

REPRODUCTIVE HEALTH IN WOMEN

Ovarian pathology

In contrast to those describing testicular pathology, there have been no autopsy series examining the ovaries in the setting of AIDS. Case reports of CMV oophoritis and ovarian non-Hodgkin's lymphomas suggest the ovaries are susceptible to OIs and HIV-associated neoplasms. HIV can directly infect cells and tissues from both the upper and lower female reproductive tract, including the vaginal mucosa, fallopian tubes, uterus, and cervix [40].

Ovarian function and alterations in sex hormones

The menstrual cycle may have an effect on viremia, as HIV-1 RNA levels decline from the early follicular phase to the luteal phase. Conversely, several studies suggest that HIV infection has little effect on the menstrual cycle. Narcotics, marijuana, and chronic alcohol consumption are known to affect menstrual function and ovulation and should be addressed in HIV-infected women with menstrual irregularities. As expected with any chronic illness, amenorrhea is more common in women with AIDS wasting. Menopause does not appear to alter the progression of HIV or response to therapy. It is uncertain whether HIV has an effect on the onset of menopause and the severity of related symptoms. Similar to findings in men, women with AIDS wasting demonstrate reduced androgen levels. This hypoandrogenism appears to be a result of shunting of adrenal steroid metabolism away from androgenic pathways toward cortisol production and is not due to decreased ovarian androgen production [41]. Hypoandrogenism in women may be associated with decreases in energy, libido, mood, strength, and BMD.

Although a small initial study linking hyperandrogenemia and hyperinsulinemia in HIV-infected women with HIV-associated lipodystrophy suggested these patients may have features of polycystic ovary syndrome, later reports from the same group found reduced free testosterone levels and LH-to-FSH ratios, normal menstrual function, and normal ovarian morphology by ultrasound [42]. Serum testosterone in the range of an androgen-secreting tumor was reported in one HIV-infected woman with peripheral lipoatrophy and central lipohypertrophy [43].

Effects of antiretroviral and other therapies

Several PIs and some NNRTIs alter the metabolism of the estrogen component of hormonal contraceptives. Nevirapine and ritonavir accelerate ethinyl estradiol metabolism, reducing contraceptive efficacy. Rifabutin, rifampicin, and itraconazole—when used in the treatment of HIV-related infections—may do the same. Fluconazole and voriconazole may inhibit exogenous estrogen metabolism, resulting in a hyperestrogenic state. Although ketoconazole has little effect on estrogen, it may interfere with early pregnancy by decreasing the production of progesterone and reducing early uterine implantation and the subsequent decidual response [15].

Treatment considerations

Contraception for HIV-infected women should include a combination of barrier method and another form of acceptable contraception. Treatment with oral contraceptives may increase cervical and vaginal shedding of HIV [35].

Though many women with AIDS-wasting syndrome may have symptoms and signs of hypoandrogenism, laboratory diagnosis of androgen deficiency is difficult in women. Further, the lack of long-term studies of the efficacy and side effects of testosterone treatment in women with AIDS-wasting limits the ability to advocate its use at present.

Fertility and reproduction

Studies of HIV-infected women who did not receive prenatal ART showed a threefold higher risk of fetal loss as a result of HIV transmission and fetal thymic dysfunction [44]. Lower pregnancy and birth rates in HIV-infected women may be partially due to knowledge of HIV seropositivity, as rates of therapeutic abortion are also higher. Even though effective ART is available during pregnancy and at delivery for prevention of mother-to-child transmission, there are complex ethical and social issues regarding conception in women with HIV infection.

Pregnancy does not appear to have an effect on the progression of HIV, though it may increase HIV-1 expression in the genital tract, thus increasing the risk of vertical disease transmission. ART in the perinatal period reduces this risk. HIV-1 RNA levels may increase in early postpartum, though the significance of this is unclear.

THE PITUITARY

Pituitary pathology

Systematic postmortem examination of pituitary glands in patients with AIDS, performed before the introduction of HAART, found direct infectious involvement in 12% of adenohypophyses by either CMV or *P. jiroveci*, rarely involving the neurohypophyses [45]. Since pituitary involvement was always accompanied by generalized and/or cerebral infection, these results may not apply to patients who do not yet have significant immunosuppression or who are effectively treated with ART. Additional patients have presented with panhypopituitarism resulting from cerebral toxoplasmosis, and central diabetes insipidus has been reported in an AIDS patient with herpetic meningoencephalitis. Neoplastic infiltration of the pituitary gland is very rare, although one case of pituitary lymphoma in a patient with AIDS has been reported [46]. Hypopituitarism, independent of cause, is treated with physiologic hormone replacement.

Alterations in pituitary function

Studies employing GnRH or thyrotropin-releasing hormone (TRH) have consistently found the functional reserve of the anterior pituitary is normal. Prolactin levels, in the absence of medication effect, are usually normal and respond to TRH stimulation appropriately [46]. Posterior pituitary function, however, may be abnormal, as hyponatremia and the syndrome of inappropriate antidiuretic hormone (SIADH) secretion was reported in hospitalized AIDS patients. A primary pituitary disorder cannot be concluded from this study, however, because there were other factors influencing the development of hyponatremia, including pulmonary infection (most notably, *P. jiroveci* pneumonia) and treatment with medications (e.g. trimethoprim) [47].

Somatotropic axis

HIV infection per se does not appear to affect the somatotropic axis, based on frequent sampling studies among men with asymptomatic HIV infection, clinically stable AIDS, and healthy controls [48]. GH and insulin-like growth factor-1 (IGF-1) secretion and action, however, are influenced by nutritional status and body composition; therefore, distinct abnormalities have been observed in patients with AIDS wasting or central lipohypertrophy.

AIDS wasting may resemble an acquired GH-resistant state, explaining the decreased levels of IGF-1 and IGF-1 binding protein-3 that have been found in the setting of increased GH. In contrast, patients with HIV-associated central lipohypertrophy demonstrate an inverse correlation between GH levels and visceral obesity, consistent with the reduced GH levels found in generalized obesity [49].

Effects of antiretroviral and other therapies

Effects of specific antiretroviral drugs on the somatotropic axis have not been investigated. Galactorrhea and marked hyperprolactinemia were reported in four patients following initiation of PIs for ART or post-HIV exposure prophylaxis [50]. Although three of these patients had received medications that may increase serum prolactin levels (metoclopramide or fluoxetine), symptoms resolved only after the PIs were discontinued. Amphotericin B is associated with a reduction in renal tubular sensitivity to antidiuretic hormone and may result in reversible nephrogenic diabetes insipidus (DI). Nephrogenic DI occurs, though far less commonly, with use of liposomal formulations of amphotericin B.

WASTING SYNDROME

Although the incidence of AIDS wasting has declined since the introduction of ART, weight loss and muscle wasting remain significant problems for individuals with HIV infection, particularly patients without access to ART. Increased mortality, accelerated disease progression, loss of muscle protein mass, and impairment of strength and functional status occur with wasting [51]. Weight loss that does not meet the CDC case definition of AIDS wasting (>10% of baseline body weight with clinical symptoms) still predicts increased morbidity and mortality in this setting. Wasting is multifactorial and may represent the common endpoint of several pathophysiologic processes related to the progression of HIV infection, including reduced caloric intake due to anorexia or malabsorption and cachexia, a state marked by disproportionate loss of muscle. Increased resting energy expenditure (REE) in HIV-infected individuals indicates the presence of a hypermetabolic state. AIDS wasting appears to be an episodic process, exacerbated by acute secondary infections or gastrointestinal disease that may result in anorexia and diminished caloric intake. Failure of the normal homeostatic response to decrease REE with reduced food intake synergistically contributes to loss of LBM. Hypogonadism may also be involved in the pathogenesis of wasting syndrome, as it is present in up to 50% of men and women with wasting and has been directly correlated with decreases in both LBM and fat.

Treatment considerations

In light of the poor prognosis associated with wasting, clinicians should emphasize the prevention of weight loss by addressing weight and nutritional status as a routine part of HIV care. Patients should be weighed at each visit and encouraged to maintain a nutritional diet with adequate caloric intake while engaging in moderate exercise. Those with active weight loss require comprehensive assessment of the potential co-morbidities described above, including ruling out secondary infection and optimizing ART. Nutritional counseling should consider psychosocial factors, as access to food, depression, and socioeconomic standing can affect both the quantity and quality of food intake.

Randomized, placebo-controlled trials have investigated approaches to the treatment of AIDS-associated weight loss such as progressive resistance training, nutritional supplementation, cytokine suppression, and the administration of appetite stimulants, androgenic steroids, and GH [51]. Dronabinol improves subjective appetite but results in little or no weight gain. Megestrol acetate effectively stimulates appetite and achieves weight gain but predominantly increases fat tissue rather than LBM. When given in conjunction with testosterone, changes in body composition are no different [52]. Among men with AIDS wasting and hypogonadism, physiologic testosterone replacement, which induces gain of LBM, may be instituted. However, treatment with supraphysiologic doses of testosterone is controversial due to concerns about its effects on lipid profile and cardiovascular risk. Treatment with anabolic steroids, including nandrolone decanoate and oxandrolone, also increases LBM but is frequently complicated by the development of abnormal liver enzymes and dyslipidemia. These changes occur particularly with oral preparations. In randomized, placebo-controlled trials, 3 months of recombinant GH treatment at high doses (0.1 mg/kg/day) induced significant increases in LBM with reductions in fat [53]. In other studies, treatment of similar duration with lower doses of GH showed little to no change in body composition. Side effects of GH include arthralgias, myalgias, edema, diarrhea, carpal tunnel compression, and perhaps most importantly, glucose intolerance. Though GH is the only treatment specifically FDA-approved for AIDS-wasting syndrome that increases LBM, it remains an expensive therapy for which long-term side effects are unclear. Its use may be considered for rapid weight loss associated with acute infection or for persistent wasting refractory to other therapies [51].

REFERENCES

[1] Lima MK, Freitas LL, Montandon C, et al. The thyroid in acquired immunodeficiency syndrome. Endocr Pathol 1998;9(3):217–23.

[2] Hofbauer LC, Heufelder AE. Endocrine implications of human immunodeficiency virus infection. Medicine (Baltimore) 1996;75 (5):262–78.

[3] Desailloud R, Hober D. Viruses and thyroiditis: an update. Virol J 2009;6:5.

[4] Manfredi R, Sabbatani S, Chiodo F. Advanced acute myelogenous leukaemia (AML) during HAART-treated HIV disease, manifesting initially as a thyroid mass. Scand J Infect Dis 2005;37(10):781–3.

[5] Grunfeld C, Pang M, Doerrler W, et al. Indices of thyroid function and weight loss in human immunodeficiency virus infection and the acquired immunodeficiency syndrome. Metabolism 1993;42 (10):1270–6.

[6] Hommes MJ, Romijn JA, Endert E, et al. Hypothyroid-like regulation of the pituitary–thyroid axis in stable human immunodeficiency virus infection. Metabolism 1993;42 (5):556–61.

[7] Hoffmann CJ, Brown TT. Thyroid function abnormalities in HIV-infected patients. Clin Infect Dis 2007;45(4):488–94.

[8] Carella C, Mazziotti G, Amato G, et al. Clinical review 169: interferon-alpha-related thyroid disease: pathophysiological, epidemiological, and clinical aspects. J Clin Endocrinol Metab 2004;89(8):3656–61.

[9] Jubault V, Penfornis A, Schillo F, et al. Sequential occurrence of thyroid autoantibodies and Graves' disease after immune restoration in severely immunocompromised human immunodeficiency virus-1-infected patients. J Clin Endocrinol Metab 2000;85(11):4254–7.

[10] Membreno L, Irony I, Dere W, et al. Adrenocortical function in acquired immunodeficiency syndrome. J Clin Endocrinol Metab 1987;65 (3):482–7.

[11] Mayo J, Collazos J, Martinez E, Ibarra S. Adrenal function in the human immunodeficiency virus-infected patient. Arch Intern Med 2002;162(10):1095–8.

[12] Piketty C, Jayle D, Leplege A, et al. Double-blind placebo-controlled trial of oral dehydroepiandrosterone in patients with advanced HIV disease. Clin Endocrinol (Oxf) 2001;55 (3):325–30.

[13] Abrams DI, Shade SB, Couey P, et al. Dehydroepiandrosterone (DHEA) effects on HIV replication and host immunity: a randomized placebo-controlled study. AIDS Res Hum Retroviruses 2007;23(1):77–85.

[14] Lo JC, Mulligan K, Tai VW, et al. "Buffalo hump" in men with HIV-1 infection. Lancet 1998;351 (9106):867–70.

[15] Lionakis MS, Samonis G, Kontoyiannis DP. Endocrine and metabolic manifestations of invasive fungal infections and systemic antifungal treatment. Mayo Clin Proc 2008;83(9):1046–60.

[16] Cooper OB, Brown TT, Dobs AS. Opiate drug use: a potential contributor to the endocrine and metabolic complications in human immunodeficiency virus disease. Clin Infect Dis 2003;37(Suppl. 2): S132–6.

[17] Chehter EZ, Longo MA, Laudanna AA, Duarte MI. Involvement of the pancreas in AIDS: a prospective study of 109 post-mortems. AIDS 2000;14 (13):1879–86.

[18] Keaveny AP, Karasik MS. Hepatobiliary and pancreatic infections in AIDS: Part one. AIDS Patient Care STDS 1998;12 (5):347–57.

[19] Gimeno-Garcia AZ, Alonso MM, Garcia Castro C, et al. Primary pancreatic lymphoma diagnosed by endoscopic ultrasound-guided fine needle aspiration biopsy. Gastroenterol Hepatol 2010;33 (9):638–42.

[20] Menges M, Pees HW. Kaposi's sarcoma of the pancreas mimicking pancreatic cancer in an HIV-infected patient. Clinical diagnosis by detection of HHV 8 in bile and complete remission following antiviral and cytostatic therapy with paclitaxel. Int J Pancreatol 1999;26 (3):193–9.

[21] Noor MA, Seneviratne T, Aweeka FT, et al. Indinavir acutely inhibits insulin-stimulated glucose disposal in humans: a randomized, placebo-controlled study. AIDS 2002;16(5): F1–8.

[22] Lee GA, Lo JC, Aweeka F, et al. Single-dose lopinavir-ritonavir acutely inhibits insulin-mediated glucose disposal in healthy volunteers. Clin Infect Dis 2006;43 (5):658–60.

[23] Lee GA, Rao M, Mulligan K, et al. Effects of ritonavir and amprenavir on insulin sensitivity in healthy volunteers. AIDS 2007;21 (16):2183–90.

[24] Taylor SA, Lee GA, Pao VY, et al. Boosting dose ritonavir does not alter peripheral insulin sensitivity in healthy HIV-seronegative volunteers. J Acquir Immune Defic Syndr 2010;55(3):361–4.

[25] Noor MA, Lo JC, Mulligan K, et al. Metabolic effects of indinavir in healthy HIV-seronegative men. AIDS 2001;15(7):F11–18.

[26] Lee GA, Seneviratne T, Noor MA, et al. The metabolic effects of lopinavir/ritonavir in HIV-negative men. AIDS 2004;18(4):641–9.

[27] Lee GA, Schwarz JM, Patzek S, et al. The acute effects of HIV protease inhibitors on insulin suppression of glucose production in healthy HIV-negative men. J Acquir Immune Defic Syndr 2009;52(2):246–8.

[28] Pao VY, Lee GA, Taylor S, et al. The protease inhibitor combination lopinavir/ritonavir does not decrease insulin secretion in healthy, HIV-seronegative volunteers. AIDS 2010;24(2):265–70.

[29] Schambelan M, Benson CA, Carr A, et al. Management of metabolic complications associated with antiretroviral therapy for HIV-1 infection: recommendations of an

International AIDS Society-USA panel. J Acquir Immune Defic Syndr 2002;31(3):257–75.

[30] Tehranzadeh J, Ter-Oganesyan RR, Steinbach LS. Musculoskeletal disorders associated with HIV infection and AIDS. Part I: infectious musculoskeletal conditions. Skeletal Radiol 2004;33 (5):249–59.

[31] Tehranzadeh J, Ter-Oganesyan RR, Steinbach LS. Musculoskeletal disorders associated with HIV infection and AIDS. Part II: non-infectious musculoskeletal conditions. Skeletal Radiol 2004;33 (6):311–20.

[32] Miller KD, Masur H, Jones EC, et al. High prevalence of osteonecrosis of the femoral head in HIV-infected adults. Ann Intern Med 2002;137 (1):17–25.

[33] Thomas J, Doherty SM. HIV infection—a risk factor for osteoporosis. J Acquir Immune Defic Syndr 2003;33(3):281–91.

[34] Salehian B, Jacobson D, Swerdloff RS, et al. Testicular pathologic changes and the pituitary–testicular axis during human immunodeficiency virus infection. Endocr Pract 1999;5 (1):1–9.

[35] Lo JC, Schambelan M. Reproductive function in human immunodeficiency virus infection. J Clin Endocrinol Metab 2001;86 (6):2338–43.

[36] Teichmann J, Stephan E, Lange U, et al. Evaluation of serum and urinary estrogen levels in male patients with HIV-infection. Eur J Med Res 1998;3(11):533–7.

[37] Dobs A. Role of testosterone in maintaining lean body mass and bone density in HIV-infected patients. Int J Impot Res 2003;15 (Suppl. 4):S21–5.

[38] Kegg S, Lau R. Tamoxifen in antiretroviral-associated gynaecomastia. Int J STD AIDS 2002;13(8):582–3.

[39] Sauer MV. Sperm washing techniques address the fertility needs of HIV-seropositive men: a clinical review. Reprod Biomed Online 2005;10(1):135–40.

[40] Howell AL, Edkins RD, Rier SE, et al. Human immunodeficiency virus type 1 infection of cells and tissues from the upper and lower human female reproductive tract. J Virol 1997;71(5):3498–506.

[41] Grinspoon S, Corcoran C, Stanley T, et al. Mechanisms of androgen deficiency in human immunodeficiency virus-infected women with the wasting syndrome. J Clin Endocrinol Metab 2001;86 (9):4120–6.

[42] Johnsen S, Dolan SE, Fitch KV, et al. Absence of polycystic ovary syndrome features in human immunodeficiency virus-infected women despite significant hyperinsulinemia and truncal adiposity. J Clin Endocrinol Metab 2005;90(10):5596–604.

[43] Dahan MH, Lyle LN, Wolfsen A, Chang RJ. Tumor-level serum testosterone associated with human immunodeficiency virus lipodystrophy syndrome. Obstet Gynecol 2004;103(5 Pt 2):1094–6.

[44] Shearer WT, Langston C, Lewis DE, et al. Early spontaneous abortions and fetal thymic abnormalities in maternal-to-fetal HIV infection. Acta Paediatr Suppl 1997; 421:60–4.

[45] Sano T, Kovacs K, Scheithauer BW, et al. Pituitary pathology in acquired immunodeficiency syndrome. Arch Pathol Lab Med 1989;113 (9):1066–70.

[46] Sellmeyer DE, Grunfeld C. Endocrine and metabolic disturbances in human immunodeficiency virus infection and the acquired immune deficiency syndrome. Endocr Rev 1996;17(5):518–32.

[47] Agarwal A, Soni A, Ciechanowsky M, et al. Hyponatremia in patients with the acquired immunodeficiency syndrome. Nephron 1989;53 (4):317–21.

[48] Heijligenberg R, Sauerwein HP, Brabant G, et al. Circadian growth hormone secretion in asymptomatic human immune deficiency virus infection and acquired immunodeficiency syndrome. J Clin Endocrinol Metab 1996;81(11): 4028–32.

[49] Bhasin S, Singh AB, Javanbakht M. Neuroendocrine abnormalities associated with HIV infection. Endocrinol Metab Clin North Am 2001;30(3):749–64.

[50] Hutchinson J, Murphy M, Harries R, Skinner CJ. Galactorrhoea and hyperprolactinaemia associated with protease-inhibitors. Lancet 2000;356(9234):1003–4.

[51] Grinspoon S, Mulligan K. Weight loss and wasting in patients infected with human immunodeficiency virus. Clin Infect Dis 2003;36 (Suppl. 2):S69–78.

[52] Mulligan K, Zackin R, Von Roenn JH, et al. Testosterone supplementation of megestrol therapy does not enhance lean tissue accrual in men with human immunodeficiency virus-associated weight loss: a randomized, double-blind, placebo-controlled, multicenter trial. J Clin Endocrinol Metab 2007;92(2):563–70.

[53] Schambelan M, Mulligan K, Grunfeld C, et al. Recombinant human growth hormone in patients with HIV-associated wasting: a randomized clinical trial. Ann Intern Med 1996;125:873–82.

Chapter | 23 |

Renal complications of HIV infection

Jula K. Inrig, Lynda A. Szczech, Trevor E. Gerntholtz, Paul E. Klotman

INTRODUCTION

In the early 1980s, a unique form of kidney disease was described among HIV-infected patients [1, 2]. Patients usually presented with significant proteinuria and rapid progression to end-stage renal disease (ESRD) [2]. When initially described, this renal failure was attributed to heroin nephropathy, as it clinically appeared similar. As clinicians continued to see renal disease associated with HIV infection, the existence of a distinct disease called HIV-associated nephropathy (HIVAN) was debated. As more patients with HIV infection without a history of heroin use were noted to have renal disease, HIVAN was established as a unique entity [2]. From a once rare complication of HIV infection, HIVAN has emerged as the most common cause of ESRD in HIV-infected patients [3]. In addition, as patients with HIV/AIDS are surviving longer, the prevalence of HIV-infected patients with chronic kidney disease continues to rise [4]. With up to 33 million people infected with HIV/AIDS worldwide and a prevalence of renal disease in HIV-infected black patients of 3.5–12%, up to 4 million people worldwide may be affected by HIV-related kidney disease [2, 5]. This chapter will review the epidemiology and clinical course of HIV-related renal disease using US, European, and African studies to compare results based on regions of the world. Such a comparison requires initial insight into methods and infrastructure for delivery of healthcare within regions to provide a framework for the understanding of study comparisons.

OVERVIEW OF GLOBAL HEALTHCARE/DELIVERY

Healthcare and its delivery vary drastically around the world. In the USA and Europe, healthcare is available to a greater proportion of the population than in many other parts of the world. In Africa, unfortunately, the availability of health services is considerably more limited. Despite the growing AIDS epidemic, limited resources are available for the majority of patients needing therapy. Due to limited preventive services in Africa, screening for renal disease is essentially non-existent and because of more pressing and immediate health concerns, screening assumes a lower priority. As a result, patients are often diagnosed late in the course of their disease after presenting to a hospital with another illness or overt nephrotic syndrome. Thus, treatment is limited by late diagnosis, co-morbid conditions, and shortage of resources. In contrast, patients in the USA and Europe with known HIV may undergo screening for renal involvement and thus may be offered therapy earlier in the course of their disease.

EPIDEMIOLOGY

One of the first clinical reports of HIVAN occurred in 1984 in the USA [1]. Not surprisingly, the initial description engendered a debate that was focused mainly on whether this was a different entity from heroin nephropathy. As children and patients without a history of heroin use were identified with renal disease and the disease became better defined histologically, the term HIVAN emerged to describe the combination of clinical and histological findings. In the early era of HIV, patients with HIVAN were diagnosed late in the course of HIV infection, usually after they had been diagnosed with AIDS. Predictably, renal survival for those diagnosed with HIVAN was 1–4 months without therapy [1, 2, 6, 7]. With the advent of potent antiretroviral therapy (ART) and the decline in mortality from AIDS, kidney diseases have become major contributors to HIV morbidity and mortality [8].

While no data on global prevalence exist, HIVAN is likely to have the highest prevalence in Africa. According to the 2009 report on the global AIDS epidemic, almost 33 million people are living with AIDS in the world [5]. Within sub-Saharan Africa alone, nearly 22.5 million people are currently infected. In the USA, the prevalence of renal disease has been noted to be between 3.5 and 12% in HIV-infected African Americans [2, 9]. If one assumes a similar prevalence among persons of African descent, then up to 2.7 million patients may have renal disease in sub-Saharan Africa alone. Any estimate of prevalence, however, needs to account for the different mortality rates among HIV-infected patients and its variation by country. Without having an exact estimate, the prevalence of renal disease could be hypothesized to be quite high. One report in 2003 in the *Nigerian Journal of Medicine* assessing the prevalence of renal disease in consecutive patients with AIDS seen in the infection unit suggested that these estimates are conservative. Of 79 patients with AIDS, renal disease was present in 51.8% (41 patients) as compared with 12.2% (7 patients) of non-HIV-infected controls. Of these 79 patients, 19% (n = 15) had azotemia, 25% had proteinuria alone, and 7.6% had both proteinuria and azotemia [10].

The current leading cause of death from AIDS worldwide is infection; but as ART becomes more available and survival is prolonged, renal disease is likely to become a major secondary cause of mortality and morbidity as it has in the USA. As the mortality rate from AIDS declined in the early 1990s, the number of black patients living with HIV increased significantly. As a result, this at-risk group lived longer, and HIVAN became one of the most rapidly growing causes of end-stage renal disease in the USA [3].

Racial distribution of HIVAN

As demonstrated by US and European epidemiologic and pathologic data, HIVAN has an overwhelmingly higher prevalence in HIV-infected patients of African descent than in Caucasians [9, 11–15]. With the emergence of HIV throughout the world in the 1980s, a change in the pathologic findings in African patients with nephrotic syndrome

was described. A study from Zaire in 1993 reported the pathologic findings of 92 patients with documented nephrotic syndrome systematically biopsied between 1986 and 1989. A total of 41% of these patients were found to have focal and segmental glomerulosclerosis (FSGS), a sevenfold increase from previous prevalence rates of only 6%. The investigators were uncertain as to the cause of the increase in FSGS but proposed that AIDS might be responsible [16]. This study cannot assess the predisposition of blacks to HIVAN but does suggest that HIVAN has become an increasing health problem in this population. Early in the HIV epidemic, epidemiologic data from the USA and Europe found that HIVAN was diagnosed primarily in areas with large populations of HIV-infected black patients [14]. Two series from France and London have reported that 97/102 and 17/17 of patients diagnosed with HIVAN were black, respectively [17, 18].

In contrast to the high rate of HIVAN in predominantly black-populated regions, Caucasians are noted to have a much lower prevalence of classic HIVAN. A postmortem analysis of 239 consecutive Swiss patients who died from AIDS between 1981 and 1989 demonstrated pathologic renal findings in 43% of patients, with HIVAN in only 1.7% (4/239) of the patients [13]. Given that 95% of the patients were Caucasians, this study emphasizes the low prevalence of classic HIVAN in Caucasians.

Another study reviewed the pathologic features of 120 consecutively autopsied HIV-infected Caucasian patients in Italy. Of these patients, 68% had pathologic renal changes, and none of the renal specimens had classic HIVAN. The most common pathologic abnormality was immune-mediated glomerular diseases (25 patients) and tubulointerstitial lesions (19 patients) [15]. A similar study of 26 Caucasian patients in northern Italy with HIV who underwent renal biopsy failed to reveal any lesions of HIVAN. The majority of diagnoses were immune complex-mediated glomerulonephritis [11]. While patients of African descent are at the highest risk for HIVAN, other ethnic groups have renal disease related to other pathologic entities.

Patterns of renal disease in Africa

There is a large variation in the patterns of renal diseases reported in different geographic regions of Africa. Unfortunately, accurate and comprehensive statistics are not available [19]. For example, a single available study of 368 patients with chronic kidney disease (CKD) in Nigeria demonstrated that 62% had an undetermined etiology of renal failure [20]. The prevalence of CKD in sub-Saharan Africa is not known. Data from the South African Dialysis and Transplant registry regarding etiologies of ESRD reflect only patients selected for dialysis. As only patients eligible for transplantation are offered dialysis, and few patients with diabetic ESRD are offered dialysis or transplantation due to co-morbid conditions, the available data are unlikely to reflect the spectrum of renal diseases in the population as a whole.

In North Africa, the incidence of renal disease appears to be much higher than in the USA, but the prevalence is lower due to higher mortality and fewer available treatment options [21]. The reported annual incidence of ESRD ranges between 34 and 200 patients per million population (pmp), and the respective prevalence ranges from 30 to 430 patients pmp. Despite the high mortality from ESRD, the prevalence of CKD appears to be increasing. The principal causes of CKD are interstitial nephritis (14–32%), glomerulonephritis (11–24%), diabetes (5–20%), and nephrosclerosis (5–31%). Trends in Egypt suggest an increasing prevalence of interstitial nephropathies and diabetes [14]. FSGS is reported in 23–34% of the glomerulonephritides (GN) and is mostly clustered in black patients [21].

Overall, glomerular disease appears to be more prevalent and more severe in Africa than in Western countries. It has been estimated that between 0.2 and 2.4% of medical admissions in tropical countries are due to renal disease (0.5% Zimbabwe; 0.2% Kwa Zulu Natal, South Africa; 2.0% in Uganda; and 2.4% Nigeria) [22]. It has been observed that the majority of these admissions are related to glomerulonephritis, which responds poorly to treatment and progresses to ESRD. In addition, glomerulonephritis in South Africa is more frequent in blacks and less frequent in Indians and Caucasians. This is a similar pattern to the distribution of HIVAN. Given the high prevalence of HIV/AIDS in South Africa, it can be postulated that some of these renal disorders may be caused by HIVAN or other HIV-related renal diseases.

NATURAL HISTORY

Among patients with HIVAN, severe proteinuria (often in the nephrotic range >3 g/day) with progression to ESRD within 1–4 months of diagnosis was initially described [1, 2, 6, 7, 23]. Subsequent data in the setting of monotherapy with zidovudine and ART suggest a much slower progression [23–25]. While early reports suggested that HIVAN was a late manifestation of AIDS, occurring when CD4 counts were well below 200 copies/mL, subsequent data suggest that a lower CD4 count may be associated with a faster progression and greater likelihood of biopsy [17, 24]. A case report of HIVAN demonstrates its presence as early as the time of acute HIV seroconversion [26].

PATHOGENESIS

Early in the description of HIVAN, it was uncertain whether HIV caused injury through a direct effect on renal cells or an indirect effect from immune dysregulation. Studies by Bruggeman and co-workers using a murine model of HIVAN demonstrated that HIV-1 expression in renal epithelial cells is necessary for the development of the HIVAN phenotype [27]. They went on to demonstrate that both tubular and glomerular epithelial cells are infected by HIV in patients with HIVAN [28]. Furthermore, Marras and co-workers demonstrated that the renal tubular epithelial cells support viral replication and subsequent divergence, and act as a separate compartment from blood [29]. According to a study by Winston and co-workers, renal parenchymal cells can serve as a reservoir for HIV, and the presence of the virus can persist in glomerular and tubular epithelial cells despite ART [30].

The mechanisms by which HIV gains entry into epithelial cells remain unclear. The major co-receptors for HIV-1 have not been detected using immunocytochemistry, but more sensitive methods including PCR suggest that CD4 and CXCR4 can be detected in cultured renal epithelial cells [31]. The data are less clear for the other co-receptors. Whether the receptors are in sufficiently high density or functional enough to mediate entry into the cell also remains unknown [31].

The observation that HIV DNA has been found in glomeruli of HIV-infected patients without HIVAN suggests that some additional factor (such as a genetic predisposition) may be required [32]. The pathologic findings of collapsing focal glomerulosclerosis combined with tubular microcystic disease have been thought to be specific to HIVAN. However, a recent report of collapsing GN in seven HIV-uninfected Caucasian patients who were treated with high-dose pamidronate suggests that other environmental agents can also induce collapse [33]. Thus, Caucasian patients can develop a collapsing phenotype, but the mechanism appears to be different from those observed in response to HIV infection in blacks.

The racial predilection for HIVAN in blacks strongly suggests that genetic factors play an important role in the pathogenesis of HIVAN. In support of this, Gharavi and co-workers assessed the influence of genetic background on the development or progression of HIVAN by crossing the HIVAN transgenic mouse with mice of different genetic backgrounds [34]. These investigators found that the HIVAN phenotype varied from severe renal disease to no renal disease based on the background strain of the mice. In addition, genome-wide analysis of linkage in 185 heterozygous transgenic backcross mice identified a locus on chromosome 3A1-3, *HIVAN1*, which showed highly significant linkage to renal disease. This locus, *HIVAN1*, is syntenic to human chromosome 3q25-27, which is an interval showing suggestive evidence of linkage to various nephropathies [34]. More recent investigations have identified 2 genomic loci that regulate podocyte gene expression and which confer an increased susceptibility in mice to HIVAN [35].

PATHOLOGY

HIV-associated nephropathy has pathologic findings similar to idiopathic and heroin-related FSGS; however, there are several unique findings suggestive of HIV infection [12]. First, in HIVAN there is a tendency for the entire glomerular

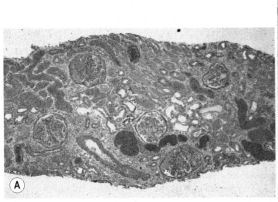

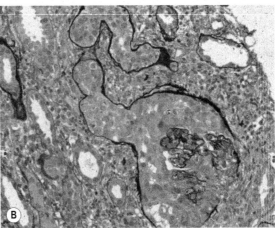

Figure 23.1 Kidney biopsy specimens. (A) Low-power view of a biopsy specimen from a patient with HIVAN in the USA. There are 5 glomeruli with collapsing sclerosis and podocyte hyperplasia. The tubules are separated by edema, mild fibrosis, and patchy interstitial inflammatory infiltrates. Some tubules show degenerative changes with focal tubular microcysts containing large casts. (B) High-power view of a biopsy specimen from a patient with HIVAN in Brazil. Note the collapsing sclerotic glomerulus, tubular atrophy, and interstitial inflammation.
(Courtesy of CE Poli de Figueiredo, MD, DPhil, Medical School PUCRS, Porto Alegre, Brazil.)

tuft to sclerose and collapse rather than finding only a segmental glomerular lesion (Fig. 23.1). In the tubules, there is often severe injury with proliferative microcyst formation and tubular degeneration. The tubular disease is characterized by the development of tubular dilation accompanied by flattening and atrophy of the tubular epithelial cells. Electron microscopy can reveal the presence of numerous tubuloreticular structures in the glomerular endothelial cells. The tubuloreticular inclusions are composed of ribonucleoprotein and membrane structures; their synthesis is stimulated by α-interferon. The only other disorder in which these structures are prominently seen is lupus nephritis, which is also associated with chronically high levels of circulating α-interferon. The finding of tubuloreticular inclusion had been noted to be a common pathologic abnormality in the pre-ART era; however, this pathologic abnormality is now found less frequently. This is potentially related to the advent of effective ART, resulting in reduced levels of plasma interferon [12, 36]. In HIV-infected patients with kidney disease, several different glomerular syndromes have been described (Box 23.1). The most common pathologic finding is HIVAN. In the USA, the second most common pathologic findings are membranoproliferative GN (often with HCV coinfection) or mesangioproliferative GN, followed by immune complex GN, membranous, and IgA nephropathy [12, 24]. Less commonly, HIV-infected patients have been found to have thrombotic microangiopathy, minimal change disease, and amyloidosis [24, 37]. This is in comparison to patients seen in Baragwanath, South Africa. Among 99 HIV-infected patients, 27% had classic HIVAN; 21% had immune complex rich "lupus-like" disease; 41% had other GN including 13% membranous, 8% post-infectious GN, 5% IgA

> **Box 23.1 Diagnosis in HIV-infected patients with proteinuria**
>
> - HIV-associated nephropathy[a]
> - Membranoproliferative GN (often with HCV)[a]
> - Mesangioproliferative GN
> - Immune complex GN
> - Membranous nephropathy
> - IgA nephropathy
> - Post-infectious GN
> - Minimal change disease
> - Diabetic nephropathy
> - Tubulointerstitial nephritis
> - Thrombotic microangiopathy
> - Amyloidosis
>
> [a]Most common pathologic findings.

nephropathy, and 6% mesangioproliferative GN, and 9% other nonspecified GN; 3% had tubulointerstitial nephritis; 3% had acute tubular necrosis; and 4% had other [38]. However, among hospitalized HIV-infected patients with acute renal failure, the most common diagnosis is acute tubular necrosis.

CLINICAL FEATURES

HIVAN typically presents in the setting of poorly controlled HIV infection with high viral loads. Rarely, HIVAN can present as part of the acute retroviral syndrome (primary HIV infection) or within the first few months of infection. HIVAN typically presents with a rapid decline in renal function with significant proteinuria. Typically the proteinuria is in the nephrotic range with >3 g protein per 24 hours or a spot protein/creatinine ratio of >3 mg/g. Most patients with HIVAN do not have significant peripheral edema, and despite the high prevalence of hypertension in blacks, patients with HIVAN are not usually hypertensive. Laboratory data are non-specific. Serologic studies for glomerular diseases (i.e. ANA, dsDNA, complements, antistreptolysin O antibodies, ANCA, anti-GBM, hepatitis B surface antigen, hepatitis C AB, cryoglobulins) are usually negative except in patients with hepatitis C co-infection. Urinalysis is typically bland without hematuria but with varying numbers of hyaline casts and renal tubular epithelial cells. Ultrasonography typically reveals bilaterally echogenic and enlarged kidneys, in contrast to other conditions, in which the kidneys shrink in size as function deteriorates. Diagnosis of specific histology requires a renal biopsy; it is difficult to distinguish HIVAN from other pathologic lesions on clinical grounds alone. There are no valid non-invasive surrogate markers for HIVAN. For example, nephrotic range proteinuria even in the presence of a low CD4 count does not reliably predict HIVAN. Detectable viremia is a typical feature of HIVAN, and the diagnosis is unlikely if the HIV viral load is <400 copies/mm^3 [39]. Therefore, if there are no contraindications to a renal biopsy, it should be performed for histologic diagnosis.

Patient evaluation, diagnosis, and differential diagnosis

Figure 23.2 proposes a screening algorithm for kidney disease in HIV-infected patients.

TREATMENT

Despite the high prevalence of kidney disease in HIV-infected patients, no prospective randomized controlled trials have been performed to assess the effect of various treatments on outcome. However, a number of retrospective analyses for assessing the association effects of ART, angiotensin-converting enzyme inhibitors, and steroids on outcomes have been performed (Box 23.2).

Antiretroviral therapy

Initial reports of the efficacy of monotherapy with zidovudine on HIVAN were conflicting. FSGS was noted to develop in many patients despite treatment with zidovudine and thus was suggested to be of little benefit [40]. Other studies suggested that zidovudine might delay the progression of HIV nephropathy if begun when patients had mild proteinuria and near-normal renal function [23]. In a retrospective

cohort of 19 patients with a clinical diagnosis of HIVAN, protease inhibitor (PI) treatment was associated with a slower decline in creatinine clearance (−0.08 mL/min per month versus −4.30 mL/min per month for those not treated with a PI) [25]. In another analysis, among patients with HIVAN, the use of ART was associated with a slower progression to end-stage renal disease (HR 0.24, $p = 0.03$) [24]. In a cohort of 36 patients with biopsy-confirmed HIVAN, patients receiving ART had a significantly lower odds of developing end-stage renal disease (odds ratio 0.30, $p < 0.05$) [41]. In this cohort, those with complete virologic response to ART also had better renal survival. In a study of 3,313 patients enrolled in a randomized antiretroviral trial in Uganda and Zimbabwe, there was stabilization or slight improvement in glomerular filtration rate (GFR) following initiation of ART, and very few patients (1.6%) developed severe reductions in GFR during 96 weeks of follow-up [42]. Recent evidence also suggests that classic HIVAN is unlikely among patients with viral loads <400 copies/mm^3 [39]. Despite a variety of study designs, it would appear that these reports are generally consistent in that either suppression of viral replication or ART significantly slowed the progression of renal disease among patients with HIVAN. Among HIV-infected patients with renal disease other than HIVAN, a single study suggests that ART may not be associated with a similar benefit [24]. Additional studies to confirm this are required.

Angiotensin-converting enzyme inhibitors

Angiotensin-converting enzyme inhibitors (ACE-I) have been shown to be efficacious in a variety of renal disorders associated with proteinuria, such as diabetes mellitus. In patients with HIVAN, retrospective analyses suggest that the use of ACE-I is associated with improved renal survival. Kimmel and co-workers reported delayed progression of renal failure in a retrospective cohort of nine patients with HIVAN compared with a group of controls [7]. Burns and co-workers prospectively evaluated 20 patients with "early" HIVAN (baseline creatinine <2.0 mg/dL, 177 micromol/L), all of whom were offered fosinopril [6]. In the 12 patients who were adherent with treatment, renal function remained stable at 12 and 24 weeks of follow-up. In the eight untreated patients, serum creatinine increased from 88.4 to 433.2 micromol/L. Long-term effects have also been reported with ACE inhibitors. In a single-center prospective study, 44 patients with biopsy-proven HIVAN and early renal disease (mean serum creatinine <2.0 mg/dL, <177 micromol/L, <50% with proteinuria >3 g/day) were all offered treatment with fosinopril [43]. In the 28 patients who consented to fosinopril, serum creatinine remained stable after a median of 479.5 days of follow-up in all but one patient, who progressed to ESRD. All of the 16 patients who refused treatment progressed to

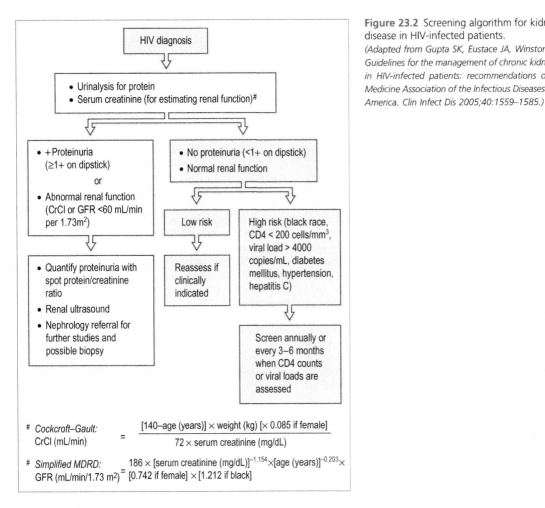

Figure 23.2 Screening algorithm for kidney disease in HIV-infected patients.
(Adapted from Gupta SK, Eustace JA, Winston JA, et al. Guidelines for the management of chronic kidney disease in HIV-infected patients: recommendations of the HIV Medicine Association of the Infectious Diseases Society of America. Clin Infect Dis 2005;40:1559–1585.)

Box 23.2 Management of kidney disease in HIV-infected patients[a]

- Control blood pressure to < 130/80, initial agents should be ACE inhibitors for patients with proteinuria
- Prepare for dialysis by placing dialysis access
- Discuss renal transplantation
- If proven HIVAN, treat with ART
- If patient with HIVAN fails to respond to ART, consider adding ACE inhibitor (if not already initiated) and/or prednisone

[a]Adapted from Gupta SK, Eustace JA, Winston JA, et al. Guidelines for the management of chronic kidney disease in HIV-infected patients: recommendations of the HIV Medicine Association of the Infectious Diseases Society of the America. Clin Infect Dis 2005; 40:1559–1585.

ESRD after a median period of 146 days. Initial serum creatinine and proteinuria were similar in both groups but exposure to ART prior to the study appeared different (57% in the ACE-I group versus 31%, $p = 0.12$) as was CD4 count (172 versus 120 cells/mm^3, $p = 0.06$).

The potential benefit of ACE-I on HIVAN was also demonstrated by Gerntholtz among 99 HIV-infected patients who underwent renal biopsy in South Africa [38]. In 27 patients with HIVAN, use of an ACE-I was associated with improved renal survival (personal communication). All patients progressed to ESRD by 15 weeks of follow-up in the absence of ACE-I compared with 30% with ESRD at 160 weeks of follow-up in the ACE-I-treated group. As patients were not randomized to treatment groups, baseline characteristics were different and included a lower creatinine (448 micromol/L versus 1082 micromol/L), higher albumin, and higher cholesterol level in the ACE-I group. ACE-I therapy appeared to have no effect on proteinuria.

As only 8 patients in this cohort were taking antiretrovirals, further research is required to define the benefit of ACE-I among patients using ART.

Steroids

Initial observations in children with HIVAN suggested that corticosteroids were ineffective. However, later research has found that some patients may respond to steroid therapy [44, 45]. In a retrospective cohort, 13 of 21 patients with biopsy-proven HIVAN received corticosteroids for one month followed by a taper over several months. Seven patients treated with corticosteroids remained off dialysis at 6 months of follow-up compared with only one of the non-corticosteroid group ($p = 0.06$) [44]. A second group reported a series of 20 patients (17 with biopsy-proven HIVAN) who were treated with prednisone 60 mg/day for 2–11 weeks followed by a slow taper. After a mean follow-up of 44 weeks, 8 patients required maintenance dialysis, 11 died from AIDS-related complications, and 7 were alive and free from dialysis [45]. Unfortunately, in both groups, infection-related complications were high. Gerntholtz retrospectively analyzed HIV-infected patients in South Africa with kidney disease and found that prednisone had no effect on outcome [38]. Szczech and co-workers retrospectively studied 19 patients with suspected HIVAN or other HIV-related kidney disease. The 5 patients who received prednisone experienced an increase in creatinine clearance of 5.57 mL/min per month, whereas the 14 patients who did not receive prednisone experienced a decline in creatinine clearance of 3.32 mL/min per month ($p = 0.003$) [25]. Given the small number of observational studies, the short follow-up, and the likelihood of relapse and adverse events, definitive conclusions cannot be made regarding the efficacy or safety of steroids for the treatment of HIVAN.

Renal replacement therapy

With the rapid progression of renal failure in patients with HIVAN, renal replacement therapy (RRT) becomes the major therapeutic option. Unfortunately, the availability of RRT to patients with ESRD is not uniform globally. In the USA, the survival of HIV-infected ESRD patients is similar to that of HIV-uninfected patients with ESRD, and increasing numbers of transplant centers are performing kidney transplantation in stable HIV-infected patients. However, the availability of dialysis and transplantation are particularly variable in Africa. According to the Dialysis Registry, only 30 patients were on renal replacement therapy in Rwanda, 290 in Kenya, and >3,000 in South Africa [46]. Treatment rates in Africa are 99 pmp and of 30–186.5 pmp in North Africa [19, 22]. This is in contrast to treatment rates of 1,090 and 800 pmp in the USA and Germany, respectively [46]. Dialysis services are predominantly available only in

urban regions in Africa and are thus inaccessible to patients living in poorer, rural areas [19].

In South Africa, there is strict rationing of dialysis due to the lack of resources and funding. The National Health Department has formalized a protocol for the management of ESRD: state facilities will only offer long-term dialysis if patients are eligible for a kidney transplant. Currently, HIV-infected patients with acute renal failure may be supported by dialysis on a short-term basis, but HIV-infected patients are not candidates for renal transplantation and thus are not offered long-term dialysis [19].

Dialysis and transplant programs in the rest of Africa are dependent on the availability of funding and donors. Nigeria, Tanzania, Ethiopia, Cote d'Ivoire, and Cameroon offer limited dialysis to a small number of patients for short time periods. Peritoneal dialysis is limited due to the high cost of peritoneal fluids and the high rate of peritonitis [21].

In the USA and Europe, renal transplantation has increasingly become an option for HIV-infected patients with ESRD. A recent comprehensive review that included 12 case series of renal transplants among 254 HIV-infected patients demonstrated 1-year patient survival at 93% [47]. While 1-year renal allograft was slightly lower at 87% (compared to national averages of 91%), these data suggest that among stable HIV-infected individuals on ART, renal transplantation is a viable option [47].

COURSE AND OUTCOME

In the absence of treatment with ART, reports from the early 1990s suggested that patients progress to ESRD within 1–4 months of diagnosis [6, 7, 23]. Subsequent data in the setting of zidovudine monotherapy and later with ART suggest a much slower progression [23–25]. Clinical variables associated with increased risk of progressive renal failure include decreased CD4 count [17, 24], elevated serum creatinine [24], increased proteinuria [17], higher viral load [17, 24], and the presence of hepatitis C co-infection [24].

Patients with a pathologic diagnosis of HIVAN had worse renal survival than patients with lesions other than HIVAN. In a cohort of 89 HIV-infected patients with renal disease biopsied between 1995 and 2000, 17 of 47 patients with lesions other than HIVAN required the institution of RRT at an average time of 731 days ($\pm$642 days) from renal biopsy as compared to 25/42 patients with HIVAN who required initiation of RRT at an average time of 254 days ($\pm$31 days) from renal biopsy ($p = 0.0003$ comparing time with initiation of RRT) [24]. The prolonged renal survival of patients with HIVAN as compared to earlier reports is arguably related to a number of factors, including the use of ART.

In a retrospective review of 99 HIV-infected patients in Baragwanath, South Africa, who underwent renal biopsy, the investigators could not distinguish a difference in renal or overall survival between patients with HIVAN and those with other pathologic findings. In the 27 South African patients with biopsy-proven HIVAN at 17 weeks of follow-up, 13/27 (48%) died, 9/27 (33%) were lost to follow-up, and the remaining 5/27 (19%) were free of dialysis. In 72 HIV-infected patients with other pathologic diagnosis at an average of 14–28 weeks of follow-up, 31/72 (43%) died, 14/72 (19%) were lost to follow-up, and the remaining 27/72 (38%) were free of dialysis [38]. However, very few of the patients were treated with ART. Further research on international differences is required to reconcile these conflicting results.

In the USA, ESRD patients with HIVAN have decreased overall survival compared with other patients with ESRD. In an analysis of 3,374 patients with incident ESRD in 1996, those with a diagnosis of HIVAN ($n =36$) had a 4.74-fold increased risk of mortality after adjusting for clinical variables other than HIV. The 1-year survival in this cohort of patients with HIVAN was 53%. However, more recent data from 1999–2000 report a 1-year survival of up to 74% in dialysis patients with HIVAN, which presumably reflects the benefit of ART in this patient population [48]. Unfortunately, dialysis is not always available for HIV-infected patients with renal failure; thus, in the absence of other life-threatening illnesses, life expectancy can be dramatically shortened.

CONCLUSION

Kidney disease in HIV-infected patients is common, and HIVAN is the leading cause of CKD, particularly in patients of African descent. Patients with HIVAN are often diagnosed late in the course of their HIV illness and present with proteinuria and renal insufficiency. Without treatment, renal survival is only a few months. However, small clinical trials and epidemiologic data strongly suggest a benefit of ART therapy in the treatment of HIVAN [23–25]. In addition, similar studies have noted that ACE-I therapy is associated with improved renal survival [6, 7, 38, 43]. Based on the best available data, if ACE-I and ART are available, they should be utilized to try to prolong renal survival. As ART becomes more widely available in resource-limited settings, patients can be expected to live longer, and an increasing number of HIV-infected patients will have advanced kidney failure. Decisions regarding RRT, including transplantation, will become significant issues, especially in resource-limited settings.

REFERENCES

[1] Gardenswartz MH, Lerner CW, Seligson GR, et al. Renal disease in patients with AIDS: a clinicopathologic study. Clin Nephrol 1984;21:197–204.

[2] Rao TK, Filippone EJ, Nicastri AD, et al. Associated focal and segmental glomerulosclerosis in the acquired immunodeficiency syndrome. N Engl J Med 1984;310:669–73.

[3] US Renal Data Systems. USRDS 2009 Annual Data Report: Atlas of End-Stage Renal Disease in the United States. Bethesda, MD: National Institutes of Health, National Institute of Diabetes and Digestive and Kidney Diseases; 2009.

[4] Evans K, Reddan DN, Szczech LA. Nondialytic management of hyperkalemia and pulmonary edema among end-stage renal disease patients: an evaluation of the evidence. Semin Dial 2004;17:22–9.

[5] WHO. Global summary of the HIV/AIDS epidemic. Global Report. Geneva: World Health Report; 2009.

[6] Burns GC, Paul SK, Toth IR, Sivak SL. Effect of angiotensin-converting enzyme inhibition in HIV-associated nephropathy. J Am Soc Nephrol 1997;8:1140–6.

[7] Kimmel PL, Mishkin GJ, Umana WO. Captopril and renal survival in patients with human immunodeficiency virus nephropathy. Am J Kidney Dis 1996;28:202–8.

[8] Collaboration TATC. Causes of death in HIV-1 infected patients treated with antiretroviral therapy, 1996–2006: collaborative analysis of 13 HIV cohort studies. Clin Infect Dis 2010;50:1387–96.

[9] Shahinian V, Rajaraman S, Borucki M, et al. Prevalence of HIV-associated nephropathy in autopsies of HIV-infected patients. Am J Kidney Dis 2000;35:884–8.

[10] Agaba EI, Agaba PA, Sirisena ND, et al. Renal disease in the acquired immunodeficiency syndrome in north central Nigeria. Niger J Med 1993;12:120–5.

[11] Casanova S, Mazzucco G, Barbiano di Belgiojoso G, et al. Pattern of glomerular involvement in human immunodeficiency virus-infected patients: an Italian study. Am J Kidney Dis 1995;26:446–53.

[12] D'Agati V, Suh JI, Carbone L, et al. Pathology of HIV-associated nephropathy: a detailed morphologic and comparative study. Kidney Int 1989;35:1358–70.

[13] Hailemariam S, Walder M, Burger HR, et al. Renal pathology and premortem clinical presentation of Caucasian patients with AIDS: an autopsy study from the era prior to antiretroviral therapy. Swiss Med Wkly 2001;131:412–17.

[14] Monahan M, Tanji N, Klotman PE. HIV-associated nephropathy: an urban epidemic. Semin Nephrol 2001;21:394–402.

[15] Monga G, Mazzucco G, Boldorini R, et al. Renal changes in patients with acquired immunodeficiency syndrome: a post-mortem study on an unselected population in northwestern Italy. Mod Pathol 1997;10:159–67.

[16] Pakasa M, Mangani N, Dikassa L. Focal and segmental glomerulosclerosis in nephrotic

syndrome: a new profile of adult nephrotic syndrome in Zaire. Mod Pathol 1993;6:125–8.

[17] Laradi A, Mallet A, Beaufils H, et al. HIV-associated nephropathy: outcome and prognosis factors. Groupe d' Etudes Nephrologiques d'Ile de France. J Am Soc Nephrol 1998;9:2327–35.

[18] Williams DI, Williams DJ, Williams IG, et al. Presentation, pathology, and outcome of HIV associated renal disease in a specialist centre for HIV/AIDS. Sex Transm Infect 1998;74:179–84.

[19] Department of Health. Nephrology Report 1 and 2: MTS meeting. South Africa: Department of Health; 2003.

[20] Mabayoje MO, Bamgboye EL, Odutola TA, Mabadeje AF. Chronic renal failure at the Lagos University Teaching Hospital: a 10-year review. Transplant Proc 1992;24:1851; discussion 1852.

[21] Barsoum RS. End-stage renal disease in North Africa. Kidney Int Suppl 2003;83:S111–14.

[22] Naicker S. End-stage renal disease in sub-Saharan and South Africa. Kidney Int Suppl 2003; S119–22.

[23] Ifudu O, Rao TK, Tan CC, et al. Zidovudine is beneficial in human immunodeficiency virus associated nephropathy. Am J Nephrol 1995;15:217–21.

[24] Szczech LA, Gupta SK, Habash R, et al. The clinical epidemiology and course of the spectrum of renal diseases associated with HIV infection. Kidney Int 2004;66:1145–52.

[25] Szczech LA, Edwards LJ, Sanders LL, et al. Protease inhibitors are associated with a slowed progression of HIV-related renal diseases. Clin Nephrol 2002;57:336–41.

[26] Levin ML, Palella F, Shah S, et al. HIV–associated nephropathy occurring before HIV antibody seroconversion. Am J Kidney Dis 2001;37:E39.

[27] Bruggeman LA, Dikman S, Meng C, et al. Nephropathy in human immunodeficiency virus-1 transgenic mice is due to renal transgene expression. J Clin Invest 1997;100:84–92.

[28] Bruggeman LA, Ross MD, Tanji N, et al. Renal epithelium is a previously unrecognized site of HIV-1 infection. J Am Soc Nephrol 2000;11:2079–87.

[29] Marras D, Bruggeman LA, Gao F, et al. Replication and compartmentalization of HIV-1 in kidney epithelium of patients with HIV-associated nephropathy. Nat Med 2002;8:522–6.

[30] Winston JA, Bruggeman LA, Ross MD, et al. Nephropathy and establishment of a renal reservoir of HIV type 1 during primary infection. N Engl J Med 2001;344:1979–84.

[31] Conaldi PG, Biancone L, Bottelli A, et al. HIV-1 kills renal tubular epithelial cells in vitro by triggering an apoptotic pathway involving caspase activation and Fas upregulation. J Clin Invest 1998;102:2041–9.

[32] Kimmel PL, Ferreira-Centeno A, Farkas-Szallasi T, et al. Viral DNA in microdissected renal biopsy tissue from HIV infected patients with nephrotic syndrome. Kidney Int 1993;43:1347–52.

[33] Markowitz GS, Appel GB, Fine PL, et al. Collapsing focal segmental glomerulosclerosis following treatment with high-dose pamidronate. J Am Soc Nephrol 2001;12:1164–72.

[34] Gharavi AG, Ahmad T, Wong RD, et al. Mapping a locus for susceptibility to HIV-1-associated nephropathy to mouse chromosome 3. Proc Natl Acad Sci U S A 2004;101:2488–93.

[35] Papeta N, Chan KT, Prakash S, et al. Susceptibility loci for murine HIV-associated nephropathy encode trans-regulators of podocyte gene expression. J Clin Invest 2009;119:1178–88.

[36] Stylianou E, Aukrust P, Bendtzen K, et al. Interferons and interferon (IFN)-inducible protein 10 during highly active anti-retroviral therapy (HAART)—possible immunosuppressive role of IFN-alpha in HIV infection. Clin Exp Immunol 2000;119:479–85.

[37] ERA-EDTA Registry. 2002 Annual Report. Amsterdam, The Netherlands: Academic Medical Center; May 2004.

[38] Gerntholtz TE, Goetsch SJ, Katz I. HIV-related nephropathy: a South African perspective. Kidney Int 2006;69:1885–91.

[39] Estrella M, Fine DM, Gallant JE, et al. HIV type 1 RNA level as a clinical indicator of renal pathology in HIV-infected patients. Clin Infect Dis 2006;43:377–80.

[40] Rao TK. Clinical features of human immunodeficiency virus associated nephropathy. Kidney Int Suppl 1991;35:S13–18.

[41] Atta MG, Gallant JE, Rahman MH, et al. Antiretroviral therapy in the treatment of HIV-associated nephropathy. Nephrol Dial Transplant 2006;21:2809–13.

[42] Reid A, Stohr W, Walker AS, et al. Severe renal dysfunction and risk factors associated with renal impairment in HIV-infected adults in Africa initiating antiretroviral therapy. Clin Infect Dis 2008;46:1271–81.

[43] Wei A, Burns GC, Williams BA, et al. Long-term renal survival in HIV-associated nephropathy with angiotensin-converting enzyme inhibition. Kidney Int 2003;64:1462–71.

[44] Eustace JA, Nuermberger E, Choi M, et al. Cohort study of the treatment of severe HIV-associated nephropathy with corticosteroids. Kidney Int 2000;58:1253–60.

[45] Smith MC, Austen JL, Carey JT, et al. Prednisone improves renal function and proteinuria in human immunodeficiency virus-associated nephropathy. Am J Med 1996;101:41–8.

[46] Katz IJ, Gerntholtz T, Naicker S. Africa and nephrology: the forgotten continent. Nephron Clin Pract 2011;117:c320–7.

[47] Landin L, Rodriguez-Perez JC, Garcia-Bello MA, et al. Kidney transplants in HIV-positive recipients under HAART. A comprehensive review and meta-analysis of 12 series. Nephrol Dial Transplant 2010;25:3106–15.

[48] Ahuja TS, Grady J, Khan S. Changing trends in the survival of dialysis patients with human immunodeficiency virus in the United States. J Am Soc Nephrol 2002;13:1889–93.

Chapter | 24 |

Pneumocystis pneumonia

Robert J. Blount, J. Lucian Davis, Laurence Huang

INTRODUCTION

Prior to the HIV/AIDS epidemic, *Pneumocystis* pneumonia (PCP) was an unusual cause of pneumonia, occurring almost exclusively in immunocompromised persons. The causative organism, previously known as *Pneumocystis carinii*, was long thought to be a protist on the presumption that cystic and trophic forms represented distinctive phases of a protozoan life cycle. However, mounting evidence, including the identification of genetic sequence homologies with fungi, led to the recategorization of this pathogen as a fungus, and its renaming as *Pneumocystis jiroveci*. In 1981, the description of PCP in previously healthy men who either had sex with men (MSM) and/or who were injection drug users (IDUs) heralded the onset of the HIV/AIDS epidemic that currently affects greater than 33 million people worldwide. Since these initial reports, tremendous advances have occurred in our understanding of HIV infection and PCP. This chapter focuses on the clinical aspects of PCP, our current understanding, and emerging concepts of clinical importance to the global community.

EPIDEMIOLOGY

Although its incidence has declined dramatically, PCP remains a leading AIDS-defining opportunistic infection in the USA and in the countries that comprise the World Health Organization (WHO) Western European Region [1]. PCP is also a frequent opportunistic infection in HIV-infected patient cohorts, and it is an important cause of HIV-associated mortality [2]. Of concern, PCP is described in Africa, Asia, and Latin America, regions of the world where >90% of the estimated people living

with HIV/AIDS reside and where access to combination antiretroviral therapy and even PCP prophylaxis with trimethoprim-sulfamethoxazole (TMP/SMX) is more limited (Table 24.1). At present, most of the data on PCP in these regions is limited to single institution studies [3]. These studies include different study designs, study populations, diagnostic procedures, and specific criteria for defining PCP (clinical versus microscopic confirmation) that limit firm conclusions. Nevertheless, PCP appears to be a significant opportunistic infection in HIV-infected people throughout the world. Importantly, a substantial proportion of these HIV-infected patients with PCP have been found to have concurrent tuberculosis, a finding that complicates the diagnosis and treatment [4]. As the HIV/AIDS epidemic progresses in these regions, it is increasingly important to develop diagnostic and treatment algorithms that can be used in settings where resources, diagnostic tests, and medications are limited.

RISK FACTORS FOR *PNEUMOCYSTIS* PNEUMONIA

A CD4 count < 200 cells/mm^3, a history of oropharyngeal candidiasis, and prior PCP are all well-established risk factors for PCP [5]. PCP was the first disease to illustrate the role of the CD4-lymphocyte count as a tool for assessing the risk for the development of an HIV-associated opportunistic infection [6]. Several studies demonstrate that the risk of PCP is increased in persons with a CD4 count < 200 cells/mm^3 and that the majority of PCP cases occur in patients whose CD4 count is < 200 cells/mm^3 [6, 7]. Thus, a CD4 count that is significantly > 200 cells/mm^3 argues against the presence of PCP. Unfortunately, CD4-lymphocyte determination is unavailable in some

Table 24.1 Clinical and autopsy studies of undifferentiated pneumonia in HIV-infected individuals in Africa, Asia, and Latin America

REFERENCE	SUBJECTS	SPECIMEN(S)	STAIN	FREQUENCY OF PCP	FREQUENCY OF OTHER LUNG DISEASES
Autopsy studies of pneumonia in HIV-infected children in Africa					
Ansari NA et al., Pediatr Infect Dis J 2003	Cross-sectional autopsy study of 35 children who died in hospital in Francistown, Botswana, 1997–1998	Lung	MS	31%	CMV 23% TB 11% RSV 11%
Rennert WP et al., Clin Infect Dis 2002	Cross-sectional study of 93 children (CDC AIDS category B & C) dying of lung disease in Soweto, South Africa, 1998–1999	Core Bx	MS IF Ab	11%	CMV 32% BPNA 14% TB 4.3%
Chintu C et al., Lancet 2002	Cross-sectional autopsy study of 180 children dying in hospital in Lusaka, Zambia, 1997–2000	Lung	MS	29%	BPNA 41% CMV 22% TB 18%
Nathoo KJ et al., Trans R Soc Trop Med Hyg 2001	Cross-sectional autopsy study of 24 children dying of pneumonia in Harare, Zimbabwe, 1995	FNA Core Bx	Giemsa MS PCR	67%	BPNA 33% CMV 10%
Ikeogu MO et al., Arch Dis Child 1997	Cross-sectional autopsy study of 122 children dying on arrival to hospital in Bulawayo, Zimbabwe, 1992–1993	Lung	MS	16%	BPNA 86% TB 4%
Lucas SB et al., BMJ 1996	Cross-sectional autopsy study of 78 children dying in hospital in Abdijan, Ivory Coast, 1991–1992	Lung	N/A	14%	BPNA 42% CMV 31% TB 1.3%
Jeena PM et al., Ann Trop Paediatr 1996	Prospective case-control autopsy study of 31 infants dying in intensive care units in Durban, South Africa, 1993–1994	ETA Core Bx	MS IF Ab PCR	52%	CMV 29% BPNA 26% TB 3.2%
Clinical studies of pneumonia in HIV-infected children in Africa					
Ferrand RA et al., PLoS Med 2010	Prospective study of 139 adolescents admitted to a hospital in Harare, Zimbabwe, 2007–2008	IS	MS	0.7%	TB 8.6% BPNA 17%
Morrow BM et al., Pediatr Infect Dis J 2010	Prospective study of 124 children with pneumonia admitted to a children's hospital in Cape Town, South Africa, 2006–2008	IS BAL Lung	IF Ab MS	27%	CMV 36% RSV 8.1% TB 3%
Rabie H et al., J Trop Pediatr 2007	Retrospective chart review of 47 consecutive children admitted to an intensive care unit in Cape Town, South Africa, 2003	NPA ETA	IF Ab	33%	CMV 8.5% TB 2.1%
Bii CC et al., Int J Tuberc Lung Dis 2006	Cross-sectional study of 30 infants and toddlers with severe pneumonia in Nairobi, Kenya, 2002–2003	IS	IF Ab	17%	N/A

Reference	Study description	Specimen	Method	PCP rate	Other pathogens
Kouakoussui A et al., Paed Resp Rev 2004	Prospective study of 98 ART-naïve children in a clinic in Abdijan, Ivory Coast, 2000–2003	N/A	N/A	0.36 per 100 child-months	LRTI 6.07, TB 0.71 per 100
Ruffini DD et al., AIDS 2002	Prospective study of 105 hospitalized infants with severe pneumonia, 18 undergoing autopsy in Soweto, South Africa, 1999	IS NPA Core Bx	MS IF Ab	49%	CMV 44% Viral 8.3% TB 2.9%
Madhi SA et al., Clin Infect Dis 2002	Cross-sectional study of 231 episodes of pneumonia in 185 children in hospital in Soweto, South Africa, 2000–2001	IS NPA	IF Ab	44% of all episodes	Viral 12% BPNA 8.1%
Zar HJ et al., Acta Paediatr 2001	Cross-sectional study of 151 children admitted to an intensive care unit with pneumonia in Soweto, South Africa, 1998	NPA IS Lavage	MS IF Ab	9.9%	BPNA 47% CMV 14% TB 7.3%
Madhi SA et al., Clin Infect Dis 2000	Cross-sectional study of 548 infants in hospital with severe LRTI in Soweto, South Africa, 1997–1998	Clinical	N/A	15%	BPNA 15%
Graham SM et al., Lancet 1999	Cross-sectional study of 93 children in hospital with severe pneumonia by WHO criteria in Blantyre, Malawi, 1996	NPA	IF Ab	17%	BPNA 13%
Kamiya Y et al., Arch Dis Child 1997	Cross-sectional study of 19 infants with clinical AIDS and acute LRTI in Lilongwe, Malawi, 1995	NPA	IF Ab	16%	N/A
Autopsy studies of pneumonia in HIV-infected adults in Africa					
Garcia-Jardon et al., Trop Doct 2010	Retrospective (2000–2005) and prospective (2006–2008) autopsy study of 86 patients dying at a tertiary care hospital in rural South Africa	Lung	Giemsa	8.9%	TB 13% BPNA 22% KS 1.3%
Murray et al., AIDS 2007	Retrospective autopsy study including 89 HIV-infected gold miners in South Africa, 1990–2002	Lung	MS	13%	TB 35% BPNA 8% KS 2%
Martinson NA et al., AIDS 2007	Prospective autopsy study of 47 adults with a premortem diagnosis of tuberculosis in Soweto, South Africa, 2003–2005	Lung	MS	11%	TB 79% BPNA 26% CMV 66%
Ansari NA et al., Int J Tuberc Lung Dis 2002	Cross-sectional autopsy study of 104 adults dying in hospital in Francistown, Botswana, 1997–1998	Lung	MS	11%	TB 40% BPNA 23% KS 11%
Lucas SB et al., AIDS 1993	Cross-sectional autopsy study of 247 adults dying in hospital in Abdijan, Ivory Coast, 1991–1992	Lung	MS	2.8%	TB 38% Nocardia 4%
Abouya YL et al., Am Rev Respir Dis 1992	Cross-sectional autopsy study of 53 adults dying on a pulmonary ward in Abdijan, Ivory Coast, 1989	Lung	MS	9.4%	TB 40% KS 5.7%

Continued

Table 24.1 Clinical and autopsy studies of undifferentiated pneumonia in HIV-infected individuals in Africa, Asia, and Latin America—cont'd

Clinical studies of pneumonia in HIV-infected adults in Africa

REFERENCE	SUBJECTS	SPECIMEN(S)	STAIN	FREQUENCY OF PCP	FREQUENCY OF OTHER LUNG DISEASES
Kyeyune R et al., J Acquir Immun Defic Syndr 2010	Prospective cohort study of 353 adults with cough > 2 weeks admitted to a referral hospital in Kampala, Uganda, 2007–2008	BAL	Giemsa	3%	TB 56% Crypto 1% KS 4%
Aderaye G et al., Scand J Infect Dis 2007	Prospective cohort study of 131 AFB smear-negative adults presenting with respiratory symptoms to a referral hospital in Addis Ababa, Ethiopia, 2004–2005	BAL	IF Ab	30%	TB 24% BPNA 34% KS 3.1%
Zouiten F et al., AIDS 2002	Cross-sectional study of 92 women seen in a specialty clinic in Tunis, Tunisia, 1986–2001	N/A	N/A	12%	BPNA 25% TB 6.5%
Corbett EL et al., Clin Infect Dis 2002	Prospective study of 1792 adult men in Welkom, South Africa, 599 in hospital, 1998–1999	N/A	MS	1.3%	TB 21% BPNA 17%
Karstaedt AS et al., Trans R Soc Trop Med Hyg 2001	Retrospective case series of 120 adults with AIDS in hospital with PCP in Soweto, South Africa, 1996–1998	IS 54% ES 42% BAL 4%	IF Ab	N/A	TB 19% BPNA 12%
Daley CL et al., Am J Respir Crit Care Med 1996	Cross-sectional study of 127 adults in hospital with respiratory symptoms in Dar es Salaam, Tanzania, 1991–1993	BAL 25%	N/A	0.8%	TB 75% BPNA 14%
Sow PS et al., AIDS 1993	Cross-sectional study of 27 adults in hospital in Dakar, Senegal, 1992	IS	Tol Blue	22%	N/A
Cheval P et al., Med Trop (Mars) 1993	Cross-sectional study of 307 patients in hospital in Pointe-Noire, Republic of Congo, 1989–1991	N/A	N/A	4.9%	N/A
Atzori C et al., Trans R Soc Trop Med Hyg 1993	Cross-sectional study of 83 adults in hospital for respiratory symptoms in Malenga Makali, Tanzania, 1991	IS	Tol Blue MS	6%	TB 39%
Karstaedt AS, S Afr Med J 1992	Cross-sectional study of 181 adults in Soweto, South Africa, 1987–1990	N/A	N/A	0.5%	TB 15% BPNA 12%
Serwadda D et al., AIDS 1989	Cross-sectional study of 40 patients with fever, pulmonary infiltrates in Kampala, Uganda, 1987–1988	BAL	Giemsa MS	0%	TB 15%

Clinical studies of pulmonary disease of undetermined etiology in HIV-infected adults in Africa

Reference	Description	Sample	Method	PCP	Other
Worodria W et al., Int J Tuberc Lung Dis 2003	Cross-sectional study of 83 adults with 3-week history of undiagnosed lung disease in hospital in Kampala, Uganda, 1999–2000	BAL	IF Ab	39%	TB 24% BPNA 19%
Aderaye G et al., AIDS 2003	Cross-sectional study of 199 adults in hospital for undiagnosed lung disease, in Addis Ababa, Ethiopia, 1996	ES	IF Ab PCR	30%	N/A
Lockman S et al., Int J Tuberc Lung Dis 2003	Cross-sectional study of 121 adults, most in hospital, with undiagnosed lung disease in Gaborone and Francistown, Botswana, 1997	IS	Tol Blue MS PCR	3.3%	TB 50% BPNA 25%
Chakaya JM et al., East Afr Med J 2003	Cross-sectional study of 51 adults in hospital with undiagnosed lung disease in Nairobi, Kenya, 1999–2000	BAL	Tol Blue IF Ab	37%	BPNA 37%
Hargreaves NJ et al., Trans R Soc Trop Med Hyg 2001	Cross-sectional study of 164 adults with undiagnosed lung disease in Lilongwe, Malawi, 1997–1999	BAL	IF Ab PCR	9.1%	TB 39%
Mahomed AG et al., East Afr Med J 1999	Cross-sectional study of 67 adults with undiagnosed lung disease, IS negative for PCP, in Johannesburg, South Africa, 1985–1992	BAL TBBx	Tol Blue MS	43%	TB 13%
Dieng Y et al., Dakar Med 1999	Cross-sectional study of 29 adults in hospital for undiagnosed lung disease in Dakar, Senegal, 1996–1997	BAL	Tol Blue Giemsa	6.9%	N/A
Malin AS et al., Am J Respir Crit Care Med 1994	Cross-sectional study of 64 adults (median CD4 183) in hospital with undiagnosed lung disease in Harare, Zimbabwe, 1992–1993	BAL	Tol Blue Giemsa MS, PCR	33%	TB 39% KS 9.3% CMV 1.6%
Batungwanayo J et al., Am J Respir Crit Care Med 1994	Prospective cohort study of 111 adults (42% with AIDS by WHO criteria) with undiagnosed lung disease in Kigali, Rwanda, 1990	BAL TBBx	Giemsa MS	5%	TB 23% Crypto 11% KS 8.1%

Autopsy studies of pneumonia in HIV-infected adults and children in Asia

Reference	Description	Sample	Method	PCP	Other
Bychkov AV et al., Int J Collab Res Int Med Pub Health 2009	Cross-sectional autopsy study of 32 adults who died in Smolensk, Russia, 2003–2008	Lung	MS	13%	TB 72% BPNA 24% CMV 6% Asp 3%
Hsiao CH et al., J Microbiol Immunol Infect 1997	Cross-sectional autopsy study of 16 adults who died in hospital in Taipei, Taiwan, 1986–1996	Lung	N/A	50%	CMV 88% TB 44%

Continued

Table 24.1 Clinical and autopsy studies of undifferentiated pneumonia in HIV-infected individuals in Africa, Asia, and Latin America—cont'd

REFERENCE	SUBJECTS	SPECIMEN(S)	STAIN	FREQUENCY OF PCP	FREQUENCY OF OTHER LUNG DISEASES
Bhoopat L et al., Asia Pac J Aller Imm 1994	Cross-sectional autopsy study of 29 children who died with AIDS in Chiang Mai, Thailand, up to 1994	Lung	N/A	66%	CMV 48% TB 3.4%
Clinical studies of pneumonia in HIV-infected adults and children in Asia					
Gautam H et al., J Int Assoc Physicians AIDS Care (Chic) 2009	Cross-sectional study of 46 ART-naïve adults with CD4 < 200 presenting for the first time to a tertiary care center in New Delhi, India, 2006	IS	IF Ab	45%	TB 42% BPNA 13%
Mishra M et al., Indian J Med Microbiol 2006	Cross-sectional study of 1101 hospitalized adults in Nagpur, India, 1999–2005	IS	Giemsa Tol Blue MS	25%	N/A
Knauer A et al., Wien Klin Wochenschr 2005	Cross-sectional study of 59 adolescents and adults in hospital with interstitial lung disease in Nonthaburi, Thailand, 2002–2003	Clinical	N/A	25%	TB 44% BP NA 20% Crypto 8.5%
Udwadia ZF et al., J Assoc Physicians India 2005	Cross-sectional study of 119 adults in hospital with lung disease in Mumbai, India, 2000–2003	N/A BAL	N/A	32%	N/A
Sharma SK et al., BMC Infect Dis 2004	Cross-sectional study of 135 adults in hospital for opportunistic disease in New Delhi, India, 2000–2003	Clinical IS	N/A	7.4%	TB 71% (All sites)
Kay Thwe H et al., SE Asian J Trop Med Pub Health 2003	Cross-sectional study of 60 adults (mean CD4 132, not on PCP prophylaxis) with >2 weeks of dry cough in Waibargi, Myanmar, 2000–2001	IS	Giemsa MS	30%	TB 17%
Usha MM et al., Indian J Pathol Microbiol 2000	Cross-sectional study of 32 adults with AIDS and a respiratory complaint in Chennai, India, up to 1997	IS	Tol Blue Giemsa IF Ab	28%	TB 47%
Mathews MS et al., Indian J Chest Dis Allied Sci 2000	Cross-sectional study of 15 adults with AIDS in Vellore, India, 1992–1997	ETA IS	Tol Blue Giemsa IF Ab	33%	N/A
Lumbiganon P et al., J Med Assoc Thai 2000	Prospective cohort study of 90 children with AIDS (WHO criteria) in Khon Kaen, Thailand, 1989–1998	N/A	N/A	36 cases	TB 8 cases

Reference	Study description	Specimen	Method	%	Other
Tansuphasawadikul S et al., AIDS 1999	Cross-sectional study of 2261 hospitalized adults in Nonthaburi, Thailand, 1993–1996	Clinical	N/A	4.8%	TB 37% Pen 3.2%
Autopsy studies of pneumonia in HIV-infected adults and children in Latin America					
Soeiro AM et al., Clinics (São Paulo) 2008	Retrospective autopsy study of 250 children and adults who died at a tertiary care center in São Paulo Brazil, 1990–2000	Lung	MS	27%	TB 14% BPNA 36% KS 4.4% Histo 1.3% CMV 13%
Eza D et al., Pathol Res Pract 2006	Retrospective autopsy study of 16 adults who died at a public hospital in Lima, Peru, 1999–2004	Lung	MS	13%	TB 13% Histo 19% Crypto 6% KS 6% Asp 6%
Cury PM et al., Pathol Res Pract 2003	Cross-sectional autopsy study of 92 adults who died with AIDS in São Paulo, Brazil, 1993–2000	Lung	MS	17%	TB 27% Histo 5.4% Crypto 4.3%
Drut R et al., Pediatr Pathol Lab Med 1997	Retrospective autopsy case series of 74 children registered in a database after dying of AIDS throughout Latin America, 1992–1994	Lung	N/A	20%	BPNA 15% CMV 5.4% Histo 2.7%
Mohar A et al., AIDS 1992	Cross-sectional autopsy study of 177 adults who died with AIDS in Mexico City, Mexico, 1984–1989	Lung	MS	24%	TB 25% (all sites)
Michalany J et al., Ann Pathol 1987	Cross-sectional autopsy study of 15 adults who died with AIDS in São Paulo, Brazil, 1981–1985	Lung	Giemsa MS	13%	CMV 47% TB 20%
Clinical studies of pneumonia in HIV-infected adults in Latin America					
Chernilo S et al., Rev Med Chile 2005	Cross-sectional study of 236 cases of lung disease in 171 hospitalized adults in Santiago, Chile, 1999–2003. Two or more conditions were present in 14% of subjects	BAL	PCR	38%	BPNA 24% TB 12% KS 3.3%
Villasis-Keever A et al., Arch Med Res 2001	Cross-sectional study of 909 adults in an outpatient clinic in Mexico City, Mexico, 1984–1995	N/A	N/A	18%	TB 18% Histo 1.4% (all sites)
Lambertucci JR et al., Rev Inst Med Trop São Paulo 1999	Cross-sectional study of 55 hospitalized adults with AIDS with fever of undetermined etiology in Minas Gerais, Brazil 1989–1997	Clinical	N/A	15%	TB 33% (all sites) Histo 3.6% (all sites)
Fonseca L et al., Int J Epidemiol 1999	Prospective study of 145 asymptomatic adults in São Paulo, Brazil, followed for 4 years between 1985 and 1997	N/A	N/A	17%	TB 19%

Continued

Table 24.1 Clinical and autopsy studies of undifferentiated pneumonia in HIV-infected individuals in Africa, Asia, and Latin America—cont'd

REFERENCE	SUBJECTS	SPECIMEN(S)	STAIN	FREQUENCY OF PCP	FREQUENCY OF OTHER LUNG DISEASES
Clinical studies of pneumonia in HIV-infected adults in Latin America—cont'd					
Santoro-Lopes G et al., J AIDS Hum Retrovirol 1998	Cross-sectional study of 124 hospitalized adults with newly developed AIDS in Rio de Janeiro, Brazil, 1991–1995	N/A	N/A	14%	N/A
Rodriguez French A et al., Rev Med Panama 1996	Cross-sectional study of 55 hospitalized adults with AIDS in Panama City, Panama, 1995	ES or IS TTA BAL	Giemsa MS	45%	N/A
Santos B et al., Int J STD AIDS 1994	Cross-sectional study of 224 adults with AIDS in a referral center in Porto Alegre, Brazil, 1986–1991	N/A	N/A	17%	TB 19% (all sites)
Weinberg A et al., Rev Inst Med Trop São Paulo 1993	Cross-sectional study of 35 adults with respiratory complaints in São Paulo, Brazil, 1988–1989	ES BAL TBBx	Tol Blue MS	55%	TB 41% CMV 7.4%
Moreira ED Jr et al., Am J Trop Med Hyg 1993	Cross-sectional study of 111 adults with AIDS in an outpatient clinic in Salvador, Brazil, 1989–1991	Clinical TBBx	MS	22%	TB 24% BPNA 22%

Specimen(s): BAL, bronchoalveolar lavage; BW, bronchial wash; Core Bx, core biopsy; ES, expectorated sputum; ETA, endotracheal aspirate; IS, induced sputum; Lavage, blind BW; Lung, fixed lung tissue; NPA, nasopharyngeal aspirate; TBBx, transbronchial biopsy; TTA, transtracheal aspirate.
Stains: MS, methenamine silver; Tol Blue, toluidine blue O; IF Ab, immunofluorescence antibody; PCR, polymerase chain reaction.
Other lung diseases: BPNA, bacterial pneumonia; CMV, cytomegalovirus; Crypto, cryptococcosis; Histo, histoplasmosis; KS, Kaposi's sarcoma; LRTI, lower respiratory tract infection; PCP, *Pneumocystis jiroveci* pneumonia; Pen, penicilliosis; RSV, respiratory syncytial virus; TB, tuberculosis; Viral, other viral infection; Asp, bronchopulmonary aspergillosis.
All categories: AFB, acid-fast bacilli; ART, antiretroviral therapy; N/A, not available.

parts of the world, and clinicians are left to infer the degree of immunocompromise from indirect measures such as the absolute lymphocyte count.

CLINICAL FEATURES

The clinical presentation of PCP in HIV-infected persons differs from the presentation in other immunocompromised persons. In general, HIV-infected patients present with a subacute onset and longer symptom duration than other immunocompromised patients [8]. Compared with HIV-negative patients, HIV-infected patients with PCP present with a higher arterial oxygen tension and a lower alveolar-arterial oxygen gradient. In addition, bronchoscopy with bronchoalveolar lavage (BAL) examination reveals significantly greater numbers of *Pneumocystis* organisms and fewer neutrophils in HIV-infected patients [9].

SYMPTOMS AND SIGNS

Classically, patients with PCP present with fever, cough, and dyspnea of 2–4 weeks' duration [10]. The cough is usually dry and non-productive unless a concurrent bacterial infection is present. Fatigue is a frequent complaint, whereas chest pain (unless due to an associated pneumothorax), chills, and night sweats are less common. Symptoms are often subtle at the onset but are gradually progressive and may be present for weeks and occasionally months before diagnosis.

Physical examination is non-specific. Vital signs often reveal an oral temperature $>38.5°C$, tachypnea, and a decreased oxygen saturation. Typically, the pulmonary examination is unremarkable, even in the presence of significant disease and hypoxemia. One maneuver that has been reported to be sensitive for PCP is the elicitation of a cough after deep inspiration. Bilateral fine inspiratory crackles are the most frequent abnormal finding on lung auscultation, although the chest exam is often normal.

LABORATORY TESTS

No current laboratory test is specific for PCP. The serum lactate dehydrogenase (LDH) is usually elevated in patients with PCP [11]. Published studies report the sensitivity of an elevated serum LDH for PCP to range from 82 to 100%. Unfortunately, the serum LDH is a non-specific test, and elevations are seen in many pulmonary and non-pulmonary conditions. The arterial blood gas (ABG) is an essential laboratory test in patients with PCP. A patient with PCP will usually have a decreased arterial oxygen tension, an increased alveolar-arterial oxygen gradient, and a respiratory alkalosis. The ABG should be used to decide whether to admit a patient to the hospital to receive supplemental oxygen, whether to administer adjunctive corticosteroids (PaO_2 <70 mmHg or an alveolar-arterial oxygen gradient >35 mmHg), and to assess response to PCP therapy.

CHEST RADIOGRAPH

The chest radiograph is the cornerstone of the diagnostic evaluation of patients with suspected PCP. Classically, patients with PCP present with bilateral, diffuse, symmetric reticular (interstitial) or granular opacities on their chest radiograph (Fig. 24.1) [12]. PCP often begins with central or perihilar opacities and a middle-lower lung zone predominance. As with the classic radiographic presentation, these opacities are bilateral and symmetric and can progress to diffuse involvement if the disease is left undiagnosed and untreated. However, patients with PCP can occasionally present with unilateral, focal, or asymmetric opacities on their chest radiograph, and the specific pattern seen is often more important than the exact distribution. Thus, PCP must be considered in any HIV-infected patient who is at risk for PCP, has a compatible clinical presentation, and presents with reticular or granular opacities on chest radiograph, regardless of whether the findings are unilateral or bilateral, focal or diffuse, asymmetric or symmetric. Clearly though, the presence of bilateral, diffuse, and symmetric reticular (interstitial) or granular opacities increases the probability of PCP significantly. In one study, patients who had

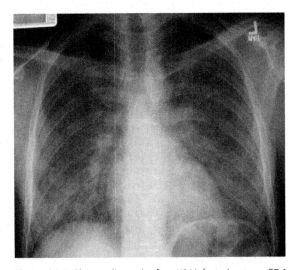

Figure 24.1 Chest radiograph of an HIV-infected person, CD4 count <200 cells/mm^3 demonstrating the characteristic bilateral, diffuse, symmetric reticular-granular opacities of PCP. Bronchoscopy with bronchoalveolar lavage (BAL) fluid examination revealed *Pneumocystis* organisms.

interstitial infiltrates noted on their radiograph had a 4.4 greater odds of having PCP than those without this pattern, and patients who had interstitial infiltrates that involved five or six of the six defined lung zones (upper, middle, and lower lung zones on the right and left lungs) had a 5.3 greater odds of having PCP [13].

Thin-walled cysts or pneumatoceles were reported in 7% of PCP cases in one large radiology series [12]. Pneumatoceles may be present at the time of diagnosis, may develop while on therapy, and may persist despite successful therapy. The pneumatoceles may be single or multiple in number and small or large in size. Usually, pneumatoceles are multiple in number and located in the upper lobes. Importantly, the presence of pneumatoceles predisposes patients to the development of pneumothorax, a difficult management problem for clinicians caring for PCP patients. However, pneumothoraces may also occur in the absence of radiographically demonstrable pneumatoceles.

Less commonly, patients with PCP may present with a lobar or segmental consolidation, and with cavitary and non-cavitary nodules of varying size. Apical or upper lung zone disease that resembles tuberculosis has been associated with aerosolized pentamidine prophylaxis, although this presentation can also occur in patients receiving other forms of PCP prophylaxis or no preventive therapy. While reported, intrathoracic adenopathy and pleural effusions are rarely due to PCP. The presence of these radiographic findings should prompt a search for an alternate or coexisting process such as bacterial pneumonia, tuberculosis, fungal pneumonia, or pulmonary Kaposi's sarcoma.

Patients with PCP may present with a normal chest radiograph, which has been reported in 0–39% of cases in published studies. While patients with PCP and a normal chest radiograph have a better prognosis than patients with bilateral diffuse opacities, they often represent a diagnostic challenge and require a timely evaluation before their disease progresses.

There are a few studies on the course of respiratory symptoms and chest radiographic abnormalities in patients successfully treated for PCP [12, 14]. Patients with PCP often experience a transient clinical and radiographic worsening in the first 3–5 days of PCP therapy. In one study of 104 patients with PCP, 46% experienced a deterioration in radiographic findings at 1 week [12]. In this same study, approximately one-third of the patients showed no change in their radiograph over the first 3 weeks. A general rule is that the more severe the PCP, the more prolonged the time to clinical and chest radiographic resolution.

OTHER TESTS

Tests including high-resolution computed tomography (HRCT) of the chest, typically demonstrating ground-glass opacities (Fig. 24.2), pulmonary function tests demonstrating

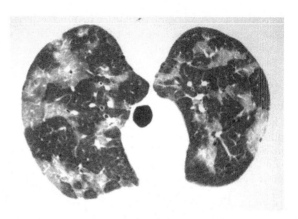

Figure 24.2 Chest high-resolution computed tomographic (HRCT) scan of an HIV-infected person, CD4 count <200 cells/mm^3, whose chest radiograph was normal. Because of a clinical suspicion for PCP, the patient underwent HRCT, which demonstrated the characteristic patchy ground-glass opacities of PCP. Induced sputum examination revealed *Pneumocystis* organisms.

decreased diffusing capacity for carbon monoxide (DLCO), and gallium scanning showing increased pulmonary uptake can all be used in the diagnostic evaluation of patients with suspected PCP [11]. Typically, these studies are performed in patients whose clinical presentation is strongly suggestive of PCP but whose chest radiograph is normal or minimally abnormal. However, these tests are relatively expensive and typically unavailable in many parts of the world. One simple test for PCP is non-invasive exercise oximetry, since patients with PCP will often have a decline in their oxygen saturation with exertion.

DIAGNOSIS

There is no universally agreed upon approach to the diagnostic evaluation of suspected PCP. Some institutions treat patients with suspected PCP empirically, while others pursue a definitive microscopic diagnosis (Fig. 24.3) [15]. In patients with suspected PCP, it is generally advantageous to make a definitive diagnosis. A false presumptive diagnosis of PCP may lead to failure or delay in making the correct diagnosis. Additionally, the drugs used to treat PCP have significant side effects, incurring unnecessary risk in the PCP-negative patient (see Treatment below). As *Pneumocystis* cannot be routinely cultured, the diagnosis of PCP traditionally relies on microscopic visualization of the characteristic cysts and/or trophic forms on stained respiratory specimens. Typically, these respiratory specimens are obtained from sputum induction or bronchoscopy. However, institutions report different degrees of success with sputum induction and bronchoscopy with BAL with and

Figure 24.3 Diagnostic algorithm for the evaluation of HIV-infected persons with suspected PCP in high-resource settings. CDC, Centers for Disease Control; COPD, chronic obstructive pulmonary disease; DLCO, single-breath diffusing capacity for carbon monoxide; HRCT, high-resolution computed tomography; GGO, ground-glass opacities; BAL, bronchoalveolar lavage; MTB, *Mycobacterium tuberculosis*; OI, opportunistic infection.

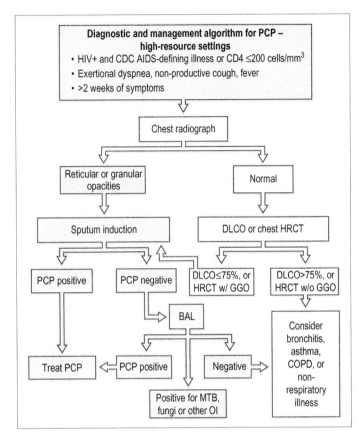

Diagnostic and management algorithm for PCP – high-resource settings
- HIV+ and CDC AIDS-defining illness or CD4 ≤200 cells/mm³
- Exertional dyspnea, non-productive cough, fever
- >2 weeks of symptoms

Chest radiograph

Reticular or granular opacities | Normal

Sputum induction | DLCO or chest HRCT

PCP positive | PCP negative | DLCO≤75%, or HRCT w/ GGO | DLCO>75%, or HRCT w/o GGO

BAL

Consider bronchitis, asthma, COPD, or non-respiratory illness

Treat PCP ⟵ PCP positive | Negative

Positive for MTB, fungi or other OI

without transbronchial biopsiy (TBBx). Advances in polymerase chain reaction (PCR) technology have enabled the use of rapid, non-invasive procedures such as oropharyngeal washing as a method for specimen acquisition. In one study, a non-invasive, 60-s gargle (oropharyngeal wash) specimen paired with a PCR-based quantitative assay had a sensitivity of 88% and specificity of 85% [16]. However, in the absence of prospective studies comparing various management and diagnostic strategies, the specific approach to a patient with suspected PCP is often based on the prevalence of PCP, clinician and institutional preferences and experiences, and availability of diagnostic procedures and microbiologic techniques and assays. In areas of the world where tuberculosis is prevalent and where resources are limited, the examination of sputum for acid-fast bacilli may be a prudent diagnostic and public health practice (Fig. 24.4). Studies designed to examine practical, cost-effective diagnostic approaches to the patient with suspected PCP in a resource-limited setting are needed.

Blood-based plasma and serum assays have also been studied for the diagnosis of PCP and may be a more practical option in resource-limited settings. Plasma S-adenosylmethionine (SAM or AdoMet) has been studied as a potential biomarker for PCP. SAM is an important biochemical intermediate involved in methylation reactions and also polyamine synthesis [17, 18]. *Pneumocystis* was thought to lack a SAM synthetase to synthesize its own SAM; therefore, it needed to scavenge this intermediate from its host (a subsequent study has demonstrated that *Pneumocystis* has a functional SAM synthetase) [19]. Thus, patients with PCP might be expected to have low SAM levels. A series of studies from New York found that plasma AdoMet levels could be used to distinguish between HIV-infected patients with PCP and those with non-PCP pneumonia and healthy controls [17, 18]. Patients with PCP had significantly lower plasma AdoMet levels compared to patients with non-PCP pneumonia and there was no overlap in AdoMet levels between these two groups of patients in one study [18]. A subsequent study that measured serum SAM found overlapping levels between HIV-infected patients with PCP and those with non-PCP pneumonia [20]. Whether the differing results from these studies relates to differences between plasma and serum SAM levels, as has been hypothesized, or to other factors is unclear, and further studies are needed. Serum (1-3)-beta-D-glucan, a cell wall component of all fungi including

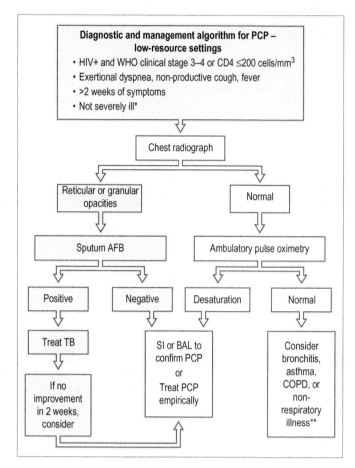

**Diagnostic and management algorithm for PCP –
low-resource settings**
- HIV+ and WHO clinical stage 3–4 or CD4 ≤200 cells/mm^3
- Exertional dyspnea, non-productive cough, fever
- >2 weeks of symptoms
- Not severely ill*

Chest radiograph

Reticular or granular opacities → Sputum AFB → Positive → Treat TB → If no improvement in 2 weeks, consider

Negative → SI or BAL to confirm PCP or Treat PCP empirically

Normal → Ambulatory pulse oximetry → Desaturation / Normal → Consider bronchitis, asthma, COPD, or non-respiratory illness**

Figure 24.4 Algorithm for evaluation of HIV-infected persons with suspected PCP in resource-limited settings. AFB, acid-fast bacilli; COPD, chronic obstructive pulmonary disease; SI, sputum induction; BAL, bronchoalveolar lavage; TB, tuberculosis; NAAT, nucleic acid amplification test; WHO, World Health Organization. *For patients with severe illness (temperature >39 C, HR>120, RR>30, inability to walk) consider empiric TB treatment. **If patient has negative workup but symptoms persist, consider repeating algorithm.

Pneumocystis, has also been investigated as a potential bio-marker for PCP, as patients with PCP might be expected to have high levels [21, 22]. Patients with PCP with and without underlying HIV infection had significantly higher serum (1-3)-beta-D-glucan levels compared to patients without PCP in one early study [21]. Using a 100 pg/mL cutoff, another study reported a diagnostic sensitivity of 100% and a specificity of 96.4% [22]. Of note, (1-3)-beta-D-glucan is elevated in a number of fungal pneumonias, and this test cannot distinguish among fungal etiologies (e.g., PCP and *Aspergillus* species). Thus, although results from these non-invasive diagnostic or bio-marker tests are promising, additional validation is needed, and bronchoscopy with BAL remains the gold standard diagnostic test for PCP at the present time.

TREATMENT

The standard treatment duration for HIV-infected patients with PCP is 21 days [5]. Trimethoprim-sulfamethoxazole is recommended as first-line treatment for PCP (Table 24.2).

Trimethoprim and sulfamethoxazole each inhibit an important enzyme in folate metabolism; trimethoprim inhibits dihydrofolate reductase, while sulfamethoxazole inhibits dihydropteroate synthase. Since many microorganisms cannot transport folate into cells as mammalian cells can, most prokaryotes and lower eukaryotes must synthesize folates *de novo*. Thus, the fixed-dose combination of trimethoprim-sulfamethoxazole offers excellent activity against *Pneumocystis* and many other important HIV-associated bacterial and protozoan pathogens. The availability of trimethoprim-sulfamethoxazole in both intravenous and oral formulations, its favorable toxicity profile (compared to intravenous pentamidine), and its low cost are all additional advantages. However, the use of trimethoprim-sulfamethoxazole for PCP prophylaxis has led to concerns about the possible development of drug-resistant *Pneumocystis* as mutations in the dihydropteroate synthase gene are reported in association with prophylaxis use and, in some studies, are associated with increased mortality and increased PCP treatment failure using trimethoprim-sulfamethoxazole [23–26]. Since trimethoprim-sulfamethoxazole is often the only PCP treatment available in many regions of the world, the development of high-level drug resistance may have

Table 24.2 Treatment options for *Pneumocystis* pneumonia[a,b]

TREATMENT REGIMEN	DOSE(S), ROUTE, FREQUENCY	SIDE EFFECTS
Trimethoprim (TMP)-sulfamethoxazole (SMX)[c]	15–20 mg/kg/day TMP and 75–100 mg/kg/day SMX, IV divided every 6–8 h or 2 DS tabs PO thrice daily for adults and adolescents with mild to moderate disease	Nausea, vomiting, rash, fever, cytopenia, elevated liver transaminases, hyperkalemia
Pentamidine	3–4 mg/kg IV daily (infused slowly over >60 min)	Nephrotoxicity, electrolyte disturbances, pancreatitis, hypo- and hyperglycemia, cardiac arrhythmias
Clindamycin plus primaquine	clindamycin 600–900 mg IV every 6–8 h or 300–450 mg PO every 6–8 h plus primaquine 15–30 mg base PO once daily	Nausea, vomiting, diarrhea, rash, hemolytic anemia (screen for G6PD deficiency prior to primaquine use), methemoglobinemia
Trimethoprim plus dapsone	trimethoprim 5 mg/kg PO every 8 h plus dapsone 100 mg PO daily	Nausea, vomiting, rash, hemolytic anemia (when possible, screen for G6PD deficiency prior to dapsone use in African and Mediterranean populations), methemoglobinemia
Atovaquone	750 mg PO twice daily (suspension, take with food)	Nausea, vomiting, diarrhea, rash

DS, double-strength (160 mg TMP/800 mg SMX); IV, intravenous; PO, oral; G6PD, glucose-6-phosphate dehydrogenase.
[a]Standard treatment duration is 21 days for all regimens.
[b]Patients with moderate to severe PCP (oxygen saturation <93%, PaO_2 <70 mmHg OR an alveolar-arterial oxygen gradient >35 mmHg) should receive adjunctive corticosteroids—either prednisone 40 mg po twice daily × 5 days, then 40 mg PO once daily × 5 days, then 20 mg PO once daily × 11 days or methylprednisolone equivalent—as soon as possible and within 72 h of treatment onset.
[c]TMP-SMX is recommended first-line treatment for PCP.

severe consequences for patients with PCP residing in these resource-limited areas [27–29].

There are several treatment alternatives in patients who are allergic to, intolerant of, or failing trimethoprim-sulfamethoxazole [5]. Intravenous pentamidine isethionate and clindamycin plus primaquine are the main alternatives in patients with moderate to severe PCP. Compared with trimethoprim-sulfamethoxazole, pentamidine has comparable efficacy but is associated with more frequent and severe toxicities that relegate it to second-line status. Clindamycin plus primaquine is reported to be an excellent salvage therapy option for PCP. In patients with mild to moderate PCP, widely used alternatives to trimethoprim-sulfamethoxazole include trimethoprim plus dapsone, atovaquone, or clindamycin plus primaquine.

Finally, patients with moderate to severe PCP, demonstrated by an oxygen saturation $\leq 93\%$, a PaO_2 <70 mmHg or an alveolar-arterial oxygen gradient > 35 mmHg, should receive corticosteroid therapy in addition to specific PCP treatment [30]. Adjunctive corticosteroids, either oral prednisone or intravenous methylprednisolone, should be started at the same time that specific PCP treatment is begun. Several studies document a reduction in respiratory failure and

mortality rates in patients randomized to corticosteroids [30]. Thus, the potential survival benefits associated with corticosteroid therapy outweigh the risks of this additional immunosuppressive therapy potentially unmasking an occult opportunistic infection such as tuberculosis.

The ideal time to start antiretroviral therapy (ART) in patients with PCP who are not yet taking ART is not clear, but growing evidence supports starting ART early rather than waiting until after completion of PCP treatment. A randomized controlled trial compared early ART versus delayed ART in 282 HIV-infected patients diagnosed with opportunistic infections (63% had PCP) [31]. Early ART was associated with a significant decrease in AIDS progression and death, with no increase in immune reconstitution syndrome.

PROPHYLAXIS

Perhaps the single most effective PCP prevention strategy is the use of combination ART to increase the CD4 count to above the threshold associated with an increased risk of

PCP (i.e., 200 cells/mm^3). Multiple studies conclusively demonstrate that the risk of PCP is low in patients whose CD4 count has risen from below to above 200 cells/mm^3 as a result of ART [5]. In these persons, both primary and secondary PCP prophylaxis can be safely discontinued once the CD4 count has remained > 200 cells/mm^3 for at least 3 months [32, 33]. One exception is that those with a history of PCP that occurred at a CD4 count > 200 cells/mm^3 should remain on PCP prophylaxis for life, regardless of the degree of antiretroviral-associated rise in CD4 count [5].

In regions where ART is unavailable or in persons who are unable or unwilling to use combination ART or who are unresponsive to these therapies, PCP prophylaxis is effective at decreasing rates of PCP. Current guidelines recommend that HIV-infected adults and adolescents who have a CD4 count < 200 cells/mm^3 or a history of oropharyngeal candidiasis receive primary PCP prophylaxis and that those with a history of PCP receive secondary prophylaxis [5]. Adults and adolescents who do not meet these criteria but who have a CD4 percentage of < 14% or a prior AIDS-defining illness should be considered for PCP prophylaxis. These recommendations also apply to HIV-infected women who are pregnant. Infants born to HIV-infected mothers should receive prophylaxis starting at 4–6 weeks of age, until the infant's HIV serostatus can be conclusively determined. Those infants who are subsequently determined to be uninfected with HIV can discontinue prophylaxis. HIV-infected infants and any infant whose HIV serostatus remains unknown should continue to receive prophylaxis for the first year of life. After the first year, the need for subsequent prophylaxis is based on age-specific CD4 count thresholds: for children 1–5 years of age, CD4 count < 500 cells/mm^3 or CD4 percentage < 15%; children ≥ 6 years of age, CD4 count < 200 cells/mm^3 (as for adults and adolescents) or CD4 percentage < 15% [34]. Once started, persons should remain on prophylaxis for life, unless their CD4 counts increase from below to above 200 cells/mm^3 for at least 3 months as a result of ART. As with PCP treatment, trimethoprim-sulfamethoxazole is recommended as first-line prophylaxis against PCP (Table 24.3). Dapsone, atovaquone, and aerosolized pentamidine are alternatives in patients who are allergic to or intolerant of trimethoprim-sulfamethoxazole.

One final aspect of PCP prevention that warrants additional study is the prevention of exposure to the source of human *Pneumocystis*. Serologic studies suggest that exposure to *Pneumocystis* occurs early in life [35–37]. Unfortunately, the natural reservoir for human *Pneumocystis* remains unknown, although emerging studies in humans indicate that humans are one reservoir [38]. In well-controlled laboratory experiments, animal-to-animal transmission of *Pneumocystis* via aerosol has been conclusively demonstrated to occur under a variety of different conditions [39–41]. Furthermore, immunocompromised laboratory animals may develop PCP after a brief exposure to a same-species animal with PCP. Thus, recommendations for immunocompromised persons to avoid contact with patients with PCP may be reasonable. However, studies in humans also suggest that immunocompetent as well as immunocompromised persons without clinical PCP may be colonized with human *Pneumocystis* and may

Table 24.3 Prophylaxis options for *Pneumocystis* pneumonia

PROPHYLAXIS REGIMEN	DOSE(S), ROUTE, FREQUENCY	COMMENT
Trimethoprim (TMP)-sulfamethoxazole (SMX)	Preferred: 1 SS or DS tablet PO daily Other options: 1 DS tablet PO thrice weekly	Recommended first-line prophylaxis against PCP
Dapsone	100 mg PO daily or 50 mg PO twice daily	—May also be combined with pyrimethamine and leucovorin for dual protection against toxoplasmosis —When possible, screen for G6PD deficiency prior to use in African and Mediterranean populations
Atovaquone	1500 mg PO daily	
Aerosolized pentamidine	300 mg aerosolized monthly	Via Respirgard II nebulizer

DS, double-strength (160 mg TMP/800 mg SMX); SS, single-strength (80 mg TMP/400 mg SMX); PO, oral; G6PD, glucose-6-phosphate dehydrogenase.

serve as an additional source of infection to unsuspecting immunocompromised persons [42–46]. Thus, even if an immunocompromised person avoids contact with a patient with PCP, the person may still be exposed to *Pneumocystis* through someone who is colonized or subclinically infected with the organism. Studies for defining the epidemiology and transmission of human *Pneumocystis* are needed to identify the potential methods of disease prevention.

CONCLUSION

The HIV/AIDS epidemic brought prominence and clinical importance to PCP, a previously uncommon pneumonia. In the past 30 years, tremendous advances have occurred in our understanding of HIV infection and PCP. However, gaps in our knowledge remain and continued study of this important disease is still needed.

REFERENCES

[1] Serraino D, Puro V, Boumis E, et al. Epidemiological aspects of major opportunistic infections of the respiratory tract in persons with AIDS: Europe, 1993–2000. AIDS 2003;17:2109–16.

[2] Morris A, Lundgren JD, Masor H, et al. Current epidemiology of *Pneumocystis* pneumonia. Emerg Infect Dis 2004; 10:1713–20.

[3] Worodria W, Okot-Nwang M, Yoo SD, et al. Causes of lower respiratory infection in HIV-infected Ugandan adults who are sputum AFB smear-negative. Int J Tuberc Lung Dis 2003;7:117–23.

[4] Fisk DT, Meshnick S, Kazanjian PH. *Pneumocystis carinii* pneumonia in patients in the developing world who have acquired immunodeficiency syndrome. Clin Infect Dis 2003;36:70–8.

[5] Kaplan JE, Benson C, Holmes KK. Guidelines for prevention and treatment of opportunistic infections in HIV-infected adults and adolescents. Recommendations from CDC, the National Institutes of Health, and the HIV Medicine Association of the Infectious Diseases Society of America. MMWR Recomm Rep 2009;58 (RR04):1–198.

[6] Phair J, Munoz A, Detels R, et al. The risk of *Pneumocystis carinii* pneumonia among men infected with human immunodeficiency virus type 1. Multicenter AIDS Cohort Study Group. N Engl J Med 1990;322:161–5.

[7] Stansell JD, Osmond DH, Charlebois E, et al. Predictors of *Pneumocystis carinii* pneumonia in HIV-infected persons. Pulmonary Complications of HIV Infection Study Group. Am J Respir Crit Care Med 1997;155:60–6.

[8] Kovacs JA, Hiemenz JW, Macher AM, et al. *Pneumocystis carinii* pneumonia: a comparison between patients with the acquired immunodeficiency syndrome and patients with other immunodeficiencies. Ann Intern Med 1984;100:663–71.

[9] Thomas Jr CF, Limper AH. *Pneumocystis* pneumonia. N Engl J Med 2004;350:2487–98.

[10] Kales CP, Murren JR, Torres RA, et al. Early predictors of in-hospital mortality for *Pneumocystis carinii* pneumonia in the acquired immunodeficiency syndrome. Arch Intern Med 1987;147:1413–17.

[11] Huang L, Stansell JD. AIDS and the lung. Med Clin North Am 1996;80:775–801.

[12] DeLorenzo LJ, Huang CT, Maguire GP, et al. Roentgenographic patterns of *Pneumocystis carinii* pneumonia in 104 patients with AIDS. Chest 1987;91:323–7.

[13] Huang L, Stansell J, Osmond D, et al. Performance of an algorithm to detect *Pneumocystis carinii* pneumonia in symptomatic HIV-infected persons. Pulmonary Complications of HIV Infection Study Group. Chest 1999;115:1025–32.

[14] Datta D, Ali SA, Henken EM, et al. *Pneumocystis carinii* pneumonia: the time course of clinical and radiographic improvement. Chest 2003;124:1820–3.

[15] Huang L, Hecht FM, Stansell JD, et al. Suspected *Pneumocystis carinii* pneumonia with a negative induced sputum examination. Is early bronchoscopy useful? Am J Respir Crit Care Med 1995;151:1866–71.

[16] Larsen HH, Huang L, Kovacs JA, et al. A prospective, blinded study of quantitative touch-down polymerase chain reaction using oral-wash samples for diagnosis of *Pneumocystis* pneumonia in HIV-infected patients. J Infect Dis 2004;189:1679–83.

[17] Skelly M, Hoffman J, Fabbri M, et al. S-adenosylmethionine concentrations in diagnosis of *Pneumocystis carinii* pneumonia. Lancet 2003;361:1267–8.

[18] Skelly MJ, Holzman RS, Merali S. S-adenosylmethionine levels in the diagnosis of *Pneumocystis carinii* pneumonia in patients with HIV infection. Clin Infect Dis 2008;46:467–71.

[19] Kutty G, Hernandez-Novoa B, Czapiga M, et al. *Pneumocystis* encodes a functional S-adenosylmethionine synthetase gene. Eukaryot Cell 2008;7:258–67.

[20] Wang P, Huang L, Davis JL, et al. A hydrophilic-interaction chromatography tandem mass spectrometry method for quantitation of serum S-adenosylmethionine in patients infected with human immunodeficiency virus. Clin Chim Acta 2008;396:86–8.

[21] Tasaka S, Hasegawa N, Kobayashi S, et al. Serum indicators for the diagnosis of *Pneumocystis* pneumonia. Chest 2007;131:1173–80.

[22] Desmet S, Van Wijngaerden E, Maertens J, et al. Serum (1-3)-beta-D-glucan as a tool for diagnosis of *Pneumocystis jiroveci* pneumonia in

patients with human immunodeficiency virus infection or hematologic malignancy. J Clin Microbiol 2009;47:3871–4.

[23] Huang L, Crothers K, Atzori C, et al. Dihydropteroate synthase gene mutations in *Pneumocystis* and sulfa resistance. Emerg Infect Dis 2004;10:1721–8.

[24] Beard CB, Roux P, Nevez G, et al. Strain typing methods and molecular epidemiology of *Pneumocystis* pneumonia. Emerg Infect Dis 2004;10: 1729–35.

[25] Stein CR, Poole C, Kazanjian P, et al. Sulfa use, dihydropteroate synthase mutations, and *Pneumocystis jirovecii* pneumonia. Emerg Infect Dis 2004;10:1760–5.

[26] Crothers K, Beard CB, Turner J, et al. Severity and outcome of HIV-associated *Pneumocystis* pneumonia containing *Pneumocystis jirovecii* dihydropteroate synthase gene mutations. AIDS 2005;19:801–5.

[27] Kazanjian PH, Fisk D, Armstrong W, et al. Increase in prevalence of *Pneumocystis carinii* mutations in patients with AIDS and *P. carinii* pneumonia, in the United States and China. J Infect Dis 2004;189:1684–7.

[28] Zar HJ, Alvarez-Martinez MJ, Harrison A, et al. Prevalence of dihydropteroate synthase mutants in HIV-infected South African Children with *Pneumocystis jiroveci* pneumonia. Clin Infect Dis 2004;39:1047–51.

[29] Iliades P, Meshnick SR, Macreadie IG. Mutations in the *Pneumocystis jirovecii* DHPS gene confer cross-resistance to sulfa drugs. Antimicrob Agents Chemother 2005; 49:741–8.

[30] The National Institutes of Health—University of California Expert Panel for Corticosteroids as Adjunctive Therapy for *Pneumocystis* Pneumonia. Consensus statement on the use of corticosteroids as adjunctive therapy for *Pneumocystis* pneumonia in the acquired immunodeficiency syndrome. N Engl J Med 1990;323:1500–4.

[31] Zolopa A, Andersen J, Powderly W, et al. Early antiretroviral therapy reduces AIDS progression/death in individuals with acute opportunistic infections: a multicenter randomized strategy trial. PLoS One 2009;4:e5575.

[32] Lopez Bernaldo de Quiros JC, Miro JM, Pena JM, et al. A randomized trial of the discontinuation of primary and secondary prophylaxis against *Pneumocystis carinii* pneumonia after highly active antiretroviral therapy in patients with HIV infection. Grupo de Estudio del SIDA 04/98. N Engl J Med 2001;344:159–67.

[33] Ledergerber B, Mocroft A, Reiss P, et al. Discontinuation of secondary prophylaxis against *Pneumocystis carinii* pneumonia in patients with HIV infection who have a response to antiretroviral therapy. Eight Eur Study Groups. N Engl J Med 2001;344:168–74.

[34] Mofenson LM, Brady MT, Danner SP, et al. Guidelines for the prevention and treatment of opportunistic infections among HIV-exposed and HIV-infected children. Recommendations from CDC, the National Institutes of Health, the HIV Medicine Association of the Infectious Diseases Society of America, the Pediatric Infectious Diseases Society, and the American Academy of Pediatrics. MMWR Recomm Rep 2009;58:1–166.

[35] Bishop LR, Kovacs JA. Quantitation of anti-*Pneumocystis jirovecii* antibodies in healthy persons and immunocompromised patients. J Infect Dis 2003;187:1844–8.

[36] Daly KR, Koch J, Levin L, et al. Enzyme-linked immunosorbent assay and serologic responses to *Pneumocystis jiroveci*. Emerg Infect Dis 2004;10:848–54.

[37] Respaldiza N, Medrano FJ, Medrano AC, et al. High seroprevalence of *Pneumocystis* infection in Spanish children. Clin Microbiol Infect 2004;10:1029–31.

[38] Kovacs JA, Gill VJ, Meshnick S, et al. New insights into transmission, diagnosis, and drug treatment of *Pneumocystis carinii* pneumonia. JAMA 2001;286:2450–60.

[39] An CL, Gigliotti F, Harmsen AG. Exposure of immunocompetent adult mice to *Pneumocystis carinii* f. sp. muris by cohousing: growth of *P. carinii* f. sp. muris and host immune response. Infect Immun 2003;71:2065–70.

[40] Gigliotti F. Harmsen AG. Wright TW. Characterization of transmission of *Pneumocystis carinii* f. sp. muris through immunocompetent BALB/c mice. Infect Immun 2003;71:3852–6.

[41] Vestereng VH, Bishop LR, Hernandez B, et al. Quantitative real-time polymerase chain-reaction assay allows characterization of *Pneumocystis* infection in immunocompetent mice. J Infect Dis 2004;189:1540–4.

[42] Maskell NA, Waine DJ, Lindley A, et al. Asymptomatic carriage of *Pneumocystis jiroveci* in subjects undergoing bronchoscopy: a prospective study. Thorax 2003;58:594–7.

[43] Morris A, Kingsley LA, Groner G, et al. Prevalence and clinical predictors of *Pneumocystis* colonization among HIV-infected men. AIDS 2004;18:793–8.

[44] Morris A, Sciurba FC, Lebedeva IP, et al. Association of chronic obstructive pulmonary disease severity and *Pneumocystis* colonization. Am J Respir Crit Care Med 2004;170:408–13.

[45] Totet A, Latouche S, Lacube P, et al. *Pneumocystis jirovecii* dihydropteroate synthase genotypes in immunocompetent infants and immunosuppressed adults, Amiens, France. Emerg Infect Dis 2004;10:667–73.

[46] Medrano FJ, Montes-Cano M, Conde M, et al. *Pneumocystis jirovecii* in general population. Emerg Infect Dis 2005;11:245–50.

Chapter 25

Other HIV-related pneumonias

John G. Bartlett

INTRODUCTION

The lower respiratory tract has been and continues to be a major site of opportunistic infections in patients with HIV infection. The infections that are encountered are quite different in the developed world and in the developing world, based on availability of antiretroviral therapy (ART), diagnostic testing, and the epidemiology of tuberculosis. There is a substantial spectrum of pathogens that are involved in pulmonary infections, although the great majority of cases are presumably bacterial or viral but are never definitively diagnosed. The purpose of this chapter is to review pneumonia, with emphasis on appropriate diagnostic studies and treatment. Emphasis will also be placed on the experiences in distinct geographic areas. *Pneumocystis jiroveci* and mycobacteria are discussed elsewhere. The focus of attention here will be on bacterial pathogens and fungi other than *P. jiroveci* and *Mycobacterium tuberculosis*.

FREQUENCY

Bacterial pneumonia was a common cause of HIV-related complications in the era before the availability of highly active ART (HAART) and has continued to be a major problem in the developing world. A prospective study of 1,100 HIV-infected patients from 1988 through 1994 in the USA found an incidence of approximately 100 cases per 1,000 person-years (PY), approximately eight times higher than for an age-matched control population [1, 2]. The major pathogens encountered in this study of 521 cases of pneumonia (in which the likely pathogen was identified) were bacterial infection, 44%; *P. jiroveci*, 42%; tuberculosis, 5%; and other opportunistic infections, 8%. Of the

bacterial causes, the most frequent were *Streptococcus pneumoniae*, *Haemophilus influenzae*, *Pseudomonas aeruginosa*, and *Staphylococcus aureus*. Atypical agents (*Legionella*, *Mycoplasma pneumoniae*, and *Chlamydophila pneumoniae*) were rarely encountered [3].

BACTERIAL PNEUMONIA

There are four bacterial agents that have been associated with HIV infection and immunodeficiency: *S. pneumoniae*, *H. influenzae*, *P. aeruginosa*, and *Nocardia*. This listing does not include mycobacteria, which are discussed elsewhere. Of these, pneumococcal pneumonia is clearly the most frequent and most important cause of pulmonary consolidation.

Pneumococcal pneumonia

The frequency of pneumococcal bacteremia is estimated to be 150–300 times higher in HIV-infected individuals than in those seronegative for HIV. The increased rate appears to apply to all CD4 cell strata, but is most common in those with low CD4 counts [3, 5]. This frequency has changed substantially in developed countries due to the notable impact of HAART, the induction of herd immunity due to the use of the Prevnar 7 vaccine in children, and the demonstrated impact of PCP prophylaxis in reducing bacterial infections [4, 7].

The clinical presentation of pneumococcal pneumonia is similar for patients with or without HIV infection, except for the high rates of bacteremia in HIV-infected patients. Extrapulmonary involvement (meningitis, septic arthritis, and endocarditis) are infrequent. The classic presentation is the acute onset of chills and fever, usually accompanied by cough, dyspnea, and pleurisy. These symptoms clearly

Table 25.1 Correlation of chest X-ray changes and causes

CHANGE	COMMON	UNCOMMON
Consolidation	Pyogenic bacteria, Kaposi's sarcoma, cryptococcosis	*Nocardia, M. tuberculosis, M. kansasii, Legionella, Bordetella bronchiseptica*
Reticulonodular infiltrates	*Pneumocystis jiroveci, M. tuberculosis,* histoplasmosis, coccidioidomycosis	Kaposi's sarcoma, toxoplasmosis, CMV, leishmaniasis, lymphoid interstitial pneumonitis
Nodule	*M. tuberculosis,* cryptococcosis	Kaposi's sarcoma, *Nocardia*
Cavity	*M. tuberculosis, S. aureus* (IDU), *Nocardia, P. aeruginosa,* cryptococcosis, coccidioidomycosis, histoplasmosis, aspergillosis, anaerobes	*M. kansasii,* MAC, *Legionella, Pneumocystis jiroveci,* lymphoma, *Klebsiella, Rhodococcus equi*
Hilar nodes	*M. tuberculosis,* histoplasmosis, coccidioidomycosis, lymphoma, Kaposi's sarcoma	*M. kansasii,* MAC
Pleural effusion	Pyogenic bacteria, Kaposi's sarcoma, *M. tuberculosis* (congestive heart failure, hypoalbuminemia)	Cryptococcosis, MAC, histoplasmosis, coccidioidomycosis, aspergillosis, anaerobes, *Nocardia,* lymphoma, toxoplasmosis, primary effusion lymphoma

distinguish this pulmonary infection from Pneumocystis pneumonia (PCP) and tuberculosis (TB). The chest radiograph demonstrates the usual focal infiltrate (Table 25.1). Cavity formation, atypical infiltrates, and hilar adenopathy are rare and suggest an alternative diagnosis. Most patients produce sputum, which becomes a diagnostic resource using Gram stain, Quellung tests, and culture [9]. As noted, blood cultures are often positive. The urinary antigen assay has a sensitivity of approximately 80% and a specificity of 95% in adults with pneumococcal bacteremia [10]. The treatment of pneumococcal pneumonia is the same for persons with HIV infection as for others.

The preferred drugs are summarized in Table 25.2. In Africa, most strains of *S. pneumoniae* appear to respond to beta-lactams, which are the preferred drugs. In the USA ceftriaxone or cefotaxime are active against about 94% of strains; if there is a reason to suspect resistance or if the patient is critically ill, most experts recommend a fluoroquinolone, either alone or in combination with one of the preferred beta-lactams. One curious observation is that patients who are critically ill with bacteremic pneumococcal pneumonia involving penicillin-sensitive strains appear to do better with a beta-lactam combined with a macrolide than with a beta-lactam alone [11]. The reason is unclear, but some suspect a role of the anti-inflammatory activity of the macrolide. The duration of therapy is arbitrary; the usual recommended duration is 5–7 days after the patient becomes afebrile. The rate of recurrent pneumococcal bacteremia is high: 8–25% within 6 months. These are generally infections involving new strains rather than relapses, so longer treatment does not appear to be beneficial [12, 13].

Administration of the 23-valent pneumococcal vaccine is recommended in HIV-infected patients, although data demonstrating clinical benefit are sparse. In other populations, the only benefit convincingly shown was a 50% reduction in the frequency of pneumococcal bacteremia, suggesting that patients with AIDS may continue to be a high priority for vaccination, especially when the CD4 count is high enough to allow for an immunologic response [14]. More recent data suggest that the new Prevnar 13 vaccine may be useful in adults at high risk for pneumococcal bacteremia [15].

Haemophilus influenzae

This organism is second to the pneumococcus as a cause of bacterial pneumonia in patients with HIV infection [16, 17]. The frequency of *H. influenzae* bacteremia is 10- to 100-fold higher in HIV-infected patients. Most cases involve non-typeable strains [17]. This infection is similar to that of pneumococcal pneumonia, with an acute onset of fever, cough, sputum production, and dyspnea. Chest X-rays usually show a bronchopneumonia. The diagnosis is best established by Gram stain and culture of sputum and culture of blood. Approximately 40% of these strains produce beta-lactamase, so amoxicillin is often ineffective. The preferred drugs are a third-generation cephalosporin, a beta-lactam/beta-lactamase inhibitor, fluoroquinolone, azithromycin, or sulfamethoxazole-trimethoprim [18]. The response is generally good, and treatment is continued for 5–7 days after the patient becomes afebrile. Trimethoprim-sulfamethoxazole prophylaxis should prevent this infection, but other forms of PCP prophylaxis will not. *Haemophilus influenzae* vaccine is not indicated in adults because the rates of this infection are relatively low and the majority involve non-typeable strains not included in the vaccine.

Table 25.2 Bacterial infections

AGENT	COURSE	FREQUENCY, SETTING	TYPICAL FINDINGS	DIAGNOSIS	TREATMENT
Gram-negative bacilli	Acute, purulent sputum	Uncommon, except with nosocomial infection or neutropenia. *Pseudomonas aeruginosa* is relatively common in late-stage disease, cavitary disease, or chronic antibiotic exposure (median CD4 count 50 cells/mm³)	Lobar or bronchopneumonia	Sputum Gram Stain (GS) and culture (sensitivity is >80%, but specificity is poor)	Need *in vitro* susceptibility tests. Long-term ciprofloxacin usually results in relapse and resistance to *P. aeruginosa*.
Haemophilus influenzae	Acute, purulent sputum	Incidence is 100-fold higher than in healthy controls; most infections are caused by unencapsulated strains	Bronchopneumonia	Sputum GS and culture (sensitivity of culture is 50%; prior antibiotics usually preclude growth)	Oral: amoxicillin/clavulanate, azithromycin, TMP-SMX, fluoroquinolone, cephalosporin. Intravenous: cefotaxime, ceftriaxone
Legionella	Acute mucopurulent sputum	Uncommon, HIV-associated risk is debated	Bronchopneumonia; sometimes multiple infiltrates in non-contiguous segments	Sputum culture; urinary antigen (*Legionella pneumophila* serogroup 1)	Fluoroquinolone, macrolide, doxycycline
Nocardia	Chronic or asymptomatic; sputum production	Uncommon; frequency higher with chronic corticosteroid use (median CD4 count 50 cells/mm³)	Nodule or cavity	Sputum or fiberoptic bronchoscopy (FOB); GS, modified acid-fast bacillus (AFB) stain and culture; should alert lab if suspected	Sulfonamide or TMP-SMX
Staphylococcus aureus	Acute, subacute, or chronic, purulent sputum	Uncommon, except with injection drug use and tricuspid valve endocarditis with septic emboli	Bronchopneumonia, cavitary disease, septic emboli with cavities ± effusion	Blood sputum GS and culture (sputum culture is sensitive, but specificity is poor). Blood cultures are nearly always positive with endocarditis	MSSA: nafcillin or oxacillin, cefuroxime, TMP-SMX, clindamycin MRSA: TMP-SMX or clindamycin if sensitive; vancomycin
Streptococcus pneumoniae	Acute, purulent sputum ± pleurisy	Common, all stages HIV infection; incidence is 100-fold higher than in healthy controls; recurrence rate at 6 months is 6–24%; higher with low CD4 counts and with smoking	Lobar or bronchopneumonia ± pleural effusion	Blood cultures often positive, sputum GS Quellung, culture (sensitivity of culture is 50%; prior antibiotics usually preclude growth)	Oral: amoxicillin, macrolide, cefdinir, cefprozil, cefpodoxime, fluoroquinolone. Intravenous: cefotaxime, ceftriaxone, fluoroquinolone

Staphylococcus aureus

Patients with HIV infection have not been clearly defined as being at higher risk for infections involving *S. aureus*. Those infected with HIV as a result of injection drug use have increased rates of infections involving *S. aureus* that appear to be independent of HIV. Most of these infections are soft tissue infections at injection sites or pyomyositis [18, 19]. There is a relatively new form of staphylococcal pneumonia that is at present quite rare, but might become more prevalent and is important to recognize. This is the strain that has the Panton-Valentine leukocidin (PVL) recognized in the late 1990s that is often resistant to all beta-lactams, but sensitive to most other drugs active against *S. aureus*, including trimethoprim-sulfamethoxazole, clindamycin, and doxycycline. It is most frequently associated with severe soft tissue infections, including necrotizing fasciitis and furunculosis. HIV-infected patients infected through homosexual sex or injection drug use are at higher risk for these soft tissue infections. This organism may also cause pneumonia characterized by a fulminant course, with shock, necrosis of the lung, and empyema. As noted, the unique strain of *S. aureus* involved in these cases in the USA is usually referred to USA 300, although similar strains with similar properties are found in other parts of the world. The pathogenic mechanism is not clear, but a characteristic feature of these strains is that they possess the genes for the PVL as well as the *mec*IV mechanism of methicillin resistance [20, 21]. Optimal treatment of pneumonia is not clear, but many authorities recommend the use of vancomycin or linezolid, often in combination with other drugs such as rifampin or clindamycin [21].

Pseudomonas aeruginosa

Pneumonia with this organism is infrequent, but it is a serious complication of late-stage disease indicating profound immunosuppression [22–24]. Most patients have a CD4 count <50 cells/mm^3, and some have additional risk factors such as neutropenia or corticosteroid therapy. Many have bacteremia, and the mortality rate is relatively high. The organism is usually easy to recover from sputum and refractory to eradication despite aggressive antimicrobial therapy. The usual treatment is a combination of antipseudomonal beta-lactams combined with tobramycin. Treatment with an oral fluoroquinolone such as levofloxacin or ciprofloxacin often results in relapse with a fluoroquinolone-resistant strain.

Atypical agents

Chlamydophila (formerly *Chlamydia*) *pneumoniae* and *Mycoplasma pneumoniae* appear to be relatively uncommon in patients with HIV infection [1–3, 16]. A major problem is the limited accuracy of the diagnostic test for these two atypical agents [9]. One study reported results with the standard microimmunofluorescence (MIF) serology; nevertheless, *C. pneumoniae* accounted for only 13 of 319 (2.5%) of pneumonias in patients with HIV infection [25]. *Chlamydophila pneumoniae* and *M. pneumoniae* have not been generally associated with infections in compromised hosts, which presumably accounts for the paucity of cases. By contrast, *Legionella* has a clear association with compromised cell-mediated immunity, so one would expect more cases with HIV infection [26–29]. One early report indicated a 50-fold increase in the frequency of Legionnaires' disease with HIV infection, but this has remained an isolated report not substantiated by others. Blatt and co-workers [26] reviewed eight cases of Legionnaires' disease encountered in the HIV Natural History Study of the US Air Force; the median CD4 count was 83 cells/mm^3; five cases were nosocomial; six had coexisting pulmonary pathogens; none acquired this infection while receiving prophylaxis with trimethoprim-sulfamethoxazole; and all responded well to standard therapy with a macrolide. The conclusion is that atypical agents play a minimal role in the etiology of bacterial pneumonia in patients with HIV infection or AIDS.

Miscellaneous pathogens

Rhodococcus equi is a relatively rare cause of pneumonia in HIV-infected patients with late-stage disease (CD4 count usually <50 cells/mm^3). Cavitation is common, and bacteremia is found in 50–80% of cases with an established diagnosis. Standard treatment is vancomycin or imipenem; one of these is usually combined with rifampin, a fluoroquinolone, or erythromycin.

Mycobacteria other than tuberculosis (MOTT) are occasional pulmonary pathogens in this population. *Mycobacterium avium* complex (MAC) is an important cause of pneumonia in selected patients without HIV infection, but seems to cause disseminated disease involving nearly all organs other than the lungs in patients with late-stage HIV. The major MOTT pathogen in patients with HIV is *Mycobacterium kansasii*, which can present like *M. tuberculosis* with pulmonary infiltrates, a chronic course, and positive AFB smears. As with tuberculosis, it can occur in patients with relatively high CD4 counts. An important clue to early diagnosis is a negative rapid molecular diagnostic test in a patient with a positive AFB smear or culture. The usual treatment is isoniazid plus ethambutol plus either rifampin or rifabutin. Immune reconstitution inflammatory syndrome (IRIS) has been reported.

Norcardia is an important pathogen in patients with defective defenses, especially defective cell-mediated immunity. However, *Nocardia* is a relatively rare pathogen in HIV-infected patients for unclear reasons. The organism is weakly acid fast, looks like *Actinomyces* on Gram stain, and causes an indolent pneumonia, consolidation, abscess formation, or fibronodular infiltrates. Trimethoprim-sulfamethoxazole (10 mg/kg/day TMP) is the preferred treatment.

Diagnostic approach

Key clues to the probability of a bacterial pneumonia in a patient with HIV infection are the features that characterize bacterial pneumonia in other populations: the acute onset and rapid progression, the usual clinical features of cough, sputum, and dyspnea, and the radiographic findings, which almost invariably include a pulmonary infiltrate. Key factors in the assessment are the CD4 count (to evaluate susceptibility to opportunistic pathogens), measures of oxygenation and vital signs (to assess severity of illness), and the characteristic features of the infiltrate [23]. Radiographic features that suggest specific etiologic causes are summarized in Table 25.1. In many cases, this will be the initial presentation, and the CD4 count may be pending when diagnostic and therapeutic decisions need to be made. The absolute lymphocyte count (ALC) may be helpful: an ALC of <1200 cells/mm^3 correlates roughly with a CD4 count of <200 cells/mm^3. Patients with advanced HIV infection may also demonstrate evidence of chronic disease with anemia, hypoalbuminemia, weight loss, etc. If HIV infection is suspected but has not been diagnosed, a rapid serologic test can be helpful. This test and the CBC are generally available in virtually all parts of the world.

To establish an etiologic diagnosis, standard tests for patients sufficiently sick to require hospitalization are blood cultures and, in many centers, Gram stain and culture of expectorated sputum [9]. Although emphasis has been placed on the probability of bacterial pneumonia in patients with acute onset of symptoms and other characteristic features, there must be a continued concern for the possibility of PCP in any patient who has a low CD4 count, substantial reduction in oxygenation, lack of PCP prophylaxis, and/or characteristic features on chest radiograph. In these cases, it is important that the diagnostic evaluation include bronchoscopy or induced sputum examination, or, if the probability is sufficiently great, empiric treatment that may or may not include agents active against common bacterial pathogens. The same vigilance applies to TB, particularly in countries where this is highly endemic. The expectorated sputum needs to be evaluated by stain and culture for AFB. Since AFB smears have a sensitivity of only about 50% in HIV-infected patients, it may be important to consider empiric treatment here as well. This problem will diminish with availability of polymerase chain reaction (PCR) assays to rapidly detect *M. tuberculosis* and multidrug resistant tuberculosis (MDR-TB) [25].

Treatment

The standard practice in the USA for treatment of hospitalized patients with bacterial pneumonia is treatment with a fluoroquinolone or a cephalosporin (ceftriaxone or cefotaxime), combined with a macrolide (azithromycin or clarithromycin or erythromycin) (Table 25.3)

[26]. Treatment should be initiated rapidly, preferably within 6 hours of registration. Pathogen-directed treatment is always preferred but often unrealistic due to time delays in establishing the etiologic agent. Recommendations based on the pathogen are provided in Table 25.3. Note that HIV infection with a CD4 count <200/mm^3 must raise concerns for an opportunistic infection, as discussed below.

In HIV-infected patients the diagnosis of community-acquired pneumonia should be established radiographically and empiric therapy should be started with a macrolide or doxycycline. In the UK the recommended treatment is amoxicillin, which should be equally effective. The assumption is that most of these cases are caused by *S. pneumoniae*, other streptococci, or *H. influenzae*. In HIV-infected patients, the concern is for other conditions that may present in a slowly progressive form such as PCP or tuberculosis, but these can usually be distinguished based on radiographic findings, time course, symptoms, and CD4 count. For hospitalized patients with community-acquired pneumonia, the standard treatment in most of the world is with a penicillin. In the USA the standard is to cover *S. pneumoniae*, *H. influenza*, and atypical pathogens.

FUNGAL PNEUMONIA

Aspergillosis

Aspergillosis previously accounted for 1–4% of pneumonias in patients with AIDS [30–34]. This was a relatively late complication, usually in patients with a CD4 count <50 cells/mm^3 who often had additional risk factors, such as neutropenia or use of chronic corticosteroid therapy. There are two distinct clinical forms of pulmonary infection (Table 25.4). The first is invasive parenchymal aspergillosis, in which the chest radiograph shows either a diffuse interstitial pneumonitis or the more characteristic pleural-based wedge-shaped infiltrate. These patients present with fever, cough, dyspnea, pleurisy, hypoxemia, hemoptysis, and the radiographic features noted [30, 31]. The second form of pulmonary aspergillosis is tracheobronchial disease with ulcers or pseudomembranes, often with obstruction from mucus plugs [30, 31]. The diagnosis of aspergillosis is established by the presence of typical clinical features combined with demonstration of the organism by histopathology; a presumptive diagnosis can be made by positive cultures for *Aspergillus* from respiratory secretions or a positive galactomanin assay when accompanied by the characteristic clinical features [32, 33]. The standard treatment is voriconazole or amphotericin B (Table 25.5), usually at high dose, preferably using a lipid formulation of amphotericin. Itraconazole may also be used. In more recent years, voriconazole has become the preferred agent [16, 34, 35]. It has not been studied in clinical trials in

Table 25.3 Treatment of bacterial pneumonia (based on guidelines of IDSA)

Outpatient

Empiric

No antibiotics × 3 months: doxycycline or macrolide[a]
Antibiotics within 3 months: fluoroquinolone,[b] telithromycin, or beta-lactam + macrolide

Hospitalized patient

Non-ICU: fluoroquinolone[b] or beta-lactam[c] + macrolide[a]

ICU beta-lactam + macrolide or beta-lactam + fluoroquinolone[b]

Aspiration

Beta-lactam/beta-lactamase inhibitor or clindamycin
Alternative: carbapenem[d]

Influenza + superinfection

Beta-lactam[c] ± antiviral agent

Healthcare-associated

Ceftriaxone, fluoroquinolone,[b] ampicillin-sulbactam or ertapenem

Pathogen-specific

S. pneumoniae

Penicillin MIC <2 μg/mL: penicillin or amoxicillin; alternatives—macrolide,[a] telithromycin, cephalosporin-cefpodoxime, cefprozil, cefuroxime, cefdinir, cefditoren, ceftriaxone or cefotaxime, doxycycline, clindamycin, fluoroquinolone[b]
Penicillin MIC ≥2 μg/mL: cefotaxime, ceftriaxone, fluoroquinolone,[b] telithromycin
Alternatives: linezolid, amoxicillin (3 g/day—if MIC ≤4 μg/mL)

H. influenzae

Non-beta-lactamase- producing: amoxicillin
Beta-lactamase-producing: cephalosporin, amoxicillin-clavulanate
Alternatives: fluoroquinolones,[b] doxycycline, azithromycin, clarithromycin

Mycoplasma pneumoniae

Macrolide[a] or tetracycline
Alternative: fluoroquinolone[b]

Chlamydophila pneumoniae

Macrolide[a] or tetracycline
Alternative: fluoroquinolone[b]

Legionella

Fluoroquinolone,[b] azithromycin, clarithromycin
Alternative: doxycycline

S. aureus

MSSA: nafcillin, oxacillin. Alternative: clindamycin, cefazolin, trimethoprim-sulfamethoxazole
MRSA: vancomycin or linezolid

P. aeruginosa

Anti-pseudomonal beta-lactam (ticarcillin, piperacillin, ceftazidime, cefepime, aztreonam, imipenem, meropenem) + (ciprofloxacin or levofloxacin) or aminoglycoside
Alternative: aminoglycoside plus ciprofloxacin or levofloxacin

---

[a]Macrolide: azithromycin or clarithromycin.
[b]Fluoroquinolone: levofloxacin (750 mg/day), moxifloxacin, gemifloxacin.
[c]Beta-lactam: ceftriaxone, cefotaxime.
[d]Carbapenem: imipenem, meropenem, ertapenem.

Table 25.4 Fungal infections

AGENT	COURSE	FREQUENCY, SETTING	TYPICAL FINDINGS	DIAGNOSIS	TREATMENT
Aspergillus	Acute or subacute	Up to 4% of AIDS patients; usually with advanced HIV infection (med. CD4 count 30 cells/mm³); ~60% have severe neutropenia (ANC <500 cells/mm³) ± chronic steroids; disseminated disease uncommon	Focal infiltrate; cavity-often pleural-based diffuse infiltrates or reticulonodular infiltrates	Sputum stain and culture; false-positive and false-negative cultures common. Best tests: tissue pathology or sputum smear and typical CT and clinical features	Amphotericin B or itraconazole or caspofungin
Candida	Chronic or subacute	Common isolate, rare cause of pulmonary disease (med. CD4 count 50 cells/mm³)	Bronchitis; rare cause of pneumonia (some say it does not exist)	Recovery in sputum or FOB specimen is meaningless (up to 30% of all expectorated sputum and FOB cultures in unselected patients yield *Candida* sp.); must have histologic evidence of invasion on biopsy	Fluconazole or amphotericin B
Coccidioides immitis±	Chronic or subacute	Up to 10% of AIDS patients in endemic area; usually advanced HIV infection (med. CD4 count 50 cells/mm³); disseminated disease in 20–40%	Diffuse nodular infiltrates, focal infiltrate, cavity; hilar adenopathy [26]	Sputum, induced sputum, or FOB stain and culture; KOH of expectorated sputum is rarely positive; PAP stain or silver stain of BAL positive in 40%, culture of BAL usually positive; serology (CF) positive in 70%; skin test positive in <10%; blood cultures positive in 10%	Fluconazole, itraconazole, or amphotericin B
Cryptococcus	Chronic, subacute, or symptomatic	Up to 8–10% in AIDS patients; late-stage HIV infection (med. CD4 count 50 cells/mm³); 80% have cryptococcal meningitis	Nodule, cavity, diffuse or nodular infiltrates	Sputum, induced sputum, or FOB stain and culture; serum cryptococcal antigen usually positive; CSF analysis indicated if antigen or organism found at any site	Fluconazole without CNS involvement; amphotericin B
Histoplasma capsulatum±	Chronic or subacute	Up to 15% of AIDS patients in endemic area; usually advanced HIV infection with disseminated histoplasmosis (med. CD4 count 50 cells/mm³). Common features: fever, weight loss, hepatosplenomegaly, lymphadenopathy	Diffuse nodular infiltrates, nodule, focal infiltrate, cavity, hilar adenopathy [27, 28]	Best test for diagnosis and follow-up of treatment is serum and urine polysaccharide antigen assay, with yield of 85% (blood) and 97% (urine). Available only through J. White (Indianapolis, IN) 800-HISTO-DG for US $70/assay; serology positive in 50–70%; yield with culture of sputum, 80%; marrow, 80%; blood cultures positive in 60–85%	Itraconazole or amphotericin B

Table 25.5 Treatment of fungal infection of the lung

Aspergillosis		
Preferred	Voriconazole 400 mg IV or PO q12h × 2 days, then 200 mg q12h	
Duration	Based on clinical response	
Alternative	Amphotericin B 1 mg/kg IV or lipid formulations of amphotericin B 5 mg/kg per day	
Cryptococcosis: disseminated disease		
Preferred	Acute	Amphotericin B 0.7 mg/kg IV ± flucytosine 25 mg PO 4 times daily × 14 days, or liposomal amphotericin × 14 days
	Consolidation	Fluconazole 400 mg/day PO × 8 weeks.
	Maintenance	Fluconazole 200 mg/day PO until CD4 count >100–200/mm^3 + asymptomatic × 6 months
Alternatives	Acute	Fluconazole 400–800 mg/day IV or PO ± flucytosine 25 mg PO 4 times daily × 14 days
	Consolidation	Itraconazole 200 mg/day PO × 8 weeks
	Maintenance	Itraconazole 400 mg PO or IV once daily
Cryptococcosis: pulmonary without disseminated disease		
Preferred	Fluconazole 200–400 mg/day PO or itraconazole 200–400 mg/day or amphotericin B 0.5–1.0 mg/kg per day IV (serious disease)	
Duration	Until asymptomatic + CD4 count >100–200 cells/mm^3 × 6 months	
Histoplasmosis: severe disseminated		
Preferred	Acute	Amphotericin B 0.7 mg/kg per day IV or liposomal amphotericin B 4 mg/kg per day × 3–10 days
	Continuation	Itraconazole 200 mg caps PO twice daily
Alternative	Acute	Itraconazole 400 mg/day IV
	Continuation	Itraconazole oral solution 200 mg PO twice daily or fluconazole 800 mg/day PO
Histoplasmosis: mild disseminated disease		
Preferred	Itraconazole 200 mg cap PO 3 times daily × 3 day, then 200 mg PO twice daily × 12 weeks, then 200 mg/day PO	
Alternative	Fluconazole 800 mg/day PO	

HIV-infected patients, but it appears to be superior to amphotericin B in other populations. Particularly important in the management is to reverse the predisposing factors as much as possible, including increasing CD4 count with ART, reversing of neutropenia, and discontinuing or reducing the dose of corticosteroids. The prognosis has been poor, with a mortality rate exceeding 90% in the pre-HAART era [28]. The prognosis is presumably substantially better with ART-mediated immune reconstitution.

Cryptococcosis

Cryptococcosis is a relatively common complication of late-stage HIV infection. This was previously a common AIDS-defining diagnosis in the developed world and is well recognized as a major cause of severe disease in resource-limited countries. This is best known as a cause of meningitis, but the lung is the portal of entry, and many patients have pulmonary involvement concurrently or in the absence of meningitis. Prior to HAART there were reports that approximately 5–8% of all persons with late-stage

HIV infection acquired disseminated cryptococcosis [36–40]. Typical pulmonary symptoms are fever, cough, and dyspnea that evolve over a period of weeks [35–37]. The chest radiograph usually shows interstitial infiltrates that may suggest PCP [36–38]; other radiographic findings include focal infiltrates, cavities that may be clinically silent, hilar adenopathy, pleural effusions, and/or reticulonodular infiltrates. The disease in the central nervous system may be clinically silent, so the diagnosis of cryptococcal pulmonary infection should always prompt a lumbar puncture to detect cryptococcal meningitis, the most common recognized clinical form of the disease. Most patients with cryptococcosis have a positive serum antigen assay for *C. neoformans* [38]. The organism can also often be found in respiratory secretions, including sputum or bronchoscopic aspirates [40].

The standard treatment for cryptococcal meningitis is amphotericin B, often combined with flucytosine for 2 weeks followed by the consolidation phase of fluconazole at 400 mg/day for 8 weeks and then fluconazole at 200 mg/day, until there is immune reconstitution [41, 42]. For patients with pulmonary cryptococcosis, the recommendation for mild disease restricted to the lung is fluconazole 400 mg/day × 6 months [42]. Itraconazole (400 mg/day) is the alternative. More serious pulmonary disease should be managed like cryptococcal meningitis [42].

Histoplasmosis

Histoplasma capsulatum is endemic in the Mississippi, Ohio, and St Lawrence River valleys. Histoplasmosis was previously diagnosed in over 5% of persons living in these endemic areas [42–45]. The frequency has declined during the HAART era. The disease is acquired by inhalation of

H. capsulatum microconidia. Infection generally remains localized in the lung in patients with CD4 counts >300 cells/mm^3, but disseminated disease is common when the CD4 count is <150 cells/mm^3. Common clinical features of pulmonary disease include cough, fever, and dyspnea that are usually indolent in onset. With disseminated disease, there are often typical lesions of the skin and mucosal surfaces, weight loss with wasting, bone marrow suppression with pancytopenia, hepatosplenomegaly with abnormal liver function tests in a cholangitic pattern, lymphadenopathy, and/or diarrhea [37]. The chest radiograph usually shows a diffused interstitial infiltrate or a reticulonodular infiltrate; other less common findings are focal infiltrates, hilar adenopathy, and pleural effusions [27, 43, 44]. A septic shock-like syndrome occurs in $<10\%$ of patients. Detection of the *Histoplasma* antigen in blood or urine is useful for the diagnosis of disseminated disease, but these tests are relatively insensitive when the infection is restricted to the lung [34, 44]. The fungus can often be isolated from blood cultures, bone marrow, or respiratory secretions, but recovery requires 2–4 weeks [45].

Patients with severe disseminated disease should be treated with liposomal amphotericin B, which has proven superior to deoxycholate amphotericin B with respect to therapeutic response and toxicity [42, 43]. Amphotericin is usually given for 7–14 days, and treatment is then changed to itraconazole 200 mg twice daily for at least 12 weeks and until there is immune reconstitution. Chronic pulmonary histoplasmosis is treated with itraconazole (200 mg twice daily) for 12–24 months until the CD4 count is >100 cells/mm^3 [34, 44]. Patients with acute pulmonary histoplasmosis and a CD4 count >500 cells/mm^3 may not require therapy and can be managed in a fashion similar to patients without HIV infection.

REFERENCES

[1] Caiaffa WT, Graham NM, Vlahov D. Bacterial pneumonia in adult populations with human immunodeficiency virus (HIV) infection. Am J Epidemiol 1993;138:909–22.

[2] Wallace JM, Rao AV, Glassroth J, et al. Respiratory illness in persons with human immunodeficiency virus infection. Am Rev Respir Dis 1993;148:1523–9.

[3] Mundy LM, Auwaerter PC, Oldach D, et al. Community-acquired pneumonia: impact of immune status. Am J Respir Crit Care Med 1995;152:1309–15.

[4] Murray JF. Pulmonary complications of HIV-1 infection among adults living in Sub-Saharan

Africa. J Tuberc Lung Dis 2005;9:826–35.

[5] Kourtis AP, Ellington S, Bansil P, et al. Hospitalizations for invasive pneumococcal disease among HIV-1-infected adolescents and adults in the United States in the era of highly active antiretroviral therapy and the conjugate pneumococcal vaccine. J Acquir Immune Defic Syndr 2010;55:128–31.

[6] French N, Gordon SB, Mwalukomo T, et al. A trial of a 7-valent pneumococcal conjugate vaccine in infected adults. N Engl J Med 2010;362:812–22.

[7] Boyton RJ. Infectious lung complications in patients with HIV/

AIDS. Curr Opin Pulm Med 2005;11:203–7.

[8] Mwenya DM, Charalambous BM, Phillips PP, et al. Impact of cotrimoxazole on carriage and antibiotic resistance of *Streptococcus pneumoniae* and *Haemophilus influenzae* in HIV-infected children in Zambia. Antimicrob Agents Chemother 2010;54:3756–62.

[9] Bartlett JG. Diagnostic tests for agents of community-acquired pneumonia. Clin Infect Dis 2011;52 (Suppl. 4):S296–304.

[10] Grau I, Pallares R, Tubau F, et al. Epidemiologic changes in bacteremic pneumococcal disease in patients with human

immunodeficiency virus in the era of highly active antiretroviral therapy. Arch Intern Med 2005;165:1533–40.

[11] Ishida T, Hashimoto T, Arita M, et al. A 3-year prospective study of a urinary antigen-detection test for *Streptococcus pneumoniae* in community acquired pneumonia. J Infect Chemother 2004;10:359–63.

[12] Lopez-Palomo C, Martin-Zamorano M, Beitez E, et al. Pneumonia in HIV-infected patients in the HAART era: incidence, risk, and impact of the pneumococcal vaccination. J Med Virol 2004;72:517–24.

[13] Schuchat A, Broome CV, Hightower A, et al. Use of surveillance for invasive pneumococcal disease to estimate the size of the immunosuppressed HIV-infected population. JAMA 1991;265:3275–9.

[14] Baddour LM, Klugman KP, Feldman C, et al. Combination antibiotic therapy lowers mortality among severely ill patients with pneumococcal bacteremia. Am J Respir Crit Care Med 2004;170:440–4.

[15] French N, Gordon SB, Mwalukomo T, et al. A trial of 7-valent pneumococcal conujugate vaccine in HIV-infected adults. N Engl J Med 2010;362:812–22.

[16] USPHS/IDSA Prevention of Opportunistic Infections Working Group. USPHS/IDSA guidelines for the prevention of opportunistic infections in persons infected with human immunodeficiency virus: disease-specific recommendations. MMWR Morb Mortal Wkly Rep 1997;51:RR–6.

[17] Munoz P, Miranda ME, Llacaqueo A, et al. *Haemophilus* species bacteremia in adults. Arch Intern Med 1997;157:1869–73.

[18] Fowler Jr VG, Miro JM, Hoen B, et al. *Staphylococcus aureus* endocarditis: a consequence of medical progress. JAMA 2005;293:3012–21.

[19] Francis J, Doherty M, Lopatin U, et al. Severe community-onset pneumonia in healthy adults caused by methicillin-resistant *Staphylococcus aureus* carrying the Panton-Valentine leukocidin genes. Clin Infect Dis 2005;40:100–7.

[20] DeLeo FR, Chambers HF. Reemergence of antibiotic-resistant *Staphylococcus aureus* in the genomics era. J Clin Invest 2009;119:2464–71.

[21] Liu C, Bayer A, Cosgrove SE, et al. Clinical practice guidelines by the Infectious Diseases Society of America for the treatment of methicillin-resistant *Staphylococcus aureus* infections in adults and children: executive summary. Clin Infect Dis 2011;52:285–92.

[22] Mendelson MH, Gurtman A, Szabo S, et al. *Pseudomonas aeruginosa* bacteria in patients with AIDS. Clin Infect Dis 1994;18:886–95.

[23] Hirschtick RE, Glassroth J, Jordan MC, et al. Bacterial pneumonia in persons infected with the human immunodeficiency virus. N Engl J Med 1995;333:845–51.

[24] Shepp DH, Tang IT, Ramundo MB, et al. Serious *Pseudomonas aeruginosa* infection in AIDS. J Acquir Immune Defic Syndr 1994;7:823–31.

[25] Boschini A, Smacchia C, DiFine M, et al. Community-acquired pneumonia in a cohort of former injection drug users with and without human immunodeficiency virus infection: incidence, etiologies, and clinical aspects. Clin Infect Dis 1996;23:107–13.

[26] Blatt SP, Dolan MJ, Hendrix CW, et al. Legionnaires' disease in human immunodeficiency virus-infected patients: eight cases and review. Clin Infect Dis 1994;18:227–32.

[27] Marston BJ, Lipman HB, Breiman RF. Surveillance for Legionnaires' disease: risk factors for morbidity and mortality. Arch Intern Med 1994;154:2417–22.

[28] Rosen MJ, Clayton K, Schneider RF, et al. Intensive care of patients with HIV infection: utilization, critical illnesses and outcomes. Pulmonary complications of HIV Infection Study Group. Am J Respir Crit Care Med 1997;155:67–71.

[29] Stout JE, Yu VL. Legionellosis. N Engl J Med 1997;337:682–7.

[30] Miller Jr WT, Sais GJ, Frank I, et al. Pulmonary aspergillosis in patients with AIDS: clinical and radiographic correlations. Chest 1994;105:37–44.

[31] Denning DW, Follansbee SE, Scolaro M, et al. Pulmonary aspergillosis in the acquired immunodeficiency syndrome. N Engl J Med 1991;324:654–62.

[32] Pervex NK, Kleinerman J, Kattan M, et al. Pseudomembranous necrotizing bronchial aspergillosis: A variant of invasive aspergillosis in patients with hemophilia and acquired immune deficiency syndrome. Am Rev Respir Dis 1985;131:961–3.

[33] Kemper CA, Hostetler JS, Follansbee SE, et al. Ulcerative and plaque-like tracheobronchitis due to infection with *Aspergillus* in patients with AIDS. Clin Infect Dis 1993;17:344–52.

[34] Limper AH, Knox KS, Sarosi GA, et al. An official American thoracic society statement: treatment of fungal infections in adult pulmonary and critical care patients. Am J Respir Crit Care Med 2011;183:96–128.

[35] Wieland T, Liebold A, Jagiello M, et al. Superiority of voriconazole over amphotericin B in the treatment of invasive aspergillosis after heart transplantation. J Heart Transplant 2005;24:102–4.

[36] Mirza SA, Phelan M, Rimaldn D, et al. The changing epidemiology of cryptococcosis: an update from population-based active surveillance in 2 large metropolitan areas, 1992–2000. Clin Infect Dis 2003;36:789–94.

[37] Chuck SL, Sande MA. Infectious with *Cryptococcus neoformans* in the acquired immunodeficiency syndrome. N Engl J Med 1989;321:794–9.

[38] Clark RA, Greer D, Atkinson W, et al. Spectrum of *Cryptococcus neoformans* infection in 68 patients infected with human immunodeficiency virus. Rev Infect Dis 1990;12:768–77.

[39] Eng RH, Bishburg E, Smith SM, et al. Cryptococcal infections in patients with acquired immunodeficiency syndrome. Am J Med 1986;81:19–23.

[40] Malabonga VM, Basti J, Kamholz SL. Utility of bronchoscopic sampling techniques for cryptococcal

disease in AIDS. Chest 1991;99:370–2.

[41] Perfect JR, Dismukees WE, Dromer F, et al. Clinical practice guidelines for the management of cryptococcal disease: 2010 update by the Infectious Diseases Society of America. Clin Infect Dis 2010;50:291–322.

[42] Limper AH, Knox KS, Sarosi GA, et al. An official American Thoracic Society statement of fungal infections in adult pulmonary and critical care patients. Am J Crit Care Med 2011;183:96–128.

[43] Salzman SH, Smith RL, Aranda CL. Histoplasmosis in patients at risk for the acquired immunodeficiency syndrome in a nonendemic

setting. Chest 1988;93: 916–21.

[44] Wheat JL, Sarosi G, McKinsey D, et al. Practice guidelines for the management of patients with histoplasmosis. Clin Infect Dis 2000;30:688–95.

[45] Wheat JL. Current diagnosis of histoplasmosis. Trends Microbiol 2003;11:488–94.

Chapter | 26 |

HIV-associated tuberculosis

Leyla Azis, Edward C. Jones-López, Jerrold J. Ellner

INTRODUCTION

Over the last three decades, tuberculosis (TB) and HIV epidemics have become inextricably connected in a bidirectional interaction, often seen as a deadly association or "the cursed duet" [1]. TB remains a major cause of morbidity and mortality in HIV-infected individuals, especially in countries with a high burden of both infections. The HIV pandemic has changed TB epidemiology, natural history, and pathogenesis, affecting its clinical and radiographic presentation, diagnosis, treatment, and prognosis.

In general, people living with HIV are 20 to 37 times more likely to develop TB disease during their lifetimes than HIV-uninfected individuals [2]. Patients with advanced HIV disease who develop TB are more likely to manifest atypical radiographic findings and develop extrapulmonary and disseminated disease. The diagnosis of TB in HIV-infected patients is more difficult, and the treatment is often complicated by drug interactions, cumulative toxicities and decreased efficacy. Furthermore, mortality rates are remarkably higher. Among individuals treated for TB, HIV-infected individuals have higher rates of recurrent TB than those who are HIV-uninfected. Conversely, active TB is associated with increased viral replication in HIV-infected patients, contributing to HIV progression and shortening survival in dually-infected patients.

The goal of this chapter is to provide a general review of TB, focusing on the unique features of HIV-associated TB and addressing specific issues of co-infection management and control strategies.

EPIDEMIOLOGY

TB is a major global health problem, ranking as the leading cause of death from an infectious agent and the seventh cause of death in the world [3]. The combined burden of disease caused by HIV and TB is daunting. More than 33 million people were living with HIV at the end of 2009, and the death toll from HIV/AIDS in the same year was 1.8 million. It is estimated that one-third of the HIV-infected population is co-infected with *Mycobacterium tuberculosis*, the majority harboring latent TB infection.

In 2009, there were 9.4 million incident cases of TB globally, equivalent to 137 cases per 100,000 population. TB prevalence was estimated at 14 million cases, equivalent to 200/100,000 [2]. Most of the estimated number of cases in 2009 occurred in Asia (55%) and Africa (30%), and smaller proportions of cases occurred in the Eastern Mediterranean region (7%), the European region (4%), and the Americas (3%). Approximately 80% of all estimated cases worldwide were concentrated in 22 high–burden countries (HBCs), among which India alone accounts for an estimated one-fifth (21%), and China and India combined account for 35% of all TB cases worldwide (Fig. 26.1A).

Of the 9.4 million incident cases in 2009, an estimated 1.1 million (12%) were HIV-infected, with approximately 80% of the TB-HIV cases occurring in Africa. In some southern and eastern African countries, more than 50% of TB patients are co-infected with HIV (Fig. 26.1B). Approximately 1.7 million people died of TB in 2009, including an

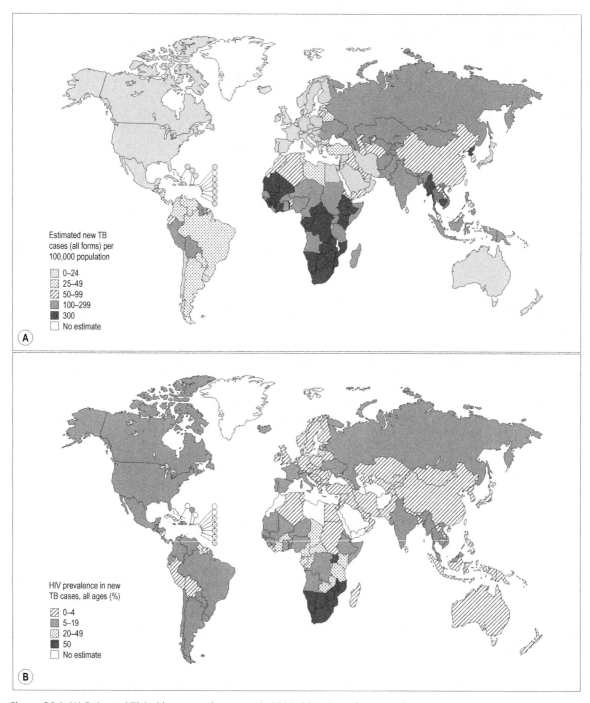

Figure 26.1 (A) Estimated TB incidence rates by country in 2009. (B) Estimated HIV prevalence in new TB cases in 2009.
Reproduced from World Health Organization. Global Tuberculosis Control. [online]. 2010. Available from: http://whqlibdoc.who.int/publications/2010/9789241564069_eng.pdf

estimated 0.4 million people with HIV, amounting to about one in four of the deaths occurring among HIV-infected individuals.

TB drug resistance, including multi-drug resistant TB (MDR-TB) and extensively-drug resistant TB (XDR-TB) is an increasing global problem. MDR-TB is defined as resistance to at least isoniazid and rifampicin, and XDR-TB is defined as an MDR isolate that is also resistant to any fluoroquinolone and at least one of the injectable second-line drugs (capreomycin, amikacin and kanamycin). There were an estimated 440,000 cases of MDR-TB in 2008, of which 85% occurred in 27 high MDR-TB burden countries; 150,000 deaths from MDR-TB occurred in 2008. The global epidemiology of drug-resistant TB in HIV-infected persons is not known. A systematic review that included 32 studies from 17 countries failed to demonstrate an overall association between MDR-TB and HIV infection [4]. However, HIV is a potent risk factor for institutional outbreaks of MDR-TB. In outbreak settings the case mortality rate has been extremely high.

Since HIV was first recognized 3 decades ago, TB incidence and notification rates have remained tightly associated with HIV prevalence rates. The global incidence of TB per capita appears to have peaked in 2004 and is now in decline, following a similar pattern to the trend in HIV prevalence in the general population, but with a 6-year delay.

Globally, the absolute number of cases is increasing slowly, reflecting population growth, although the number of cases per capita (expressed as the number of cases per 100,000 population) is falling by around 1% per year. In 2009, the per capita TB incidence rate was stable or falling in five of the six World Health Organization (WHO) regions, with the exception of the South-East Asia region, where the incidence rate is stable, largely explained by apparent stability in the TB incidence rate in India. The most recent assessment for the 22 HBCs suggests that incidence rates are falling or stable in all countries except South Africa. Mortality rates (excluding TB deaths among HIV-infected people) are falling in all six WHO regions. Among the 22 HBCs, mortality rates appear to be falling, with the possible exception of Afghanistan and Uganda.

Since monitoring of the scale-up of integrated TB/HIV activities began in 2003, considerable progress has been made. By 2009, 1.6 million TB patients knew their HIV status, equivalent to 22% of notified cases, up from 4% in 2003. In 2009, there were 55 countries in which >75% of TB patients knew their HIV status, including 16 African countries. Of the HIV-infected TB patients, 75% were receiving co-trimoxazole preventive therapy (CPT), and 37% were enrolled on antiretroviral therapy (ART) in 2009. Despite the progress achieved over the past several years, the epidemic of HIV-associated-TB continues to rage in many parts of the world and greatly increased collaboration between programs and services is needed.

PATHOGENESIS AND NATURAL HISTORY

TB is caused by one of the pathogenic mycobacteria belonging to *Mycobacterium tuberculosis* complex, most commonly *Mycobacterium tuberculosis* and rarely *M. bovis* or *M. africanum*.

HIV infection is the most significant risk factor for TB progression, accelerating the development of TB at all stages that follow the deposition of *M. tuberculosis* in the pulmonary alveoli.

TB stages are conventionally viewed as "primary TB," "progressive primary TB," "latent TB," and "secondary or post-primary TB". There is, however, evidence supporting the paradigm that the interaction between *M. tuberculosis* and the human host represents a continuum of immune responses, pathologic manifestations, mycobacterial metabolic activity and clinical disease [5]. Nonetheless, this chapter will utilize the classical presentation for simplicity.

Transmission of *M. tuberculosis*

The chain of host–pathogen interactions begins with the inhalation into the pulmonary alveoli of droplet aerosols containing *M. tuberculosis*. When a patient with active pulmonary or laryngeal tuberculosis coughs, speaks, sings or sneezes, he or she generates respiratory droplets that transform into small droplet nuclei through water evaporation. The infected aerosols can remain dispersed in the air for prolonged periods of time. Particles smaller than 5 μm reach the pulmonary alveoli, a process that is necessary for *M. tuberculosis* transmission.

Environmental characteristics such as ventilation, humidity or presence of UV light influence the likelihood of transmission. The likelihood of TB transmission also depends on the infectiousness of the source case as measured by the cough strength [6] and the grade of acid-fast bacilli (AFB) sputum smear results. Patients with cavitary lesions and intensely positive sputum smears have a higher risk of TB transmission. Bacterial factors such as virulence and viability also influence *M. tuberculosis* transmission, as evidenced by the Beijing strain family of *M. tuberculosis* that has been associated with increased transmission, dissemination and outbreaks. Transmission of MDR-TB is comparable to that of drug-susceptible *M. tuberculosis*.

In general, TB transmission occurs as a consequence of household exposure, the prolonged and frequent contact with an active TB patient being much more likely to transmit *M. tuberculosis* than a brief contact. This pattern is observed in both low- and high-prevalence countries, irrespective of HIV status and can be demonstrated by traditional epidemiological studies and confirmed by molecular approaches [7, 8]. Occasionally, *M. tuberculosis* transmission has been reported after casual contact with an infectious case. Transmission after brief exposure has been linked more often to outbreaks in shelters, nursing homes, hospitals, prisons or air travel. In such cases, transmission may be related to increased virulence of the involved strain, environmental factors or patient characteristics. There is, in fact, evidence that some patients with pulmonary TB are "super-transmitters."

Remarkably, only about one-half of the household contacts of active TB patients become infected [9], suggesting that in addition to the type of exposure, host-related factors may influence susceptibility to *M. tuberculosis*. The existence of innate immunity to TB is a certainty, although the immunologic mechanisms that render some populations susceptible and others resistant to TB remain largely uncharacterized. Several studies have demonstrated the association of various human leukocyte antigens (HLA) with disease susceptibility in different ethnic populations [10, 11]. Genetic susceptibility to TB has also been associated with polymorphisms in the human *SLC11A1* (formerly *NRAMP1*) gene, some toll-like receptor (*TLR*) genes, the genes for the vitamin D receptor and components of the interferon (IFN) gamma-signaling pathways.

The interplay between these multiple factors and possibly others, still unknown, will determine the likelihood that the inhaled mycobacteria reach the alveoli and initiate a host–bacterial interaction that culminates in *M. tuberculosis* infection.

The effect of HIV on *M. tuberculosis* transmission has been studied extensively with contradictory results. A meta-analysis concluded that HIV infection does not significantly increase the risk of *M. tuberculosis* transmission, as patients with HIV-1 infection and TB are no more infectious than HIV–uninfected patients with TB [12].

M. tuberculosis infection

In most cases, the first lesion that develops as a result of *M. tuberculosis* infection (primary focus) is located in the lung, whereas the initial inoculation of *M. tuberculosis* at extra-pulmonary sites is uncommon.

Transmitted *M. tuberculosis* bacilli are usually deposited in the mid-lung, subpleural alveoli and are first ingested by resident alveolar macrophages, dendritic cells and recruited monocytes. Within the alveolar macrophages, *M. tuberculosis* bacilli multiply, destroy the macrophages (and are taken up by monocytes recruited to the inflammatory focus), giving rise to an initial exudative primary pulmonary focus. The infected macrophages are transported to the regional hilar and mediastinal lymph nodes, where bacilli continue to multiply, events that define the primary TB infection. A discrete lympho-hematogenous dissemination may occur before the development of acquired immunity, giving rise to small, micronodular pulmonary foci (apical Simon foci) or extra-pulmonary foci that can harbor viable bacilli for prolonged periods of time. These are considered to be the origin of the future secondary pulmonary or extra-pulmonary TB (endogenous reactivation).

Adaptive immunity and delayed-type hypersensitivity (DTH) develop after 3–8 weeks. Adaptive immunity is characterized by decreased bacillary multiplication, macrophage apoptosis, and granuloma formation at the site of the primary focus and disseminated areas. The immune response usually controls the infection. Most often, the lesions of primary TB undergo fibrosis and calcification and may be observed radiographically as calcified peripheral lung nodules (Ghon lesion), calcified adenopathy, or both (Ranke complex), hallmarks of primary TB infection. Caseous necrosis at the center of the lesion, tissue destruction, and cavity formation are the result of DTH.

Primary TB in HIV-infected individuals may occasionally progress directly to disease without an intervening period of clinical latency. This is termed progressive primary tuberculosis, a condition characterized by exudative, caseous and ulcerative pulmonary lesions as a result of pneumonic progression of the primary focus. The host adaptive T cell-mediated response, mainly mediated by interleukin (IL)-12 and interferon (IFN)-γ production by Th1 cells and the local expression of tumor necrosis factor (TNF)-α, is important in the control of *M. tuberculosis* infection, granuloma formation and prevention of mycobacterial dissemination. HIV infection causes CD4 T cell depletion and impairment of cytokine expression, which accounts for poor granuloma formation and TB dissemination (extrapulmonary/miliary forms) in co-infected patients.

TB disease

The reactivation of pulmonary TB in the host with pre-existing immunity leads to a vigorous inflammatory response with the development of caseating granulomas and ultimately cavitary lesions. Pathologically, the lungs of HIV-infected patients dying with TB are frequently characterized by caseous lesions containing tubercle bacilli; however, the type of lesion is correlated with the degree of immunosuppression. In patients with high CD4 counts, typical caseating granulomas can be seen, while in patients with low CD4 counts, the lesions tend to be diffuse, with more extensive caseous necrosis, poor granuloma formation, reduced fibrosis and less frequent cavity formation, reflecting the impaired immune activation.

In HIV-infected individuals, post-primary TB most commonly develops through the endogenous reactivation of the small foci of hematogenous dissemination occurring in the course of primary infection, as in HIV-uninfected populations. In both HIV-infected and uninfected individuals, the most common site of TB reactivation is the lung. Extrapulmonary TB, which may occur in any organ, is more common in HIV-infected patients. In contrast to HIV-uninfected individuals, active TB occurring as a result of TB re-infection, proved through restriction fragment length polymorphism (RFLP) analysis of strains, has been observed frequently in HIV-infected patients, especially in countries where the prevalence of TB is high [13, 14].

In HIV-uninfected individuals, the lifetime risk of developing TB disease by reactivating latent TB infection is approximately 5–10%. In HIV-infected individuals, this risk increases to 5–15% annually, rising as immune deficiency worsens. The increased risk is manifest even in the absence of immunodeficiency. In South African gold miners, the risk of active TB was increased two- to three-fold within the first 2 years of HIV infection despite the absence of significant CD4 cell depletion [15]. In general, the risk of TB progression correlates with the CD4 count. In an African cohort, the TB incidence rate was 17.5 cases/100 person-years in HIV-infected patients with CD4 counts <200/mm^3 versus 3.6 cases/100 person-years for CD4 counts >350/mm^3 [16].

Immunologic aspects

Multiple distinct receptors, such as complement receptors CR1, CR3, CR4, the mannose receptor, CD14, surfactant protein A (Sp-A) receptors and scavenger receptors, have the potential to recognize and bind *M. tuberculosis in vitro*. *M. tuberculosis* can activate the alternative pathway of complement and become opsonized by complement products that facilitate uptake by complement receptors. *M. tuberculosis* also expresses surface polysaccharides that can directly interact with complement receptors.

Besides expressing traditional phagocytic receptors for antibody and complement, macrophages and dendritic cells also express Toll-like receptors (TLRs) that recognize conserved antigens expressed on pathogens. Binding of TLRs to these pathogen-specific ligands initiates a signal transduction pathway in the host cell that culminates in the activation of NFκB and the induction of cytokines and chemokines that are crucial to eliciting the adaptive immune response against *M. tuberculosis*. The sequence of the initial immune events following interaction of *M. tuberculosis* with TLRs and other receptors is not completely understood. Nevertheless, it is clear that in the vast majority of individuals, the interaction culminates in the development of a protective Th1 dominant immune response [17]. Th1 lymphocytes are characterized by expression of IL-2 and IFN-γ.

Several mechanisms, including induction of Th2 and T-regulatory cells, contribute to host susceptibility to TB. Th2 cells are characterized by secretion of IL-4 and IL-10. T-regulatory cells are a distinct subset of T cells that suppress Th1 responses and are characterized by the cell surface expression of CD25, cytoplasmic expression of FOXP3, and secretion of IL-10 and transforming growth factor-β. TB disease and particularly disease with a poor prognosis have been associated with increased production of IL-4 and IL-10. IL-10-secreting CD8 T cells have also been described in anergic TB patients, and increased levels of CD4 CD25 regulatory T cells have been reported in

bronchoalveolar lavage of untreated TB patients. These studies imply that an imbalance in effector cell populations and modulation by regulatory T cells may determine progression from latent infection to disease.

Although the precise immune mechanisms engendering protection in the acute or latent phase of TB remain incompletely defined, current evidence supports the notion that effective acquired cellular immunity to *M. tuberculosis* is critically dependent on the activation of the Th1 subset of CD4 T cells.

Impact of TB infection on HIV

Several studies indicate that active TB accelerates HIV progression, shortening survival, although the underlying mechanisms are not completely understood.

Immunologic activation induced by *M. tuberculosis* is associated with an overproduction of cytokines, such as TNF that increases HIV replication in latently-infected cells. One study demonstrated a 5- to 160-fold increase in viral replication during the acute phase of untreated TB [18]. It is also observed that active TB sometimes induces a transient CD4 T cell depletion, which may contribute to HIV progression.

CLINICAL MANIFESTATIONS

TB is a complex, dynamic and multifaceted disease, with protean manifestations in both HIV-uninfected and HIV-infected individuals. Depending on the involved organ and the underlying immunological state (reflected by the CD4 count), TB may present as a myriad of clinical syndromes ranging from asymptomatic disease to fever of unknown origin to a fulminant presentation mimicking septic shock. In general, HIV-infected patients with high CD4 counts tend to present with clinical and radiographic manifestations of secondary TB disease similar to those seen in HIV-uninfected individuals, whereas HIV-infected patients with advanced degrees of immunosuppression are more likely to present with findings consistent with progressive primary TB. Patients with low CD4 counts often present with atypical radiographic findings or extrapulmonary and disseminated TB, reflecting the inability of their immune system to contain the infection.

Primary tuberculosis

Occult primary tuberculosis

In general, primary TB is asymptomatic in adults, and the radiographic findings are entirely normal, primary TB being diagnosed through the detection of tuberculin skin test (TST) conversion. In contrast to normal hosts, HIV-infected patients with advanced immunosuppression are less likely to have occult primary TB and are more likely to present with symptoms that will allow clinical recognition.

Uncomplicated primary tuberculosis

Occasionally, the radiologic examination can identify elements of the primary complex. The primary focus (Ghon lesion) appears as a millimetric opacity located peripherally, especially subpleural, often in the mid-lower pulmonary fields, with a reported predilection for right lung involvement. It is difficult to observe on conventional chest X-ray and thus rarely identified. The predominant radiographic finding of primary tuberculosis is hilar and/or mediastinal (paratracheal) lymphadenopathy, usually unilateral (with right predilection), sometimes bilateral. On contrast-enhanced CT scan, tuberculous lymph nodes, often measuring more than 2 cm, show a characteristic, but not pathognomonic "rim sign" consisting of a low-density center surrounded by a peripheral enhancing rim. HIV-infected patients may have more prominent lymphadenopathy associated with primary TB.

The clinical manifestations associated with these radiographic findings are subtle or absent in a host with normal immunity. HIV-infected patients are more likely to have prolonged fever and constitutional symptoms of fatigue, anorexia, weight loss, and respiratory symptoms such as persistent non-productive cough. The physical examination may reveal no abnormalities.

Primary tuberculosis with complications

The primary TB complex may be associated with relatively benign local complications, such as sero-fibrinous pleural effusion, epituberculosis, bronchial compression or bronchial perforation by lymph nodes, complications that may regress spontaneously in the absence of advanced immunosuppression.

A transient small sero-fibrinous pleural effusion associated with DTH may complicate primary TB, resolving without specific treatment in patients able to develop an adaptive immune response. Patients may experience pleuritic chest pain, and a pleural rub may be noted on the physical exam.

Epituberculosis is characterized radiographically by an extensive pneumonic opacity, related to the inflammatory changes associated with DTH and/or compression atelectasis from enlarged lymphadenopathy and with additional components related to bronchogenic spread. In contrast to the extensive radiologic changes, the clinical symptoms may be mild and include fever, cough, and dyspnea. The physical findings may reveal signs consistent with lung consolidation.

Upper or middle lobe collapse due to bronchial compression by enlarged lymph nodes may also be seen. Bronchial stenosis may be manifested clinically by non-productive cough, dyspnea, and localized wheezing. The enlarged lymph nodes may perforate into the adjacent bronchus, causing a fistula, through which the infectious caseous material can be expectorated. Clinical symptoms include low-grade fever, productive cough with muco-purulent sputum and rarely hemoptysis. Radiologic examination is not revealing. Fistulas may be diagnosed through bronchoscopic examination, and AFB smear may be positive, allowing bacteriologic confirmation.

The spectrum of progressive primary TB includes extensive lobar consolidation or bronchopneumonia, miliary TB and TB meningitis, and is a syndrome clinically indistinguishable from secondary (active) TB. It represents a severe complication of primary TB, more likely to manifest in patients with advanced immunosuppression. The extensive parenchymal involvement may lead to tissue destruction with cavity formation, fibrosis, and bronchiectasis, similar to secondary TB. Caseous bronchopneumonia evolves rapidly with altered general status, fever, weight loss, productive cough, often with hemoptysis, and the physical exam may reveal findings of consolidation or show other HIV stigmata such as oral thrush or wasting. Sputum may be positive for AFB. Radiographically, there are extensive bilateral dense, bronchopneumonic infiltrates. Miliary TB and TB meningitis are discussed below.

Secondary tuberculosis

Pulmonary tuberculosis

Classically, the onset of post-primary pulmonary TB is insidious, with non-specific constitutional symptoms such as fever, malaise, anorexia, weight loss, and nocturnal sweats that are often the earliest indicator of disease. Respiratory symptoms such as cough, dyspnea, or pleuritic chest pain develop subsequently. A pattern of onset with flu-like symptoms with fever, and upper respiratory tract congestion, may be more common in HIV-infected patients. An acute onset with hemoptysis or pleuritic chest pain is sometimes seen.

Cough, fever, fatigue, weight loss, and night sweats are the most frequent symptoms of pulmonary TB used in clinical algorithms for TB screening in both HIV-infected and HIV-uninfected individuals. Several studies were conducted to determine the performance of these symptoms in predicting the diagnosis of TB in HIV-infected patients. Screening algorithms that combine multiple symptoms have demonstrated higher sensitivity, but lower specificity. A Southeast Asian study of HIV-infected individuals has shown that the presence of cough, fatigue, fever or weight loss in the previous 4 weeks had a sensitivity greater than 70% for each of the individual symptoms, with relatively lower specificities. However, the performance of clinical indicators was greatly increased if a combination of these symptoms was used for TB screening [19]. Although the presence of cough for 2–3 weeks has traditionally served as a criterion for identifying the TB suspects, this duration was found to have a relatively low (22–33%) sensitivity in this study, whereas a cough of any duration in the previous 4 weeks had a sensitivity greater than 70%. The combination of cough of any duration, fever of any duration and night sweats lasting 3 or more weeks in the preceding 4 weeks was 93% sensitive for TB and had a negative predictive value of 97%. A subsequent WHO meta-analysis of 12 studies that included more than 8,000 HIV-infected patients concluded that the absence of current cough, fever, night sweats, and weight loss (all inclusive) had a negative predictive value of ~98% in a setting with TB prevalence >5% [20].

If present, cough is usually characterized by mucopurulent sputum production, reflecting the expectoration of caseous material. If present, hemoptysis is usually mild, manifested as bloody-streaked sputum. Moderate or severe hemoptysis may occur secondary to arterial rupture in the wall of a cavity (Rasmussen's aneurysm) or in the setting of bronchiectasis associated with fibrotic changes, as well as secondary to the development of a mycetoma or fungus ball within an old cavity (aspergilloma). Occasionally, patients may have dysphonia, suggesting laryngeal involvement, often associated with active pulmonary TB, as a result of laryngeal contamination with highly contagious caseous sputum. Pulmonary TB may often remain asymptomatic, particularly in the setting of HIV co-infection.

The contribution of physical examination to the diagnosis of TB is inferior to the radiologic examination. Fever, tachypnea, tachycardia, clubbing, or cyanosis may be seen. The chest examination may be normal or reveal rhonchi, rales, wheezing, or altered breath sounds. Occasionally, amphoric (hollow, resonant) breath sounds may be heard in large cavitary disease. Dullness to percussion or decreased breath sounds may be present over pleural effusions. The chest examination is often completely normal, contrasting with the advanced anatomic and radiographic abnormalities.

Laboratory evaluation may reveal mild leukocytosis with monocytosis. HIV-infected patients may show lymphopenia. Normochromic, normocytic anemia is often associated with TB. Elevation of ESR and CRP is nonspecific. Hyponatremia secondary to SIADH is associated with extensive lung involvement. ABG usually shows normal PaO_2, except for extensive parenchymal disease or miliary TB, which can be associated with hypoxia. Findings of hypercapnia and respiratory acidosis can be encountered in the post-tuberculous syndrome or chronic pulmonary TB, in relation to chronic structural lung disease. Pulmonary function testing is non-specific in active TB, although a restrictive pattern with decreased DLCO may be seen in patients with chronic disease.

Radiographically, the typical lesions are located in the apico-posterior lung segments or in the apical segments of the lower lobes, most commonly manifesting as heterogeneous opacities. Early stages are usually characterized by ill-defined areas of increased opacity often associated with nodular and linear opacities. If the disease is minimal it

may be best seen on apical lordotic chest radiographs or CT scan. HRCT scan may reveal early bronchogenic spread as 2- to 4-mm centrilobular nodules and linear branching opacities that represent caseous necrosis containing bacilli around terminal and respiratory bronchioles ("tree-in-bud"). This pattern is not specific to mycobacterial infection and may be seen in other infectious or inflammatory conditions. As the disease progresses, additional opacities develop that may coalesce and include small areas of increased lucency. These areas may establish communication with the tracheobronchial tree to form cavities. Aspergilloma may form within old cavities. Coughing may result in bronchogenic spread in the ipsi- or contralateral lower lung zones (apico-caudal dissemination). There may be an associated pleural effusion or pyopneumothorax if the cavities rupture into the pleural space. A marked fibrotic response may be associated with atelectasis of the upper lobe, retraction of the hilum toward the apex, compensatory lower lobe hyperinflation, and mediastinal shift towards the fibrotic lung. Complete destruction of a whole lung can be seen in advanced cases.

In TB associated with HIV infection, radiographic manifestations correlate with the level of immunosuppression. In patients with CD4 counts >350 cells/mm³, TB presents with classical radiographic findings of reactivation disease. In patients with fewer CD4 cells, the likelihood of atypical radiographic findings increases, and up to 20% of patients may have a normal or near-normal chest radiograph. In a study of radiographic patterns of TB in HIV-infected patients, diffused or localized infiltration were more frequent, as well as hilar or mediastinal lymphadenopathy. Pleural disease, cavitation, and normal radiography were the least common findings [21]. However, studies conducted in Africa demonstrated a greater frequency of cavitation in HIV-infected patients with TB, possibly related to the high incidence of TB in this region. Several radiographical forms of pulmonary TB are illustrated in Fig. 26.2.

Extrapulmonary tuberculosis

HIV infection is associated with a higher frequency of extrapulmonary disease, including the more serious forms, disseminated (miliary) TB and TB meningitis.

Miliary TB

Miliary TB usually presents with fever, weight loss, night sweats, and minimal or absent localizing symptoms or signs. Physical examination may show pathognomonic choroidal tubercles in 15% of cases (bilateral, raised white-yellow plaques on funduscopic examination), lymphadenopathy, and hepatomegaly. Chest radiograph may show multiple bilateral small opacities resembling millet seeds (miliary infiltrates). The yield of sputum AFB microscopy and culture is low, averaging 30% and 50%, respectively, with variations across the reported series. The diagnosis can be improved

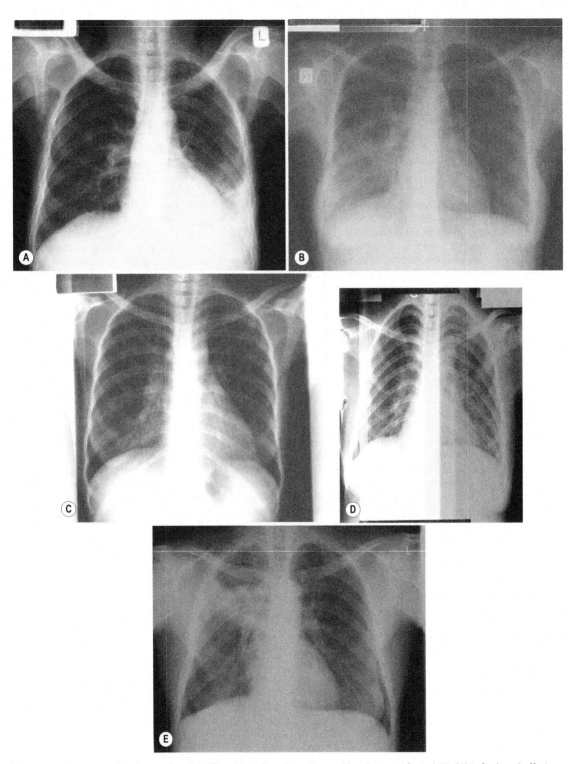

Figure 26.2 Representative chest radiographs from Ugandan HIV patients with culture-confirmed TB: (A) Left pleural effusion; (B) right cavitary disease; (C) right lower lobe infiltrate; (D) miliary infiltrate; (E) right upper lobe infiltrate.

by using a combination of smear and culture from sputum, bronchoalveolar lavage, CSF, bone marrow, gastric aspirate and biopsies from multiple sites: transbronchial, pleural, bone marrow, liver or lymph nodes. In the HIV-infected patients with advanced immunodeficiency, blood cultures are positive for *M. tuberculosis* in 20–40% of patients.

TB meningitis

TB meningitis usually presents with fever, headache, and meningismus and occasionally depressed levels of consciousness, diplopia or hemiparesis. Physical examination shows stiff neck and occasionally cranial neuropathy (nerves VI, III, IV, VII) and long tract signs. Chest radiograph may be consistent with primary or miliary TB. Brain imaging may show contrast enhancement over the basilar meninges, hypodense areas consistent with infarcts, hydrocephalus and occasionally focal inflammatory lesions (tuberculomas). CSF shows elevated protein level, low glucose concentration, and pleocytosis with lymphocytosis. The AFB smear and culture are rarely positive, with less than one-third of patients having a positive CSF smear or culture. Nucleic acid amplification tests (PCR) can be used if available, although the use of this technology for non-respiratory specimens has not been validated.

TB lymphadenitis

The supraclavicular and posterior cervical lymph nodes are most frequently involved, in contrast to scrofula due to atypical mycobacteria or *M. bovis*, which usually involves the submandibular and high anterior cervical lymph nodes. The lymphadenitis is not painful, and aspiration of the lymph node with the finding of AFB or biopsy with findings of caseating granulomas can establish the diagnosis in 25–50% of the patients.

Pleural TB

Pleural TB occurs by direct extension from an adjacent subpleural pulmonary focus or through hematogenous seeding. Typical presentation is the abrupt onset of fever, pleuritic chest pain, and cough. Occasionally there is an insidious presentation with fever, weight loss, and malaise. If the pleural effusion is large enough, there may be shortness of breath. Physical examination shows dullness to percussion and decreased breath sounds. Egophony is a helpful sign if present. Chest radiograph typically shows unilateral pleural effusion more frequently in the right hemithorax. Bilateral disease is seen in 10% of cases. Pleural fluid analysis demonstrates high protein concentration, low glucose concentration, and lymphocytosis. The presence of >5% mesothelial cells in the pleural fluid usually argues against a diagnosis of TB pleural effusion, as the chronic pleural inflammation is thought to prevent the exfoliation of mesothelial cells in the pleural cavity. The AFB smear is positive in less than 10% of cases, and the yield of culture has been less than 30% in most series, with a range

between 12% and 70%. In patients co-infected with HIV, the yield of pleural fluid and pleural biopsy culture may be higher than in HIV-uninfected individuals with TB pleurisy [22]. Pleural biopsy may show granulomas in approximately half of the cases, and the yield is higher on pleural biopsy culture. An elevated concentration (>70 U/L) of pleural fluid adenosine deaminase (ADA) may suggest the diagnosis of TB.

TB peritonitis

TB peritonitis may present with abdominal pain, fever, night sweats, and weight loss. The physical examination shows ascites, and abdominal tenderness may be present. The classic sign is a "doughy abdomen," because matted loops of bowel may be palpable. The peritoneal fluid analysis reveals an exudative fluid with elevated cell count, typically with lymphocytic predominance. The AFB smear is rarely positive, and culture yield is generally low, averaging 25–30%. The best method for diagnosis is a laparoscopic-guided peritoneal biopsy, which has a diagnostic yield of 65–68% with culture and a histopathologic yield of 85–97%. In areas endemic for TB and HIV, the finding of intra-abdominal lymphadenopathy on abdominal ultrasound or CT scan is often used to support the diagnosis of abdominal TB.

Gastrointestinal TB

The ileo-cecal area is the site most typically involved in gastrointestinal TB, although any other part of the gastrointestinal tract may be affected. The patient usually presents with fever, abdominal pain, diarrhea, gastrointestinal bleeding or obstruction. Radiologic examination of the small bowel and abdominal CT scan show involvement of the terminal ileum resembling Crohn's disease. The diagnosis is made on clinical suspicion in areas endemic for TB and HIV or by the finding of TB elsewhere. Occasionally intra-luminal biopsy of the terminal ileum or other involved sites is used to establish the diagnosis.

TB pericarditis

The usual presentation is chronic but may occasionally be subacute, with fever, night sweats, chest pain, shortness of breath, pedal edema, and other signs of right heart failure reflecting pericardial restriction. Physical examination shows signs of pericardial disease, right-sided heart failure or tamponade. Pulsus paradoxus, defined as an exaggeration of the normal inspiratory fall of systolic blood pressure, may be an extremely helpful sign. Pericardial aspiration and biopsy are the diagnostic procedures of choice. Pericardial fluid is characterized by low bacterial burden, with frequent negative smear microscopy (yield of 0–40% in different series) and culture (yield averaging 50% with Lowenstein–Jensen media, higher with liquid media or BACTEC). Histopathologic examination of pericardial tissue may show caseating granulomas and/or AFB, with a widely variable diagnostic yield (10–60%).

Renal TB

The patient may be asymptomatic or manifest dysuria, hematuria, and flank pain. The diagnosis often is suggested by the finding of sterile pyuria or hematuria as presenting abnormalities that trigger evaluation. Physical examination is usually unremarkable. Intravenous pyelography or CT scan shows cortical scarring, occasionally with mass or cavitary lesions, papillary necrosis with caliceal and ureteral dilation, and "beading" of the ureter due to ureteral strictures.

Vertebral osteomyelitis

The lower thoracic and lumbar vertebrae are involved most commonly. The disk space is initially spared, but involved later in the course of disease, with spread to adjacent vertebrae. Paravertebral "cold abscesses" may dissect through tissue planes. Patients present with back and sometimes radicular pain. Physical examination may show a gibbus deformity due to anterior compression fractures and paraparesis may be present occasionally. Radiographic evaluation of the spine including CT scan and MRI may show abnormalities in adjacent vertebrae with anterior compression or paravertebral inflammatory collections/abscesses. Vertebral biopsy for microbiological and histopathological examination assists in the diagnosis.

DIAGNOSIS

The worldwide distribution of *M. tuberculosis* and its potential to involve most body organs should remind clinicians to keep TB in the differential diagnosis for a long list of acute, subacute, and chronic clinical syndromes. In the setting of HIV the risk of TB is higher and diagnosis potentially more difficult.

Diagnosis of latent TB infection (LTBI)

By definition, LTBI refers to asymptomatic *M. tuberculosis* infection with no evidence of active disease; however, the distinction between LTBI and early TB disease may be difficult in clinical practice. The rates of subclinical TB are higher in HIV-infected individuals [23]. Therefore, the WHO recommends that adults and adolescents living with HIV should be screened for TB at every medical visit to facilitate either isoniazid preventive therapy (IPT) in people unlikely to have active TB or additional diagnostic evaluation for TB in symptomatic people [24].

No direct methods for the identification of patients who are latently infected with *M. tuberculosis* are currently available. Consequently, the diagnosis of LTBI relies on the quantification of immune responses induced by the infection with *M. tuberculosis*, using tuberculin skin tests (TSTs) or interferon-gamma releasing assays (IGRAs), and the exclusion of active TB.

Tuberculin skin test

TST positivity is a marker of DTH directed towards antigens of *M. tuberculosis* and other mycobacteria.

Until recently, the only available tool to diagnose *M. tuberculosis* infection was TST, a well-validated, but 100-year-old test with multiple limitations, including instability over time, poor specificity due to cross-reactivity with antigens present in environmental mycobacteria and bacille Calmette-Guérin (BCG) vaccine strains, as well as decreased sensitivity in certain clinical conditions such as advanced stages of HIV infection. In addition, the TST does not distinguish TB disease from LTBI, and a single determination of TST does not indicate the time *M. tuberculosis* infection occurred, which is important, as recent TST converters are at higher risk of disease progression.

TST is performed using the Mantoux technique, consisting of the intradermal injection of purified protein derivative (PPD) or RT-23 on the inner surface of the forearm and measuring the induration (not erythema) 48 to 72 hours later.

Interpretation of the tuberculin test depends on the epidemiological context, age, co-morbidities, and general health of the skin-tested individuals, which could affect T cell-mediated immunity. The tuberculin reaction can be boosted by repeated tuberculin tests, BCG vaccination or infection with environmental mycobacteria. In defining a positive TST in HIV-infected individuals, guidelines generally recommend the use of a lower cutoff, such as the presence of an induration ≥5 mm in diameter at 48 hours [25].

TST, when feasible, remains a useful tool to detect *M. tuberculosis* infection. In resource-constrained settings, TST should not be a requirement for initiating IPT for people living with HIV; however, TST-positive patients benefit more from IPT than those who are TST negative [24].

Interferon-gamma releasing assays (IGRAs)

IGRAs, QuantiFERON-TB Gold, QuantiFERON-TB Gold In-Tube (both from Cellestis, Victoria, Australia), and T-SPOT.TB (Oxford Immunotec, Oxford, United Kingdom) measure the amount of IFN-γ released from sensitized human T cells after exposure to *M. tuberculosis*. The development of IGRAs significantly improved the specificity of the diagnosis of *M. tuberculosis* infection because the assay is based on early secretory antigenic target-6 (ESAT-6) and culture filtrate protein 10 (CFP-10) antigens which are specific to *M. tuberculosis* and not present in most environmental mycobacteria or BCG strains.

A recent systematic review and meta-analysis that included over 5,700 HIV-infected individuals reported that pooled sensitivity was higher for T-SPOT than for

QuantifERON-Gold (72 vs 61%, respectively); however, neither IGRA was more sensitive than TST [26]. The performance of IGRAs is decreased in HIV-infected individuals, especially if the CD4 counts are low. Other limitations include the limited experience with IGRA use and the uncertainty in result interpretation, especially when there is discordance between IGRA and TST, and discordance between different IGRA types or serial IGRA results (reversion/conversion). The WHO does not recommend IGRA to screen for eligibility to receive IPT for HIV-infected patients living in resource-constrained settings.

The Centers for Disease Control and Prevention (CDC) states that IGRAs can be used interchangeably with TST in all circumstances in which TST is indicated, including contact investigation, evaluation of recent immigrants who have had BCG vaccination, and TB screening of healthcare workers and others undergoing serial evaluation. The CDC suggests that an IGRA might be preferred for testing persons who will be unlikely to return for TST reading or those who have received BCG vaccine [27].

Although routine testing with both TST and an IGRA is not generally recommended, performance of both tests may be considered when the initial test (TST or IGRA) is negative in several situations associated with an increased risk for infection, progression or poor outcome, such as HIV infection.

Diagnosis of active pulmonary tuberculosis

Clinical symptoms

Several studies evaluated the performance of different clinical predictors of TB and proposed symptom-based algorithms for TB screening in people living with HIV, as discussed above. TB screening is potentially relevant to the diagnosis of active TB, but also to exclude TB in candidates for preventive therapy.

At extremely high TB prevalence rates, symptomatic screening is inadequate and ideally should be supplemented with sputum culture. In this setting, consideration should be given to empirical TB treatment, particularly if ART is to be initiated, given the inherent risk of "unmasking TB," as discussed below.

Chest radiography

Chest radiography is a sensitive but non-specific test to detect pulmonary TB. Radiographic examination of the thorax may be useful to identify persons for further evaluation, but a diagnosis of TB should never be established by radiography alone. Reliance on the chest radiograph as the only diagnostic test for TB will result in both over-diagnosis and missed diagnosis of TB. HIV-infected patients who present with an abnormal chest radiograph but no respiratory symptoms may still have significant pulmonary disease [28].

TB may also present with respiratory symptoms and a normal chest radiograph. Similarly, active pulmonary TB cannot be distinguished from inactive disease on the basis of radiography alone, and readings of "fibrosis" or "scarring" do not exclude active disease.

Sputum microscopy

The microscopic examination of stained sputum is the most frequently relied upon diagnostic test, as it is feasible in nearly all settings, and the diagnosis of TB can be strongly inferred by finding AFB by microscopic examination. In high prevalence areas, finding AFB in stained sputum is highly specific for TB and, thus is the equivalent of a confirmed diagnosis. Identification of AFB by microscopic examination has multiple advantages: it is the most rapid method for determining if a person has TB, identifies persons who are at greatest risk of dying from the disease (although the case-fatality rate is high in smear-negative HIV-infected TB patients), and identifies the most likely transmitters of infection. The main limitations of smear microscopy include its low sensitivity (50–60% in most studies), inability to allow species identification and drug susceptibility testing, and inability to distinguish viable from dead bacteria while monitoring the response to treatment. Moreover, the prevalence of smear-negative TB may vary between 30% and 50% and increases in HIV co-infection proportional to the magnitude of immunodeficiency [29].

Smear-negative pulmonary TB constitutes a significant public health problem leading to delays in diagnosis, over- or under-treatment and increased *M. tuberculosis* transmission. A diagnosis of smear-negative pulmonary TB can be made if two sputum specimens are smear-negative but chest radiography findings suggest TB and the clinician decides to treat with a full course of TB therapy. Response to therapy may provide confirmatory evidence. In addition, a diagnosis of smear-negative TB can be established if a patient with AFB smear-negative sputum has a culture positive for *M. tuberculosis*.

The probability of finding AFB in sputum smears by microscopy is directly proportional to the density of bacilli in the sputum. Sputum microscopy is likely to be positive when there are at least 5000–10,000 organisms/mL of sputum. At densities below 1000 organisms/mL of sputum, the chance of observing AFB in a smear is less than 10%. In contrast, properly performed culture can detect far lower numbers AFB (detection limit is 100 organisms/mL).

Several studies have examined the optimum number of sputum specimens to establish a diagnosis of pulmonary TB. It has been conclusively shown that microscopy of two consecutive sputum specimens identifies the vast majority (95–98%) of smear-positive TB patients, whereas a third sputum specimen adds minimally to the diagnosis. Therefore, in 2007 the WHO recommended reduction in the number of specimens examined from three to two, in settings of good quality of microscopy.

Fluorescence microscopy, in which auramine-based staining causes the AFB to fluoresce against a dark background, may be 10% more sensitive than conventional Ziehl–Neelsen (ZN) staining with light microscopy and have equivalent specificity. These characteristics make fluorescence microscopy a more accurate test, although the increased cost and complexity make it less applicable in many settings.

Light-emitting diode (LED) microscopy is a novel diagnostic tool that has demonstrated accuracy equivalent to international reference standards, increase in sensitivity 6% over conventional ZN microscopy, and qualitative, operational and cost advantages relative to both conventional fluorescent and ZN microscopy.

Mycobacterial culture

Mycobacterial culture also improves TB detection, increasing the number of diagnosed cases by 30–50%. Conventional drug susceptibility testing (DST), in turn, allows a definitive diagnosis of drug-resistant TB.

Traditional solid culture media (Lowenstein–Jensen or Ogawa) are more sensitive than AFB microscopy, but require from 2–3 weeks to several months to yield colonies of *M. tuberculosis* and may have a high rate of contamination. Other solid media techniques (7 H9, 7 H10, and 7 H11) have lower contaminations rates but are, in general, too onerous for low-income laboratory settings. Newer liquid culture automated systems for mycobacteria detection and susceptibility testing can provide faster culture results (7–21 days) and are currently considered the gold-standard approach for isolating mycobacteria. The most commonly used automated liquid culture systems are BACTEC 460 TB which detects radiolabeled CO_2 from replicating mycobacteria and the BACTEC MGIT 960 system which relies on a fluorescent, non-radiometric method (both from Becton Dickinson, Franklin Lakes, NJ, USA). Other non-radiometric automated liquid culture systems include the BacT/ALERT MB system (bioMerieux Inc., Durham, NC, USA) and the VersaTREK system (Trek Diagnostic Systems, West Lake, OH, USA). Studies have shown that liquid systems increase the yield by 10% compared with solid media and significantly reduce time to results. For DST, the delay may be reduced to 10 days, compared to 28–42 days with conventional solid media. The WHO endorses the use of liquid TB culture and drug susceptibility testing in low-resource settings.

DST techniques include phenotypic methods on solid and liquid media (culturing *M. tuberculosis* in the presence of anti-TB drugs to detect growth which indicates drug resistance) and genotypic methods that identify specific molecular mutations associated with resistance against individual drugs. DST is most accurate for rifampicin and isoniazid and less reliable and reproducible for streptomycin, ethambutol and pyrazinamide. Rifampicin resistance is a valid and reliable indicator of MDR-TB. Once MDR-TB

has been confirmed, additional first- and second-line drug susceptibility results should be obtained. The WHO recommends several non-commercial culture and DST methods such as microscopically observed drug susceptibility (MODS), nitrate reductase assay (NRA), and colorimetric redox indicator (CRI) methods to be used in resource-constrained settings in patients suspected of having MDR-TB. In general, these methods are not subjected to optimal levels of standardization and quality control.

Nucleic acid amplification tests (NAATs)

Multiple NAATs have been developed to detect mycobacterial nucleic acid using polymerase chain reaction (PCR) amplification, molecular beacons, transcription-mediated amplification (TMA), strand displacement amplification (SDA), ligase chain reaction (LCR) amplification, and loop-mediated isothermal amplification (LAMP).

Conventional NAATs have been used for several years, and they have high specificity, but limited sensitivity, especially for smear-negative pulmonary TB and for non-respiratory specimens. The accuracy of both commercial and non-commercial (in house- or "home brew") assays was found to be highly variable in meta-analyses.

CDC recommends that NAAT be performed on at least one respiratory specimen from each patient with suspected TB to aid in the initial diagnosis, and in persons for whom the test result would alter case management or TB control activities [30].

The newly approved Xpert MTB/RIF assay (Cepheid, Sunnyvale, CA, USA) is a fully automated NAAT platform that can simultaneously detect TB and rifampicin resistance. A validation study involving over 1,700 individuals with suspected TB showed a sensitivity of 98.2% for smear-positive, culture-confirmed cases with a single test and 90.2% for smear-negative cases with 3 tests, with a specificity of 99.2%. The test correctly identified 97.6% of rifampicin-resistant bacteria [31]. The assay allows identification of *M. tuberculosis* and detects resistance to rifampicin within 90 minutes, is not prone to cross-contamination, requires minimal biosafety, and offers multiple advantages over conventional NAATs. In 2010, the WHO endorsed this test, strongly recommending its use as the initial diagnostic test in individuals suspected of MDR-TB or HIV-TB. The limitation is cost of the equipment and the sputum cartridges.

Line probe assays (LPAs)

LPAs are used for molecular detection of drug resistance from smear-positive specimens or cultures, allowing the detection of resistance to rifampicin, isoniazid, fluoroquinolones, aminoglycosides or ethambutol. In 2008, WHO endorsed the use of LPAs for rapid detection of MDR-TB at the country level.

Phage-based assays

Phage-amplification assays have high specificity, but lower sensitivity for the diagnosis of active pulmonary TB and can be used for the detection of rifampicin resistance on culture isolates. However, studies evaluating this technology have shown inconsistent results.

Serologic, antibody detection tests

Available serologic tests have shown inconsistent results and thus are of low clinical value. Marketing and use of sub-standard serodiagnostics in some resource-limited environments is problematic.

Antigen detection tests

Studies evaluating the detection of urinary lipoarabino-mannan (LAM), a lipoglycan in the mycobacterial cell wall, found variable test performance. However, recent data suggest that LAM performance may be better in HIV-infected individuals. It may have a place in the diagnosis of TB in the setting of advanced immunodeficiency.

Serum biomarkers

There is an enormous need for biomarkers for TB, such as biomarkers that predict protection induced by vaccination, distinguish between latent or active disease or predict relapse or durable cure. Unfortunately, clinically relevant biomarkers are not currently available. A recent study reported the identification of a gene expression signature dominated by a neutrophil-driven IFN-inducible gene profile that differentiates between latent and active TB [32]. Research on biomarkers needs additional evaluation and validation, especially in people living with HIV.

TREATMENT

The treatment of TB focuses on both the patient and the community and should be designed to cure the patient without relapse, prevent transmission to others, and prevent the development of resistant organisms. The decision to initiate anti-tuberculous therapy should be based on clinical and radiographic findings and epidemiological data. It is sometimes necessary to initiate treatment before the results of smear and culture are known, particularly in high HIV prevalence settings, where the prevalence of smear-negative TB is increased. The threshold for initiation of empirical therapy must be low in patients with potentially life-threatening infections such as meningitis, pericarditis, and miliary disease.

Several national and international organizations have recommended treatment regimens for TB [33, 34].

All recommendations comprise two phases. WHO-recommended treatment regimens are summarized in Table 26.1.

For smear-positive pulmonary TB patients treated with first-line drugs, sputum smear microscopy may be performed at completion of the intensive phase of treatment: the end of the second month for the 6-month regimen or the end of the third month for the 8-month retreatment regimen (conditional/high and moderate grade of evidence). If the specimen obtained at the end of the second month is smear-positive, sputum smear microscopy should be obtained at the end of the third month (strong/high grade of evidence) and, if positive, sputum culture and DST should be performed (strong/high grade of evidence). The available evidence shows that sputum positivity at the end of the intensive phase is a poor predictor of relapse and failure in individual patients. Therefore, the WHO is no longer recommending the extension of the intensive phase if a positive sputum smear is found at completion of the intensive phase in patients treated with a regimen containing rifampicin throughout treatment (strong/high grade of evidence). However, the WHO continues to recommend performing smear microscopy at this stage because a positive smear should trigger an assessment of the patient, as well as additional sputum monitoring.

The WHO recommends obtaining sputum specimens for smear microscopy at the end of months 5 and 6 for all new pulmonary TB patients who were smear-positive at the start of treatment. Patients whose sputum smears are positive at month 5 or 6 are considered to have failed treatment.

Previously treated TB is a strong risk factor for resistance, 15% of previously treated TB patients having MDR-TB at a global level. For previously treated patients, the WHO recommends performing culture and DST for at least isoniazid and rifampicin before the start of treatment. In settings where rapid molecular-based DST is available, the results should guide the choice of regimen, whereas in settings where testing is not routinely available, empirical treatment should be started. TB patients whose treatment has failed or other patient groups with high likelihood of MDR-TB should be started on an empirical MDR regimen, in accordance with country-specific resistance data. Empirical regimens for MDR-TB are often inadequate, contributing to disease progression and propagation of drug-resistant disease. TB patients returning after defaulting or relapsing from their first treatment course may receive the retreatment regimen containing first-line drugs 2HRZES/1HRZE/5HRE (H = isoniazid, R = rifampicin, Z = pyrazinamide, E = ethambutol, S = streptomycin) if country-specific data show low or medium levels of MDR in these patients.

Patients with extrapulmonary TB should be treated with the same regimen as patients with pulmonary TB. Some experts recommend 9–12 months of treatment for TB meningitis given the serious risk of disability and mortality, and 9 months of treatment for TB of bones or joints because of the difficulties of assessing treatment response. Unless drug

Table 26.1 WHO-recommended treatment regimens

TREATMENT CATEGORY	TREATMENT		COMMENTS (GRADE OF EVIDENCE)
	Intensive phase	Continuation phase	
New TB (presumed, or known, to have drug-susceptible TB)	2 months of HRZE[a] daily	4 months of HR[b] daily	Optimal (strong/high grade of evidence)
	2 months of HRZE[a] daily	4 months of HR[b] three times per week	Acceptable alternative provided that the patient is receiving directly observed therapy (conditional/high or moderate grade of evidence)
	2 months of HRZE[a] three times per week	4 months of HR[b] three times per week	Acceptable alternative provided that the patient is receiving directly observed therapy and is not living with HIV or living in an HIV-prevalent setting (conditional/high or moderate grade of evidence)
Retreatment regimen with first-line drugs (relapse or default/low or medium likelihood of MDR)	2 months of HRZES and 1 month HRZE	5 months of HRE	Regimen should be modified once DST results are available
MDR regimen (failure/high likelihood of MDR)	Empirical MDR regimen (country specific)		Regimen should be modified once DST results are available

H = isoniazid, R = rifampicin, Z = pyrazinamide, E = ethambutol, S = streptomycin.
[a]In tuberculous meningitis, ethambutol should be replaced by streptomycin (2 months of HRZS in the intensive phase)
[b]In populations with known or suspected high levels of isoniazid resistance, new TB patients may receive HRE as therapy in the continuation phase as an acceptable alternative to HR (Weak/Insufficient evidence, expert opinion).
Based on World Health Organization. Treatment of tuberculosis guidelines-Fourth edition [online]. 2010. Available from— http://whqlibdoc.who.int/publications/2010/9789241547833_eng.pdf

resistance is suspected, adjuvant corticosteroid treatment is recommended for TB meningitis and pericarditis.

The first-line drugs should be employed preferentially; the use of second-line therapies should be restricted to patients with documented resistance or patients with limiting conditions. The recommended dosing for the first- and second-line drugs is presented in Table 26.2 and Table 26.3, respectively. Discussion of the treatment of MDR-TB is complex and beyond the scope of this chapter. It should be restricted to referral treatment centers.

Treatment of TB in special populations

Pregnancy or breastfeeding

The WHO recommends the treatment of TB in pregnant women using isoniazid, rifampicin, pyrazinamide, and ethambutol, whereas US guidelines do not recommend pyrazinamide unless there is no alternative. Streptomycin is ototoxic to the fetus and should not be used during pregnancy. The risks of untreated TB in a pregnant woman far outweigh the risks of the medications. A breastfeeding woman who has TB should receive a full course of TB treatment and she can continue to breastfeed. After active TB is excluded, the baby should receive 6 months of IPT, followed by BCG vaccination. Most anti-TB drugs are safe for breastfeeding and are not significantly concentrated in breast milk.

Liver disease

The presence of concomitant liver disease has to be evaluated before TB treatment is initiated. Whereas hepatotoxicity due to isoniazid is more likely as age increases, this should not preclude treatment of TB. Any signs of liver toxicity should be investigated promptly. WHO recommends reducing the number of hepatotoxic drugs in patients with advanced or unstable liver disease. Guidelines recommend monitoring of liver enzymes in all patients with pre-existing liver disease (viral hepatitis, alcoholism, etc.). If a patient with liver failure requires treatment for TB, ethambutol, streptomycin, and a fluoroquinolone may be used. The most important risk factor for isoniazid-induced hepatotoxicity is alcohol consumption. Patients receiving isoniazid should be counseled to abstain from alcohol use.

Table 26.2 Routes of administration, normal and adjusted doses for first-line TB drugs in adults and children

DRUG	ROUTE	NORMAL DOSES						ADJUSTED DOSES	
		Daily dose (range)			Three times per week				
		Children mg/kg (range)	Adults mg/kg (range)	Max mg	Children mg/kg (range)	Adults mg/kg (range)	Max mg	Renal impairment	Hepatic impairment
Isoniazid	p.o, i.m, i.v.	10 (10–15)	5 (4–6)	300	10	10 (8–12)	900	No change	No change
Rifampicin	p.o, i.v.	15 (10–20)	10 (8–12)	600	10	10 (8–12)	600	No change	No change, frequent monitoring
Rifabutin	p.o	—	5	300	—	5	300	No change	No change, frequent monitoring
Pyrazinamide	p.o.	35 (30–40)	25 (20–30)	—	35	35 (30–40)	—	25–35 mg/kg 3×/week, not daily if creatinine clearance <30 mL/min	No change, frequent monitoring
Ethambutol	p.o.	20 (15–25)	15 (15–20)	—	30	30 (25–35)	—	15–25 mg/kg 3×/week, not daily if creatinine clearance <70 mL/min	No change
Streptomycin	i.m, i.v.	NR	15 (12–18)		NR	15 (12–18)	1000	15 mg/kg 3×/week, not daily	No change

Based on American Thoracic Society, CDC, and Infectious Diseases Society of America. Treatment of Tuberculosis [online]. 2007. Available from: http://www.cdc.gov/mmwr/preview/mmwrhtml/rr5211a1.htm#tab15 and World Health Organization. Treatment of tuberculosis guidelines, 4th edn [online]. 2010. Available from: http://whqlibdoc.who.int/publications/2010/9789241547833_eng.pdf

Renal disease

Isoniazid, rifampicin, and pyrazinamide are metabolized by the liver and thus safe to use in patients with renal disease. Ethambutol is excreted through urine and consideration should be given to replacing it with a second-line drug. Streptomycin should be avoided in patients with renal failure because of nephrotoxicity. Patients should receive their medications after hemodialysis. Patients with renal disease are at risk for neuropathy and should receive pyridoxine.

Pyridoxine

All patients with HIV infection, diabetes, renal failure, malnutrition, pregnant and breastfeeding women, and persons with seizures should receive pyridoxine 25 mg/day for prevention of neuropathy while receiving isoniazid. In patients with established neuropathy, higher doses of pyridoxine should be used for neuropathy treatment (75–100 mg/day).

New drugs

Fluoroquinolones

Several fluoroquinolones, such as ciprofloxacin, levofloxacin; and ofloxacin, have been used as second-line drugs for the treatment of MDR-TB. Gatifloxacin and moxifloxacin, the most recently developed fluoroquinolones showed better *in vitro* activity against *M. tuberculosis* than the older compounds and better rates of sputum conversion at 2 months when substituted for ethambutol or isoniazid in phase 2 trials; they are being evaluated in phase 3 trials for possible use in treatment of drug-susceptible TB to shorten duration of therapy to 4 months.

Table 26.3 Routes of administration, normal and adjusted doses for the second-line TB drugs in adults and children

DRUG	ROUTE	NORMAL DOSES			ADJUSTED DOSES	
		Daily dose (range)				
		Children	Adults (usual dose)	Max	Renal impairment	Hepatic impairment
Cycloserine	p.o.	10–15 mg/kg/day	10–15 mg/kg/day (500 mg twice daily)	1000 mg	Contraindicated if creatinine clearance <50 mL/min unless on hemodialysis 500 mg/dose, 3×/week if on hemodialysis	No change
Ethionamide, prothionamide	p.o.	15–20 mg/kg/day	15–20 mg/kg/day (500–750 mg daily or 2 divided doses)	1000 mg	250–500 mg daily if creatinine clearance <30 mL/min or on hemodialysis	No change, but use with caution
Amikacin, kanamycin	i.m, i.v.	15–30 mg/kg/day	15 mg/kg/day	1000 mg	12–15 mg/kg/dose, 3×/week, not daily	No change
Capreomycin	i.m, i.v.	15–30 mg/kg/day	15 mg/kg/day	1000 mg	12–15 mg/kg/dose, 3×/week, not daily	No change
P-aminosalicylic acid	p.o.	200–300 mg/kg/day in 2–4 divided doses	8–12 g/day (4 g thrice daily)		Contraindicated in severe renal impairment unless on hemodialysis 4 g twice daily after hemodialysis	No change
Levofloxacin	p.o, i.v.	NR	500–1000 mg/day		750–1000 mg/dose, 3×/week, not daily	No change
Moxifloxacin	p.o.	NR	400 mg/day		Decrease dose/increase interval	No change
Gatifloxacin	p.o.	NR	400 mg/day		Decrease dose/increase interval	No change

Based on American Thoracic Society, CDC, and Infectious Diseases Society of America. Treatment of Tuberculosis [online]. 2007. Available from: http://www.cdc.gov/mmwr/preview/mmwrhtml/rr5211a1.htm#tab15

Diarylquinolines

TMC 207 is a new ATP-synthase inhibitor that was shown to be highly potent against both drug-susceptible and drug-resistant strains of *M. tuberculosis*. The agent showed favorable 2-month culture conversion rates for MDR-TB therapy in a phase 2 trial. The second stage of the study is in progress to evaluate the microbiological outcomes at 6 months with the addition of TMC 207 to the individualized treatment for MDR-TB.

Nitroimidazoles

Nitroimidazoles are agents that exert their antimycobacterial activity through a novel mechanism of bioreduction, shown to be active against drug-susceptible and drug-resistant strains of *M. tuberculosis*. In addition, nitroimidazoles are active against replicating and non-replicating bacteria, suggesting their potential to shorten the duration of treatment for active disease and a possible role in the management of latent infection. Two nitroimidazoles are in phase 2 clinical development: OPC-67683 and PA-824.

Ethylenediamines

SQ-109 is a derivative of ethambutol that inhibits mycobacterial cell wall synthesis and acts synergistically with isoniazid and rifampicin, suggesting its potential to shorten the duration of TB treatment. The compound has demonstrated excellent *in vitro* activity against drug-susceptible and drug-resistant bacteria, including XDR-TB, as well as potent *in vivo* activity against pulmonary TB. A phase 2 trial for treatment of drug-susceptible pulmonary TB is currently recruiting subjects.

Oxazolidinones

Linezolid has modest *in vitro* activity against *M. tuberculosis*, exerting its effect through the inhibition of ribosome synthesis. It has been used off-label in combination regimens for the treatment of MDR-TB, but its effectiveness remains uncertain. It is presently evaluated in two distinct phase 2 trials for treatment of XDR-TB and MDR-TB. A close analogue of linezolid, PNU-100480, demonstrated slightly better activity *in vitro* and significantly improved bactericidal activity *in vivo* when added to first-line TB drugs or used in combination with moxifloxacin and pyrazinamide and a phase 2 trial for treatment of drug-susceptible TB is under way.

Rifamycins

Rifamycins are potent inhibitors of bacterial RNA polymerase. Rifapentine is a more potent analogue of rifampicin and has a longer half-life, characteristics that make it an attractive candidate for shortening the duration of treatment and for intermittent treatment. In a trial of once-weekly rifapentine and isoniazid in the continuation phase of treatment, efficacy was suboptimal, especially in HIV-infected patients who were at increased risk of relapse secondary to acquired rifamycin resistance. Several phase 2 trials are in progress to assess the effects of daily rifapentine in the intensive phase of treatment from the perspective of shortening treatment of drug-susceptible TB.

A number of other novel TB drugs are in preclinical development.

Special issues of treatment in HIV-infected individuals

Rifamycins are a key component of anti-tuberculous treatment in HIV-infected patients. A systematic review of treatment of TB in the setting of HIV co-infection found lower relapse rates in people living with HIV treated with 8 or more months of rifampicin-containing regimens compared with using 2 months of rifamycin [35]. The review showed that, compared with daily therapy in the initial phase, thrice-weekly therapy was associated with higher rates of failure and relapse.

Rifapentine, a long-acting rifamycin, is not recommended in HIV-infected patients due to increased risks of development of drug resistance.

Thiacetazone should never be given to HIV-infected patients because of its diminished efficacy and association with severe skin reactions.

Low serum concentrations of antimycobacterial drugs in HIV-infected patients may contribute to treatment failures.

A study of 91 patients in Botswana (68% HIV-infected) found low serum drug concentrations in a significant proportion of patients undergoing TB treatment: rifampicin (78%), isoniazid (30%), and ethambutol (41%). Only 1% of patients had low levels of pyrazinamide. Importantly, 26% had low plasma levels of both rifampicin and isoniazid, a factor that may contribute to poor outcomes and the emergence of resistance in a clinical setting [36]. Clinical studies of high-dose rifampicin are planned.

Co-administration of TB and HIV treatment

The rifamycins are a key component of TB regimen, but their use in patients with HIV co-infection is complicated by drug interactions with ART. Rifampicin, a potent stimulator of the cytochrome P450 CYP3A4 system is prone to drug–drug interactions with several antiretroviral drugs including non-nucleoside reverse transcriptase inhibitors (NNRTIs) and protease inhibitors (PIs). Nucleoside reverse transcriptase inhibitors (NRTIs) are not metabolized by the cytochrome P450 system and thus are not susceptible to drug interactions with the rifamycins. Rifampicin is also a potent inducer of UGT1A1 involved in the metabolism of raltegravir, an HIV-integrase inhibitor, and therefore has the potential to reduce raltegravir concentrations.

The preferred first-line ART in treatment-naive adults with HIV-TB co-infection is zidovudine/lamivudine/efavirenz or tenofovir/emtricitabine/efavirenz. In patients starting ART while on TB treatment, the preferred NNRTI is efavirenz because of less drug interaction with rifampicin compared with nevirapine. For co-infected individuals who are unable to tolerate efavirenz, a nevirapine-based regimen is an alternative. Similarly, a triple NRTI regimen, either zidovudine/lamivudine/abacavir, or zidovudine/lamivudine/tenofovir, can be administered safely with standard TB therapy as an acceptable alternative when efavirenz cannot be used. However, this strategy should be weighed against the risk of HIV drug resistance to NRTIs resulting from suboptimal virologic suppression, as triple NRTI regimens have been shown to be inferior to NNRTI or PI-based regimens. Other triple NRTI regimens (abacavir/lamivudine/tenofovir or tenofovir/didanosine/lamivudine) have demonstrated unacceptably high rates of virologic failure and should not be used.

If rifabutin is available, the second-line ART regimens for co-infected patients include the same agents used in adults without TB, such as an NRTI backbone tenofovir/emtricitabine or zidovudine/lamivudine and a ritonavir-boosted PI such as atazanavir/ritonavir or lopinavir/ritonavir. With PI use, the dose of rifabutin should be adjusted as recommended below. If rifabutin is not available, second-line ART will include same NRTI backbones recommended for adults plus lopinavir/ritonavir or saquinavir/ritonavir with adjusted doses of ritonavir.

Drug–drug interactions

Rifampicin and efavirenz

Rifampicin causes an approximately 20% decrease in efavirenz concentration, which led some authorities to recommend increasing the dose of efavirenz from 600 to 800 mg daily in patients concomitantly treated with rifampicin. The optimal dose of efavirenz in the presence of rifampicin-containing therapy remains controversial; however, there is insufficient evidence to support increasing efavirenz dose in this setting and CDC recommends the use of standard dose of efavirenz in patients with HIV-related tuberculosis [37].

Rifampicin and nevirapine

Rifampicin decreases serum concentrations of nevirapine by 20–55%, and some investigators have suggested using an increased dose of nevirapine in patients on rifampicin; however, an increased risk of nevirapine hypersensitivity was observed in patients receiving higher doses of nevirapine. Therefore, the CDC recommends the use of the standard dose of nevirapine in patients on rifampicin, starting with 200 mg daily for 2 weeks (lead-in dosing), followed by 200 mg twice daily [37]. Although it has been suggested that efavirenz should be preferred over nevirapine for eligible patients if both NNRTIs are available, nevirapine-based ART remains a reasonably effective option if efavirenz administration is contraindicated.

Rifampicin and protease inhibitors

Rifampicin decreases serum concentrations of indinavir, lopinavir, atazanavir boosted with standard dose of ritonavir (100 mg) by >90%, rendering them ineffective. Therefore, administration of standard doses of PIs with rifampicin is contraindicated. The effects of rifampicin on serum concentrations of PIs can be overcome with high doses of ritonavir (400 mg twice-daily, "super-boosted" lopinavir or saquinavir) or by doubling the dose of co-formulated protease inhibitors such as lopinavir/ritonavir (800/200 mg ritonavir twice daily). However, this approach is associated with high rates of hepatotoxicity and gastrointestinal intolerance and should only be used with close clinical and laboratory monitoring [37].

Rifampicin and other antiretroviral agents

Rifampicin decreases the trough concentrations of etravirine, raltegravir, and maraviroc, and caution is advised when rifampicin is co-administered with these antiretroviral agents given the limited clinical experience.

Rifabutin and ART

Rifabutin has similar *in vitro* antituberculous activity to rifampicin, with less potential for drug–drug interactions, and is currently recommended for the treatment of TB in HIV when available. The PIs, particularly if boosted with ritonavir, increase serum concentrations of rifabutin; therefore, the dose of rifabutin should be decreased from 300 mg daily to 150 mg three times per week when used with PIs. There is some concern for development of resistance to rifabutin when the rifamycin is being administered at the reduced dose of 150 mg three times a week, and some clinicians prefer to administer rifabutin at a dose of 150 mg daily. Some experts recommend monitoring rifabutin serum concentrations in patients taking PIs [38]. If rifabutin is administered with efavirenz, the rifabutin dose is increased to 450–600 mg daily. The pharmacokinetics of the nevirapine/rifabutin interaction are favorable, and this would be a preferred combination. There are no data on combined use of rifabutin and either maraviroc, raltegravir or etravirine.

Immune reconstitution inflammatory syndrome (IRIS)

IRIS comprises two distinct syndromes: paradoxical IRIS and unmasking IRIS. Paradoxical IRIS refers to worsening TB in patients started on ART (TB diagnosed prior to starting ART). Unmasking IRIS refers to a new presentation of TB within 3 months after ART initiation, with heightened intensity of clinical manifestations and excessive inflammatory response.

Major and minor criteria common to both syndromes have been defined; the diagnosis of IRIS requires one major and two minor criteria. Major criteria refer to new or worsening lymphadenopathy, new or worsening radiologic features of TB, CNS TB or serositis (pleural effusion, ascites, or pericardial effusion). Minor criteria include new or worsening constitutional symptoms including fever, respiratory symptoms or abdominal pain associated with peritonitis, hepatomegaly, splenomegaly, or abdominal lymphadenopathy. Although not part of the consensus diagnosis criteria, a rapid decline in HIV RNA and an increase in the CD4 count in response to ART are two factors clearly associated with IRIS. Patients typically develop TB-IRIS symptoms 2–4 weeks after starting ART. IRIS can manifest with different levels of severity. The duration of IRIS symptoms is typically 2–3 months, although there were reports of IRIS symptoms lasting more than 1 year. IRIS remains a diagnosis of exclusion, as similar symptoms may reflect progression of TB disease or treatment failure as a result of TB drug resistance or poor adherence, drug toxicity or the development of a new opportunistic infection or malignancy. Clinicians should screen for TB prior to ART initiation, because patients with severe immunosuppression may have subclinical, unrecognized active TB and develop unmasking IRIS during early ART.

Although the immunopathogenesis of IRIS remains insufficiently characterized, it is generally thought that both forms of TB-IRIS result from increased recognition of mycobacterial antigens by a recovering immune system. IRIS appears to be a predominantly CD4-mediated phenomenon, with reconstituting T cells showing evidence of increased activation from antigenic exposure.

The risk of both forms of IRIS is higher with lower CD4 counts, shorter interval between the initiation of TB therapy and the initiation of ART and extrapulmonary and disseminated TB [39]. The incidence of TB-IRIS was 15.7%, and mortality of IRIS-associated TB was 3.2% in a recent systematic review [40].

In general, IRIS can be managed with NSAIDs or corticosteroids, and interruption of ART is not recommended, but may be considered with life-threatening TB-IRIS, such as in cases of severe neurological involvement. A randomized controlled clinical trial of prednisone (1.5 mg/kg/day for 2 weeks then 0.75 mg/kg/day for 2 weeks) in patients with paradoxical TB-IRIS in South Africa showed a reduced duration of hospitalization and a more rapid clinical and radiographic improvement in the steroid-treated group [41]. The role of corticosteroids in unmasking TB has not been defined.

A recent randomized controlled trial reported a greater than threefold risk of IRIS when ART was initiated during TB therapy versus sequential treatment for TB and HIV (12.4 vs 3.8%, respectively) [42]. Despite increased incidence of IRIS in patients receiving concurrent TB and HIV treatment, the risk of death was significantly lower with integrated versus sequential therapy, and new evidence supports early initiation of ART.

Timing of ART initiation

The decision regarding the optimal time to start ART during TB treatment must balance the risks of overlapping toxicities, drug interactions, and development of IRIS with early initiation of ART against the risks of increased mortality and development of other opportunistic infections with delayed ART. The current WHO guidelines recommend starting TB treatment first, followed by ART as early as possible after starting TB treatment.

Findings of recent randomized controlled studies support early initiation of ART in patients with TB. The South African SAPiT trial (Starting Antiretroviral Therapy at Three Points in Tuberculosis Therapy) compared three different strategies of starting ART in smear-positive TB patients with CD4 counts between 0 and 500 cells/mm^3: during the intensive phase of TB treatment, after the intensive phase, and after completing TB treatment. Mortality was significantly

reduced by 56% when ART was initiated before completion of TB therapy (integrated versus sequential therapy). The mortality benefit was observed in both patients with CD4 count <200/mm^3 and CD4 count >200/mm^3, suggesting that ART should not be deferred until TB treatment is completed; however, integrated therapy was associated with higher risk of IRIS [42]. Additional results from the SAPiT study comparing the early ART (within 4 weeks of starting TB therapy) versus late ART (within 4 weeks of completing the intensive phase of TB treatment) showed a 68% reduction in AIDS-defining illness and death rate with early integrated therapy in patients with CD4 counts < 50 cells/mm^3 [43]. The analysis showed no significant differences in these outcomes between the two arms for patients with CD4 counts >50 cells/mm^3.

The CAMELIA study (Cambodian Early Versus Late Introduction of Antiretrovirals) found a mortality benefit in starting ART 2 weeks after TB treatment initiation versus 8 weeks later in AFB smear-positive, HIV-infected patients with CD4 counts less than 200 cells/mm^3. Late ART increased mortality by 52% in a multivariate analysis. The majority of subjects in the CAMELIA trial had an average CD4 count of 25 cells/mm^3. Earlier initiation of ART was associated with an increased rate of IRIS; however, early initiation of ART appeared to decrease mortality in patients with advanced HIV disease [44].

An international randomized clinical trial (A5221 STRIDE study) compared the strategy of immediate (within 2 weeks) versus early (8–12 weeks) initiation of ART in HIV-infected patients with TB and CD4 counts <250 cells/mm^3 and found a significant reduction in AIDS-related death with immediate ART (15.5 vs 26.6%) at 48 weeks in the group of HIV-infected patients with CD4 counts <50 cells/mm^3 [45]. The study showed no significant difference in AIDS-defining illness and death with immediate versus early ART for patients with higher CD4 counts. These findings, together with the recent data from the SAPiT trial, support the initiation of ART immediately after starting TB therapy in patients with CD4 counts < 50 cells/mm^3. However, the same studies suggest that initiation of ART could be deferred to the start of the continuation phase of TB treatment (8–12 weeks) in patients with CD4 counts >50 cells/mm^3. Pending the official recommendations, the determination of the optimal timing for ART initiation should rely on the current evidence and clinical judgment, balancing the risks of AIDS progression/death against risks of IRIS and cumulative drug toxicities.

Mortality in HIV-associated tuberculosis

HIV-infected individuals who develop TB are at higher risk of dying during treatment for TB than patients with TB without HIV infection, the death usually being secondary to complications of HIV infection rather than to TB itself. The mortality is higher in the group of HIV-infected patients with smear-negative pulmonary and extrapulmonary TB, reflecting their more advanced degree of immunosuppression. The impact TB has on the mortality of HIV-infected individuals is higher at lower CD4 counts. Moreover, people living with HIV who develop TB have an approximately twofold greater risk of death from all causes compared with HIV-infected patients without TB [46].

ART reduces the mortality risk of HIV-infected patients with TB by 64–95%, substantially improving the prognosis [47]. Therefore, the WHO recommends ART for all HIV-infected patients who develop TB, irrespective of the CD4 count and ART be initiated as soon as possible after the start of TB treatment. As detailed above, recent studies support this recommendation for patients with CD4 counts <50 cells/mm^3.

In addition to the mortality benefit, ART has a positive impact on other TB outcomes, reducing the smear and culture conversion time [48] and decreasing the rates of TB recurrence by 50% [49]. Moreover, ART initiated in HIV-infected individuals prior to TB development can reduce the risk of TB by up to 90% at the individual level and by approximately 60% at the population level.

The outcomes of HIV-infected patients with TB can be additionally improved with the use of CPT, a strategy shown to be effective in decreasing the mortality rates by 45–50%, with the greatest impact seen in the first 12 weeks and sustained at 72 weeks, with possible waning of the effect subsequently [50, 51]. CPT also improves the quality of life across a broad range of levels of immunodeficiency. The exact mechanism that makes co-trimoxazole beneficial in this setting is not well characterized, but it may be related to prevention of *Pneumocystis jiroveci* infection, malaria or other bacterial infections in HIV-infected patients. The WHO recommends that all HIV-infected patients with TB should be initiated on CPT as soon as possible, and this therapy should be given throughout TB treatment.

The deleterious effect TB has on HIV mortality suggests that a substantial benefit could be derived from TB prevention strategies.

TB PREVENTION

Treatment of latent tuberculosis and secondary prevention

A recent meta-analysis of efficacy of treatment of LTBI in HIV-infected persons showed that preventive therapy reduced the risk of active TB by 32% compared to placebo [52]. Efficacy was similar for all regimens, regardless of the drug type, frequency, or duration of treatment; however, compared to isoniazid (INH) monotherapy, short-course multi-drug regimens were much more likely to require discontinuation of treatment due to adverse effects.

Therefore, the WHO recommends INH as the drug of choice for chemotherapy to prevent TB in adults living with HIV, administered at a dose of 300 mg/day in adults and 10 mg/kg/day in children more than 12 months of age [24].

The WHO strongly recommends a minimum of 6 months of IPT, regardless of the degree of immunosuppression. Recognizing the potential benefit of extended IPT, and preliminary data from the CDC-Botswana trial, the WHO conditionally recommends 36 months of IPT for people living with HIV in settings with high TB prevalence and transmission. The CDC recommends a 9-month course of INH as the preferred regimen and a second-line regimen of 4 months of rifampicin in patients intolerant of INH. However, this regimen is not as widely studied and may be associated with an increased risk of relapse.

The risk of TB recurrence after completion of treatment is high in HIV-infected patients, and secondary prevention with INH may be an effective strategy to prevent TB recurrence in high-transmission areas. The WHO strongly recommends that HIV-infected adults and adolescents who successfully complete TB treatment should continue to receive INH for another six months, with the possibility of continuing INH for up to 36 months. However, this strategy should be carefully evaluated.

BCG vaccination

Bacille Calmette-Guérin vaccine (BCG), the only currently available TB vaccine, provides protection against life-threatening TB, such as TB meningitis and disseminated (miliary) TB in children, but it does not prevent TB transmission, infection or reactivation of latent TB.

The efficacy of BCG vaccination has been variable by age and geographic location, possibly influenced by exposure to environmental mycobacteria or helminthic infections. A meta-analysis found an overall efficacy of 50%, with approximately 80% efficacy in preventing the severe forms of TB in childhood [53].

Despite BCG vaccine limitations, the WHO continues to recommend that a single dose of BCG should be given to neonates or as soon as possible after birth in countries with a high prevalence of TB for protection against TB meningitis and miliary TB [54]. Most high-burden countries use BCG vaccination as part of the national childhood immunization programs, whereas in low-prevalence countries, vaccination is limited to defined high-risk groups. BCG vaccination is contraindicated in HIV-infected children with symptomatic disease; however, the WHO continues to recommend BCG vaccination in asymptomatic HIV-infected infants living in highly endemic TB areas. Children infected with HIV are at higher risk of developing disseminated BCG disease.

The development of efficient, safe, and affordable vaccines against TB is seen as a global research priority, and 12 vaccine candidates were in different phases of clinical trials in 2009 [55]. The strategies to improve TB vaccination include substituting primary immunization with recombinant BCG strains (rBCG) that improve antigen presentation and/or over-express immunodominant antigens or an attenuated strain of *M. tuberculosis*. There is interest as well in boosting BCG with an attenuated vaccinia or adenovirus vector over-expressing immunogenic antigens or a subunit vaccine composed of highly immunogenic proteins in adjuvant. A heat-inactivated *M. vaccae (environmental saprophyte mycobacteria) vaccine administered to* HIV-infected Tanzanian adults (previously immunized with BCG) with CD4 counts >200 cells/mm^3 reduced TB by 39% [56]. This can be considered a useful proof-of-concept with respect to both the prime-boost strategy and the potential for safely immunizing individuals even with advanced HIV disease.

CONTROL STRATEGIES

Over the past years, the international community has developed comprehensive strategies to fight the HIV and TB pandemics. Building on previously implemented DOTS strategy, the WHO launched a new six-point Stop TB Strategy in 2006, aiming to ensure universal access to high-quality diagnosis and treatment for all TB patients, including those co-infected with HIV, and supporting the development of effective tools to prevent, detect, and treat TB. In the same year, with its Global Plan to Stop TB 2006–2015, the Stop TB Partnership published a comprehensive assessment of the action and resources needed to implement the Stop TB Strategy, with the UN Millennium Development Goal of halting and beginning to reverse the epidemic by 2015 and halving TB prevalence and death rates by 2015, compared with 1990 levels. In 2010, taking into account the progress made since 2006, the Stop TB partnership has updated the plan, focusing on the 2015 targets and adding the commitment to eliminate TB as a public health problem by 2050. The plan emphasizes the need

for laboratory strengthening as a major component, includes goals and targets for research and sets strategic frameworks for each major component in the plan [55].

TB/HIV collaborative activities have been incorporated as major components of the Stop TB Strategy and the Global Plan to Stop TB to reduce the burden of TB and HIV in populations affected by both diseases [57]. The "3Is" (intensified case finding, INH prophylaxis, and improved infection control) strategy has been proposed to HIV control programs to reduce the burden of TB in people living with HIV. Just as HIV programs should implement TB prevention and control interventions, TB programs should also implement HIV testing and prevention methods, ART and CPT as standard of care for patients affected by both diseases.

Integration of TB and HIV responses is viewed as a key strategy to control the dual epidemic. However, despite clear guidelines, interventions known to be effective have not been implemented. By 2008, only 4% of HIV-infected individuals were actively screened for TB and only 48,000 individuals (less than 0.2% of the eligible HIV-infected population) were offered IPT, data that reflect a minimal level of implementation of TB prevention activities. Similarly, the HIV care provided by TB programs is far from reaching the proposed targets. Almost 80% of patients who develop TB are not tested for HIV, and a large proportion of HIV-infected individuals do not have access to CPT and ART. By 2008, approximately 30% of HIV-infected TB patients were not receiving CPT, and only 32% of the HIV-infected patients who developed TB started ART. These data highlight the need for a more aggressive approach to implementing integrated HIV and TB activities.

Globally, TB/HIV control efforts are hampered by multiple challenges at different levels: scientific, political, economic, and cultural. Their implications should be taken into account by the international community to find effective solutions for a successful response to HIV/TB co-infection in the new millennium.

REFERENCES

[1] Chretien J. Tuberculosis and HIV. The cursed duet. Bull Int Union Tuberc Lung Dis 1990;65(1):25–8.

[2] World Health Organization. Global tuberculosis control. WHO/HTM/TB/2010.7. Geneva: WHO; 2010.

[3] World Health Organization. The global burden of disease: 2004 update. Geneva: WHO; 2008.

[4] Suchindran S, Brouwer E, Van Rie A. Is HIV infection a risk factor for multi-drug resistant tuberculosis? A systematic review. PLoS ONE 2009;4:e5561.

[5] Lawn S, Wood R, Wilkinson R. Changing concepts of "latent tuberculosis infection" in patients living with HIV infection. Clin Dev Immunol 2011; Epub doi:10.1155/2011/980594.

[6] Fennelly K, Martyny J, Fulton K, et al. Cough-generated aerosols of *Mycobacterium tuberculosis*: a new method to study infectiousness. Am J Respir Crit Care Med 2004;169:604–9.

[7] Guwatudde D, Nakakeeto M, Lopez-Jones E. Tuberculosis in household

contacts of infectious cases in Kampala, Uganda. Am J Epidemiol 2003;158:887–98.

[8] Crampin A, Glynn J, Traore H, et al. Tuberculosis transmission attributable to close contacts and HIV status, Malawi. Emerg Infect Dis 2006;12(5):729–35.

[9] Morrison J, Madhukar P, Hopewell P. Tuberculosis and latent tuberculosis infection in close contacts of people with pulmonary tuberculosis in low-income and middle-income countries: a

systematic review and meta-analysis. Lancet Infect Dis 2008;8 (6):359–68.

[10] Yim J, Selvaraj P. Genetic susceptibility in tuberculosis. Respirology 2010;15(2):241–56.

[11] Duarte R, Carvalho C, Pereira C, et al. HLA class II alleles as markers of tuberculosis susceptibility and resistance. Rev Port Pneumol 2011;17(1):15–19.

[12] Cruciani M, Malena M, Bosco O, et al. The impact of human immunodeficiency virus type 1 on infectiousness of tuberculosis: a meta-analysis. Clin Infect Dis 2001;33(11):1922–30.

[13] Charalambous S, Grant A, Moloi V, et al. Contribution of reinfection to recurrent tuberculosis in South African gold miners. Int J Tuberc Lung Dis 2008;12(8):942–8.

[14] Crampin A, Mwaungulu J, Mwaungulu F, et al. Recurrent TB: relapse or reinfection? The effect of HIV in a general population cohort in Malawi. AIDS 2010;24 (3):417–26.

[15] Glynn J, Murray J, Bester A. Effects of duration of HIV infection and secondary tuberculosis transmission on tuberculosis incidence in the South African gold miners. AIDS 2008;22 (14):1859–67.

[16] Badri M, Douglas W, Wood R. Effect of highly active antiretroviral therapy on incidence of tuberculosis in South Africa: a cohort study. Lancet 2002;359:2059–64.

[17] Flynn J. Immunology of tuberculosis. Annu Rev Immunol 2001;19:93–129.

[18] Goletti D, Weissman D, Jackson R, Fauci A. Effect of Mycobacterium tuberculosis on HIV replication. Role of immune activation. J Immunol 1996;157(3):1271–8.

[19] Cain K, McCarthy K, Heilig C, et al. An algorithm for tuberculosis screening and diagnosis in people with HIV. N Engl J Med 2010;362:707–16.

[20] Getahun H, Kittikraisak W, Heilig C, et al. Development of a standardized screening rule for tuberculosis in people living with HIV in resource-constrained settings: individual participant data metaanalysis of obervational

studies. PLoS Med 2011;8(1): e1000391.

[21] Perlman D, El-Sadr W, Nelson E, et al. Variation of chest radiographic patterns in pulmonary tuberculosis by degree of human immunodeficiency virus-related immunosuppression. Clin Infect Dis 1997;25:242–6.

[22] Luzze H, Elliott A, Joloba L, et al. Evaluation of suspected tuberculous pleurisy: clinical and diagnostic findings in HIV-1-positive and HIV-negative adults in Uganda. Int J Tuberc Lung Dis 2001;5(8):746–53.

[23] Mtei L, Matee M, Herfort O, et al. High rates of clinical and subclinical tuberculosis among HIV-infected ambulatory subjects in Tanzania. Clin Infect Dis 2005;40:1500–7.

[24] World Health Organization (WHO). Guidelines for intensified tuberculosis case finding and isoniazid preventive therapy for people living with HIV in resource constrained settings. Geneva: WHO; 2011.

[25] Centers for Disease Control and Prevention. Targeted tuberculin testing and treatment of latent tuberculosis infection. MMWR 2000;49(No. RR-6).

[26] Cattamanchi A, Smith R, Steingart K, et al. Interferon-gamma release assays for the diagnosis of latent tuberculosis infection in HIV-infected individuals—a systematic review and meta-analysis. J Acquir Immune Defic Syndr 2011;56 (3):230–8.

[27] Centers for Disease Control and Prevention. Updated guidelines for using interferon gamma release assays to detect Mycobacterium tuberculosis infection—United States, 2010. MMWR 2010;59:10–12.

[28] Gold J, Rom W, Harkin T. Significance of abnormal chest radiograph findings in patients with HIV-1 infection without respiratory symptoms. Chest 2002;121:1472–7.

[29] Elliott A, Namaambo K, Allen B. Negative sputum smear results in HIV-positive patients with pulmonary tuberculosis in Lusaka, Zambia. Tuber Lung Dis 1993;74:191–4.

[30] Centers for Disease Prevention and Control. Updated Guidelines for the

use of nucleic acid amplification tests in the diagnosis of tuberculosis. MMWR 2009;(1):7–10.

[31] Boehme C, Nabeta P, Hillemann D, et al. Rapid molecular detection of tuberculosis and rifampin resistance. N Engl J Med 2010;363:1005–15.

[32] Berry M, Graham C, O'Garra A, et al. An interferon-inducible neutrophil-driven blood transcriptional signature in human tuberculosis. Nature 2010;466:973–7.

[33] World Health Organization. Treatment of tuberculosis: guidelines—4th edn. WHO/HTM/ TB/2009.420. Geneva: WHO; 2010.

[34] American Thoracic Society. Centers for Disease Control and Prevention, and Infectious Diseases Society of America. Treatment of tuberculosis. MMWR 2003;1–77.

[35] Khan FA, Minion J, Pai M, et al. Treatment of active tuberculosis in HIV-coinfected patients: a systematic review and meta-analysis. Clin Infect Dis 2010;50 (9):1289–99.

[36] Tappero J, Bradford W, Agerton T, et al. Serum concentrations of antimycobacterial drugs in patients with pulmonary tuberculosis in Botswana. Clin Infect Dis 2005;41:461–9.

[37] Centers for Disease Control and Prevention. Managing drug interactions in the treatment of HIV-related tuberculosis, Available from: http://www.cdc.gov/tb/TB_HIV_ Drugs/default.htm; 2007.

[38] Boulanger C, Hollender E, Farrell K, et al. Pharmacokinetic evaluation of rifabutin in combination with lopinavir-ritonavir in patients with HIV infection and active tuberculosis. Clin Infect Dis 2009;49(9):1305–11.

[39] Leone S, Nicastri E, Giglio S, et al. Immune reconstitution inflammatory syndrome associated with Mycobacterium tuberculosis infection: a systematic review. Int J Infect Dis 2010;14:283–91.

[40] Muller M, Wandel S, Colebunders R, et al. Immune reconstitution inflammatory syndrome in patients starting antiretroviral therapy for HIV infection: a systematic review and meta-analysis. Lancet Infect Dis 2010;10(4):251–61.

[41] Meintjes G, Wilkinson R, Maartens G, et al. Randomized placebo-controlled trial of prednisone for paradoxical tuberculosis-associated immune reconstitution inflammatory syndrome. AIDS 2010;24 (15):2381–90.

[42] Abdool Karim S, Naidoo K, Grobler A, et al. Timing of initiation of antiretroviral drugs during tuberculosis therapy. N Engl J Med 2010;362(8):697–706.

[43] Abdool Karim S, et al. SAPiT: early versus late ART initiation during integrated TB/ART therapy. In: 18th Conference on Retroviruses and Opportunistic Infections; 2011. Boston Abstract 39.

[44] Blanc F, Sok T, Laureillard D, et al. Significant enhancement in survival with early (2 weeks) vs. late (8 weeks) initiation of highly active antiretroviral treatment (HAART) in severely immunosuppressed HIV-infected adults with newly diagnosed tuberculosis. In: Program and abstracts of the XVIII International AIDS Conference; 2010 Vienna, Austria.

[45] Havlir D, et al. International randomized trial of immediate versus early ART in HIV-positive patients treated for TB: ACTG 5221 STRIDE study. In: 18th Conference on Retroviruses and Opportunistic Infections. Boston: 2011. Abstract 38.

[46] Straetemans M, Bierrenbach A, Nagelkerke N, et al. The effect of tuberculosis on mortality in HIV positive people: a meta-analysis. PLoS ONE 2010;5(12):e15241.

[47] Lawn S, Kranzer K, Wood R. Antiretroviral therapy for control of the HIV-associated tuberculosis epidemic in resource-limited settings. Clin Chest Med 2009;30 (4):685–99.

[48] Nahid P, Gonzalez L, Rudoy I, et al. Treatment outcomes of patients with HIV and tuberculosis. Am J Respir Crit Care Med 2007;175 (11):1199–1206.

[49] Golub J, Durovni B, King B, et al. Recurrent tuberculosis in HIV-infected patients in Rio de Janeiro, Brazil. AIDS 2008;22(18):2527–33.

[50] Nunn A, Mwaba P, Chintu C, et al. Role of co-trimoxazole prophylaxis in reducing mortality in HIV infected adults being treated for tuberculosis: randomised clinical trial. BMJ 2008;337:a257.

[51] Walker A, Ford D, Gilks C, et al. Daily co-trimoxazole prophylaxis in severely immunosuppressed HIV-infected adults in Africa started on combination antiretroviral therapy: an observational analysis of the DART cohort. Lancet 2010;375:1278–86.

[52] Akolo C, Adetifa I, Shepperd S, Volmink J. Treatment of latent tuberculosis infection in HIV infected persons (review). Cochrane Database Syst Rev 2010;(1) CD000171.

[53] Colditz G, Berkey C, Mosteller F, et al. The efficacy of bacillus Calmette-Guérin vaccination of newborns and infants in the prevention of tuberculosis: meta-analyses of the published literature. Pediatrics 1995;1:29–35.

[54] World Health Organization. WHO position paper on BCG. Wkly Epidemiol Rec 2004;79(4):25–40.

[55] World Health Organization. The global plan to stop TB 2011–2015: transforming the fight towards elimination of tuberculosis. Geneva: WHO; 2010.

[56] von Reyn C, Mtei L, Arbeit R, et al. Prevention of tuberculosis in Bacille Calmette-Guérin-primed, HIV-infected adults boosted with an inactivated whole-cell mycobacterial vaccine. AIDS 2010;24(5):675–85.

[57] World Health Organization. A guide to monitoring and evaluation for collaborative TB/HIV activities—2009 revision. Geneva: WHO; 2009.

Chapter 27

Disseminated *Mycobacterium avium* complex and other atypical mycobacterial infections

Mark A. Jacobson

EPIDEMIOLOGY

Prior to the AIDS epidemic, disseminated *Mycobacterium avium* complex (MAC) infection had been reported only rarely, yet after 1981 this infection became one of the most important opportunistic infections associated with the AIDS in many parts of the world. Disseminated MAC occurs almost exclusively in AIDS patients with an absolute CD4 count <50 cells/mm^3 [1]. Localized MAC infection can occur at higher CD4 counts, especially among patients with advanced AIDS who have experienced immune reconstitution on highly active antiretroviral therapy (HAART, or ART) [2].

Disseminated MAC in industrialized countries

In the era prior to the widespread availability of HAART in North America, Western Europe and Australia, one-third to one-half of AIDS patients in these regions developed disseminated MAC infection. In the USA, a study reported in 1986 that 53% of 79 autopsies of AIDS patients showed evidence of disseminated MAC [3]. In another study from the late 1980s, conducted in patients with advanced HIV disease who had serial blood specimens cultured for mycobacteria over a median 1-year period, the 2-year actuarial incidence of MAC bacteremia was 40% [1]. In Australia during this same time period, 50% of AIDS patients developed disseminated MAC [4]. Similarly, an autopsy study conducted in Japan in the pre-HAART era reported evidence of disseminated MAC in 40% of 43 autopsies [5]. The risk among European patients was more variable, with patients in northern Europe having a similar risk to US

patients, whereas those in southwestern Europe had one-sixth that risk [6]. After HAART became available, the incidence of disseminated MAC dramatically decreased and has subsequently stabilized at a much lower level.

Disseminated MAC in resource-poor countries

Disseminated MAC has been less common in parts of the world where tuberculosis is more prevalent, perhaps because of cross-reactive immunity or perhaps because end-organ disease caused by tuberculosis tends to occur earlier in the course of HIV than disease caused by MAC. In the pre-HAART era, MAC was isolated from the blood of 18% of febrile AIDS patients in a study conducted in Brazil [7]. The point prevalence of disseminated MAC in hospitalized AIDS patients in South Africa has been reported to be only 10% [8], and in Thailand, only 1% [9].

Effect of MAC prophylaxis and ART on incidence

With the advent of MAC prophylaxis in the early 1990s, the incidence of the infection began to decline in Western industrialized countries. Between 1993 and 1994, a 40% decrease in the incidence of adult AIDS-defining disseminated MAC was noted by the US Centers for Disease Control (CDC) that almost certainly resulted from the widespread introduction of rifabutin and macrolide MAC prophylaxis into clinical practice during this time period. After early 1996, when HAART became widely available in North America and Western Europe, the incidence decreased by more than 80% compared with the period before 1994. More recently, a similar decrease in MAC bacteremia has been reported in Brazil after the widespread introduction of HAART in that country [10]. In a recently published prospective cohort study of 8,070 HIV-infected patients from the USA with a median CD4 count of 298 cells/mm^3, the incidence of disseminated MAC was only 2.5 new cases per 1,000 patient-years between 2003 and 2007 [11].

Acquisition of MAC infection

MAC is a ubiquitous soil and water saprophyte, and epidemiologic data suggest that disseminated MAC infection results from new environmental acquisition of the organism (rather than reactivation of quiescent, endogenous infection). As an example, a common water source nosocomial outbreak of MAC disease was reported in an AIDS ward [12]. The route of MAC infection in AIDS patients may be through the gastrointestinal or respiratory tract. The presence of large clusters of mycobacteria within macrophages of the small bowel lamina propria suggests that the bowel might be the portal of entry. However, respiratory isolation of MAC frequently precedes disseminated infection, suggesting that MAC infection may begin in the lungs as well [13].

PATHOGENESIS

In AIDS, the key host defect allowing dissemination of MAC is macrophage dysfunction, specifically the failure of macrophages to kill phagocytized MAC. The organism is able to survive within macrophages unless intracellular killing mechanisms, which become defective with advanced HIV infection, are activated. Defects in the activity of cytokines that are essential for intracellular killing of pathogens, such as interferon-gamma, tumor necrosis factor, interleukin-12 and interleukin-2, have all been implicated in the pathogenesis of disseminated MAC infection among patients with rare heritable immune deficiencies and probably have a role in the pathogenesis of this opportunistic infection in AIDS patients. However, cytokine therapy has shown benefit in AIDS patients with disseminated MAC to date.

In AIDS, MAC causes high-grade, widely disseminated infection. Nearly all AIDS patients with invasive MAC infection (as opposed to stool, urine, or respiratory colonization) have positive mycobacterial blood cultures. In the majority of cases autopsied, MAC has been isolated from the spleen, lymph nodes, liver, lung, adrenals, colon, kidney, and bone marrow. The magnitude of mycobacteremia can range from 1 to 10,000 colony-forming units per mL of blood. Tissue specimens from bone marrow, spleen, lymph nodes, and liver have yielded even higher amounts of the microbe. Histopathologic studies of involved organs typically have shown absent or poorly formed granulomas and acid-fast bacteria within macrophages. In AIDS

patients who have experienced immune reconstitution on ART, there have been reports of localized, non-disseminated, MAC infection associated with granuloma formation, tissue destruction, and abscess formation in lymph nodes or skin. These cases of MAC immune reconstitution inflammatory syndrome (IRIS) have usually occurred soon after antiretroviral therapy was initiated, suggesting that reconstitution of either MAC-specific T-cell responses or of some innate, cytokine-related functions may have occurred.

CLINICAL MANIFESTATIONS

Effect of disseminated MAC infection on survival in AIDS

Because most AIDS patients with disseminated MAC infection have other concomitant infections or neoplasms, and because systemic MAC infection appears to cause little inflammatory response or tissue destruction in patients with advanced AIDS, the relationship between constitutional symptoms, organ dysfunction, and MAC infection was initially uncertain. Nevertheless, several large retrospective studies from the pre-HAART era strongly suggested that disseminated MAC increased mortality and morbidity in AIDS patients. Horsburgh and co-workers noted a median 4-month survival among 39 patients with untreated disseminated MAC infection compared with 11 months among 39 controls matched for CD4 lymphocyte count, prior AIDS status, history of antiretroviral therapy, history of *Pneumocystis* pneumonia (PCP) prophylaxis, and year of diagnosis ($p<0.0001$) [14]. At San Francisco General Hospital, among 137 consecutive patients who had a sterile body site cultured for mycobacteria within 3 months of their first AIDS-defining episode of PCP, median survival was significantly shorter in those with disseminated MAC infection than in those who had negative cultures (107 vs 275 days; $p < 0.01$), even after controlling for age, absolute lymphocyte count, and hemoglobin concentration [13].

Clinical presentation of disseminated MAC

The clinical presentation of disseminated MAC infection almost always includes fever and malaise. Weight loss is common, and anemia and/or neutropenia are often present. Diarrhea and malabsorption may occur as a result of MAC invasion of the gut wall. Abdominal pain may be present and can be severe as a result of bulky retroperitoneal adenopathy. Rarely, extrabiliary obstructive jaundice caused by periportal lymphadenopathy occurs. In a prospective natural history study of MAC bacteremia conducted at San Francisco General Hospital in the pre-HAART era, we observed, among patients with CD4 count <50 cells/mm^3, that a history of fever for >30 days, a hematocrit <30%, or a serum albumin level <3.0 g/dL were all sensitive predictors of MAC bacteremia [15]. However, neither severe fatigue, diarrhea, weight loss, nor neutropenia discriminated between those who were subsequently found to be blood culture positive or negative for MAC.

MAC immune reconstitution inflammatory syndrome

As noted above, localized, non-disseminated MAC infection associated with granuloma formation, tissue destruction, and abscess formation in lymph nodes or skin can occur in AIDS patients who have recently initiated antiretroviral therapy [2]. The clinical course is sometimes explosive, with large abscess formations and high fever. In general, these MAC IRIS cases have occurred in patients who had an absolute CD4 count <50 cells/mm^3 before initiating ART and have presented soon after the absolute CD4 count rises to >100 cells/mm^3. MAC IRIS sometimes involves the bone or lungs, with infiltrates apparent on chest X-ray. Mycobacterial blood cultures are usually negative at the time of presentation. MAC IRIS can present either as a recrudescence of a clinically resolved infection (paradoxical IRIS) or as the new clinical appearance of MAC infection that was previously subclinical (unmasking IRIS). In some observational studies, IRIS has occurred in up to one-third of patients who had a diagnosis of disseminated MAC prior to initiating ART and in up to 4% of all patients who initiate ART with a pre-treatment absolute CD4 count <100 cells/mm^3. Unlike disseminated infection, these lesions have responded remarkably well to drainage and antimycobacterial therapy, although a short course of prednisone is sometimes needed before fever resolves. There is no need to discontinue ART in such patients.

DIAGNOSIS

Special blood culture techniques for isolating mycobacteria, such as the broth-based BACTEC system or agar-based Dupont Isolator system, are sensitive methods for diagnosing disseminated MAC infection [16]. Specific DNA probes for MAC are also available and make it possible to differentiate MAC from other mycobacteria within hours when there is sufficient mycobacterial growth in broth or agar [17]. Time to culture positivity ranges from 5 to 51 days. It is uncommon for blood cultures to be negative when there is a positive histologic diagnosis from lymph node, liver, or bone marrow biopsies. However, one advantage of obtaining biopsied specimens is that stains may demonstrate acid-fast bacteria (AFB) or granuloma immediately, thus confirming a clinical suspicion of the diagnosis weeks before the blood culture turn positive. A single blood culture for mycobacteria is approximately 90% sensitive in diagnosing disseminated MAC infection; this sensitivity can

be increased to 95% by obtaining a second blood culture on a separate day.

The clinical significance of MAC isolated from sputum or stool remains controversial. In our prospective natural history study, we found that only two-thirds of patients with negative blood cultures but positive stool or sputum cultures for MAC subsequently developed disseminated MAC infection [18]. Hence, neither stool nor sputum culture can be recommended as a screening test to identify patients likely to develop MAC bacteremia.

THERAPY

MAC is not killed by standard antituberculous drugs at concentrations achievable in plasma. However, at least half of MAC strains can be inhibited by achievable plasma concentrations of rifabutin, rifampin, clofazimine, cycloserine, amikacin, ethionamide, ethambutol, azithromycin, clarithromycin, ciprofloxacin, or sparfloxacin. Unfortunately, drug levels necessary to kill MAC *in vitro* (minimum bactericidal concentration) have been 8 to >32 times that of inhibitory levels. While combinations of antimycobacterial agents have shown *in vitro* inhibitory synergism, bactericidal synergism has been more difficult to demonstrate. In addition, for *in vivo* killing, drugs must penetrate macrophages as well as the MAC cell wall. Nevertheless, in animal models of disseminated MAC infection, both single and combination antimycobacterial regimens have reduced mycobacterial colony counts by several logs and improved survival.

Results of several sequential trials reported by the California Collaborative Treatment Group (CCTG) highlight the caution needed when interpreting results of treatment trials that have no control arm. In 1990, this group reported striking microbiologic and clinical effects in previously untreated patients with disseminated MAC who were given a combination regimen that included intravenous amikacin and oral rifampin, ethambutol, and ciprofloxacin [19]. Given the modest results that had previously been reported with oral antimycobacterial agents, many drew the conclusion from this uncontrolled trial that the amikacin was primarily responsible for the efficacy of this regimen. Subsequently, the CCTG reported similar microbiologic and clinical results in another similarly designed uncontrolled trial in which intravenous amikacin was replaced by oral clofazimine [20]. To address the question of amikacin's clinical utility, a randomized controlled trial was then conducted by the AIDS Clinical Trials Group (ACTG) in which 72 patients with previously untreated disseminated MAC were all given a combination oral regimen of rifampin, ethambutol, ciprofloxacin, and clofazimine and were also randomly assigned to receive or not receive intravenous amikacin. In this controlled trial, there were no significant differences in microbiologic or clinical outcomes, demonstrating that the cost, inconvenience, and risk of toxicity of intravenous amikacin were not balanced by increased clinical benefit [21]. After the uncontrolled CCTG study of a clofazimine-containing regimen, data from a subsequent study found that this drug added no clinical benefit and may actually be harmful when used in macrolide-based combination regimens. A trial assigned 106 patients with MAC bacteremia to receive clarithromycin and ethambutol with or without clofazimine. Clofazimine was not associated with any benefit in microbiologic response, and the patients assigned to the clofazimine arm had significantly higher mortality. Clearly, neither clofazimine nor amikacin should be used in the initial treatment of disseminated MAC.

Macrolides: clarithromycin and azithromycin

In vivo data on microbiologic efficacy against MAC have been most impressive with two macrolides, clarithromycin and azithromycin. A multicenter, randomized, placebo-controlled, dose-ranging trial of clarithromycin monotherapy in patients with previously untreated disseminated MAC reported a median decrease of >2 log in blood colony-forming units—a more potent microbiologic effect than reported in any earlier treatment trials [22]. This microbiologic effect was accompanied by significant clinical improvement in symptoms and quality of life. However, unacceptably high gastrointestinal toxicity occurred at a dose of 2,000 mg twice daily. Although a 1,000 mg twice-daily dose had greater microbiologic efficacy than 500 mg twice daily, there was actually a trend toward increased mortality with the higher dose. This paradoxical dose–response relationship was subsequently confirmed in another study, indicating that the optimal dose for this drug is 500 mg twice daily. Not surprisingly, drug resistance emerged after 2 months of monotherapy in this trial, affecting approximately half of patients in all dosing arms. Hence, one or more other antimycobacterial agents must be co-administered with the macrolide in an attempt to prevent or at least delay emergence of resistance, which is likely to result in relapse and clinical deterioration. On the other hand, these data should reassure clinicians that inadvertently initiating MAC prophylaxis with clarithromycin in patients who already have subclinical MAC infection is unlikely to lead to drug resistance as long as blood cultures are obtained at the time that clarithromycin is started (i.e. blood cultures will be positive and additional medication can be added before the development of macrolide resistance).

Azithromycin is another effective macrolide for the treatment of MAC. The antimycobacterial efficacy of azithromycin or clarithromycin, when combined with other agents, has been compared in two randomized trials. In one study, 246 patients were randomized to an ethambutol-based regimen combined with either azithromycin 250 mg daily, azithromycin 600 mg daily, or clarithromycin 500 mg twice daily [23]. The low-dose azithromycin arm was terminated early in the trial due to poor microbiologic efficacy. There was no significant difference in either microbiologic or survival outcomes between the high-dose azithromycin and the clarithromycin arms; however, there were non-significant trends toward better survival, greater clearance of bacteremia, and lower relapse rates with clarithromycin in this trial. In another trial, 59 patients with disseminated MAC were randomized to receive an ethambutol-based regimen with either clarithromycin 500 mg twice daily or azithromycin 600 mg once daily. Clearance of bacteremia occurred in 86% of subjects assigned to clarithromycin versus only 38% assigned to azithromycin ($p < 0.007$) [24]. However, only 37 of the 59 patients were evaluable microbiologically, and only two deaths occurred during the short follow-up period, making it difficult to generalize the results of this trial.

Ethambutol

In order to determine which of the orally bioavailable non-macrolide antimycobacterial agents was the most potent *in vivo*, a randomized, controlled trial was conducted in which patients with previously untreated disseminated MAC were assigned to receive a 4-week regimen of rifampin, ethambutol, or clofazimine monotherapy [25]. In this trial, only ethambutol resulted in a statistically significant reduction in blood MAC colony-forming units. A subsequent trial confirmed the clinical benefit of ethambutol when combined with clarithromycin [26]. A total of 80 patients with newly diagnosed disseminated MAC infection received clarithromycin and clofazimine and were randomized to receive or not receive ethambutol 800 mg daily. Although 69% of patients in both groups initially cleared their bacteremia, the subsequent microbiological relapse rate at 36 weeks was 50% with ethambutol versus 91% without ethambutol ($p = 0.014$).

Rifabutin

When rifabutin was initially evaluated in the 1980s as a treatment for MAC at doses of 100–300 mg/day, it was found to be ineffective. However, a subsequent randomized, placebo-controlled trial demonstrated clinical benefit. Among patients with newly diagnosed disseminated MAC randomized to receive either clofazimine/ethambutol or clofazimine/ethambutol/rifabutin (600 mg/day), half of the patients receiving the rifabutin-containing regimen had a >2-log decrease in blood MAC colony-forming units or sterilization of the blood compared with none of those receiving only clofazimine/ethambutol [27].

Optimal combination treatment regimens

The long-term clinical benefit of combination regimens that include both macrolide and non-macrolide agents for treatment of disseminated MAC were confirmed in a randomized multicenter trial conducted by the Canadian MAC Study Group in which 187 evaluable patients with disseminated MAC were randomized to receive a regimen of clarithromycin 1,000 mg twice daily, rifabutin 600 mg once daily, and ethambutol 15 mg/kg/day versus ciprofloxacin 750 mg twice daily, rifampin 600 mg once daily, clofazimine 100 mg once daily, and ethambutol 15 mg/kg/day. The *in vivo* quantitative antimycobacterial effect was significantly better with the macrolide-containing regimen, as was median survival (8.6 vs 5.2 months; $p < 0.001$) [28].

Currently, the best option for the treatment of disseminated MAC is to combine one of the macrolides (clarithromycin 500 mg twice daily or azithromycin 500–600 mg once daily) with either ethambutol 15 mg/kg once-daily or rifabutin 150–450 mg once daily (dose dependent on concurrent medications, Table 27.1), or both (Table 27.2). To address the issue of whether it is more effective to use one or both of these two drugs, in combination with a macrolide,

Table 27.1 Recommended dosing adjustments when rifabutin is combined with antiretroviral drug

ANTIRETROVIRAL DRUG	ANTIRETROVIRAL DOSE	RIFABUTIN DOSE
Protease inhibitors		
Fosamprenavir	No change	150 mg daily
Nelfinavir	No change	150 mg daily
Indinavir	1000 mg t.i.d.	150 mg daily
Atazanavir	No change	150 mg daily
Any ritonavir-boosted protease inhibitor	No change	150 mg daily
Saquinavir	Contraindicated	Contraindicated
Non-nucleoside reverse transcriptase inhibitors		
Efavirenz	No change	450 mg daily
Nevirapine	No change	No change
Etravirine	Contraindicated with darunavir/ritonavir and etravirine combination	No change unless given with a ritonavir-boosted protease inihibitor

Table 27.2 Treatment regimen for disseminated *M. avium* complex infection

FOR PATIENTS LIKELY TO INITIATE ART SOON	FOR PATIENTS UNLIKELY TO RECEIVE ART WITHIN THE NEXT FEW MONTHS
Clarithromycin 500 mg twice daily (or clarithromycin extended release formulation 1000 mg once daily)[a]	Clarithromycin 500 mg twice daily (or clarithromycin extended release formulation 1000 mg once daily)[a]
plus	*plus*
Ethambutol 15 mg/kg once daily[b]	Ethambutol 15 mg/kg once daily and rifabutin 300 mg once daily[c]

[a]For patients intolerant of clarithromycin, azithromycin 500 or 600 mg once daily can be substituted.
[b]For patients intolerant of ethambutol, rifabutin 300 mg once daily can be substituted (450–600 mg daily if co-administered with azithromycin rather than clarithromycin; 450 mg daily if co-administered with efavirenz; 150 mg daily if co-administered with a ritonavir-boosted protease inhibitor).
[c]Rifabutin dose should be dosed at 450–600 mg daily if co-administered with azithromycin rather than clarithromycin, 450 mg daily if co-administered with efavirenz, 150 mg daily if co-administered with indinavir or nelfinavir or a ritonavir-boosted protease inhibitor.

Benson and co-workers randomized patients with disseminated MAC to receive clarithromycin and ethambutol, clarithromycin and rifabutin, or clarithromycin plus ethambutol and rifabutin [29]. A similar microbiologic response, defined as a sterile blood culture at 12 weeks, occurred in all three arms: 40, 42, and 51%, respectively ($p = 0.45$). However, higher survival was observed in the three-drug arm (hazard ratio of death approximately halved). There was no significant difference in dose-limiting toxicity between the three arms. This difference in survival may not be generalizable to patients who initiate ART soon after diagnosis of MAC, and who are likely to experience immune reconstitution and thus have a far lower risk of mortality than during the pre-HAART era when this trial was conducted.

MANAGEMENT OF TREATMENT FAILURE

Since disseminated MAC infection has become a curable disease for AIDS patients who experience immune reconstitution on ART, treatment failure is now a rare event. However, in patients who remain immunosuppressed, progressive resistance to first-line drugs can eventually occur. Other than testing for macrolide resistance, resistance testing of blood culture isolates has not been correlated with clinical outcome and thus cannot be reliably used to guide treatment in patients. Since few drugs have demonstrated clinical efficacy in randomized treatment trials (i.e. the macrolides, ethambutol, and rifabutin) and some drugs with *in vitro* activity against MAC have been of no benefit (e.g. amikacin) or harmful (e.g. clofazimine), there are limited salvage options for patients who are clinically failing treatment. It is not known whether continuing macrolide treatment is beneficial for such failing patients, but there is evidence that increasing the clarithromycin dose above 500 mg twice daily is harmful. The only evidence-based options for salvage therapy are to increase doses of drugs with established clinical efficacy: for example, (1) increasing the ethambutol dose to 25 mg/kg/day while monitoring the patient for signs of retrobulbar neuritis, and/or (2) increasing the rifabutin dose until clinical toxicity occurs (most commonly manifested as painful anterior uveitis, which typically resolves with rifabutin dose reduction). Fluoroquinolones such as ciprofloxin and moxifloxacin have demonstrated *in vitro* activity and have not been shown to harm patients with disseminated MAC, so one might consider adding such a drug.

Drug interactions with antiretroviral medications

Azithromycin and ethambutol do not have clinically important drug interactions with antiretroviral medications. Ritonavir can increase clarithromycin plasma levels enough that clarithromycin dosing should be reduced to 500 mg/day in patients on ritonavir-boosted protease inhibitor regimens who also have moderate renal insufficiency (estimated creatinine clearance <60 mL/min). Efavirenz accelerates clarithromycin metabolism and lowers drug levels; combining this drug with clarithromycin is contraindicated. Rifabutin has clinically significant drug interactions with some antiretroviral protease inhibitors and non-nucleoside reverse transcriptase inhibitors that require dosage adjustment (Table 27.1).

Initiating antiretroviral therapy and stopping MAC treatment after immune restoration

During the pre-HAART era, relapse of disseminated MAC typically occurred rapidly when chronic suppressive therapy was discontinued. However, since the widespread availability of ART, there have been several reports describing a series of patients who had taken prolonged therapy for disseminated MAC infection, then experienced immune reconstitution on ART with a rise in CD4 count to >100 cells/mm^3, with resolution of all MAC-related symptoms. After blood culture negativity was documented, these individuals discontinued MAC therapy and had no relapse during long-term follow-up. It now appears to be safe for

such patients who have completed at least one year of an appropriate MAC regimen to discontinue chronic suppressive therapy.

These observations underscore the importance of initiating effective ART and suppressing HIV replication as soon as possible after diagnosing disseminated MAC. While some observational studies have shown that a shorter time interval between initiatiation of MAC therapy and ART was associated with an increased risk of MAC IRIS [30], this is outweighed by the results of a randomized controlled trial that demonstrated that in AIDS patients with newly diagnosed opportunistic infections, early initiation of ART (i.e. within two weeks versus at least four weeks) reduces the risk of AIDS progression and death [31].

Empiric treatment for disseminated MAC and tuberculosis

Distinguishing tuberculosis from MAC disease in patients with advanced HIV disease can be difficult. Therefore, empiric antituberculous therapy should be considered when acid-fast bacteria are demonstrated in a specimen from an HIV-infected patient with clinical evidence of mycobacterial disease while awaiting speciation of the organism. MAC and tuberculosis can both be empirically treated by adding clarithromycin to standard tuberculosis treatment regimens.

PROPHYLAXIS

In countries where the incidence of AIDS-related disseminated MAC is high (e.g. Europe and the United States), prophylaxis should be given to at-risk AIDS patients (i.e. those with CD4 counts <50 cells/mm^3).

Clarithromycin

The most convincing data regarding the efficacy of MAC prophylaxis have been obtained with clarithromycin in a placebo-controlled study in which 667 patients with advanced HIV disease were randomized to receive either clarithromycin 500 mg twice daily or placebo. During a median 10-month follow-up, only 6% of clarithromycin-assigned patients versus 16% of placebo-assigned patients developed mycobacteremia ($p<0.001$) [32]. More importantly, median survival was significantly longer in clarithromycin- than placebo-assigned patients (32 vs 41% mortality, $p = 0.026$). However, among the clarithromycin-assigned patients who did develop disseminated MAC infection, 58% had mycobacteremia with MAC isolates that were highly resistant to clarithromycin (minimum inhibitory concentration [MIC] $\geq$512 μg/mL). Clarithromycin at this same dose has also been compared with rifabutin and to the combination of clarithromycin and rifabutin in a large randomized trial involving 1,216 patients with absolute CD4 counts <100 cells/mm^3. In this trial, clarithromycin was significantly more effective than rifabutin in preventing MAC (9 vs 15% of patients, $p = 0.01$), but the addition of rifabutin to clarithromycin provided no significant increase in efficacy compared with clarithromycin alone [33].

Azithromycin

A regimen of weekly azithromycin prophylaxis was evaluated in a placebo-controlled, double-blind trial in which 10.6% of 85 azithromycin recipients and 24.7% of 89 placebo recipients developed MAC infection (hazard ratio, 0.34; $p = 0.004$) [34]. There was no difference between the groups in survival or in the macrolide susceptibility of breakthrough MAC isolates. In another trial, 693 patients with CD4 count <100 cells/mm^3 were randomized to azithromycin 1,200 mg once weekly, daily rifabutin or both. Azithromycin was more effective than rifabutin in preventing MAC (7.6 vs 15.3%, $p = 0.008$), and the combination of both agents was more effective than either one alone (2.8%, $p = 0.03$) [35]. Among the patients in whom azithromycin prophylaxis was not successful, only 11% of MAC isolates were resistant to azithromycin. Both clarithromycin and azithromycin prophylaxis are well-tolerated. The main adverse effects of clarithromycin are nausea and altered taste and the main effect of azithromycin is diarrhea.

Rifabutin

Rifabutin alone at a dose of 300 mg once daily also has been compared with placebo for MAC prophylaxis in two randomized trials conducted in over 1,000 patients with advanced HIV disease. Rifabutin demonstrated efficacy by reducing the incidence of MAC by half. Patients who received rifabutin and subsequently developed MAC had blood isolates that retained susceptibility to rifabutin. However, neither trial alone, nor the combined analysis, demonstrated that rifabutin significantly reduced mortality. In addition, rifabutin requires dose adjustment when used in combination with some antiretroviral agents (Table 27.1).

Discontinuation of primary prophylaxis

Two randomized, placebo-controlled trials have addressed the question of whether chronic prophylaxis is needed for patients who at one time had a CD4 count <50 cells/mm^3 but now have absolute CD4 counts above 100 cells/mm^3 on ART [36, 37]. Among the 583 patients who were assigned to receive placebo in these combined trials, there were only two cases of MAC infection, both localized to the vertebral spine. Thus, MAC prophylaxis should be discontinued in patients on ART who maintain CD4 counts >100 cells/mm^3.

OTHER ATYPICAL MYCOBACTERIAL INFECTIONS IN HIV-INFECTED PATIENTS

Disseminated and localized infections caused by *M. kansasii*, *M. celatum*, *M. xenopi*, *M. simiae*, *M. haemophilum*, *M. marinum*, *M. scrofulaceum*, *M. gordonae*, *M. genavense*, *M. fortuitum*, *M. chelonae*, *M. malmoense*, *M. abscessus*, *M. triplex*, and *M. terrae* also have been reported in patients with AIDS. Those with disseminated disease generally have had clinical presentations similar to that of disseminated MAC infection, although pulmonary involvement is more common with *M. kansasii* infection. The *in vitro* sensitivity of isolates to standard antituberculous drugs has been variable. Of note, cases of disseminated *M. simiae-avium* infection have been reported in Thailand and Malawi.

M. kansasii

M. kansasii has been the most frequently reported of the other atypical mycobacteria. A trend toward increased incidence of HIV-related *M. kansasii* was noted in Northern California in the mid-1990s. *M. kansasii* lung infection is also an emerging problem among HIV-infected people in South Africa, especially miners, and has been reported to occur at high CD4 counts [38]. This organism, like MAC, is acquired from the environment, and no cases of human-to-human transmission have been documented. In three published series from New Orleans, Kansas City, and Miami, the clinical features of 119 cases of AIDS-related *M. kansasii* infection have been reported [39–41]. A total of 91% of these cases involved pulmonary disease; 32% had disseminated disease. The median CD4 count at diagnosis was <50 cells/mm^3 in all three series. Fever, cough and weight loss were common. Radiographic manifestations of *M. kansasii* infection can include cavitation, consolidation or nodular densities. Patients with AIDS-related *M. kansasii* infection have been reported to respond to therapy with combinations of agents, including isoniazid, rifampin, ethambutol, clarithromycin and ciprofloxacin. Although the American Thoracic Society recommends a combination of isoniazid, rifampin, and ethambutol as therapy for this disease, clinicians must substitute clarithromycin and/or rifabutin for rifampin in patients receiving protease inhibitors. The recommended duration of therapy is a minimum of 18 months. The *in vitro*, isoniazid resistance and clarithromycin sensitivity is commonly observed. Rifampin resistance is also an emerging problem. Thus, multi-drug therapy should be tailored to the results of *in vitro* sensitivities of a culture isolate.

M. genavense

M. genavense can cause disseminated infection that is clinically similar to disseminated MAC in patients with CD4 counts <50 cells/mm^3 [42]. This fastidious organism is difficult to detect and does not grow on conventional solid media. Small colonies can be detected in specially supplemented Middlebrook media, and low growth index can be observed in BACTEC broth. Since susceptibilities to drugs cannot be reliably determined, an empiric treatment choice must be made. Clinical reports indicate that clarithromycin-containing combination regimens may be effective therapy.

M. haemophilum

M. haemophilum is an atypical mycobacterium with a propensity to cause joint, bone, and ulcerative skin lesions (perhaps related to the lower temperature it requires for optimal growth). In addition, disseminated infection can occur in patients with advanced AIDS. A cluster of cases was reported in the New York City area. Clarithromycin and rifabutin appear to be the most active therapeutic agents.

REFERENCES

[1] Nightingale SD, Byrd LT, Southern PM, et al. Incidence of *Mycobacterium avium-intracellulare* complex bacteremia in human immunodeficiency virus-positive patients. J Infect Dis 1992;165:1082–5.

[2] Race EM, Adelson-Mitty J, Kriegel GR, et al. Focal mycobacterial lymphadenitis following initiation of protease inhibitor therapy in patients with advanced HIV-1 disease. Lancet 1998;351:252–5.

[3] Hawkins CC, Gold JWM, Whimbey E, et al. *Mycobacterium avium* complex infections in patients with the acquired immunodeficiency syndrome. Ann Intern Med 1986;105:184–8.

[4] Dore GJ, Hoy JF, Mallal SA, et al. Trends in incidence of AIDS illnesses in Australia from 1983 to 1994: the Australian AIDS cohort. J AIDS 1997;16:39–43.

[5] Ohtomo K, Wang S, Masunaga A, et al. Secondary infections of AIDS autopsy cases in Japan with special emphasis on *Mycobacterium avium-intracellulare* complex infection. Tohoku J Exp Med 2000;192:99–109.

[6] Blaxhult A, Fox Z, Colebunders R, et al. Regional and temporal changes in AIDS in Europe before HAART. Epidemiol Infect 2002;129:565–76.

[7] Barreto JA, Palaci M, Ferrazoli L, et al. Isolation of *Mycobacterium avium* complex from bone marrow aspirates of AIDS patients in Brazil. J Infect Dis 1993;168:777–9.

[8] Pettipher CA, Karstaedt AS, Hopley M. Prevalence and clinical manifestations of disseminated *Mycobacterium avium* complex infection in South Africans with acquired immunodeficiency syndrome. Clin Infect Dis 2001;33:2068–71.

[9] Anekthananon T, Ratanasuwan W, Techasathit W, et al. HIV infection/acquired immunodeficiency syndrome at Siriraj Hospital, 2002: time for secondary prevention. J Med Assoc Thai 2004;87:173–9.

[10] Hadad DJ, Palaci M, Pignatari AC, et al. Mycobacteraemia among HIV-1-infected patients in Sao Paulo, Brazil: 1995 to 1998. Epidemiol Infect 2004;132:151–5.

[11] Buchacz K, Baker RK, Palella Jr. FJ, et al. HOPS Investigators. AIDS-defining opportunistic illnesses in US patients, 1994–2007: a cohort study. AIDS 2010;24:1549–59.

[12] C.F. Von Reyn, Maslow JN, Barber TW, et al. Persistent colonisation of potable water as a source of *Mycobacterium avium* infection in AIDS. Lancet 1994;343:1137–41.

[13] Jacobson MA, Hopewell PC, Yajko DM, et al. Natural history of disseminated *Mycobacterium avium* complex infection in AIDS. J Infect Dis 1991;164:994–8.

[14] Horsburgh CR, Havlik JA, Ellis DA, et al. Survival of patients with acquired immune deficiency syndrome and disseminated *Mycobacterium avium* complex infection with and without antimycobacterial chemotherapy. Am Rev Respir Dis 1991;144:557–9.

[15] Chin DP, Reingold AL, Horsburgh CR Jr, et al. Predicting *Mycobacterium avium* complex bacteremia in patients with the human immunodeficiency virus: a prospectively validated model. Clin Infect Dis 1994;19:668–74.

[16] Young LS. *Mycobacterium avium* complex infection. J Infect Dis 1988;157:863–7.

[17] Evans KD, Nakasone AS, Sutherland PA, et al. Identification of *Mycobacterium tuberculosis* and *Mycobacterium avium-M. intracellulare* directly from primary BACTEC cultures by using acridinium-ester labelled DNA probes. J Clin Microbiol 1992;30:2427–31.

[18] Chin DP, Hopewell PC, Yajko DM, et al. *Mycobacterium avium* complex in the respiratory or gastrointestinal tract and the risk of *M. avium* complex bacteremia in patients with the human immunodeficiency virus. J Infect Dis 1994;169:289–95.

[19] Chiu J, Nussbaum J, Bozzette S, et al. Treatment of disseminated *Mycobacterium avium* complex infection in AIDS with amikacin, ethambutol, rifampin, and ciprofloxacin. Ann Intern Med 1990;113:358–61.

[20] Kemper CA, Meng TC, Nussbaum J, et al. Treatment of *Mycobacterium avium* complex bacteremia in AIDS with a four-drug oral regimen. Ann Intern Med 1992;116:466–72.

[21] Parenti D, Williams PL, Hafner R, et al. A phase II/III trial of antimicrobial therapy with or without amikacin in the treatment of disseminated *Mycobacterium avium* infection in HIV-infected individuals. AIDS Clinical Trials Group Protocol 135 Study Team. AIDS 1998;12:2439–46.

[22] Chaisson RE, Benson C, Dube M, et al. Clarithromycin therapy for bacteremic *Mycobacterium avium* complex disease. Ann Intern Med 1994;121:905–11.

[23] Dunne M, Fessel J, Kumar P, et al. A randomized, double-blind trial comparing azithromycin and clarithromycin in the treatment of disseminated *Mycobacterium avium* infection in patients with human immunodeficiency virus. Clin Infect Dis 2000;31:1245–52.

[24] Ward TT, Rimland D, Kauffman C, et al. Randomized, open-label trial of azithromycin plus ethambutol vs. clarithromycin plus ethambutol as therapy for *Mycobacterium avium* complex bacteremia in patients with human immunodeficiency virus infection. Veterans Aff HIV Res Consortium Clin Infect Dis 1998;27:1278–85.

[25] Kemper C, Havlir D, Haghighat D, et al. The individual microbiologic effect of three antimycobacterial agents, clofazimine, ethambutol, and rifampin, on *Mycobacterium avium* complex bacteremia in patients with AIDS. J Infect Dis 1994;170:157–64.

[26] Dube MP, Sattler FR, Torriani FJ, et al. A randomized evaluation of ethambutol for prevention of relapse and drug resistance during treatment of *Mycobacterium avium* complex bacteremia with clarithromycin-based combination therapy. Calif Collab Treat Group J Infect Dis 1997;176:1225–32.

[27] Sullam P, Gordin F, Wynne B. The Rifabutin Treatment Group. Efficacy of rifabutin in the treatment of disseminated infection due to *Mycobacterium avium* complex. Clin Infect Dis 1994;19:84–6.

[28] Shafran SD, Singer J, Zarowny DP, et al. A comparison of two regimens for the treatment of *Mycobacterium avium* complex bacteremia in AIDS: rifabutin, ethambutol, and clarithromycin versus rifampin, ethambutol, clofazimine, and ciprofloxacin. N Engl J Med 1996;335:377–83.

[29] Benson CA, Williams PL, Currier JS, et al. A prospective, randomized trial examining the efficacy and safety of clarithromycin in combination with ethambutol, rifabutin, or both for the treatment of disseminated *Mycobacterium avium* complex disease in persons with acquired immunodeficiency syndrome. Clin Infect Dis 2003;37:1234–43.

[30] Shelburne SA, Visnegarwala F, Darcourt J, et al. Incidence and risk factors for immune reconstitution inflammatory syndrome during highly active antiretroviral therapy. AIDS 2005;19:399–406.

[31] Zolopa A, Andersen J, Powderly W, et al. Early antiretroviral therapy reduces AIDS progression/death in individuals with acute opportunistic infections: a multicenter randomized strategy trial. PLoS One 2009;4:e5575.

[32] Pearce M, Crampton S, Henry D, et al. A randomized trial of clarithromycin as prophylaxis against disseminated *Mycobacterium avium* complex infection in patients with advanced acquired immunodeficiency syndrome. N Engl J Med 1995;335:384–91.

[33] Benson CA, Williams PL, Cohn DL, et al. Clarithromycin or rifabutin alone or in combination for primary prophylaxis of *Mycobacterium avium* complex disease in patients with AIDS. A randomized, double-blind, placebo-controlled trial. The AIDS Clinical Trials Group 196/Terry Beirn Community Programs for Clinical Research on AIDS 009 Protocol Team. J Infect Dis 2000;181:1289–97.

[34] Oldfield EC, Fessel WJ, Dunne MW, et al. Once weekly azithromycin therapy for prevention of *Mycobacterium avium* complex infection in patients with AIDS: a randomized, double-blind, placebo-controlled multicenter trial. Clin Infect Dis 1998;26:611–19.

[35] Havlir DV, Dube MP, Sattler FR, et al. Prophylaxis against disseminated *Mycobacterium avium* complex with weekly azithromycin, daily rifabutin or both. N Engl J Med 1996;335:392–8.

[36] Currier JS, Williams PL, Koletar SL, et al. Discontinuation of *Mycobacterium avium* complex prophylaxis in patients with antiretroviral therapy-induced increases in CD4+ cell count. A randomized, double-blind, placebo-controlled trial. AIDS Clinical Trials Group 362 Study Team. Ann Intern Med 2000;133:493–503.

[37] El-Sadr WM, Burman WJ, Grant LB, et al. Discontinuation of prophylaxis for *Mycobacterium avium* complex disease in HIV-infected patients who have a response to antiretroviral therapy. Terry Beirn Community Programs for Clinical Research on AIDS. N Engl J Med 2000;342:1085–92.

[38] Corbett EL, Churchyard GJ, Hay M, et al. The impact of HIV infection on *Mycobacterium kansasii* disease in South African gold miners. Am J Respir Crit Care Med 1999;160:10–14.

[39] Campo RE, Carlos CE. *Mycobacterium kansasii* disease in patients infected with human immunodeficiency virus. Clin Infect Dis 1997;24:1233–8.

[40] Bamberger DM, Driks MR, Gupta MR, et al. *Mycobacterium kansasii* among patients infected with human immunodeficiency virus in Kansas City. Clin Infect Dis 1994;18:395–400.

[41] Witzig RS, Fazal BA, Mera RM, et al. Clinical manifestations and implications of coinfection with *Mycobacterium kansasii* and human immunodeficiency virus type 1. Clin Infect Dis 1995;21:77–85.

[42] Bessesen MT, Shlay J, Stone-Venohr B, et al. Disseminated *Mycobacterium genavense* infection: clinical and microbiological features and response to therapy. AIDS 1993;7:1357–61.

Chapter | 28 |

Candida in HIV infection

William G. Powderly

EPIDEMIOLOGY

Candidiasis is caused by fungi of the *Candida* species, which are yeasts that are ubiquitous in the environment. *Candida* species are common human commensal organisms on skin and mucous membranes; between 30% and 80% of adults and children are colonized with *Candida* species [1, 2]. The point prevalence of carriage is higher in at-risk groups, such as cancer patients and HIV-infected persons [3–5]. In general, such colonization with *Candida* does not cause infection. The primary defense mechanisms involved in protection against local infection with *Candida* involve the cell-mediated immune system. Progressive loss of T-cell function associated with HIV disease leads to an increased risk of direct local invasion of *Candida* and localized infection. Other host factors important in the defense against *Candida* infections include blood group secretor status, salivary flow rates, epithelial barrier, antimicrobial constituents of saliva, and the presence of normal bacterial flora. Several studies suggest that HIV infection is associated with impairment in a number of these local mucosal defense mechanisms.

Mucosal candidiasis is a common opportunistic infection in HIV-infected individuals. Oropharyngeal candidiasis (OPC) usually occurs with low CD4 counts, but tends to be one of the earliest opportunistic infections and may be seen in patients with CD4 counts $<200/mm^3$. The finding of oropharyngeal candidiasis should never be dismissed in an HIV-infected patient; it indicates progressive immune deficiency and should prompt the institution of effective antiretroviral therapy.

Prior to the era of highly active antiretroviral therapy (HAART, or ART), between 50 and 75% of HIV-infected individuals developed at least one episode of mucosal candidiasis. Recurrent episodes are frequent with progressive immune deficiency. The incidence has declined since the introduction of ART in the late 1990s. Higher HIV viral load is significantly associated with increased oral or vaginal colonization and candidiasis, an association that has been reduced by ART [6]. However, in parts of the world where ART is not widely available, mucosal candidiasis continues to represent a significant cause of morbidity. Esophageal candidiasis affects between 10% and 20% of patients with AIDS. *Candida* infection is the most common cause of esophageal disease in persons with HIV infection.

The epidemiology of mucocutaneous candidiasis has changed in the last 10 years primarily because of two factors. The first is the widespread use of antifungal agents, particularly the azoles. Continuous use of azoles has led to a decline in the prevalence of mucosal candidiasis but also led to the emergence of refractory infections caused by azole-resistant *Candida*. The second factor influencing *Candida* epidemiology in AIDS has been the introduction of potent ART, which has resulted in a significant decline in the incidence of all opportunistic illnesses, including mucosal candidiasis. It is reasonable to expect that the incidence of mucocutaneous candidiasis in HIV-infected patients will continue to decline as more patients receive effective ART.

The majority of cases of candidiasis in the setting of HIV infection are confined to mucosal surfaces i.e. oropharyngeal, esophageal, and vulvovaginal; systemic candidiasis is rare and usually occurs in patients with advanced HIV/AIDS (often in the setting of neutropenia) or occurs as a result of nosocomial acquisition. While oropharyngeal and esophageal candidiasis are clearly HIV-associated illnesses, it is likely that vulvovaginal candidiasis (VVC) is not. HIV-seropositive women have a higher prevalence of vaginal colonization with *Candida* compared with seronegative women. However, the incidence of vulvovaginal candidiasis is unrelated to HIV serostatus and tends to reflect other risk factors for vulvovaginal *Candida* infection such as sexual activity and socioeconomic status. The prevalence of vulvovaginal disease is also independent of CD4 count and does not increase with advancing immunodeficiency. However, the severity and frequency of recurrence of vulvovaginal candidiasis may be linked to progressive HIV infection, and, as a consequence, this remains an important source of morbidity in infected women. This may indicate a difference in pathogenesis of *Candidal* infection at the two sites, oropharynx and vagina [7].

The most common causative organism is *Candida albicans* [8], found in over 90% of isolates from patients with their first episode of oropharyngeal candidiasis. In patients with recurrent disease, the same strain causes the relapse in approximately half of cases, but other strains or species may also be implicated. The majority of disease is caused by organisms that are part of the normal flora of an individual, although rare cases of person-to-person transmission have been documented. In patients with prolonged or recurrent antifungal use, non-*albicans* species with different antimicrobial susceptibilities become more commonly isolated. These include *C. glabrata*, *C. tropicalis*, *C. krusei*, and *C. dubliniensis* [9, 10]. Some of these species are more likely to be associated with decreased susceptibility to azole antifungals [11].

CLINICAL MANIFESTATIONS

Oropharyngeal candidiasis

Almost all patients with OPC are symptomatic, complaining of a sore mouth or oropharyngeal pain with swallowing. On inspection, OPC is usually associated with visible creamy white plaques on the tongue, hard or soft palate. If scraped, these plaques have an erythematous base (this is the pseudomembranous form of OPC, often referred to as thrush). Other clinical manifestations include angular cheilitis, which is a non-specific inflammation of the angles of the mouth, and acute or chronic atrophic candidiasis, which can present as erythematous tongue and/or thinning of the mucous membranes. Although usually associated with mild morbidity, OPC can be clinically significant. Severe OPC can interfere with the administration of medications and adequate nutritional intake, and may spread to the esophagus.

The differential diagnosis of oropharyngeal candidiasis includes:

1. *Oral hairy leukoplakia (OHL)*. OHL is characterized by raised white lesions in the oral mucosa, usually found on the sides of the tongue. It is associated with herpes viruses in the epithelial cells, particularly Epstein–Barr virus (EBV). It can be differentiated from candidiasis by inability to scrape off the plaque or by lack of response to antifungal therapy. Antiviral therapy with acyclovir

can be used for treatment, although specific antiviral treatment is not usually required as the condition is typically asymptomatic. OHL is an indication for ART.

2. *Oral ulcers*. Extensive oral ulceration can be seen in the setting of HIV infection. It has many causes, including herpes simplex virus (HSV) type I and II, cytomegalovirus (CMV), drug toxicities (e.g. Stevens–Johnson syndrome due to co-trimoxazole or antiretrovirals). However, the most common cause is idiopathic aphthous ulceration. Patients typically have single or multiple discrete ulcers that are usually painful and may coalesce or become secondarily infected. Treatment involves identifying the cause and discontinuing the causative agent if relevant. In the case of viral ulceration, systemic antivirals such as acyclovir may be useful. With aphthous ulceration, topical steroids or analgesic mouthwashes are helpful, and oral thalidomide therapy has been shown to be effective in severe cases [12].

3. *Gingivitis and periodontitis*. Severe oral cavity disease has been seen in HIV infection. It usually presents with painful bleeding gums, halitosis, and dental loosening. There may be ulceration of gums. It is caused by mixed aerobic and anaerobic infection and responds to topical agents; systemic therapy with metronidazole may be required.

4. *Kaposi's sarcoma*. When present in the oral cavity, the typical purple lesions of KS are usually seen on the palate. If large, the lesions may ulcerate due to local trauma. Biopsy establishes the diagnosis.

5. *Non-Hodgkin's lymphoma* can cause oral cavity disease in HIV patients. It may present as a mass lesion, tonsillar in origin, or as ulceration of the mucosa. Biopsy establishes the diagnosis.

Esophageal candidiasis

Patients are usually symptomatic with dysphagia and/or odynophagia. Retrosternal pain or discomfort may be present. There may or may not be concurrent oropharyngeal involvement. Severe symptoms can lead to considerable difficulty in eating or swallowing liquids, which can interfere with nutrition or hydration. In a patient with OPC, complaints of swallowing difficulty or retrosternal symptoms, should prompt a high clinical suspicion of esophageal candidiasis, and empiric antifungal therapy should be initiated. In atypical cases or those refractory to empiric antifungal therapy, direct visualization of the esophagus by endoscopy is the best way to make the diagnosis. The epithelial lining of the esophagus is coated in a pseudomembrane consisting of yeasts, epithelial cells, leukocytes, and necrotic debris. Erosions or ulcers may be seen. An experienced endoscopist will often make the diagnosis on macroscopic appearance. Definitive diagnosis is made by brushings or biopsy of the mucosa. The differential diagnosis includes viral esophagitis caused by CMV or HSV types I and II and severe aphthous ulceration. A helpful clinical clue in differentiating the different infectious causes of esophagitis in HIV-infected patients is that esophagitis due to *C. albicans* often results in complaints of food 'sticking in the throat,' whereas esophagitis due to HSV or CMV more often produces complaints of actual pain with swallowing.

Vulvovaginal candidiasis

As noted previously, this is a common clinical syndrome in women irrespective of HIV status or immune function. There are many additional predisposing factors to the development of genital *Candida* infection, including diabetes, oral contraceptive use, pregnancy, and systemic antibiotic therapy.

VVC generally presents with itching, a vaginal discharge (which may be watery or thick), vaginal erythema with adherent white discharge, dyspareunia, dysuria, and erythema and swelling of the labia and vulva. The cervix usually appears normal. Initial episodes tend to be uncomplicated, mild to moderate in severity, and sporadic, usually caused by *C. albicans*. More complicated VVC tends to occur in more immunocompromised hosts, is often recurrent, and is more likely to be caused by non-*albicans* species.

Unprotected intercourse with a partner with VVC may lead to *Candida* balanitis in the male partner, manifested by pruritic, erythematous patches on the glans penis.

Disseminated candidiasis and candidemia

In HIV-infected individuals, this is a rare and usually late event, typically occurring in patients with advanced immunosuppression. It is most often a hospital-acquired infection, with non-*albicans Candida* playing a significant role in pathogenesis. There has been a significant reduction in the incidence of nosocomial candidemia in HIV-infected patients in the post-HAART era [13]. Risk factors are those of nosocomial acquisition, including presence of a central venous catheter, use of gastric acid suppressants, nasogastric tubes, antibiotics, ICU admission [14], severe esophageal mucosal disease, advanced AIDS, concomitant opportunistic infections, non-*albicans* species, and neutropenia. Virtually every body organ can be affected by *Candida* infection. Involvement of the eyes (endophthalmitis), central nervous system (meningitis [15], encephalitis), and heart (endocarditis) are described but rare in the setting of HIV infection.

Community-acquired candidemia and disseminated candidiasis in HIV is sometimes seen in countries where injection drug users make up a significant proportion of the HIV-infected population. This can present as end-organ disease such as endocarditis, endophthalmitis or skin lesions [16–18].

DIAGNOSIS

The diagnosis of mucosal candidiasis is usually a clinical one. The presence of characteristic symptoms with or without clinical findings in an HIV-infected patient is often enough to warrant treatment. In many ways, this constitutes a therapeutic trial, with lack of response to empiric antifungal therapy prompting further diagnostic testing. Oropharyngeal cultures often demonstrate *Candida* species but are not diagnostic because colonization is common. The diagnosis of OPC can be confirmed by examining a 10% potassium hydroxide (KOH) slide preparation of a scraping of an active lesion. Pseudohyphae and budding yeast are characteristic findings. Culture is usually not necessary with initial episodes of OPC unless the lesions fail to clear with appropriate antifungal therapy. In patients with poorly responsive OPC, a culture should be obtained to look for drug-resistant yeast or those that respond poorly to certain azoles (e.g. *C. krusei* or *C. glabrata*).

The diagnosis of *Candida* vaginitis is made by the presence of a characteristic clinical appearance and observation of yeast forms on microscopic examination. A KOH preparation from vaginal lesions can confirm the diagnosis of candidiasis and differentiate it from other conditions that can be similar in appearance (e.g. trichomoniasis). Routine fungal cultures are rarely helpful in the absence of KOH-positive lesions because yeasts are normal inhabitants of the vaginal mucosa. A fungal culture should be obtained if a patient fails to respond to standard antifungal therapy to determine whether azole resistance is contributing to the therapeutic failure.

In the microbiology laboratory *Candida* spp. are relatively easy to culture. They grow rapidly on simple media at 25–37°C. *Candida* colonies are smooth and creamy white in color on agar plates. Specialized media can differentiate between species by colony color (CHROMagar *Candida*) and are very useful. Germ tube testing is a relatively quick method of determining whether the organism is *Candida albicans* or a non-*albicans* species. Many microbiology laboratories report yeast cultures as either *C. albicans* or non-*albicans* species based upon the germ tube test; if specific identification is required, further discussion with the microbiologist is often necessary.

Efforts to develop a standardized reproducible and clinically relevant method of susceptibility testing for yeasts have resulted in development of the NCCLS M27-A2 methodology [19], which has data-driven interpretive breakpoints for susceptibility of *Candida* spp. to antifungal agents (Table 28.1). Data relating to fluconazole and itraconazole are more readily available than for other antifungals. Susceptibility testing of *Candida* spp. is not routinely used in most laboratories. The identification of the species is often enough to predict likely antifungal susceptibility, and further testing is not required. However, in the setting

Table 28.1 Definition of *in vitro* resistance for *Candida* species. Range of MICs (μg/mL)

ANTIFUNGAL AGENT	SUSCEPTIBLE	SUSCEPTIBLE—DOSE DEPENDENT	RESISTANT
Itraconazole	≤0.125	0.25–0.5	≥1.0
Fluconazole	≤8.0	16–32	>64
Amphotericin B	≤1.0	–	≥2.0

Adapted from NCCLS standard definitions for antifungal susceptibilities using microbroth or macrotube dilution methodology.

of recurrent infection, failure to respond to initial therapy or systemic infection with non-*albicans* species, susceptibility testing may contribute to clinical decision making and can also be used to support a decision to switch from a parenteral to oral agent. The dose and delivery of the antifungal agent are important in interpreting the data, and host factors play a significant role in the clinical response to a particular agent irrespective of laboratory susceptibility data [20].

TREATMENT

Many antifungal agents with activity against *Candida* spp. are now available. In general, therapy for mucosal candidiasis can be given as local preparations (usually as mouthwashes, troches, or suspensions for oropharyngeal disease or as creams or suppositories for vaginal disease), or as systemic preparations for more severe infections (Table 28.2). Treatment of OPC is usually straightforward. In trials, response rates vary from 34 to 95%. However, most studies of antifungal treatment for mucocutaneous candidiasis suffer from one or more weaknesses, such as small numbers of patients, heterogeneous populations, short follow-up, and non-blinded designs. In the case of HIV-associated *Candida* infection, studies have not stratified patients by CD4 counts. This is important because persons with low CD4 counts respond more slowly to treatment, have lower rates of fungal eradication, and higher relapse rates than persons with less advanced disease.

Azoles

The azoles are the most commonly used drugs and are available as local (topical) and systemic products. They act as inhibitors of the demethylase enzyme involved in ergosterol synthesis, ergosterol being the essential sterol on the fungal cell membrane. Drugs in this class include clotrimazole, ketoconazole, itraconazole, voriconazole, and posoconazole.

Fluconazole

Fluconazole is a triazole antifungal and is the most widely available and commonly used agent to treat *Candida* infection. It is available in oral and intravenous forms. It has good bioavailability, with the same doses being administered both orally and intravenously (100–800 mg/day). It is generally well tolerated but may cause headache (up to 13%), GI upset (<10%) or liver enzyme abnormalities, especially at higher doses. It requires dose adjustment in severe renal impairment. It is a CYP450 inhibitor and can interact with other drugs metabolized by these enzymes, but there are few important interactions described for the drugs commonly used in HIV infection. Rifampin can decrease the concentrations of fluconazole and may lead to treatment failure. Nevirapine can also reduce fluconazole levels, but the clinical significance is unknown. Fluconazole is FDA category C for use in pregnancy and should be used with caution. It can be used for treatment of mucosal and disseminated candidiasis and for prophylaxis. Resistance to fluconazole has been seen in patients who receive continuous or intermittent fluconazole [21]. It is active against most *C. albicans* strains; primary resistance is rare but strains with decreased susceptibility emerge over time at rates varying between 5 and 30% in patients with prolonged exposure to fluconazole [22]. *C. glabrata and C. krusei* often have decreased susceptibility to fluconazole [23].

Itraconazole

Itraconazole is another triazole agent. It is available in oral capsules, pastilles, suspension, and intravenous infusion (100–200 mg/day). Oral bioavailability is not as good as that of fluconazole, and it requires gastric acidity for absorption. It has a similar side-effect profile to fluconazole, but drug interactions are more frequent. It is also category C for use in pregnancy. It is active against mucosal candidiasis. There is cross-resistance with fluconazole, particularly in non-*albicans* species [24–26], but there are strains of *C. albicans* with reduced susceptibility to fluconazole that may respond to itraconazole.

Table 28.2 Treatment guide

CLINICAL SYNDROME	DRUGS	MODE OF DELIVERY	PREPARATION	DOSE	DURATION
Vulvovaginal candidiasis	Clotrimazole; Miconazole; Butoconazole; Tioconazole	Topical	Cream, pessary		3–5 days
	Boric acid	PV	Gelatin capsules	600 mg once daily	14 days
	Fluconazole	PO	Capsule	150 mg	Single dose
Oropharyngeal candidiasis	Clotrimazole	Topical	Troche	10 mg 5/day	7–14 days
	Nystatin	Topical	Suspension or pastilles	4–6 mL q.i.d 1–2 pastilles 4–5 times/day	7–14 days
	Amphotericin B	Topical	Suspension	1 mL = 100 mg q.i.d.	7–14 days
	Fluconazole	PO	Capsule	100–400 mg once daily	7–14 days
	Itraconazole	PO	Capsule or solution	200 mg once daily	7–14 days
Esophageal candidiasis	Fluconazole	PO/IV	Capsule or infusion	200 mg once daily	14–21 days
	Itraconazole	PO	Solution	200 mg once daily	14–21 days
	Caspofungin	IV	Infusion	70 mg loading then 50 mg/day	14–21 days
	Micafungin	IV	Infusion	150 mg/day	14–21 days
	Anidulafungin	IV	Infusion	100 mg load then 50 mg/day	14–21 days
	Amphotericin B deoxycholate; lipid-associated AmB	IV	Infusion	0.6–1 mg/kg per day; 3–5 mg/kg per day	14–21 days
	Voriconazole	PO/IV	Tablet or infusion	100–200 mg twice daily	14–21 days
	Posaconazole	PO	Solution	400 mg once daily	14–21 days
Candidemia	Fluconazole[a]	IV	Infusion	400–800 mg once daily	14–21 days; # from negative cultures
	Amphotericin B deoxycholate	IV	Infusion	0.5–0.6 mg/kg per day	
	Lipid-associated AmB	IV	Infusion	3–5 mg/kg per day	
	Caspofungin	IV	Infusion	70 mg loading then 50 mg/day	
	Anidulafungin	IV	Infusion	100 mg load then 50 mg/day	
	Micafungin	IV	Infusion	150 mg/day	

[a]Consider switch to oral dosing towards end of treatment.

Voriconazole and posoconazole

Voriconazole and posoconazole are newer azole agents available in oral and parenteral forms Although they are effective for the treatment of oral and esophageal candidiasis, they are significantly more costly. Voriconazole is associated with reversible visual disturbances (23%) [27]. Both drugs have significant interactions with efavirenz, ritonavir, and rifampin; concurrent use is not recommended. These agents are rarely indicated as initial therapy but may be effective in patients with fluconazole-resistant disease, including infection caused by *C. krusei* [28].

Cell wall synthesis inhibitors (caspofungin, anidulafungin, and micafungin)

These are a new class of antifungal agents, of which caspofungin was the first to become readily available. They are only available in intravenous formulation. The dose of caspofungin is 70 mg as a loading dose, followed by 50 mg/day, anidulafungin is given as a 100 mg load followed by 50 mg/day, and the micafungin dose is 150 mg/day. A dosage increase of caspofungin to 70 mg/day is required with concomitant use of enzyme inducers such as rifampin, NNRTIs, phenytoin, etc. These agents have been shown to be effective and well tolerated in the treatment of esophageal candidiasis [29–31], including fluconazole-resistant infection.

Polyenes

Previously the mainstay of antifungal therapy, the polyenes are increasingly regarded as second-line therapies because of issues of toxicity and bioavailability. Polyenes are not well-absorbed after oral administration. This characteristic makes them potentially useful as topical therapy in the management of mucosal disease, and oral suspensions of nystatin and amphotericin B are available. However, they must be administered frequently (4–5 times daily) and in relatively large volumes to be most effective, and these characteristics, in addition to their bitter taste, has made them less popular than the azoles for local therapy. Several formulations of amphotericin B are available for systemic use, including amphotericin B deoxycholate (dose 0.6–1 mg/kg per day), amphotericin B lipid complex (ABLC) (5 mg/kg per day), amphotericin B colloidal dispersion (3–6 mg/kg per day), and liposomal amphotericin B (3–5 mg/kg per day). Most experience in the treatment of systemic candidiasis is with the traditional form of amphotericin B. The three newer lipid-associated formulations have not been shown to be superior to traditional amphotericin but have less nephrotoxicity and are better tolerated. With the advent of better tolerated agents such as fluconazole and caspofungin, amphotericin B is now regarded as second-line therapy in proven candidiasis; the lipid formulations are preferred in patients felt to be at high risk of toxicities (renal, infusion reactions) from the traditional formulation.

Treatment of oropharyngeal and esophageal candidiasis

Oropharyngeal candidiasis

Initial episodes of oropharyngeal candidiasis usually respond well to any antifungal agent: topical azoles (clotrimazole one 10 mg troche 5 times/day); oral azoles (fluconazole 100 mg/day for 7–14 days; itraconazole solution 100 mg/day 7–14 days or ketoconazole) or oral polyenes (nystatin suspension/pastilles or oral amphotericin B). Patients with mild OPC, especially those with less advanced immunosuppression can be treated with topical agents, as these are less likely to have systemic side effects. Of the systemic agents, fluconazole has been well studied and is as effective or superior to topical therapy. Doses can range from 50 to 200 mg daily for uncomplicated OPC, but higher doses should be used if there is a suspicion of esophageal involvement or if the patient has more advanced HIV disease. In general, the first episode of OPC will

resolve within 2–3 days of starting fluconazole. Recurrent episodes often require higher doses and a more prolonged therapy.

The best way to prevent further episodes of candidiasis is with ART. However, recurrent symptomatic episodes may prompt the need for suppressive therapy in selected patients. Prophylactic therapy for patients with frequent symptomatic recurrences limited to the oral mucosa should be tailored to suit the clinical situation, and either intermittent or continuous therapy can be considered. Oral fluconazole 100-400 mg daily is usually the treatment of choice. The risk of developing azole-resistant disease appears to be the same with either continuous or intermittent therapy [32]. If resistance develops, doses of up to 800 mg/day may be effective in some cases. Fluconazole resistance is often (but not always) associated with cross-resistance to the other azole antifungal agents. About half of patients with fluconazole-unresponsive esophageal candidiasis respond to itraconazole cyclodextrin solution at 100 mg twice daily.

If antifungal resistance seems likely, a variety of alternative strategies can be employed. First, as noted, azole cross-resistance is not universal, and a trial of itraconazole at 200 mg twice daily is warranted. Use of itraconazole solution is preferred, due both to its local effects and its better absorption. Second, individuals with refractory esophageal candidiasis have had response rates of approximately 50% with voriconazole at its standard dosage of 200 mg twice daily. Third, topical solutions of polyenes may be used. Fourth, the echinocandins have had response rates of 70–80% for esophageal candidiasis, including fluconazole-resistant cases.

Esophageal candidiasis

Esophageal candidiasis requires systemic treatment. Oral fluconazole at 200 mg/day for 14–21 days will resolve symptoms in over 80% of patients within a week. Initial therapy with intravenous preparations may be needed in patients who have severe odynophagia or dysphagia. Azoles, echinocandins, and amphotericin B are the agents of choice in descending order. Itraconazole solution and voriconazole are as effective as fluconazole but are generally reserved for refractory cases. Patients with advanced AIDS patients who are not taking ART are likely to suffer from recurrent infections, and long-term suppressive therapy with fluconazole 200 mg daily may be required.

Treatment of vulvovaginal candidiasis

Symptomatic relief is the aim of treatment. Topical agents are often most effective, with systemic therapy needed for severe or recurrent cases. Uncomplicated VVC usually responds well to topical agents such as clotrimazole, miconazole, butoconazole, tioconazole creams, and pessaries or boric acid 600 mg gelatin capsules administered intra-vaginally daily for 2 weeks. Oral fluconazole 150 mg as a single dose orally is very effective. Alternatively, itraconazole (200 mg twice daily for 1 day or 200 mg/day for 3 days) or ketoconazole (400 mg twice daily for 5 days) can be used.

More complicated vaginitis requires longer duration of therapy, either topical treatment for 7 days or oral therapy with two doses of fluconazole 150 mg 72 h apart. Non-*albicans Candida* infection may not respond as well to azole therapy but is an infrequent cause of vulvovaginal candidiasis.

Recurrent disease is usually due to azole-susceptible *C. albicans* and may require prolonged therapy or even long-term prophylaxis with weekly fluconazole. This may select for non-*albicans* strains, but the significance of this is not certain [33].

Treatment of candidemia

This is a serious infection with a significant mortality and propensity to disseminate and cause end-organ disease. Along with definitive antifungal therapy, removal of an infected intravascular catheter and evaluation for metastatic disease (i.e. ophthalmologic evaluation, echocardiography) are advised. Parenteral therapy is usually indicated initially with intravenous fluconazole, caspofungin or amphotericin B. The choice of agent should be based on the individual patient's status, prior antifungal exposure, likely causative organism or definitive microbiological data. Most patients can be switched to high-dose oral fluconazole (800 mg/day) when clinically stable. Therapy for candidemia should be given for at least 14 days after sterilization of the blood cultures.

Candida and ART

Since the introduction of HAART in the late 1990s, the incidence and prevalence of opportunistic infections (OIs) in HIV-infected individuals on therapy has declined. This is true not only for initial episodes of mucosal or esophageal candidiasis but also for more advanced disease. For example, fluconazole-resistant candidiasis, which once had a prevalence of over 20% in cohort studies, is now extremely uncommon. However, in the resource-limited setting where ART is not widely available, candidiasis is still prevalent.

A large number of studies published after the availability of ART showed a decline in the incidence and prevalence of mucosal candidiasis. Although this can largely be

attributed to the restoration of cell-mediated immunity, as reflected in the rise in CD4 count, there have been some interesting data suggesting a direct anti-candidal effect exhibited by HIV protease inhibitors both *in vitro* [34, 35] and *in vivo* [36]. This has been attributed to inhibition of secreted aspartic proteinases (Saps) by HIV protease inhibitors [37]. Saps are key virulence factors of *C. albicans*. Inhibition of Sap expression is not seen with other antiretroviral classes [38, 39]; however, there are little data to suggest that PIs are associated with better control of mucosal candidiasis than other antiretrovirals.

One manifestation of the successful treatment of HIV-infected persons with effective ART is a risk of developing immune reconstitution inflammatory syndrome (IRIS). This manifests as the development of an acute inflammatory reaction to opportunistic pathogens as the immune system recovers. This is most commonly seen with mycobacterial disease; however, cases describing IRIS with candidiasis (OPC) [40, 41] have been reported.

Candidiasis is a sign of the failure of the immune system, which is usually well controlled with effective ART. The development of candidiasis should therefore be taken as an indication to initiate ART or to look for evidence of virologic failure. The development of candidiasis in a patient already taking ART suggests treatment failure due either to non-adherence, the development of resistant HIV, or both.

PREVENTION OF *CANDIDA* INFECTIONS

As previously noted, several studies have shown that fluconazole, given daily or even weekly, could significantly reduce the incidence of mucosal candidiasis in patients with advanced HIV disease. Fluconazole has also been shown to be effective in reducing the prevalence of other invasive fungal infections. However, in the developed world, routine prophylaxis for candidiasis has not been routinely recommended, largely because of cost and fears of resistance. Prophylaxis can be used in certain recurrent cases [42], especially with esophageal disease. However, the availability of potent antiretroviral therapy has eliminated the need for specific antimicrobial prophylaxis, an observation that is as true for *Candida* infection as it is for other opportunistic diseases.

REFERENCES

[1] Schmidt-Westhausen AM, Bendick C, Reichart PA, et al. Oral candidosis and associated *Candida* species in HIV-infected Cambodians exposed to anti-mycotics. Mycoses 2004;47:435–41.

[2] Tekeli A, Dolapci I, Emral R, et al. *Candida* carriage and *Candida dubliniensis* in oropharyngeal samples of type 1 diabetes mellitus patients. Mycoses 2004;47:315–18.

[3] Al-Abeid HM, Abu-Elteen KH, Elkarmi AZ, et al. Isolation and characterization of *Candida* spp. in Jordanian cancer patients: prevalence, pathogenic determinants and antifungal

sensitivity. Jpn J Infect Dis 2004;57:279–84.

[4] Gugnani HC, Becker K, Fegeler W, et al. Oropharyngeal carriage of *Candida* species in HIV-infected patients in India. Mycoses 2003;46:299–306.

[5] Pongsiriwet S, Iamaroon A, Sriburee P, et al. Oral colonization of *Candida* species in perinatally HIV-infected children in northern Thailand. J Oral Sci 2004;46: 101–15.

[6] Schuman P, Sobel JD, Ohmit SE, et al. Mucosal candidal colonization and candidiasis in women with or at risk for human immunodeficiency virus infection. HIV Epidemiology Research Study (HERS) Group. Clin Infect Dis 1998;27:1161–7.

[7] Ohmit SE, Sobel JD, Schuman P, et al. Longitudinal study of mucosal *Candida* species colonization and candidiasis among human immunodeficiency virus (HIV)-seropositive and at-risk HIV-seronegative women. J Infect Dis 2003;188:118–27.

[8] Powderly WG, Mayer K, Perfect J. Diagnosis and treatment of oropharyngeal candidiasis in patients infected with HIV: a critical reassessment. AIDS Res Hum Retroviruses 1999;15:1405–12.

[9] Cartledge JD, Midgley J, Gazzard BG. Non-*albicans* oral candidosis in HIV-positive patients. J Antimicrob Chemother 1999;43:419–22.

[10] Melo NR, Taguchi H, Jorge J, et al. Oral candida flora from Brazilian human immunodeficiency virus-infected patients in the highly active antiretroviral therapy era. Mem Inst Oswaldo Cruz 2004;99:425–31.

[11] Martinez M, Lopez-Ribot JL, Kirkpatrick WR, et al. Replacement of *Candida albicans* with *C. dubliniensis* in human immunodeficiency virus-infected patients with oropharyngeal candidiasis treated with fluconazole. J Clin Microbiol 2002;40:3135–9.

[12] Paterson DL, Georghiou PR, Allworth AM, et al. Thalidomide as treatment of refractory aphthous

ulceration related to human immunodeficiency virus infection. Clin Infect Dis 1995;20:250–4.

[13] Bertagnolio S, de Gaetano Donati K, Tacconelli E, et al. Hospital-acquired candidemia in HIV-infected patients. Incidence, risk factors and predictors of outcome. J Chemother 2004;16:172–8.

[14] Puzniak L, Teutsch S, Powderly W, et al. Has the epidemiology of nosocomial candidemia changed? Infect Control Hosp Epidemiol 2004;25:628–33.

[15] Casado JL, Quereda C, Corral I. Candidal meningitis in HIV-infected patients. AIDS Patient Care STDS 1998;12:681–6.

[16] Bisbe J, Miro JM, Latorre X, et al. Disseminated candidiasis in addicts who use brown heroin: report of 83 cases and review. Clin Infect Dis 1992;15:910–23.

[17] Miro JM, del Rio A, Mestres CA. Infective endocarditis in intravenous drug abusers and HIV-1 infected patients. Infect Dis North Am 2002;16:vii–viii, 273–95.

[18] Kim RW, Juzych MS, Eliott D. Ocular manifestations of intravenous drug use. Infect Dis Clin North Am 2002;16:607–22.

[19] Pappas PG, Rex JH, Sobel JD, et al. Guidelines for the treatment of candidiasis. Clin Infect Dis 2004;38:161–89.

[20] Rex JH, Pfaller MA. Has antifungal susceptibility testing come of age? Clin Infect Dis 2002;35:982–9.

[21] Revankar SG, Kirkpatrick WR, McAtee RK, et al. A randomized trial of continuous or intermittent therapy with fluconazole for oropharyngeal candidiasis in HIV-infected patients: clinical outcomes and development of fluconazole resistance. Am J Med 1998;105:7–11.

[22] Martins MD, Lozano-Chiu M, Rex JH. Point prevalence of oropharyngeal carriage of fluconazole-resistant *Candida* in human immunodeficiency virus-infected patients. Clin Infect Dis 1997;25:843–6.

[23] Ostrosky-Zeichner L, Rex JH, Pappas PG, et al. Antifungal susceptibility survey of 2,000 blood

stream *Candida* isolates in the United States. Antimicrob Agents Chemother 2003;47:3149–54.

[24] Goldman M, Cloud GA, Smedema M, et al. Does long-term itraconazole prophylaxis result in in vitro azole resistance in mucosal *Candida albicans* isolates from persons with advanced human immunodeficiency virus infection? The National Institute of Allergy and Infectious Diseases Mycoses study group. Antimicrob Agents Chemother 2000;44:1585–7.

[25] Vazquez JA, Peng G, Sobel JD, et al. Evolution of anti-fungal susceptibility among *Candida* species isolates recovered from human immunodeficiency virus-infected women receiving fluconazole prophylaxis. Clin Infect Dis 2001;33:1069–75.

[26] Barchiesi F, Colombo AL, McGough DA, et al. In vitro activity of itraconazole against fluconazole-susceptible and -resistant *Candida albicans* isolates from oral cavities of patients infected with human immunodeficiency virus. Antimicrob Agents Chemother 1994;38:1530–3.

[27] Ally R, Schurmann D, Kreisel W, et al. Esophageal Candidiasis Study Group. A randomized, double blind, double dummy, multi-center trial of voriconazole and fluconazole in the treatment of esophageal candidiasis in immunocompromised patients. Clin Infect Dis 2001;33:1447–54.

[28] Ostrosky-Zeichner L, Oude Lashof AM, Kullberg BJ, et al. Voriconazole salvage treatment of invasive candidiasis. Eur J Clin Microbiol Infect Dis 2003;22:651–5.

[29] Villanueva A, Gotuzzo E, Arathoon EG, et al. A randomized double-blind study of caspofungin versus fluconazole for the treatment of esophageal candidiasis. Am J Med 2002;113:294–9.

[30] Vazquez J, Schranz JA, Clark R, et al. A phase 2, open-label study of the safety and efficacy of intravenous anidulafungin as a treatment for azole-refractory mucosal candidiasis. J Acquir Immune Defic Syndr 2008;48:304–9.

[31] de Wet N, Llanos-Cuentas A, Suleiman J, et al. A randomized, double-blind, parallel-group, dose–response study of micafungin compared with fluconazole for the treatment of esophageal candidiasis in HIV-positive patients. Clin Infect Dis 2004;39:842–89.

[32] Goldman M, Cloud GA, Wade KD, et al. A randomized study of the use of fluconazole in continuous versus episodic therapy in patients with advanced HIV infection and a history of oropharyngeal candidiasis: AIDS Clinical Trials Group Study 323/Mycoses Study Group Study 40. Clin Infect Dis 2005;41:1473–80.

[33] Vazquez JA, Sobel JD, Peng G, et al. Evolution of vaginal *Candida* species recovered from human immunodeficiency virus-infected women receiving fluconazole prophylaxis: the emergence of *Candida glabrata*? Clin Infect Dis 1999;28:1025–31.

[34] Tacconelli E, Bertagnolio S, Posteraro B, et al. Azole susceptibility patterns and genetic relationship among oral *Candida* strains isolated in the era of

highly active antiretroviral therapy. J Acquir Defic Syndr 2002;31:38–44.

[35] Cassone A, De Bernardis F, Torosantucci A, et al. In vitro and in vivo anticandidal activity of human immunodeficiency virus protease inhibitors. J Infect Dis 1999;180:448–53.

[36] Mata-Essayag S, Magaldi S, Hartung de Capriles C, et al. "In vitro" antifungal activity of protease inhibitors. Mycopathologica 2001;152:135–42.

[37] Cauda R, Tacconelli E, Tumbarello M, et al. Role of protease inhibitors in preventing recurrent oral candidosis in patients with HIV infection: a prospective case-control study. J Acquir Immune Defic Syndr 1999;21:20–5.

[38] Bektic J, Lell CP, Fuchs A, et al. HIV protease inhibitors attenuate adherence of *Candida albicans* to epithelial cells in vitro. FEMS Immunol Med Microbiol 2001;31:65–71.

[39] De Bernardis F, Tacconelli E, Mondello F, et al. Anti-retroviral therapy with protease inhibitors decreases virulence enzyme expression in vivo by *Candida*

albicans without selection of avirulent strains or decreasing their anti-mycotic susceptibility. FEMS Immunol Med Microbiol 2004;41:27–34.

[40] Cassone A, Tacconelli E, De Bernardis F, et al. Antiretroviral therapy with protease inhibitors has an early, immune reconstitution-independent beneficial effect on *Candida* virulence and oral candidiasis in human immunodeficiency virus-infected subjects. J Infect Dis 2002;185:188–95.

[41] Jevtovic DJ, Salemovic D, Ranin J, et al. The prevalence and risk of immune restoration disease in HIV-infected patients treated with highly active antiretroviral therapy. HIV Med 2005;6:140–3.

[42] Kaplan JE, Benson C, Holmes KH, et al., Centers for Disease Control and Prevention (CDC), National Institutes of Health, HIV Medicine Association of the Infectious Diseases Society of America. Guidelines for prevention and treatment of opportunistic infections in HIV-infected adults and adolescents. MMWR Recomm Rep 2009;58 (RR-4):1–207.

Chapter | 29 |

Cryptococcosis and other fungal infections (histoplasmosis and coccidioidomycosis) in HIV-infected patients

Kathleen R. Page, Richard E. Chaisson, Merle Sande

INTRODUCTION

Systemic fungal infections are generally late manifestations of HIV disease. Overall, cryptococcal infection is the most common systemic fungal infection in HIV-infected patients. However, in certain endemic regions, histoplasmosis or coccidioidomycosis are more prevalent. These diseases can affect patients without HIV, but among HIV-infected patients, they tend to occur when the CD4 count is < 200 cells/mm³. Immune reconstitution with antiretroviral therapy (ART) has led to significant declines in the incidence of fungal disease among HIV-infected individuals. However, among patients with limited access to ART, opportunistic infections with fungal pathogens remain a major cause of death. This chapter reviews the approach to diagnosis and management of the most commonly occurring systemic mycosis in HIV-infected patients: cryptococcosis, histoplasmosis, and coccidioidomycosis.

CRYPTOCOCCUS

Microbiology

Cryptococcus neoformans is a round or oval yeast (4–6 μm in diameter), surrounded by a capsule that can be up to 30 μm thick. The organism grows readily on fungal or bacterial culture media and is usually detectable within 1 week after inoculation, although in some circumstances up to 4 weeks are required for growth. It grows well at 37°C, does not form pseudomycelin on cornmeal or rice-Tween agar, and hydrolyzes urea, a property that allows rapid presumptive identification [1].

On the basis of antigenic differences in the capsule, biochemical use of nutrients, and distinct DNA base sequences, four serotypes (A, B, C, and D) of *Cryptococcus* have been delineated. Serotypes A and D are classified as *C. neoformans* var. *neoformans*, and serotypes B and C are classified as *C. neoformans* var. *gatii* [2]. *Cryptococcus neoformans* var. *neoformans* is the major cause of cryptococcal disease worldwide. Serotype A is the most common serotype infecting AIDS patients [3, 4].

Epidemiology

Before the onset of the AIDS epidemic, cryptococcal infection occurred in a small number of immunocompetent individuals, but most often in patients with a compromised immune system, such as diabetics, transplant recipients, patients with lymphoma, or patients requiring chronic steroid therapy [5]. In the AIDS era, cryptococcal disease became a leading opportunistic infection, affecting 6–10% of HIV-infected patients [6–10]. It is the third most common central nervous system (CNS) disorder in AIDS patients after toxoplasmosis and HIV dementia [11].

In the past decade the incidence of disease caused by *C. neoformans* in developed countries has decreased dramatically, in part due to more widespread use of azole therapy [12], but primarily resulting from the introduction of highly active antiretroviral therapy (HAART). Surveillance and clinical studies in the USA and Europe have shown a 2- to 10-fold decrease in the incidence of cryptococcosis since the introduction of HAART [9, 11, 13, 14]. Demographic characteristics of patients with cryptococcosis show that poor access to medical care is a major risk factor for developing cryptococcal disease in the HAART era [14-17].

However, in areas of the world with limited access to ART, cryptococcosis remains a major cause of morbidity and mortality. It is estimated that there are approximately 1 million cases of HIV-associated cryptococcosis annually, the majority occurring in resource-limited settings [18]. Studies from sub-Saharan Africa and Southeast Asia show that up to one-third of patients infected with HIV develop cryptococcal disease [19-21], which is a major cause of death among HIV-infected patients [22]. Despite antifungal therapy, mortality from cryptococcal disease in these settings is exceedingly high [18, 22, 23], with an average survival of <6 months after diagnosis [24, 25]. In sub-Saharan Africa, the estimated mortality attributed to cryptococcal meningoencephalitis (~500,000 deaths per year) is higher that the mortality attributed to tuberculosis (350,000 deaths/year) [18]. Poor outcomes may be related to the late presentation of disease and suboptimal management of raised intracranial pressure.

Natural history, pathogenesis, and pathology

Cryptococcus neoformans infection is acquired from the environment. Because it is ubiquitous in soil and dust, exposure to the organisms is practically unavoidable. The organism, most likely in an encapsulated form, is inhaled into the lungs and deposited in the small airways. Once there, yeast multiply and compress the surrounding tissue but cause little damage, and pulmonary infection is often asymptomatic. Indeed, in 85–95% of patients with cryptococcal meningoencephalitis, no evidence of pneumonitis is present [7, 26]. The organism has a strong propensity for dissemination to the CNS but also may infect skin, bone, and the genitourinary tract.

Clinical features

The onset of cryptococcal disease usually is insidious. The most common symptoms are headache, malaise, and a prolonged febrile prodrome that may be indistinguishable from symptoms caused by other opportunistic infections [7, 26–28]. The median time between the onset of symptoms and the diagnosis of cryptococcal disease is 30 days [7, 26, 27]. Diagnosis is often delayed by the waxing and waning course of the disease and the absence of specific symptoms.

CRYPTOCOCCAL MENINGOENCEPHALITIS

CNS involvement is the most serious and common manifestation of cryptococcal disease in HIV-infected patients. Over 75% of HIV-associated cryptococcal meningoencephalitis occurs in patients with CD4 counts <50 cells/mm^3. In general, CNS disease presents as a chronic meningoencephalitis, with headaches, nausea, and photophobia,

but occasionally can present with focal neurologic signs associated with mass lesions (cryptococcomas). In a prospective study conducted in Uganda, 20% of HIV-infected patients presenting with headaches were diagnosed with cryptococcal meningoencephalitis [29]. Classic signs of meningeal irritation are uncommon. HIV-infected patients presenting with seizures, altered mental status, psychosis, and dementia should be evaluated for cryptococcal meningoencephalitis. Pulmonary or disseminated disease may be associated, but usually CNS disease presents in isolation.

The physical examination in patients with cryptococcal disease is non-specific, with fevers in approximately half the cases, but less than one-third with nuchal rigidity or other neurologic deficits [7]. Altered mental status, which is the most important predictor of poor outcome, is present in 20–30% of patients with cryptococcal disease. Papilledema is seen in < 10% of patients. Raised, sometimes umbilicated, typical skin lesions that resemble those caused by molluscum contagiosum or *Penicillium marneffei* are reported in 3–10% of patients with cryptococcal meningoencephalitis.

Immune reconstitution syndrome (IRIS) occurs in 8-49% of patients with cryptococcosis treated with ART [30]. The syndrome is characterized by a paradoxical clinical deterioration resulting from an exuberant inflammatory response that may manifest itself as worsening or new lymphadenopathy, mediastinitis, pneumonitis, new headache and stiff neck, CNS lesions, increased intracranial pressure, or subcutaneous abscesses [30–35]. The onset of IRIS usually occurs between the first and tenth month of ART initiation [30]. Several factors have been associated with the risk of IRIS, including high baseline viral load, initiation of ART during induction therapy, rapid rise in CD4 count, high cryptococcal titers, and lack of CSF inflammation at baseline [30, 36–38]. Usually *C. neoformans* cultures are negative.

Patient evaluation, diagnosis, and differential diagnosis

Cryptococcal meningoencephalitis is by far the most common manifestation of cryptococcosis in HIV-infected patients. The most common symptoms are fever, malaise, and worsening headaches over the course of a few weeks, but the indolent and non-specific presentation requires a high index of suspicion to diagnose the disease in a timely manner. Although the presentation is subacute, and not usually suggestive of bacterial meningoencephalitis, in a study from Malawi, 10% of suspected bacterial meningoencephalitis cases turned out to be cryptococcal meningoencephalitis [39]. The CD4 count can help guide the work-up and differential diagnosis. While cryptococcal meningoencephalitis is rare in patients with a CD4 count > 100 cells/mm^3, it is the leading diagnosis for HIV-infected patients with low CD4 counts presenting with fever and headache.

The differential diagnosis depends to some extent on local epidemiology. Central nervous system (CNS) tuberculosis

Table 29.1 Differential diagnosis of HIV-associated fungal infections

CRYPTOCOCCAL MENINGO-ENCEPHALITIS	SPECIFIC FEATURES	DISSEMINATED HISTOPLASMOSIS	SPECIFIC FEATURES	COCCIDIOIDOMYCOSIS
Non-focal examination:		Tuberculosis		Tuberculosis
CNS tuberculosis	Basilar involvement	*Pneumocystis* pneumonia		*Pneumocystis* pneumonia
Coccidioidomycosis	SW USA, Central and South America	Coccidioidomycosis	SW USA, Central and South America	Community-acquired pneumonia
Histoplasmosis	Ohio/Mississippi river valleys, Central America	Paracoccidioidomycosis	Central and South America	Histoplasmosis
Penicilliosis	Southeast Asia	Blastomycosis	Ohio/Mississipi river valleys, Central America	Paracoccidioidomycosis
Focal examination, also includes:		Penicilliosis	Southeast Asia	Blastomycosis
Toxoplasmosis	Usually no headache	Melioidosis (*Burkholderia pseudomallei*)	Southeast Asia, Australia	Penicilliosis
CNS lymphoma		*Rhodococcus equi*	Rural exposure	Melioidosis (*B. pseudomallei*)
Cysticercosis (non-USA)				*Rhodococcus equi*

(TB) is a major concern in patients from TB-endemic areas. Other considerations include chronic fungal infections such as penicillosis in patients from Southeast Asia and histoplasmosis or coccidioidomycosis in patients from Latin America. In patients who present with focal neurologic deficits or seizures, the differential diagnosis can also include toxoplasmosis, CNS lymphoma, and other non-HIV related conditions, such as cysticercosis or CNS malignancy. Despite an extensive differential diagnosis, the diagnosis of cryptococcal meningoencephalitis is generally straightforward due to the characteristic elevation in intracranial pressure and the high sensitivity and specificity of cryptococcal antigen tests (Table 29.1).

If available, the serum cryptococal antigen (CRAG) test is an excellent starting point for the evaluation of cryptococcal meningoencephalitis. Serum CRAG tests are positive in over 99% of patients with cryptococcosis and can be used to rule out cryptococcal meningoencephalitis in HIV-infected patients with a fever and a headache (Fig. 29.1) [40]. In the USA, a lumbar puncture is recommended if the serum CRAG is positive to evaluate for the presence of CNS involvement and to measure intracranial pressure [41]. However, in resource-limited settings lumbar punctures may only be practically available for patients with advanced disease. In such scenarios, it is appropriate to screen ambulatory HIV-infected patients presenting with headaches with a serum CRAG and a chest radiograph to rule out tuberculosis. Patients with a positive CRAG, negative chest radiograph, and no focal neurologic signs, headache, or altered consciousness can be successfully treated with oral fluconazole. In Uganda, screening with serum CRAG detected cryptococcal infection 20 days before the onset of frank meningoencephalitis, and early therapy with fluconazole reduced mortality rates and was cost-effective [29, 42]. However, patients with altered mental status or focal neurologic signs must have a lumbar puncture performed to confirm the diagnosis and to appropriately manage elevated intracranial pressure [41]. The CSF CRAG has high sensitivity (93–99%) and specificity (93–98%) [7, 26, 43] and can expedite or exclude the diagnosis of cryptococcal meningoencephalitis (Table 29.2).

The CSF profile of HIV-infected patients with cryptococcal meningoencephalitis is normal in 25–50% of patients [7, 26, 44–46]. Over 50% of patients have a low CSF white blood count ($<20/mm^3$), and the India ink preparation is positive in 74–88% of cases [7, 26, 45–47]. Interpretation of the India ink stain should be performed by an

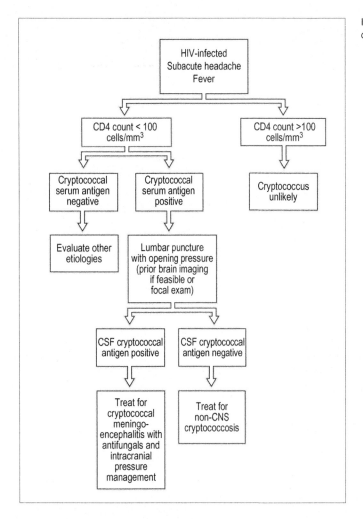

Figure 29.1 Algorithm for the work-up of cryptococcal meningoencephalitis.

experienced technician since false-positive tests have been reported. After staining, *C. neoformans* is visible as round cells 4–6 μm in diameter surrounded by a characteristic thick polysaccharide capsule (Fig. 29.2). Budding forms can usually be detected with viable *C. neoformans*.

The gold standard diagnostic test for cryptococcal meningoencephalitis is a positive CSF culture for *C. neoformans*. CSF fungal cultures require a minimum of 2 mL to obtain maximum sensitivity. By definition, 100% of cases of cryptococcal meningoencephalitis have positive CSF fungal cultures. Approximately 50–80% of HIV-infected patients with cryptococcal meningoencephalitis have positive blood cultures for *C. neoformans* [27, 47, 48].

Prognosis

Left untreated, cryptococcal meningoencephalitis is uniformly fatal [29]. Although survival in HIV-infected patients with cryptococcal meningoencephalitis has improved with better therapeutic management and ART, 10–20% of patients die or fail therapy despite access to tertiary care [28, 47]. In areas with limited medical resources, mortality rates are even higher [22, 25, 33, 48]. In the post-HAART era in Uganda, 20% of hospitalized patients with CSF-confirmed cryptococcal meningoencephalitis died within the first two weeks of therapy and only 41% survive 6 months [25]. The most important baseline prognostic factor is mental status at the time of presentation. Individuals with altered sensorium have a much worse prognosis than those who are awake and alert [27, 47, 49]. High fungal burden, a positive India ink test, elevated intracranial pressure, and lack of inflammatory cells in the CSF are also associated with poor outcomes [25, 27, 28, 47, 49, 50]. Early detection of cryptococcal infection with serum CRAG testing and treatment with fluconazole can decrease the rate of progression and mortality from cryptococcal disease in resource-limited settings [42].

Table 29.2 Sensitivity of commercially available non-culture-based diagnostic methods

DISEASE	SEROLOGY		ANTIGEN DETECTION			
Cryptococcosis						
Disseminated	N/A		Serum:	99% [49]		
Pulmonary	N/A		Serum:	96% [59]		
Meningeal	N/A		Serum: CSF:	99%,[a] [54] 93–100% [49]		
Histoplasmosis						
Disseminated	Serum:	67–70%,[b] [108]	Serum:	80%	Urine:	90% [108, 112]
Pulmonary	Serum:	90–100% [108]			Urine:	15% [108]
Meningeal	CSF:	70–88% [98, 107–109]	CSF:	40–70% [108, 109]		
Coccidioidomycosis						
Disseminated	Serum:	75–94% [133, 135, 145, 149]	N/A			
Pulmonary	Serum:	<10% [133]	N/A			
Meningeal	CSF:	50% [147]	N/A			

[a]Not specific for meningoencephalitis; must evaluate CSF.
[b]Does not distinguish active disease from prior infection.

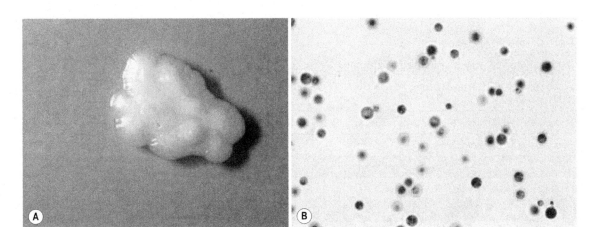

Figure 29.2 (A) Mature *Cryptococcus neoformans* colony. (B) Microscopic appearance of *C. neoformans*.
Photographs courtesy of Dr William Merz, Department of Pathology, Johns Hopkins University School of Medicine.

Treatment

Early diagnosis is crucial to improving treatment outcomes for HIV-infected patients with cryptococcosis. Other key factors for providing optimal care include early induction therapy for meningoencephalitis followed by suppressive regimens, early recognition and management of elevated intracranial pressure and IRIS, and the use of lipid formulations of amphotericin B in patients with renal impairment [41]. However, in many settings, management options may be limited by the medical resources available. In all cases, treatment of the underlying immunosuppression from HIV infection is critical to managing cryptococcosis

The treatment of cryptococcal meningoencephalitis in AIDS patients requires initial induction therapy with a fungicidal regimen, preferably amphotericin B and flucytosine, followed by suppressive therapy with fluconazole (Table 29.3). Amphotericin B is more effective than azole therapy during the initial phase of treatment, leading to faster sterilization of the CSF and fewer relapses [47, 51, 52]. The addition of flucytosine increases the efficacy of amphotericin [28, 41, 52]. A randomized study from Thailand showed that the combination of amphotericin B and flucytosine cleared *Cryptococcus* from the CSF faster than amphotericin B alone, amphotericin B and fluconazole, or triple therapy with amphotericin B, flucytosine, and fluconazole [53]. The prospective multicenter study CryptoA/D also showed that flucytosine therapy was associated with

mycologic clearance at 2 weeks of therapy [48]. Therefore, amphotericin and flucytosine combination therapy is recommended in the USA. Of note, flucytosine causes significant hematologic toxicity, and levels and hematologic parameters should be monitored closely. Patients who develop amphotericin-related nephrotoxicity or infusion reactions can be treated with lipid formulations of amphotericin, which are associated with less toxicity and similar efficacy, but are more costly [54–56].

In resource-limited settings, optimal induction therapy with amphotericin B and flucytosine may not be feasible due to lack of medications or inability to monitor toxicity, and oral fluconazole is an alternative for the treatment of cryptococcal meningoencephalitis in patients with mild symptoms and normal sensorium. Results from

Table 29.3 Therapy of HIV-associated cryptococcal meningoencephalitis

REGIMEN	DURATION	EVIDENCE[a]
Induction therapy[b]		
Preferred		
Amphotericin B (0.7–1.0 mg/kg/day)[c] + flucytosine (100 mg/day)[d]	2 weeks	**1**
If flucytosine intolerant:		
Amphotericin B (0.7–1.0 mg/kg/day) or liposomal amphotericin B (3–4 mg/kg/day or amphotericin B lipid complex (5 mg/kg/day)	4–6 weeks	**2**
Alternatives for resource-limited settings		
Amphotericin B (0.7-1.0 mg/kg/day) + fluconazole (800 mg/day)	2 weeks	1
Fluconazole (>800 mg/day) + flucytosine	6 weeks	2
Fluconazole (>1200 mg/day)	10–12 weeks	**2**
Consolidation therapy		
Fluconazole (400–800 mg/day)[e]	8 weeks	**1**
Maintenance therapy		
Fluconazole (200 mg/day)	Until CD4 count > 100 cells/mm^3 and/or viral load undetectable for > 3 months with at least 1 year of total therapy	1
Primary prophylaxis	Not recommended[f]	

[a]Evidence 1 = randomized clinical study, 2 = clinical trial > 20 patients
[b]Manage elevated intracranial pressure with serial lumbar puncture if necessary.
[c]Alternative: liposomal amphotericin B (3–4 mg/kg/day) for patients with renal dysfunction.
[d]Monitor renal function on amphotericin, and flucytosine blood levels and/or hematologic parameters.
[e]Use higher-dose fluconazole (800 mg/day) during consolidation if using alternative induction regimen.
[f]Consider checking serum cryptococcal antigen in areas with high incidence of cryptococcemia prior to ART initiation.

several studies evaluating the efficacy of fluconazole monotherapy for cryptococcal meningoencephalitis have been mixed [57, 58], but a recent study found treatment success rates over 60% using higher doses of fluconazole (1,600–2,000 mg daily) [59]. Nausea and vomiting are common, but may be alleviated by administering 3 to 4 divided doses daily. Therefore, patients with cryptococcal meningoencephalitis without neurologic complications may be appropriately treated with 10 weeks of oral high-dose (>800 mg daily, 1,200 mg/day preferred) fluconazole followed by lower-dose maintenance therapy (200–400 mg daily) [41]. Primary and secondary fluconazole resistance may be an issue in patients treated with fluconazole alone, and MIC testing may be indicated in some cases. In a small retrospective study of HIV-infected African patients with cryptococcal meningoencephalitis treated with fluconazole monotherapy, 76% of the isolates recovered during treatment failure had reduced susceptibility to fluconazole [60]. If flucytosine is not available, fluconazole (800 mg/day) can be used as a substitute in combination with amphotericin B during the first two weeks of induction therapy [41].

Following the 2-week induction phase with parenteral therapy, patients can be switched to oral fluconazole (400 mg/day) for 8 weeks (consolidation therapy). It is commonly recommended that CSF be evaluated for sterility after this period. The cryptococcal CSF antigen may remain positive for up to 1 year after successful therapy, so fungal cultures of the CSF should be performed. Prolongation of induction therapy is appropriate in patients who remain comatose, have persistently elevated intracranial pressures, or are clinically deteriorating [41].

Persistent infection is generally defined as persistently positive CSF cultures after 4 weeks of adequately dosed therapy [41]. Due to a paucity of relevant trials, recommendations for "salvage therapy" are predominantly based on expert opinion. Patients with persistently positive cultures should have their immune status optimized with ART and induction therapy should be reinitiated, usually with higher doses of amphotericin. If possible, drug resistance should be evaluated in persistent isolates. Small open-label salvage trials have reported treatment success with voriconazole or posaconazole as salvage therapy in 40–50% of patients with persistent cryptococcosis [41, 61, 62].

Cerebral cryptococcomas

Cerebral cryptococcomas are rare but require prolonged courses of induction and maintenance therapy. Induction therapy with amphotericin B and flucytosine is recommended for at least 6 weeks, followed by consolidation therapy with fluconazole (400–800 mg daily) for 6 to 18 months, depending on clinical response. Corticosteroid therapy may be necessary in cases of mass effect surrounding the lesions, and surgery may be appropriate for large accessible lesions associated with mass effect [41].

Management of elevated intracranial pressure

Elevated intracranial pressure is a common and potentially life-threatening complication of cryptococcal meningoencephalitis [7, 63]. Early recognition and treatment of increased intracranial pressure is a key principle for optimal management [41]. In contrast to the usual pathophysiology of chronic meningoencephalitis, in which pro-inflammatory responses play an important role, cryptococcal meningoencephalitis in HIV-infected patients is notable for a lack of inflammatory cells and seems to be directly related to high fungal titers which cause an outflow obstruction. However, immune reconstitution in patients receiving ART may lead to an inflammatory response that increases intracranial pressure.

In a retrospective study of 211 HIV-infected patients with cryptococcal meningoencephalitis, 60% were found to have initial opening pressures of ≥ 250 mmH$_2$O, and 30% had a pressure ≥ 350 mmH$_2$O [49]. Those with opening pressures ≥ 350 mmH$_2$O had a significantly higher fungal burden and were more likely to have papilledema, hearing loss, and meningismus [49]. Interestingly, this group was less likely to have fever and night sweats, perhaps reflecting an impaired ability to mount an inflammatory response. However, clinical findings were not sensitive or specific predictors of intracranial pressure elevation, and opening pressures should be measured in all patients with cryptococcal meningoencephalitis without contraindication to a lumbar puncture. If available, radiologic imaging of the brain is recommended prior to lumbar puncture in patients with focal neurologic signs or impaired mentation [63]. In resource-limited settings where imaging is not available, no adverse outcomes have occurred in patients without focal neurologic deficits undergoing lumbar puncture with adequate monitoring of opening and closing pressures [64].

The best intervention for elevated intracranial pressure associated with cryptococcal meningoencephalitis is drainage of the CSF. This can usually be accomplished by large-volume lumbar punctures removing up to 30 mL of CSF at one time, which should be repeated daily until the intracranial pressure normalizes and symptoms have been stabilized for at least 2 days [41]. Patients who require frequent lumbar punctures or whose opening pressure is >400 mm H$_2$O may benefit from a lumbar drain. Ventriculoperitoneal shunting may be indicated for persistently elevated pressures or progressive neurologic deficits [41, 65–68]. Patients with rising intracranial pressure while on treatment are at high risk of adverse outcomes and death [49].

Perhaps due to the sparse cellular infiltrate and limited host response, corticosteroids do not improve clinical outcomes in HIV-associated cryptococcal meningoencephalitis [49]. However, patients experiencing major complications from ART-associated IRIS may benefit from corticosteroids. A 2- to 4-week course of steroids is reasonable, but may be extended depending on the clinical scenario and patient response. There is not enough experience to recommend non-steroidal anti-inflammatory agents or thalidomide for the treatment of IRIS.

Relapses

Over one-third of patients successfully treated for cryptococcal meningoencephalitis will relapse without maintenance therapy [69]. Relapse rates are even higher in patients treated only with fluconazole during induction therapy [60]. Therefore, following the 8 weeks of 400 mg/day fluconazole, patients must be placed on suppressive antifungal therapy [69]. Lower-dose fluconazole (200 mg/day) is the preferred maintenance regimen. Fluconazole maintenance therapy is superior to amphotericin or itraconazole for preventing relapses [70]. Another major strategy to prevent relapses is the initiation of ART. Several studies in patients with a history of cryptococcal meningoencephalitis have shown that maintenance therapy can be safely discontinued in patients on ART with sustained immunologic and virologic responses (CD4 counts > 100 cells/mm^3 or undetectable viral load for more than 3 months) [71–75]. In a retrospective multicenter study of 100 patients with a history of cryptococcal meningoencephalitis, the incidence of relapse after discontinuation of fluconazole was only 1.5/100 person-years among patients on ART with a CD4 counts > 100 cells/mm^3 [73]. In a small trial of 42 patients with cryptococcal meningoencephalitis randomized to continue or discontinue fluconazole maintenance therapy when the CD4 count increased to greater than 100 cells/mm^3 and the viral load was undetectable, there were no relapses in the discontinuation arm after 48 weeks of follow-up [75].

Timing of ART and IRIS

There are no large studies that definitively establish the best timing for ART initiation in patients with cryptococcal meningoencephalitis. In a retrospective study from France, 10 out of 120 patients with cryptococcal meningoencephalitis who initiated ART developed IRIS, and 3 of the 10 died. Development of IRIS was associated with initiating ART within 2 months of the diagnosis of cryptococcosis [37]. In contrast, a recent prospective cohort study of 101 AIDS patients with cryptococcal meningoencephalitis found an association between high cryptococcal antigen titers and the risk of IRIS, but not with the timing of ART [38]. In a study of 282 AIDS patients with opportunistic infections, early ART (within 14 days of starting opportunistic infections treatment) improved survival/AIDS progression compared to delayed ART (after completion of acute opportunistic infections therapy), and there was no association between timing of ART and IRIS [76, 77]. Although only 35 patients in this trial had cryptococcal meningoencephalitis, there was a trend towards improved survival in patients receiving early ART [77]. The most recent guidelines from the Infectious Disease Society of America recommend initiating ART within 2 to 10 weeks of diagnosis of

cryptococcal meningoencephalitis [41]. Prolonged delays in ART initiation should be avoided to prevent other complications and mortality from untreated HIV infection. Screening for asymptomatic antigenemia should be considered in patients with CD4 counts < 100 cells/mm^3 living in high incidence areas, such as sub-Saharan Africa or Southeast Asia. Subclinical antigenemia can successfully be treated with fluconazole, but without therapy is a major risk factor for IRIS [42, 78–80].

EXTRANEURAL CRYPTOCOCCOSIS

The incidence of extraneural cryptococcal disease in AIDS patients ranges between 20 and 60% [7, 26, 81, 82]. Despite entry through the lung, evidence of pulmonary symptoms is present in only 20–30% of cases. Other sites of extraneural involvement include the joints, oral cavity, pericardium, myocardium, skin, mediastinum, and genitourinary tract.

Diagnosis

The serum CRAG test has excellent sensitivity and specificity for the diagnosis of disseminated cryptococcosis without CNS involvement. Serum CRAF ≥ 1:8 should always be treated regardless of symptoms. Fungal blood cultures are often positive and bone marrow examination does not increase the diagnostic yield [83]. In contrast to immunocompetent patients with cryptococcal pneumonia, in whom the serum CRAG is often negative, HIV-infected patients with pulmonary cryptococcosis usually have a positive test [84]. HIV-infected patients with pneumonia and a CD4 count ≤ 100 cells/mm^3 should also have fungal cultures of sputum performed. *C. neoformans* can be readily identified using methenamine silver, mucicarmine, and periodic acid-Schiff stains, but cannot be detected with regular Gram's stain of tissue.

Treatment

In immunocompetent patients, asymptomatic pulmonary cryptococcosis often resolves spontaneously and does not require antifungal therapy. In HIV-infected patients, however, pulmonary cryptococcosis should always be treated to prevent disseminated disease [41]. Isolated cryptococcemia indicates deep tissue invasion and should also be treated. In any presentation of extraneural disease, a lumbar puncture should be performed to rule out CNS involvement.

The treatment of extraneural cryptococcosis does not usually require parenteral therapy except in cases of severe pneumonia (acute respiratory distress syndrome) which should be treated like CNS disease. Most cases of mild to moderate disease are treated with daily oral fluconazole (400 mg/day) [57]. The length of therapy has not been well established in clinical trials, though most experts advocate continuing lifelong therapy. In patients on ART, therapy may be discontinued after 1 year of treatment if the CD4 count rises over 100 cells/mm^3 and the cryptococcal antigen titer is < 1:512 [41, 85].

Primary fungal prophylaxis

Three studies have evaluated the role of primary prophylactic antifungal therapy for HIV-infected patients with low CD4 counts [86–88]. Two studies conducted in the USA showed that fluconazole prophylaxis decreased the incidence of cryptococcosis, and itraconazole prophylaxis decreased the incidence of both cryptococcosis and histoplasmosis, especially in patients with CD4 counts < 50 cells/mm^3, but there was no survival benefit [87, 88]. Given the relatively low prevalence of systemic fungal infections in the USA, the widespread use of ART, and the risk of promoting drug resistance, routine antifungal primary prophylaxis is not routinely advocated. However, it may be considered in HIV-infected patients with CD4 counts < 100 cells/mm^3 in areas where there is limited availability of ART and the incidence of cryptococcosis or other fungal infections, such as histoplasmosis or coccidioidomycosis, is high. Asymptomatic cryptococcal antigenemia has been associated with increased mortality in patients initiating ART. Screening patients with CD4 counts < 100 cells/mm^3 with CRAG testing and offering preemptive therapy for patients with a positive result is cost-effective in settings with high incidence of cryptococcosis [42, 89].

HISTOPLASMOSIS

Microbiology

Histoplasma capsulatum (Fig. 29.3) is a dimorphic fungus that exists as a mold in soil and as a yeast in humans. There are two varieties of *Histoplasma* which cause disease in humans: *H. capsulatum* var. *capsulatum* and *H. capsulatum* var. *duboisii*. The former is smaller (1–4 μm) and is found in the Americas, parts of Africa, Asia, and Australia. The latter measures 10–12 μm, is found only in Africa, and is the cause of African histoplasmosis [90].

Epidemiology

Histoplasmosis is endemic in the central and south regions of the USA [90]. The endemic area extends along the Ohio and Mississippi river valleys north into the Canadian provinces of Quebec and Ontario and south into Mexico, Central and South America.

HIV-infected patients often serve as sentinel markers for histoplasmosis outbreaks [91]. During an outbreak in Indianapolis before the HAART era, the incidence of histoplasmosis in HIV-infected individuals was 27%, and among those afflicted, histoplasmosis was the initial AIDS-defining illness in 50% [92]. The incidence of disseminated histoplasmosis has declined with the introduction of HAART [93].

H. capsulatum prefers moderate, humid climates and is found in soil and droppings from birds and bats [94]. The organism has never been cultured from birds, but it can infect bats, and rarely dogs, cats, horses, swine, and a variety of rodents [90]. Certain areas, such as caves, chicken coops, bird roosts, and old buildings, are notorious for having high burdens of *H. capsulatum*, and histoplasmosis can be an occupational hazard [90, 94].

Natural history, pathogenesis, and pathology

As with other systemic fungal infections, initial primary infection occurs in the lung after inhalation of arthroconidia (spores), which are rapidly converted into yeast at

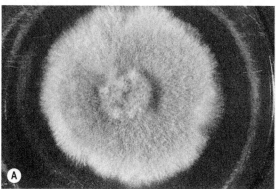
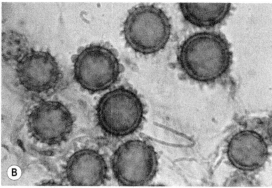

Figure 29.3 (A) *Histoplasma capsulatum* colonies on Saboraud's dextrose agar. (B) Microscopic appearance of *H. capsulatum* showing tuberculate chlamydospores.
Photographs courtesy of Dr William Merz, Deparment of Pathology, Johns Hopkins University School of Medicine.

body temperature. The yeasts are phagocytosed by the reticuloendothelial cells in the lung. Dissemination probably occurs within the first 2 weeks of infection, prior to the onset of adaptive cell-mediated immunity. In immunocompetent individuals, the infection is often controlled by the host response, and the patient may be minimally symptomatic. Reactivation disease is a common form of disseminated histoplasmosis, especially in patients with defective T-cell immunity. In HIV-infected patients, histoplasmosis usually occurs when the CD4 count is <100 cells/mm^3 [95, 96].

Clinical features

In immunocompetent individuals, infection with *H. capsulatum* is usually self-limited, while HIV-infected patients usually develop disseminated disease [91]. The median CD4 count at the time of diagnosis is 50 cells/mm^3 [91]. Fever, weight loss, and other constitutional symptoms are present in over 95% of patients with disseminated disease [91, 95, 97]. Pulmonary symptoms are present in 50–60% of cases. On physical examination, approximately 30% have hepatosplenomegaly, 20% have lymphadenopathy, and 5–15% develop a rash [91, 95, 97]. Neurologic manifestations are reported in 10% of disseminated histoplasmosis cases [92, 98]. Most patients develop a subacute meningoencephalitis, which may be basilar, one-third present with focal brain lesions [92, 98]. Up to 18% of HIV-infected patients with disseminated histoplasmosis present with septic shock and acute respiratory distress syndrome (ARDS) [91, 99]. Renal insufficiency and low albumin at presentation are associated with a worse prognosis, and the mortality for patients with severe symptoms is 70% [99]. On rare occasions, histoplasmosis may present as retinitis, pericarditis, endocarditis, prostatitis, pancreatitis, adrenal insufficiency, or nephritis [91, 95, 100, 101]. There are few reports of immune reconstitution syndrome associated with histoplasmosis in patients initiating ART, with various manifestations such as splenic and liver abscesses, pulmonary nodules, lymphadenitis, uveitis, and skin lesions [102–104]. In endemic areas, initiation of ART may unmask previously undiagnosed histoplasmosis [105].

Routine laboratory test results are generally non-specific. Approximately one-third of patients present with leukopenia and anemia [106]. Occasionally the organism can be seen on peripheral blood mononuclear cells. Liver function test abnormalities are common in HIV-infected patients, but lactate dehydrogenase (LDH) levels >600 mm^3 may suggest histoplasmosis in patients presenting with fevers [107]. Chest radiographs are abnormal in approximately 50% of patients [91, 107, 108]. The most common abnormalities include diffuse interstitial or reticulonodular infiltrates. Mediastinal lymphadenopathy is evident in 20% of cases, and cavitation is rare.

Patient evaluation, diagnosis, and differential diagnosis

Owing to the non-specific symptoms of disseminated histoplasmosis, the disease may be difficult to diagnose. This is especially true in non-endemic areas, where clinicians may not consider the diagnosis, or pathologists may be unaccustomed to identifying *H. capsulatum* in tissue specimens. Clinicians should remember that very transient exposures in an endemic area can lead to infection, so that a history of previous residence is not particularly useful in excluding histoplasmosis.

The gold standard is a positive culture of the organism from peripheral blood or tissue specimens. Blood cultures are positive in 50–70% of cases of disseminated histoplasmosis [91, 106, 109]. Lysis-centrifugation systems and BACTEC cultures have similar sensitivity, but the latter may take longer to become positive [109]. Culture of lymph nodes, liver, skin, and bronchoalveolar lavage is less sensitive, but may be useful in establishing the diagnosis. CSF cultures are positive in 65% of patients with *Histoplasma* meningoencephalitis [92, 110].

Histopathologic examination of tissues is more rapid than culture and establishes the diagnosis in 50% of patients. The most accessible site to biopsy is the bone marrow and skin in patients with dermatologic manifestations. The organism can be identified within macrophages with methenamine silver stains or periodic acid–Schiff stains. An experienced pathologist should review the samples since the organism may be confused with *Cryptococcus*, *Blastomyces*, *Penicillium*, *Toxoplasma*, *Leishmania*, or *Pneumocystis jiroveci* [94].

Serodiagnostic studies are positive in over 80% of all patients with disseminated disease and 90% of those with pulmonary disease, but the sensitivity may decrease with profound immunosuppression and the presence of antibody does not differentiate active from past infection (Table 29.2) [106, 111, 112]. Furthermore, the antibody may cross-react with *Blastomyces*, *Coccidioides*, or *Paracoccidioides* antigens [111, 113]. Nonetheless, a negative antibody test in a patient with histoplasmosis is rare and should prompt further diagnostic work-up.

A rapid and sensitive test for histoplasmosis is antigen detection [114]. The urine antigen test is more sensitive than the serum antigen test for disseminated histoplasmosis (80 vs 90%, respectively) (Table 29.2) [107]. The overall specificity of the test is good, but the antigen test may cross-react with *Penicillium*, *Paracoccidioides*, and *Blastomyces* antigens [111]. Importantly, the test is useful in following the response to therapy [91, 115–117]. Persistent antigenuria implies ongoing infection and increased titers (≥2-fold) suggest relapse and should be treated [117].

Treatment

Untreated progressive disseminated histoplasmosis has a mortality of 80%. Amphotericin B is the drug of choice for HIV-infected patients with moderate to severe disease, but treatment failure occurs in approximately 20–35% of patients [91, 118]. In a randomized study of 81 HIV-infected patients with disseminated histoplasmosis, treatment with liposomal amphotericin resulted in higher success rates (88%) compared with regular amphotericin B (64%) and was associated with less toxicity [118]. Amphotericin lipid complex is a cheaper and adequate alternative, and non-lipid formulations of amphotericin B can be used in patients at low risk for nephrotoxicity [119]. For mild disease, itraconazole therapy is successful in 85% of cases [120, 121]. Fluconazole is less effective than itraconazole, with 74% response rate at a dose of 800 mg per day, but relapses occur frequently and are associated with fluconazole resistance [121–123]. In experimental models, the newer triazoles posaconazole, ravuconazole, and voriconazole have good activity against *H. capsulatum* [124, 125]. Voriconazole may be less effective against isolates resistant to fluconazole and should be used with caution in patients with prior fluconazole exposure [125]. Posaconazole and voriconazole have been used effectively in a few patients with histoplasmosis [126, 127]. The role of the echinocandins in the treatment of histoplasmosis has not been established.

Current practice guidelines for HIV-infected patients with histoplasmosis recommend an initial 12-week intensive phase of therapy to induce remission, followed by chronic maintenance therapy to prevent relapse (Table 29.4) [128]. Liposomal amphotericin B (3 mg/kg/day) or amphotericin B lipid complex (0.7–1 mg/kg/day) should be used for induction in hospitalized patients, and itraconazole (200 mg three times a day for 3 days, then twice a day) can be used upon discharge or in ambulatory patients. Itraconazole is also effective against severe disease and is commonly used in patients who cannot tolerate amphotericin B. Itraconazole absorption is highly variable and blood levels need to be monitored. Itraconazole capsules should be taken with food or cola to increase gastric acidity and absorption, or liquid formulations can be used. Itraconazole is a potent inhibitor and substrate of CYP3A4, and drug interactions are common [129–131]. In selecting an ART regimen, non-nucleoside reverse transcriptase inhibitors (NNRTI's) should be used with caution since they can significantly decrease itraconazole levels. Ritonavir-boosted protease inhibitors increase itraconazole levels [132].

Fluconazole (800 mg daily for 12 weeks, followed by 400 mg daily) can be used cautiously in patients who cannot tolerate itraconazole, but clinical response should be closely monitored since it is less effective than itraconazole and resistance can develop [122, 123]. Ketoconazole is more affordable than itraconazole but has a worse toxicity profile and should only be used for mild cases [128]. Patients with CNS involvement should be treated with 4–6 weeks of liposomal amphotericin B (5 mg/kg/day; total 175 mg/kg), followed by itraconazole (200 mg two to three times daily) for at least one year with resolution of CSF abnormalities.

As with other systemic mycoses, the relapse rate in HIV-infected patients treated for histoplasmosis is high. Therefore, itraconazole maintenance therapy should be prescribed following induction therapy [133]. Maintenance therapy can be discontinued in patients with a CD4 count > 150 cells/mm^3 who have received > 12 months of antifungal therapy, have been on ART for more than 6 months, and have a *Histoplasma* urinary antigen level < 2 ng/ml (if available)

Table 29.4 Therapy for HIV-associated progressive disseminated histoplasmosis

PHASE OF THERAPY	SEVERITY OF DISEASE	PREFERRED DRUG	DURATION OF THERAPY	EVIDENCE[a]
Induction	Mild	Itraconazole[b] (200 mg twice daily)	12 weeks	2
	Moderate to severe	Liposomal amphotericin B[c] (3.0 mg/kg/day)	1–2 weeks	1
	Meningoencephalitis	Liposomal amphotericin B (5.0 mg/kg; day; total 175 mg/kg)	10–12 weeks	5
Maintenance		Itraconazole (200 mg twice daily)	At least 12 months[d]	1
Primary prophylaxis		Itraconazole (200 mg once daily)	Consider in endemic area if CD4 < 100	1

[a]Evidence 1 = randomized clinical study, 2 = clinical trial > 20 patients, 3 = clinical trial < 20 patients, 4 = case series, 5 = expert opinion, expert committees.
[b]Monitor itraconazole blood levels. If possible, avoid concomitant use with efavirenz.
[c]Amphotericin B lipid complex (5.0 mg/kg per day) may be a cheaper alternative. Deoxycholate formulations of amphotericin B (0.7–1.0 mg/kg daily) are an alternative for patients at low risk of nephrotoxicity.
[d]Can discontinue after 12 months of therapy if CD4 > 200 cells/mm^3 for > 6 months.

[128, 134]. The timing of ART in patients with histoplasmosis has not been extensively studied, but IRIS related to histoplasmosis is generally mild. Concern over unmasking or worsening histoplasmosis should not delay initiation of ART [34, 77, 103, 105, 135]. Primary prophylaxis with itraconazole for patients with low CD4 counts is not routinely recommended, but should be considered in endemic areas where the risk of histoplasmosis is > 10/100 patient years [87, 128].

COCCIDIOIDOMYCOSIS

Epidemiology

Coccidioides immitis is endemic in the southwestern USA, northern Mexico, and portions of Central and South America. HIV-associated coccidioidal disease can occur in non-endemic regions due to reactivation disease [136, 137]. Before the era of HAART, coccidioidomycosis was an important opportunistic infection, accounting for 10% of hospitalizations among HIV-infected patients in Arizona between 1990 and 1995 [138]. In the post-HAART era, the incidence and severity of coccidioidal disease in HIV-infected patients has decreased dramatically [140–142].

Natural history, pathogenesis, and pathology

C. immitis is a soil-dwelling dimorphic fungi that is inhaled in the form of arthroconidia (spores). The organism lives in the soil in the mycelial phase, and, when inhaled, aerosolized infectious particles are inhaled into the lungs of potential hosts. Once in the alveolar space, the organism multiplies, resulting in a giant spherule (Fig. 29.4). Histopathologically, HIV-associated pulmonary coccidioidomycosis is characterized by poor granuloma formation and high organism burden [142]. Dissemination of the organism can occur in people with impaired cellular immune responses. The major risk factor for developing HIV-associated coccidioidomycosis is a CD4 count < 250 cells/mm^3 [139, 144–146].

Clinical features

Coccidioidal infection may occur in a wide variety of forms, ranging from positive serologic tests to life-threatening pneumonitis and meningoencephalitis [144, 145]. Patients usually present with fevers, chills, and night sweats [145]. Pulmonary involvement occurs in 66–80% of all HIV-associated cases [144, 145]. The most common radiologic finding is a dramatic, diffuse reticulonodular infiltrate which may mimic *Pneumocystis* pneumonia and sometimes tuberculosis. Co-infection with coccidioidomycosis and tuberculosis has been reported in Hispanic patients living in Texas [146]. The mortality associated with bilateral pulmonary disease from coccidioidomycosis is exceeding high, ranging from 40 to 85% [144, 145, 147, 148].

In HIV-infected patients with high CD4 counts or patients on ART, pulmonary coccidioidomycosis is less severe, presenting with fever, cough, and focal infiltrates [141]. Mediastinal lymphadenopathy, peripheral eosinophilia, and lack of response to antibiotics can help distinguish it from community-acquired pneumonia [149]. In patients on ART and with suppressed viral load, mild cases of coccidioidomycosis may resolve without antifungal therapy or with shortened courses of therapy [141].

Following pulmonary infection, *C. immitis* can disseminate to skin, bone, and CNS. Unique manifestations in HIV-infected patients include liver, intestinal, genitourinary, and extrathoracic lymph node involvement [144]. For unclear reasons, skeletal coccidioidomycosis is distinctly unusual in HIV-infected individuals.

A subacute meningoencephalitis occurs in approximately 15% of HIV-infected patients with coccidioidomycosis, and is associated with high morbidity and mortality (~40%) [145, 150]. Headache is the most common

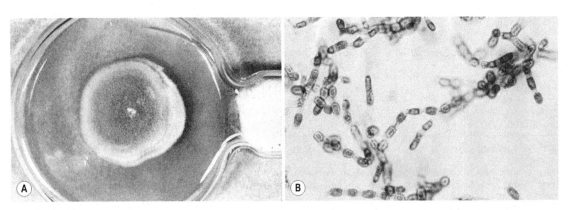

Figure 29.4 (A) *Coccidioides immitus* colony. (B) Arthrospores in colonies from a patient with *C. immitus* infection.

presenting symptom, followed by symptoms of increased intracranial pressure, such as nausea and vomiting. CSF findings include hypoglycorrhachia, high protein, and a moderate leukocytosis, which may have a polymorphonuclear predominance, or less commonly, can be eosinophilic [151, 152]. Imaging studies may reveal hydrocephalus, basilar enhancement, or cerebral infarction [153]. Hydrocephalus associated with arachnoid fibrosis and meningeal inflammation is a serious complication that can develop rapidly and should be considered in patients with worsening symptoms, even if they are receiving appropriate antifungal therapy [150].

Patient evaluation, diagnosis, and differential diagnosis

Definitive evidence of *C. immitis* infection is obtained through direct visualization or culture of the organism from respiratory or other tissues using standard histochemical staining techniques, such as the hematoxylin-eosin stain. The organism grows easily and relatively rapidly (< 5 days) on nearly any laboratory media, and a nucleic acid probe is available to rapidly identify *C. immitis* once isolated in culture [154]. The sensitivity of culture is high for pulmonary disease but low for extrapulmonary disease, with $<30\%$ of blood culture positivity for disseminated disease, and $<15\%$ recovery from the CSF in cases of meningoencephalitis. In tissue, *Coccidioides* can be easily identified by its characteristic large (20–70 μm) spherules which can be seen at 100–400 magnification with methenamine silver or Papanicolaou stain [148]. However, cytological staining has low sensitivity for the diagnosis of pulmonary disease. *C. immitis* can be an occupational hazard and is listed by the Centers for Disease Control and Prevention (CDC) as a potential agent of bioterrorism. Therefore, the laboratory should be notified if coccidioidomycosis is suspected so that appropriate biohazard precautions are taken.

Serologic tests are commonly used to diagnose coccidioidomycosis [155]. Anti-coccidioidal antibodies are quite specific and tend to reflect active disease [156]. IgM antibodies are detectable 1 or 2 weeks after infection and persist up to 6 months. IgG antibodies appear later and persist until the infection is resolved. Quantitation of coccidioidal IgG titers is useful to assess prognosis and response to therapy [155]. Complement fixation serologic tests can be performed on CSF samples, with high specificity and moderate sensitivity [157]. Asymptomatic HIV-infected patients with positive serologies have a high risk ($\sim 40\%$) of developing coccidioidomycosis within 2 years [158]. However, serology can be negative in 20–40% of HIV-infected patients with coccidioidomycosis, especially in those with diffuse pulmonary disease (Table 29.2) [144, 145, 159]. Therefore, a positive test can be diagnostic, but a negative test does not exclude coccidioidal disease. Concentration of serum can

increase the sensitivity of serologic tests in HIV-infected patients with disseminated coccidioidomycosis to $>90\%$ (Pappagianis, personal communication) [160]. The majority of patients with CNS coccidioidomycosis have positive serologies, usually with a titer greater than 1:16 [150].

Treatment

In immunocompetent individuals, infection with *C. immitis* often resolves spontaneously and does not require therapy. HIV-infected patients, however, have a high risk of dissemination and should always be treated if infected with *C. immitis* [158, 161]. Even with therapy (Table 29.5), coccidioidomycosis has a poor prognosis in HIV-infected patients who are not receiving ART [137, 144, 145]. Outcomes are much better in patients receiving ART, and no cases of IRIS associated with coccidioidomycosis have been reported [141]. Therefore, antifungal therapy should be complemented with control of HIV infection with ART.

There has only been one controlled trial of antifungal therapy for coccidioidomycosis, which found no significant difference in efficacy between fluconazole and itraconazole in primarily HIV-uninfected individuals with non-meningeal coccidioidomycosis [162]. Given the sparcity of data, treatment recommendations are primarily based on expert opinion [148, 149]. For diffuse pulmonary disease, which can be particularly severe, a combination of amphotericin B (0.7 mg/kg/day) and a triazole (itraconazole or fluconazole) antifungal is recommended. After a total dose of 500–1,000 mg of amphotericin B is administered, the triazole can be continued alone indefinitely [148, 149]. Fluconazole is usually preferred over itraconazole because of fewer drug–drug interactions with ART [162].

Other manifestations of coccidioidomycosis, including focal pneumonia, disseminated disease, and meningoencephalitis, can be treated with triazole antifungal monotherapy (usually fluconazole 400–800 mg/day) [163]. Several clinical trials have evaluated the efficacy of various azoles, but none have specifically addressed outcomes in HIV-infected patients. In HIV-negative individuals, the efficacy of fluconazole ranges from 55% in patients with chronic pulmonary disease to 86% in those with skeletal involvement [164]. The overall efficacy of itraconazole (200 mg twice daily) and ketoconazole (400 mg once daily) is approximately 50% [162, 165, 166]. In a randomized study comparing fluconazole with itraconazole for progressive, non-meningeal coccidioidomycosis, there was not a statistically significant difference between the two regimens, except for slightly improved outcomes in patients receiving itraconazole for bone disease [162].

CNS coccidioidomycosis does not respond to amphotericin B and is generally treated with fluconazole [148, 149]. In a study of 49 patients (9/49 HIV infected) with coccidioidal meningoencephalitis, 79% responded to fluconazole (400 mg/day) [157]. Therapy was continued for 37 months (mean)

Table 29.5 Therapy for HIV-associated coccidioidomycosis

TYPE OF DISEASE	PREFERRED DRUG	DURATION OF THERAPY	EVIDENCE[a]
Diffuse pneumonia	Amphotericin B[b] (0.7 mg/kg/day)	Until clinical improvement, followed by azole	5
	Fluconazole[c] (40 mg/day)	Lifelong	5
Meningoencephalitis	Fluconazole (400–800 mg/day)	Lifelong	2
Other (focal pulmonary, skin, disseminated)	Fluconazole[c] (400 mg/day)	Lifelong	2

Note: Maintenance therapy should be continued even in patients with CD4 counts < 200 cells/mm^3. Primary prophylaxis is controversial; consider in endemic area with CD4 count < 100 cells/mm^3.
[a]Evidence 1 = randomized clinical study, 2 = clinical trial > 20 patients, 3 = clinical trial < 20 patients, 4 = case series, 5 = expert opinion, expert committees.
[b]Alternative: liposomal amphotericin B (4 mg/kg/day).
[c]Alternative: itraconazole (400–600 mg/day).

and clinical response was apparent after 4–8 months of therapy. In a small study ($n = 10$), itraconazole was reported to have comparable efficacy [167]. For refractory cases, some authorities recommend intrathecal amphotericin B [148, 150, 168]. Hydrocephalus usually requires ventricular shunt placement. Voriconazole and posaconazole are active against *C. immitis in vitro* and have been successfully used in a few cases of coccidioidal meningoencephalitis [150, 169, 170].

Response to therapy should be monitored by serial coccidioidal IgG titers. The risk of relapse after therapy for coccidioidomycosis is high even in immunocompetent patients, ranging from 20 to 39% [162, 164]. Lifelong therapy is generally recommended for all patients with progressive pulmonary, disseminated, or meningeal disease [161, 171]. HIV-infected patients on ART can relapse despite immune reconstitution; therefore, discontinuation of secondary prophylaxis is not recommended even in patients with a CD4 count >250 cells/mm^3, except for patients with focal pulmonary disease [148, 172]. There are no data to support primary prophylaxis for the prevention of coccidioidomycosis, but ART may be the best preventive measure against severe disease [141].

REFERENCES

[1] Sabetta JR, Andriole VT. Cryptococcal infection of the central nervous system. Med Clin North Am 1985;69(2):333–44.

[2] Wilson DE, Bennett JE, Bailey JW. Serologic grouping of *Cryptococcus neoformans*. Proc Soc Exp Biol Med 1968;127(3):820–3.

[3] Rinaldi MG, Drutz DJ, Howell A, et al. Serotypes of *Cryptococcus neoformans* in patients with AIDS. J Infect Dis 1986;153(3):642.

[4] Shimizu RY, Howard DH, Clancy MN. The variety of *Cryptococcus neoformans* in patients with AIDS. J Infect Dis 1986;154 (6):1042.

[5] Speed B, Dunt D. Clinical and host differences between infections with the two varieties of *Cryptococcus neoformans*. Clin Infect Dis 1995;21 (1):28–34; discussion 35–6.

[6] CDC. HIV/AIDS Surveillance Report. Atlanta: CDC; 1991.

[7] Chuck SL, Sande MA. Infections with *Cryptococcus neoformans* in the acquired immunodeficiency syndrome. N Engl J Med 1989;321 (12):794–9.

[8] Currie BP, Casadevall A. Estimation of the prevalence of cryptococcal infection among patients infected with the human immunodeficiency virus in New York City. Clin Infect Dis 1994;19 (6):1029–33.

[9] Dromer F, Mathoulin S, Dupont B, Laporte A. Epidemiology of cryptococcosis in France: a 9-year survey (1985–1993). French Cryptococcosis Study Group. Clin Infect Dis 1996;23(1):82–90.

[10] Selik RM, Karon JM, Ward JW. Effect of the human immunodeficiency virus epidemic on mortality from opportunistic infections in the United States in 1993. J Infect Dis 1997;176 (3):632–6.

[11] Sacktor N, Lyles RH, Skolasky R, et al. HIV-associated neurologic disease incidence changes: Multicenter AIDS Cohort Study, 1990–1998. Neurology 2001;56 (2):257–60.

[12] Hajjeh RA, Conn LA, Stephens DS, et al. Cryptococcosis: population-based multistate active surveillance and risk factors in human immunodeficiency virus-infected persons. Cryptococcal Active Surveillance Group. J Infect Dis 1999;179(2):449–54.

[13] Kaplan JE, Hanson D, Dworkin MS, et al. Epidemiology of human immunodeficiency

virus-associated opportunistic infections in the United States in the era of highly active antiretroviral therapy. Clin Infect Dis 2000;30(Suppl. 1):S5–14.

[14] Mirza SA, Phelan M, Rimland D, et al. The changing epidemiology of cryptococcosis: an update from population-based active surveillance in 2 large metropolitan areas, 1992–2000. Clin Infect Dis 2003;36(6): 789–94.

[15] Adeyemi OM, Pulvirenti J, Perumal S, et al. Cryptococcosis in HIV-infected individuals. AIDS 2004;18(16):2218–19.

[16] Dromer F, Mathoulin-Pelissier S, Fontanet A, et al. Epidemiology of HIV-associated cryptococcosis in France (1985–2001): comparison of the pre- and post-HAART eras. AIDS 2004;18(3):555–62.

[17] Tintelnot K, Lemmer K, Losert H, et al. Follow-up of epidemiological data of cryptococcosis in Austria, Germany and Switzerland with special focus on the characterization of clinical isolates. Mycoses 2004;47(11–12):455–64.

[18] Park BJ, Wannemuehler KA, Marston BJ, et al. Estimation of the current global burden of cryptococcal meningitis among persons living with HIV/AIDS. AIDS 2009;23(4):525–30.

[19] Bogaerts J, Rouvroy D, Taelman H, et al. AIDS-associated cryptococcal meningitis in Rwanda (1983–1992): epidemiologic and diagnostic features. J Infect 1999;39(1):32–7.

[20] Hakim JG, Gangaidzo IT, Heyderman RS, et al. Impact of HIV infection on meningitis in Harare, Zimbabwe: a prospective study of 406 predominantly adult patients. AIDS 2000;14 (10):1401–7.

[21] Tansuphasawadikul S, Amornkul PN, Tanchanpong C, et al. Clinical presentation of hospitalized adult patients with HIV infection and AIDS in Bangkok, Thailand. J Acquir Immune Defic Syndr 1999;21 (4):326–32.

[22] Corbett EL, Churchyard GJ, Charalambos S, et al. Morbidity and mortality in South African gold miners: impact of untreated

disease due to human immunodeficiency virus. Clin Infect Dis 2002;34(9):1251–8.

[23] Moosa MY, Coovadia YM. Cryptococcal meningitis in Durban, South Africa: a comparison of clinical features, laboratory findings, and outcome for human immunodeficiency virus (HIV)-positive and HIV-negative patients. Clin Infect Dis 1997;24(2):131–4.

[24] Mwaba P, Mwansa J, Chintu C, et al. Clinical presentation, natural history, and cumulative death rates of 230 adults with primary cryptococcal meningitis in Zambian AIDS patients treated under local conditions. Postgrad Med J 2001;77(914):769–73.

[25] Kambugu A, Meya DB, Rhein J, et al. Outcomes of cryptococcal meningitis in Uganda before and after the availability of highly active antiretroviral therapy. Clin Infect Dis 2008;46(11): 1694–701.

[26] Clark RA, Greer D, Atkinson W, et al. Spectrum of *Cryptococcus neoformans* infection in 68 patients infected with human immunodeficiency virus. Rev Infect Dis 1990;12(5):768–77.

[27] Dismukes WE. Cryptococcal meningitis in patients with AIDS. J Infect Dis 1988;157(4):624–8.

[28] van der Horst CM, Saag MS, Cloud GA, et al. Treatment of cryptococcal meningitis associated with the acquired immunodeficiency syndrome. National Institute of Allergy and Infectious Diseases Mycoses Study Group and AIDS Clinical Trials Group. N Engl J Med 1997;337 (1):15–21.

[29] French N, Gray K, Watera C, et al. Cryptococcal infection in a cohort of HIV-1-infected Ugandan adults. AIDS 2002;16(7):1031–8.

[30] Haddow LJ, Colebunders R, Meintjes G, et al. Cryptococcal immune reconstitution inflammatory syndrome in HIV-1-infected individuals: proposed clinical case definitions. Lancet Infect Dis 2010;10(11):791–802.

[31] Boelaert JR, Goddeeris KH, Vanopdenbosch LJ, Casselman JW. Relapsing meningitis caused by persistent cryptococcal antigens

and immune reconstitution after the initiation of highly active antiretroviral therapy. AIDS 2004;18(8):1223–4.

[32] Cattelan AM, Trevenzoli M, Sasset L, et al. Multiple cerebral cryptococcomas associated with immune reconstitution in HIV-1 infection. AIDS 2004;18 (2):349–51.

[33] Lortholary O, Fontanet A, Memain N, et al. Incidence and risk factors of immune reconstitution inflammatory syndrome complicating HIV-associated cryptococcosis in France. AIDS 2005;19(10):1043–9.

[34] Shelburne SA, Visnegarwala F, Darcourt J, et al. Incidence and risk factors for immune reconstitution inflammatory syndrome during highly active antiretroviral therapy. AIDS 2005;19(4):399–406.

[35] Woods 2nd ML, MacGinley R, Eisen DP, Allworth AM. HIV combination therapy: partial immune restitution unmasking latent cryptococcal infection. AIDS 1998;12(12):1491–4.

[36] Boulware DR, Bonham SC, Meya DB, et al. Paucity of initial cerebrospinal fluid inflammation in cryptococcal meningitis is associated with subsequent immune reconstitution inflammatory syndrome. J Infect Dis 2010;202(6):962–70.

[37] Lortholary O, Fontanet A, Memain N, et al. Incidence and risk factors of immune reconstitution inflammatory syndrome complicating HIV-associated cryptococcosis in France. AIDS 2005;19(10):1043–9.

[38] Sungkanuparph S, Filler SG, Chetchotisakd P, et al. Cryptococcal immune reconstitution inflammatory syndrome after antiretroviral therapy in AIDS patients with cryptococcal meningitis: a prospective multicenter study. Clin Infect Dis 2009;49(6):931–4.

[39] Scarborough M, Gordon SB, Whitty CJ, et al. Corticosteroids for bacterial meningitis in adults in sub-Saharan Africa. N Engl J Med 2007;357(24):2441–50.

[40] Asawavichienjinda T, Sitthi-Amorn C, Tanyanont V. Serum cryptococcal antigen: diagnostic

value in the diagnosis of AIDS-related cryptococcal meningitis. J Med Assoc Thai 1999;82 (1):65–71.

[41] Perfect JR, Dismukes WE, Dromer F, et al. Clinical practice guidelines for the management of cryptococcal disease: 2010 update by the Infectious Diseases Society of America. Clin Infect Dis 2010;50 (3):291–322.

[42] Meya DB, Manabe YC, Castelnuovo B, et al. Cost-effectiveness of serum cryptococcal antigen screening to prevent deaths among HIV-infected persons with a CD4+ cell count < or = 100 cells/microL who start HIV therapy in resource-limited settings. Clin Infect Dis 2010;51(4):448–55.

[43] Tanner DC, Weinstein MP, Fedorciw B, et al. Comparison of commercial kits for detection of cryptococcal antigen. J Clin Microbiol 1994;32(7):1680–4.

[44] Darras-Joly C, Chevret S, Wolff M, et al. *Cryptococcus neoformans* infection in France: epidemiologic features of and early prognostic parameters for 76 patients who were infected with human immunodeficiency virus. Clin Infect Dis 1996;23(2):369–76.

[45] Garlipp CR, Rossi CL, Bottini PV. Cerebrospinal fluid profiles in acquired immunodeficiency syndrome with and without neurocryptococcosis. Rev Inst Med Trop Sao Paulo 1997;39 (6):323–5.

[46] Zuger A, Louie E, Holzman RS, et al. Cryptococcal disease in patients with the acquired immunodeficiency syndrome. Diagnostic features and outcome of treatment. Ann Intern Med 1986;104(2):234–40.

[47] Saag MS, Powderly WG, Cloud GA, et al. Comparison of amphotericin B with fluconazole in the treatment of acute AIDS-associated cryptococcal meningitis. The NIAID Mycoses Study Group and the AIDS Clinical Trials Group. N Engl J Med 1992;326(2):83–9.

[48] Dromer F, Mathoulin-Pelissier S, Launay O, Lortholary O. Determinants of disease presentation and outcome during cryptococcosis: the CryptoA/D study. PLoS Med 2007;4(2):e21.

[49] Graybill JR, Sobel J, Saag M, et al. Diagnosis and management of increased intracranial pressure in patients with AIDS and cryptococcal meningitis. The NIAID Mycoses Study Group and AIDS Cooperative Treatment Groups. Clin Infect Dis 2000;30 (1):47–54.

[50] Bicanic T, Muzoora C, Brouwer AE, et al. Independent association between rate of clearance of infection and clinical outcome of HIV-associated cryptococcal meningitis: analysis of a combined cohort of 262 patients. Clin Infect Dis 2009;49(5):702–9.

[51] de Gans J, Portegies P, Tiessens G, et al. Itraconazole compared with amphotericin B plus flucytosine in AIDS patients with cryptococcal meningitis. AIDS 1992;6 (2):185–90.

[52] Larsen RA, Leal MA, Chan LS. Fluconazole compared with amphotericin B plus flucytosine for cryptococcal meningitis in AIDS. A randomized trial. Ann Intern Med 1990;113(3):183–7.

[53] Brouwer AE, Rajanuwong A, Chierakul W, et al. Combination antifungal therapies for HIV-associated cryptococcal meningitis: a randomised trial. Lancet 2004;363 (9423):1764–7.

[54] Baddour LM, Perfect JR, Ostrosky-Zeichner L. Successful use of amphotericin B lipid complex in the treatment of cryptococcosis. Clin Infect Dis 2005;40(Suppl. 6): S409–13.

[55] Coker RJ, Viviani M, Gazzard BG, et al. Treatment of cryptococcosis with liposomal amphotericin B (AmBisome) in 23 patients with AIDS. AIDS 1993;7 (6):829–35.

[56] Leenders AC, Reiss P, Portegies P, et al. Liposomal amphotericin B (AmBisome) compared with amphotericin B both followed by oral fluconazole in the treatment of AIDS-associated cryptococcal meningitis. AIDS 1997;11 (12):1463–71.

[57] Bicanic T, Meintjes G, Wood R, et al. Fungal burden, early fungicidal activity, and outcome in cryptococcal meningitis in antiretroviral-naive or antiretroviral-experienced patients treated with amphotericin B or fluconazole. Clin Infect Dis 2007;45(1):76–80.

[58] Nussbaum JC, Jackson A, Namarika D, et al. Combination flucytosine and high-dose fluconazole compared with fluconazole monotherapy for the treatment of cryptococcal meningitis: a randomized trial in Malawi. Clin Infect Dis 2010;50 (3):338–44.

[59] Milefchik E, Leal MA, Haubrich R, et al. Fluconazole alone or combined with flucytosine for the treatment of AIDS-associated cryptococcal meningitis. Med Mycol 2008;46(4):393–5.

[60] Bicanic T, Harrison T, Niepieklo A, et al. Symptomatic relapse of HIV-associated cryptococcal meningitis after initial fluconazole monotherapy: the role of fluconazole resistance and immune reconstitution. Clin Infect Dis 2006;43(8):1069–73.

[61] Perfect JR, Marr KA, Walsh TJ, et al. Voriconazole treatment for less-common, emerging, or refractory fungal infections. Clin Infect Dis 2003;36(9):1122–31.

[62] Pitisuttithum P, Negroni R, Graybill JR, et al. Activity of posaconazole in the treatment of central nervous system fungal infections. J Antimicrob Chemother 2005;56(4):745–55.

[63] Denning DW, Armstrong RW, Lewis BH, Stevens DA. Elevated cerebrospinal fluid pressures in patients with cryptococcal meningitis and acquired immunodeficiency syndrome. Am J Med 1991;91(3):267–72.

[64] Bicanic T, Brouwer AE, Meintjes G, et al. Relationship of cerebrospinal fluid pressure, fungal burden and outcome in patients with cryptococcal meningitis undergoing serial lumbar punctures. AIDS 2009;23 (6):701–6.

[65] Coplin WM, Avellino AM, Kim DK, et al. Bacterial meningitis associated with lumbar drains: a retrospective cohort study.

J Neurol Neurosurg Psychiatry 1999;67(4):468–73.

[66] Lindvall P, Ahlm C, Ericsson M, et al. Reducing intracranial pressure may increase survival among patients with bacterial meningitis. Clin Infect Dis 2004;38 (3):384–90.

[67] Macsween KF, Bicanic T, Brouwer AE, et al. Lumbar drainage for control of raised cerebrospinal fluid pressure in cryptococcal meningitis: case report and review. J Infect 2005;51(4):e221–4.

[68] Park MK, Hospenthal DR, Bennett JE. Treatment of hydrocephalus secondary to cryptococcal meningitis by use of shunting. Clin Infect Dis 1999;28 (3):629–33.

[69] Bozzette SA, Larsen RA, Chiu J, et al. A placebo-controlled trial of maintenance therapy with fluconazole after treatment of cryptococcal meningitis in the acquired immunodeficiency syndrome. California Collaborative Treatment Group. N Engl J Med 1991;324(9):580–4.

[70] Saag MS, Cloud GA, Graybill JR, et al. A comparison of itraconazole versus fluconazole as maintenance therapy for AIDS-associated cryptococcal meningitis. National Institute of Allergy and Infectious Diseases Mycoses Study Group. Clin Infect Dis 1999;28(2):291–6.

[71] Aberg JA, Price RW, Heeren DM, Bredt B. A pilot study of the discontinuation of antifungal therapy for disseminated cryptococcal disease in patients with acquired immunodeficiency syndrome, following immunologic response to antiretroviral therapy. J Infect Dis 2002;185(8):1179–82.

[72] Martinez E, Garcia-Viejo MA, Marcos MA, et al. Discontinuation of secondary prophylaxis for cryptococcal meningitis in HIV-infected patients responding to highly active antiretroviral therapy. AIDS 2000;14 (16):2615–17.

[73] Mussini C, Pezzotti P, Miro JM, et al. Discontinuation of maintenance therapy for cryptococcal meningitis in patients with AIDS treated with highly

active antiretroviral therapy: an international observational study. Clin Infect Dis 2004;38 (4):565–71.

[74] Rollot F, Bossi P, Tubiana R, et al. Discontinuation of secondary prophylaxis against cryptococcosis in patients with AIDS receiving highly active antiretroviral therapy. AIDS 2001;15(11):1448–9.

[75] Vibhagool A, Sungkanuparph S, Mootsikapun P, et al. Discontinuation of secondary prophylaxis for cryptococcal meningitis in human immunodeficiency virus-infected patients treated with highly active antiretroviral therapy: a prospective, multicenter, randomized study. Clin Infect Dis 2003;36(10):1329–31.

[76] Grant PM, Komarow L, Andersen J, et al. Risk factor analyses for immune reconstitution inflammatory syndrome in a randomized study of early vs. deferred ART during an opportunistic infection. PLoS One 2010;5(7):e11416.

[77] Zolopa A, Andersen J, Powderly W, et al. Early antiretroviral therapy reduces AIDS progression/death in individuals with acute opportunistic infections: a multicenter randomized strategy trial. PLoS One 2009;4(5):e5575.

[78] Jarvis JN, Lawn SD, Vogt M, et al. Screening for cryptococcal antigenemia in patients accessing an antiretroviral treatment program in South Africa. Clin Infect Dis 2009;48(7):856–62.

[79] Micol R, Lortholary O, Sar B, et al. Prevalence, determinants of positivity, and clinical utility of cryptococcal antigenemia in Cambodian HIV-infected patients. J Acquir Immune Defic Syndr 2007;45(5):555–9.

[80] Micol R, Tajahmady A, Lortholary O, et al. Cost-effectiveness of primary prophylaxis of AIDS associated cryptococcosis in Cambodia. PLoS One 2010;5(11):e13856.

[81] Eng RH, Bishburg E, Smith SM, Kapila R. Cryptococcal infections in patients with acquired immune deficiency syndrome. Am J Med 1986;81(1):19–23.

[82] Kovacs JA, Kovacs AA, Polis M, et al. Cryptococcosis in the acquired immunodeficiency syndrome. Ann Intern Med 1985;103(4):533–8.

[83] Ker CC, Hung CC, Huang SY, et al. Comparison of bone marrow studies with blood culture for etiological diagnosis of disseminated mycobacterial and fungal infection in patients with acquired immunodeficiency syndrome. J Microbiol Immunol Infect 2002;35(2):89–93.

[84] Meyohas MC, Roux P, Bollens D, et al. Pulmonary cryptococcosis: localized and disseminated infections in 27 patients with AIDS. Clin Infect Dis 1995;21 (3):628–33.

[85] CDC. Guidelines for preventing opportunistic infections among HIV-infected persons—2002. Recommendations of the U.S. Public Health Service and the Infectious Diseases Society of America. MMWR 2002;14(51(RR-8)):1–52.

[86] Chariyalertsak S, Supparatpinyo K, Sirisanthana T, Nelson KE. A controlled trial of itraconazole as primary prophylaxis for systemic fungal infections in patients with advanced human immunodeficiency virus infection in Thailand. Clin Infect Dis 2002;34(2):277–84.

[87] McKinsey DS, Wheat LJ, Cloud GA, et al. Itraconazole prophylaxis for fungal infections in patients with advanced human immunodeficiency virus infection: randomized, placebo-controlled, double-blind study. National Institute of Allergy and Infectious Diseases Mycoses Study Group. Clin Infect Dis 1999;28 (5):1049–56.

[88] Powderly WG, Finkelstein D, Feinberg J, et al. A randomized trial comparing fluconazole with clotrimazole troches for the prevention of fungal infections in patients with advanced human immunodeficiency virus infection. NIAID AIDS Clinical Trials Group. N Engl J Med 1995;332 (11):700–5.

[89] Liechty CA, Solberg P, Were W, et al. Asymptomatic serum

cryptococcal antigenemia and early mortality during antiretroviral therapy in rural Uganda. Trop Med Int Health 2007;12(8):929–35.

[90] Cano MV, Hajjeh RA. The epidemiology of histoplasmosis: a review. Semin Respir Infect 2001;16(2):109–18.

[91] Wheat LJ, Connolly-Stringfield PA, Baker RL, et al. Disseminated histoplasmosis in the acquired immune deficiency syndrome: clinical findings, diagnosis and treatment, and review of the literature. Medicine (Baltimore) 1990;69(6):361–74.

[92] Wheat LJ, Batteiger BE, Sathapatayavongs B. *Histoplasma capsulatum* infections of the central nervous system. A clinical review. Medicine (Baltimore) 1990;69(4):244–60.

[93] Jones JL, Hanson DL, Dworkin MS, et al. Trends in AIDS-related opportunistic infections among men who have sex with men and among injecting drug users, 1991–1996. J Infect Dis 1998;178(1):114–20.

[94] Wheat LJ, Kauffman CA. Histoplasmosis. Infect Dis Clin North Am 2003;17(1):1–19, vii.

[95] Gutierrez ME, Canton A, Sosa N, et al. Disseminated histoplasmosis in patients with AIDS in Panama: a review of 104 cases. Clin Infect Dis 2005;40(8):1199–202.

[96] Hajjeh RA. Disseminated histoplasmosis in persons infected with human immunodeficiency virus. Clin Infect Dis 1995;21(Suppl. 1):S108–10.

[97] Sarosi GA, Johnson PC. Disseminated histoplasmosis in patients infected with human immunodeficiency virus. Clin Infect Dis 1992;14(Suppl. 1):S60–7.

[98] Wheat LJ, Musial CE, Jenny-Avital E. Diagnosis and management of central nervous system histoplasmosis. Clin Infect Dis 2005;40(6):844–52.

[99] Wheat LJ, Chetchotisakd P, Williams B, et al. Factors associated with severe manifestations of histoplasmosis in AIDS. Clin Infect Dis 2000;30(6):877–81.

[100] Burke DG, Emancipator SN, Smith MC, Salata RA. Histoplasmosis and kidney disease in patients with AIDS. Clin Infect Dis 1997;25(2):281–4.

[101] Goodwin Jr RA, Shapiro JL, Thurman GH, et al. Disseminated histoplasmosis: clinical and pathologic correlations. Medicine (Baltimore) 1980;59(1):1–33.

[102] Thompson GR 3rd, LaValle CE 3rd, Everett ED. Unusual manifestations of histoplasmosis. Diagn Microbiol Infect Dis 2004;50(1):33–41.

[103] Breton G, Adle-Biassette H, Therby A, et al. Immune reconstitution inflammatory syndrome in HIV-infected patients with disseminated histoplasmosis. AIDS 2006;20(1):119–21.

[104] Shelburne SA 3rd, Visnegarwala F, Adams C, et al. Unusual manifestations of disseminated histoplasmosis in patients responding to antiretroviral therapy. Am J Med 2005;118(9):1038–41.

[105] Nacher M, Sarazin F, El Guedj M, et al. Increased incidence of disseminated histoplasmosis following highly active antiretroviral therapy initiation. J Acquir Immune Defic Syndr 2006;41(4):468–70.

[106] Sathapatayavongs B, Batteiger BE, Wheat J, et al. Clinical and laboratory features of disseminated histoplasmosis during two large urban outbreaks. Medicine (Baltimore) 1983;62(5):263–70.

[107] Corcoran GR, Al-Abdely H, Flanders CD, et al. Markedly elevated serum lactate dehydrogenase levels are a clue to the diagnosis of disseminated histoplasmosis in patients with AIDS. Clin Infect Dis 1997;24(5):942–4.

[108] Conces Jr DJ, Stockberger SM, Tarver RD, Wheat LJ. Disseminated histoplasmosis in AIDS: findings on chest radiographs. AJR Am J Roentgenol 1993;160(1):15–19.

[109] Fuller DD, Davis Jr TE, Denys GA, York MK. Evaluation of BACTEC MYCO/F Lytic medium for recovery of mycobacteria, fungi, and bacteria from blood. J Clin Microbiol 2001;39(8):2933–6.

[110] Wheat J, French M, Batteiger B, Kohler R. Cerebrospinal fluid *Histoplasma* antibodies in central nervous system histoplasmosis. Arch Intern Med 1985;145(7):1237–40.

[111] Wheat LJ. Laboratory diagnosis of histoplasmosis: update 2000. Semin Respir Infect 2001;16(2):131–40.

[112] Wheat LJ, Kohler RB, Tewari RP, et al. Significance of *Histoplasma* antigen in the cerebrospinal fluid of patients with meningitis. Arch Intern Med 1989;149(2):302–34.

[113] Wheat J, French ML, Kohler RB, et al. The diagnostic laboratory tests for histoplasmosis: analysis of experience in a large urban outbreak. Ann Intern Med 1982;97(5):680–5.

[114] Wheat LJ, Kohler RB, Tewari RP. Diagnosis of disseminated histoplasmosis by detection of *Histoplasma capsulatum* antigen in serum and urine specimens. N Engl J Med 1986;314(2):83–8.

[115] Wheat LJ, Connolly P, Haddad N, et al. Antigen clearance during treatment of disseminated histoplasmosis with itraconazole versus fluconazole in patients with AIDS. Antimicrob Agents Chemother 2002;46(1):248–50.

[116] Wheat LJ, Connolly-Stringfield P, Blair R, et al. Effect of successful treatment with amphotericin B on *Histoplasma capsulatum* variety *capsulatum* polysaccharide antigen levels in patients with AIDS and histoplasmosis. Am J Med 1992;92(2):153–60.

[117] Wheat LJ, Connolly-Stringfield P, Kohler RB, et al. *Histoplasma capsulatum* polysaccharide antigen detection in diagnosis and management of disseminated histoplasmosis in patients with acquired immunodeficiency syndrome. Am J Med 1989;87(4):396–400.

[118] Johnson PC, Wheat LJ, Cloud GA, et al. Safety and efficacy of liposomal amphotericin B compared with conventional amphotericin B for induction therapy of histoplasmosis in

patients with AIDS. Ann Intern Med 2002;137(2):105–9.

[119] Perfect JR. Treatment of non-*Aspergillus* moulds in immunocompromised patients, with amphotericin B lipid complex. Clin Infect Dis 2005;40 (Suppl. 6):S401–8.

[120] Wheat J, Hafner R, Korzun AH, et al. Itraconazole treatment of disseminated histoplasmosis in patients with the acquired immunodeficiency syndrome. AIDS Clinical Trial Group. Am J Med 1995;98(4):336–42.

[121] Wheat LJ, Cloud G, Johnson PC, et al. Clearance of fungal burden during treatment of disseminated histoplasmosis with liposomal amphotericin B versus itraconazole. Antimicrob Agents Chemother 2001;45(8):2354–7.

[122] Wheat J, MaWhinney S, Hafner R, et al. Treatment of histoplasmosis with fluconazole in patients with acquired immunodeficiency syndrome. National Institute of Allergy and Infectious Diseases Acquired Immunodeficiency Syndrome Clinical Trials Group and Mycoses Study Group. Am J Med 1997;103(3):223–32.

[123] Wheat LJ, Connolly P, Smedema M, et al. Emergence of resistance to fluconazole as a cause of failure during treatment of histoplasmosis in patients with acquired immunodeficiency disease syndrome. Clin Infect Dis 2001;33(11):1910–13.

[124] Connolly P, Wheat LJ, Schnizlein-Bick C, et al. Comparison of a new triazole, posaconazole, with itraconazole and amphotericin B for treatment of histoplasmosis following pulmonary challenge in immunocompromised mice. Antimicrob Agents Chemother 2000;44(10):2604–8.

[125] Wheat LJ, Connolly P, Smedema M, et al. Activity of newer triazoles against *Histoplasma capsulatum* from patients with AIDS who failed fluconazole. J Antimicrob Chemother 2006;57 (6):1235–9.

[126] Freifeld A, Proia L, Andes D, et al. Voriconazole use for endemic fungal infections. Antimicrob

Agents Chemother 2009;53 (4):1648–51.

[127] Restrepo A, Tobon A, Clark B, et al. Salvage treatment of histoplasmosis with posaconazole. J Infect 2007;54(4):319–27.

[128] Wheat LJ, Freifeld AG, Kleiman MB, et al. Clinical practice guidelines for the management of patients with histoplasmosis: 2007 update by the Infectious Diseases Society of America. Clin Infect Dis 2007;45(7):807–25.

[129] Koo HL, Hamill RJ, Andrade RA. Drug–drug interaction between itraconazole and efavirenz in a patient with AIDS and disseminated histoplasmosis. Clin Infect Dis 2007;45(6):e77–9.

[130] Huet E, Hadji C, Hulin A, et al. Therapeutic monitoring is necessary for the association itraconazole and efavirenz in a patient with AIDS and disseminated histoplasmosis. AIDS 2008;22(14):1885–6.

[131] Andrade RA, Evans RT, Hamill RJ, et al. Clinical evidence of interaction between itraconazole and nonnucleoside reverse transcriptase inhibitors in HIV-infected patients with disseminated histoplasmosis. Ann Pharmacother 2009;43 (5):908–13.

[132] Crommentuyn KM, Mulder JW, Sparidans RW, et al. Drug–drug interaction between itraconazole and the antiretroviral drug lopinavir/ritonavir in an HIV-1-infected patient with disseminated histoplasmosis. Clin Infect Dis 2004;38(8):e73–5.

[133] Wheat J, Hafner R, Wulfsohn M, et al. Prevention of relapse of histoplasmosis with itraconazole in patients with the acquired immunodeficiency syndrome. Ann Intern Med 1993;118(8):610–6.

[134] Goldman M, Zackin R, Fichtenbaum CJ, et al. Safety of discontinuation of maintenance therapy for disseminated histoplasmosis after immunologic response to antiretroviral therapy. Clin Infect Dis 2004;38 (10):1485–9.

[135] Tobon AM, Agudelo CA, Rosero DS, et al. Disseminated

histoplasmosis: a comparative study between patients with acquired immunodeficiency syndrome and non-human immunodeficiency virus-infected individuals. Am J Trop Med Hyg 2005;73(3):576–82.

[136] Hernandez JL, Echevarria S, Garcia-Valtuille A, et al. Atypical coccidioidomycosis in an AIDS patient successfully treated with fluconazole. Eur J Clin Microbiol Infect Dis 1997;16 (8):592–4.

[137] Jones JL, Fleming PL, Ciesielski CA, et al. Coccidioidomycosis among persons with AIDS in the United States. J Infect Dis 1995;171 (4):961–6.

[138] CDC . Coccidioidomycosis—Arizona, 1990–1995. MMWR 1996;45(49):1069–73.

[139] Ampel NM. Coccidioidomycosis among persons with human immunodeficiency virus infection in the era of highly active antiretroviral therapy (HAART). Semin Respir Infect 2001;16 (4):257–62.

[140] Woods CW, McRill C, Plikaytis BD, et al. Coccidioidomycosis in human immunodeficiency virus-infected persons in Arizona, 1994–1997: incidence, risk factors, and prevention. J Infect Dis 2000;181 (4):1428–34.

[141] Masannat FY, Ampel NM. Coccidioidomycosis in patients with HIV-1 infection in the era of potent antiretroviral therapy. Clin Infect Dis 2010;50(1):1–7.

[142] Graham AR, Sobonya RE, Bronnimann DA, Galgiani JN. Quantitative pathology of coccidioidomycosis in acquired immunodeficiency syndrome. Hum Pathol 1988;19(7):800–6.

[143] Ampel NM, Dols CL, Galgiani JN. Coccidioidomycosis during human immunodeficiency virus infection: results of a prospective study in a coccidioidal endemic area. Am J Med 1993;94 (3):235–40.

[144] Fish DG, Ampel NM, Galgiani JN, et al. Coccidioidomycosis during human immunodeficiency virus infection. A review of 77 patients.

Medicine (Baltimore) 1990;69 (6):384–91.

[145] Singh VR, Smith DK, Lawerence J, et al. Coccidioidomycosis in patients infected with human immunodeficiency virus: review of 91 cases at a single institution. Clin Infect Dis 1996;23(3):563–8.

[146] Cadena J, Hartzler A, Hsue G, Longfield RN. Coccidioidomycosis and tuberculosis coinfection at a tuberculosis hospital: clinical features and literature review. Medicine (Baltimore) 2009;88 (1):66–76.

[147] Bronnimann DA, Adam RD, Galgiani JN, et al. Coccidioidomycosis in the acquired immunodeficiency syndrome. Ann Intern Med 1987;106(3):372–9.

[148] Ampel NM. Coccidioidomycosis in persons infected with HIV type 1. Clin Infect Dis 2005;41 (8):1174–8.

[149] Galgiani JN, Ampel NM, Blair JE, et al. Coccidioidomycosis. Clin Infect Dis 2005;41(9):1217–23.

[150] Mathisen G, Shelub A, Truong J, Wigen C. Coccidioidal meningitis: clinical presentation and management in the fluconazole era. Medicine (Baltimore) 2010;89 (5):251–84.

[151] Ismail Y, Arsura EL. Eosinophilic meningitis associated with coccidioidomycosis. West J Med 1993;158(3):300–31.

[152] Lo Re, V 3rd, Gluckman SJ. Eosinophilic meningitis. Am J Med 2003;114(3):217–23.

[153] Arsura EL, Johnson R, Penrose J, et al. Neuroimaging as a guide to predict outcomes for patients with coccidioidal meningitis. Clin Infect Dis 2005;40(4):624–7.

[154] Sandhu GS, Kline BC, Stockman L, Roberts GD. Molecular probes for diagnosis of fungal infections. J Clin Microbiol 1995;33 (11):2913–19.

[155] Pappagianis D. Serologic studies in coccidioidomycosis. Semin Respir Infect 2001;16(4):242–50.

[156] Pappagianis D, Zimmer BL. Serology of coccidioidomycosis. Clin Microbiol Rev 1990;3 (3):247–68.

[157] Galgiani JN, Catanzaro A, Cloud GA, et al. Fluconazole therapy for coccidioidal meningitis. The NIAID-Mycoses Study Group. Ann Intern Med 1993;119(1):28–35.

[158] Sobonya RE, Barbee RA, Wiens J, Trego D. Detection of fungi and other pathogens in immunocompromised patients by bronchoalveolar lavage in an area endemic for coccidioidomycosis. Chest 1990;97(6):1349–55.

[159] Antoniskis D, Larsen RA, Akil B, et al. Seronegative disseminated coccidioidomycosis in patients with HIV infection. AIDS 1990;4 (7):691–3.

[160] Wolf JE, Little JR, Pappagianis D, Kobayashi GS. Disseminated coccidioidomycosis in a patient with the acquired immune deficiency syndrome. Diagn Microbiol Infect Dis 1986;5 (4):331–6.

[161] Galgiani JN, Ampel NM, Catanzaro A, et al. Practice guideline for the treatment of coccidioidomycosis. Infectious Diseases Society of America. Clin Infect Dis 2000;30 (4):658–61.

[162] Galgiani JN, Catanzaro A, Cloud GA, et al. Comparison of oral fluconazole and itraconazole for progressive, nonmeningeal coccidioidomycosis. A randomized, double-blind trial. Mycoses Study Group. Ann Intern Med 2000;133 (9):676–86.

[163] Galgiani JN, Ampel NM. Coccidioidomycosis in human immunodeficiency virus-infected patients. J Infect Dis 1990;162 (5):1165–9.

[164] Catanzaro A, Galgiani JN, Levine BE, et al. Fluconazole in the treatment of chronic pulmonary

and nonmeningeal disseminated coccidioidomycosis. NIAID Mycoses Study Group. Am J Med 1995;98(3):249–56.

[165] Brass C, Galgiani JN, Campbell SC, Stevens DA. Therapy of disseminated or pulmonary coccidioidomycosis with ketoconazole. Rev Infect Dis 1980;2(4):656–60.

[166] Diaz M, Puente R, de Hoyos LA, Cruz S. Itraconazole in the treatment of coccidioidomycosis. Chest 1991;100(3):682–4.

[167] Tucker RM, Denning DW, Dupont B, Stevens DA. Itraconazole therapy for chronic coccidioidal meningitis. Ann Intern Med 1990;112 (2):108–12.

[168] Chiller TM, Galgiani JN, Stevens DA. Coccidioidomycosis. Infect Dis Clin North Am 2003;17 (1):41–57, viii.

[169] Proia LA, Tenorio AR. Successful use of voriconazole for treatment of Coccidioides meningitis. Antimicrob Agents Chemother 2004;48(6):2341.

[170] Catanzaro A, Cloud GA, Stevens DA, et al. Safety, tolerance, and efficacy of posaconazole therapy in patients with nonmeningeal disseminated or chronic pulmonary coccidioidomycosis. Clin Infect Dis 2007;45(5): 562–8.

[171] Dewsnup DH, Galgiani JN, Graybill JR, et al. Is it ever safe to stop azole therapy for Coccidioides immitis meningitis? Ann Intern Med 1996;124(3):305–10.

[172] Mathew G, Smedema M, Wheat LJ, Goldman M. Relapse of coccidioidomycosis despite immune reconstitution after fluconazole secondary prophylaxis in a patient with AIDS. Mycoses 2003;46(1–2):42–4.

Chapter | 30 |

Infection due to *Penicillium marneffei*

Thira Sirisanthana, Khuanchai Supparatpinyo

INTRODUCTION

Penicillium marneffei infection is one of the most common opportunistic infections in persons with advanced human immunodeficiency virus (HIV) infection in Southeast Asia, northeastern India, southern China, Hong Kong, and Taiwan. In northern Thailand. It is one of the four most common opportunistic infections, which include tuberculosis, cryptococcal infection, and *Pneumocystis jiroveci* pneumonia [1]. Cases have also been reported in HIV-infected patients from the USA, Europe, Japan, and Australia following visits to the endemic area [2]. Diagnosis depends on familiarity with the clinical syndrome and a high index of suspicion. This can be problematic when the patient presents for medical care outside the endemic area. As in other systemic fungal infections, confirmation of the diagnosis requires demonstration of the fungus in the infected organ and culturing the organism from clinical specimens. The response to antifungal treatment is good if the treatment is started early. After the initial treatment, the patients need prolonged suppressive therapy to prevent relapse at least until their immune system is sufficiently restored by antiretroviral therapy.

EPIDEMIOLOGY

Penicillium marneffei was first isolated from a bamboo rat in Vietnam in 1956 [2]. It is the only known *Penicillium* species that exhibits temperature-dependent dimorphic growth. At temperatures below 37°C, the fungus grows as mycelia with the formation of septate hyphae, bearing conidiophores and conidia typical of the genus *Penicillium*.

At 37°C on artificial medium or in human tissue, the fungus grows in a yeast-like form with the formation of fission arthroconidium cells. The fission yeast cells represent the parasitic form of *P. marneffei*. This form is seen in the intracellular infection of the macrophages as well as extracellularly.

The first naturally infected case was reported in 1973 in an American missionary with Hodgkin's disease who had been living in Southeast Asia. Between 1973 and 1988 less than 40 cases of *P. marneffei* infection had been reported in the literature [3]. The rarity of *P. marneffei* infection changed when the global HIV/AIDS epidemic arrived in Southeast Asia. The first case of *P. marneffei* infection in an HIV-infected native of Southeast Asia was reported in 1989 from Bangkok. The number of cases has markedly increased since then. At one tertiary hospital in Chiang Mai, northern Thailand, a total of 1,592 patients with *P. marneffei* infection were seen between January 1991 and December 2000; almost all of these patients were also infected with HIV. Patients would typically be in the late stage of HIV disease with CD4 count <100 cells/mm^3. Common manifestations were fever, anemia, weight loss, lymphadenopathy, hepatosplenomegaly, and skin lesions. Cases had been reported in 21 children with perinatally acquired HIV infection from the same hospital. The clinical manifestations in these children were similar to those in adults [4]. There is extensive seasonal variation in the incidence of *P. marneffei* infection, with increased number of cases in the rainy season [5]. Between 1991 and 2003, more than 6,000 cases of *P. marneffei* infection in HIV-infected patients were reported to the Thai Ministry of Public Health (MOPH). However, between 2006 and 2010, when the Thai MOPH free access to antiretroviral program was fully implemented, the average number of cases reported to the MOPH fell to 148 cases per year. As the HIV/AIDS epidemic spread in the region, the

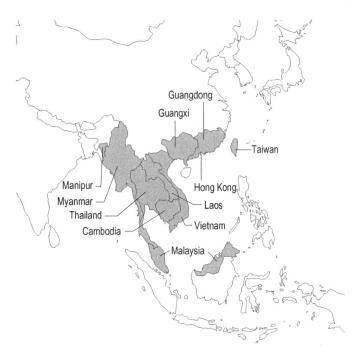

Figure 30.1 Geographic regions of *Penicillium marneffei* infection. The endemic area of *P. marneffei* infection includes Southeast Asia, northeastern India, the Guangxi and Guangdong provinces of China, Taiwan, and Hong Kong.
With kind permission from Springer Science + Business Media. From Supparatpinyo K, Sirisanthana T. Penicillium marneffei infections. In: Kauffman CA, ed. Atlas of Fungal Infections, 2nd edn. Philadelphia; Springer, 2006:191–201.

incidence of *P. marneffei* infection has also increased in other countries, including Vietnam [6], India [7, 8], China [9, 10], Hong Kong [11], and Taiwan [12]. Figure 30.1 shows the endemic area of this fungal pathogen.

NATURAL HISTORY AND PATHOGENESIS

Many important features of the natural history and pathogenesis of *P. marneffei* infection remain unknown. Humans and bamboo rats are the only known animal hosts. The fungus can infect four species of bamboo rats: namely, *Rhyzomys sinensis*, *R. pruinosus*, *R. sumatraensis*, and the reddish-brown subspecies of *Cannomys badius* [13]. These infected animals showed no signs of illness. The geographic ranges of these bamboo rats (*Cannomys* spp. and *Rhizomys* spp.) broadly follow the distribution of human cases of *P. marneffei* infection: namely, Southeast Asia, northeastern India, and southern China [14]. This suggests that bamboo rats may be an obligate stage in the life cycle of the fungus. However, an attempt to epidemiologically link bamboo rats and human infection was not successful. Chariyalertsak and colleagues compared 80 patients with AIDS who had *P. marneffei* infection with 160 AIDS patients who did not have *P. marneffei* infection, in a case–control study [15]. The main risk factor found was a recent history of occupational or other exposures to soil, especially during the rainy season. Both cases and controls were often

familiar with and had seen bamboo rats; 31.3% of cases and 28.1% of controls had eaten bamboo rats but this difference was not statistically significant. Reported cases of *P. marneffei* in HIV-infected infants also suggest that human and bamboo rat infection are not connected [4]. Bamboo rats live in the wild and have limited or no contact with these infants. In another study from Chiang Mai, it was found that disseminated *P. marneffei* infections have been markedly seasonal, with a doubling of cases during the rainy season [5]. This suggested that there might be an expansion of the environmental reservoir with favorable conditions for growth during these rainy seasons and that both humans and bamboo rats are infected with *P. marneffei* from this common reservoir. A recent genotypic study of *P. marneffei* isolated from humans and bamboo rats in China also supports the existence of a common reservoir [16]. However, attempts in culturing the fungus from environmental sources, for example, soil samples, air samples (using high-volume air samplers), domestic animals, and vegetation including bamboo, have been unsuccessful [17, 18].

The mode of transmission of *P. marneffei* to humans is not known. Analogous to other endemic fungal pathogens, such as *Coccidioides immitis* and *Histoplasma capsulatum*, it is likely that *P. marneffei* conidia are inhaled from an environmental reservoir. Also by analogy to histoplasmosis, it is likely that subclinical infections with *P. marneffei* may occur commonly in persons living in endemic areas who are exposed to the fungus in nature. The existence of subclinical infection in humans is supported by a case report from Australia of an HIV-infected patient who had a latent period of more than a decade between exposure in an endemic area and the subsequent onset of clinical infection in Australia [19]. However, in many other instances, the clinical appearance of disseminated infection occurred within a few weeks of exposure to the organism. The seasonal variation of cases with disseminated *P. marneffei* infection, as well as cases of *P. marneffei* in HIV-infected infants reported from northern Thailand [4], also suggest that progress from infection to clinical dissemination is usually brisk. There is no evidence of person-to-person spread.

CLINICAL FEATURES

Penicillium marneffei infection occurs late in the course of HIV infection. The Thai MOPH as well as the health authority of Hong Kong have included *P. marneffei* infection as one of the AIDS-defining illnesses in those countries [11, 20]. The CD4 count at the time of the diagnosis of *P. marneffei* infection is usually <100 cells/mm³. Cases were reported in which *P. marneffei* infection occurred with other late HIV-related infections, such as cryptococcal meningitis, *Pneumocystic jiroveci* pneumonia, cerebral toxoplasmosis, tuberculosis or *Salmonella* bacteremia. Table 30.1 shows the more common clinical presentations of HIV-infected patients with *P. marneffei* infection from case series from Thailand [20, 21], India [7], Hong Kong [11], and Vietnam [6]. Patients commonly present with symptoms and signs of

infection of the reticuloendothelial system. These include fever, generalized lymphadenopathy, hepatomegaly, and splenomegaly. Clinical manifestations associated with late HIV infection such as anorexia, asthenia, anemia, diarrhea, weight loss, and cachexia are also seen in the majority of the patients. Other presentations, such as skin lesions, mucosal lesions, and bone and joint infection [22], are secondary to dissemination of the fungus via the bloodstream. Skin lesions are seen in more than 70% of the patients in most case series and, when present, are the best clues to the diagnosis (see Fig. 30.2). They are usually found as papules on the face, chest, and extremities. The center of the papule subsequently becomes necrotic, giving the appearance of an umbilicated papule (also called papulonecrotic skin lesion or molluscum-contagiosum-like skin lesion). Biochemical and hematologic laboratory values are non-specific and may include elevation of liver enzymes and bilirubin, anemia, and leukocytosis or leukopenia. In patients with symptoms and signs of the respiratory system, the chest radiograph may show diffuse reticular infiltration, diffuse or localized alveolar infiltrates, or pleural effusion [23].

As the HIV epidemic spread and more patients were seen, other less common clinical presentations of *P. marneffei* infection in HIV-infected patients were encountered. Cases with chest radiographs showing lung mass or single or multiple cavitary lesions have been reported [24, 25]. Bone infections have been reported in the ribs, long bones, flat bone of the skull, mandible, lumbar vertebrae, scapula, and small bones of the fingers. Arthritis involving both large peripheral joints and small joints of the fingers has

Table 30.1 Clinical features of HIV-infected patients with *Penicillium marneffei* infection from 5 case series

	THAILAND [20] AUG 87–JUN 92 (*n* = 80)	THAILAND [21] JUN 90–AUG 97 (*n* = 74)	INDIA [7] APR 98–OCT 99 (*n* = 36)	HONG KONG [11] JAN 94–FEB 04 (*n* = 47)[a]	VIETNAM [6] JUL 05–JUN 08 (*n* = 94)
Clinical features					
Fever	93%	96%	97%	96%	99%
Skin lesion	71%	85%	81%	28%	86%
Anemia	78%	76%	86%	79%	77%
Hepatomegaly	51%	65%	39%[b]	28%	69%[c]
Splenomegaly	16%	23%	—	15%	—
Lymphadenopathy	58%	84%	33%	62%	68%
CD4 count (cells/mm³)	NA	Mean: 63.8 SD: 47	NA	Median: 20 IQR: 8.0–43.5	Mean: 29 Range: 2-196

NA, not available; SD, standard deviation; IQR, interquartile range.
[a]44 of the 47 subjects are confirmed HIV-infected.
[b]Hepatosplenomegaly.
[c]Hepatomegaly and/or splenomegaly.

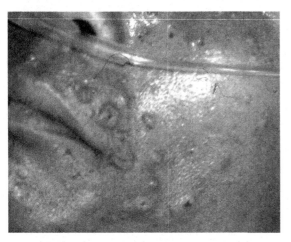

Figure 30.2 Skin lesions of HIV-positive patient with
P. marneffei infection. Some of the papules had central
umbilication resembling lesions of molluscum contagiosum.
*Reprinted from the Lancet. From Supparatpinyo K, Khamwan C,
Baosoung V, et al. Disseminated* Penicillium marneffei *infection in
southeast Asia. Lancet 1994; 344:110–113. Copyright Elsevier 1994.*

been seen [22]. Ukarapol and colleagues reported three
children who presented with fever, mesenteric lymphadenitis, and abdominal pain. Two of the patients had had
unnecessary abdominal operations for the diagnosis of
peritonitis and acute appendicitis, respectively. All three
cases had positive blood and bone marrow cultures for
P. marneffei [26]. Kantipong and colleagues reported six patients who presented with fever, hepatomegaly, and markedly elevated serum alkaline phosphatase levels. *Penicillium
marneffei* was demonstrated in the liver and cultured from
the blood [27]. Mucosal lesions in the oral cavity, oropharynx, hypopharynx, stomach, colon, and genitalia have
been reported [20, 28–30]. *Penicillium marneffei* could be
demonstrated in or cultured from these lesions. Twenty-
one patients from Vietnam whose cerebrospinal fluid
(CSF) culture grew *P. marneffei* have been reported. They
presented with fever and symptoms of altered mentation
including confusion, agitation, or drowsiness. Symptoms
of increased intracranial pressure and signs of meningeal
inflammation were uncommon. CSF pleocytosis was seen
in only one-third of the cases. A total of 71% of the cases
had elevated CSF protein and 24% had a CSF glucose/se-
rum glucose ratio <0.5. The disease course was rapidly
progressive with a high mortality rate [31].

PATIENT EVALUATION, DIAGNOSIS, AND DIFFERENTIAL DIAGNOSIS [32]

In evaluating an HIV-infected patient with the possible
diagnosis of *P. marneffei* infection, it is important to keep
in mind that the majority of the patients were first

diagnosed to have HIV infection at the time of diagnosis
of *P. marneffei* infection [11, 20]. Taking time to explain
and answer the patient's questions about HIV infection,
the course of the disease, and what it means to them is important to ensure the patient's trust and cooperation in
the process of establishing the diagnosis and management.
Also, because the disease is usually seen in the advanced
stage of HIV infection, the majority may have other
concurrent opportunistic infections such as cryptococcal
meningitis, *Pneumocystic jiroveci* pneumonia, cerebral toxoplasmosis, tuberculosis, or *Salmonella* bacteremia. These
should be watched out for. For physicians who are not in
the endemic area, a high degree of suspicion and a careful
travel history are essential. Antinori et al. have reviewed
the literature and found reports of 36 HIV-infected patients
whose diagnosis of *P. marneffei* infection were made in European countries, the USA, the UK, Japan, and Australia.
Practically all patients had a clear history of exposure in
the endemic area before their subsequent diagnosis [33].

The diagnosis of *P. marneffei* infection rests on the microscopic demonstration of the fungus in the tissues and/or isolation of the fungus from clinical specimens. *Penicillium
marneffei* can be seen in histopathological sections stained
with Grocott methenamine silver or periodic–acid Schiff.
The organisms appear as unicellular round to oval cells that
divide by cross-wall formation in macrophages or histiocytes.
Extracellular elongated or sausage-shaped cells with one or
two septa may also be seen. Neither the cell wall nor the cytoplasm of *P. marneffei* cells takes up the hematoxylin-eosin
stain well (see Fig. 30.3).

Penicillium marneffei can be readily cultured from various
clinical specimens. Both automated blood culture system and
blood culture medium for mycobacteria (for example, BD

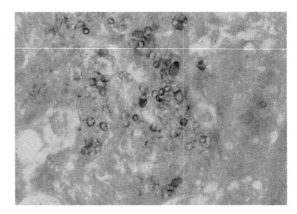

Figure 30.3 Photomicrograph of a tissue section stained with
Gomori methenamine silver, showing the black fungal elements
in subcutaneous tissue underneath the skin lesion. Note the
typical yeast-like organism with central septation. (×1000)
*From Hay RJ. Fungal infections. Clin Dermatol 2006; 24:201–212.
Copyright Elsevier 2006.*

Table 30.2 Sources of isolation in 80 HIV-infected patients with disseminated *Penicillium marneffei* infection in northern Thailand [20]

SPECIMEN TYPE	NUMBER OF SPECIMENS	
	Total	Positive (%)
Blood	78	59 (76)
Skin biopsy	52	47 (90)
Bone marrow	26	26 (100)
Sputum	41	14 (34)
Lymph node biopsy	9	9 (100)

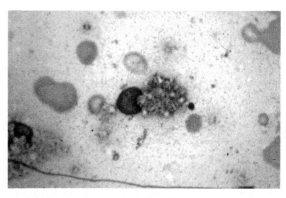

Figure 30.4 Photomicrograph of Wright's-stained touch smear of skin-biopsy specimen from patient infected with HIV and *P. marneffei*. Note spherical, oval, and elliptical yeast-like organisms with central septation in a macrophage. (×1000) *Reprinted from the Lancet. From Supparatpinyo K, Khamwan C, Baosoung V, et al. Disseminated* Penicillium marneffei *infection in southeast Asia. Lancet 1994; 344:110–113. Copyright Elsevier 1994.*

BACTEC Myco/F Lytic Medium) support the growth of *P. marneffei*. Bone marrow culture is the most sensitive, followed by culture of a specimen obtained from skin biopsy, and blood culture (Table 30.2). At 25–30°C on Sabouraud dextrose agar, the colonies of *P. marneffei* are granular with shades of greenish-yellow color and a characteristic red diffusible pigment. The fungus grows as mycelia with the formation of septate hyphae, bearing conidiophores and conidia typical of the genus *Penicillium*. Mold-to-yeast conversion is achieved by subculturing the fungus on to brain–heart-infusion agar and incubating at 35–37°C. Demonstration of this conversion is required before concluding that the isolate is *P. marneffei*.

Several methods of obtaining cytology specimens such as fine-needle aspiration of lymph nodes, bone-marrow aspiration, touch-smears of skin, or lymph-node biopsy specimens allow rapid presumptive diagnosis of *P. marneffei* infection. In one such method, a knick of the skin lesion is made with a surgical blade or the tip of a hypodermic needle, and a small amount of tissue is scraped from under the skin and smeared on a glass slide. The slide is stained with Wright's stain. Examination under the microscope shows intracellular and extracellular basophilic, spherical, oval, and elliptical yeast cells. Some of these cells have clear central septation, which is a characteristic feature of *P. marneffei* (see Fig. 30.4) [20]. In addition, in patients with fulminant infection, *P. marneffei* can be seen in the peripheral blood smear [34].

Several tests that detect antigen or antibody specific to *P. marneffei*, as well as molecular tests such as PCR, have been described [2]. However, these tests are not widely used because commercial reagents are not available. Also, large clinical trials are needed to show the usefulness of these tests in the diagnosis of active *P. marneffei* infection or to predict relapses, as well as to identify individuals who are infected with *P. marneffei* but who are still asymptomatic. This latter group of individuals may then benefit from pre-emptive treatment with an antifungal agent similar to isoniazid treatment in asymptomatic persons with a positive tuberculin skin test.

In the endemic area when a patient in late-stage HIV infection presents with fever, generalized lymphadenopathy, hepatosplenomegaly, and papular lesions of the skin, the differential diagnoses include *P. marneffei* infection, cryptococcosis, and histoplasmosis. If the patient does not have skin lesions, additional differential diagnoses should include tuberculosis, *Salmonella* bacteremia, and lymphoma. Evaluation should include blood culture, skin and/or lymph node biopsy for histopathology, fungal culture, and cytology.

TREATMENT

The mortality rate of patients with disseminated *P. marneffei* infection has been high, mostly because of a lack of timely diagnosis [20]. The outcome has been much better in the hospital where physicians have been aware of the clinical features of the infection and the diagnosis has been made early. Although there is no standardized technique for susceptibility testing for dimorphic fungus, a study of 30 clinical isolates from northern Thailand revealed that all were susceptible to amphotericin B, itraconazole, ketoconazole, and miconazole [35]. Sirisanthana and colleagues conducted an open-label non-comparative study to evaluate the combination of 0.6 mg/kg/day of amphotericin B given intravenously for 2 weeks followed by 400 mg/day of itraconazole taken orally for 10 weeks [36]. Of the 74 patients treated, 72 (97.3%) responded. No serious adverse drug effects were observed. This regimen is recommended as the treatment of choice in HIV-infected patients with disseminated *P. marneffei* infection [37]. However, in a report of 46 patients from northeastern India treatment with oral itraconazole alone was effective in all but one patient [7]. Thus, oral treatment with 400 mg/day of itraconazole for 8 weeks is an alternative recommendation in patients with less severe disease [37]. A new antifungal drug, voriconazole, has been evaluated, but further study involving more patients is needed [38].

Relapses of *P. marneffei* infection are common. In one study, 12 out of 40 patients who responded to initial treatment relapsed within 6 months [35]. Secondary prophylaxis is required for as long as a significant immunocompromised status persists. Supparatpinyo and colleagues conducted a controlled trial of 71 patients in northern Thailand [39]. A total of 20 of the 35 patients (57%) assigned to the placebo group relapsed, whereas none of the 36 patients given itraconazole 200 mg orally once daily relapsed. The drug was well tolerated.

With the increased access to combination antiretroviral treatment for patients in the endemic area, the immune restoration inflammatory syndrome (IRIS) has increasingly been reported in patients with *P. marneffei* infection [40]. It usually occurs within a few weeks or months after starting combination antiretroviral treatment. Antifungal therapy should be started or continued (if the patient is already taking it). Antiretroviral therapy should not be stopped. Short-course glucocorticosteroids may be given in patients with severely symptomatic IRIS [37].

No controlled study exists that demonstrates the safety of discontinuation of secondary prophylaxis for *P. marneffei* infection. However, in an open-label historical-controlled study, no relapse of *P. marneffei* infection occurred after discontinuation of itraconazole in patients receiving combination antiretroviral treatment and a CD4 count >100/mm^3 [41]. Thus, discontinuation of secondary prophylaxis is recommended for patients who receive combination antiretroviral treatment and have a CD4 count >100/mm^3 for ≥6 months [37].

Primary prophylaxis with an antifungal agent should be considered in areas where fungal infections are common AIDS-associated opportunistic infections. In northern Thailand, disseminated fungal infections due to *P. marneffei*, *Cryptococcus neoformans*, and *Histoplasma capsulatum* as well as other fungal infections, such as candidiasis, are common, accounting for over one-third of the reported AIDS-defining illnesses [1]. Chariyalertsak and colleagues evaluated the efficacy of primary prophylaxis with 200 mg/day of itraconazole given orally in a controlled study [42]. The trial was conducted in 129 HIV-infected patients who had CD4 counts <200/mm^3 and had not experienced a systemic fungal infection. In the intention-to-treat analysis, disseminated *P. marneffei* infection developed in 1 of 63 patients (1.6%) assigned to receive itraconazole and a systemic fungal infection developed in 11 of 66 patients (16.7%) given placebo (7 patients had cryptococcal meningitis, and 4 patients had disseminated *P. marneffei* infection). However, there was no survival advantage of being on itraconazole when compared to placebo.

REFERENCES

[1] Chariyalertsak S, Sirisanthana T, Saengwonloey O, et al. Clinical presentation and risk behaviors of patients with acquired immunodeficiency syndrome in Thailand, 1994–1998: regional variation and temporal trends. Clin Infect Dis 2001;32:955–62.

[2] Vanittanakom N, Cooper Jr. CR, Fisher MC, Sirisanthana T. *Penicillium marneffei* infection and recent advances in the epidemiology and molecular biology aspects. Clin Microbiol Rev 2006;19:95–110.

[3] Sirisanthana T, Supparatpinyo K. Epidemiology and management of penicilliosis in human immunodeficiency virus-infected patients. Int J Infect Dis 1998;3:48–53.

[4] Sirisanthana V, Sirisanthana T. Disseminated *Penicillium marneffei* infection in human immunodeficiency virus-infected children. Pediatr Infect Dis J 1995;14:935–40.

[5] Chariyalertsak S, Sirisanthana T, Supparatpinyo K, et al. Seasonal variation of disseminated *Penicillium marneffei* infections in northern Thailand: a clue to the reservoir? J Infect Dis 1996;173:1490–3.

[6] Vu Hai V, Ngo AT, Ngo VH, et al. Penicilliosis in Vietnam: a series of 94 patients. Rev Med Interne 2010;31:812–18.

[7] Ranjana KH, Priyokumar K, Singh TJ, et al. Disseminated *Penicillium marneffei* infection among HIV-infected patients in Manipur state, India. J Infect 2002;45:268–71.

[8] Devi SB, Devi TS, Ningshen R, et al. *Penicillium marneffei*, an emerging AIDS-related pathogen—a RIMS study. J Indian Med Assoc 2009;107:208–10.

[9] Liyan X, Changming L, Xianyi Z, et al. Fifteen cases of penicilliosis in Guangdong, China. Mycopathologia 2004; 158:151–5.

[10] Lu PX, Zhu WK, Liu Y, et al. Acquired immunodeficiency syndrome associated disseminated *Penicillium marneffei* infection; report of 8 cases. Chin Med J (Engl) 2005;118:1395–9.

[11] Wu TC, Chan JW, Ng CK, et al. Clinical presentations and outcomes of *Penicillium marneffei* infections: a series from 1994 to 2004. Hong Kong Med J 2008;14:103–9.

[12] Sun HY, Chen MY, Hsiao CF, et al. Endemic fungal infections caused by *Cryptococcus neoformans* and *Penicillium marneffei* in patients infected with human immunodeficiency virus and treated with highly active anti-retroviral therapy. Clin Microbiol Infect 2006;12:381–8.

[13] Gugnani HC, Fisher MC, Paliwal-Johsi A, et al. *Cannomys badius* as a natural animal host of *Penicillium marneffei* in India. J Clin Microbiol 2004;42:5070–5.

[14] Corbet GB, Hill JE, editors. Subfamily Rhizomyinae: bamboo rats. The mammals of the Indo Malaya region: a systematic review. Oxford: Oxford University Press; 1992. pp. 404–7.

[15] Chariyalertsak S, Sirisanthana T, Supparatpinyo K, et al. Case–control study of risk factors for *Penicillium marneffei* infection in human immunodeficiency virus-infected patients in northern Thailand. Clin Infect Dis 1997;24:1080–6.

[16] Cao C, Liang L, Wang W, et al. Common reservoirs for *Penicillium marneffei* infection in humans and rodents, China. Emerg Infect Dis 2011;17:209–14.

[17] Chariyalertsak S, Vanittanakom P, Nelson KE, et al. *Rhizomys sumatrensis* and *Cannomys badius*, new natural animal hosts of *Penicillium marneffei*. J Med Vet Mycol 1996;34:105–10.

[18] Chaiwun B, Vanittanakom N, Jiviriyawat Y, et al. Investigations of dogs as a reservoir of *Penicillium marneffei* in northern Thailand. Int J Infect Dis 2011;15:e236–9.

[19] Jones PD, See J. *Penicillium marneffei* infection in patients infected with human immunodeficiency virus: late presentation in an area of nonendemicity (letter). Clin Infect Dis 1992;15:744.

[20] Supparatpinyo K, Khamwan C, Baosoung V, et al. Disseminated *Penicillium marneffei* infection in southeast Asia. Lancet 1994;344:110–13.

[21] Vanittanakom N, Sirisanthana T. *Penicillium marneffei* infection in patients infected with human immunodeficiency virus. Curr Top Med Mycol 1997;8:35–42.

[22] Louthrenoo W, Thamprasert K, Sirisanthana T. Osteoarticular penicilliosis marneffei. A report of eight cases and review of the literature. Br J Rheumatol 1994;33:1145–50.

[23] Deesomchok A, Tanprawate S. A 12-case series of *Penicillium marneffei* pneumonia. J Med Assoc Thai 2006;89:441–7.

[24] McShane H, Tang CM, Conlon CP. Disseminated *Penicillium marneffei* infection presenting as a right upper lobe mass in an HIV positive patient. Thorax 1998;53:905–6.

[25] Cheng NC, Wong WW, Fung CP, et al. Unusual pulmonary manifestations of disseminated *Penicillium marneffei* infection in three AIDS patients. Med Mycol 1998;36:429–32.

[26] Ukarapol N, Sirisanthana V, Wongsawasdi L. *Penicillium marneffei* mesenteric lymphadenitis in human immunodeficiency virus-infected children. J Med Assoc Thai 1998;81:637–40.

[27] Kantipong P, Panich V, Pongsurachet V, et al. Hepatic penicilliosis in patients without skin lesions. Clin Infect Dis 1998;26:1215–17.

[28] Tong AC, Wong M, Smith NJ. *Penicillium marneffei* infection presenting as oral ulcerations in a patient infected with human immunodeficiency virus. J Oral Maxillofac Surg 2001;59:953–6.

[29] Kronauer CM, Schar G, Barben M, et al. HIV-associated *Penicillium marneffei* infection. Schweiz Med Wochenschr 1993;123:385–90.

[30] Leung R, Sung JY, Chow J, et al. Unusual cause of fever and diarrhea in a patient with AIDS: *Penicillium marneffei* infection. Dig Dis Sci 1996;41:1212–15.

[31] Le T, Huu Chi N, Kim Cuc NT, et al. AIDS-associated *Penicillium marneffei* infection of the central nervous system. Clin Infect Dis 2010;51:1458–62.

[32] Wong SY, Wong KF. *Penicillium marneffei* infection in AIDS. Patholog Res Int 2011;2011: 764293.

[33] Antinori S, Gianelli E, Bonaccorso C, et al. Disseminated *Penicillium marneffei* infection in an HIV-positive Italian patient and a review of cases reported outside endemic regions. J Travel Med 2006;13:181–8.

[34] Supparatpinyo K, Sirisanthana T. Disseminated *Penicillium marneffei* infection diagnosed on examination of a peripheral blood smear of a patient with human immunodeficiency virus infection. Clin Infect Dis 1994;18:246–7.

[35] Supparatpinyo K, Nelson KE, Merz WG, et al. Response to antifungal therapy by human immunodeficiency virus-infected patients with disseminated *Penicillium marneffei* infections and in vitro susceptibilities of isolates from clinical specimens. Antimicrob Agents Chemother 1993;37:2407–11.

[36] Sirisanthana T, Supparatpinyo K, Perriens J, et al. Amphotericin B and itraconazole for treatment of disseminated *Penicillium marneffei* infection in human immunodeficiency virus-infected patients. Clin Infect Dis 1998;26:1107–10.

[37] Kaplan JE, Benson C, Holmes KH, et al. Guidelines for prevention and treatment of opportunistic infections in HIV-infected adults and adolescents: recommendations from CDC, the National Institutes of Health, and the HIV Medicine Association of the Infectious Diseases Society of America. MMWR Report 2009;58:RR.4.

[38] Supparatpinyo K, Schlamm HT. Voriconazole as therapy for systemic *Penicillium marneffei* infections in AIDS patients. Am J Trop Med Hyg 2007;77:350–3.

[39] Supparatpinyo K, Perriens J, Nelson KE, et al. A controlled trial of itraconazole to prevent relapse of *Penicillium marneffei* infection in patients infected with the human immunodeficiency virus. N Engl J Med 1998;339:1739–43.

[40] Gupta S, Mathur P, Maskey D, et al. Immune restoration syndrome with disseminated *Penicillium marneffei* and cytomegalovirus co-infections in an AIDS patient. AIDS Res Ther 2007;4:21.

[41] Chaiwarith R, Charoenyos N, Sirisanthana T, Supparatpinyo K. Discontinuation of secondary prophylaxis against penicilliosis marneffei in AIDS patients after HAART. AIDS 2007; 21:365–7.

[42] Chariyalertsak S, Supparatpinyo K, Sirisanthana T, et al. A controlled trial of itraconazole as primary prophylaxis for systemic fungal infections in patients with advanced human immunodeficiency virus infection in Thailand. Clin Infect Dis 2002;34:277–84.

Chapter | **31** |

AIDS-associated toxoplasmosis

Pablo A. Moncada, Jose G. Montoya

INTRODUCTION AND EPIDEMIOLOGY

Toxoplasma gondii is among the most prevalent causes of latent infection of the central nervous system (CNS) throughout the world. After an acute infection, cysts of *T. gondii* persist in the CNS and in multiple extraneural tissues. Although normal human hosts maintain infection in a quiescent state, immunocompromised individuals may be at risk for reactivation and dissemination of chronic (latent) infection. Defective T cell-mediated immunity in HIV-infected patients results in loss of the primary arm of host defense against this parasite. Reactivation of latent infection in patients with AIDS may lead to clinically apparent disease (toxoplasmosis), which most frequently manifests as life-threatening toxoplasmic encephalitis (TE) [1].

Seroprevalence varies among geographic locales and even within subpopulations of the same locale [2, 3]. The seroprevalence of the infection with the parasite in HIV-infected individuals usually reflects the seroprevalence of the population they come from. Studies performed in the United States reveal an age-adjusted seroprevalence of approximately 10% [4], with a higher prevalence (>25%) among certain ethnic groups. Early studies indicated that 20–47% of *T. gondii*-seropositive patients with AIDS ultimately developed TE [5]. The risk of toxoplasmosis has significantly decreased since the introduction of primary prophylaxis against *T. gondii* and antiretroviral therapy (ART). The incidence in the USA among patients who had developed AIDS declined from 2.1/100 person-years (PY) in 1992 to 0.7/100 PY in 1997 [6]. However, TE remains a prevalent opportunistic infection in patients with signs and symptoms of central nervous system involvement even in the late ART era, particularly among severely immunosuppressed patients whose CD4 counts

decline <50 cells/mm^3 and who are not taking anti-*Toxoplasma* prophylaxis. TE can be the presenting illness in patients with AIDS [7]. In two European studies TE still was the most prevalent central nervous system infection in HIV-infected patients during the past decade [8, 9].

Primary infection is rarely symptomatic in HIV-infected patients or in those with AIDS. However, *Toxoplasma*-seronegative individuals infected with HIV should be counseled about how to avoid exposure to the parasite. Ingestion of undercooked or raw meat containing tissue cysts and of vegetables or other food products contaminated with oocysts is a major means of transmission of the parasite, as is direct contact with contaminated cat feces. Although cats are the definitive host for *T. gondii*, antibody seroconversion in adult HIV-infected individuals appears unrelated to cat ownership or exposure [10]. Recently, drinking of unfiltered drinking water and ingestion of raw mussels, oysters, and clams have also been implicated as a source of acute *T. gondii* infection [11].

CLINICAL PRESENTATION

AIDS patients who develop TE can do so after the diagnosis of AIDS has been made [12, 13]. Because multifocal involvement of the CNS frequently occurs in TE in AIDS patients, there may be a wide spectrum of clinical findings, including alteration of mental status, seizures, motor weakness, sensory abnormalities, cerebellar dysfunction, meningismus, movement disorders, and neuropsychiatric manifestations [14]. The characteristic presentation is usually one of subacute onset, with focal neurologic abnormalities in 58–89% of patients. Altered mental status, manifested by confusion, lethargy, delusional behavior, frank psychosis, global cognitive impairment, anomia, or coma, may be present initially in as many as 60% of patients. Seizures are the reason for seeking medical attention in approximately one-third of AIDS patients with TE. Focal neurologic deficits are evident on neurologic examination in approximately 60% of patients. Although hemiparesis is the most common focal neurologic finding, patients may have evidence of aphasia, ataxia, visual field loss, cranial nerve palsies dysmetria, hemichorea-hemiballismus, tremor, parkinsonism, akathisia, or focal dystonia [10]. In addition, infection of the spinal cord with *T. gondii* has been described in cases of transverse myelitis, conus medullaris syndrome [15], and of ventriculitis accompanied by hydrocephalus [16].

A rapidly fatal panencephalitis form of diffuse cerebral toxoplasmosis has also been described [17]. Unfortunately, computed tomography (CT) of the head was unrevealing in these cases [17, 18]. In case reports involving HIV-uninfected, severely immunocompromised patients with biopsy-proven diffuse TE, no changes were reported on magnetic resonance imaging (MRI) with gadolinium in the majority of patients, and only minimal changes were detected in one patient (e.g. minimal enhancement of the cortex and subcortical white matter) [19, 20]. Hence, although rare, diffuse TE should be suspected as a possible cause of severe encephalitis in patients with advanced immunosuppression (e.g. those with CD4 count below 50 cells/mm^3) in whom other causes have been ruled out and the suspicion for TE is high despite the lack of brain-occupying lesions in MRI. Extracerebral sites with or without concomitant TE may be involved in HIV-infected individuals. As is true for TE, extracerebral toxoplasmosis usually occurs in patients with CD4 counts of <100 cells/mm^3 [21–23]. In patients with extracerebral toxoplasmosis, ocular and pulmonary sites are most commonly involved (50 and 26% of patients, respectively) [10].

Significant pulmonary disease, including acute respiratory distress syndrome caused by toxoplasmosis, has been reported. Mortality, even in the presence of treatment for toxoplasmosis, is high in these patients [24]. The most common clinical syndrome is a prolonged febrile illness with cough, hypoxemia, and dyspnea that is clinically indistinguishable from *Pneumocystis* pneumonia. This presentation has also been reported as a manifestation of an undiagnosed HIV infection [25]. Associated extrapulmonary disease caused by *T. gondii* has been reported in approximately 50% of the patients at the time of clinical presentation. TE may precede or follow pulmonary toxoplasmosis if maintenance therapy is not instituted. A highly lethal syndrome of disseminated toxoplasmosis has been described in AIDS patients that present with fever and a sepsis-like syndrome with hypotension, disseminated intravascular coagulation, elevated lactate dehydrogenase, and pulmonary infiltrates [23]. This syndrome is usually not associated with clinical or radiologic evidence of TE [21].

Ocular disease caused by toxoplasmosis occurs relatively infrequently in AIDS patients (compared with the incidence of cytomegalovirus retinitis) [26]. Ocular pain and loss of visual acuity are typical complaints, and funduscopic examination typically reveals findings consistent with necrotizing retinochoroiditis. The lesions are yellow-white areas of retinitis with fluffy borders. In reported series, the lesions were multifocal in 17–50%, bilateral in 18–40%, and accompanied by optic neuritis in approximately 10% of the cases. Scant retinal inflammation is frequently observed in AIDS-associated toxoplasmic retinochoroiditis [26]. Thus the features of toxoplasmic retinochoroiditis commonly observed in the immunocompetent host may be absent in patients with AIDS. Vitreal inflammation may vary from mild localized vitreal haze to extensive vitreous inflammation. Vasculitis and hemorrhage are uncommon. In most patients the ocular lesions are located away from areas of pre-existing scars. This suggests that the pathogenesis of these lesions may be secondary to hematogenous seeding rather than local reactivation of infection. The presence of concurrent TE in AIDS patients with ocular toxoplasmosis has varied from 29 to 63% [27, 28].

Most AIDS patients with TE (80–95%) have CD4 counts of <100 cells/mm^3. Cerebrospinal fluid (CSF) may be normal or reveal mild pleocytosis (predominantly lymphocytes and monocytes) and an elevated protein level, whereas the glucose content usually is normal [13].

Congenital toxoplasmosis and the HIV-infected woman

As with HIV-uninfected women, women infected with HIV are at risk for transmission of *T. gondii* infection to their fetus if they are seronegative for *Toxoplasma* and acquire infection during pregnancy [29]. In addition, maternal–fetal transmission can occur in HIV-infected pregnant women who are chronically infected with *T. gondii*; however, the risk of transmission is low (less than 4%) [30, 31]. Studies that addressed this problem were conducted in cohorts of primarily asymptomatic women, most of whom had a CD4 count >200 cells/mm^3 [32, 33]. The risk of transmission may be higher in severely immunocompromised HIV-infected women, particularly in those in whom clinical reactivation occurs (e.g. TE) [34]. However, there are insufficient data to accurately estimate this risk. In one study, one of the three dually infected mothers with CD4 counts <100 cells/mm^3 transmitted *T. gondii* infection to her baby [32]. When dually infected women developed toxoplasmosis during pregnancy, 75% of their infants were born with congenital toxoplasmosis and HIV infection [3]. All infants with congenital toxoplasmosis born to mothers who were HIV-infected were also infected with HIV. The initial clinical presentation of congenital toxoplasmosis in the HIV-infected infant is similar to that in HIV-uninfected infants but appears to run a more rapid and progressive course. The infants often appear normal at birth. In the ensuing months, they fail to gain weight or develop appropriately. The majority develop multisystem organ involvement, including the CNS, heart, and lungs [30].

DIAGNOSIS

At present, the definitive diagnosis of toxoplasmosis in AIDS patients can only be made by demonstration of the organism in tissues or amplification of *T. gondii* DNA from body fluids (i.e. CSF, BAL, vitreous fluid, peripheral blood, urine) (Box 31.1). In cases where TE is highly likely (see Management), brain biopsy can be deferred while awaiting results of empiric anti-*T. gondii* therapy. The likelihood of TE is high in AIDS patients who are seropositive for *T. gondii*, whose CD4 count is <200 cells/mm^3 (risk is greater when it is <100 cell/mm^3 [35]), have multiple ring-enhancing lesions on MRI of the brain, and who are not taking anti-*Toxoplasma* prophylaxis. In this clinical scenario, an optimal response to anti-*Toxoplasma* therapy further supports the diagnosis of TE. In these patients an inadequate clinical response to treatment (e.g. lack of 50% improvement in the patient's neurological exam by day 7) makes the diagnosis less likely and should prompt a lumbar puncture, if safe and feasible, for examination of the CSF by polymerase chain reaction (PCR), and/or a brain biopsy. The morbidity associated with brain biopsy for the evaluation of focal brain lesions in HIV-infected patients is less than that from an erroneous diagnosis [36].

Thus, a brain biopsy should be strongly considered in cases where the likelihood of TE is low if lumbar puncture is not possible or if PCR testing is non-diagnostic. In addition to TE, examination of the CSF by PCR can also be diagnostic for JCV-associated progressive multifocal leukoencephalopathy (PML), EBV-associated central nervous system lymphoma, and CMV ventriculitis. The likelihood of TE is low in *Toxoplasma*-seronegative patients, those with CD4 counts >200 cells/mm^3, those with single space-occupying lesions on brain MRI, and those who have been compliant with anti-*Toxoplasma* prophylaxis [10].

Serology

Because TE in patients with AIDS almost always represents reactivation of chronic (latent) infection, the presence of *T. gondii*-specific IgG antibodies in an HIV-infected patient must be regarded as a marker for the potential development of toxoplasmosis. If the serologic status of an HIV-infected patient with suspected TE is unknown, the IgG and IgM antibody status should be determined.

Although almost all AIDS patients with TE have detectable IgG *T. gondii* in their serum, published series have reported a 0–3% seronegativity rate [14].

Toxoplasma gondii IgM antibodies, routinely measured in an attempt to diagnose acute toxoplasmosis in non-AIDS patients, are rarely demonstrable in AIDS patients with TE. In HIV-infected patients whose *Toxoplasma* serology results are unknown, both IgG and IgM should be measured initially. Positive results on both tests should suggest recently acquired infection, though this is not diagnostic of toxoplasmosis [3]. Positive or equivocal IgM results are not necessarily diagnostic of an acute infection; in fact they may be false positive or observed in chronically infected individuals. Thus, HIV-infected patients with equivocal or positive *Toxoplasma* IgM results should undergo confirmatory testing at a reference laboratory when feasible (e.g. in the USA, at the Palo Alto Medical Foundation Toxoplasma Serology Laboratory [PAMF-TSL]).

Isolation studies

Isolation of *T. gondii* from body fluids or from tissue in the appropriate clinical setting, obtained from a patient with AIDS, should be considered diagnostic of active infection. Because isolation of the organism may not be evident for 6 days to 6 weeks after mice or tissue cultures are inoculated, the results are rarely helpful in initial management of the patient. Nevertheless, isolation of the organism may obviate the future need for brain biopsy.

Toxoplasma gondii readily forms plaques in tissue cultures of human foreskin fibroblasts and most other cultured cells [37, 38]. It has been isolated from the blood in 14–38% of AIDS patients with toxoplasmosis [39, 40]. *Toxoplasma gondii* may also be isolated from bronchoalveolar lavage (BAL) fluid in patients with toxoplasmic pneumonitis [41].

> **Box 31.1 Methods for the diagnosis of *T. gondii* infection and toxoplasmosis in patients with HIV infection or AIDS**
>
> - Serology (including titer in differential agglutination assay, IgG, IgM[a])
> - Visual demonstration of *T. gondii* in body fluids (CSF, BAL) by microscopic examination (i.e. using Wright-Giemsa stain)
> - Amplification of *T. gondii* DNA by PCR examination of body fluids (i.e. CSF, peripheral blood, BAL, vitreous fluid) or tissue biopsies
> - Histologic evaluation, including immunoperoxidase staining of tissue biopsies
> - Isolation of *T. gondii* from tissue biopsies or body fluids (i.e. CSF, blood, BAL)
> - CT scans and/or MR images of the brain in an attempt to demonstrate the presence of multiple ring-enhancing lesions
>
> BAL, bronchoalveolar lavage; CSF, cerebrospinal fluid; CT, computed tomography; Ig, immunoglobulin; MR, magnetic resonance; PCR, polymerase chain reaction.
> [a]Useful, mainly in areas of high seroprevalence, IgM positive results should undergo confirmatory testing at a reference laboratory (e.g. in the USA, at the Palo Alto Medical Foundation Toxoplasma Serology Laboratory [PAMF-TSL]; Palo Alto, CA; http://www.pamf.org/serology/; telephone number (650) 853-4828; e-mail toxolab@pamf.org).

DNA detection (PCR)

The high specificity of PCR testing for *T. gondii* DNA makes this method of diagnosis useful when positive. The use of the PCR has enabled detection of *T. gondii* DNA in brain tissue [42, 43], CSF [44, 45], BAL fluid [46, 47], peripheral blood [44, 48, 49], aqueous humor [42, 46], and vitreous fluid [50] of AIDS patients with toxoplasmosis. Because *T. gondii* cysts persist in certain organs (i.e. brain, skeletal and heart muscle, and eyes) for years after infection, a positive PCR in these tissues does not necessarily reflect active infection.

Of note, attempts to use PCR from amniotic fluid to make a prenatal diagnosis of congenital infection have been hampered by concerns about potential of transmission of HIV to the fetus during amniocentesis [51]. However, in a recent study by Mandelbrot and colleagues, the risk of mother-to-child transmission was negligible in mothers taking ART. Thus, in HIV-infected women who acquired primary *T. gondii* infection during gestation or in women with AIDS who develop toxoplasmosis, amniocentesis can be performed, if they are taking effective ART [52].

Neuroimaging studies

Imaging studies of the brain are essential for diagnosis and management of patients with TE [53]. Typically, multiple, bilateral, hypodense, enhancing mass lesions are found on CT scan. Lesions have a predilection for, but are not limited to, the basal ganglia and hemispheric corticomedullary junction. Significant enhancement of intracerebral lesions is usually seen on CT scan. However, *Toxoplasma* abscesses may fail to enhance or may be solitary and located anywhere in the brain. MRI is more sensitive than CT scan for detection of brain lesions in patients with TE. Masses demonstrated by MRI may be absent on CT scan [54], whereas the converse is not true. Abnormal contrast-medium enhancement, both on CT and MRI, appears to correlate with the CD4 count: pathological uptake may be absent or mild with CD4 count <50 cells/mm^3 and increases accordingly with increasing CD4 count [55, 56].

The neuroradiologic response of TE to specific treatment is seen on CT as a reduction in mass effect, number and extent of lesions, and enhancement. Although the time to resolution of lesions may vary from 20 days to 6 months, the vast majority of patients who respond clinically will also show radiographic improvement [57, 58]. The MRI response to therapy also varies with the location and complexity of the mass lesion. Persistent enhancement on CT scans or MRI after treatment for TE has been associated with a higher incidence of subsequent relapse. Findings on MRI and CT scans are not pathognomonic for TE. Primary CNS lymphoma cannot be distinguished from toxoplasmosis solely on the basis of neuroradiologic criteria, as both present as contrast-enhancing lesions with mass effect. However, the presence of hyperattenuation on non-enhanced CT scans, subependymal location, and crossing of the corpus callosum suggest the possibility of lymphoma [59]. Other imaging techniques appear to be useful for distinction between CNS lymphoma and infectious processes in HIV-infected patients with focal brain lesions. Magnetic resonance techniques, positron emission tomography scanning and radionuclide scanning have been used to evaluate AIDS patients with focal CNS lesions, specifically to differentiate between toxoplasmosis and primary CNS lymphoma. Magnetic resonance spectroscopy (MRS), although widely available, is not usually performed; differences between CNS lymphoma and TE in levels of lipids and lactate have been reported. However, the improper choice of voxel positions in clinical practice may have contributed to the failure to accurately distinguish differences between the spectra of lymphoma and toxoplasmosis [60–62]. Fluoro-deoxyglucose [18F]-positron emission tomography (FDG-PET) is used for the diagnosis of tumors in the CNS; uptake of [18F] is significantly higher in patients with CNS lymphoma compared to patients with TE [63–66]. Although the studies reported high sensitivity and specificity for the diagnosis of CNS lymphoma, the number of patients was small, patients were receiving empirical treatment for TE, and the procedures were performed several days after treatment was initiated, which can decrease the uptake of the lesions. Similarly, several studies demonstrated increased uptake by thallium-201 single-photon emission computer tomography (201Tl SPECT) as highly sensitive and specific for the diagnosis of CNS lymphoma in HIV-infected patients [67–69]. It has also been used as a complementary imaging procedure for MRI with improved diagnostic accuracy [70]. 201Tl SPECT may have decreased diagnostic utility in HIV-infected patients receiving ART [71].

Although MRS, FDG-PET, and 201Tl SPECT, have demonstrated usefulness in the diagnosis of brain lesions in HIV-infected patients, they are infrequently utilized in clinical practice due to variability in uptake, high cost, and low availability.

HISTOPATHOLOGY

Definitive diagnosis of TE often requires demonstration of the organism on histopathologic section of brain tissue obtained at biopsy. Some evidence suggests the superiority of open excisional biopsy compared to needle biopsy in making the histopathologic diagnosis of TE. The response of the brain to *T. gondii* infection can vary from a granulomatous reaction with gliosis and microglial nodule formation to a severe focal or generalized necrotizing encephalitis [72]. Perivascular and intimal inflammatory cell infiltrates can lead to fibrosis necrosis, which can result in hemorrhage or thrombosis, accounting for neurologic signs and symptoms.

The presence of numerous *T. gondii* tachyzoites or cysts surrounded by an inflammatory reaction is diagnostic.

Cysts or free organisms (tachyzoites) not demonstrable on routine histopathologic examination can be identified using the peroxidase-antiperoxidase method [73]. Thus, when routine histopathologic studies fail to provide a definitive diagnosis, appropriately fixed brain tissue should be stained by the immunoperoxidase technique in an attempt to identify *T. gondii* antigens or organisms.

Wright–Giemsa-stained smears or touch preparations should be made as soon as is feasible from tissue obtained at surgery. Similarly, Wright–Giemsa stain of a cytocentrifuge preparation of CSF or BAL may reveal the presence of tachyzoites.

DIFFERENTIAL DIAGNOSIS

The main differential diagnosis of HIV-infected patients with focal brain lesions is between CNS lymphoma and TE. In *Toxoplasma*-seropositive, HIV-infected patients with a CD4 count of <200 cells/mm³ who are not receiving anti-*T. gondii* prophylaxis, the presence of multiple enhancing lesions is strongly suggestive of TE. In patients with a low probability of having TE, the initial differential diagnosis should also include PML, fungal abscess (e.g. cryptococcoma), tuberculosis, pyogenic brain abscess, syphilitic lesions (gummas) [74] or cytomegalovirus disease, and Kaposi's sarcoma in addition to TE. Because therapy is available for most of these disorders, brain biopsy for histopathologic diagnosis in patients with low likelihood of having TE (e.g. single lesion by MRI, negative anti-*Toxoplasma* IgG, CD4 count >200 cells/mm³, use of anti-*Toxoplasma* prophylaxis, lack of response to therapy) may be necessary for successful management of the patient. The characteristic appearance of PML on neuroimaging studies often facilitates differentiation of this disorder from other causes of intracerebral mass lesions. Generally, lesions are multifocal and asymmetric at presentation, predominantly involve white matter, and progress in size and number. Ring enhancement, edema and mass effect are rare [74–76] and more often seen with immune reconstitution inflammatory syndrome (IRIS) [77]. However, brain biopsy remains the gold standard for definitive diagnosis.

MANAGEMENT

General principles

Because TE generally reflects reactivation of a latent infection, all HIV-infected individuals should be tested for anti-*Toxoplasma* IgG antibody. For those who are seronegative, we recommend periodic repeat testing. Those who are seropositive are at risk for development of TE (Fig. 31.1). Studies have associated TE with a more rapid progression of HIV, high TE mortality 16–40%, and persistent neurologic impairment 40% [78, 79]. Therefore, prevention of the disease is critical.

Primary prophylaxis is recommended for those who are seropositive with CD4 counts of <200 cells/mm³ [35, 80, 81]. It is important to emphasize that the threshold suggested in this chapter is different than the threshold of <100 cells/mm³ suggested by Guidelines for Prevention and Treatment of Opportunistic Infections in HIV-infected Adults and Adolescents [35]. We suggest using a threshold of 200 cells/mm³ because all of the North American studies demonstrating the efficacy of primary prophylaxis were evaluating the efficacy of PCP prophylaxis, in which the threshold for intervention was CD4 counts <200 cells/mm³. Using different CD4 thresholds for the primary prophylaxis of PCP and TE may also be confusing for non-expert physicians, and might make it more difficult for physicians in resource-limited settings, where frequent CD4 testing is unavailable. Several authors have reported that in South America [82, 83] and in some areas of the United States, more aggressive strains of *T. gondii* circulate that may reactivate at higher CD4 count thresholds.

MRI is more sensitive than a CT scan and thus is the preferred imaging technique, especially in patients without focal neurologic abnormalities. Patients with a solitary lesion or no lesions on CT scan should undergo MRI to determine whether more than one lesion is present. Because a single lesion on MRI is uncharacteristic of TE, CNS lymphoma and other causes of focal brain lesions should be suspected. Early brain biopsy should be considered in this situation. CSF examination by PCR for *T. gondii*, EBV, JC, and CMV viruses should also be considered if lumbar puncture is deemed safe.

TE used to be the most common cause of focal brain lesions in AIDS patients. Therefore, empiric therapy was considered appropriate for all *Toxoplasma*-seropositive HIV-infected patients with multiple focal brain lesions, *Toxoplasma* IgG antibodies, and CD4 counts <200 cells/mm³. Brain biopsy was recommended in those who did not improve clinically within 7–10 days of initiation of specific therapy. However, the incidence of TE in AIDS patients has decreased in recent years due to the use of primary prophylaxis and ART. In contrast, the primary CNS lymphoma is now a more common cause of focal brain lesions [84]. Thus, empiric therapy for all patients with focal brain lesions without an aggressive diagnostic work-up may delay initiation of appropriate therapy and expose patients to potentially unnecessary and toxic regimens.

CSF for PCR should be obtained in patients with a low likelihood of TE, provided that these tests are available and it is safe to perform a lumbar puncture. Patients who may benefit from these studies include those with negative *T. gondii* IgG antibodies, CD4 counts of >200 cells/mm³, single lesions on MRI, or multiple lesions on MRI/CT scan while receiving primary *T. gondii* prophylaxis. If these tests are not available, early brain biopsy without awaiting response to therapy should be considered. The presence

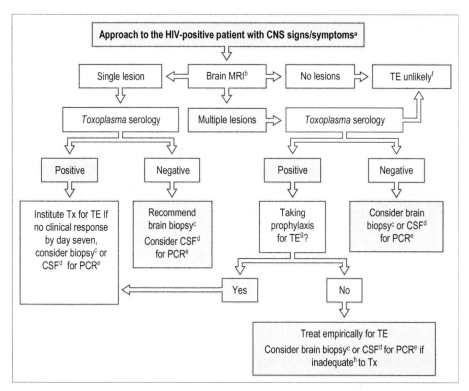

Figure 31.1 Guidelines for the evaluation and management of patients with suspected toxoplasmic encephalitis (TE). (a) Patients with TE may present with a non-focal neurological examination. (b) MRI is superior to CT scan. (c) *T. gondii*-specific immunoperoxidase stain is both highly sensitive and specific for the diagnosis of TE. (d) CSF should be obtained only if safe to perform a lumbar puncture. (e) In addition to PCR for *T. gondii*, consider PCR for EBV (PCNSL), JCV (PML), and CMV. (f) If CD4 T count <50 cells/mm³, *Toxoplasma* IgG is positive, and no other cause of encephalitis has been identified, suspect diffuse TE. (g) For regimens considered to be effective for TE prophylaxis see Table 31.2. (h) Inadequate response to therapy is defined as deterioration of the neurological findings within 3 to 5 days of institution of an appropriate anti-*Toxoplasma* regimen or no significant clinical response (less than 50% improvement in neurological examination) within 7 to 10 days. CMV, cytomegalovirus; CSF, cerebrospinal fluid; CT, computed tomography; EBV, Epstein–Barr virus; JC virus; MRI, magnetic resonance imaging; PCNSL, primary central nervous system lymphoma; PCR, polymerase chain reaction; PML, progressive multifocal leukoencephalopathy; Tx, treatment.

of multiple brain lesions in a *Toxoplasma*-seropositive, HIV-infected patient with a CD4 count <200 cells/mm³ who is not receiving prophylaxis is still considered highly predictive of TE. Thus, awaiting clinical response to empiric anti-*Toxoplasma* therapy still appears to be an appropriate approach in this setting.

Diffuse TE is rare but it frequently goes under-diagnosed and should be suspected when a patient with severe CD4 cell depletion and a positive *T. gondii* serology experiences unexplained fever and neurologic disease. When diagnostic investigations fail to disclose a specific cause in these cases, a trial of empiric therapy should be urgently considered.

A prospective study demonstrated that 71% of patients with TE had a complete or partial response [57]. The neurologic response was rapid, with 51% of patients showing signs of improvement by day 3 and 91% by day 14 [57]. Thus, brain biopsy with or without change of therapy

should be considered in patients whose condition worsens early in the course of therapy or in patients who do not show clinical improvement by 10–14 days [57]. Repeat neuroradiologic study by the same modality as originally selected should be performed 2–4 weeks after initiation of therapy in patients who demonstrate a satisfactory clinical response (or earlier if response is poor). Lesions should have diminished in size and possibly in number. Patients with extraneurologic toxoplasmosis should be evaluated for CNS disease, because a significant number of them will also have intracerebral involvement.

Corticosteroids should be considered in patients with intracranial hypertension caused by the mass effect from *T. gondii* abscesses. A study reported that there was no difference in the response rate and the time to response in patients who received corticosteroids when compared with those who did not [57]. At present, AIDS patients with

TE should receive corticosteroids only when necessary, preferably for no more than 2 weeks. Anticonvulsant agents should be administered to those patients with TE and seizures during initial therapy but are not recommended for routine prophylaxis [35].

It is important to distinguish between two forms of therapy for TE in patients with AIDS: primary therapy and maintenance therapy. Primary therapy is administered during the acute disease. Maintenance therapy is administered after an adequate clinical and neuroradiologic response has been observed. Unless ART-induced immune reconstitution takes place, maintenance therapy should be continued for life, because the rate of relapse is prohibitively high when treatment is discontinued.

Once the CD4 T count has increased to >200 cells/mm^3 and the HIV viral load has been non-detectable for 3 months or longer, maintenance therapy can be safely discontinued in clinically stable patients.

Primary (induction) therapy

Pyrimethamine, a potent dihydrofolate reductase inhibitor, is the cornerstone of current treatment of AIDS-associated TE. It is standard practice to administer the combination of pyrimethamine plus sulfadiazine or pyrimethamine plus clindamycin (Table 31.1).

Prospective, randomized studies of treatment of TE showed that pyrimethamine plus clindamycin and pyrimethamine plus sulfadiazine were equally efficacious during the acute phase of therapy. Several studies have found that trimethoprim-sulfamethoxazole (TMP-SMX) may also be effective for acute therapy of TE [85–87]. A randomized, prospective study revealed that the clinical response rate to TMP-SMX (10 mg/kg per day of the trimethoprim component) was similar to that of pyrimethamine (50 mg/day) plus sulfadiazine (60 mg/kg per day) [86]. In a recent observational retrospective cohort study, improvement was observed in 71 patients (85.5%) [88].

A study of the combination of atovaquone (administered orally as a suspension) plus either pyrimethamine or sulfadiazine as treatment for acute disease reported 6-week response rates of 75 and 82%, respectively [89]. Thus, atovaquone/pyrimethamine can be used as an alternative treatment for patients intolerant of sulfonamides, and atovaquone/sulfadiazine for patients who are intolerant of pyrimethamine. However, large variation among individuals in the absorption of atovaquone has been reported. Levels above 18.5 μg/mL are ideal, although measurements are not usually available in general practice [90]. Primary or induction therapy is recommended for at least 6 weeks assuming the patient experiences clinical and radiological improvement. Longer treatment duration should be considered in patients with an incomplete clinical or radiological response. Changes in anti-*Toxoplasma* IgG titers are not useful for monitoring response to treatment.

Table 31.1 Guidelines for acute or primary treatment of AIDS patients with TE

DRUGS	DOSAGE
Recommended regimens	
Pyrimethamine	PO: 200 mg loading followed by 50 (<60 kg) to 75 (>60 kg) mg once daily
Folinic acid	PO, IV, or IM: 10–20 mg once daily (max. 50 mg)
plus sulfadiazine (preferred)	PO: 1000 (<60 kg) to 1500 (>60 kg) mg q6h
or clindamycin	PO or IV: 600 mg q6h (up to 1200 mg IV q6h recommended in severe cases with altered mental status as an IV medication)
Alternative regimens	
TMP-SMX	PO or IV: 10 mg/kg/day (TMP component) divided in two doses (15–20 mg/kg per day has been used).
Pyrimethamine plus folinic acid	As in recommended regimen
plus one of the following:	
• Atovaquone • Clarithromycin • Azithromycin • Dapsone	PO: 1500 mg twice daily PO: 500 mg twice daily PO: 900–1200 mg once daily PO: 100 mg once daily
Atovaquone	PO: 1500 mg twice daily ± sulfadiazine PO: 1000 (<60 kg) to 1500 (>60 kg) mg q6h

In view of the dramatic immune reconstitution observed as a result of ART, it is critical that HIV be treated to add antiretroviral drug regimens as soon as possible after the diagnosis of toxoplasmosis. Although *Toxoplasma* IRIS has been reported, including IRIS-mediated TE [91–93] and IRIS-mediated placental toxoplasmosis with fetal loss [34], prompt institution of ART is warranted in the setting of acute TE [94].

Almost all the studies on the use of antimicrobial agents for the treatment of toxoplasmosis have focused on patients with TE. Limited data suggest that patients with extracerebral toxoplasmosis also respond to therapy with pyrimethamine-sulfadiazine or pyrimethamine-clindamycin, but the mortality rate in patients with pulmonary or disseminated toxoplasmosis may be higher than in patients with TE alone.

Maintenance treatment (secondary prophylaxis)

While the combination of pyrimethamine plus sulfadiazine is highly active against the proliferative form of *T. gondii*, neither it, nor any of the other currently used drugs is effective in eradicating the cyst form of *T. gondii*. It is believed that persistence of the cyst form accounts for relapse of TE after therapy is discontinued. The relapse rate of TE in patients who are not receiving ART and maintenance therapy for toxoplasmosis is 50–80% at 12 months [95]. The CT scans or MRI images in patients who relapse often demonstrate mass lesions in the same location as at initial presentation. Thus it is essential that patients who complete a course of primary therapy and who have had a favorable clinical and radiologic response to therapy for TE receive lifelong anti-*Toxoplasma* therapy unless they experience ART-induced immune reconstitution (e.g. CD4 count >200 cells/mm^3 and undetectable HIV viral load for at least 3 months) [96].

After successful primary therapy, drug dosages are generally decreased for maintenance therapy (Table 31.2). There is no single regimen that is both effective and has an acceptable safety profile. Although TE can recur during maintenance therapy, it is important to be aware that some of these failures are due to non-adherence.

The regimen of pyrimethamine plus sulfadiazine appears to have a lower rate of relapse than other regimens and is recommended. Patients on maintenance therapy with pyrimethamine-sulfadiazine do not require additional *Pneumocystis* prophylaxis. Although most investigators favor the daily use of pyrimethamine-sulfadiazine, many patients requiring alternative regimens continue this regimen because of drug toxicity (Table 31.2).

Relapse rates with pyrimethamine plus clindamycin have been reported to be relatively high (e.g. 22%) [97]. Whether the high relapse rate was due to the low dose of clindamycin (1.2 g/day) used remains to be determined. In addition, it is important to be aware that pyrimethamine-clindamycin does not prevent *Pneumocystis* pneumonia. Pyrimethamine-sulfadoxine (*Fansidar*), administered as a single tablet twice weekly, has been reported to be effective as maintenance therapy. Side effects were relatively common (40%), with 7% of patients discontinuing therapy because of adverse effects [98]. Atovaquone may be an alternative for secondary prophylaxis in patients with intolerance to standard therapy or for whom such therapy failed.

Considerations during pregnancy

Women who are co-infected with HIV and *T. gondii* and who have developed AIDS are at risk of reactivating their *T. gondii* infection, developing severe toxoplasmosis (i.e. toxoplasmic encephalitis, pneumonia, etc.), and/or transmitting the parasite to the fetus [51].

Pregnant HIV-infected women should receive the same treatment for TE as non-pregnant adults [35]. Although pyrimethamine has been associated with birth defects in animals, limited human data have not suggested an increased risk of birth defects. However, the use of pyrimethamine should be limited to the second and third trimesters [3, 51].

Acute maternal *Toxoplasma* infection in HIV-infected women can result in the transplacental transmission of *Toxoplasma*. There have been case reports of congenital transmission of the parasite in HIV-infected women with significant immunosuppression who develop symptoms due to toxoplasmosis. At present, data are insufficient to determine the effectiveness of treatment intended to prevent vertical transmission of *T. gondii* in an HIV-infected woman. We suggest that asymptomatic *Toxoplasma*-seropositive pregnant women whose CD4 count is below 200 cells/mm^3 receive trimethoprim-sulfamethoxazole (160 mg trimethoprim and 800 mg sulfamethoxazole in a double-strength tablet, 1 tablet per day), which is also used to prevent *Pneumocystis* pneumonia. The goal is to prevent both reactivation of latent *Toxoplasma* infection and transmission of the parasite to their offspring. Trimethoprim can increase the risk of kernicterus and should be avoided in the first trimester, because it is a

Table 31.2 Guidelines for maintenance treatment of AIDS patients with TE (secondary prophylaxis)

	ORAL DOSE	FREQUENCY
Recommended regimens		
Pyrimethamine[a]	25–50 mg PO	once daily
plus sulfadiazine	2000–4000 mg PO	2-4 divided doses daily
Pyrimethamine[a]	25–50 mg PO	once daily
plus clindamycin	600 mg PO	3 times daily
Alternative regimens		
Pyrimethamine[a]	25–50 mg PO	once daily
plus one of the following:		
Dapsone	50 mg PO	once daily
Atovaquone	1500 mg PO	once daily
Clarithromycin	500 mg PO	once daily
Azithromycin	600 mg PO	once daily

[a]Folinic acid (leucovorin calcium) 10–25 mg once daily (can increase up to 50 mg) is recommended for all patients receiving pyrimethamine to help ameliorate the hematologic side effects associated with pyrimethamine. The dose of folinic acid is titrated against the patient's hematologic indices.

folic acid antagonist. In asymptomatic women with evidence of acute toxoplasmosis infection during pregnancy whose CD4 count is above 200 cells/mm^3, spiramycin, a macrolide reported to decrease the frequency of vertical transmission treatment, is suggested for the duration of the pregnancy [35, 51].

The fetus should be examined monthly by ultrasound to detect evidence of congenital infection (hydrocephalus) [51].

Prevention (primary prophylaxis)

Serologic testing for *T. gondii* antibodies will distinguish those HIV-infected individuals who are at risk for reactivation of infection from those at risk for acquisition of infection. All patients who are seronegative for *T. gondii* antibodies, and especially patients with deficient cellular immunity, should be educated about appropriate precautions to take to prevent acquisition of *T. gondii* infection (Box 31.2). Seroconversion to *T. gondii* positivity in

HIV-infected individuals has been reported to occur in 2% after a mean follow-up of 2 years.

Despite the availability of effective antimicrobial regimens, toxoplasmosis in AIDS patients is associated with a mortality rate of 70% by 12 months after the diagnosis of TE if ART is not instituted [99]. Among AIDS patients the 1-year probability of HIV disease progression or death after a diagnosis of TE has been reported to be 40 and 23%, respectively [79]. Numerous studies have reported the efficacy of TMP-SMX, pyrimethamine-dapsone or pyrimethamine-sulfadoxine, in the prevention of TE in HIV-infected patients (Table 31.3). It must be emphasized that among patients receiving primary prophylaxis with TMP-SMX [100], pyrimethamine-dapsone [101], or pyrimethamine-sulfadoxine, 40–60% will have untoward side effects, and 2–12% of the total number of patients will require discontinuation of therapy.

Pyrimethamine alone is not recommended as primary prophylaxis against TE in patients who cannot tolerate TMP-SMX [102].

Although there are no data available on the use of prophylaxis against congenital toxoplasmosis in HIV-infected women who are seropositive for *T. gondii* antibodies and whose *T. gondii* infection was acquired prior to pregnancy and in the distant past, administration of TMP/SMX 1 double-strength tablet daily throughout pregnancy for women with CD4 count <200 cells/mm^3 has been

---

Box 31.2 Methods for preventing toxoplasmosis in patients with HIV infection*

Individuals should take the following precautions:
- Cook meat to "well done" or thoroughly to 67 °C (153 °F).
- Meat should not be "pink" in the center.
- Freeze meat to −20 °C (−4 °F) for at least 24 hours.
- Note that meat that is smoked, cured in brine or dried may still be infectious.
- Avoid touching mucous membranes of mouth and eyes while handling raw meat.
- Wash hands thoroughly after handling raw meat.
- Wash kitchen surfaces that come into contact with raw meat, wearing gloves.
- Wash fruits and vegetables before consumption.
- Avoid drinking unpasteurized goat's milk.
- Avoid eating raw oysters, clams, or mussels.
- Prevent access of flies, cockroaches, and the like to fruits and vegetables.
- Avoid contact with materials that are potentially contaminated with cat feces (e.g. cat litter boxes) or wear gloves when handling such materials or when gardening.
- Wearing gloves is recommended when these activities cannot be avoided.
- Avoid drinking untreated water, including that from wells or reservoirs that have not been secured from potential contamination by feces from wild or domestic cats.

*Note that up to 50% of individuals can get infected with *T. gondii* even if they do not occur in behaviors associated with the acute infection [108].

Table 31.3 Regimens used for primary prophylaxis against toxoplasmosis

DRUG	DOSAGE SCHEDULE
TMP-SMX	1 DS tab PO once daily 1 SS tab PO once daily
Pyrimethamine^a + dapsone	Pyrimethamine 50 mg PO once weekly + dapsone 50 mg PO once daily Pyrimethamine 75 mg once weekly + dapsone 200 mg once weekly
Pyrimethamine-sulfadoxine (Fansidar)^{a,b}	3 tabs PO every 2 weeks 1 tab PO twice weekly
Atovaquone	Atovaquone 1500 mg once daily ± pyrimethamine 25 mg plus folinic acid 10 mg PO once daily

DS, double strength; SS, single strength.
^{a}Folinic acid (leucovorin) 25 mg weekly is recommended for all patients receiving pyrimethamine to help ameliorate the hematologic side effects associated with pyrimethamine. The dose of folinic acid is titrated against the patient's hematologic indices.
^{b}Each tablet contains pyrimethamine 25 mg, sulfadoxine 500 mg.

recommended. Pyrimethamine-sulfadiazine after the seventeenth week of pregnancy should be considered for those who are more severely immunosuppressed and in whom fetal infection is highly suspected or documented.

Discontinuation of primary and secondary prophylaxis

Although *in vitro* studies indicate that ART does not fully restore cell-mediated immunity against *T. gondii* in all HIV-infected patients, the use of ART has been associated with a decline in mortality and incidence of opportunistic infections, including TE, in HIV-infected patients [9, 103]. These findings prompted studies that explored the safety of discontinuing prophylaxis against opportunistic pathogens in patients receiving ART. According to a recent study on the restoration of T cell responses to *T. gondii* antigens in patients with AIDS and *T. gondii* infection, similar lymphocyte proliferative response against *T. gondii* antigens and interferon gamma production were observed among HIV-infected patients on ART whose CD4 count is >200 cells/mm^3, and those who were HIV-uninfected. However, HIV-infected patients on ART whose CD4 counts were <200 cells/mm^3 had significantly lower lymphocyte proliferative and functional responses. These data are consistent with previous studies indicating that TE secondary prophylaxis can be safely withdrawn after ART-mediated recovery of the CD4 count to >200 cells/mm^3 [96, 104].

Observational and randomized studies indicate that it is safe to discontinue primary prophylaxis against *T. gondii* in adults and adolescents whose CD4 counts increase to >200 cells/mm^3 for at least 3 months in response to ART. It is important to note that the majority of these patients were on protease inhibitor-containing regimens, had a CD4 count >200 cells/mm^3 for an average of 8 months, had a median CD4 count at study entry of more than 300 cells/mm^3, and had undetectable plasma viral load [105].

It appears reasonable to consider stopping maintenance therapy in patients who have completed acute-phase treatment for TE, are free of signs and symptoms attributable to this disease, and have experienced sustained (>3 month) increase in CD4 count to >200 cells/mm^3 [35, 80, 96, 106, 107].

Although no studies have directly addressed criteria for restarting prophylaxis, it would be prudent to reinitiate primary and secondary prophylaxis in patients whose CD4 count decreases to <200 cells/mm^3.

REFERENCES

[1] Montoya JG, Liesenfeld O. Toxoplasmosis. Lancet 2004;363:1965–76.

[2] Rosso F, Les JT, Agudelo A, et al. Prevalence of infection with *Toxoplasma gondii* among pregnant women in Cali, Colombia, South America. Am J Trop Med Hyg 2008;78:504–8.

[3] Remington J, McLeod R. Toxoplasmosis. In: Remington J, Klein JO, Wilson CB, et al., Infectious Disease of the Fetus and Newborn Infant. 7th ed. Philadelphia: Saunders; 2011. pp. 918–1041.

[4] Jones JL, Kruszon-Moran D, Sanders-Lewis K, Wilson M. *Toxoplasma gondii* infection in the United States, 1999 2004, decline from the prior decade. Am J Trop Med Hyg 2007;77:405–10.

[5] Israelski DM, Chmiel JS, Poggensee L, et al. Prevalence of *Toxoplasma* infection in a cohort of homosexual men at risk of AIDS and toxoplasmic encephalitis. J Acquir Immune Defic Syndr 1993;6:414–18.

[6] Jones JL, Hanson DL, Dworkin MS, et al. Surveillance for AIDS-defining opportunistic illnesses, 1992-1997. MMWR CDC Surveill Summ 1999;48:1–22.

[7] Girardi E, Sabin CA, Monforte AD. Late diagnosis of HIV infection: epidemiological features, consequences and strategies to encourage earlier testing. J Acquir Immune Defic Syndr 2007;46 (Suppl. 1):S3–8.

[8] Bonnet F, Lewden C, May T, et al. Opportunistic infections as causes of death in HIV-infected patients in the HAART era in France. Scand J Infect Dis 2005;37:482–7.

[9] Abgrall S, Rabaud C, Costagliola D. Incidence and risk factors for toxoplasmic encephalitis in human immunodeficiency virus-infected patients before and during the highly active antiretroviral therapy era. Clin Infect Dis 2001;33:1747–55.

[10] Montoya JG, Remington J. *Toxoplasma gondii*. In: Mandell, Douglas, and Bennett's Principles and Practice of Infectious Diseases. 7th ed. Philadelphia: Elsevier; 2010.

[11] Jones JL, Dargelas V, Roberts J, et al. Risk factors for *Toxoplasma gondii* infection in the United States. Clin Infect Dis 2009;49:878–84.

[12] Luft BJ, Conley F, Remington JS, et al. Outbreak of central-nervous-system toxoplasmosis in western Europe and North America. Lancet 1983;1:781–4.

[13] Navia BA, Petito CK, Gold JW, et al. Cerebral toxoplasmosis complicating the acquired immune deficiency syndrome: clinical and neuropathological findings in 27 patients. Ann Neurol 1986;19:224–38.

[14] Porter SB, Sande MA. Toxoplasmosis of the central nervous system in the acquired immunodeficiency syndrome. N Engl J Med 1992;327: 1643–8.

[15] Garcia-Gubern C, Fuentes CR, Colon-Rolon L, Masvidal D. Spinal cord toxoplasmosis as an unusual presentation of AIDS: case report

and review of the literature. Int J Emerg Med 2010;3:439–42.

[16] Sell M, Klingebiel R, Di Iorio G, Sampaolo S. Primary cerebral toxoplasmosis: a rare case of ventriculitis and hydrocephalus in AIDS. Clin Neuropathol 2005;24:106–11.

[17] Gray F, Gherardi R, Wingate E, et al. Diffuse "encephalitic" cerebral toxoplasmosis in AIDS. Report of four cases.. J Neurol 1989;236:273–7.

[18] Grant IH, Gold JW, Rosenblum M, et al. Toxoplasma gondii serology in HIV-infected patients: the development of central nervous system toxoplasmosis in AIDS. AIDS 1990;4:519–21.

[19] Ionita C, Wasay M, Balos L, Bakshi R. MR imaging in toxoplasmosis encephalitis after bone marrow transplantation: paucity of enhancement despite fulminant disease. Am J Neuroradiol 2004;25:270–3.

[20] de Medeiros BC, de Medeiros CR, Werner B, et al. Disseminated toxoplasmosis after bone marrow transplantation: report of 9 cases. Transpl Infect Dis 2001;3:24–8.

[21] Lucet JC, Bailly MP, Bedos JP, et al. Septic shock due to toxoplasmosis in patients infected with the human immunodeficiency virus. Chest 1993;104:1054–8.

[22] Rabaud C, May T, Amiel C, et al. Extracerebral toxoplasmosis in patients infected with HIV. A French National Survey. Medicine (Baltimore) 1994;73:306–614.

[23] Rabaud C, May T, Lucet JC, et al. Pulmonary toxoplasmosis in patients infected with human immunodeficiency virus: a French National Survey. Clin Infect Dis 1996;23:1249–54.

[24] Derouin F, Sarfati C, Beauvais B, et al. Prevalence of pulmonary toxoplasmosis in HIV-infected patients. AIDS 1990;4:1036.

[25] Kovari H, Ebnother C, Schweiger A, et al. Pulmonary toxoplasmosis, a rare but severe manifestation of a common opportunistic infection in late HIV presenters: report of two cases. Infection 2010;38:141–4.

[26] Holland GN, Engstrom Jr. RE, Glasgow BJ, et al. Ocular toxoplasmosis in patients with the acquired immunodeficiency syndrome. Am J Ophthalmol 1988;106:653–67.

[27] Friedman DI. Neuro-ophthalmic manifestations of human immunodeficiency virus infection. Neurol Clin 1991;9:55–72.

[28] Cochereau-Massin I, LeHoang P, Lautier-Frau M, et al. Ocular toxoplasmosis in human immunodeficiency virus-infected patients. Am J Ophthalmol 1992;114:130–5.

[29] Lago EG, Conrado GS, Piccoli CS, et al. Toxoplasma gondii antibody profile in HIV-infected pregnant women and the risk of congenital toxoplasmosis. Eur J Clin Microbiol Infect Dis 2009;28:345–51.

[30] Mitchell CD, Erlich SS, Mastrucci MT, et al. Congenital toxoplasmosis occurring in infants perinatally infected with human immunodeficiency virus 1. Pediatr Infect Dis J 1990;9:512–18.

[31] Bachmeyer C, Mouchnino G, Thulliez P, Blum L. Congenital toxoplasmosis from an HIV-infected woman as a result of reactivation. J Infect 2006;52: e55–7.

[32] Minkoff H, Remington JS, Holman S, et al. Vertical transmission of toxoplasma by human immunodeficiency virus-infected women. Am J Obstet Gynecol 1997;176:555–9.

[33] Low incidence of congenital toxoplasmosis in children born to women infected with human immunodeficiency virus. European Collaborative Study and Research Network on Congenital Toxoplasmosis. Eur J Obstet Gynecol Reprod Biol 1996; 68:93–6.

[34] Caby F, Lemercier D, Coulomb A, et al. Fetal death as a result of placental immune reconstitution inflammatory syndrome. J Infect 2010;61:185–8.

[35] Kaplan JE, Benson C, Holmes KH, et al. Guidelines for prevention and treatment of opportunistic infections in HIV-infected adults and adolescents: recommendations from CDC, the National Institutes of Health, and the HIV Medicine Association of the Infectious Diseases Society of America. MMWR Recomm Rep 2009;58:1–207. quiz CE1-4.

[36] Cimino C, Lipton RB, Williams A, et al. The evaluation of patients with human immunodeficiency virus-related disorders and brain mass lesions. Arch Intern Med 1991;151:1381–4.

[37] Derouin F, Mazeron MC, Garin YJ. Comparative study of tissue culture and mouse inoculation methods for demonstration of Toxoplasma gondii. J Clin Microbiol 1987;25:1597–600.

[38] Hofflin JM, Remington JS. Tissue culture isolation of Toxoplasma from blood of a patient with AIDS. Arch Intern Med 1985;145:925–6.

[39] Dannemann B, McCutchan JA, Israelski D, et al. Treatment of toxoplasmic encephalitis in patients with AIDS. A randomized trial comparing pyrimethamine plus clindamycin to pyrimethamine plus sulfadiazine. The California Collaborative Treatment Group. Ann Intern Med 1992;116:33–43.

[40] Tirard V, Niel G, Rosenheim M, et al. Diagnosis of toxoplasmosis in patients with AIDS by isolation of the parasite from the blood. N Engl J Med 1991;324:634.

[41] Derouin F, Sarfati C, Beauvais B, et al. Laboratory diagnosis of pulmonary toxoplasmosis in patients with acquired immunodeficiency syndrome. J Clin Microbiol 1989;27:1661–3.

[42] van de Ven E, Melchers W, Galama J, et al. Identification of Toxoplasma gondii infections by B1 gene amplification. J Clin Microbiol 1991;29:2120–4.

[43] Burg JL, Grover CM, Pouletty P, Boothroyd JC. Direct and sensitive detection of a pathogenic protozoan, Toxoplasma gondii, by polymerase chain reaction. J Clin Microbiol 1989;27:1787–92.

[44] Dupon M, Cazenave J, Pellegrin JL, et al. Detection of Toxoplasma gondii by PCR and tissue culture in cerebrospinal fluid and blood of human immunodeficiency virus-seropositive patients. J Clin Microbiol 1995;33:2421–6.

[45] Correia CC, Melo HR, Costa VM. Influence of neurotoxoplasmosis characteristics on real-time PCR sensitivity among AIDS patients in Brazil. Trans R Soc Trop Med Hyg 2010;104:24–8.

[46] Chakroun M, Meyohas MC, Pelosse B, et al. Ocular toxoplasmosis in AIDS. Ann Med Interne (Paris) 1990;141:472–4.

[47] Bretagne S, Costa JM, Fleury-Feith J, et al. Quantitative competitive PCR with bronchoalveolar lavage fluid for diagnosis of toxoplasmosis in AIDS patients. J Clin Microbiol 1995;33:1662–4.

[48] Parmley SF, Goebel FD, Remington JS. Detection of *Toxoplasma gondii* in cerebrospinal fluid from AIDS patients by polymerase chain reaction. J Clin Microbiol 1992;30: 3000–2.

[49] Pelloux H, Dupouy-Camet J, Derouin F, et al. A multicentre prospective study for the polymerase chain reaction detection of *Toxoplasma gondii* DNA in blood samples from 186 AIDS patients with suspected toxoplasmic encephalitis. Bio-Toxo Study Group. AIDS 1997;11:1888–90.

[50] Montoya JG, Parmley S, Liesenfeld O, et al. Use of the polymerase chain reaction for diagnosis of ocular toxoplasmosis. Ophthalmology 1999;106:1554–63.

[51] Montoya JG, Remington JS. Management of *Toxoplasma gondii* infection during pregnancy. Clin Infect Dis 2008;47:554–66.

[52] Mandelbrot L, Jasseron C, Ekoukou D, et al. Amniocentesis and mother-to-child human immunodeficiency virus transmission in the Agence Nationale de Recherches sur le SIDA et les Hepatites Virales French Perinatal Cohort. Am J Obstet Gynecol 2009;200(160): e1–9.

[53] Levy RM, Breit R, Russell E, Dal Canto MC. MRI-guided stereotaxic brain biopsy in neurologically symptomatic AIDS patients. J Acquir Immune Defic Syndr 1991;4:254–60.

[54] Levy RM, Mills CM, Posin JP, et al. The efficacy and clinical impact of brain imaging in neurologically symptomatic AIDS patients: a prospective CT/MRI study. J Acquir Immune Defic Syndr 1990;3:461–71.

[55] Offiah CE, Turnbull IW. The imaging appearances of intracranial CNS infections in adult HIV and AIDS patients. Clin Radiol 2006;61:393–401.

[56] Suzuki K, Masuya M, Matsumoto T, et al. High-intensity signals in the basal ganglia from gadolinium-enhanced T1-weighted MRI as an early change in toxoplasma encephalitis in an AIDS patient. J Infect Chemother 2010;16:135–8.

[57] Luft BJ, Hafner R, Korzun AH, et al. Toxoplasmic encephalitis in patients with the acquired immunodeficiency syndrome. Members of the ACTG 077p/ANRS 009 Study Team. N Engl J Med 1993;329:995–1000.

[58] Levy RM, Rosenbloom S, Perrett LV. Neuroradiologic findings in AIDS: a review of 200 cases. AJR Am J Roentgenol 1986;147:977–83.

[59] Dina TS. Primary central nervous system lymphoma versus toxoplasmosis in AIDS. Radiology 1991;179:823–8.

[60] Kingsley PB, Shah TC, Woldenberg R. Identification of diffuse and focal brain lesions by clinical magnetic resonance spectroscopy. NMR Biomed 2006;19:435–62.

[61] Hegde AN, Mohan S, Lath N, Lim CC. Differential diagnosis for bilateral abnormalities of the basal ganglia and thalamus. Radiographics 2011;31: 5–30.

[62] Ramsey RG, Gean AD. Neuroimaging of AIDS. I. Central nervous system toxoplasmosis. Neuroimaging Clin N Am 1997;7:171–86.

[63] Rosenfeld SS, Hoffman JM, Coleman RE, et al. Studies of primary central nervous system lymphoma with fluorine-18-fluorodeoxyglucose positron emission tomography. J Nucl Med 1992;33:532–6.

[64] Hoffman JM, Waskin HA, Schifter T, et al. FDG-PET in differentiating lymphoma from nonmalignant central nervous system lesions in patients with AIDS. J Nucl Med 1993;34:567–75.

[65] Pierce MA, Johnson MD, Maciunas RJ, et al. Evaluating contrast-enhancing brain lesions in patients with AIDS by using positron emission tomography. Ann Intern Med 1995;123:594–8.

[66] O'Doherty MJ, Barrington SF, Campbell M, et al. PET scanning and the human immunodeficiency virus-positive patient. J Nucl Med 1997;38:1575–83.

[67] Lorberboym M, Wallach F, Estok L, et al. Thallium-201 retention in focal intracranial lesions for differential diagnosis of primary lymphoma and nonmalignant lesions in AIDS patients. J Nucl Med 1998;39:1366–9.

[68] Lorberboym M, Estok L, Machac J, et al. Rapid differential diagnosis of cerebral toxoplasmosis and primary central nervous system lymphoma by thallium-201 SPECT. J Nucl Med 1996;37:1150–4.

[69] O'Malley JP, Ziessman HA, Kumar PN, et al. Diagnosis of intracranial lymphoma in patients with AIDS: value of ^{201}Tl single-photon emission computed tomography. AJR Am J Roentgenol 1994;163:417–21.

[70] Kita T, Hayashi K, Yamamoto M, et al. Does supplementation of contrast MR imaging with thallium-201 brain SPECT improve differentiation between benign and malignant ring-like contrast-enhanced cerebral lesions? Ann Nucl Med 2007;21:251–6.

[71] Giancola ML, Rizzi EB, Schiavo R, et al. Reduced value of thallium-201 single-photon emission computed tomography in the management of HIV-related focal brain lesions in the era of highly active antiretroviral therapy. AIDS Res Hum Retroviruses 2004;20:584–8.

[72] Post MJ, Chan JC, Hensley GT, et al. *Toxoplasma* encephalitis in Haitian adults with acquired

immunodeficiency syndrome: a clinical-pathologic-CT correlation. AJR Am J Roentgenol 1983;140:861–8.

[73] Conley FK, Jenkins KA, Remington JS. Toxoplasma gondii infection of the central nervous system. Use of the peroxidase-antiperoxidase method to demonstrate Toxoplasma in formalin fixed, paraffin embedded tissue sections. Hum Pathol 1981;12:690–8.

[74] Walot I, Miller BL, Chang L, Mehringer CM. Neuroimaging findings in patients with AIDS. Clin Infect Dis 1996;22:906–19.

[75] Skiest DJ. Focal neurological disease in patients with acquired immunodeficiency syndrome. Clin Infect Dis 2002;34:103–15.

[76] Whiteman ML, Post MJ, Berger JR, et al. Progressive multifocal leukoencephalopathy in 47 HIV-seropositive patients: neuroimaging with clinical and pathologic correlation. Radiology 1993;187:233–40.

[77] Tan K, Roda R, Ostrow L, et al. PML-IRIS in patients with HIV infection: clinical manifestations and treatment with steroids. Neurology 2009;72:1458–64.

[78] Pedrol E, Gonzalez-Clemente JM, Gatell JM, et al. Central nervous system toxoplasmosis in AIDS patients: efficacy of an intermittent maintenance therapy. AIDS 1990;4:511–17.

[79] Antinori A, Larussa D, Cingolani A, et al. Prevalence, associated factors, and prognostic determinants of AIDS-related toxoplasmic encephalitis in the era of advanced highly active antiretroviral therapy. Clin Infect Dis 2004;39:1681–91.

[80] Jacobson JM, Hafner R, Remington J, et al. Dose-escalation, phase I/II study of azithromycin and pyrimethamine for the treatment of toxoplasmic encephalitis in AIDS. AIDS 2001;15:583–9.

[81] Mallolas J, Zamora L, Gatell JM, et al. Primary prophylaxis for Pneumocystis carinii pneumonia: a randomized trial comparing cotrimoxazole, aerosolized pentamidine and dapsone plus pyrimethamine. AIDS 1993;7:59–64.

[82] Demar M, Ajzenberg D, Maubon D, et al. Fatal outbreak of human toxoplasmosis along the Maroni River: epidemiological, clinical, and parasitological aspects. Clin Infect Dis 2007;45: e88–95.

[83] Vaudaux JD, Muccioli C, James ER, et al. Identification of an atypical strain of Toxoplasma gondii as the cause of a waterborne outbreak of toxoplasmosis in Santa Isabel do Ivai, Brazil. J Infect Dis 2010;202:1226–33.

[84] Ammassari A, Scoppettuolo G, Murri R, et al. Changing disease patterns in focal brain lesion-causing disorders in AIDS. J Acquir Immune Defic Syndr Hum Retrovirol 1998;18: 365–71.

[85] Canessa A, Del Bono V, De Leo P, et al. Cotrimoxazole therapy of Toxoplasma gondii encephalitis in AIDS patients. Eur J Clin Microbiol Infect Dis 1992;11:125–30.

[86] Torre D, Casari S, Speranza F, et al. Randomized trial of trimethoprim-sulfamethoxazole versus pyrimethamine-sulfadiazine for therapy of toxoplasmic encephalitis in patients with AIDS. Italian Collaborative Study Group. Antimicrob Agents Chemother 1998;42:1346–9.

[87] Arens J, Barnes K, Crowley N, Maartens G. Treating AIDS-associated cerebral toxoplasmosis - pyrimethamine plus sulfadiazine compared with cotrimoxazole, and outcome with adjunctive glucocorticoids. S Afr Med J 2007;97:956–8.

[88] Beraud G, Pierre-Francois S, Foltzer A, et al. Cotrimoxazole for treatment of cerebral toxoplasmosis: an observational cohort study during 1994-2006. Am J Trop Med Hyg 2009; 80:583–7.

[89] Chirgwin K, Hafner R, Leport C, et al. Randomized phase II trial of atovaquone with pyrimethamine or sulfadiazine for treatment of toxoplasmic encephalitis in patients with acquired immunodeficiency syndrome: ACTG 237/ANRS 039 Study. AIDS Clinical Trials Group 237/Agence Nationale de Recherche sur le SIDA, Essai 039. Clin Infect Dis 2002;34:1243–50.

[90] Kovacs JA. Efficacy of atovaquone in treatment of toxoplasmosis in patients with AIDS. The NIAID-Clinical Center Intramural AIDS Program. Lancet 1992;340:637–8.

[91] Tsambiras PE, Larkin JA, Houston SH. Case report. Toxoplasma encephalitis after initiation of HAART. AIDS Read 2001;11(608–10):615–16.

[92] Pfeffer G, Prout A, Hooge J, Maguire J. Biopsy-proven immune reconstitution syndrome in a patient with AIDS and cerebral toxoplasmosis. Neurology 2009;73:321–2.

[93] Tremont-Lukats IW, Garciarena P, Juarbe R, El-Abassi RN. The immune inflammatory reconstitution syndrome and central nervous system toxoplasmosis. Ann Intern Med 2009;150:656–7.

[94] Grant PM, Komarow L, Andersen J, et al. Risk factor analyses for immune reconstitution inflammatory syndrome in a randomized study of early vs. deferred ART during an opportunistic infection. PLoS ONE 2010;5:e11416.

[95] Haverkos HW. Assessment of therapy for Toxoplasma encephalitis. The TE Study Group. Am J Med 1987;82:907–14.

[96] Miro JM, Lopez JC, Podzamczer D, et al. Discontinuation of primary and secondary Toxoplasma gondii prophylaxis is safe in HIV-infected patients after immunological restoration with highly active antiretroviral therapy: results of an open, randomized, multicenter clinical trial. Clin Infect Dis 2006;43:79–89.

[97] Katlama C, De Wit S, O'Doherty E, et al. Pyrimethamine-clindamycin vs. pyrimethamine-sulfadiazine as acute and long-term therapy for toxoplasmic encephalitis in patients with AIDS. Clin Infect Dis 1996;22:268–75.

[98] Ruf B, Schurmann D, Bergmann F, et al. Efficacy of pyrimethamine/ sulfadoxine in the prevention of toxoplasmic encephalitis relapses

and *Pneumocystis carinii* pneumonia in HIV-infected patients. Eur J Clin Microbiol Infect Dis 1993;12:325–9.

[99] Oksenhendler E, Charreau I, Tournerie C, et al. *Toxoplasma gondii* infection in advanced HIV infection. AIDS 1994;8:483–7.

[100] Podzamczer D, Santin M, Jimenez J, et al. Thrice-weekly cotrimoxazole is better than weekly dapsone-pyrimethamine for the primary prevention of *Pneumocystis carinii* pneumonia in HIV-infected patients. AIDS 1993;7:501–6.

[101] Girard PM, Landman R, Gaudebout C, et al. Dapsone-pyrimethamine compared with aerosolized pentamidine as primary prophylaxis against *Pneumocystis carinii* pneumonia and toxoplasmosis in HIV infection. The PRIO Study Group. N Engl J Med 1993;328:1514–20.

[102] Leport C, Chene G, Morlat P, et al. Pyrimethamine for primary prophylaxis of toxoplasmic encephalitis in patients with human immunodeficiency virus infection: a double-blind, randomized trial. ANRS 005-ACTG 154 Group Members. Agence Nationale de Recherche sur le SIDA. AIDS Clinical Trial Group. J Infect Dis 1996;173:91–7.

[103] Belanger F, Derouin F, Grangeot-Keros L, Meyer L. Incidence and risk factors of toxoplasmosis in a cohort of human immunodeficiency virus-infected patients: 1988–1995. HEMOCO and SEROCO Study Groups. Clin Infect Dis 1999;28:575–81.

[104] Lejeune M, Miro JM, De Lazzari E, et al. Restoration of T cell responses to *Toxoplasma gondii* after successful combined antiretroviral therapy in patients with AIDS with previous toxoplasmic encephalitis. Clin Infect Dis 2011;52:662–70.

[105] Mussini C, Pezzotti P, Govoni A, et al. Discontinuation of primary prophylaxis for *Pneumocystis carinii* pneumonia and toxoplasmic encephalitis in human immunodeficiency virus type I-infected patients: the changes in opportunistic prophylaxis study. J Infect Dis 2000;181:1635–42.

[106] Kirk O, Lundgren JD, Pedersen C, et al. Can chemoprophylaxis against opportunistic infections be discontinued after an increase in CD4 cells induced by highly active antiretroviral therapy? AIDS 1999;13:1647–51.

[107] Soriano V, Dona C, Rodriguez-Rosado R, et al. Discontinuation of secondary prophylaxis for opportunistic infections in HIV-infected patients receiving highly active antiretroviral therapy. AIDS 2000;14:383–6.

[108] Boyer KM, Holfels E, Roizen N, et al. Risk factors for *Toxoplasma gondii* infection in mothers of infants with congenital toxoplasmosis: implications for prenatal management and screening. Am J Obstet Gynecol 2005;192:564–71.

Chapter | 32 |

Hepatitis virus infections

Marion G. Peters, Monika Sarkar

INTRODUCTION

Viral hepatitis has become one of the major causes of morbidity and mortality in HIV-infected individuals worldwide [1]. For those on antiretroviral therapy (ART), co-infection with either hepatitis B (HBV) or hepatitis C (HCV) leads to accelerated progression to chronic hepatitis, cirrhosis, and hepatocellular carcinoma [2]. For those initiating ART, co-infection is associated with higher rates of hepatotoxicity and immune recovery may be associated with reactivation of viral hepatitis, especially with HBV [3]. For these reasons, understanding the basic epidemiology, natural history, and therapy of viral hepatitis is essential in HIV-infected individuals. Since the introduction of ART, immune restoration has prolonged the lives of HIV-infected patients. As a result, morbidity and mortality associated with chronic liver disease have emerged as a significant problem facing HIV and viral hepatitis co-infected patients and their caregivers. Hepatotoxicity associated with ART complicates the treatment of HBV/HCV-HIV-co-infected patients, and anti-HCV treatment is complicated by lower response rates and toxic drug interactions.

EPIDEMIOLOGY

Hepatitis A virus (HAV) is an RNA virus that occurs worldwide in sporadic or epidemic forms. It is transmitted almost exclusively by the fecal–oral route, but can also be transmitted from person to person as a sexually transmitted disease, described primarily among homosexual men [4]. Risk factors for HAV infection in homosexual men include high numbers of sexual partners and sexual practices that involve oro–anal contact [5].

Hepatitis B is a partially double-stranded DNA virus and a member of the Hepadnaviridae family. Worldwide, over 400 million individuals are infected with HBV, approximately two-thirds of cases in Asia and 25% in Africa [6]. The majority of individuals in these areas acquire HBV infection vertically at birth or in infancy, but infections can also be acquired by parenteral or sexual routes in adults. After exposure, the risk of development of chronic disease varies with age and immune status. While over 95% of neonates, compared to 5% of adults exposed to HBV, develop chronic hepatitis, approximately 20% of HIV-infected individuals who are exposed as adults develop chronic HBV [7]. The eight known genotypes vary in distribution geographically: predominantly genotypes B and C in Asia; genotype A in Northern Europe; genotype D in the Mediterranean and Middle East; genotype F in South America; and genotypes A and E in Africa [6]. Because of the diversity of the population in the United States, genotypes A through D are commonly found. Co-infection with HBV in seen in two distinct settings: in regions of high endemicity (Asia and Africa), HIV may affect populations with a high background incidence of HBV; or both HIV and HBV infection may be acquired in adulthood through similar modes of transmission (USA, Europe). Thus, co-infection with HBV and HIV varies geographically, with high rates in sub-Saharan Africa (up to 25.9% of HIV positive Nigerians in Nigeria are HBsAg positive) compared to 6–10% of HIV positive individuals in the United States [8].

Hepatitis C virus is an RNA flavivirus that infects approximately 4.1 million persons in the United States and an estimated 170 million persons worldwide. HCV is mainly transmitted parenterally, with the highest prevalence of HCV infection found among injection drug users, hemophiliacs who received pooled clotting factor concentrates, and recipients of multiple blood transfusions prior to testing. The recent epidemic of acute HCV in men who have sex with men (MSM) is associated with traumatic sex and sexually transmitted diseases and likely predominantly transmitted via blood contact [9]. Due to the shared modes of transmission, co-infection with HCV and HIV is common; there are an estimated 150,000 to 300,000 HIV–HCV co-infected individuals in the United States. Twenty-five to 30% of HIV-infected persons in the United States and Europe are infected with HCV, while 5 to 10% of HCV-infected persons are also infected with HIV [10]. The prevalence of HCV-HIV-co-infection differs by the population studied. Approximately 50–90% of HIV-infected injection drug users, the majority of HIV-infected hemophiliacs, but only 4–8% of HIV-infected homosexual men are infected with HCV, which is similar to the prevalence found in HIV-uninfected homosexuals [11]. Sexual and vertical transmission of HCV is, at best, inefficient (see earlier comment about MSM epidemic) but co-infection with HIV and HCV increases the risk of perinatal transmission of either virus. Percutaneous exposure to infected blood carries a 30% risk of HBV transmission and a 3% risk of HCV transmission, compared to <0.3% risk of HIV transmission. HCV HIV-co-infection is associated with higher HCV RNA levels and an accelerated rate of progression to cirrhosis [10]. In the United States, HIV individuals are usually infected with genotype 1, but in Europe, genotypes 2 and 3 are also found in HIV co-infection, and genotype 4 is frequent in some injection drug user populations [10].

Hepatitis D (HDV) infection occurs in the setting of HBV. HDV is a defective RNA virus that requires HBV for replication and utilizes the hepatitis B surface antigen (HBsAg) as its envelope protein. It occurs most commonly in HIV-infected drug users [12].

Hepatitis E (HEV) is a zoonotic, single-stranded RNA virus with an incidence of approximately 7/100,000 in the US [13]. HEV is most commonly transmitted through fecally contaminated water and consumption of undercooked or raw meats, and is less readily transmitted between humans. The most common animals reservoirs of HEV include fish, swine, deer, chicken, wild rats, and shellfish. There are four HEV genotypes: genotypes 1 and 2 infect humans almost exclusively while genotypes 3 and 4 infect animals and humans. The incubation period ranges from 15 to 60 days and the clinical presentation ranges from asymptomatic disease to subacute and acute liver failure. Chronic HEV has been reported in HIV-infected patients and after organ transplantation.

NATURAL HISTORY

Hepatitis A

Hepatitis A virus is an RNA virus that occurs worldwide in sporadic or epidemic forms and does not cause chronic disease. Risk factors for HAV infection in MSM include high numbers of sexual partners and sexual practices that involve oro-anal contact [5]. A case-control study MSM found that during a prolonged outbreak of acute HAV, the HAV viral load was higher and the duration of viremia was longer in HIV-infected patients as compared to those without HIV during a single, prolonged outbreak of acute HAV. It also found that, at the onset of symptoms, HAV viral load was higher and the duration of HAV viremia was longer in HIV-infected subjects compared to HIV-uninfected subjects [4]. In this study, the alanine transaminose (ALT) level in the HIV-infected subjects was also lower than in HIV-uninfected subjects, corresponding to a less severe illness in HIV-infected individuals. Since hepatic injury in HAV is the result of host immune response, immunosuppression in HIV may result in a less severe and more prolonged HAV infection. Though this study was conducted after the introduction of ART, no information on ART use was provided and no correlation between duration or severity of HAV infection and CD4 counts were noted.

Hepatitis B

Co-infection with hepatitis B and HIV leads to increased chronicity [14], accelerated progression of liver disease to end-stage liver disease, and higher mortality [15]. In addition, HIV infection can lead to reactivation of HBV and higher HBV DNA levels, likely due to immunosuppression as is seen after organ transplantation and chemotherapy. Serum aminotranferases are usually lower in HIV co-infected individuals and are less useful in determining the need for therapy. The majority of patients with HBV worldwide have immune-controlled and inactive disease with HBsAg positivity but normal liver enzymes and low HBV DNA titers. Reactivation of HBV can occur at any time and is manifest by the presence of HBeAg, elevated serum aminotransferases and elevated serum HBV DNA (2,000 IU/mL). Mutations in the core gene may lead to inability to produce HBeAg in the presence of active viral replication (elevated HBV DNA and serum aminotransferases with no HBeAg in serum), so-called "precore mutant" HBV infection. This type of infection is increasing worldwide, particularly in those infected since birth with genotypes B and C (Asia) and D (Mediterranean). In immune suppressed patients, serum HBV DNA is higher and reactivation of HBV (with flares in serum aminotransferases) may occur with recovery of immune control, usually 8–12 weeks after starting ART therapy. In addition, seroconversion to anti-HBe and anti-HBs are less commonly achieved with HIV co-infection, therefore long-term therapy is the rule.

Hepatitis C

Co-infection with HIV is associated with increased levels of HCV RNA and accelerated progression of HCV-related liver disease [16]. HIV seropositivity, alcohol consumption, older age at the time of HCV infection, and CD4 count <200 cells/mm^3 are associated with a higher rate of fibrosis progression [17]. Prior to the widespread use of

ART, HIV-HCV co-infection was associated with more rapid progression to cirrhosis by 1–2 decades [17, 18]. Overall progression to cirrhosis is three-fold higher in HIV-infected patients, and more than a third progress to cirrhosis in less than 20 years [19]. ART has improved liver-related outcomes in patients with HIV and HCV but they are still increased over those with HCV alone [19, 20]. The risk of hepatocellular carcinoma is also increased in patients with HIV–HCV co-infection and occurs at a younger age [21]. Liver-related deaths are now the most common cause of non-AIDS-related mortality among HIV-infected patients, an observation that is mainly due to concurrent HCV infection [1].

The effect of HCV infection on the natural history of HIV is controversial. The Swiss HIV Cohort Study [22], a prospective cohort study of 3,111 HIV-infected subjects receiving ART, demonstrated an increased risk of progression to AIDS and death, as well as decreased CD4 cell recovery, in co-infected individuals compared with HCV-uninfected individuals. Even among those with well-controlled HIV–HCV-infected people had over three times the risk of developing AIDS-defining opportunistic illnesses and death compared with those without HCV infection. Though the study initially reported delayed CD4 cell recovery one year after the start of ART among HCV-infected compared with HCV-uninfected people, further data showed no difference in recovery of CD4 cells after four years of follow-up [23]. A prospective cohort study of 1,955 patients in an urban HIV clinic in Baltimore, Maryland, found no difference in progression to AIDS, death, or decline in CD4 count below 200 cells/mm^3 when comparing HCV-infected with HCV-uninfected patients, even after controlling for ART use and well-controlled HIV replication [24]. A 20-year prospective study of IV drug using HIV-infected and HIV-uninfected individuals also found that despite ART, liver-related deaths were significantly higher among these HIV-infected individuals [25]. These and other data suggest that HCV may affect the natural history of HIV disease and supports early introduction of HCV therapy in HIV-infected patients.

Hepatitis D

HDV is the most aggressive viral hepatitis. Its poor prognosis is accentuated in HIV patients [26]. The prevalence of HDV antibodies in HIV and HBV patients ranges from 15 to 50%, depending on geographical region and risk group category. In Western countries, HDV is more frequent in intravenous drug users than persons sexually infected with HIV. HDV viremia is common in HIV positive patients with detectable antibodies to HDV.

Hepatitis E

HEV is most commonly manifest as an acute, self-limited icteric hepatitis, though fulminant hepatic failure occurs at disproportionally high rates among pregnant women, particularly those in the third trimester. Severe presentations are also more common in individuals with underlying liver disease. Although chronic HEV is less common than an acute self-limited hepatitis, this chronic carrier state does afflict immunocompromised patients. HEV seroprevalence is actually higher among HIV-infected than HIV negative patients, and chronic HEV has been reported in HIV-infected individuals [27].

PATIENT EVALUATION

Patients with viral hepatitis and HIV co-infection should be evaluated for the presence of chronic liver disease (Table 32.1). This includes history and physical examination for signs of chronic liver disease, as well as measurement of serum albumin, aminotransferases (AST and ALT), bilirubin, prothrombin time, and platelet count. Histologic evaluation by liver biopsy is at present the most reliable method to determine disease activity and fibrosis stage. However, discordance of at least one stage of fibrosis has been noted in up to 30% of paired liver biopsies [28]. Sampling error, heterogeneity of liver fibrosis and associated procedural risks have encouraged investigation of non-invasive measures of fibrosis. These measures include ultrasound-based images such a transient elastometry (FibroScan) [29] and serological measures of fibrosis markers. FibroScan is not currently available in the USA. Serum markers of fibrosis that are available include APRI [30], FIB-4 [31], and fibrotest [32]. These tools are generally accurate in identifying patients with no fibrosis or existing advanced fibrosis/cirrhosis but do not distinguish between moderate stages of fibrosis. Screening for hepatocellular carcinoma with abdominal imaging, with or without alpha feta protein, is recommended for all cirrhotic patients. In addition, for those with HBV, HCC screening should start in Asian males at age 40 years, asian females at age 50 years,

Table 32.1 Monitoring clinical status of patients with liver disease

SYNTHETIC FUNCTION	PROTHROMBIN TIME, SERUM ALBUMIN
Inflammation	AST, ALT, liver biopsy
Fibrosis	Liver biopsy, serum markers, transient elastography
Hepatocellular carcinoma	Alpha-fetoprotein, imaging studies
Check HAV (HAV IgG) and HBV status (HBsAg, anti-HBc, anti-HBs)	Vaccinate to HAV and HBV if not immune
Check HCV Ab	

sub-Saharan African males over age 20 years, and those with a family history of HCC [33]. It is not clear how frequently to image HIV/HCV or HIV/HBV patients who acquire infection as adults and do not have cirrhosis.

Patients should also be vaccinated against hepatitis A and hepatitis B if they are susceptible [34]. Vaccination against HAV is safe and well-tolerated and confers protective immunity in virtually all healthy recipients. However, lower responses are noted in older subjects, patients with liver disease, and immune suppressed individuals [34]. Prior to the introduction of ART, vaccination with two double doses of HAV vaccine, given either 1 or 6 months apart, resulted in a protective serologic response in 88% of HIV-infected MSM compared with 100% response in HIV-uninfected MSM [5]. A CD4 count >200 cells/mm^3 correlated with an increased chance of seroconversion and a higher titer of anti-HAV antibody, but those initiating ART after a nadir CD4 count of >50 cells/mm^3 demonstrated even lower response rates to HAV vaccination, with only 46% seroconverting after two vaccinations. For HBV vaccination, the responses are low (47%): even using double dose (40 μg), in those with CD4 counts ≥ 350 cells/mm^3, only 64% of individuals responded [35]. This suggests that, even with ART-induced restoration of immune function, HIV-infected patients may have an inadequate response to HAV and HBV vaccinations. Two large randomized clinical trials of HEV vaccines are promising, with efficacy rates of 95–100% [36, 37]. These vaccines have not been studied in HIV-infected individuals and are not commercially available.

DIAGNOSIS

Given the high prevalence of co-infection in certain populations, all HIV-infected persons should be screened for HCV and HBV infection. For diagnosis of acute HBV infection, hepatitis B surface antigen (HBsAg) and IgM antibody to hepatitis B core antigen (anti-HBc) are used. For chronic HBV infection, both HBsAg and total anti-HBc should be tested. If either is positive, then serum HBV DNA should be tested as atypical serologies occur with HBV and HIV co-infection. Some studies have shown HBV viremia in subjects whose only marker for HBV in the serum was total anti-HBc for over 2 years [38]. The prevalence of serum HBV DNA in HIV individuals whose sole marker for HBV is total anti-HBc varies from 2 to 45% depending on the study, but viremia is rare in HBV mono-infected individuals [39, 40].

For chronic HCV infection, serum HCV antibody should be tested using an enzyme immunoassay (EIA). Positive EIA results should be confirmed by quantitative testing for HCV RNA. There is a 4 to 6% false-negative rate with EIA in HIV infection, especially in those with low CD4 counts [10]. HIV-infected patients with undetectable HCV antibody should undergo HCV RNA testing if there is unexplained liver disease, such as elevated liver enzymes.

Acute hepatitis A is diagnosed with IgM antibody to hepatitis A (HAV IgM). HAV IgG is evidence of immunity. Acute hepatitis E infection is diagnosed with IgM antibody to hepatitis E (HEV IgM).

TREATMENT

The goal of treatment of viral hepatitis is to decrease viral replication, to lessen symptoms, to improve histology with decrease in inflammation and fibrosis, and thus to decrease progression to cirrhosis and hepatocellular carcinoma and ultimately to improve long-term survival.

HBV therapy

Current recommendations are to start ART regardless of HBV DNA level in co-infected individuals who have HBV [41]. Two anti-HBV drugs must be included as part of the ART regimen. Currently licensed therapies for the treatment of HBV infection are interferon-alpha (IFN-α) an immunomodulatory agent, and nucleos(t)ide analogs lamivudine (3TC), adefovir dipivoxil, entecavir, and tenofovir. In addition, emtricitabine (FTC) is licensed for HIV but has activity against HBV. Tenofovir, entecavir, lamivudine, emtricitabine, and telbivudine should not be used in HIV-infected patients in the absence of ART because of the development of resistance to HIV [3, 42].

Recombinant IFN-α's were the first drugs approved for the treatment of hepatitis B infection. However, their use in HIV co-infection is limited, as response rates have generally been poor. Studies of newer pegylated interferons in HBV are limited to those without HIV infection and show benefit of pegylated forms over standard conventional IFN in both HBV HBeAg positive and negative disease, with control of HBV DNA in 41–73% of cases [43]. Predictors of response are female gender, low serum HBV DNA levels, and high serum ALT. The latter two are uncommonly found in HBV-HIV co-infection, limiting its use. In addition to the goals of therapy noted above, goals specific for the management of HBV infection are seroconversion from HBeAg to anti-HBe and ultimately loss of HBsAg with seroconversion to anti-HBs [6].

Nucleos(t)ides are competitive inhibitors of HBV DNA polymerase (reverse transcriptase), causing premature termination of DNA chain elongation, resulting in inhibition of viral replication. However, the inhibition of polymerases is not entirely specific, and can also bind to human DNA polymerase. Thus, there is a potential to induce mitochondrial toxicity and multi-organ failure, and mitochondrial toxicity has been implicated in the etiology of some of the dose-limiting adverse effects such as peripheral neuropathy, lactic acidosis, and steatosis associated with nucleoside analogs. Entecavir and tenofovir are potent antivirals with a high barrier of resistance. Tenofovir is active against both wild-type HBV and HBV with lamivudine (3TC)/emtricitabine resistance mutations (YMDD and other compensatory mutations). Resistance to lamivudine increases with time on therapy and is more rapid in patients co-infected with HIV, with 90% of subjects who have HIV and HBV developing HBV resistance to lamivudine by 4 years [44]. Adefovir has been used successfully in co-infected individuals for up to 4 years with no reports as yet of resistance [44]. However, resistance up to 18% after 4 years has been reported in mono-infected HBV individuals who have HBeAg-negative disease [3].

Acute HCV

Indications for treatment of acute HCV in HIV infection are the same as those in HIV-uninfected individuals. Treatment is generally not initiated until 12 weeks after initial HCV infection to allow for possible spontaneous clearance, which occurs in 30–50% of mono-infected patients, and in 15–20% of HIV-infected individuals. Sustained virologic response (SVR: absence of detectable HCV RNA 6 months after cessation of therapy) occurs in 60–80% of subjects with acute HCV [45, 46]. Delaying treatment after this time is associated with progressively reduced rates of SVR. Robust studies of pegylated interferon without ribavirin have not been conducted in HIV-infected patients with acute HCV. Many experts use combination pegylated interferon and weight-based ribavirin for 48 weeks. In contrast, ribavirin is not used with acute HCV in HIV-uninfected patients and only 24 weeks of pegylated interferon is recommended. Recent studies have suggested that in patients who achieve a rapid virologic response, defined by undetectable HCV viral load by week 4 of treatment, a shortened 24-week course of treatment may be appropriate [45].

Chronic HCV

Treatment of chronic HCV in HIV-infected patients is more complex and less algorithmic than treatment of acute HCV. The general approach involves weighing the morbidity associated with pegylated interferon and ribavirin (PEG/R) with the benefits of therapy, while considering the likelihood that an individual patient may actually respond to treatment. Given improved response to HCV therapy in those with well-controlled HIV, treatment of HIV is generally initiated prior to treatment of HCV. However, in cases where ART-related toxicity precludes continuation of ART, HCV may need to be treated first, allowing for improved tolerability of ART. The benefits of HCV treatment in HIV infection include decreased ART-associated hepatotoxicity, regression of liver fibrosis, decreased risk of decompensated liver disease, decreased liver-related death, and as decreased all-cause mortality [47].

Predictors of response to HCV therapy in HIV-infected patients include younger age, lower baseline HCV viral load, HCV genotype 2/3 compared to genotype 1/4, and higher CD4 count [41]. Ideally, CD4 counts over 350 cells/mm^3 should be achieved to optimize response to interferon/ribavirin. A recently discovered single nucleotide polymorphism (SNP) near the *IL28B* gene on chromosome 13 also correlates highly with spontaneous HCV clearance and is one of the strongest predictors of treatment response in HIV-uninfected patients, particularly with HCV genotype 1 [48]. This susceptibility allele is more common in Caucasians and Asians compared to African Americans and may explain much of the racial/ethnic discrepancies in response to HCV therapy. IL28B studies in HIV/HCV co-infected patients also suggest a prognostic utility of IL-28B in predicting interferon-based response to HCV treatment.

Treatment of chronic HCV in HIV-infected patients has traditionally included pegylated interferon and ribavirin for 48 weeks, regardless of HCV genotype. Pegylated interferon (PEG/R) has documented superiority over standard interferon [3]. Guidelines recommend 48 weeks of treatment in HIV treatment experienced HCV patients, regardless of genotype. However, in those who achieve a negative HCV RNA at week 4 of therapy, treatment may be shortened to 24 weeks [49]. In patients who fail to achieve an early virologic response (EVR), defined by < 2 log drop in HCV viral load by week 12 of treatment, or who have detectable HCV RNA at week 24, HCV treatment should be discontinued. Patients with evidence of decompensated liver disease, including ascites, hepatic encephalopathy, and liver-related gastrointestinal bleeding, should generally not initiate HCV therapy due to the risk of further liver decompensation related to interferon therapy. Select patients that are concurrently listed for liver transplantation may be treated with caution.

The introduction of direct-acting antivirals (DAAs) has opened a new era of therapy in HCV, including studies of HCV protease inhibitors and polymerase inhibitors in patients with HCV genotype 1. PEG/R remains the standard of care for non-genotype 1 HCV patients. Studies in HCV genotype 1 HCV mono-infection show that combination DAA and PEG/R have yielded higher SVR rates than PEG/R alone, in both treatment-naïve and treatment-experienced patients [50]. Two HCV NS3 protease inhibitors, telaprevir and boceprevir, were FDA approved in 2011 for use in combination with PEG/R in genotype 1 HCV mono-infected patients [51, 52]. These drugs cannot be used as monotherapy to the rapid emergence of drug resistance. These drugs are currently approved for genotype 1, although studies including genotypes 2/3 are underway. Ribavirin remains essential to prevent relapse. Both protease inhibitors markedly improve the response rates in both naïve and treatment-experienced patients with chronic HCV.

Boceprevir (Merck, PA, USA) 800 mg must be administered every 8 hours with food in combination with PEG/R. For HCV mono-infected patients, response-guided therapy is recommended: IFN/R is given for a 4-week lead-in, followed by IFN/R and boceprevir. If HCV RNA is undetectable at weeks 8 and 24, therapy is stopped at week 28 in treatment-naïve patients and week 36 in treatment-experienced patients [53]. If HCV RNA is not undetectable until week 24, then triple therapy is continued for 36 weeks followed by 12 additional weeks of PEG/R [51]. Treatment should be stopped for futility if HCV RNA is ≥ 100 IU/mL at week 12 or confirmed detectable at week 24. SVR rates were increased from 38% (PEG/R) to 63–66% (triple therapy) in treatment-naïve HCV genotype 1 patients and from $\sim 20\%$ (PEG/R) to 59–66% (triple therapy) in treatment-experienced patients [51, 52]. Among patients with an undetectable HCV RNA level at week 8, the SVR rate was 88%. Limited data show that triple therapy increases response rates most in those with unfavorable IL28B genotypes (CT or TT) although CC patients have the overall highest response. However, SVR rates still increased from 28 to 65–71% in patients with CT and to 55–59% in patients with TT genotype [53]. Anemia is significantly more common and erythropoietin must be administered more frequently in those receiving PEG/R and boceprevir than in those on PEG/R alone [51, 52].

The second protease inhibitor, telaprevir, (Vertex, MA, USA) is a 750 mg dose administered every 8 hours with food in combination with PEG/R for 12 weeks followed by PEG/R alone for 24–48 weeks. If HCV RNA is undetectable at weeks 4 and 12, the total duration of PEG/R therapy is 24 weeks. If HCV RNA is detectable but $\leq 1,000$ IU/mL at weeks 4 and 12, the total duration of PEG/R therapy is 48 weeks (12 weeks of triple therapy and 48 weeks of PEG/R). Reported SVR rates with triple therapy are 79%, compared to 46% in patients receiving PEG/R in treatment-naïve HCV genotype 1 patients; 86% in prior relapsers; 59% in prior partial responders; and 32% in prior null responders [54, 55]. The most common side effects are rash, pruritus, and anemia.

Studies in HIV/HCV-infected subjects with genotype 1 HCV have not been completed as yet. An interim analysis of telaprevir in combination with PEG/R was presented in abstract form at CROI 2011 (Sulkowski et al., CROI 2011). Sixty patients received 12 weeks of triple therapy (telaprevir and PEG/R), followed by 36 weeks of PEG/R. Undetectable HCV RNA was noted at weeks 4 and 12 in 70 and 68% of those receiving triple therapy, compared to 5 and 14%, respectively, of those who received PEG/R alone. Similar results were noted in those not on ART as in those receiving efavirenz/tenofovir/emtricitabine but a lower response was noted in those receiving atazanavir/tenofovir/emtricitabine.

These protease inhibitors have not been approved for use in HIV/HCV co-infected patients. Caution is required as drug–drug interactions are predicted between ART and HCV protease inhibitors but few drug–drug interactions have been performed (updated information is available at www.hep-druginteractions.org and package inserts

for each drug). Telaprevir is a substrate of and inhibitor of CYP3A and P-glycoprotein. Contraindicated drugs include rifampin, lovastatin, simvastatin, atorvastatin, triazolam, and St John's wort [55]. Limited data were presented in abstract form of *in vitro* studies between telaprevir and ART. Telaprevir is not recommended for use with fosamprenavir, darunavir, and lopinavir. Use with atazanavir, efavirenz, and tenofovir lead to changes in both telaprevir and ART levels (Van Heeswijk R et al. Abstract 119 CROI 2011).

Boceprevir is a strong inhibitor of CYP3A4/5 and is partially metabolized by CYP3A4/5. Multiple drugs require dose adjustment because of drug–drug interactions and are listed in the package insert [53]. Other drugs and herbs utilized in HIV patients are contraindicated with boceprevir, including rifampin, phenytoin, carbamazepine, lovastatin, simvastatin, and St John's wort [53]. Studies of interactions of boceprevir and ART [56] are limited. Efavirenz appears to decrease boceprevir levels and boceprevir increases efavirenz levels. Interactions with many HIV protease inhibitors are not yet available.

Despite promising results of DAAs in HIV-uninfected individuals, several issues unique to HIV-infected patients must be considered. HIV patients have higher baseline HCV viral loads than HIV-uninfected patients, contributing to their overall lower response rates. Drug interactions may adversely affect ART and DAA serum levels as well as many other medications in HIV patients and further studies are needed to investigate these interactions. Limited available data on DAA effects on ART show that interactions are not entirely predictable (see PI interactions above) such that each drug may need careful study with individual DAAs to elucidate interactions. In addition more HIV-infected genotype 1 patients are infected with genotypes 1a than 1b, and genotype 1a is associated with higher resistance rates to current HCV protease inhibitors [57]. This is because only one nucleoside substitution is required for HCV resistance to HCV genotype 1a, compared to two substitutions required for HCV resistance to genotype 1b. Toxicities of PEG/R are significant in HIV/HCV co-infected patients such that all oral DAA regimens are eagerly awaited in the next few years.

HCV therapy should be monitored closely for side effects of interferon and ribavirin therapy (Table 32.2). Side effects include flu-like symptoms; interferon-associated thyroid dysfunction; neuropsychiatric disorders such as depression, irritability, and insomnia; and cytopenias, such as neutropenia, lymphopenia, anemia, and thrombocytopenia. The frequency of IFN- and RBV-related side effects in the treatment of HCV-HIV-co-infected patients does not differ significantly from that observed in the treatment of HCV-monoinfected subjects [3]. As seen in the major pegylated interferon treatment trials, lymphopenia may be associated with a decrease in absolute CD4 count; however, CD4 cell percentage is typically unchanged or increased, with no observed additional risk for infection [58]. In addition

Table 32.2 Monitor therapy in HIV patients co-infected with HCV or HBV

	THERAPY	MONITOR
HBV	• Nucleos(t)ide analogs • Long-term therapy the rule • Always use with ART • Need 2 anti-HBV drugs with ART • Monitor for resistance	• AST, ALT for inflammation • HBV DNA 3–4 monthly
HCV	• Pegylated IFN and ribavirin • 48 weeks for all genotypes • Stopping rule: HCV RNA decrease is < 2 log at 12 weeks or HCV RNA detected at 24 weeks • Cytokine support for cytopenias	• CBC closely for pancytopenia • AST, ALT monthly • ANA, TSH 3-monthly • If ≥ 2 log drop in HCV RNA from baseline, continue for 48 weeks

potential drug–drug interactions between ribavirin and nucleoside reverse transcriptase inhibitors may be an issue in HIV/HCV co-infection. Ribavirin, a guanosine nucleoside analogue, interferes with the intracellular phosphorylation of pyrimidine 2', 3'-dideoxynucleosides, including zidovudine, zalcitibine, and stavudine. Ribavirin also increases the phosphorylation of didanosine and may lead to increased toxicity, including pancreatitis and mitochondrial dysfunction [59, 60]. The combination of didanosine and ribavirin should be avoided, and the combination of zidovudine or stavudine with ribavirin should be used with caution.

HDV

Treatment of chronic HDV in HIV patients with interferon is rarely effective [61]. Whether long-term PEG/R is safe and efficacious in HIV-uninfected persons is unknown.

HEV

Due to its typically self-limited course, few studies have investigated HEV treatment. However, case reports have documented successful treatment of chronic HEV using pegylated interferon and ribavirin [62].

ANTIRETROVIRAL-ASSOCIATED HEPATOTOXICITY

All classes of antiretroviral drugs have been associated with the development of hepatotoxicity, defined by significant elevations in liver enzymes [63, 64]. Hepatotoxicity may be dose-dependent or idiosyncratic (unpredictable due to hypersensitivity or a metabolic abnormality). In studies of hepatotoxicity associated with ART, the risk of hepatotoxicity has been consistently associated with elevated baseline transaminases and the presence of HBV or HCV co-infection. Proposed mechanisms of hepatotoxicity include decreased drug metabolism, immune restoration, and mitochondrial dysfunction. Despite the increased risk of hepatotoxicity in the setting of HCV or HBV co-infection, most (80–90%) co-infected patients do not develop hepatotoxicity [63, 65]. Studies that have followed subjects after the onset of biochemical hepatotoxicity have demonstrated that significant clinical hepatotoxicity is rare, and transaminases return to baseline in the majority of cases even if the offending medication is continued (adaptation) [66, 67]. Therefore, it is probably not necessary to discontinue ART if hepatotoxicity develops, unless the patient is symptomatic, has associated hypersensitivy (fever, lymphadenopathy, rash), is jaundiced or there are significant elevations in the aminotransferases.

Although the incidence of antiretroviral-associated hepatotoxicity increased with the introduction of HIV protease inhibitors (PIs), establishing a direct link between PIs and liver impairment has been difficult. High-dose ritonavir is associated with increased hepatotoxicity compared to boosted ritonavir [63]. While there are reported associations between indinavir use and liver toxicity, the risk of developing severe liver impairment with saquinavir, nelfinavir, lopinavir, and amprenavir is low [63].

Of the non-nucleoside reverse transcriptase inhibitors (NNRTIs), nevirapine (NVP) is consistently associated with an increased risk of hepatotoxicity [63]. Cases of severe liver toxicity, some fatal, are associated with NVP use for post-exposure prophylaxis [68]. Risk factors proposed for NVP-induced hepatotoxicity are conflicting but have included higher baseline CD4 count, female sex, HBV or HCV co-infection, alcohol consumption, wasting, concomitant use of stavudine, and abnormal baseline liver function abnormalities. Nevirapine hepatotoxicity commonly occurs early in treatment, suggesting an idiosyncratic mechanism. However, later-onset hepatotoxicity of NVP-containing regimens occurs > 120 days, with the risk increasing with an increasing duration of treatment and in cirrhotic patients. Some studies have shown a direct correlation between plasma NVP concentrations and hepatotoxicity independent of the presence of HCV co-infection, while others have shown higher NVP levels in subjects with higher transaminase levels and in HBV- or HCV-co-infected subjects [63].

Efavirenz (EFV) is generally considered to have a lower risk of hepatotoxicity compared with NVP [63]. There is clearly an increased risk of hepatotoxicity with the use of both NVP and EFV compared with the use of either drug alone. The NNRTIs are substrates for cytochrome P450 metabolic pathways, so variability in drug metabolism between individuals may explain hepatotoxicity. It remains unclear whether NNRTI-associated hepatotoxicity is dose-dependent or idiosyncratic.

The majority of nucleoside reverse transcriptase inhibitors (NRTIs) can cause mitochondrial toxicity and have the potential to cause liver injury [63]. NRTIs inhibit γ-DNA polymerase, the enzyme responsible for mitochondrial DNA replication. Cases of lactic acidosis and steatosis are more frequently reported with didanosine, stavudine, or zidovudine. It is believed that cumulative exposure to NRTI is a factor in the development of lactic acidosis.

LIVER TRANSPLANTATION

Liver transplantation is now considered a therapeutic option for HIV-infected patients. In the post-HAART era, initial studies of liver transplant in HIV-infected patients reported no significant differences in patient or graft survival when compared to HIV-uninfected patients [69–71]. HIV/HBV patients do as well as HBV mono-infected patients after liver transplantation [72]. However, data focusing on liver transplant in HIV/HCV co-infected patients are less encouraging, with higher rates of graft failure due to HCV re-infection and greater mortality among co-infected as compared to mono-infected patients [71, 73]. Given the additional complexity of liver transplant in HIV-infected patients, careful selection of transplant candidates is critical, and multidisciplinary care, including pharmacologists, infectious disease specialists, hepatologists, and transplant surgeons, is crucial.

SUMMARY

Viral hepatitis is increasingly being recognized in HIV-infected individuals and has become one of the major causes of morbidity and mortality. Co-infection with either HBV or HCV leads to accelerated progression to chronic hepatitis, cirrhosis, and hepatocellular carcinoma. In addition, co-infection with either HBV or HCV is associated with higher rates of hepatotoxicity. Immune recovery may be associated with reactivation of viral hepatitis, especially with HBV. Selection of therapy for HIV mandates understanding the HBV and HCV status of the individual. All individuals should be evaluated for co-infections and vaccinations for HAV and HBV performed if needed. Our understanding of the natural history of viral hepatitis and HIV in the current ART era and the response to anti-HCV and HIV treatment has improved significantly over recent years.

REFERENCES

[1] Weber R, Sabin CA, Friis-Moller N, et al. Liver-related deaths in persons infected with the human immunodeficiency virus: the D:A:D study. Arch Intern Med 2006;166:1632–41.

[2] Bica I, McGovern B, Dhar R, et al. Increasing mortality due to end-stage liver disease in patients with human immunodeficiency virus infection. Clin Infect Dis 2001;32:492–7.

[3] Koziel MJ, Peters MG. Viral hepatitis in HIV infection. N Engl J Med 2007;356:1445–54.

[4] Ida S, Tachikawa N, Nakajima A, et al. Influence of human immunodeficiency virus type 1 infection on acute hepatitis A virus infection. Clin Infect Dis 2002;34:379–85.

[5] Neilsen GA, Bodsworth NJ, Watts N. Response to hepatitis A vaccination in human immunodeficiency virus-infected and -uninfected homosexual men. J Infect Dis 1997;176:1064–7.

[6] Lai CL, Ratziu V, Yuen MF, Poynard T. Viral hepatitis B. Lancet 2003;362:2089–94.

[7] Hadler SC, Judson FN, O'Malley PM, et al. Outcome of hepatitis B virus infection in homosexual men and its relation to prior human immunodeficiency virus infection. J Infect Dis 1991;163:454–9.

[8] Thio CL. Hepatitis B in the human immunodeficiency virus-infected patient: epidemiology, natural history, and treatment. Semin Liver Dis 2003;23:125–36.

[9] Danta M, Brown D, Bhagani S, et al. Recent epidemic of acute hepatitis C virus in HIV-positive men who have sex with men linked to high-risk sexual behaviours. AIDS 2007;21:983–91.

[10] Rockstroh JK, Spengler U. HIV and hepatitis C virus co-infection. Lancet Infect Dis 2004;4: 437–44.

[11] Sulkowski MS, Thomas DL. Hepatitis C in the HIV-infected person. Ann Intern Med 2003;138:197–207.

[12] Sheldon J, Ramos B, Toro C, et al. Does treatment of hepatitis B virus (HBV) infection reduce hepatitis delta virus (HDV) replication in HIV-HBV-HDV-coinfected patients? Antivir Ther 2008;13:97–102.

[13] Teshale EH, Hu DJ, Holmberg SD. The two faces of hepatitis E virus. Clin Infect Dis 2010;51:328–34.

[14] Hadler SC. The treatment of chronic type B viral hepatitis. Ann Int Med 1988;109:89–94.

[15] Thio CL, Seaberg EC, Skolasky, R Jr, et al. HIV-1, hepatitis B virus, and risk of liver-related mortality in the

Multicenter Cohort Study (MACS). Lancet 2002;360:1921–6.

[16] Sherman K, Rouster S, Chung R, Rajicic N. Hepatitis C prevalence in HIV-infected patients: a cross sectional analysis of the US Adult AIDS Clinical Trials Group. Antivir Ther 2000;5:64.

[17] Benhamou Y, Di MV, Bochet M, et al. Factors affecting liver fibrosis in human immunodeficiency virus- and hepatitis C virus-coinfected patients: impact of protease inhibitor therapy. Hepatology 2001;34:283–7.

[18] Soto B, Sanchez-Quijano A, Rodrigo L, et al. Human immunodeficiency virus infection modifies the natural history of chronic parenterally-acquired hepatitis C with an unusually rapid progression to cirrhosis [see comments]. J Hepatol 1997; 26:1–5.

[19] Pineda JA, Romero-Gomez M, Diaz-Garcia F, et al. HIV coinfection shortens the survival of patients with hepatitis C virus-related decompensated cirrhosis. Hepatology 2005;41:779–89.

[20] Qurishi N, Kreuzberg C, Luchters G, et al. Effect of antiretroviral therapy on liver-related mortality in patients with HIV and hepatitis C virus coinfection. Lancet 2003;362:1708–13.

[21] Salmon-Ceron D, Rosenthal E, Lewden C, et al. Emerging role of hepatocellular carcinoma among liver-related causes of deaths in HIV-infected patients: The French national Mortalité 2005 study. J Hepatol 2009;50:736–45.

[22] Greub G, Ledergerber B, Battegay M, et al. Clinical progression, survival, and immune recovery during antiretroviral therapy in patients with HIV-1 and hepatitis C virus coinfection: the Swiss HIV Cohort Study. Lancet 2000;356:1800–5.

[23] Kaufmann GR, Perrin L, Pantaleo G, et al. CD4 T-lymphocyte recovery in individuals with advanced HIV-1 infection receiving potent antiretroviral therapy for 4 years: the Swiss HIV Cohort Study. Arch Intern Med 2003;163:2187–95.

[24] Sulkowski MS, Moore RD, Mehta SH, et al. Hepatitis C and

progression of HIV disease. JAMA 2002;288:199–206.

[25] Smit C, van den Berg C, Geskus R, et al. Risk of hepatitis-related mortality increased among hepatitis C virus/HIV-coinfected drug users compared with drug users infected only with hepatitis C virus: a 20-year prospective study. J Acquir Immune Defic Syndr 2008;47:221–5.

[26] Housset C, Pol S, Carnot F, et al. Interactions between human immunodeficiency virus-1, hepatitis delta virus and hepatitis B virus infections in 260 chronic carriers of hepatitis B virus. Hepatology 1992;15:578–83.

[27] Pischke S, Wedemeyer H. Chronic hepatitis E in liver transplant recipients: a significant clinical problem? Minerva Gastroenterol Dietol 2010;56:121–8.

[28] Regev A, Berho M, Jeffers LJ, et al. Sampling error and intraobserver variation in liver biopsy in patients with chronic HCV infection. Am J Gastroenterol 2002;97:2614–18.

[29] Ganne-Carrie N, Ziol M, de Ledinghen V, et al. Accuracy of liver stiffness measurement for the diagnosis of cirrhosis in patients with chronic liver diseases. Hepatology 2006;44: 1511–17.

[30] Wai CT, Greenson JK, Fontana RJ, et al. A simple noninvasive index can predict both significant fibrosis and cirrhosis in patients with chronic hepatitis C. Hepatology 2003;38:518–26.

[31] Sterling RK, Lissen E, Clumeck N, et al. Development of a simple noninvasive index to predict significant fibrosis in patients with HIV/HCV coinfection. Hepatology 2006;43:1317–25.

[32] Poynard T, Imbert-Bismut F, Munteanu M, et al. Overview of the diagnostic value of biochemical markers of liver fibrosis (FibroTest, HCV FibroSure) and necrosis (ActiTest) in patients with chronic hepatitis C. Comp Hepatol 2004;3:8.

[33] Lok AS, McMahon BJ. Chronic hepatitis B. Hepatology 2007;45:507–39.

[34] Murdoch DL, Goa K, Figgitt DP. Combined hepatitis A and B vaccines: a review of their

immunogenicity and tolerability. Drugs 2003;63:2625–49.

[35] Fonseca MO, Pang LW, de Paula CN, et al. Randomized trial of recombinant hepatitis B vaccine in HIV-infected adult patients comparing a standard dose to a double dose. Vaccine 2005;23:2902–8.

[36] Shrestha MP, Scott RM, Joshi DM, et al. Safety and efficacy of a recombinant hepatitis E vaccine. N Engl J Med 2007;356:895–903.

[37] Zhu FC, Zhang J, Zhang XF, et al. Efficacy and safety of a recombinant hepatitis E vaccine in healthy adults: a large-scale, randomised, double-blind placebo-controlled, phase 3 trial. Lancet 2010;376:895–902.

[38] Hofer M, Joller-Jemelka HI, Grob PJ, et al. Frequent chronic hepatitis B virus infection in HIV-infected patients positive for antibody to hepatitis B core antigen only. Swiss HIV Cohort Study. Eur J Clin Microbiol Infect Dis 1998; 17:6–13.

[39] Mphahlele MJ, Lukhwareni A, Burnett RJ, et al. High risk of occult hepatitis B virus infection in HIV-positive patients from South Africa. J ClinVirol 2006;35:14–20.

[40] Shire NJ, Rouster SD, Rajicic N, Sherman KE. Occult hepatitis B in HIV-infected patients. J Acquir Immune Defic Syndr 2004;36:869–75.

[41] Rockstroh JK, Bhagani S, Benhamou Y, et al. European AIDS Clinical Society (EACS) guidelines for the clinical management and treatment of chronic hepatitis B and C coinfection in HIV-infected adults. HIV Med 2008;9:82–8.

[42] McMahon MA, Jilek BL, Brennan TP, et al. The HBV drug entecavir—effects on HIV-1 replication and resistance. N Engl J Med 2007;356:2614–21.

[43] Marcellin P, Lau GK, Bonino F, et al. Peginterferon alfa-2a alone, lamivudine alone, and the two in combination in patients with HBeAg-negative chronic hepatitis B. N Engl J Med 2004;351:1206–17.

[44] Benhamou Y, Bochet M, Thibault V, et al. Safety and efficacy of adefovir dipivoxil in patients co-infected with HIV-1 and lamivudine-resistant hepatitis B virus: an

open-label pilot study. Lancet 2001;358:718–23.

[45] Vogel M, Dominguez S, Bhagani S, et al. Treatment of acute HCV infection in HIV-positive patients: experience from a multicentre European cohort. Antivir Ther 2010;15:267–79.

[46] Boesecke C, Rockstroh JK. Treatment of acute hepatitis C infection in HIV-infected patients. Curr Opin HIV AIDS 2011;6:278–84.

[47] Soriano V, Labarga P, Ruiz-Sancho A, et al. Regression of liver fibrosis in hepatitis C virus/HIV-co-infected patients after treatment with pegylated interferon plus ribavirin. AIDS 2006;20:2225–7.

[48] Ge D, Fellay J, Thompson AJ, et al. Genetic variation in IL28B predicts hepatitis C treatment-induced viral clearance. Nature 2009;461:399–401.

[49] Soriano V, Puoti M, Sulkowski M, et al. Care of patients coinfected with HIV and hepatitis C virus: 2007 updated recommendations from the HCV-HIV International Panel. AIDS 2007;21:1073–89.

[50] Asselah T, Marcellin P. New direct-acting antivirals' combination for the treatment of chronic hepatitis C. Liver Int 2011;31(Suppl. 1):68–77.

[51] Bacon BR, Gordon SC, Lawitz E, et al. Boceprevir for previously treated chronic HCV genotype 1 infection. N Engl J Med 2011;364:1207–17.

[52] Poordad F, McCone, J Jr, Bacon BR, et al. Boceprevir for untreated chronic HCV genotype 1 infection. N Engl J Med 2011;364:1195–206.

[53] Boceprevir Package insert. In: Merck; 2011: www.vitrelis.com.

[54] Smith LS, Nelson M, Naik S, Woten J. Telaprevir: an NS3/4A protease inhibitor for the treatment of chronic hepatitis C. Ann Pharmacother 2011;45:639–48.

[55] Telaprevir product label. In; 2011: www.inciveti.com.

[56] Kasserra C, Hughes E, Treitel M, et al. Clinical Pharmacology of BOC: Metabolism, Excretion, and Drug-Drug Interactions. Merck & Co, Inc, Kenilworth, NJ, US 18th Conference on Retroviruses and Opportunistic Infections (CROI) 2001; February 27–March 2, 2011, Boston, MA.

[57] Pawlotsky JM. Treatment failure and resistance with direct-acting antiviral drugs against hepatitis C virus. Hepatology 2011;53:1742–51.

[58] Chung RT, Andersen J, Volberding P, et al. Peginterferon Alfa-2a plus ribavirin versus interferon alfa-2a plus ribavirin for chronic hepatitis C in HIV-coinfected persons. N Engl J Med 2004;351:451–9.

[59] Moreno A, Quereda C, Moreno L, et al. High rate of didanosine-related mitochondrial toxicity in HIV/HCV-coinfected patients receiving ribavirin. Antivir Ther 2004;9:133–8.

[60] Rockstroh JK, Reichel C, Hille H, et al. Pharmacokinetics of azidothymidine and its major metabolite glucuronylazidothymidine in hemophiliacs coinfected with human immunodeficiency virus and chronic hepatitis C. Am J Ther 1998;5:387–91.

[61] Puoti M, Rossi S, Forleo MA, et al. Treatment of chronic hepatitis D with interferon alpha-2b in patients with human immunodeficiency virus infection. J Hepatol 1998;29:45–52.

[62] Mallet V, Nicand E, Sultanik P, et al. Brief communication: case reports of ribavirin treatment for chronic hepatitis E. Ann Intern Med 2010;153:85–9.

[63] Nunez M, Soriano V. Hepatotoxicity of antiretrovirals: incidence, mechanisms and management. Drug Saf 2005;28:53–66.

[64] Pol S, Lebray P, Vallet-Pichard A. HIV infection and hepatic enzyme abnormalities: intricacies of the pathogenic mechanisms. Clin Infect Dis 2004;38(Suppl. 2):S65–72.

[65] Sulkowski MS. Management of hepatic complications in HIV-infected persons. J Infect Dis 2008;197(Suppl. 3):S279–93.

[66] Stern JO, Robinson PA, Love J, et al. A comprehensive hepatic safety analysis of nevirapine in different populations of HIV infected patients. J Acquir Immune Defic Syndr 2003;34(Suppl. 1):S21–33.

[67] Sherman KE, Shire NJ, Cernohous P, et al. Liver injury and changes in hepatitis C virus (HCV) RNA load associated with protease inhibitor-based antiretroviral therapy for treatment-naive HCV-HIV-coinfected patients: lopinavir-ritonavir versus nelfinavir. Clin Infect Dis 2005;41:1186–95.

[68] Benn PD, Mercey DE, Brink N, et al. Prophylaxis with a nevirapine-containing triple regimen after exposure to HIV-1. Lancet 2001;357:687–8.

[69] Ragni MV, Belle SH, Im K, et al. Liver transplantation in HIV-seropositive individuals. Ann Intern Med 2006;144:223–4.

[70] Neff GW, Shire NJ, Rudich SM. Outcomes among patients with end-stage liver disease who are coinfected with HIV and hepatitis C virus. Clin Infect Dis 2005;41(Suppl. 1):S50–5.

[71] Tan-Tam CC, Frassetto LA, Stock PG. Liver and kidney transplantation in HIV-infected patients. AIDS Rev 2009;11:190–204.

[72] Coffin CS, Terrault NA. Management of hepatitis B in liver transplant recipients. J Viral Hepat 2007;14(Suppl. 1):37–44.

[73] de Vera ME, Dvorchik I, Tom K, et al. Survival of liver transplant patients coinfected with HIV and HCV is adversely impacted by recurrent hepatitis C. Am J Transplant 2006;6:2983–93.

Chapter | 33 |

Bartonella infections in HIV-infected individuals

Jane E. Koehler

HISTORICAL PERSPECTIVE

Bacillary angiomatosis (BA), a unique vascular proliferative lesion, was first described by Stoler and colleagues in 1983 [1] in an HIV-infected patient with multiple subcutaneous nodules. Numerous bacilli were observed by Warthin–Starry staining of the biopsied nodules, and the subcutaneous masses resolved during erythromycin therapy. Subsequently, the BA bacilli visualized using the Warthin–Starry silver stain were noted to have an appearance similar to that of the cat-scratch disease (CSD) bacillus [2, 3]. The BA bacillus remained refractory to isolation attempts for many years, impeding identification efforts. Studies of bacterial DNA extracted from BA lesions subsequently identified the bacillus as closely related to *Bartonella* (*Rochalimaea*) *quintana* [4], and after isolation of the bacillus from the blood of two HIV-infected patients without BA [5], the organism was further characterized and named *B. henselae* in 1992 [6, 7]. The BA bacillus was directly cultivated from cutaneous BA lesions for the first time in 1992, which led to the identification of two species of the genus *Bartonella* as causative agents of BA: *B. henselae* and *B. quintana* [8].

The *Bartonella* genus has expanded from a single species in 1993 to 29 officially recognized species (http://www.bacterio.cict.fr/b/bartonella.html) [9, 10], and at least six unofficial *Bartonella* species. Of these, eight *Bartonella* species have been isolated from humans: *B. henselae, B. quintana, B. elizabethae, B. bacilliformis, B. rochalimae, B. washoensis, B. tamiae,* and *B. vinsonii* subsp. *arupensis.* Although the *Bartonella* species causing BA has been identified in more than 60 AIDS patients, only two species have been found to cause BA or bacillary peliosis hepatis [8, 11]. Interestingly, the two different species differ in their predilection to form a specific type of lesion. *B. henselae,* but never *B. quintana,* has been associated with peliosis of the liver or spleen, or both

[11]. *B. henselae* also is associated with lymphadenopathy, and *B. quintana* with subcutaneous nodules in late-stage HIV infection [11].

CLINICAL PRESENTATION OF *BARTONELLA* INFECTIONS

In patients with severe immunosuppression due to HIV infection, organ transplantation or chemotherapy, infection with *B. henselae* or *B. quintana* can produce focal BA lesions composed of proliferating endothelial cells [12, 13]. BA occurs as a late manifestation of HIV infection; in a study of 42 patients with BA, the median CD4 count was 21 cells/mm^3 [14]. These vascular proliferative lesions can form in many different organs, including skin, bone, brain parenchyma, lymph nodes, bone marrow, and the gastrointestinal and respiratory tract. A histopathologically different vascular proliferative response to *Bartonella* infection, known as bacillary peliosis hepatis (BP), is seen in the liver and spleen [15]. One notable aspect of focal *Bartonella* infection, especially cutaneous BA, is the chronic, indolent nature of the disease: lesions can be present for as long as one year before a diagnosis is made [14, 16].

HIV-infected individuals also can develop manifestations of *Bartonella* infection other than vascular proliferation. Bacteremia with [17] or without [5, 18] endocarditis has been reported in HIV-infected individuals, in the absence of focal BA or BP involvement. Patients with higher CD4 counts can develop focal necrotizing infections due to *B. henselae* in lymph nodes, liver or spleen that have an appearance similar to that of CSD in immunocompetent individuals. Rarely, HIV-infected individuals with CD4 counts <50 cells/mm^3 can develop this necrotizing lymphadenitis without vascular proliferation [19].

A case-control study comparing clinical findings of 42 patients with BA and/or BP compared with 84 control patients found that cases were significantly more likely than controls to have fever, abdominal pain, lymphadenopathy, hepatomegaly, splenomegaly, a low CD4 count, anemia and/or an elevated serum alkaline phosphatase [14]. With the exception of cutaneous lesions, many of the clinical findings are not specific, and the major obstacle to diagnosis of *Bartonella* infection in the presence of concomitant HIV infection is recognition of the disease by the physician. BP and BA can be indistinguishable from a number of other infectious or malignant conditions, and the diagnosis can usually be made only after biopsy and careful histopathological evaluation of tissue, or by direct culture of *Bartonella* species from blood or the affected organ [20].

Cutaneous bacillary angiomatosis

The most frequently diagnosed BA lesions are those affecting the skin [20]. Cutaneous BA lesions can have myriad presentations, including vascular proliferative lesions with a smooth red or eroded surface (Fig. 33.1, groin BA lesion) or papules that enlarge to form friable, exophytic lesions (Fig. 33.1, finger BA lesion). These vascular lesions of cutaneous BA are particularly difficult to distinguish clinically from Kaposi's sarcoma (KS), and thus histopathological examination of biopsied tissue is essential. BA may appear as a cellulitic plaque, usually overlying an osteolytic lesion (Fig. 33.2). Less vascular-appearing lesions can be dry and scaly (Fig. 33.3) and some lesions are subcutaneous, with or without overlying erythema (Fig. 33.4). BA lesions

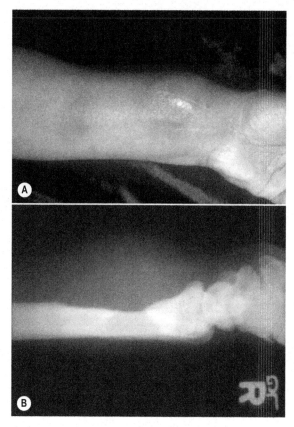

Figure 33.2 (A) A tense, firm, erythematous wrist mass due to BA. (B) A radiograph of the wrist of the same patient, demonstrating cortical bone erosion of the radius, with active periostitis, adjacent to the vascular soft-tissue mass.
(Reproduced with permission from Koehler JE, LeBoit PE, Egbert BM, Berger TG. Cutaneous vascular lesions and disseminated cat-scratch disease in patients with the acquired immunodeficiency syndrome (AIDS) and AIDS-related complex. Ann Intern Med 1988; 109:449–455.)

also can develop as very deep, highly vascular soft-tissue masses (Fig. 33.5) [16].

Osseous bacillary angiomatosis

Bartonella infection of the bone causes osteolytic lesions that are extremely painful. The long bones, including tibia, fibula, and radius, are most commonly involved [20, 21], although osseous BA has occurred in a rib [21] and vertebra [22, 23]. A radiograph usually demonstrates well-circumscribed osteolysis and deep soft-tissue swelling (Fig. 33.2B). The BA lytic lesions can be detected by technetium-99m methylene diphosphonate bone scans, and bone scintigraphy allows screening of the entire skeleton for multifocal osteomyelitis [24]. Osseous BA should be a primary consideration in the differential diagnosis of a lytic bone lesion in HIV-infected patients.

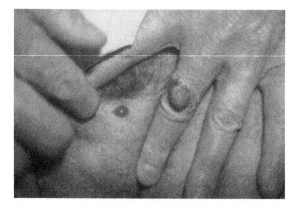

Figure 33.1 A friable, exophytic angiomatous BA nodule of the finger and an evolving dome-shaped vascular papule in the same patient.
(Reproduced with permission from Koehler JE, LeBoit PE, Egbert BM, Berger TG. Cutaneous vascular lesions and disseminated cat-scratch disease in patients with the acquired immunodeficiency syndrome (AIDS) and AIDS-related complex. Ann Intern Med 1988; 109:449–455.)

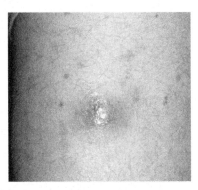

Figure 33.3 Unusual appearing erythematous, dry, scaling plaque of cutaneous BA mimicking staphylococcal pyoderma. *Bartonella quintana* was cultured from this lesion.
(Reproduced with permission from Koehler JE, Tappero JW. Bacillary angiomatosis and bacillary peliosis in patients infected with human immunodeficiency virus. Clin Infect Dis 1993; 17:612–624.)

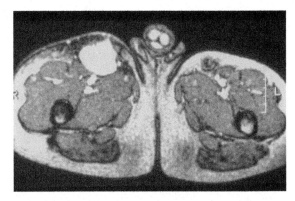

Figure 33.5 Magnetic resonance imaging showing a deep, highly vascular subcutaneous soft-tissue mass of BA in the anterior right thigh.
(Reproduced with permission from Koehler JE, Tappero JW. Bacillary angiomatosis and bacillary peliosis in patients infected with human immunodeficiency virus. Clin Infect Dis 1993; 17:612–624.)

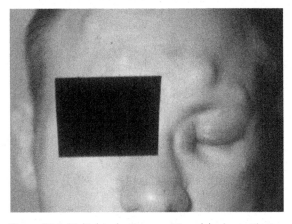

Figure 33.4 Multiple subcutaneous BA nodules in a patient with concomitant KS of the medial left eye canthus.
(Reproduced with permission from Koehler JE, Tappero JW. Bacillary angiomatosis and bacillary peliosis in patients infected with human immunodeficiency virus. Clin Infect Dis 1993; 17:612–624.)

Splenic and hepatic bacillary peliosis

Bacillary peliosis hepatis, a vascular lesion of the liver associated with infiltration of *Bartonella* bacilli, was first described in eight HIV-infected individuals by Perkocha and co-workers [15]. The symptoms of patients with BP hepatis usually include abdominal pain and fever. All eight patients had hepatomegaly, and six also had splenomegaly [15]. Two of the patients underwent splenectomy, and histopathological examination revealed BP of the spleen. One-quarter of the patients also had cutaneous BA lesions. The serum alkaline phosphatase was more prominently elevated than the hepatic transaminases in these patients with BP hepatis. In one HIV-infected patient, BP presented as

massive hemoperitoneum and hypotension, and bleeding from the liver was the only source of hemorrhage that could be identified during laparotomy [25]. Abdominal CT of the peliotic liver usually reveals numerous hypodense lesions [20, 26] as shown in Figure 33.6, but this appearance is not specific for BP; thus the diagnosis of *Bartonella* infection must be confirmed by histopathological evaluation. Additionally, some HIV-infected patients with hepatic *Bartonella* infection develop inflammatory nodules in the liver without the vascular proliferative characteristics of peliosis hepatis [27]. Patients with splenic BP can have thrombocytopenia or pancytopenia and abdominal ascites [28, 29].

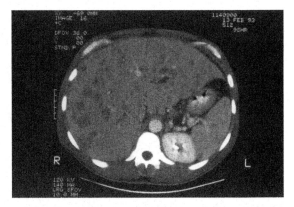

Figure 33.6 Computed tomography of the abdomen, showing hepatosplenomegaly with numerous low-density hepatic parenchymal lesions, in addition to pelvic ascites and pulmonary effusions. Percutaneous biopsy of the liver demonstrated peliosis hepatis by histopathology.
(Reproduced with permission from Koehler JE, Tappero JW. Bacillary angiomatosis and bacillary peliosis in patients infected with human immunodeficiency virus. Clin Infect Dis 1993; 17:612–624.)

Gastrointestinal and respiratory tract bacillary angiomatosis

Histopathologically proven BA of the gastrointestinal tract has been described by several groups [30–32]. The lesions can involve oral, anal, peritoneal, and gastrointestinal tissue appearing as raised, nodular, ulcerated intraluminal mucosal abnormalities of the stomach and large and small intestine during endoscopy [31]. Extraluminal, intra-abdominal BA presenting with massive upper gastrointestinal hemorrhage has also been described [32]. Hemorrhage in this patient occurred when the highly vascular mass eroded through the small intestine; B. quintana was cultured from tissue obtained by transabdominal needle biopsy of the mass.

Bacillary angiomatosis lesions of the respiratory tract have been observed in the larynx [30, 33]; in one of these patients, the BA lesions enlarged to cause an asphyxiative death [30]. Endobronchial BA lesions have been visualized during bronchoscopy, and described as polypoid lesions located in the segmental bronchi and the trachea [34, 35]. Several of these patients also had cutaneous BA. Bartonella infection can also cause pulmonary nodules in the immunocompromised patient: a renal transplant patient with chemotherapy-induced immunocompromise developed high fever (41°C) and bilateral pulmonary nodules [36]. Bartonella henselae DNA was demonstrated in parenchymal lung nodule biopsy specimens.

Lymph node bacillary angiomatosis

Lymph node involvement has been described frequently in association with cutaneous lesions or peliosis of the liver or spleen [20]. In these cases, the lymph nodes most commonly affected are those draining the BA lesion, and histopathological examination may reveal angiomatous changes within the lymph node. In other cases, however, BA involves only a single or several lymph nodes, in the absence of cutaneous or other organ involvement.

Central nervous system manifestations of *Bartonella* infection

Bartonella infection has been associated with aseptic meningitis [19] or parenchymal brain masses [37] in HIV-infected individuals. A left temporal lobe mass due to BA developed in an HIV-infected patient with new onset of seizures and facial nerve deficit [37]. The etiology of the mass remained undetermined for 8 months until the patient developed a cutaneous BA lesion. Treatment with erythromycin led to resolution of the cutaneous lesion and neurologic deficit; the parenchymal mass decreased in size during antibiotic treatment. Another patient developed fever, headache, diabetes insipidus, and altered mental status with multiple, small contrast-enhancing brain lesions, including a single suprasellar lesion [38]. Examination of biopsied brain tissue revealed an inflammatory infiltrate primarily involving the leptomeninges, and clumps of bacillary organisms by Warthin–Starry staining. B. henselae DNA was amplified from the biopsy material. The lesions and symptoms resolved after treatment with doxycycline and rifampin.

Retinal disease can occur in patients with AIDS and infection with B. henselae. The manifestations are often more severe than those seen in immunocompetent patients and can include neuroretinitis and retinochoroiditis [39]. Warren and co-workers [40] described an HIV-infected patient who developed severe and progressive retinal disease that did not respond to treatment for Toxoplasma or CMV. Retinal biopsy revealed vascular proliferation consistent with BA. Sequencing of amplified DNA extracted from the biopsy specimen identified B. henselae DNA. The patient was treated with minocycline or doxycycline, with resolution of the retinitis and improvement in his visual acuity.

Unusual bacillary angiomatosis presentations

Several cases of BA involving the bone marrow have been reported [4, 28, 41]. Hepatosplenomegaly and thrombocytopenia were noted in both of these patients, and both resolved with antibiotic treatment. Venous thrombosis of the left upper extremity occurred in an AIDS patient with B. quintana bacteremia during relapse [16]. This was characterized by multiple non-contiguous, erythematous, tender superficial thromboses in the absence of trauma or intravenous drug use. All rapidly resolved after institution of antibiotic therapy.

Cutaneous BA complicating pregnancy in an HIV-infected woman was reported by Riley and co-workers [42]. Cutaneous lesions resolved after antibiotic treatment, and the subsequent pregnancy and delivery were uneventful. BA lesions have been described in several pediatric patients: one patient was immunocompromised due to chemotherapy [43]; the other was 3.5 years old and had been infected with HIV perinatally [44].

Bacteremia with *Bartonella* species and fever of unknown origin

Many patients with BA and BP also have Bartonella bacteremia. One-half of our patients with culture-positive focal BA or BP also had the corresponding Bartonella species simultaneously isolated from the blood [11]. Bartonella bacteremia in the absence of focal BA disease has been reported by a number of groups [5, 6, 45], and may be more common than focal Bartonella disease. In a study of 382 patients with fever of undetermined etiology, 68 patients (18%) had evidence of Bartonella infection by serology and/or culture. A total of 12 patients had bacteremia with B. henselae or B. quintana (six each) [45]. When examined carefully by a healthcare provider experienced in the recognition of BA, six of the 12 bacteremic patients were found to have lesions suspicious for BA, and the other six had isolated bacteremia without focal *Bartonella* disease. The median CD4 count was 33 cells/mm^3 for the case patients in this study, indicating that both BA and *Bartonella*-related fever with bacteremia are usually identified in late-stage HIV infection. Also of note, endocarditis was described in one patient with HIV infection and culture-proven *B. quintana* [17].

DIAGNOSIS OF *BARTONELLA* INFECTIONS

Histopathological diagnosis

Obtaining tissue for diagnosis

Biopsy is the principal procedure available for the diagnosis of cutaneous BA. Because KS lesions can be clinically indistinguishable from those of BA, any new vascular lesion should be biopsied. In patients with previously diagnosed KS, any vascular lesion that has a different appearance or rate of growth should also be biopsied, because KS and cutaneous BA can occur simultaneously in the same patient [46]. Pedunculated lesions can be biopsied by shave excision, and smaller, papular, or subcutaneous lesions should be examined by punch biopsy. Biopsy of the cellulitic plaque that frequently overlies osteolytic lesions may be sufficient to yield a diagnosis of BA, but in some patients, open excisional bone biopsy is necessary [16]. Fine needle aspiration of BA lymph nodes has not been useful in diagnosis of BA in our center; thus, open excisional or incisional biopsy remains the optimal technique for diagnosis. For BP of the liver or spleen, the diagnostic procedure with greatest

yield appears to be excisional wedge biopsy of the liver or splenectomy; however, peliosis hepatis has been diagnosed by either transvenous liver biopsy [47] or percutaneous liver biopsy [29]. As with cutaneous lesions, several opportunistic infections and malignancies can have a similar appearance on computed tomography of the abdomen; thus, biopsy is extremely important to direct specific treatment. No case of hemorrhage following percutaneous biopsy of a peliotic liver has been reported, although this remains a theoretical concern.

Histopathological characteristics

A characteristic vascular proliferation is seen on routine hematoxylin and eosin staining of BA or BP tissue (Fig. 33.7A). Numerous bacilli also can be demonstrated in these lesions by modified silver staining (e.g. Warthin–Starry, Steiner, Dieterle) or electron microscopy (Fig. 33.7B) [13, 15]. Other stains, such as those for tissue Gram-staining, fungi or acid-fast mycobacteria do not stain *Bartonella* bacilli.

Cutaneous BA lesions can be misdiagnosed histopathologically, most often as KS [2, 3, 34, 48], angiosarcoma [22, 23, 30, 48], and pyogenic granuloma [33, 49]. The histopathological appearance of cutaneous BA lesions can be indistinguishable from pyogenic granuloma (lobular capillary hemangioma) and verruga peruana, the late, chronic phase of infection with *B. bacilliformis* [3]. A histopathological diagnosis of pyogenic granuloma, angiosarcoma or peliosis of the liver or spleen in an HIV-infected patient should prompt further evaluation of the tissue for bacilli to determine whether the lesion may actually be due to *Bartonella* infection. The presence of bacillary organisms is the diagnostic feature that distinguishes cutaneous BA, extracutaneous BA, and parenchymal BP from these other

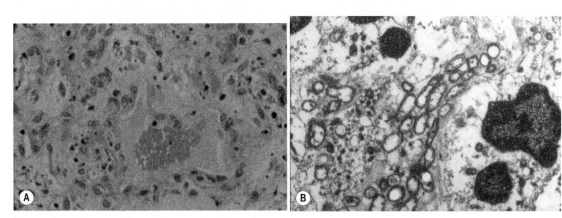

Figure 33.7 (A) Hematoxylin and eosin staining of a biopsied cutaneous BA lesion demonstrating a dermal vessel. The vessel is lined with protuberant endothelial cells surrounded by myxoid connective tissue containing neutrophils and amphophilic granular material in close proximity to the vascular lumen. (B) Transmission electron micrograph of cutaneous tissue showing multiple trilaminar cell-walled bacillary organisms.
(Reproduced with permission from Koehler JE, LeBoit PE, Egbert BM, Berger TG. Cutaneous vascular lesions and disseminated cat-scratch disease in patients with the acquired immunodeficiency syndrome (AIDS) and AIDS-related complex. Ann Intern Med 1988; 109:449–455.)

diagnoses (with the exception of the cutaneous lesions of verruga peruana, which are associated with *B. bacilliformis* bacilli).

Serological diagnosis

Bartonella antibodies can be detected in patients with CSD by an indirect fluorescence antibody (IFA) test developed at the Centers for Disease Control and Prevention [18]. This test also detects *Bartonella* antibodies in serum from patients with BA [50]. Antibodies to *Bartonella* were detected in seven HIV-infected patients with biopsy-confirmed cutaneous BA, and no antibodies were detected in seven HIV-infected patients without BA. For three of the patients with *Bartonella* antibodies, examination of banked serum revealed the presence of *Bartonella* antibodies as long as 7 years prior to the development of BA disease, suggesting infection with this bacterium occurred years before the diagnosis of BA. Prior to the diagnosis of BA in these three patients, a fourfold rise in titer occurred, raising the possibility of either relapse or reinfection. Culture-proven relapse in another BA patient [16] was also predicted by a rising serum antibody titer [50]. This IFA is useful for the diagnosis of BA and other *Bartonella*-associated infections in HIV-infected patients, as well as in following the response to antibiotic treatment.

Culture of *Bartonella* species from blood and tissue of patients with BA

Slater and co-workers [5] first reported isolation of *Bartonella* species from blood using lysis-centrifugation tubes (Isostat; Wampole, Cranbury, New Jersey) and plating onto chocolate agar or fresh heart infusion agar with 5% rabbit blood without antibiotics. Blood collection tubes containing EDTA also were used to isolate *B. henselae* from the blood of an HIV-infected patient [6]; this standard CBC collection tube is much less expensive and more readily available. *Bartonella* bacteremia can be detected using acridine orange staining of aliquots removed from Bactec blood culture bottles [51]. The use of semi-quantitative cultures demonstrates that immunocompromised patients can have a high-grade bacteremia with *Bartonella*, with blood cultures yielding >1,000 colony-forming units/mL of blood [16].

Isolation of *Bartonella* species directly from cutaneous BA lesions is difficult due to the fastidious growth characteristics of this genus. Both *B. quintana* or *B. henselae* can be isolated by mincing a sterilely obtained skin [16], lymph node [52], splenic [29], or hepatic biopsy specimen in inoculation media [16], and then spreading onto both fresh heart infusion agar with 5% rabbit blood and chocolate agar, and incubating for 3 weeks in a humid, 5% CO_2 environment [16]. The highest recovery rate of *Bartonella* species from cutaneous BA lesions has been accomplished using an endothelial cell monolayer co-cultivation system [16] or shell

vial culture assay [53], but these systems are not readily available to most microbiology labs. Because culture of *Bartonella* species from biopsied cutaneous or hepatic tissue remains difficult, blood culture represents the most accessible method of isolating *Bartonella* species; however, bacteremia is not always present in patients with cutaneous BA or BP.

TREATMENT OF *BARTONELLA* INFECTIONS

Choice of antibiotics

There have been no controlled trials for antibiotic treatment of BA. The first patient diagnosed with BA was treated empirically with erythromycin, with complete resolution of subcutaneous nodules [1]. From subsequent reports and our experience at San Francisco General Hospital, it is evident that doxycycline or erythromycin are the drugs of first choice for patients with BA and BP (Fig. 33.8). Oral doxycycline (100 mg twice daily) or oral erythromycin (500 mg four times daily) are standard, but intravenous therapy should be given to patients with severe disease or those unable to tolerate oral medication. Resolution of BA due to *B. henselae* was reported in one HIV-infected patient following oral tetracycline treatment [16] and two immunocompetent patients with *B. henselae* bacteremia [5]; an immunocompetent patient with cutaneous BA was successfully treated with minocycline [54]. In several retrospective descriptions of patients with cutaneous BA, resolution of lesions was noted to be temporally related to institution of antimycobacterial therapy [2, 3, 55–57], presumably due to the rifampin component.

A summary of recommended treatment for patients with *Bartonella* infection, in the presence or absence of immunocompromise, has been published [58]. In addition, treatment recommendations for HIV-infected adults [59] and children [60] with *Bartonella* infections are available. Although immunocompetent patients with *B. henselae* infection (CSD) usually do not need to be treated with antibiotics [58], all immunocompromised patients with *Bartonella* infection should be treated with an appropriate antibiotic for at least 3 months, regardless of the degree of immunosuppression. Note that some patients develop a Jarisch–Herxheimer reaction after the first several doses of antibiotic, with exacerbation of systemic symptoms and fever [16]. This response may be attenuated by pretreatment with an antipyretic, but severely ill AIDS patients should be monitored closely after the first 48 hours of treatment.

The clinical response of patients with BA to treatment with erythromycin, doxycycline, and tetracycline usually corresponds to the *in vitro* susceptibilities of *B. quintana* and *B. henselae* to these antibiotics [5, 61–63]. However,

Figure 33.8 Algorithm for treatment of *Bartonella* infections in HIV-infected individuals. MAC, *Mycobacterium avium* complex; TMP-SMX, trimethoprim-sulfamethoxazole.

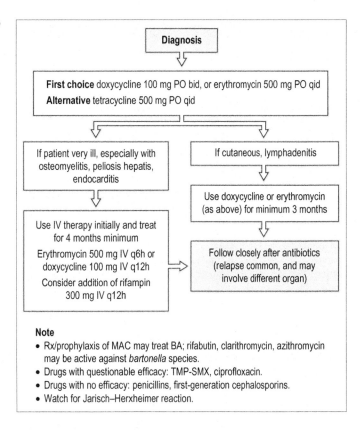

there is little correlation between the *in vivo* and *in vitro* antibiotic susceptibilities for other antibiotics, especially those that target steps in cell wall synthesis, e.g. penicillins. It is obvious from numerous reports that penicillin, penicillinase-resistant penicillins, aminopenicillins, and first-generation cephalosporins have no activity against the *B. quintana* and *B. henselae* bacilli in BA lesions [2, 3, 16, 33, 46, 49, 64]. An apparent initial response to some antibiotics, e.g. vancomycin [33] or a first-generation cephalosporin [49], likely represents the treatment of superinfecting skin flora. We pretreated one patient who had superinfected cutaneous BA lesions with cephradine to successfully isolate *Bartonella* organisms selectively from the lesions [16], and *B. quintana* was isolated from the BA lesions of another patient who had received nafcillin and gentamicin for several days prior to biopsy [11]. The discrepancies between *in vitro* and *in vivo* sensitivities may occur because the bacilli present in BA lesions have different cell wall characteristics from those grown on agar; these *in vivo* changes in composition could alter susceptibility to cell wall-active antibiotics. Additionally, the fastidious nature of *Bartonella* species makes accurate susceptibility testing difficult to perform.

Rifampin appears to have clinical efficacy in treating *Bartonella* infections (Table 33.1), but use of this drug alone

Table 33.1 Clinical efficacy of antibiotics in the treatment of BA and BP

DEFINITE	POSSIBLE	INCONCLUSIVE	NONE
Erythromycin	Rifampin	Ceftriaxone	Penicillin
Doxycycline	Gentamicin	Ceftizoxime	Ceph [1]
Tetracycline		Ciprofloxacin	PCN-D
Minocycline		TMP/SMX	

Ceph [1], first-generation cephalosporins; PCN-D, penicillin derivatives (PCNase-resistant penicillins and aminopenicillins); TMP-SMX, trimethoprim-sulfamethoxazole.

is not recommended due to the rapid development of resistance. For severely ill patients, we administer rifampin in addition to a first-line drug (erythromycin or doxycycline) during the initial several weeks of therapy. For some other antibiotics listed in Table 33.1 with possible clinical efficacy, single case reports have been associated with improvement in lesions or symptoms, but the response to these antibiotics is not consistent enough to warrant their recommendation at present. It also is difficult to directly attribute improvement of symptoms to treatment with a specific antibiotic when many patients have concomitant infection with other pathogens. The clinical efficacy of ciprofloxacin, trimethoprim-sulfamethoxazole and third-generation cephalosporins remains inconclusive. One pregnant patient received 2 weeks of ceftizoxime treatment for cutaneous BA and experienced complete resolution of lesions [42]. Of note, we observed progression of BA lesions in patients treated with ciprofloxacin in our study of patients with BA [65]. Although one patient reportedly improved with trimethoprim-sulfamethoxazole [34], most patients demonstrated no improvement or had progression of lesions [14, 17, 42, 44, 64], and we have isolated *B. henselae* from the tissue of two patients taking prophylactic oral trimethoprim-sulfamethoxazole[11]. In contrast, no *Bartonella* isolate was recovered from any BA patient treated with a tetracycline or erythromycin (even after a single dose) [66], and prior treatment with a macrolide has been found to be significantly protective against development of BA [11].

Treatment of cutaneous bacillary angiomatosis lesions

Immunocompromised patients with cutaneous BA should be evaluated for parenchymal and osseous disease before beginning treatment, because presence of either of these requires treatment for a longer duration. For cutaneous disease alone, antibiotic therapy can be given orally. Response of cutaneous lesions is usually rapid, with improvement in 1 week and complete resolution by 1 month, although hyperpigmentation may persist at the site of the lesion. As a result of our experience, we treat patients with cutaneous lesions for 3 months, and if relapse occurs we extend treatment for an additional 4 months and occasionally treat indefinitely.

Treatment of osseous bacillary angiomatosis lesions

Duration of antibiotic therapy for patients with *Bartonella* osteomyelitis is not well established. We treated one patient (Fig. 33.2) with oral erythromycin 500 mg six times a day for 2 months, followed by 500 mg four times a day for an additional 2 months [2]. This patient experienced complete resolution of the osteolytic lesion without relapse during the subsequent 24 months, when he died of another opportunistic infection. Relapse occurred in another patient with osseous BA [16] despite 4 months of oral treatment with 500–1,000 mg erythromycin four times a day; the osseous BA healed but relapse with *B. quintana* bacteremia occurred 1 month after stopping erythromycin. For patients with osseous BA, it may be most appropriate to treat initially with several weeks of intravenous antibiotics (erythromycin or doxycycline) followed by prolonged, and

perhaps indefinite, oral antimicrobial therapy. Serial technetium-99m methylene diphosphonate bone scans or radiographs can be used to monitor treatment efficacy, although resolution of osseous lesions is delayed, as seen with other causes of osteomyelitis.

Treatment of hepatic and splenic bacillary peliosis

Most patients with BP have severe systemic symptoms, including nausea and vomiting that may substantially decrease absorption of oral antibiotics. Additionally, oral erythromycin or doxycycline may not be tolerated by these patients; thus, initial treatment should be with intravenous antibiotics for several weeks, followed by oral therapy for at least 4 months, possibly indefinitely. For severely ill patients, rifampin can be added to the initial treatment regimen. Treatment progress can be monitored by following hepatic transaminases and by serial computed tomography, if peliotic lesions are visualized at the time of diagnosis (Fig. 33.6).

Treatment of *Bartonella* bacteremia

If possible, *Bartonella* blood cultures should be performed for patients with all forms of BA, prior to antibiotic treatment. For bacteremia, an initial period of intravenous antibiotic therapy with doxycycline 100 mg IV q12h (with or without oral rifampin 300 mg twice daily) is probably appropriate for bacteremia, followed by at least 3 months of oral antibiotic therapy with oral doxycycline 100 mg twice daily. Fever and constitutional symptoms typically resolve within 1 week of institution of antibiotic treatment, although one patient did not have permanent remission of fever until he had received 8 weeks of treatment [5].

Because endocarditis can develop during infection with *B. quintana* [17, 67], *B. henselae* [68], and rarely other *Bartonella* species, all patients with *Bartonella* bacteremia and a cardiac murmur or relapsing bacteremia should be evaluated with echocardiography. Patients with *Bartonella* endocarditis should receive 6 weeks of intravenous antibiotic therapy, probably with two drugs (doxycycline plus rifampin or erythromycin plus rifampin), because neither first-line drug is bactericidal. Although gentamicin has been shown to be a useful adjunctive antibiotic when added to doxycycline in the first 2 weeks of therapy [58], we have found that the majority of patients do not tolerate gentamicin due to the renal insufficiency that frequently accompanies *Bartonella* endocarditis.

Relapse

Both *B. quintana* [69] and *B. henselae* [70] produce relapsing illness in immunocompetent hosts; therefore, it is thus not surprising that immunocompromised patients with BA or BP frequently experience relapse despite prolonged antibiotic therapy [5, 6, 16, 33, 46, 49, 64, 71]. It should be noted that reinfection remains a possibility in these patients, but the majority of these cases probably represent relapse. The frequency of relapse appears to be increased when patients are treated with antibiotics for a shorter duration. Over the years, we have increased the duration of treatment for all presentations of BA as the result of our increased experience, and we currently recommend that all patients with BA be treated for a minimum of 3 months, and those with peliosis hepatis be treated for a minimum of 4 months [58]. If relapse of *Bartonella* infection occurs after a first or second full course of an appropriate antibiotic, prophylactic treatment with a macrolide or doxycycline should be administered as long as the CD4 count remains < 200 cells/mm^3.

EPIDEMIOLOGY AND PREVENTION OF *BARTONELLA* INFECTIONS

Arthropods serve as vectors of *Bartonella* species. *Bartonella quintana* is known to be transmitted from the human reservoir to other humans via the body louse [69], and the cat flea is the vector that transmits *B. henselae* from cat to cat. However, at present the vector most strongly implicated in transmission of *B. henselae* to humans is the domestic cat. Ticks are also possible vectors of *Bartonella* species: two patients reported tick bites preceding the diagnosis of *B. henselae* bacteremia [7, 70]. However, there are no definitive data supporting direct transmission of *Bartonella* species from ticks to humans.

Serological studies initially revealed that *B. henselae* is the principal bacterial agent causing CSD in immunocompetent individuals [18]. Subsequent, corroborating data included the direct culture of *B. henselae* from lymph nodes that had histopathological characteristics suggestive of CSD [52] and the demonstration of *Bartonella* DNA (but not *A. felis* DNA) in the CSD skin test antigen [72]. Similarly, an association between cat exposure and the development of BA was noted in many case reports [20]. The first systematic evaluation of the relationship between cat contact, numerous other environmental exposures, and development of BA was conducted by Tappero and co-workers [65]. This case-control study found a significant epidemiological association between development of BA and traumatic cat exposure (cat bite or cat scratch). Both CSD and BA due to *B. henselae* are statistically associated with cat exposure [11, 65, 73]. The association between *B. henselae*-infected cats and development of BA in the cat owners was demonstrated in 1994, when bacteremia was detected in all seven cat contacts of four patients with BA due to *B. henselae* [74]. It was further found that about 40% of the domestic cat population sampled in the greater San Francisco Bay Area was bacteremic with *B. henselae*

[74, 75], providing compelling evidence that the domestic cat is the major reservoir for *B. henselae*.

The cat flea has been established as a vector of *B. henselae* among cats [76]. Initially, an epidemiological association between owning a kitten with fleas and development of CSD was described [73]. Also, a seroprevalence survey of *B. henselae* antibodies in pet cats throughout regions of North America revealed that the regions with the highest average prevalence of antibodies coincided with the geographic areas predicted to have the highest prevalence of the cat flea (e.g. Hawaii, coastal California, the Pacific Northwest, and south central plains) [77]. Viable *B. henselae* bacilli were isolated from several fleas combed from a bacteremic cat [74], and *B. henselae* transmission from cat to cat via the cat flea was demonstrated in 1996 [76]. Finally, Foil and co-workers [78] demonstrated that the feces of fleas fed on bacteremic cats are infectious and capable of transmitting *B. henselae* to uninfected cats.

According to the Humane Society, there are 93.6 million owned cats in the USA. Despite this large number, and the high percentage of cats with *B. henselae* infection, transmission of *B. henselae* to humans is relatively rare; thus, the benefit of these companion animals far outweighs the risk of *B. henselae* infection [79]. We suggest that several practical measures be followed to reduce the risk of *B. henselae* infection in HIV-infected individuals: (1) wash hands after petting and handling pets; (2) wash bites and scratches immediately with soap and water; (3) never allow any pet to lick an open wound; and (4) minimize flea infestation of pets (keep pets indoors and use flea protection products).

Although the domestic cat has been identified as the major reservoir and vector for *B. henselae*, it is evident that *B. quintana*, which causes nearly half of the BA infections in San Francisco, is not associated with cat contact. In a study of 49 patients and 96 matched controls, patients with BA caused by *B. quintana* infection were significantly more likely than controls to be homeless, have low socioeconomic status, and have had recent infestation with head or body lice [11]. Physicians should consider *B. quintana* infection as a cause of fever in homeless patients, whether cutaneous lesions are present or absent. Strategies to prevent infection with *B. quintana* are currently limited to reducing homelessness and exposure to body lice.

ACKNOWLEDGMENTS

Dr Koehler received funding support from a California HIV/AIDS Research Program Award, a Burroughs Wellcome Fund Clinical Scientist Award in Translational Research, and from NIH R01AI52813 and NIH U54AI065359 from the National Institute of Allergy and Infectious Diseases.

REFERENCES

[1] Stoler MH, Bonfiglio TA, Steigbigel RT, Pereira M. An atypical subcutaneous infection associated with acquired immune deficiency syndrome. Am J Clin Pathol 1983;80:714–18.

[2] Koehler JE, LeBoit PE, Egbert BM, Berger TG. Cutaneous vascular lesions and disseminated cat-scratch disease in patients with the acquired immunodeficiency syndrome (AIDS) and AIDS-related complex. Ann Intern Med 1988;109:449–55.

[3] LeBoit PE, Berger TG, Egbert BM, et al. Epithelioid haemangioma-like vascular proliferation in AIDS: manifestation of cat-scratch disease bacillus infection? Lancet 1988; i:960–3.

[4] Relman DA, Loutit JS, Schmidt TM, et al. The agent of bacillary angiomatosis: an approach to the identification of uncultured pathogens. N Engl J Med 1990;323:1573–80.

[5] Slater LN, Welch DF, Hensel D, Coody DW. A newly recognized fastidious gram-negative pathogen as a cause of fever and bacteremia. N Engl J Med 1990;323:1587–93.

[6] Regnery RL, Anderson BE, Clarridge JE, et al. Characterization of a novel Rochalimaea species, R. henselae sp. nov., isolated from blood of a febrile, human immunodeficiency virus-positive patient. J Clin Microbiol 1992;30:265–74.

[7] Welch DF, Pickett DA, Slater LN, et al. Rochalimaea henselae sp. nov., a cause of septicemia, bacillary angiomatosis, and parenchymal bacillary peliosis. J Clin Microbiol 1992;30:275–80.

[8] Koehler JE. Bartonella species. In: Nataro JP, Blaser MJ, Cunningham-Rundles S, editors. Persistent bacterial infections. Washington, DC: American Society for Microbiology Press; 2000. p. 339–53.

[9] Gundi V, Taylor C, Raoult D, La Scola B. Bartonella rattaustraliani sp. nov., Bartonella queenslandensis sp. nov. and Bartonella coopersplainsensis sp. nov., identified in Australian

rats. Int J Syst Evol Microbiol 2009;59:2956–61.

[10] Inoue K, Kabeya H, Hiratori H, et al. Bartonella japonica sp. nov. and Bartonella silvatica sp. nov., isolated from Apodemus mice. Int J Syst Evol Microbiol 2010;60:759–63.

[11] Koehler JE, Sanchez MA, Garrido CS, et al. Molecular epidemiology of bartonella infections in patients with bacillary angiomatosis-peliosis. N Engl J Med 1997;337:1876–83.

[12] Cockerell CJ, LeBoit PE. Bacillary angiomatosis: A newly characterized, pseudoneoplastic, infectious, cutaneous vascular disorder. J Am Acad Dermatol 1990;22:501–12.

[13] LeBoit PE, Berger TG, Egbert BM, et al. Bacillary angiomatosis: the histopathology and differential diagnosis of a pseudoneoplastic infection in patients with human immunodeficiency virus disease. Am J Surg Pathol 1989;13:909–20.

[14] Mohle-Boetani JC, Koehler JE, Berger TG, et al. Bacillary angiomatosis and bacillary peliosis in patients infected with human immunodeficiency virus: clinical characteristics in a case-control study. Clin Infect Dis 1996;22:794–800.

[15] Perkocha LA, Geaghan SM, Yen TSB, et al. Clinical and pathological features of bacillary peliosis hepatis in association with human immunodeficiency virus infection. N Engl J Med 1990;323:1581–6.

[16] Koehler JE, Quinn FD, Berger TG, et al. Isolation of Rochalimaea species from cutaneous and osseous lesions of bacillary angiomatosis. N Engl J Med 1992;327:1625–31.

[17] Spach DH, Callis KP, Paauw DS, et al. Endocarditis caused by Rochalimaea quintana in a patient infected with human immunodeficiency virus. J Clin Microbiol 1993;31:692–4.

[18] Regnery RL, Olson JG, Perkins BA, Bibb W. Serological response to "Rochalimaea henselae" antigen in suspected cat-scratch disease. Lancet 1992;339:1443–5.

[19] Wong MT, Dolan MJ, Lattuada Jr. CP, et al. Neuroretinitis, aseptic meningitis, and lymphadenitis associated with Bartonella (Rochalimaea) henselae infection in immunocompetent patients and patients infected with human immunodeficiency virus type 1. Clin Infect Dis 1995;21:352–60.

[20] Koehler JE, Tappero JW. Bacillary angiomatosis and bacillary peliosis in patients infected with human immunodeficiency virus. Clin Infect Dis 1993;17:612–24.

[21] Baron AL, Steinbach LS, LeBoit PE, et al. Osteolytic lesions and bacillary angiomatosis in HIV infection: radiologic differentiation from AIDS-related Kaposi sarcoma. Radiology 1990;177:77–81.

[22] Herts BR, Rafii M, Spiegel G. Soft-tissue and osseous lesions caused by bacillary angiomatosis: unusual manifestations of cat-scratch fever in patients with AIDS. Am J Radiol 1991;157:1249–51.

[23] Schinella RA, Greco MA. Bacillary angiomatosis presenting as a soft-tissue tumor without skin involvement. Hum Pathol 1990;21:567–9.

[24] Tehranzadeh J, Ter-Oganesyan RR, Steinbach LS. Musculoskeletal disorders associated with HIV infection and AIDS. Part I: infectious musculoskeletal conditions. Skeletal Radiol 2004;33:249–59.

[25] Lozano F, Corzo JE, Leon EM, et al. Massive hemoperitoneum: a new manifestation of bacillary peliosis in human immunodeficiency virus infection. Clin Infect Dis 1999;28:911–12.

[26] Wyatt SH, Fishman EK. Hepatic bacillary angiomatosis in a patient with AIDS. Abdom Imaging 1993;18:336–8.

[27] Slater LN, Pitha JV, Herrera L, et al. Rochalimaea henselae infection in acquired immunodeficiency syndrome causing inflammatory disease without angiomatosis or peliosis. Demonstration by immunocytochemistry and

corroboration by DNA amplification. Arch Pathol Lab Med 1994;118:33–8.

[28] Milam M, Balerdi MJ, Toney JF. Epithelioid angiomatosis secondary to disseminated cat scratch disease involving the bone marrow and skin in a patient with acquired immune deficiency syndrome: a case report. Am J Med 1990;88:180–3.

[29] Slater LN, Welch DF, Min KW. *Rochalimaea henselae* causes bacillary angiomatosis and peliosis hepatis. Arch Intern Med 1992;152:602–6.

[30] Cockerell CJ, Whitlow MA, Webster GF, Friedman-Kien AE. Epithelioid angiomatosis: a distinct vascular disorder in patients with the acquired immunodeficiency syndrome or AIDS-related complex. Lancet 1987;2:654–6.

[31] Tuur SM, Macher AM, Angritt P, et al. AIDS case for diagnosis series, 1988. Milit Med 1988;153:M57–64.

[32] Koehler JE, Cederberg L. Intra-abdominal mass associated with gastrointestinal hemorrhage: a new manifestation of bacillary angiomatosis. Gastroenterology 1995;109:2011–4.

[33] van der Wouw PA, Hadderingh RJ, Reiss P, et al. Disseminated cat-scratch disease in a patient with AIDS. AIDS 1989;3:751–3.

[34] Slater LN, Min KW. Polypoid endobronchial lesions. A manifestation of bacillary angiomatosis. Chest 1992;102:972–4.

[35] Foltzer MA, Guiney Jr. WB, Wager GC, Alpern HD. Bronchopulmonary bacillary angiomatosis. Chest 1993;104:973–5.

[36] Caniza MA, Granger DL, Wilson KH, et al. *Bartonella henselae*: etiology of pulmonary nodules in a patient with depressed cell-mediated immunity. Clin Infect Dis 1995;20:1505–11.

[37] Spach DH, Panther LA, Thorning DR, et al. Intracerebral bacillary angiomatosis in a patient infected with human immunodeficiency virus. Ann Intern Med 1992;116:740–2.

[38] George TI, Manley G, Koehler JE, et al. Detection of *Bartonella henselae* by polymerase chain reaction in brain tissue of an immunocompromised patient with multiple enhancing lesions. Case report and review of the literature. J Neurosurg 1998;89:640–4.

[39] Cunningham, ET Jr. Koehler JE. Ocular bartonellosis. Am J Ophthalmol 2000;130:340–9.

[40] Warren K, Goldstein E, Hung VS, et al. Use of retinal biopsy to diagnose *Bartonella* (formerly *Rochalimaea*) *henselae* retinitis in an HIV-infected patient. Arch Ophthalmol 1998;116:937–40.

[41] Kemper CA, Lombard CM, Deresinski SC, Tompkins LS. Visceral bacillary epithelioid angiomatosis: possible manifestations of disseminated cat scratch disease in the immunocompromised host: a report of two cases. Am J Med 1990;89:216–22.

[42] Riley LE, Tuomala RE. Bacillary angiomatosis in a pregnant patient with acquired immunodeficiency syndrome. Obstet Gynecol 1992;79:818–19.

[43] Myers SA, Prose NS, Garcia JA, et al. Bacillary angiomatosis in a child undergoing chemotherapy. J Pediatr 1992;121:574–8.

[44] Malane MS, Laude TA, Chen CK, Fikrig S. An HIV-1-positive child with fever and a scalp nodule. Lancet 1995;346:1466.

[45] Koehler J, Sanchez M, Tye S, et al. Prevalence of *Bartonella* infection among human immunodeficiency virus-infected patients with fever. Clin Infect Dis 2003;37:559–66.

[46] Berger TG, Tappero JW, Kaymen A, LeBoit PE. Bacillary (epithelioid) angiomatosis and concurrent Kaposi's sarcoma in acquired immunodeficiency syndrome. Arch Dermatol 1989;125:1543–7.

[47] Marullo S, Jaccard A, Roulot D, et al. Identification of the *Rochalimaea henselae* 16S rRNA sequence in the liver of a French patient with bacillary peliosis hepatis [letter]. J Infect Dis 1992;166:1462.

[48] Angritt P, Tuur SM, Macher AM, et al. Epithelioid angiomatosis in HIV infection: neoplasm or cat-scratch disease? Lancet 1988;1:996.

[49] Marasco WA, Lester S, Parsonnet J. Unusual presentation of cat scratch disease in a patient positive for antibody to the human immunodeficiency virus. Rev Infect Dis 1989;11:793–803.

[50] Tappero J, Regnery R, Koehler J. Detection of serologic response to *Rochalimaea henselae* in patients with bacillary angiomatosis (BA) by immunofluorescent antibody (IFA) testing. In: 32nd Interscience Conference on Antimicrobial Agents and Chemotherapy; 1992. American Society for Microbiology; 1992. p. 674.

[51] Larson AM, Dougherty MJ, Nowowiejski DJ, et al. Detection of *Bartonella* (*Rochalimaea*) *quintana* by routine acridine orange staining of broth blood cultures. J Clin Microbiol 1994;32:1492–6.

[52] Dolan MJ, Wong MT, Regnery RL, et al. Syndrome of *Rochalimaea henselae* adenitis suggesting cat scratch disease. Ann Intern Med 1993;118:331–6.

[53] La Scola B, Raoult D. Culture of *Bartonella quintana* and *Bartonella henselae* from human samples: a 5-year experience (1993 to 1998). J Clin Microbiol 1999;37:1899–905.

[54] Tappero JW, Koehler JE, Berger TG, et al. Bacillary angiomatosis and bacillary splenitis in immunocompetent adults. Ann Intern Med 1993;118:363–5.

[55] Knobler EH, Silvers DN, Fine KC, et al. Unique vascular skin lesions associated with human immunodeficiency virus. J Am Med Assoc 1988;260:524–7.

[56] Hall AV, Roberts CM, Maurice PD, et al. Cat-scrach disease in patient with AIDS: atypical skin manifestation. Lancet 1988;2:453–4.

[57] Lopez-Elzaurdia C, Fraga J, Sols M, et al. Bacillary angiomatosis associated with cytomegalovirus infection in a patient with AIDS. Br J Dermatol 1991;125:175–7.

[58] Rolain JM, Brouqui P, Koehler JE, et al. Recommendations for treatment of human infections caused by *Bartonella* species. Antimicrob Agents Chemother 2004;48:1921–33.

[59] Kaplan JE, Benson C, Holmes KH, et al. Guidelines for prevention and treatment of opportunistic infections in HIV-infected adults

and adolescents: recommendations from CDC, the National Institutes of Health, and the HIV Medicine Association of the Infectious Diseases Society of America. MMWR Recomm Rep 2009;58(RR-4):1–207.

[60] Mofenson LM, Brady MT, Danner SP, et al. Guidelines for the Prevention and Treatment of Opportunistic Infections among HIV-exposed and HIV-infected children: recommendations from CDC, the National Institutes of Health, the HIV Medicine Association of the Infectious Diseases Society of America, the Pediatric Infectious Diseases Society, and the American Academy of Pediatrics. MMWR Recomm Rep 2009;58(RR-11):1–166.

[61] Daly JS, Worthington MG, Brenner DJ, et al. *Rochalimaea elizabethae* sp. nov. isolated from a patient with endocarditis. J Clin Microbiol 1993;31(4):872–81.

[62] Myers WF, Grossman DM, Wisseman CLJ. Antibiotic susceptibility patterns in *Rochalimaea quintana*, the agent of trench fever. Antimicrob Agents Chemother 1984;25:690–3.

[63] Maurin M, Gasquet S, Ducco C, Raoult D. MICs of 28 antibiotic compounds for 14 *Bartonella* (formerly *Rochalimaea*) isolates. Antimicrob Agents Chemother 1995;39:2387–91.

[64] Szaniawski WK, Don PC, Bitterman SR, Schachner JR. Epithelioid angiomatosis in patients with AIDS. J Am Acad Dermatol 1990;23:41–8.

[65] Tappero JW, Mohle-Boetani J, Koehler JE, et al. The epidemiology of bacillary-angiomatosis and bacillary peliosis. JAMA 1993;269:770–5.

[66] Whitfeld MJ, Kaveh S, Koehler JE, et al. Bacillary angiomatosis associated with myositis in a patient infected with human immunodeficiency virus. Clin Infect Dis 1997;24:562–4.

[67] Drancourt M, Mainardi JL, Brouqui P, et al. *Bartonella (Rochalimaea) quintana* endocarditis in three homeless men. N Engl J Med 1995;332:419–23.

[68] Holmes AH, Greenough TC, Balady GJ, et al. *Bartonella henselae* endocarditis in an immunocompetent adult. Clin Infect Dis 1995;21:1004–7.

[69] Strong RPl. Trench Fever: Report of Commission, Medical Research Committee, American Red Cross. Oxford: Oxford University Press; 1918.

[70] Lucey D, Dolan MJ, Moss CW, et al. Relapsing illness due to *Rochalimaea henselae* in immunocompetent hosts: implication for therapy and new epidemiological associations. Clin Infect Dis 1992;14:683–8.

[71] Krekorian TD, Radner AB, Alcorn JM, et al. Biliary obstruction caused by epithelioid angiomatosis in a patient with AIDS. Am J Med 1990;89:820–2.

[72] Perkins BA, Swaminathan B, Jackson LA, et al. Case 22–1992—pathogenesis of cat scratch disease [letter]. N Engl J Med 1992;327:1599–601.

[73] Zangwill KM, Hamilton DH, Perkins BA, et al. Cat scratch disease in Connecticut. Epidemiology, risk factors, and evaluation of a new diagnostic test. N Engl J Med 1993;329:8–13.

[74] Koehler JE, Glaser CA, Tappero JW. *Rochalimaea henselae* infection. A new zoonosis with the domestic cat as reservoir. JAMA 1994;271:531–5.

[75] Chomel BB, Abbott RC, Kasten RW, et al. *Bartonella henselae* prevalence in domestic cats in California: risk factors and association between bacteremia and antibody titers. J Clin Microbiol 1995;33:2445–50.

[76] Chomel BB, Kasten RW, Floyd-Hawkins K, et al. Experimental transmission of *Bartonella henselae* by the cat flea. J Clin Microbiol 1996;34:1952–6.

[77] Jameson P, Greene C, Regnery R, et al. Prevalence of *Bartonella henselae* antibodies in pet cats throughout regions of North America. J Infect Dis 1995;172:1145–9.

[78] Foil L, Andress E, Freeland RL, et al. Experimental infection of domestic cats with *Bartonella henselae* by inoculation of *Ctenocephalides felis* (Siphonaptera: Pulicidae) feces. J Med Entomol 1998;35:625–8.

[79] Regnery RL, Childs JE, Koehler JE. Infections associated with *Bartonella* species in persons infected with human immunodeficiency virus. Clin Infect Dis 1995;21(Suppl. 1): S94–8.

Chapter 34

Management of herpesvirus infections (cytomegalovirus, herpes simplex virus, and varicella-zoster virus)

W. Lawrence Drew, Kim S. Erlich

CYTOMEGALOVIRUS

General comments

With the advent of highly active antiretroviral therapy (HAART), there has been a marked decline in cytomegalovirus (CMV) disease except in the developing world, where up to 25% of AIDS patients may develop end-organ CMV disease. Even where antiretroviral therapy (ART) is available, the syndromes discussed below still occur in the early months of therapy, because the CD4 lymphocytes require weeks to months to become fully functional [1]. CMV disease is also seen in patients who have eluded medical care and in those who fail or are intolerant of ART [2].

Serologic evidence of infection with CMV is extremely common in HIV-infected patients, and the virus can cause several clinical illnesses, including chorioretinitis, esophagitis, colitis, pneumonia, and several neurologic disorders in patients with severe immunosuppression. Even patients with blood, urine, or tissue cultures positive for CMV may not develop clinical illness related to the infection. However, in patients with advanced AIDS (CD4 counts of <50 cells/mm^3), the risk of developing CMV disease and death is directly related to the quantity of CMV nucleic acid in plasma. In a study of over 600 advanced AIDS patients, each $\log_{10}$ increase in baseline CMV DNA was associated with an approximate three-fold increase in CMV disease and a twofold increase in mortality at 1 year [3].

Diagnosis of CMV disease may require tissue biopsy with histologic evidence of viral inclusions, antigen or nucleic acid in tissue. This section reviews the most common clinical manifestations of CMV and their management (Table 34.1).

Chorioretinitis

Ocular disease caused by CMV occurs only in patients with severe immunodeficiency and was especially common in patients with AIDS prior to the advent of HAART. Clinical evidence of CMV retinitis (Fig. 34.1) occurred in as many as 40% of AIDS patients, and autopsy series revealed that CMV retinitis was present in up to 30% of patients. With the routine use of prophylaxis against *Pneumocystis* pneumonia, retinitis became a common presenting manifestation of AIDS, but it occurred more often months to years after the diagnosis of AIDS had been established. The incidence of CMV disease is currently low, primarily because of the efficacy of ART in preventing severe immunosuppression.

Decreased visual acuity, the presence of floaters, or unilateral visual field loss are the most common presenting complaints. Ophthalmologic examination typically reveals large creamy to yellowish white granular areas with perivascular exudates and hemorrhages (Fig. 34.1). These lesions initially occur more often at the periphery of the fundus and, if left untreated, progress centrally within 2–3 weeks. Retinitis usually begins unilaterally, but progression to bilateral involvement is common because of associated viremia. Systemic CMV infection involving other viscera may be present.

CMV accounts for at least 90% of HIV-related infectious retinopathies. Differentiating suspected CMV retinitis lesions from cotton-wool spots is essential. Cotton-wool spots appear as small, fluffy, white lesions with indistinct margins and are not associated with exudates or hemorrhages. They are common in AIDS patients, are usually asymptomatic, and represent areas of focal ischemia. These lesions do not progress and often undergo spontaneous regression. Toxoplasmosis is the second most common opportunistic infection of the eye but is characterized by little if any hemorrhage.

Table 34.1 Treatment of cytomegalovirus (CMV) infection in AIDS patients

	PREFERRED THERAPY	ALTERNATIVE THERAPY
CMV retinitis[a,b,c]		
Sight-threatening lesions (induction therapy)	Ganciclovir implant + valganciclovir or valganciclovir	GCV IV, foscarnet IV, cidofovir IV
Peripheral lesions (induction therapy)	Valganciclovir	Same as above
Maintenance therapy	Valganciclovir	Same as above
Relapsing and/or GCV resistant	Re-induction with ganciclovir/valganciclovir +/− ganciclovir implant; foscarnet IV +/− ganciclovir/valganciclovir	Cidofovir (if only UL97 mutation); fomivirsen
CMV gastrointestinal disease	Ganciclovir IV Foscarnet IV or valganciclovir (if absorbing)	
CMV neurological disease	Ganciclovir IV + foscarnet IV	

[a]If not already begun, ART should be initiated concurrent with anti-CMV therapy, except possibly when treating CNS disease.
[b]For retinitis, anti-CMV therapy should be continued until CD4 count has exceeded 100–150 cells/mm^3 for 3-6 months and retinitis is inactive. If anti-CMV therapy is discontinued, regular eye exams should be performed every three months.
[c]Early relapses of CMV retinitis in patients treated systemically are usually due to inadequate drug penetration; re-induction with the same drug is often effective. Drug resistance may occur in patients treated for >3 months. Therapy of these patients may be guided by antiviral susceptibility testing.

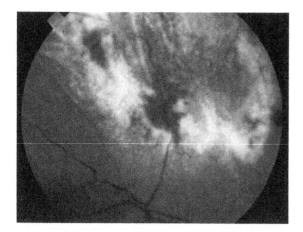

Figure 34.1 Funduscopic appearance of CMV retinitis, illustrating 'cottage cheese and catsup' appearance resulting from perivascular exudates and hemorrhages.
(Courtesy of Dr L Schwartz, San Francisco, California.)

with pupillary dilation, and ideally, indirect ophthalmoscopy, may be valuable when cell counts decline to this level. It is also important to ask about visual abnormalities, especially increased floaters or visual field defects, and to examine the fundus carefully when there are visual complaints. Patients with confirmed CMV chorioretinitis should be treated with ganciclovir, valganciclovir, foscarnet, or cidofovir [4–6]. These agents are equally effective in the treatment of CMV retinitis [7]. The toxic effects of these agents vary widely but the usual drug of choice is ganciclovir/valganciclovir. In resource-poor settings, intravitreal treatment may be employed.

Nervous system

CMV commonly involves the central nervous system (CNS) in AIDS patients. The spectrum of neurologic syndromes in AIDS patients ranges from polyradiculopathy, encephalitis with dementia, and ventriculoencephalitis to mononeuritis multiplex and painful neuropathy.

Polyradiculopathy and myelitis

The clinical syndrome of CMV polyradiculopathy and myelitis usually has an insidious onset with low back pain radiating to the perianal area and progressive lower extremity weakness, hypo- or areflexia, and variable sensory deficit,

It is associated with cerebral toxoplasmosis in the majority of patients. Syphilis, herpes simplex virus (HSV), varicella-zoster virus (VZV), and tuberculosis are other infections that may rarely involve the retina.

Virtually all patients with CMV retinitis have CD4 counts of <50 cells/mm^3. Ophthalmologic screening of patients usually with preserved proprioception and vibratory sensation. Most patients develop urinary retention and fecal incontinence due to bladder and/or anal sphincter dysfunction. The disease clinically resembles Guillain–Barré syndrome but may be differentiated by lack of sphincter involvement in the latter.

Diagnosis of CMV polyradiculopathy is based on the characteristic neurologic features described above. The cerebrospinal fluid (CSF) abnormalities are unusual for a viral infection: pleocytosis with predominant polymorphonuclear leukocytosis and hypoglycorrhachia. Culture of CSF is usually positive, but antigen or DNA assays are more sensitive methods of diagnosis. Magnetic resonance imaging (MRI) may reveal enhancement of leptomeninges and clumping of lumbosacral roots. Characteristic pathologic changes seen in CMV polyradiculopathy are demyelination and destruction of axons.

Acute CMV polyradiculopathy should be differentiated from idiopathic lumbosacral polyradiculopathy, in which CSF pleocytosis is predominantly mononuclear and clinical improvement is seen without CMV treatment. Lymphoma, tuberculosis, syphilis, and toxoplasmosis also cause similar clinical syndromes.

Encephalitis with dementia and ventriculoencephalitis

CMV encephalitis (CMVE) with dementia and ventriculoencephalitis are the two syndromes of CMVE described in AIDS patients. CMVE with dementia, the more common of the two syndromes, is well described neuropathologically [8] as a multifocal, scattered micronodular encephalitis that resembles HIV encephalitis, the cause of HIV-associated dementia (HIVD) [9]. CMV ventriculoencephalitis is a late and terminal event with acute onset of encephalitis often associated with cranial nerve involvement and nystagmus. The significance of differentiating CMVE and HIVD lies in the different drugs available for treatment.

CMVE is seen more commonly among men who have sex with men (MSM), which may reflect the increased CMV seroprevalence in that population [10]. CMVE always occurs in patients with CD4 counts of <100 cells/mm^3 and should be suspected in patients presenting with a subacute encephalopathy who have had AIDS for more than 1 year. Clinicians should suspect a diagnosis of CMVE in patients who have a history of systemic CMV infection, especially those with CMV retinitis who develop encephalopathic features and change in mental status.

Patients with dementia caused by CMVE usually have a more acute onset and rapid progression than patients with HIVD. The encephalopathic symptoms include delirium and confusion, lethargy and somnolence, apathy and withdrawal, personality changes, and focal neurologic signs with cranial nerve involvement. During the course of illness, recurrent fever episodes may occur that may be attributed to other opportunistic infections (e.g. *Mycobacterium*

avium complex). Psychomotor slowing, primitive reflexes, and peripheral neuropathy may also be seen in CMVE. Distal sensory polyneuropathy usually antedates the onset of CMVE [11].

The course of encephalopathic illness in both CMVE and HIVD includes progressive worsening in mental status until death. The median survival of CMVE patients is significantly shorter (weeks) compared with that of HIVD patients (months). Autopsies reveal a range of neuropathology, including ependymal and subependymal necrosis, areas of demyelination, and microglial nodules that are more frequently encountered than typical nuclear and cytoplasmic CMV inclusions [12]. Neuropathologic evaluations of CMVE and HIV co-infection of single cells suggests that CMV and HIV increase each other's replication in the brain [13].

It is difficult to make a definitive diagnosis of CMVE, and laboratory investigations are not helpful in distinguishing CMV from HIVD. Electrolyte abnormality, especially hyponatremia, is more commonly present in CMVE patients [14]. There are insufficient data to determine whether CMV antigen or DNA is regularly detected in CSF. Conversely, detection of CMV DNA may only reflect latent, but not active, CMV diseases. MRI scans showing meningeal enhancement consistent with ventriculitis and periventricular enhancement are helpful in differentiating CMVE from HIVD. However, periventricular enhancement may also be seen in lymphoma, toxoplasmosis, and pyogenic brain abscesses. Progressive ventriculomegaly, if seen in serial computed tomography scans, is highly suspicious for CMVE [15, 16].

Combination therapy with ganciclovir and foscarnet is commonly used, especially when disease progression is noted with single-agent therapy but trials of single versus combined therapy have not been performed.

Mononeuritis multiplex

This is the least common of all the neurologic syndromes attributed to CMV. Clinical characteristics of CMV mononeuritis are more varied than polyradiculopathy/myelitis. Patients may present with multifocal, patchy and/or asymmetrical sensory and motor deficits. Cranial nerve palsies caused by CMV, especially in the recurrent laryngeal nerve, have been reported in the setting of severe immunosuppression [17]. This symptom may occur with other manifestations of CMV (e.g. polyradiculopathy, encephalitis, or retinitis). Pathologic findings in peripheral nerve biopsies have shown endoneurial necrosis with cellular infiltrates and Schwann cells showing CMV inclusions.

Painful distal neuropathy

A syndrome of painful distal symmetrical neuropathy of subacute onset limited to the feet and associated with some numbness and weakness has been reported with CMV infection [18].

Gastrointestinal system

CMV colitis may occur in at least 5–10% of untreated AIDS patients. Diarrhea, weight loss, anorexia, and fever are often present. The differential diagnosis includes infection by other gastrointestinal pathogens, including *Cryptosporidium*, *Giardia*, *Entamoeba*, mycobacteria, *Shigella*, *Campylobacter*, and *Strongyloides stercoralis*, and involvement by lymphoma or Kaposi's sarcoma. Endoscopy usually reveals diffuse submucosal hemorrhages and mucosal ulcerations, although a grossly normal-appearing mucosa may be encountered in up to 10% of those with histologic evidence of CMV colitis (Fig. 34.2). Biopsy reveals vasculitis, neutrophilic infiltration, and non-specific inflammation, but the diagnosis is confirmed by the presence of characteristic CMV inclusions, antigen, or nucleic acid and the absence of other pathogens.

Symptomatic esophagitis in AIDS patients is most often due to *Candida albicans* but may also be caused by CMV. Patients with CMV esophagitis are apt to have pain on swallowing and distal ulceration on endoscopy. As in colitis, diagnosis should be established through endoscopic examination and biopsy. Other causes of ulcerative esophagitis include HSV and aphthous esophagitis.

The efficacy of anti-CMV treatment in patients with enterocolitis is not dramatic [19]. When compared with placebo, a significant antiviral effect was observed, but a clinical benefit was less apparent. Diarrhea and abdominal discomfort were not relieved, but in general, patients seemed to improve with this therapy [19].

Patients with symptomatic esophagitis or enterocolitis who have CMV (and no other pathogens) detected by endoscopy, histology, or culture should benefit from anti-CMV treatment for 3–6 weeks and should be considered for continued maintenance treatment, in part to prevent retinitis [20].

Pulmonary system

Isolation of CMV from pulmonary secretions or lung tissue in AIDS patients with pneumonia who undergo bronchoscopy is common, but a true pathogenic role of the virus in the disease process may be difficult to establish. Many patients with pulmonary disease and CMV isolation from the lung have concomitant infection with other pathogens, especially *Pneumocystis jiroveci*. Many of the patients respond to therapy directed at *P. jiroveci* pneumonia alone, raising the question of whether CMV is a true pulmonary pathogen in patients with AIDS. However, patients with positive CMV cultures and consistent histologic findings from lung tissue in whom no other pathogens are identified may truly have invasive CMV pneumonia.

When CMV causes pulmonary disease in AIDS patients, the syndrome is that of an interstitial pneumonitis. Patients often complain of gradually worsening shortness of breath, dyspnea on exertion, and a dry, non-productive cough. The heart and respiratory rates are elevated, but auscultation of the lungs often reveals minimal findings with no evidence of consolidation. Chest radiographs show diffuse interstitial infiltrates similar to those in patients with *P. jiroveci* pneumonia. Hypoxemia is invariably present.

Anti-CMV therapy should be considered when a patient has documented CMV pulmonary infection as the only pathogen identified and a progressive, deteriorating clinical course [21–23].

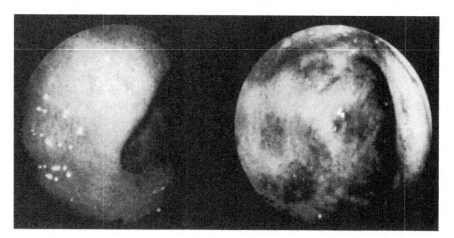

Figure 34.2 Sigmoidoscopic appearance of CMV colitis (two views), demonstrating diffuse submucosal hemorrhages and mucosal ulcerations.
(Courtesy of Dr D Dieterich, New York.)

Treatment of CMV infection

Ganciclovir/valganciclovir

Structure and mechanism of action

Ganciclovir is a nucleoside analog that differs from acyclovir by a single carboxyl side chain. This structural change confers approximately 50 times greater activity than acyclovir against CMV. Acyclovir has low activity against CMV because it is not well phosphorylated in CMV-infected cells. This is due to the absence of the gene for thymidine kinase (TK) in CMV. Ganciclovir, however, is active against CMV because it does not require TK for phosphorylation. Instead, another viral-encoded phosphorylating enzyme (UL 97) is present in CMV-infected cells [24]. It is capable of phosphorylating ganciclovir and converting it to the monophosphate. Cellular enzymes then convert the monophosphate to the active compound, ganciclovir triphosphate. Ganciclovir triphosphate acts to inhibit the viral DNA polymerase. Valganciclovir is an oral prodrug of ganciclovir, i.e. it is converted to ganciclovir after absorption.

Pharmacology and dosage

Ganciclovir is available for clinical use in intravenous formulations, as well as a sustained release intraocular implant. The oral form of ganciclovir has been replaced by valganciclovir. Intravenous ganciclovir is used for initial induction therapy, followed by either intravenous ganciclovir or oral valganciclovir for maintenance therapy.

Initial intravenous induction treatment for CMV disease consists of 5 mg/kg twice daily for 14–21 days or until there is an adequate clinical response. The standard intravenous dosage for maintenance therapy is approximately one-half the induction dose (i.e. 5 mg/kg per day, 7 days/week) or, if oral valganciclovir, 900 mg daily, with food.

When administered by intravenous infusion over 1 h in the usual dosage of 5 mg/kg, peak ganciclovir blood levels are approximately 8–9 µg/mL, and the serum half-life is 3.5 h. The absolute bioavailability of oral valganciclovir capsules is approximately 60%. When administered orally as 900 mg with food, peak serum levels approach those achieved by intravenous administration of 5 mg/kg. Oral valganciclovir may be used for induction treatment and is the drug of choice for maintenance therapy [25]. Because ganciclovir is excreted unchanged through the kidneys, dosage for intravenous ganciclovir must be reduced in patients with renal impairment. Dosage adjustments should also be considered for oral valganciclovir. The appropriate dose reductions are presented in Table 34.2. Initial response in retinitis (improvement or stabilization in vision or ophthalmoscopic appearance) occurs in approximately 75% of treated patients [6]. By comparison, the disease is relentlessly progressive in 90% of patients if left untreated. Visual-field defects present at the onset of therapy do not reverse, but a decrease in visual acuity caused by edema of the macula may improve with treatment. Retinal detachment may occur in later stages as the necrotic retina scars and thins.

Prior to the availability of HAART, maintenance therapy throughout the life of the patient was critical for CMV retinitis because the virus is only suppressed by ganciclovir and is not eliminated. Even with continued maintenance therapy, CMV retinitis eventually progressed. Why this occurred is not clearly understood, but it is likely related to suboptimal drug delivery to the retina. This hypothesis is

Table 34.2 Ganciclovir dosage adjustment in patients with impaired renal function

CREATININE CLEARANCE (mL/min)[a]	IV INDUCTION DOSE (mg/kg)	INDUCTION DOSING INTERVAL (h)	MAINTENANCE DOSE (mg/kg)	MAINTENANCE DOSING INTERVAL (h)	ORAL VALGANCICLOVIR INDUCTION DOSE
>70	5.0	12	5.0	24	900 mg twice daily every other day
50–69	2.5	1	2.5	24	900 mg twice daily every other day
25–49	2.5	24	1.25	24	450 mg once daily
10–24	1.25	24	0.625	24	450 mg three-times a week
<10	1.25	3 three times a week following hemodialysis		3 three times a week following hemodialysis	Do not use

[a]Creatinine clearance can be related to serum creatinine by the following formulas:

$$\text{For males}: \frac{140 - \text{age (years)} \times \text{weight (kg)}}{72 \times \text{serum creatinine (mg/dL)}}$$

For females: $0.85 \times$ male value.

supported by the longer times to progression achieved with the ganciclovir intraocular implant, which delivers greater concentrations of ganciclovir to the vitreous [26]. Viral resistance does not appear to be involved in most progressions of CMV retinitis [27].

With successful ART, it is possible for selected patients with CMV retinitis to discontinue maintenance therapy but not until CD4 count has exceeded 100 cells/mm³ for 3–6 months and the retinitis is inactive [28].

Intravitreal injection of ganciclovir has been used in certain special situations, such as in patients in whom neutropenia limited the systemic use of the drug, and in one series [29] appeared effective and relatively safe. Sustained intravitreal release of ganciclovir has been accomplished using a surgical implantable device [14, 30, 31]. This implant, which is designed to deliver ganciclovir into the vitreous over several months, has been shown to be highly efficacious for local control of retinitis. When the implant is used, oral valganciclovir should also be given at least until CD4 function is restored by ART. This is needed to treat or prevent contralateral eye or systemic disease. The implant delivers approximately five times as much ganciclovir compared with intravenous therapy and may be useful in treating low-level GCV-resistant CMV retinitis.

Clinical use

Administration of ganciclovir or valganciclovir is indicated for the treatment of CMV disease, but other herpesviruses, including HSV-1, HSV-2, VZV, and human herpesvirus (HHV)-6, are also susceptible to the drug *in vitro*. Because HIV-infected patients with severe CMV infection frequently have illnesses caused by other herpesviruses, a bonus of ganciclovir/valganciclovir therapy may be prevention or improvement of these infections.

Resistance

Erice and co-workers [32] reported three patients whose clinical course suggested the emergence of resistance and whose CMV isolates exhibited increases in the concentration of ganciclovir required to inhibit the virus in tissue culture over baseline determinations. In a separate report, after 3 months of continuous intravenous ganciclovir therapy, approximately 10% of patients were excreting resistant strains of CMV (arbitrarily defined as strains that are only inhibited by four times or more the median concentration of ganciclovir required to inhibit a group of pretherapy isolates) [33]. In virtually all isolates, there was a mutation in the phosphorylating gene (UL 97) [34]. These strains remain sensitive to foscarnet, which may be used as an alternative therapy. As treatment continues, a polymerase mutation (UL 54) conferring further ganciclovir resistance

may occur. Many strains with this mutation are cross-resistant to cidofovir but usually remain sensitive to foscarnet [35, 36].

The most rapid method for detecting resistance is to genotype UL 97 and UL 54, to detect resistance mutations. This may be done on a viral isolate or on body fluids directly (e.g. plasma) if sufficient CMV DNA copy numbers are present. Patients with ganciclovir-resistant disease should be switched to foscarnet, since cross-resistance to these two drugs is rare. Discontinuing ganciclovir may allow reversion to wild-type virus to occur more rapidly than if continued.

Toxicity

Toxicity may limit therapy with ganciclovir. CBCs, electrolytes and renal function should be monitored weekly while on therapy. The following adverse effects may occur.

Effects on hematopoiesis

Leukopenia and anemia may occur in up to 40 and 25%, respectively, of patients receiving intravenous ganciclovir or oral valganciclovir for treatment of CMV disease (Table 34.3). Many patients have low white blood cell counts before therapy, so the contribution of ganciclovir/valganciclovir to leukopenia is not always clear. Neutropenia may develop at any time and is usually reversible. Cytokines, such as granulocyte colony-stimulating factor (G-CSF; filgrastim), are effective in reversing ganciclovir/valganciclovir induced neutropenia. Severe neutropenia (absolute neutrophil count < 500 cells/mm³) requires a ganciclovir/valganciclovir dose interruption until evidence of marrow recovery is

Table 34.3 Selected laboratory abnormalities in patients receiving ganciclovir for treatment of CMV retinitis

CMV RETINITIS TREATMENT	IV (5 mg/kg L/d)	PLACEBO
Number of patients	175	234
Neutropenia (ANC/L)		
< 500	25	6
500–749	14	7
750–1000	26	16
Anemia (hgb, g/dL)		
< 6.5	5	< 1
6.5–7.9	16	3
8.0–9.5	26	16

Data are percentages of patients. ANC; absolute neutrophil count; hgb, hemoglobin.

observed and neutrophil counts have risen, preferably to > 1,000 cells/mm^3. Thrombocytopenia occurs in up to 6% of ganciclovir/valganciclovir-treated patients.

Toxicities in other organ systems

Gastrointestinal adverse events, most commonly diarrhea, nausea, anorexia, and vomiting, affect a substantial number of patients treated with ganciclovir. When compared to placebo, events are only modestly higher among ganciclovir-treated patients; 48% developed diarrhea (versus 42% of placebo-treated patients), 19% developed anorexia (placebo, 16%), and 14% developed vomiting (placebo, 11%) [37]. In patients receiving valganciclovir, diarrhea occurred in 41%, nausea in 30%, and vomiting in 24%. Neuropathy and paresthesia are the most frequent adverse events involving the nervous system, affecting up to 21 and 10% of patients, respectively, and only neuropathy occurred more often in ganciclovir-versus placebo-treated patients (21% versus 15%, respectively). Neuropathy occurred in 9% of patients receiving valganciclovir. A minority of ganciclovir-treated patients will experience modest elevations in serum creatinine (maximum levels of at least 1.5 mg/dL, or > 25% increases over pretreatment levels).

Gonadal toxicity

In pre-clinical animal studies, ganciclovir (and therefore valganciclovir) is a potent inhibitor of spermatogenesis and may also suppress female fertility. Sperm counts in humans before and during ganciclovir therapy, however, have been performed too infrequently to provide meaningful information on spermatogenesis. Patients wishing to have children should use ganciclovir/valganciclovir only for the strongest indications.

Teratogenesis

Because ganciclovir and valganciclovir are mutagens and teratogens in animals, effective contraception should be practiced by men and women with childbearing potential during treatment. Ganciclovir/valganciclovir should be used during pregnancy only if the potential benefit justifies the potential risk to the fetus.

Foscarnet

Foscarnet is a pyrophosphate that inhibits the DNA polymerase of CMV. Specifically, the drug blocks the pyrophosphate-binding site of the viral DNA polymerase, preventing cleavage of pyrophosphate from deoxyadenosine triphosphate [38]. This action is relatively selective in that CMV DNA polymerase is inhibited at concentrations < 1% of that required to inhibit cellular DNA polymerase. Unlike such nucleosides as acyclovir and ganciclovir, foscarnet does not require phosphorylation intracellularly to be an active inhibitor of viral DNA polymerases. This biochemical fact becomes especially important with regard to viral resistance, because the principal mode of viral resistance to nucleoside analogs is a mutation that eliminates phosphorylation of the drug in virus-infected cells. Foscarnet can be used to treat patients with ganciclovir-resistant CMV; cross-resistance to foscarnet is rare. However, patients treated with foscarnet may develop foscarnet resistance due to mutations in the viral polymerase UL54 [36].

Pharmacology

The recommended dose for initial therapy is 60 mg/kg by intravenous infusion every 8 hours or 90 mg/kg every 12 hours. A dose of 120 mg/kg per day may be superior in efficacy to 90 mg/kg/per day [39], but this dose may also be more toxic.

CSF concentrations of foscarnet are approximately 40% of serum levels. Excretion is entirely renal, without a hepatic component. Oral bioavailability is estimated at 12–22%, but it is poorly tolerated and not used.

Adverse effects include renal impairment, anemia, hypocalcemia (especially ionized calcium), hypomagnesemia, and hypophosphatemia. It is important to measure renal function frequently and adjust dosage accordingly to minimize toxicity. Daily pre-infusion of 1 L of saline may reduce nephrotoxicity during maintenance therapy.

Palestine and co-workers [5] reported the results of a randomized control trial of foscarnet in the treatment of CMV retinitis in HIV-infected patients. Patients were assigned to receive either no therapy or immediate treatment with intravenous foscarnet. The justification for the design was that the lesions were peripheral and not threatening visual acuity. The mean time to progression of retinitis was 3 weeks in the control group versus 13 weeks in the treatment group, thereby demonstrating the effectiveness of foscarnet. Also, an excellent antiviral effect was achieved in the treatment group (i.e. 9 of 13 patients had positive blood cultures for CMV at entry, and all nine had CMV cleared from their blood by the end of the 3-week induction period). Adverse effects were seizures, hypomagnesemia, hypocalcemia, and elevated serum creatinine levels.

Ganciclovir and foscarnet

The results of a Studies of Ocular Complications of AIDS (SOCA) trial of combination therapy versus monotherapy for relapsed CMV retinitis were published in early 1996 [40]. Combination therapy (5 mg/kg per day ganciclovir and 90 mg/kg per day foscarnet) was significantly superior in delaying progression than either ganciclovir alone (10 mg per day) or foscarnet alone (120 mg/kg per day). This study also found no advantage in switching monotherapy. That is, patients in whom monotherapy failed with ganciclovir who then switched to high-dose foscarnet did not do better than patients who continued ganciclovir at the higher dose. The median times to progression were: foscarnet group, 1.3 months; ganciclovir group, 2.0 months;

and combination group, 4.3 months ($p < 0.001$). Side effects were not statistically significantly different in any group, but the quality of life was poorest in the combination group as a result of the prolonged daily infusion time of 3.1 hours.

Cidofovir

Cidofovir represents a departure from previous nucleoside analogs because it appears to the cell as a nucleotide. It has a phosphonate moiety attached to a cytosine analog and does not require phosphorylation by viral-encoded enzyme. It is therefore active against the majority of ganciclovir-resistant CMV strains that only have resistance mutations in UL97, the phosphorylating gene. When polymerase, UL54, mutations occur in ganciclovir UL54 treated patients, cross-resistance to cidofovir is frequent. These UL54 resistance mutations also occur in patients treated with cidofovir *de novo* [36]. The drug also has an extremely long half-life, permitting intravenous administration as infrequently as every 2 weeks during maintenance treatment [41].

Cidofovir is nephrotoxic, especially to the proximal renal tubule, but toxicity can be diminished with prehydration and concomitant probenecid therapy. Renal function and toxicity must be monitored carefully, and proteinuria or a rising creatinine level are reasons for dosage reduction, interruption, or discontinuation. Concurrent administration of other nephrotoxic drugs must be avoided and there must be at least a 7-day period of "washout" of these drugs if their use precedes administration of cidofovir.

Immune recovery uveitis

Immune recovery uveitis is an immunologic reaction to CMV characterized by inflammation in the anterior chamber or vitreous. It occurs after the initiation of ART and typically occurs in patients who experience a substantial rise in CD4 count during the 4–12 weeks after initiation of therapy. Treatment consists of periocular corticosteroids or a short course of systemic steroids [42].

HERPES SIMPLEX VIRUS

Herpes simplex virus types 1 and 2 (HSV-1, HSV-2) cause disease in both normal and immunocompromised hosts and are responsible for substantial morbidity in patients with AIDS. Most adult patients with AIDS have been infected with one or both HSV types before the development of AIDS, and these patients are not susceptible to primary HSV infection following new exposure. During initial HSV infection, viral latency develops in the nerve root ganglia corresponding to the site of mucocutaneous inoculation. Latent virus can then reactivate at any time throughout the life of the host, and all infected persons are at risk for virus shedding and recurrent symptomatic disease. Recurrent HSV mucocutaneous eruptions are common in patients with HIV infection and can be severe, with extensive tissue destruction and prolonged viral shedding [43–45].

Recent studies confirm the high prevalence of both HSV-1 and HSV-2 in the general population [46–48]. Type-specific serologic studies conclude that up to 70% of the population are infected with HSV-1, and up to 22% are infected with HSV-2. HSV-2 infection rates are higher in women than in men and higher in African-Americans and Mexican-Americans than in Caucasians [46–48]. The presence of underlying HSV infection may increase the risk of acquiring HIV infection following exposure to HIV. This increased risk for HIV may occur as a result of the presence of susceptible CD4 T cells present in HSV ulcerations [49, 50]. The prevalence of HSV infection in homosexual AIDS patients exceeds that of the general population and likely reflects the common risk factor for transmission of both HSV and HIV (sexual contact). Serologic studies have revealed that up to 77% of HIV-infected patients have been previously infected with HSV. AIDS subgroups who did not acquire HIV infection through sexual contact, such as hemophiliacs and transfusion recipients, have rates of HSV infection that are lower than the incidence in patients with AIDS as a whole, and are likely comparable with those in the general population. The presence of latent HSV infection in this high percentage of patients with HIV infection explains the frequency of clinical disease in this population. Clinical observations suggest that the frequency and severity of HSV recurrences may increase with advancing immunosuppressions [48, 51–54].

Clinical presentation

Because most HIV-infected patients have been infected with HSV before acquiring HIV, recurrent HSV is much more common than primary HSV infection in this population. HSV infection in AIDS patients may appear similar to the typical HSV lesions observed in the normal host or, alternatively, lesions may appear quite atypical and unusual because of the immunosuppressed state associated with HIV infection. The severity of clinical illness depends on several factors, including the anatomic site of initial infection, the degree of immunosuppression, and whether the clinical episode represents initial primary infection (no previous exposure to either HSV type), initial non-primary infection (previous exposure to the heterologous HSV type), or recurrent infection [43–45].

Localized mucocutaneous ulcerative lesions, without visceral or cutaneous dissemination, is the most frequent presentation of HSV infection in HIV-infected patients. Because the lesions may appear atypical, a high index of suspicion is required by the clinician in evaluating any mucocutaneous lesion in a patient with HIV infection. Chronic or persistent HSV infection (ulcerative HSV infection present for great than one month) is an AIDS-defining condition.

Orolabial infection

Orolabial infection in adults with AIDS is usually due to recurrent disease from previously latent infection. Primary infection of the mouth or nose may occur, however, in a seronegative individual who acquires infection at this site for the first time. Primary infection is more likely to occur in children with AIDS than in adults, because HIV infection in children (especially those infected prenatally) is more likely to precede initial exposure to HSV.

The incubation period of primary HSV infection ranges between 2 and 12 days. In the normal host, primary orolabial infection may be asymptomatic or result in clinically apparent gingivostomatitis [45–48, 55]. Immunocompromised patients are at greater risk than normal hosts of developing a severe clinical illness during primary HSV-1 infection, with a painful vesicular eruption occurring along the lips, tongue, pharynx, or buccal mucosa. The vesicles rapidly coalesce and rupture to form large ulcers covered by a whitish yellow necrotic film [55, 56]. Fever, pharyngitis, and cervical lymphadenopathy are often present in adults, whereas infants may display poor feeding and persistent drooling.

Following initial or primary infection, all infected patients remain at risk for virus reactivation and recurrent disease. Recurrent HSV gingivostomatitis ("fever blisters") may occur spontaneously or as a result of external stimuli, such as a febrile illness, excessive wind or ultraviolet light exposure to the lips, surgical manipulation of the trigeminal nerve, or stress. Prodromal symptoms, consisting of tingling or numbness at the site of the impending recurrence, may be present from 12 to 24 hours before the onset of an HSV recurrence. Instituting antiviral therapy during the prodrome may shorten the duration of illness or may abort the development of visible cutaneous lesions (see Treatment of HSV Infection, below). Recurrences may increase in frequency and severity as immunosuppression worsens, although many AIDS patients will have only infrequent, mild, self-limiting recurrences throughout the course of their disease [51, 55].

In the normal host, orolabial herpes lesions usually heal in 7–10 days. By comparison, AIDS patients often have a prolonged illness with markedly delayed healing of mucocutaneous lesions. If left untreated, chronic ulcerative lesions with persistent viral shedding may last for several weeks [56].

Genital infection

After a 2- to 12-day incubation period, many individuals with primary genital herpes develop local symptoms [43–45]. Symptoms will be most apparent in patients with primary genital infection (no prior infection with the heterologous HSV type) as compared with patients with non-primary initial infection (prior infection with the heterologous HSV type). When present, signs and symptoms include small papules that rapidly evolve into fluid-filled vesicles. These lesions are usually painful and tender to palpation. The vesicles ulcerate rapidly and, in the normal host, heal over 3–4 weeks by crusting and re-epithelialization. Tender inguinal adenopathy is common, and dysuria may be present even if the urethra is not infected. Systemic symptoms, such as fever, headache, myalgias, malaise, and meningismus, may be present during primary infection [43–45].

In the normal host, recurrent genital herpes is less severe than primary infection. Compared with primary infection, recurrent herpes typically results in fewer external lesions, a shorter duration of illness, and the absence of systemic symptoms [43–45]. As with primary infection, recurrent genital herpes in patients with AIDS may be more severe and prolonged compared with that seen in the normal host. Prolonged new lesion formation, continued tissue destruction, persistent virus shedding, and severe local pain are not uncommon findings in this setting. As with orolabial herpes, the frequency and severity of genital recurrences may increase with advancing immunosuppression, and symptoms may last for several weeks if left untreated [51, 57].

Asymptomatic genital HSV shedding in non-immunocompromised patients occurs on between 1 and 6% of the days on which cultures are obtained [58, 59]. HIV-infected patients infected with HSV shed HSV at even higher rates, and asymptomatic shedding may increase with advancing immunosuppression [60]. All HSV-infected individuals (whether HIV infected or not) should be counseled about asymptomatic HSV shedding and the risk of transmission to sexual partners despite the absence of symptoms or visible lesions [61].

Anorectal infection

Chronic perianal herpes was among the first reported opportunistic infections associated with AIDS. HSV is the most frequent cause of non-gonococcal proctitis in sexually active homosexual men [62, 63]. HSV proctitis usually results from primary HSV-2 infection but may also occur as a result of HSV-1 infection or recurrent disease caused by either viral type. Severe anorectal pain, perianal ulcerations, constipation, tenesmus, and neurologic symptoms in the distribution of the sacral plexus (sacral radiculopathy, impotence, and neurogenic bladder) are common findings of HSV proctitis. These signs and symptoms help differentiate HSV proctitis from proctitis from other causes (Fig. 34.3) [62]. Anorectal or sigmoidoscopic examination in patients with HSV proctitis typically reveals a friable mucosa, diffuse ulcerations, and occasional intact vesicular or pustular lesions [62].

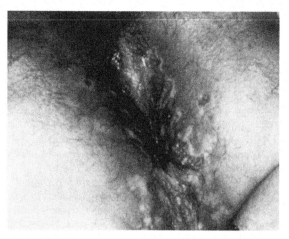

Figure 34.3 Perianal ulcerations typical of herpes simplex.

Recurrent perianal lesions caused by HSV in the absence of true proctitis is a common finding in patients with AIDS. Local pain, tenderness, itching, and pain on defecation are prominent symptoms of these lesions. Shallow ulcers in the perianal region are often visible on external examination, and ulcerative lesions frequently coalesce and extend along the gluteal crease to involve the area overlying the sacrum. These lesions are often atypical in appearance and may be confused with pressure decubiti (Fig. 34.3). To prevent misdiagnosis, perianal ulcerations and anal fissures in patients with AIDS should be examined for the presence of HSV by culture, polymerase chain reaction (PCR), or direct antigen detection whenever possible.

Esophagitis

Symptoms of HSV esophagitis typically include retrosternal pain and odynophagia. Patients may present with acute onset of dysphagia or with chronic swallowing complaints, and symptoms may be severe enough to interfere with eating and adequate nutrition. Visible herpetic lesions in the oropharynx may not be present, and the clinical picture may be confused with *Candida*, CMV, or aphthous esophagitis. Radiographic contrast studies typically reveal a cobblestone appearance of the esophageal mucosa, but this finding is non-specific and is also present with esophagitis from other causes (Fig. 34.4) [64]. Definitive diagnosis of HSV esophagitis should be made by direct endoscopic visualization of the esophageal mucosa with positive viral studies and histopathologic evidence of invasive viral infection [65].

Encephalitis

HSV encephalitis occurs rarely in AIDS but is the most life-threatening complication of HSV infection. Both HSV-1 and HSV-2 have been identified in brain tissue of AIDS

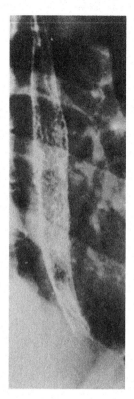

Figure 34.4 Barium esophagram revealing a cobblestone appearance of the esophageal mucosa. These findings are typical in both HSV esophagitis and *Candida* esophagitis. *(Reprinted with permission from Farthing CF, Brown SE, Staughton RCD. A Colour Atlas of AIDS and HIV Disease Slide Set. 2nd edn. London: Mosby; 1989.)*

patients, and simultaneous brain infections with HSV and CMV have been reported [66–68]. In adults with AIDS, HSV encephalitis usually occurs as a complication of primary or reactivated orolabial HSV infection. In neonates, the disease may occur as a result of primary HSV infection at the time of birth [45].

The presentation of HSV encephalitis in adults with AIDS is often highly atypical. A subacute illness with subtle neurologic abnormalities is common in AIDS patients with HSV encephalitis, suggesting that host immune responses contribute to the clinical manifestations of the disease [55, 68]. Headache, meningismus, and personality changes may develop gradually as the illness progresses. Alternatively, however, some AIDS patients with HSV encephalitis present with acute onset of symptoms. Abrupt onset of fever, headache, nausea, lethargy, and confusion may occur with temporal lobe abnormalities, cranial nerve defects, and focal seizures. Grand mal seizures, obtundation, coma, and death may eventually ensue.

The clinical diagnosis of HSV encephalitis may be extremely difficult, because other central nervous system infections (including HIV encephalopathy, *Cryptococcus neoformans*, and *Toxoplasma gondii*) may present with similar features. Studies have demonstrated the utility of detecting HSV DNA in CSF by the polymerase chain reaction technique as a method of non-invasive diagnosis of HSV encephalitis, although false-positive and false-negative results do occur [69, 70]. CSF usually reveals non-specific findings, including elevated protein and a lymphocytic pleocytosis. Viral CSF cultures are usually negative [70]. Other non-invasive diagnostic studies (such as MRI scan, CT scan, radionuclide brain scan, or electroencephalography) are rarely diagnostic but may reveal localized abnormalities (often in the temporal lobes) to guide diagnostic brain biopsy. Definitive diagnosis may require brain biopsy and the recovery of virus or demonstration of viral DNA or antigens from tissue specimens [71]. The histopathologic abnormalities typically observed in normal hosts (hemorrhagic cortical necrosis and lymphocytic infiltration) may be absent in patients with AIDS [66–68, 71]. HIV-infected patients with suspected HSV encephalitis should be treated with high-dose intravenous acyclovir pending results of diagnostic studies.

Drug-resistant HSV infection

Since the initial description of acyclovir-resistant HSV infection in patients with AIDS, numerous additional reports have appeared in the literature [72, 73]. The incidence of acyclovir-resistant HSV infections in immunocompromised hosts had been estimated as 4–5% [72], but the incidence has decreased dramatically since the advent of HAART. The most common mechanism of acyclovir resistance in patients with AIDS is the selection and overgrowth of HSV strains deficient in the enzyme thymidine kinase. These mutated TK-deficient strains do not phosphorylate acyclovir or penciclovir to the active antiviral compounds, and these viruses are resistant to standard dosages of acyclovir, valacyclovir, and famciclovir. Although these strains have reduced virulence in animal models [74] and only rarely cause clinical disease in non-immunocompromised hosts [75], they are capable of causing severe clinical illness in patients with advanced HIV disease [74]. Other mechanisms of drug resistance, including alteration of TK and DNA polymerase specificity, have been described but occur much less frequently. Most reports of drug-resistant HSV have cited localized chronic mucocutaneous infection, but cases of disseminated mucocutaneous disease [73], meningoencephalitis [76], and esophagitis [72] caused by these strains have been described.

Treatment of HSV infection

Mucocutaneous HSV infections in patients with AIDS are often symptomatic and can be a source of great discomfort. Visceral involvement or disseminated HSV disease can be life threatening, and all symptomatic HSV infections should be treated aggressively even if they are reactivations. The prompt administration of antiviral chemotherapy in patients with acute HSV infection reduces morbidity and the risk of serious complications. Currently, several effective antiviral drugs are available, and the clinician must choose the appropriate medication and the optimal route of administration (topical, oral, or intravenous).

Acyclovir

Acyclovir, a synthetic purine nucleoside analog, was the first antiviral agent approved by the FDA for treatment of mucocutaneous HSV infection. Acyclovir has been available and widely used since the early 1980s and, until recently, has been the undisputed antiviral agent of choice for HSV infections in patients with AIDS and for other immunocompromised and non-immunocompromised hosts [77] The drug has significant activity against HSV-1, HSV-2, and VZV. Despite excellent *in vitro* activity against these viruses, the bioavailability of oral acyclovir is only about 20%, resulting in relatively low serum drug levels following oral administration compared with levels achieved with intravenous therapy. Despite these findings, the serum levels of acyclovir achieved with standard acyclovir dosing (200 mg five times daily or 400 mg three times daily) exceed the levels required to inhibit the growth of HSV-1 and HSV-2,. Higher oral doses (800 mg five times daily) are needed to achieve inhibitory serum drug levels to treat VZV (see below) [77]. Acyclovir has a high therapeutic-to-toxic ratio because it undergoes selective activation and phosphorylation by virus-induced TK only in HSV- and VZV-infected cells. Acyclovir triphosphate selectively inhibits HSV DNA polymerase and results in early termination of DNA chain synthesis. The drug has slightly higher activity against HSV-1 than HSV-2.

Acyclovir distributes into all tissues, including the brain and CSF, and is cleared by renal mechanisms. The serum half-life in patients with normal renal function is 2.5–3.3 hours. The dose of intravenous acyclovir is 15 mg/kg per day in three divided doses for treatment of mucocutaneous infection and 30 mg/kg per day for HSV encephalitis. Although oral dosage adjustment is not required because of poor bioavailability, the intravenous dose should be reduced in patients with impaired renal function (Table 34.4). High-dose intravenous therapy can be associated with crystalluria, and adequate hydration should be maintained in patients on intravenous acyclovir to prevent this complication [77].

Numerous studies have shown acyclovir to be effective for treatment of primary as well as recurrent HSV infection, and as suppressive therapy for patients with frequently recurring HSV. In HIV-infected patients with symptomatic HSV infection, treatment is of great benefit in reducing symptoms, viral shedding, and the duration of illness. The drug has an excellent safety record and is usually well

Table 34.4 Dosage adjustment of intravenous acyclovir in patients with renal dysfunction

CREATININE CLEARANCE (mL/min per 1.73 m^2)	STANDARD DOSE (%)	DOSING INTERVAL (h)
>50	100	8
25–50	100	12
10–25	100	12
0–10	50	24

Usually 5 mg/kg; 10 mg/kg is used for HSV CNS infections and in some instances for VZV infections.

tolerated, although some patients may complain of headache or nausea. Acyclovir can be administered orally [78–84], intravenously [85, 86], or topically [57, 81], and the optimal route of administration, dosage, and duration of therapy depend on the site and severity of the HSV infection. Oral acyclovir is usually appropriate for outpatients with localized, non-life-threatening mucocutaneous HSV infection. Intravenous therapy should be prescribed for patients with disseminated disease, HSV encephalitis, or visceral organ involvement. Additionally, intravenous therapy is indicated for those patients who do not respond adequately to oral treatment, raising concern over issues such as poor drug absorption, poor compliance with oral therapy, or the development of drug-resistant infection. Topical acyclovir ointment is only minimally effective and should not be prescribed in the place of systemic antiviral therapy.

Valacyclovir

Valacyclovir hydrochloride is the l-valyl ester of acyclovir, and is available and effective in the treatment of HSV [87] and VZV [88] infections. Following oral administration, valacyclovir is rapidly absorbed from the gastrointestinal tract. The drug is rapidly and extensively converted to acyclovir *in vivo*, and the resulting acyclovir serum levels are much higher than those achieved with oral acyclovir. Pharmacokinetic studies reveal that a therapeutic drug level equivalent to acyclovir 800 mg five times daily can be achieved with 1000 mg valacyclovir given every 8 hours [87–89].

Because of the improved bioavailability of valacyclovir compared with acyclovir, studies have evaluated less frequent dosing for patients with HSV infection. Valacyclovir is effective in the treatment of first-episode HSV infection at a dose of 500–1000 mg to twice daily, and in the treatment of recurrent HSV infection at a dose of 500 mg twice daily if initiated within the first 24 h of signs or symptoms. Therapy should be continued until all lesions are dry and crusted. Additionally, valacyclovir is effective as suppressive therapy at a dose of 250 mg twice daily, 500 mg once daily (for patients with fewer than 10 recurrences per year), and 1 g once daily (for patients with 10 or more recurrences per year) [89]. Dosage reduction is recommended in patients with a creatinine clearance <50 mL/min (Table 34.5).

A study evaluating very high valacyclovir dosing (8 g/day) for suppression of CMV in patients with advanced HIV disease suggested a possible association between valacyclovir and the syndromes of thrombotic thrombocytopenic purpura and hemolytic-uremic syndrome (TTP/HUS). A cause-and-effect relationship has not been firmly established, however, and these findings have not been observed in patients receiving standard dosages of valacyclovir. In view of these observations, the standard recommended dosages of valacyclovir should not be exceeded [89].

Famciclovir

Famciclovir is the diacetyl 6-deoxy analog of the active antiviral compound penciclovir. When taken orally, famciclovir is readily absorbed from the upper gastrointestinal tract, and is rapidly converted into penciclovir. In a manner similar to acyclovir, penciclovir undergoes phosphorylation to the triphosphate compound by viral-induced TK and cellular enzymes. Penciclovir triphosphate acts as a

Table 34.5 Valacyclovir dosing based on indications for treatment and renal function

CREATININE CLEARANCE (mL/min)	DOSAGE FOR VARICELLA ZOSTER INFECTION (CHICKENPOX OR SHINGLES)	DOSAGE FOR INITIAL HERPES SIMPLEX VIRUS INFECTION	DOSAGE FOR RECURRENT HERPES SIMPLEX VIRUS INFECTION
≥50	1 gm every 8 hours	1 gm every 12 hours	500 mg every 12 hours
30–49	1 gm every 12 hours	1 gm every 12 hours	500 mg every 12 hours
10–29	1 gm every 24 hours	1 gm every 24 hours	500 mg every 24 hours
<10	500 mg every 24 hours	500 mg every 24 hours	500 mg every 24 hours

competitive inhibitor of the natural substrate required for viral DNA replication, but does not irreversibly terminate DNA replication. The drug has a very long half-life (10–20 h) in HSV-infected cells, ensuring prolonged antiviral activity [90–94].

Clinical studies have shown that oral famciclovir is effective in the treatment of first-episode HSV infections at a dose of 250 mg three times daily and is effective in the treatment of recurrent HSV infection at a dose of 125 mg twice daily if given within the first 6 hours of symptoms or signs. Therapy should be continued until all lesions are dry and crusted. Additionally, famciclovir is effective as suppressive therapy at a dose of 250 mg twice daily [89, 91, 92, 94]. Dosage reduction is recommended in patients with creatinine clearance less than 60 mL/min (Table 34.6).

Topical penciclovir has been approved by the FDA for the treatment of recurrent HSV gingivostomatitis. Unlike topical acyclovir, penciclovir appears to have a beneficial effect on recurrent mucocutaneous HSV infection when compared with placebo [95]. Topical penciclovir has not been extensively evaluated in patients with HIV infection, however, and may not be as effective as systemic therapy in this immunocompromised population.

Foscarnet

Foscarnet (phosphonoformic acid) is an inorganic pyrophosphate with a broad range of antiviral activities against herpesviruses as well as HIV [38]. Studies have demonstrated foscarnet to be effective in the treatment of CMV disease and in the treatment of drug-resistant HSV and VZV infections. Unlike acyclovir and famciclovir, foscarnet does not require viral enzyme-mediated phosphorylation for activity. Hence, foscarnet remains an effective antiviral agent for treatment of TK-deficient, drug-resistant HSV [96–98]. Foscarnet is superior to vidarabine in the treatment of acyclovir-resistant HSV infections in patients with AIDS, and remains a treatment of choice for this illness at a dose of 40 mg/kg three times daily [96].

Foscarnet must be given intravenously, and side effects (including nausea, fever, headache, anemia, and renal failure) are common. Because of the potential for nephrotoxic effects and electrolyte imbalances, close monitoring of renal function and serum levels of potassium, calcium, phosphate, and magnesium is required. Variable penetration into the CSF has been reported. Dosage adjustments are required in patients with renal dysfunction.

Other antiviral drugs

Cidofovir is a long-acting antiviral drug approved by the FDA for the treatment of CMV retinitis, and also appears to be effective in the treatment of drug-resistant HSV [99, 100]. Cidofovir has a prolonged serum half-life, allowing for once-weekly intravenous administration. Nephrotoxicity can occur with therapy, however, and pretreatment with intravenous fluids and probenecid is recommended. A gel form of cidofovir for topical use is effective for mucocutaneous drug-resistant HSV infections [101].

Management of patients with HSV infection

Most HIV-infected patients with primary or recurrent mucocutaneous HSV infections are not ill enough to require hospitalization and are suitable candidates for outpatient treatment. The treatment of choice for most HSV infections in AIDS is either oral acyclovir, oral valacyclovir, or oral famciclovir (Table 34.7). Because therapy with valacyclovir or famciclovir results in serum antiviral levels comparable to those with intravenous acyclovir, many HIV-infected patients with severe HSV infection who can tolerate oral therapy can be treated as outpatients.

Although the bioavailability and resultant serum drug levels with oral acyclovir are not as favorable as those with valacyclovir or famciclovir, acyclovir remains a safe,

Table 34.6 Dosage adjustment of famciclovir in patients with zoster and renal dysfunction

CREATININE CLEARANCE (mL/min)	DOSAGE REGIMEN
≥60	500 mg every 8 h
40–59	500 mg every 12 h
20–39	500 mg every 24 h

There are insufficient data to recommend a dosage for patients with creatinine clearance <20 mL/min.

Table 34.7 Management of HSV infections in AIDS

Mucocutaneous infection, mild	Acyclovir 400 mg PO three times daily, famciclovir 500 mg PO twice daily, or valacyclovir 1000 mg PO twice daily
Mucocutaneous infection, severe	Acyclovir 5 mg/kg IV three times daily, famciclovir PO 500 mg twice daily, or valacyclovir PO 1000 mg twice daily
Suppression of mucocutaneous lesions	Acyclovir 400–800 mg PO twice daily or three times daily famciclovir 500 mg PO twice daily, or valacyclovir 500 mg PO twice daily
Acyclovir-resistant infection	Foscarnet 40 mg/kg IV three times daily

effective, and well-tolerated treatment regimen in HIV-infected patients with HSV infection. Most HIV-infected patients respond well to oral acyclovir, although many clinicians use higher doses of acyclovir in HIV-infected patients than those recommended in non-immunocompromised patients.

The most recent guidelines (December 2010) from the Centers for Disease Control and Prevention (CDC) state that patients with symptomatic HSV disease should be treated as early as possible with acyclovir 400 mg three times daily, valacyclovir 1000 mg twice daily, or famciclovir 500 mg twice daily for 5 to 10 days [102]. Ideally, treatment should be continued until all mucocutaneous lesions are dry and healed. In some individuals, depending on the immune status and clinical features, higher or lower antiviral doses and durations may be more appropriate.

Patients requiring suppressive therapy because of frequent or exceptionally severe recurrence can be treated with acyclovir 400–800 mg two or three times daily, valacyclovir 500 mg twice daily or famciclovir 500 mg twice daily. These doses are higher than those used for non-HIV-infected patients with HSV, but are endorsed by the CDC [102]. As mentioned above, FDA-approved doses of valacyclovir should be used cautiously in patients with HIV infection because of the observation of TTP/HUS with high-dose (8 g/day) therapy.

Intravenous acyclovir should be reserved for patients with severe or extensive mucocutaneous HSV infection and for patients with viral dissemination, visceral organ infection (e.g. brain, esophagus, eye), or neurologic complications (atonic bladder, transverse myelitis). Intravenous therapy may also be indicated for patients who require antiviral chemotherapy but are unable to tolerate or absorb oral antiviral therapy because of nausea, dysphagia, or protracted diarrhea. The dose of intravenous acyclovir for patients with mucocutaneous HSV infection and normal renal function is 15 mg/kg per day in three divided doses [85]. Patients with life-threatening HSV infection (encephalitis, neonatal infection, disseminated infection), or visceral organ involvement (esophagitis, proctitis), should receive intravenous acyclovir 30 mg/kg per day in three divided doses [86]. Treatment should last for a minimum of 10 days, but longer therapy may be necessary if response to therapy is slow. As noted above, the dose of intravenous acyclovir should be adjusted in patients with impaired renal function (Table 34.4). Oral treatment with acyclovir, valacyclovir, or famciclovir can be substituted for intravenous acyclovir once the patient is ready for hospital discharge.

Because of their limited absorption, topical acyclovir and topical penciclovir are much less effective than either oral or intravenous therapy in the treatment of HSV infections in AIDS. Although topical therapy slightly decreases the duration of viral shedding in immunocompromised hosts with mucocutaneous HSV infection, these non-systemic therapies do not reduce new lesion formation or the risk of dissemination. There is no added benefit to combining topical therapy with either oral or intravenous antiviral therapy. Topical therapy has little, if any, usefulness in the clinical setting [81].

Systemic antiviral therapy should be continued until all mucocutaneous lesions have crusted or re-epithelialized. This may require longer treatment than the usual duration of therapy prescribed in the non-immunocompromised host, because HSV lesions may heal slowly in AIDS patients even with optimal antiviral therapy. If lesions do not heal despite standard therapy, repeat viral cultures should be obtained, high-dose oral therapy (e.g. acyclovir 800 mg five times daily, famciclovir 500 mg three times daily, valacyclovir 1 g three times daily, or intravenous acyclovir 30 mg/kg per day) should be given, and the possibility of drug-resistant HSV infection should be considered. If available, antiviral susceptibility testing should be performed in this setting to determine whether drug-resistant HSV infection is present. If antiviral testing is not available, patients who continue to have positive cultures for HSV and no evidence of clinical response despite high-dose intravenous acyclovir should be treated presumptively for drug-resistant infection with intravenous foscarnet.

Suppressive antiviral therapy for HSV infection

Many HIV-infected patients suffer from frequently recurring HSV infection or develop new HSV recurrences shortly after antiherpes therapy is discontinued. These patients can often be managed with suppressive antiviral therapy [85–87, 90, 91, 96, 98, 101, 103]. As mentioned above, the CDC states that patients requiring suppressive therapy should initially be treated with a regimen of oral acyclovir 400–800 mg two or three times daily, valacyclovir 1000 mg twice daily, or famciclovir 500 mg twice daily [102]. Increased daily dosage may be necessary to control recurrences, but gastrointestinal intolerance may limit the amount of drug that can be taken, Breakthrough recurrences that develop while the patient is receiving suppressive therapy may be controlled by increasing the daily suppressive dose. Breakthrough recurrences may or may not represent the emergence of drug-resistant strains [104]. Patients who demonstrate a good response to suppressive therapy at high doses may attempt a reduction in the daily suppressive dose [80, 105]. Some clinicians and patients choose to continue suppressive therapy longer than FDA recommendations in order to avoid development of symptomatic recurrences. Recurrences after discontinuation of antiviral suppression may be more severe than those experienced before starting suppression. Suppressive therapy has been used continuously for over 15 years without evidence of adverse reactions or cumulative toxicity. Studies have shown that the incidence of asymptomatic virus shedding is decreased while a patient is on acyclovir suppression [106]. Individuals maintained on long-term suppressive therapy should be cautioned, however, that recurrences will likely develop after discontinuation of therapy and that the first recurrence may be more severe than those previously experienced [78, 79, 83, 84]. In a study that evaluated immunocompetent, heterosexual, HSV discordant couples, the use of valacyclovir 500 mg daily as suppression reduced the risk of HSV transmission from the infected individual to the susceptible partner [107]. Acyclovir and famciclovir have also been shown to reduce asymptomatic HSV shedding and may also play a role in preventing transmission to sexual contacts [108]. Recent studies have shown that suppressive therapy for HSV results in a reduction in HIV RNA, suggesting a possible adjunctive role of treatment directed at HSV in patients co-infected with both HSV and HIV [109–112].

Management of drug-resistant HSV infection

Since the wide availability of HAART, drug-resistant HSV has become much less common. However, studies of acyclovir-resistant HSV infections in the pre-HAART era examined the utility of alternate antiviral agents and treatment regimens. Standard doses of intravenous or oral acyclovir have no clinical benefit if the HSV isolate is resistant to acyclovir (ID_{50} >3.0 µg/mL) *in vitro*. Most acyclovir-resistant strains isolated from patients with AIDS have been TK-deficient and are therefore also resistant to valacyclovir and famciclovir. These strains remain susceptible to foscarnet, which does not require phosphorylation for activity. Foscarnet is effective in the treatment of these TK-deficient, drug-resistant HSV infections, and foscarnet remains the treatment of choice in this setting [96–98]. The dosage of foscarnet used for the treatment of acyclovir-resistant HSV infections in AIDS patients is 40 mg/kg every 8 hours (with reduction in dose for renal dysfunction).

Continuous-infusion acyclovir therapy has been effective in a few AIDS patients with severe acyclovir-resistant HSV infection. Acyclovir has been administered at a dosage of 1.5–2.0 mg/kg/h for 6 weeks, and complete resolution of acyclovir-resistant HSV proctitis has been reported [113]. Other investigational agents for possible treatment of drug-resistant HSV infections include topical trifluridine [114], topical cidofovir gel [101], and intravenous cidofovir [99].

As with many opportunistic infections in AIDS patients, there is a high incidence of recurrent HSV disease after successful treatment for drug-resistant HSV. Some relapses in this setting have been due to drug-resistant strains, suggesting that these mutant viruses are capable of causing latency in the immunocompromised host. Chronic prophylaxis with daily acyclovir, valacyclovir, famciclovir, or foscarnet can be considered in patients who are treated successfully for drug-resistant HSV, although there are no data to confirm efficacy in this setting. Foscarnet-resistant strains of HSV have been reported, raising concerns over the possible selection for multi-drug-resistant HSV with suppressive therapy [100, 115].

VARICELLA ZOSTER VIRUS

Prior to widespread vaccination, primary VZV infection was typically a childhood illness, with attack rates exceeding 90% in susceptible household contacts [116]. Primary VZV is now much less common since many children are vaccinated against VZV, but primary infection still occurs. Most adults with AIDS have either been previously infected or vaccinated with VZV and (as with HSV) are not susceptible to primary infection.

HIV-infected patients develop recurrent VZV infection (zoster) more frequently than do age-matched immunocompetent hosts. A retrospective review of 300 HIV-infected patients with Kaposi's sarcoma revealed that 8% had at least one prior attack of zoster, an incidence seven times greater than expected by the age of the study group. Zoster also occurs with a higher-than-expected frequency in HIV-infected individuals who appear otherwise healthy. Additionally, some HIV-infected patients develop more than one episode of zoster in a relatively short period of time, an uncommon occurrence in immunocompetent hosts [117–121].

Primary infection varicella

Varicella in immunocompetent children is usually a benign illness. However, adults are more likely to develop complications during primary VZV infection. Viral dissemination to visceral organs occurs in up to one-third of immunocompetent adults with primary infection [116]. Although most HIV-infected adults have been previously infected or vaccinated against VZV and are not susceptible to primary infection [122], for those who are susceptible, a protracted and potentially life-threatening illness could follow [117].

Herpes zoster

Unlike primary VZV infection, herpes zoster is common in HIV-infected patients. The illness usually begins with radicular pain and is followed by a localized or segmental erythematous rash covering 1–3 dermatomes. Maculopapules develop in the dermatomal area, and the patient experiences increasing pain. The maculopapules progress to fluid-filled vesicles, and contiguous vesicles may become confluent, with true bullae formation. In most HIV-infected patients, the lesions remain confined to a dermatomal distribution and heal by crusting and re-epithelialization. Occasionally, however, widespread cutaneous or visceral dissemination may occur. Extensive cutaneous dissemination may appear identical to primary varicella. Visceral dissemination to lung, liver, or the CNS may produce a life-threatening illness [117–120, 123].

Reactivated infection involving the ophthalmic division of the trigeminal nerve often results in infection of the cornea (zoster ophthalmicus). The presence of vesicles on the tip of the nose is often associated with involvement of the eye. Although healing without sequelae may occur, untreated patients are at increased risk of developing anterior uveitis, corneal scarring, and permanent visual loss [104]. Acyclovir-resistant zoster is a rare complication, and has a peculiar dermatomal wart-like, non-healing appearance [124].

Complications

Complications of VZV infection are common in immunocompromised patients and may cause prolonged morbidity and death. Dissemination of virus to the lung, liver, and CNS has been associated with a mortality rate of 6–17%. Varicella pneumonia may occur during primary VZV infection or during reactivated infection with visceral dissemination in immunocompromised patients. Symptoms are variable. Many patients develop only mild respiratory symptoms, whereas others suffer from severe hypoxemia and succumb to respiratory failure. Radiographic abnormalities are usually out of proportion to the clinical findings, with diffuse nodular densities on chest radiograph and occasional pleural effusions [116, 125].

Encephalitis is a rare complication of VZV infection in AIDS patients but may occur with or without visceral dissemination. The illness begins 3–8 days after the onset of varicella or 1–2 weeks after the development of zoster, although occasionally AIDS patients have developed progressive neurologic disease caused by VZV up to 3 months after the onset of localized zoster [123]. Headache, vomiting, lethargy, and cerebellar symptoms (ataxia, tremors, dizziness) are prominent findings. Diagnosis based on clinical criteria alone can be difficult, because other CNS infections can present in a similar fashion. The diagnosis of VZV encephalitis is documented by finding VZV DNA by polymerase chain reaction or VZV antibody in CSF. Postherpetic neuralgia, defined as prolonged pain following resolution of the cutaneous lesions from zoster, can be severe and disabling [116, 126, 127].

Although post-herpetic neuralgia is a more common occurrence in elderly individuals with zoster, HIV-infected patients also may be at risk for this complication. Polyradiculopathy similar to that caused by CMV may rarely be due to VZV. In these cases, VZV may be isolated from CSF.

Management of VZV infection

HIV-infected patients who develop primary or VZV infection or herpes zoster should be treated promptly with an effective antiviral regimen (Table 34.8) [128]. Acyclovir, valacyclovir, and famciclovir are safe and effective in the treatment of patients with primary or recurrent VZV infection. Treatment should be started as soon as the diagnosis is made (preferably within 72 hours of rash onset), and should be continued until all the external lesions are dry and crusted (usually 7–10 days).

Table 34.8 Management of VZV infections in AIDS

CLINICAL PRESENTATION	TREATMENT
Primary infection (varicella)	Acyclovir, 30 mg/kg/day IV, or acyclovir 800 mg PO five times daily, or valacyclovir 1 g PO three times daily, or famciclovir 500 mg PO. three times daily
Recurrent infection (localized zoster)	Acyclovir 30 mg/kg/day IV, or acyclovir 800 mg PO five times daily, or valacyclovir 1 g PO three times daily, or famciclovir 500 mg PO three times daily
Recurrent infection, disseminated	Acyclovir 30 mg/kg/day IV
Severe infection caused by acyclovir-resistant VZV	Foscarnet 40 mg/kg IV three times daily (not FDA-approved)

Modified with permission from Drew WL, Buhles W, Erlich KS. Herpesvirus infections (cytomegalovirus, herpes simplex virus, varicella-zoster virus). How to use ganciclovir (DHPG) and acyclovir. Infect Dis Clin North Am 1988; 2:495–509.

Because VZV is less susceptible to acyclovir, valacyclovir, and famciclovir than HSV, the dosages of antiviral therapy used for treatment of VZV infections must be higher. Oral acyclovir in the dosage used to treat HSV does not produce serum drug levels high enough to inhibit VZV in tissue culture, and is unlikely to be effective in patients with active VZV infection. To treat VZV with oral acyclovir, a dose of 800 mg five times daily should be prescribed [125, 129–131]. This higher dose results in serum levels high enough to inhibit the growth of VZV in vitro, and this regimen has been shown to modestly decrease the incidence and severity of postherpetic neuralgia in non-immunocompromised patients [127, 132].

Valacyclovir and famciclovir (discussed in detail above) are also effective agents against VZV and are suitable for oral treatment of acute VZV infections. Because of their improved bioavailability, these drugs have the advantage of producing higher serum drug levels than that achieved with oral acyclovir. Treatment with valacyclovir 1 g three times daily [88], or famciclovir 500 mg three times daily [93, 133], reduces the severity of acute VZV infection and appears to reduce the severity and duration of postherpetic neuralgia [90, 126]. Although the favorable pharmacokinetics and higher serum drug levels achieved with these agents could be expected to offer a therapeutic advantage as compared with oral acyclovir, no comparative trials evaluating clinical outcome in HIV-infected patients have been reported.

As mentioned in the section on treatment of HSV, the possible association between valacyclovir and TTP/HUS in patients with advanced HIV disease must be kept in mind when prescribing valacyclovir. Although a cause-and-effect relationship has not been firmly established, the standard FDA-recommended dosages should not be exceeded [89].

Most HIV-infected patients with dermatomal zoster are not ill enough to require hospitalization, and can be treated on an outpatient basis with oral acyclovir, valacyclovir, or famciclovir. Intravenous acyclovir remains an available option, however, and has been shown to be effective in the treatment of patients with VZV infection. Treatment with intravenous acyclovir reduces the duration of viral shedding, new lesion formation, the incidence of dissemination, and mortality rates in immunocompromised hosts with VZV infection [129, 134]. Intravenous acyclovir should be prescribed to patients with disseminated disease or visceral organ involvement, and for those who are unable to tolerate oral therapy. The dosage for patients with VZV infection is 30 mg/kg per day in three divided doses (with dosage adjustments for renal dysfunction; see Table 34.4). Treatment should be continued for at least 7 days or until all external lesions are crusted. The decision whether to hospitalize a patient for intravenous acyclovir must be based on several factors, including the severity of the infection, the immune status of the host, and whether visceral or cutaneous dissemination has occurred.

Treatment with steroids to prevent post-herpetic neuralgia remains a controversial topic in a non-immunocompromised population, but recent studies have failed to document the efficacy of this practice [135, 136], although the general quality of life may be improved. Because of the potential for further immunosuppression and increasing the risk of VZV dissemination in HIV-infected patients, steroids should not be routinely prescribed for this indication in this population.

Treatment of drug-resistant VZV infection

Drug-resistant VZV has been reported in patients with AIDS. These patients may present with atypical-appearing cutaneous lesions that shed VZV intermittently despite ongoing high-dose antiviral therapy. All strains have been isolated from patients previously treated with acyclovir for recurrent VZV or HSV infection, and these strains may be resistant to acyclovir, valacyclovir, and famciclovir by deficiency of the enzyme thymidine kinase [137]. Foscarnet has been shown to be effective in small studies, but remains investigational for this purpose [124]. The intravenous dosage used has been 40 µg/kg three times daily.

Prevention of VZV infection

Varicella-zoster immune globulin (VZIG) is effective in preventing severe primary VZV infection in susceptible (i.e. seronegative) immunocompromised hosts if administered within 96 hours of the time of exposure. Care should be taken to ensure that an exposed individual is truly susceptible to infection (serologic testing could be performed if there is no history of chickenpox in an exposed individual) prior to administration of VZIG. VZIG is contraindicated in individuals with a history of prior chickenpox and in those who have serologic evidence of previous VZV infection. VZIG is not effective as treatment in individuals who present with acute VZV infection.

Effective vaccines are licensed in the USA for prevention of primary VZV infection (varicella) and recurrent disease (zoster) in non-immunocompromised hosts [138–140]. Both vaccines contain the live, attenuated OKA strain of VZV, although the zoster vaccine contains higher titers of virus than that found in the varicella vaccine. The efficacy and safety of these vaccines in HIV-infected patients has not been studied, and current CDC guidelines recommend the varicella vaccine for HIV-infected children greater than or equal to 8 years of age who have CD4 count ≥ 200 cells/ mm^3 (percentage > 15%) and no evidence of varicella immunity. Vaccinating younger children is also suggested by many authorities. Vaccinating HIV-infected adults to protect against herpes zoster should be done with caution, since the zoster vaccine is not licensed for use in HIV-infected patients and there is the theoretical risk of dissemination in immunocompromised hosts. A small number of patients receiving the varicella vaccine have developed a varicella-like rash after administration [141], and this rash contains live virus that is transmissible. HIV-infected patients who receive either vaccine and develop a varicella-like rash following vaccination should be treated with one of the effective antiviral drugs discussed above. Because the vaccine strain produces latency after administration, vaccinated individuals remain at risk to develop zoster later in life [138, 139, 142].

CONCLUSION

Herpesvirus (CMV, HSV, VZV) infections are common in AIDS patients and often exist in a chronic or progressive form. Oral valganciclovir prophylaxis can reduce the risk of developing CMV disease. CMV retinitis occurs in up to 40% of AIDS patients and can be treated effectively with ganciclovir, valganciclovir, or foscarnet. Perianal ulcers, proctitis, and other clinical syndromes caused by HSV can be treated effectively with acyclovir, valacyclovir, or famciclovir. These drugs can be administered daily to prevent HSV recurrences. Herpes zoster in a young adult may be the first indication of immune deficiency resulting from HIV. Because VZV is less susceptible to antiviral drugs than HSV, higher doses of acyclovir, valacyclovir, or famciclovir are required to achieve inhibitory blood levels. HSV and VZV resistant to acyclovir and related drugs are usually susceptible to foscarnet.

REFERENCES

[1] O'Sullivan C, Drew WL, McMullen D, et al. Decrease of cytomegalovirus replication in human immunodeficiency virus infected patients after treatment with highly active antiretroviral therapy. J Infect Dis 1999;180:847–9.

[2] Heiden D, Ford N, Wilson D, et al. Cytomegalovirus retinitis: the neglected disease of the AIDS pandemic. PLoS Med 2007;4(12): e334.

[3] Spector SA, Wong R, Hsia K, et al. Plasma cytomegalovirus (CMV) DNA load predicts CMV disease and survival in AIDS patients. J Clin Invest 1998;101:497.

[4] Felsenstein D, D'Amico DJ, Hirsch MS, et al. Treatment of cytomegalovirus retinitis with 9-[2-hydroxy1-(hydroxymethyl) ethoxymethyl]guanine. Ann Intern Med 1985;103:377.

[5] Palestine AG, Polis MA, DeSmet MD, et al. A randomized, controlled trial of foscarnet in the treatment of cytomegalovirus retinitis in patients with AIDS. Ann Intern Med 1991;115:665.

[6] Spector SA, Weingeist T, Pollard RB, et al. A randomized, controlled study of intravenous ganciclovir therapy for cytomegalovirus peripheral retinitis in patients with AIDS. J Infect Dis 1993;168:557.

[7] Jabs D and the Studies of Ocular Complications of AIDS Research Group, in collaboration with the AIDS Clinical Trials Group. Mortality in patients with the acquired immunodeficiency syndrome treated with either foscarnet or ganciclovir for cytomegalovirus retinitis. N Engl J Med 1992;326:213.

[8] Morgello S, Cho E, Nielsen S, et al. Cytomegalovirus encephalitis in patients with acquired immunodeficiency syndrome: an autopsy study of 30 cases and review of literature. Hum Pathol 1987;18:289.

[9] Holland NR, Power C, Mathews VP, et al. Cytomegalovirus encephalitis in AIDS. Neurology 1994;44:507.

[10] Drew WL, Mintz L, Miner RC, et al. Prevalence of cytomegalovirus infection in homosexual men. J Infect Dis 1981;143:188.

[11] Fiala M, Singer EJ, Graves MC, et al. AIDS dementia complex complicated by cytomegalovirus encephalopathy. J Neurol 1993;240:223.

[12] Vinters HV, Kwok MK, Ho HW, et al. Cytomegalovirus in the nervous system of patients with the acquired immune deficiency syndrome. Brain 1989;112:245.

[13] Casareale D, Fiala M, Chang CM, et al. Cytomegalovirus enhances lysis of HIV infected T lymphoblasts. Int J Cancer 1989;44:124.

[14] Anand R, Nightingale D, Fish RH, et al. Control of cytomegalovirus retinitis using sustained release of intraocular ganciclovir. Arch Ophthalmol 1993;111:223.

[15] Walot I, Miller BL, Chang L, et al. Neuroimaging findings in patients with AIDS. Clin Infect Dis 1996;22:906.

[16] Clough LA, Clough JA, Maciunsas RJ, et al. Diagnosing CNS mass lesions in patients with AIDS. AIDS Reader 1997;7:83.

[17] Small PM, McPhaul LW, Sooy CD, et al. Cytomegalovirus infection of the laryngeal nerve presenting as hoarseness in patients with acquired immunodeficiency syndrome. Am J Med 1989;86:108.

[18] Fuller GN, Jacobs JM, Guiloff RJ. Axonal atrophy in the painful peripheral neuropathy in AIDS. Acta Neuropathol 1990;81:198.

[19] Dieterich DT, Kotler DP, Busch DF. Ganciclovir treatment of cytomegalovirus colitis in AIDS: a randomized, double-blind, placebo-controlled multicenter study. J Infect Dis 1993;167:278.

[20] Whitley RJ, Jacobson MA, Friedberg DN, et al. Guidelines for the treatment of cytomegalovirus diseases in patients with AIDS in the era of potent antiretroviral therapy. Arch Intern Med 1998;158:957.

[21] Emanuel D, Cunningham I, Jules-Elysee K, et al. Cytomegalovirus pneumonia after bone-marrow transplantation successfully treated with the combination of ganciclovir and high-dose intravenous immune globulin. Ann Intern Med 1988;109:777.

[22] Reed EC, Bowden RA, Dandliker PS, et al. Treatment of cytomegalovirus pneumonia with ganciclovir and intravenous cytomegalovirus immunoglobulin in patients with bone marrow transplants. Ann Intern Med 1988;109:783.

[23] Shepp DH, Dandliker PS, de Miranda P, et al., Activity of 9-[2-hydroxy-1-(hydroxymethyl) ethoxymethyl]guanine in the treatment of cytomegalovirus pneumonia. Ann Intern Med 1985;103:368.

[24] Sullivan V, Taliarico CL, Stanat SC, et al. A protein kinase homologue controls phosphorylation of ganciclovir in human cytomegalovirus-infected cells. Nature 1992;358:162.

[25] Martin DF, Sierra-Madero J, Walmsley S, et al. for the Valganciclovir Study Group. A controlled trial of valganciclovir as induction therapy for cytomegalovirus. N Engl J Med 2002;346:1119–26.

[26] Musch DC, Martin DF, Gordon JF, et al. Treatment of cytomegalovirus retinitis with a sustained-release ganciclovir implant. N Engl J Med 1997;337:83.

[27] Drew WL, Ives D, Lalezari JP, et al. Oral ganciclovir as maintenance treatment for cytomegalovirus retinitis in patients with AIDS. N Engl J Med 1995;333:615.

[28] Wohl DA, Kendall MA, Owens S, et al. The safety of discontinuation of maintenance therapy for cytomegalovirus (CMV) retinitis and incidence of immune recovery uveitis following potent antiretroviral therapy. HIV Clin Trials 2005;6:136–46.

[29] Cantrill HL, Henry K, Melroe H, et al. Treatment of cytomegalovirus retinitis with intravitreal ganciclovir: long-term results. Ophthalmology 1989;96:367.

[30] Martin DF, Parks DJ, Mellow D, et al. Treatment of cytomegalovirus retinitis with an intraocular sustained-release ganciclovir implant. Arch Ophthalmol 1994;112:1531.

[31] Sanborn GE, Anand R, Torti RE, et al. Sustained-release ganciclovir therapy for treatment of cytomegalovirus retinitis. Arch Ophthalmol 1992;110:188.

[32] Erice A, Chou S, Biron K, et al. Progressive disease due to ganciclovir-resistant cytomegalovirus in immunocompromised patients. N Engl J Med 1989;320:289.

[33] Drew WL, Miner RC, Busch DF, et al. Prevalence of resistance in patients receiving ganciclovir for serious cytomegalovirus infection. J Infect Dis 1991;163:716.

[34] Chou S, Guentzel S, Michels KR, et al. Frequency of UL97 phosphotransferase mutations related to ganciclovir resistance in clinical cytomegalovirus isolates. J Infect Dis 1995;172:239–42.

[35] Jacobson MA, Drew WL, Feinberg J, et al. Foscarnet therapy for ganciclovir-resistant cytomegalovirus retinitis in patients with AIDS. J Infect Dis 1991;163:1348.

[36] Chou S, Lurain NS, Thompson KD, et al. Viral DNA polymerase mutations associated with drug resistance in human cytomegalovirus. J Infect Dis 2003;188:32–9.

[37] Spector SA, McKinley GF, Lalezari JP, et al. Oral ganciclovir for the prevention of cytomegalovirus disease in persons with AIDS. N Engl J Med 1996;334:1491.

[38] Chrisp P, Clissold SP. Foscarnet: a review of its antiviral activity, pharmacokinetic properties and therapeutic use in immunocompromised patients with cytomegalovirus retinitis. Drugs 1991;41:104.

[39] Jacobson MA, Causey D, Polsky B. A dose-ranging study of daily maintenance intravenous foscarnet therapy for cytomegalovirus retinitis in AIDS. J Infect Dis 1993;168:444.

[40] Studies of Ocular Complications of AIDS Research Group in Collaboration with the AIDS Clinical Trials Group . Combination foscarnet and ganciclovir therapy vs monotherapy for the treatment of relapsed cytomegalovirus retinitis in patients with AIDS: The Cytomegalovirus Retreatment Trial. Arch Ophthalmol 1996;114:23.

[41] Lalezari JP, Drew WL, Glutzer E, et al. (S)-I-[3-hydroxy- 2-(phosphonylmethoxy)propyl]-cytosine (cidofovir): results of a Phase I/II study of a novel antiviral nucleotide analogue. J Infect Dis 1995;171:788.

[42] Kosobucki BR, Goldberg DE, Bessho K, et al. Valganciclovir therapy for immune recovery uveitis complicated by macular edema. Am J Ophthalmol 2004;137:636–8.

[43] Corey L, Adams HG, Brown ZA, et al. Genital herpes simplex virus infections: clinical manifestations, course, and complications. Ann Intern Med 1983;98:958.

[44] Corey L, Homes KK. Genital herpes simplex virus infections: current concepts in diagnosis, therapy, and prevention. Ann Intern Med 1983;98:973.

[45] Corey L, Spear PG. Infections with herpes simplex viruses (parts 1 and 2). N Engl J Med 1986;314 (686):749.

[46] Fleming DT, McQuillan GM, Johnson RE, et al. Herpes simplex virus type 2 in the United States, 1976 to 1995. N Engl J Med 1997;337:1105.

[47] Johnson RE, Nahmias AJ, Magder LS, et al. A seroepidemiologic survey of the prevalence of herpes simplex virus type 2 infection in the United States. N Engl J Med 1989;321:7.

[48] Nahmias AJ, Keyserling H, Lee FK. Herpes simplex viruses 1 and 2. In: Evans A, editor. Viral Infections of Humans: Epidemiology and Control. 3rd ed. New York: Plenum Press; 1989. p. 393.

[49] Reynolds SJ, Risbud AR, Shepherd ME, et al. Recent herpes simplex virus type 2 infection and the risk of human immunodeficiency virus type 1 acquisition in India. J Infect Dis 2003;187:1509–12.

[50] Bartlett JG. Recent developments in the management of herpes simplex Virus Infection in HIV-infected persons. Clin Infect Dis 2004;39:237–9.

[51] Quinnan GV, Masur H, Rook AH, et al. Herpes simplex infections in the acquired immune deficiency syndrome. JAMA 1984;252:72.

[52] Safrin S, Arvin A, Mills J, et al. Comparison of the Western immunoblot assay and a glycoprotein G enzyme immunoassay for detection of serum antibodies to herpes simplex virus type 2 in patients with AIDS. J Clin Microbiol 1992;30:1312.

[53] Siegel D, Golden E, Washington E, et al. Prevalence and correlates of herpes simplex infections: the population-based AIDS in Multiethnic Neighborhoods study. JAMA 1992;268:1702.

[54] Stewart JA, Reef SE, Pellett PE, et al. Herpesvirus infections in persons infected with human immunodeficiency virus. Clin Infect Dis 1995;21(Suppl.): S114.

[55] Spruance SI, Overall JC, Kern ER, et al. The natural history of recurrent herpes simplex labialis: implications for antiviral therapy. N Engl J Med 1977;297:68.

[56] Straus SE, Smith HA, Brickman C, et al. Acyclovir for chronic mucocutaneous herpes simplex virus infection in immunosuppressed patients. Ann Intern Med 1982;96:270.

[57] Whitley RJ, Levin M, Barton N, et al. Infections caused by herpes simplex virus in the immunocompromised host: natural history and topical acyclovir therapy. J Infect Dis 1984;150:323.

[58] Brock BV, Selke S, Benedetti J, et al. Frequency of asymptomatic shedding of herpes simplex virus in women with genital herpes. JAMA 1990;263:418.

[59] Koelle DM, Benedetti J, Langenberg A, et al. Asymptomatic reactivation of herpes simplex virus in women after the first episode of genital herpes. Ann Intern Med 1992;116:433.

[60] Augenbraun M, Feldman J, Chirgwin K, et al. Increased genital shedding of herpes simplex virus type 2 in HIV-seropositive women. Ann Intern Med 1995;123:845.

[61] Wald A, Zeh J, Selke S, et al. Virologic characteristics of subclinical and symptomatic genital herpes infections. N Engl J Med 1995;333:770.

[62] Goodell SE, Quinn TC, Mkrtichian F, et al. Herpes simplex proctitis in homosexual men: clinical, sigmoidoscopic, and histopathologic features. N Engl J Med 1983;308:868.

[63] Siegel FP, Lopez C, Hammer BS, et al. Severe acquired immunodeficiency in male homosexuals, manifested by chronic perianal ulcerative herpes simplex lesions. N Engl J Med 1981;305:1439.

[64] Farthing CF, Brown SE, Staughton RCD. A Colour Atlas of AIDS and HIV Disease Slide Set. 2nd ed. London: Mosby; 1989.

[65] Genereau T, Lortholary O, Bouchaud O, et al. Herpes simplex esophagitis in patients with AIDS: report of 34 cases. Clin Infect Dis 1996;22:926.

[66] Dix RD, Bredesen DE, Davis RL, et al. Herpesvirus neurological diseases associated with AIDS: recovery of viruses from central nervous system (CNS) tissues, peripheral nerve, and cerebrospinal fluid (CSF). Atlanta: International Conference on AIDS; 1985.

[67] Dix RD, Bredesen DE, Erlich KS, et al. Recovery of herpes-viruses from cerebrospinal fluid of immunodeficient homosexual men. Ann Neurol 1985;18:611.

[68] Dix RD, Waitzman DM, Follansbee S, et al. Herpes simplex virus type 2 encephalitis in two homosexual men with persistent adenopathy. Ann Neurol 1985;17:203.

[69] Lakeman FD, Whitley RJ, and the National Institute of Allergy and Infectious Diseases Collaborative Antiviral Study Group. Diagnosis of herpes simplex encephalitis: application of polymerase chain reaction to cerebrospinal fluid from brain-biopsied patients and correlation with disease. J Infect Dis 1995;171:857.

[70] Landry ML. False-positive polymerase chain reaction results in the diagnosis of herpes simplex encephalitis. J Infect Dis 1995;172:1641.

[71] Nahmias AJ, Whitley RD, Visintine AN, et al. Herpes simplex virus type 2 encephalitis: laboratory evaluations and their diagnostic significance. J Infect Dis 1982;146:829.

[72] Englund JA, Zimmerman ME, Swierkosz EM, et al. Herpes simplex virus resistant to acyclovir: a study in a tertiary care center. Ann Intern Med 1990;112:416.

[73] Marks GL, Nolan PE, Erlich KS, et al. Mucocutaneous dissemination of acyclovir-resistant herpes simplex virus in a patient with AIDS. Rev Infect Dis 1989;11:474.

[74] Erlich KS, Mills J, Chatis P, et al. Acyclovir-resistant herpes simplex virus infections in patients with the acquired immunodeficiency syndrome. N Engl J Med 1989;320:293.

[75] Kost RG, Hill EL, Tigges M, et al. Recurrent acyclovir-resistant genital herpes in an immunocompetent patient. N Engl J Med 1993;329:1777.

[76] Gateley A, Gander RM, Johnson PC, et al. Herpes simplex type 2 meningoencephalitis resistant to acyclovir in a patient with AIDS. J Infect Dis 1990;161:711.

[77] Whitley RJ, Gnann JW. Acyclovir: a decade later. N Engl J Med 1993;327:782.

[78] Douglas JM, Critchlow C, Benedetti J, et al. Double blind study of oral acyclovir for suppression of recurrences of genital herpes simplex virus infection. N Engl J Med 1984;310:1551.

[79] Fife KH, Crumpacker CS, Mertz CJ, et al. Recurrence and resistance patterns of herpes simplex virus following cessation of 6 years of chronic suppression with acyclovir. J Infect Dis 1994;169:1338.

[80] Kaplowitz LG, Baker D, Gelb L, et al. Prolonged continuous acyclovir treatment of normal adults with frequently recurring genital herpes simplex virus infection. JAMA 1991;265:747.

[81] Kinghorn GR, Abeywickreme I, Jeavons M, et al. Efficacy of combined treatment with oral and topical acyclovir in first episode genital herpes. Genitourin Med 1986;62:186.

[82] Shepp DH, Newton BA, Dandliker PS, et al. Oral acyclovir therapy for mucocutaneous herpes simplex virus infections in immunocompromised marrow transplant recipients. Ann Intern Med 1985;102:783.

[83] Straus SE, Seidlin M, Takiff H, et al. Oral acyclovir to suppress recurring herpes simplex virus infections in immunodeficient patients. Ann Intern Med 1984;100:522.

[84] Wade JC, Newton B, Flournoy N, et al. Oral acyclovir for prevention of herpes simplex virus reactivation after marrow transplantation. Ann Intern Med 1984;100:823.

[85] Wade JC, Newton B, McLaren C, et al. Intravenous acyclovir to treat mucocutaneous herpes simplex virus infection after marrow transplantation. Ann Intern Med 1982;96:265.

[86] Whitley RJ, Alford CA, Hirsch MS, et al. Vidarabine versus acyclovir therapy in herpes simplex encephalitis. N Engl J Med 1986;314:144.

[87] Spruance SL, Tyring SK, DeGregorio B, et al. A large-scale, placebo-controlled, dose-ranging trial of peroral valacyclovir for episodic treatment of recurrent herpes genitalis. Arch Intern Med 1996;156:1729.

[88] Beutner KR, Friedman DJ, Forszpaniak C, et al. Valaciclovir compared with acyclovir for improved therapy for herpes zoster in immunocompetent adults. Antimicrob Agents Chemother 1995;39:1546.

[89] Centers for Disease Control and Prevention. Guidelines for treatment of sexually transmitted diseases. MMWR 1998;47:20.

[90] Gnann JW. New antivirals with activity against varicella-zoster virus. Ann Neurol 1994;34:S69.

[91] Mertz GJ, Loveless MO, Levin MJ, et al. Oral famciclovir for suppression of recurrent genital herpes simplex virus infection in women: a multicenter, double-blind, placebo-controlled trial. Arch Intern Med 1997;157:343.

[92] Sacks SL, Aoki FY, Diaz-Mitoma F, et al. Patient-initiated, twice-daily oral famciclovir for early recurrent genital herpes: a randomized, double-blind multicenter trial. JAMA 1996;276:44.

[93] Saltzman R, Jurewicz R, Boon R. Safety of famciclovir in patients with herpes zoster and genital herpes. Antimicrob Agents Chemother 1994;2454:38.

[94] Schacker T, Hu H, Koelle DM, et al. Famciclovir for the suppression of symptomatic and asymptomatic herpes simplex virus reactivation in HIV-infected persons: A double-blind, placebo-controlled trial. Ann Intern Med 1998;128:21.

[95] Spruance SL, Rea TL, Thoming C, et al. Penciclovir cream for the treatment of herpes simplex labialis: a randomized, multicenter, double-blind, placebo controlled trial. JAMA 1997;277:1374.

[96] Safrin S, Crumpacker C, Chatis P, et al. A controlled trial comparing foscarnet with vidarabine for acyclovir-resistant mucocutaneous herpes simplex in the acquired immunodeficiency syndrome. N Engl J Med 1991;325:551.

[97] Chatis PA, Miller CH, Schrager LE, et al. Successful treatment with foscarnet of an acyclovir resistant mucocutaneous infection with herpes simplex virus in a patient with acquired immunodeficiency syndrome. N Engl J Med 1989;320:297.

[98] Erlich KS, Jacobson MA, Koehler JE, et al. Foscarnet therapy for severe acyclovir-resistant herpes simplex virus type-2 infections in patients with the acquired immunodeficiency syndrome

(AIDS): An uncontrolled trial. Ann Intern Med 1989;110:710.

[99] Lalezari JP, Drew WL, Glutzer E, et al. Treatment with intravenous (S)-1[3-hydroxy-2-(phosphonylmethoxy)propyl)-cytosine of acyclovir-resistant mucocutaneous infection with herpes simplex virus in a patient with AIDS. J Infect Dis 1994;170:570.

[100] Snoeck R, Andrei G, Gerard M, et al. Successful treatment of progressive mucocutaneous infection due to acyclovir- and foscarnet-resistant herpes simplex virus with (S)-1-(3-hydroxy-2-phosphonylmethoxypropyl) cytosine (HPMPC). J Infect Dis 1994;18:570.

[101] Lalezari J, Schacker T, Feinberg J, et al. A randomized, double-blind placebo-controlled trial of cidofovir gel for the treatment of acyclovir-unresponsive mucocutaneous herpes simplex virus infection in patients with AIDS. J Infect Dis 1997;176:892.

[102] Centers for Disease Control and Prevention. Sexually Transmitted Disease Treatment Guidelines, 2010. MMWR Morb Mortal Wkly Rep 2010;59.

[103] DeJesus E, Wald A, Warren T, et al. Valacyclovir for the suppression of recurrent genital herpes in human immunodeficiency virus-infected subjects. J Infect Dis 2003;188:1009–16.

[104] Nusinoff-Lehrman S, Douglas JM, Corey L, et al. Recurrent genital herpes and suppressive oral acyclovir therapy: relation between clinical outcome and in vitro sensitivity. Ann Intern Med 1986;104:786.

[105] Goldberg LH, Kaufman R, Kurtz TO, et al. Long-term suppression of recurrent genital herpes with acyclovir: a 5-year benchmark study. Arch Derm 1993;129:582.

[106] Wald A, Zeh J, Barnum G, et al. Suppression of subclinical shedding of herpes simplex virus type 2 with acyclovir. Ann Intern Med 1996;124:8.

[107] Corey L, Wald AA, Patel R, et al. Once daily valacyclovir to reduce the risk of transmission of genital

herpes. N Engl J Med 2004;350:11–20.

[108] Gupta R, Wald A, Krantz E, et al. Valacyclovir and acyclovir for suppression of shedding of herpes simplex virus in the genital tract. J Infect Dis 2004;190:1374–81.

[109] Nagot N, Ouedraogo A, Foulongne V, et al. Reduction of HIV-1 RNA levels with therapy to suppress herpes simplex virus. N Engl J Med 2007;356:790–9.

[110] Corey L. Herpes simplex virus type 2 and HIV-1: the dialogue between the 2 organisms continues. J Infect Dis 2007;195:1242–4.

[111] Corey L, Wald A, Celum C, Quinn TC. The effects of herpes simplex virus-2 on HIV-1 acquisition and transmission: a review of two overlapping epidemics. J Acquir Immun Defic Syndr 2004;35:435–45.

[112] Kapiga SH, Sam NE, Bang H, et al. The role of herpes simplex virus type 2 and other genital infections in the acquisition of HIV-1 among high-risk women in northern Tanzania. J Infect Dis 2007;195:1260–9.

[113] Engel JP, Englund JA, Fletcher CV, et al. Treatment of resistant herpes simplex virus with continuous-infusion acyclovir. JAMA 1990;263:1662.

[114] Kessler HA, Hurwitz S, Farthing C, et al. Pilot study of topical trifluridine for the treatment of acyclovir resistant mucocutaneous herpes simplex disease in patients with AIDS (ACTG 172). J Acquir Immune Defic Syndr Hum Retrovirol 1996;12:147.

[115] Safrin S, Kemmerly S, Plotkin B, et al. Foscarnet resistant herpes simplex virus infection in patients with AIDS. J Infect Dis 1994;169:193.

[116] Weller TH. Varicella and herpes zoster: changing concepts of the natural history, control, and importance of a not-so-benign virus (parts 1 and 2). N Engl J Med 1983;309(1362):1434.

[117] Buchbinder SP, Katz MH, Hessol NA, et al. Herpes zoster and human immunodeficiency virus infection. J Infect Dis 1992;166:1153.

[118] Cole EL, Meisler DM, Calabrese LH, et al. Herpes zoster ophthalmicus and acquired immune deficiency syndrome. Arch Ophthalmol 1984;102:1027.

[119] Cone LA, Schiffman HA. Herpes zoster and the acquired immunodeficiency syndrome. Ann Intern Med 1984;100:462.

[120] Friedman-Kien AE, Lafleur FL, Gendler E, et al. Herpes zoster: a possible early clinical sign for development of acquired immunodeficiency syndrome in high-risk individuals. J Am Acad Derm 1986;14:1023.

[121] Gershon AA, Mervish N, LaRussa P, et al. Varicella-zoster virus infection in children with underlying human immunodeficiency virus infection. J Infect Dis 1997;176:1496.

[122] Rogers MF, Morens DM, Stewart JA, et al. National case-control study of Kaposi's sarcoma and *Pneumocystis carinii* pneumonia in homosexual men: Part 2, Laboratory results. Ann Intern Med 1983;99:151.

[123] Ryder JW, Croen K, Kleinschmidt-DeMasters BK, et al. Progressive encephalitis three months after resolution of cutaneous zoster in a patient with AIDS. Ann Neurol 1986;19:182.

[124] Safrin S, Berger TG, Gilson I, et al. Foscarnet therapy in five patients with AIDS and acyclovir-resistant varicella-zoster virus infection. Ann Intern Med 1991;115:19.

[125] Wallace MR, Katz MH, Hessol NA, et al. Treatment of adult varicella with oral acyclovir: a randomized, placebo-controlled trial. Ann Intern Med 1992;117:358.

[126] Gilden DH. Herpes zoster with postherpetic neuralgia-persisting pain and frustration. N Engl J Med 1994;330:932.

[127] Huff JC, Drucker LL, Clemmer A, et al. Effect of oral acyclovir on pain resolution in herpes zoster: a reanalysis. J Med Virol 1993;1 (Suppl.):93.

[128] Drew WL, Buhles W, Erlich KS. Herpesvirus infections (cytomegalovirus, herpes simplex virus, varicella-zoster virus). How to use ganciclovir (DHPG) and acyclovir. Infect Dis Clin North Am 1988;2:495–509.

[129] Balfour HH, Bean B, Laskin OL, et al. Acyclovir halts progression of herpes zoster in immunocompromised patients. N Engl J Med 1983;308:1448.

[130] Laskin O. Acyclovir: Pharmacology and clinical experience. Arch Intern Med 1984;144:1241.

[131] Haake DA, Zakowski PC, Haake DL, et al. Early treatment with acyclovir for varicella pneumonia in otherwise healthy adults: retrospective controlled study and review. Rev Infect Dis 1990;12:788.

[132] Huff JC, Bean B, Balfour HH, et al. Therapy of herpes zoster with oral acyclovir. Am J Med 1988;85 (Suppl.):84.

[133] Tyring S, Barbarash RA, Nahlik JE, et al. Famciclovir for the treatment of acute herpes zoster: effects on acute disease and postherpetic neuralgia. A randomized, double blind, placebo controlled trial. Ann Intern Med 1995;123:89.

[134] Shepp DH, Dandliker PS, Meyers JD. Treatment of varicella zoster virus infection in severely immunocompromised patients. N Engl J Med 1986;314:208.

[135] Whitley RJ, Weiss H, Gnann JW, et al. Acyclovir with and without prednisone for the treatment of herpes zoster: a randomized, placebo controlled trial. Ann Intern Med 1996;125:376.

[136] Wood MJ, Johnson RW, McKendrick MW, et al. A randomized trial of acyclovir for 7 days or 21 days with and without prednisolone for treatment of acute herpes zoster. N Engl J Med 1994;330:896.

[137] Jacobson MA, Berger TG, Fikrig S, et al. Acyclovir (ACV)-resistant varicella zoster virus (VZV) infection following chronic oral ACV therapy in patients with AIDS. Ann Intern Med 1990;112:187.

[138] Gershon AA, Steinberg SP, LaRussa P, et al. Immunization of healthy adults with live attenuated varicella vaccine. J Infect Dis 1988;158:132.

[139] White CJ, Kuter BJ, Hidebrand CS, et al. Varicella vaccine (VARIVAX) in healthy children and adolescents: results from clinical trials, 1987 to 1989. Pediatrics 1991;87:604.

[140] Oxman MN, Levin MJ, Johnson GR, et al. a Vaccine to prevent herpes zoster and postherpetic neuralgia in older adults. N Engl J Med 2005;352:2271–84.

[141] LaRussa P, Steinberg S, Meurice F, et al. Transmission of vaccine strain varicella-zoster virus from a healthy adult with vaccine-associated rash to susceptible household contacts. J Infect Dis 1997;176:1072.

[142] Hardy I, Gershon AA, Steinberg SP, et al. The incidence of zoster after immunization with live attenuated varicella vaccine. N Engl J Med 1991;325:1545.

Chapter | 35 |

HIV-associated malignancies

Ronald T. Mitsuyasu

INTRODUCTION

Malignancies have been a well-recognized manifestation of AIDS since the beginning of the epidemic. The increased incidence of aggressive B-cell non-Hodgkin's lymphoma and Kaposi's sarcoma led to one of the first description of this new disease in 1981 [1, 2]. Cancers considered to be AIDS-defining by the US Centers for Disease Control and Prevention (CDC) are listed in Table 35.1, and include Kaposi's sarcoma (KS), aggressive B-cell non-Hodgkin's lymphoma (NHL), primary CNS lymphoma (PCNSL), and invasive squamous carcinoma of the cervix. The relative risks of these neoplasms are listed, along with several other malignancies for which there appears to be a relationship with HIV disease based on the higher relative risk among HIV-infected patients. It is important to recognize, however, that while HIV-induced immunodeficiency clearly plays a role in the development of these cancers, many are also associated with oncogenic viruses. Some, such as squamous conjunctival cancer and leiomyosarcoma, are less commonly seen in Western countries or are seen in certain subpopulations, such as in children.

It has been suggested that loss of immune surveillance may be the most important factor in the pathogenesis of neoplasms with viral etiologies. The listing of suspected viral pathogens associated with cancers in HIV (Table 35.1) would suggest that this hypothesis is correct, although the exact mechanism by which these viruses give rise to neoplasms has not been fully elucidated.

More recently, the incidence of non-AIDS-defining cancers (NADCs) has increased in the HIV-infected population, while the incidence of AIDS-defining cancers (ADCs), specifically KS and NHL, has decreased. These NADCs now account for a significant proportion of deaths and morbidity in HIV in the era of highly active antiretroviral therapies (HAART, or ART).

EPIDEMIOLOGY OF HIV-ASSOCIATED MALIGNANCIES

The introduction of HAART in 1996 has not only extended life and reduced the incidence of AIDS in HIV but has also resulted in a change in the spectrum of HIV-associated malignancies. Several large epidemiologic studies have demonstrated a change in the distribution of cancers seen in HIV in Western countries with widespread use of ART [3–6]. An assessment by the NCI Cancer Epidemiology and Genetics Branch using data from the US cancer and HIV match registry identified 472,378 individuals with HIV and cancer from 1980 to 2006 [7]. Using non-parametric competing-risk methods, the cumulative incidence of cancer was estimated across 3 calendar periods (1980–9, 1990–5, and 1996–2006). Measured at 5 years after AIDS onset, the cumulative incidence of ADC declined from 18% in 1980–9, to 11% in 1990–5, to 4.2% in 1996–2006. This decline was seen for both KS and for NHL. The cumulative incidence of NADC increased during this same time, with the incidence of specific cancers such as anal cancer, Hodgkin's lymphoma, and liver cancer increasing steadily over this period. The incidence of lung cancer increased initially from 0.14 to 0.32% and has remained stable in the post-HAART era.

Possible reasons for this change in cancer distribution may include: the reversal of HIV-induced declines in CD4 count with ART, resulting in decreased incidence of KS and NHL, which are more closely associated with immunosuppresion; the enhanced longevity of individuals living with immune impairment; the continued exposure to carcinogenic substances such as tobacco and alcohol; decreased immune surveillance and increased immune activation; and perhaps increased susceptibility

Table 35.1 Relative risks and viral associations for neoplasms associated with HIV infection

NEOPLASM	RELATIVE RISK	VIRAL ASSOCIATION
Kaposi's sarcoma	>10,000	KSHV
B-cell NHL	100–400	EBV, KSHV
Cervical carcinoma	2.9–4	HPV
Anal carcinoma	14	HPV
Hodgkins' lymphoma	7–11	EBV
Leiomyosarcoma	10,000	EBV
Hepatoma	6–9	HBV, HCV
Squamous conjunctiva	13	HPV
Oral and head/neck squamous carcinoma	2–6	HPV
Merkle cell carcinoma	2.3–13.4	MCV

KSHV, Kaposi's sarcoma-associated herpes virus, also known as human herpesvirus-8 (HHV-8); EBV, Epstein–Barr virus; HPV, human papilloma virus; HBV, hepatitis B virus; HCV, hepatitis C virus; MCV, Merkle cell virus.

to cancer-inducing genetic mutations or to environmental toxins.

LYMPHOPROLIFERATIVE DISEASE

Non-Hodgkin's lymphoma

NHL remains one of the most common AIDS-defining conditions, occurring in approximately 16% of all new cases of AIDS [8]. All age groups and all groups at risk for HIV infection are equally likely to develop lymphoma. Systemic NHL, PCNSL, and primary effusion lymphoma (PEL) have all been described in patients with HIV infection.

Systemic NHL

Although the risk of lymphoma has decreased significantly in patients treated with ART, this decline has been smaller than that seen with KS or various opportunistic infections, resulting in a relative increase in the occurrence of lymphoma as the initial AIDS-defining illness.

Most AIDS-related lymphomas are of high-grade B-cell type. Approximately 60% are immunoblastic lymphomas or small non-cleaved lymphomas, including Burkitt or non-Burkitt

types. About 30% of patients have intermediate-grade, diffuse, large, B-cell lymphoma (DLBCL), and 10% present with more unusual form of lymphoma including low-grade B-cell lymphomas, anaplastic large-cell lymphomas, plasmablastic lymphomas, and rare T-cell lymphomas [9].

The pathogenesis of these lymphomas is not fully understood and may involve a number of different pathogenic mechanisms. Pathogenesis may involve interactions between host factors, HIV infection, chronic B-cell antigenic stimulation, and cytokine dysregulation. Between 40 and 60% of HIV-associated lymphomas are associated with the Epstein–Barr virus (EBV) [10]. EBV is more commonly associated with large-cell lymphomas and with Burkitt-type lymphomas. It is commonly believed that the excessive B-cell stimulation associated with HIV infection results in the proliferation of antigen-selected B-cell clones [9, 11], with subsequent genetic changes leading to the evolution of a transformed clonal lymphoma. The molecular pathogenesis of AIDS-NHL is characterized by distinct genetic pathways, including chromosomal rearrangements of c-MYC and BCL6 in AIDS-associated Burkitt lymphoma and AIDS-associated diffuse large B-cell lymphoma, respectively [9].

Clinical management

Most patients with HIV-associated lymphoma present with advanced-stage and extranodal disease. Two-thirds of patients have stage IV disease at the time of presentation, and 90% have extranodal lymphoma at the time of diagnosis [12]. About 80% present with B symptoms, consisting of fever, drenching night sweats, and/or weight loss. Meningeal involvement at the time of diagnosis has been observed in 3–20% of patients. Although in the pre-HAART era, the median CD4 count at the time of diagnosis had been reported to be in the range 100–180 cells/mm^3, there has been a recent trend toward earlier presentation, in patients with higher CD4 counts and fewer HIV-related complications prior to diagnosis.

Decreased survival is associated with CD4 counts <100 cells/mm^3, age >35 years, Karnofsky performance status <70%, advanced stage IV disease, elevated lactate dehydrogenase, higher International Prognostic Index (IPI) scores (2–3), and certain subtypes of lymphoma (e.g. PCNSL, PEL, and perhaps subtypes of DLBCL, such as activated B-cell phenotype) [13–17].

In the pre-HAART era, treatment outcomes were poor regardless of treatment choice, with complete response rates of approximately 50%, and median survivals in the 5- to 8-month range [12, 18].

Since the introduction of ART in 1996, several studies have demonstrated significant improvement in clinical outcome in ART-treated patients compared to historical controls. Furthermore, patients experiencing virologic failure on ART had poorer outcomes than those being treated with suppressive ART. These findings have made ART a critical component of the management of patients with HIV-associated NHL; it is now recommended that ART be administered concurrently in patients receiving chemotherapy for HIV-NHL [19].

Infusional chemotherapy

The use of infusional combination chemotherapy regimens to increase dose intensity of chemotherapy and to reduce toxicities has been evaluated in both HIV-infected and HIV-uninfected individuals with NHL. Three different infusional regimens have been studied in the HIV-NHL population. Sparano and co-workers. were the first to study the infusional regimen CDE, in which cyclophosphamide, doxorubicin, and etoposide are infused over 96 hours every 28 days [20]. This trial included patients who were treated both in the pre- and post-HAART eras, and demonstrated a 2-year overall survival of 47% in the post-HAART group with no treatment-related mortality compared with 30% in the pre-HAART-era patients, who also had a 10% treatment-related mortality.

However, the regimen that has generated the greatest interest is EPOCH. In this regimen, doxorubicin, vincristine, and etoposide are administered as a continuous 96-hour infusion, and cyclophosphamide, dose adjusted for initial CD4 count, is administered as a bolus intravenous infusion on day 5. In a phase II National Cancer Institute trial using this regimen, the overall complete remission rate was 74%, and at 53 months of follow-up, the disease-free survival was 92%, with an overall survival rate of 60%. It should be noted that 59% fell into the intermediate-high or high of risk groups by the IPI, 41% had CD4 counts ≤ 100 cells/mm^3, and none received ART until chemotherapy had been completed [21].

Use of rituximab

Rituximab is a humanized monoclonal anti-CD20 antibody currently in widespread use for treatment of a variety of B-cell non-Hodgkin's lymphomas. Its use in combination with CHOP chemotherapy for treatment of diffuse large B-cell lymphoma in HIV-uninfected patients became standard of care after publication of a randomized study demonstrating a survival advantage for patients receiving CHOP plus rituximab versus CHOP alone [22]. Initial trials of rituximab with CHOP from other groups raised concerns about the risk of treatment-related infectious deaths that occurred in a higher proportion of rituximab-receiving versus non-receiving individuals [23]. Most of these deaths occurred in patients with baseline CD4 counts <50 cells/mm^3 [23]. A larger subsequent study of EPOCH with either concurrent or sequential rituximab with use of concurrent ART, prophylactic antibiotics, and white cell growth factor conducted by the AIDS Malignancy Consortium has shown a low incidence of treatment-related infections and high response rates and disease-free survivals [24].

Hematopoietic cell transplantation for HIV-NHL

Several reports have suggested the potential value of high-dose chemotherapy with autologous stem cell transplant. In the largest of these studies, 20 (subsequently updated to 29) patients with HIV-associated lymphoma who either had relapsed or had refractory disease or high-risk first remission received high-dose chemotherapy with autologous stem cell infusion [25]. Mobilization and stem cell collection were successful in all patients. There was no engraftment failure, although one patient who was receiving zidovudine had delayed engraftment. Two patients who were not compliant with prophylaxis developed *Pneumocystis* pneumonia. Two developed disseminated herpes zoster, one developed cytomegalovirus (CMV) retinitis, and two developed asymptomatic CMV viremia. All of these patients responded to therapy. With a 31.8-month median follow-up time, 17 of the patients remained in remission. Progression-free survival was 85%, and overall survival was 85% for the entire group. Other small series have demonstrated similarly effective stem cell mobilization and collection, lack of unexpected toxicities, and significant long-term disease-free survival times [26–29]. A case-control study comparing 53 HIV-infected patients with lymphoma who underwent stem cell transplantation to HIV-uninfected matched controls demonstrated an overall survival of 61.5% (95% CI 47–76%) for HIV-infected patients and 70% for controls ($p = $ NS), with a median follow-up of 30 months [30]. In view of this experience, high-dose chemotherapy with autologous stem cell transplant may be considered the best treatment option for individuals with refractory or relapsed HIV-NHL [31].

Primary CNS lymphoma

PCNSL usually occurs in severely immunocompromised patients with advanced HIV infection, the vast majority of whom have CD4 counts <50 cells/mm^3. The incidence of PCNSL has fallen significantly since the introduction of ART [32].

PCNSL in the setting of HIV infection is universally associated with Epstein–Barr virus [11], which can be useful diagnostically. EBV is rarely detected in the cerebrospinal fluid (CSF) of HIV-infected patients without PCNSL, but it is commonly detected in the CSF of patients with this tumor. In one study EBV DNA was detected by nested polymerase chain reaction (PCR) in the CSF in 7 of 8 patients with PCNSL diagnosed by brain biopsy (87.5% sensitivity), and in none of the 11 controls with non-lymphomatous mass lesions (100% specificity). A total of 21 AIDS patients with or without neurological disorders but without focal brain lesions were PCR-negative [32]. In another study, EBV DNA was detected in the CSF from 16/20 (80%) patients with PCNSL [33]. In combination with imaging studies, EBV PCR may obviate the need for brain biopsy [34].

Most HIV-PCNSLs are characterized as diffuse large B-cell lymphomas and tend to be multifocal in the brain. Confusion, memory loss, lethargy, and focal neurologic findings are the most frequent presenting symptoms and signs.

Historically, prognosis for these individuals has been poor. Palliative whole-brain radiotherapy has been used, with survival of 1–3 months. Most patients died from opportunistic infections. High-dose methotrexate with leukovorin is now used alone or in combination with radiotherapy, especially since the advent of ART, which seems to make such therapy more tolerable. A pre-ART study in PCNSL patients with a median CD4 count of 30 cells/mm^3 found a 50% complete response rate and a median survival of 10 months [35]. Data suggest that immune recovery associated with ART can dramatically improve survival. A retrospective review of 111 patients with PCNSL found that the use of ART and radiotherapy were each associated with significantly improved survival [36].

Hodgkin's lymphoma

Hodgkin's lymphoma is not an AIDS-defining condition. However, multiple cohort studies have demonstrated an increased risk of Hodgkin's lymphoma in HIV-infected patients [2, 37]. HIV-associated Hodgkin's lymphoma has largely been associated with a predominance of two unfavorable subtypes: lymphocyte-depleted and mixed-cellularity, although nodular sclerosing and lymphocyte predominant subtypes also occur [38–40]. Clonal EBV is identified in 80–100% of cases associated with HIV infection [11].

Early clinical trials of standard chemotherapy regimens for HIV-associated Hodgkin's lymphoma showed poor long-term survival, with treatment being frequently complicated by severe and prolonged myelosuppression [41]. Significant improvement in tolerability and clinical outcome in patients with HIV-associated Hodgkin's lymphoma have been documented since the advent of ART [38]. Retrospective evaluation of 108 patients from a single institution demonstrated improvement in complete response rate from 64.5 to 74.5% and improvement in 2-year disease-free survival from 45 to 62% ($p = 0.03$) in the years following introduction of ART [42].

The best chemotherapy option for patients with HIV-HL has not yet been established. With the use of ART, it does appear that standard full-dose chemotherapy regimens such as ABVD and BEACOPP can be given and are well tolerated in this patient population [43, 44]. It is currently recommended that individuals with HIV-HL receive the same treatments that are used in the general population based on the staging of disease and other prognostic factors. An intergroup study of ABVD, with randomization to continue therapy or intensify to BEACOPP in those with persistent disease after 2 cycles of therapy, is currently being conducted in HIV-infected and HIV-uninfected patients with HL.

Other lymphoproliferative disease in HIV infection

Primary effusion lymphoma (PEL)

Primary effusion lymphoma (PEL) accounts for < 5% of all AIDS-related lymphomas. The disease is characterized by presentation as a body cavity effusion. Almost all of these cases are associated with Kaposi's sarcoma-associated herpes virus (KSHV), also known as human herpesvirus-8 (HHV-8), and EBV has been identified in the vast majority of cases. These lymphomas generally lack B- or T-cell markers, although the presence of immunoglobulin gene rearrangements in most cases suggests a B-cell origin. Most patients present with advanced HIV disease and severe immunodeficiency [45]. As a result, complete response rates using CHOP-like regimens have been < 50%, and overall survival is in the 3- to 6-month range [45, 46]. More intensive chemotherapy regimens with ART may lead to better outcomes.

Plasmablastic lymphoma

Although this disorder has been observed in immunocompetent individuals, it has been reported predominately in patients with HIV disease [47]. These lymphomas are typically negative for B- and T-cell markers and generally have a phenotype more typical of mature plasma cells. Morphologically, the malignant cells appear most like plasmablasts but carry a phenotype more typical of mature plasma cells. Monoclonal gammopathy is not commonly noted, helping to distinguish this entity from solitary plasmacytoma. Historically, these lymphomas have been associated with a poor prognosis and a median survival of approximately 9 months, although use of ART has extended life expectancy [48, 49].

Multicentric Castleman's disease

This lymphoproliferative disorder characteristically presents with polyclonal hypergammaglobulinemia, generalized lymphadenopathy, hepatosplenomegaly, constitutional symptoms, and often autoimmune hemolytic anemia [50]. Lymph node histologic findings include perifollicular vascular proliferation and germinal center angiosclerosis. Overexpression of IL-6 appears to be the hallmark of this disease [51]. The disease is associated with HHV-8 infection of the B-cells in the mantle zone of the lymph node [52]. Natural history can vary from an indolent, waxing and waning course to one that is extremely aggressive and may transform to non-Hodgkin's lymphoma in some cases. Based on several small series, rituximab with/or without etoposide seems to give the best responses [53–55]. Although some transient responses to anti-herpesvirus agents have been reported, overall results with these agents have been disappointing [54]. Standard lymphoma chemotherapy regimens have generally been associated with relatively transient responses and poor long-term outcome [56, 57].

KAPOSI'S SARCOMA

Pathogenesis

KS was one of the first opportunistic disorders recognized as an AIDS-defining condition. AIDS-related KS is seen in all HIV risk groups worldwide, although most cases in the United States have occurred in gay or bisexual men.

The epidemiology of KS has always suggested a sexually transmissible etiology and KSHV (HHV-8) has been identified in virtually all tissue specimens from individuals with KS, whether HIV-infected or not [58].

The pathogenesis of KS is believed to involve interactions between KSHV/HHV-8, HIV, and immune dysregulation [59]. KSHV is a lymphotropic gamma-2 herpesvirus whose seroprevalence correlates with the incidence rates of clinical KS in various populations. The viral genome encodes a variety of genes that are homologs of normal human cell cycle regulatory and angiogenesis proteins such as vCyclin D, vbcl-2, basic fibroblast growth factor (bFGF), vascular endothelial growth factor (VEGF), and a G protein-coupled receptor that are capable of inducing angiogenesis *in vitro* [60]. HIV may directly induce production of Tat protein, which in combination with bFGF can induce KS-like lesions. There is also evidence that platelet-derived growth factor receptor (PDGFR) may play a role in inducing KS spindle cell growth and inducing angiogenesis by upregulating production of VEGF [60].

The clear association of KS with immunodeficiency in HIV, in old age, and in transplant recipients, and its regression with restoration of better immune function, provide evidence of the close association of this tumor with underlying immunodeficiency.

Clinical presentation

AIDS-KS typically presents at multiple mucocutaneous sites. Lymphatic and visceral sites of disease have been common historically, with up to 40% of ART-untreated individuals having gastrointestinal involvement at diagnosis. GI KS is usually asymptomatic but occasionally may cause vague abdominal pain, bleeding, or obstruction. Pleuropulmonary disease is seen in some patients and is usually associated with cough, bronchospasm, dyspnea and eventually hypoxemia. The dramatic decline in the incidence of epidemic KS since the introduction of ART has resulted in fewer individuals presenting with advanced, symptomatic disease.

Clinical management

In addition to reducing the incidence of KS, there is strong evidence for an antitumor effect of ART in those with established disease. Multiple case reports and small series have documented significant regression of KS after ART therapy alone. In patients who have never taken ART before, the overall response rate of KS to ART alone is approximately 60% after 6 months (11% complete remission) and increases to 75% at 24 months, with 60% achieving complete remissions [61]. Multivariate analysis demonstrated that reduction of KSHV viral load to undetectable levels and improvement in CD4 count correlated with KS response [62, 63].

It is most important, however, to note that while ART alone may be sufficient therapy for individuals with limited cutaneous or mucocutaneous disease, it is not adequate for those with more advanced or symptomatic disease. In a study of moderate to advanced KS, those receiving liposomal doxorubicin in addition to ART had a markedly better response rate at 48 months than did those on ART alone (76 versus 20%) [64].

While ART is recommended for all HIV-infected patients with KS, individuals with advanced and/or symptomatic KS should receive some form of local or systemic therapy. Standard therapeutic approaches are summarized below.

Local therapies

These are generally appropriate for treating unsightly or locally symptomatic lesions. They may be used in those individuals with limited disease as an adjunct to ART. Surgical removal, cryotherapy, laser, local radiation therapy, local low-dose intralesional chemotherapy or topical 9-*cis*-retinoic acid gel (aliretinoin 1%) have all been use with good local responses.

Radiotherapy

At one time radiotherapy was the mainstay of local therapy. Used as a single 80 Gy or equivalent fractionated dose, it is an active treatment modality. It is less commonly used now due to local toxicities when administered over large cutaneous areas, resulting in loss of skin elasticity, discomfort, and occasionally contractures. When used, it should be administered only to small fields for treating localized mucocutaneous lesions. Lower fractionated doses are associated with less-significant long-term toxicities. Doses of 15 Gy for oral lesions, 20 Gy for lesions involving eyelids, conjunctiva, and genitals, and 30 Gy for cutaneous lesions have been shown to be sufficient to produce shrinkage of the tumor and good palliation of the symptoms [65].

Alitretinoin gel

Alitretinoin gel (1%): a randomized phase III vehicle-controlled study of topical administration of this agent demonstrated a 37% response rate compared with 7% in vehicle control patients [66]. It was particularly useful for facial lesions, although often associated with excessive local irritation.

Intralesional vinblastine

Generally used as dilute injected solution, this cytotoxic agent is a vesicant useful for treating small cosmetically unsightly mucocutaneous lesions. There is pain associated with injection and several injections may be required. It often results in residual hyperpigmentation.

Cryotherapy

Liquid nitrogen cryotherapy is commonly used by dermatologists for local treatment of small lesions. Multiple therapies may also be required with this modality, which tends to leave a hypopigmented area following therapy.

Systemic therapy

Chemotherapy

Cytotoxic therapy is still the most effective treatment for advanced, symptomatic and visceral disease (Table 35.2). First-line standard of care is liposomal doxorubicin (Doxil), which had a higher response rate than a standard three-drug combination (ABV) in a randomized phase III trial [67]. Except for some myelosuppression and occasional skin rash and desquamation, it is a well-tolerated agent with a low incidence of gastrointestinal toxicity and rare alopecia. For patients who are poorly responsive to or relapse after lipsomal doxorubicin (Doxil) therapy, paclitaxel (Taxol) has been

associated with response rates as high as 70% in previously treated patients with advanced KS [68]. The use of oral etoposide has been recommended by some due to its ease of administration. In a study from Brazil, 21 patients received daily oral etoposide at a dose of 20 mg/m^2 every 8 hours for 7 days every 21 days. This was associated with an objective response rate of 83% [69]. Paclitaxel is associated with a 44% incidence of alopecia, making it less favorable than liposomal doxorubicin as first-line therapy. It is also associated with significant myelosuppression. In a randomized study of oral etoposide compared to radiotherapy or 3-drug combination chemotherapy in Zimbabwe, oral etoposide had better improvement in quality of life scores, although there were no differences in tumor responses or survival [70]. Vinorelbine has also been evaluated for KS treatment and was associated with a 43% response rate in a group of 35 individuals with KS refractory to a variety of prior chemotherapy regimens [71]. A small retrospective study of gemcitabine therapy in previously treated patients with Kaposi's sarcoma in Kenya demonstrated good clinical responses with minimal toxicities [72].

Interferon-α

Interferon-α was documented to have activity in HIV-KS early in the AIDS epidemic. The debilitating constitutional toxicities associated with high-dose interferon limited its use. However, it may be effective at lower doses (1 million units daily by subcutaneous injection) when combined with ART [73]. This

Table 35.2 Cytotoxic therapy for Kaposi's sarcoma

AGENT	DOSE	RESPONSE (%)	TOXICITY
Liposomal doxorubicin	10–20 mg/m^2 every 21 days	46–59	Neutropenia; cardiomyopathy; hand–foot rashes
Paclitaxel	100 mg/m^2 every 14 days	59–79	Neutropenia; myalgias; neuropathy; alopecia
Vinorelbine	30 mg/m^2 every 14 days	43	Neutropenia; neuropathy
Etoposide	50 mg every day for 7 days, every 21 days	83	Neutropenia; alopecia
Bleomycin	15 mg/m^2 } every 21 days	23	Pulmonary fibrosis; peripheral neuropathy
Vincristine	2 mg		
Doxorubicin	20 mg/m^2 } every 14 days	25	Neutropenia; pulmonary fibrosis, neuropathy; cardiomyopathy
Bleomycin	10 mg/m^2		
Vincristine	1 mg		
Gemcitabine	1 g/m^2 every 14 days	48	Neutropenia, alopecia

may be an option for patients who have limited disease that is unresponsive to ART and who do not require chemotherapy. Responses to this agent are associated with higher CD4 counts. Those with a CD4 count of < 100 cells/mm^3 are unlikely to respond.

Investigational agents

Several approaches to therapy based upon the pathogenesis of the disease have also been studied in recent years. The AIDS Malignancy Consortium is actively investigating a number of these agents, and referral to local network trials sites is encouraged (http://www.aidscancer.org) [74, 75].

CERVICAL CANCER

Cervical cancer has been recognized as an AIDS-defining malignancy since 1993. In some women cervical cancer may be the first indication of HIV infection. Women constitute the fastest-growing group of new AIDS cases in much of the world. The primary risk factor for HIV infection in these individuals is heterosexual transmission, often from a partner whose HIV status was unknown to the woman.

Cervical intraepithelial neoplasia (CIN) is also seen with increased frequency in HIV infection. These premalignant lesions, also known as squamous intraepithelial lesions (SILs), have been associated with human papillomavirus (HPV) infection, particularly those subtypes with high oncogenic potential, e.g. serotypes 16, 18, 31, 32, and 35.

Epidemiology

In high-prevalence areas for HIV, among women younger than age 50 with cervical cancer, up to 19% were found to be HIV-infected [76]. Similarly, HIV-infected women have up a 10-fold higher risk of abnormal cervical cytology on Pap testing. Prevalence of abnormal cytology among HIV-infected women in some parts of the world has ranged from 30 to 60%, and cervical dysplasia incidence increases with declining CD4 count. In the USA, invasive cervical cancer was found in 1.3% of women with AIDS; this cancer constitutes up to 4% of AIDS-defining illnesses in women [77].

Etiology

There is abundant evidence that HPV infection is related to malignant and premalignant lesions in the genital tract. Immunosuppression may allow more rapid development of both *in situ* and invasive disease in the setting of infection with oncogenic HPV strains. Infection with more than one serotype of HPV and lower CD4 counts have been associated with a higher incidence of cervical cancer and CIN [78].

Screening and diagnosis

Because the majority of women with cervical dysplasia and early invasive cervical cancer are asymptomatic, cytologic screening should be performed frequently. The role of newly developed HPV vaccines in preventing HPV infection or disease progression in HIV-infected women is currently under investigation, although its clear efficacy in non-HIV-infected girls and young women suggests that its use in the HPV-uninfected, HIV-infected population may be important [79, 80].

Current screening recommendations call for women with HIV to undergo pelvic examinations and cytologic screening every 6 months during the first year after HIV diagnosis and annually thereafter if the test results are normal [81]. Pap smears demonstrating cervical SIL should be followed by colposcopy and biopsy. Although abnormalities are sometimes missed by relying solely on cytologic screening, the routine use of colposcopy has not yet been established for this population. For women who have a history of cervical SIL, more frequent evaluations and screening are indicated. Since these women are at high risk for recurrence or development of lesions in other areas of the genital tract, post-therapy monitoring with repeat colposcopy is warranted. In resource-limited settings, visual inspection with acetic acid (VIA) has been shown to be a practical and effective way of screening for high-grade cervical neoplasia, on a par with or better than cervical cytology [82, 83].

For women with invasive carcinoma, complete staging should be undertaken, including pelvic examination, CT and possibly PET scanning of the pelvis and abdomen, chest X-ray, and screening laboratory testing for hepatic and bone disease.

Treatment

The staging classification for cervical carcinoma as adopted by the American Joint Committee on Cancer (AJCC) or the International Federation of Gynecology and Obstetrics (FIGO) also applies to AIDS patients.

Cervical dysplasia in HIV-infected women is often of higher histologic grade (CIN 2–3), and should be treated with ablative therapy. Cryotherapy, laser, cone biopsy, and and loop electrosurgical excision procedures (LEEP) have all been used successfully to treat preinvasive disease in HIV-infected patients. Short-term recurrence rates of 40–60% have been reported. In resource-limited settings use of cryoablation at the time of screening allows for local treatment of abnormal-appearing lesions and helps reduce loss to follow-up when it is difficult to refer such women for more extensive colposcopy and biopsy [84].

For invasive cervical carcinoma, the same principles that guide the management of the immunocompetent patient with cancer should be utilized in HIV-infected women. Decisions about surgical intervention should be based on oncologic appropriateness rather than HIV status. As most HIV-infected women with cervical cancer present with advanced disease, radiation therapy is often indicated. For patients with advanced, stage III–IV disease, a combination of irradiation and concurrent cisplatinum-based chemotherapy is often used. At this time there is no evidence to suggest that treatment of cervical carcinoma in HIV-infected women is less effective than HIV-uninfected women with similar stage disease [76].

ANAL CANCER

Although anal cancer is not currently an AIDS-defining illness, the incidence of this cancer is increasing in the population at risk for HIV infection [84]. The incidence of anal cancer in homosexual men in a San Francisco study was estimated at between 25 and 87 cases per 100,000, compared to 0.7 per 100,000 in the general male population.

Etiology

Anal intraepithelial neoplasia (AIN), also known as anal squamous intraepithelial lesion (SIL), is generally associated with oncogenic serotypes of HPV, especially 16, 18, 31, 32, 33, and 35. Cytologic abnormalities have been noted in as many as 40% of patients with HIV, especially those with CD4 counts < 200 cells/mm^3 [85].

Screening

Studies evaluating the usefulness of yearly Pap cytologic screening with subsequent high-resolution anoscopy (HRA) and biopsy have found a high incidence of false-negative Pap tests, even in some individuals with high-grade AIN [86]. Guidelines for frequency of screening have not yet been established, but many HIV practitioners recommend 2 initial baseline Pap tests or HRAs 6 months apart, followed by yearly screening if no abnormalities are seen. Findings of low-grade SIL (AIN 1) are generally followed closely with repeat HRA and biopsies. Patients with high-grade AIN 2–3 undergo ablative therapy, either surgically or with infrared or electrocauterization [87].

Treatment

Treatment for invasive cancer requires coordinated concurrent chemoradiotherapy and in some cases surgical resection followed by radiation or chemoradiotherapy. For most patients with squamous cell carcinoma of the anus, chemotherapy consists of mitomycin (10 mg/m^2 on day 1) and fluorouracil (5-FU; 1,000 mg/m^2 by continuous infusion on days 1–4) combined with radiation therapy. Alternatively, some clinicians prefer substituting cisplatin for mitomycin in patients with HIV [88]. Despite high response rates to this combined therapy, patients with HIV have a higher risk of relapse and studies including the EGFR

antibody, cetuximab, are being conducted to determine if the addition of this agent to standard chemoradiotherapy may result in longer disease-free survival in HIV-infected and HIV-uninfected individuals.

NON-AIDS-DEFINING MALIGNANCIES

With improved HIV therapy, patients are living longer and are developing other cancers that are not AIDS-defining. A number of reports from around the world now show that other cancers are occurring with greater frequency in HIV-infected individuals [5, 89, 90]. These include: Hodgkin's lymphoma, anal cancer, liver cancer, head and neck cancers, lung cancer, non-melanomatous skin cancers, germ cell tumors, myeloid and lymphoid leukemias, squamous cell cancers of various organs, and leiomyosarcoma in pediatric patients. Rates of these NADCs suggest that these cancers are now occurring at a higher frequency overall than the ADCs in the developed world. Interestingly, the rates of some of the more common cancers, such as breast, prostate, and colon cancer, do not appear to be higher in the HIV-infected population.

Clinical features

In general, in HIV-infected individuals NADC seem to present at a younger age, with more advanced-stage disease at diagnosis and with a higher likelihood of relapse after definitive therapy. Unusual locations and presentations of some of these tumors have been reported. A high index of suspicion for cancer needs to be maintained in the HIV-infected population, and more frequent screening for the more common cancers may also be required. The routine use of screening biomarkers has not yet been evaluated in HIV-infected patients; however, periodic screening tests such as screening mammography, alpha fetoprotein, prostate-specific antigen, and routine skin exam may be warranted.

Treatment

In the absence of prospective clinical trials data for many of these cancers in HIV-infected patients, treatment strategies have generally followed the same stage-adjusted approaches as used in individuals not infected with HIV. Appreciation for the greater likelihood and/or severity of drug toxicities, the potential for drug interactions between anticancer agents and antiretroviral drugs, and the need to provide supportive treatment and prophylactic antibiotics should be incorporated into the management of HIV-infected patients with cancer.

ACKNOWLEDGMENTS

Supported in part by grants from the California HIV/AIDS Research Program (MC08-LA-710) and USPHS, NIH grants, AI-69424, AI-28697, CA-121947, and RR-00865.

REFERENCES

[1] Centers for Disease Control. Kaposi's sarcoma and *pneumocystis* pneumonia among homosexual men—New York City and California. MMWR Morb Mortal Wkly Rep 1981;30:305–8.

[2] Hymes KB, Cheung T, Greene JB, et al. Kaposi's sarcoma in homosexual men—a report of eight cases. Lancet 1981;2 (8247):598–600.

[3] Crun-Cianflone N, Hullsiek KH, Marconi V, et al. Trends in the incidence of cancers among HIV-infected persons and the impact of antiretroviral therapy; a 20-year cohort study. AIDS 2009;23:41–50.

[4] Engels EA, Biggar RJ, Hall HI, et al. Cancer risk in people infected with HIV in the Untied States. Int J Cancer 2008;123:187–94.

[5] Simard EP, Pfeiffer RM, Engels EA. Cumulative incidence of cancer among individuals with AIDS in the United States. Cancer 2011;117:1089–96.

[6] Stebbing J, Duru O, Bower M. Non-AIDS-defining cancers. Curr Opin Infect Dis 2009;22:7–10.

[7] Simard EP, Engels EA. Cancer as a cause of death among people with AIDS in the United States. Clin Infect Dis 2010;51:957–62.

[8] Matthews GV, Bower M, Mandalia S, et al. Changes in acquired immunodeficiency syndrome-related lymphoma since the introduction of highly active antiretroviral therapy. Blood 2000;96:2730–4.

[9] Knowles DM. Etiology and pathogenesis of AIDS-related non-Hodgkin's lymphoma. Hematol Oncol Clin North Am 2003;17:785–820.

[10] Carbone A, Gaidano G, Gloghini A, et al. Differential expression of BCL-6, CD138/syndecan-1, and Epstein–Barr virus-encoded latent membrane protein-1 identifies distinct histogenetic subsets of acquired immunodeficiency syndrome-related non-Hodgkin's lymphomas. Blood 1998;91:747–55.

[11] Ambinder RF. Epstein–Barr virus associated lymphoproliferations in the AIDS setting. Eur J Cancer 2001;37:1209–16.

[12] Kaplan LD, Abrams DI, Feigal E, et al. AIDS-associated non-Hodgkin's lymphoma in San Francisco. JAMA 1989;261:719–24.

[13] Straus DJ, Huang J, Testa MA, et al. Prognostic factors in the treatment of human immunodeficiency virus-associated non-Hodgkin's lymphoma: analysis of AIDS Clinical Trials Group protocol 142—low-dose versus standard-dose m-BACOD plus granulocyte-macrophage colony-stimulating factor. National Institute of Allergy and Infectious Diseases. J Clin Oncol 1998;16:3601–6.

[14] Lim S-T, Karim R, Tulpule A, et al. Prognostic factors in HIV related diffuse large cell lymphoma: before versus after highly active antiretroviral therapy. J Clin Oncol 2005;23:8477–82.

[15] Bower M, Gazzard B, Mandalia S, et al. A prognostic index for systemic AIDS-related non-Hodgkin lymphoma treated in the era of highly active antiretroviral therapy. Ann Intern Med 2005;143:265–73.

[16] Chadburn A, Chiu A, Lee JY, et al. Immunophenotypic analysis of AIDS-related diffuse large B-cell lymphoma and clinical implications in patients from AIDS Malignancy Consortium Clinical Trials 010 and 034. J Clin Oncol 2009;27:5039–48.

[17] Mounier N, Spina M, Gabarre J, et al. AIDS-related non-Hodgkin lymphoma: final analysis of 485 patients treated with risk-adapted intensive chemotherapy. Blood 2006;107:3832–40.

[18] Kaplan LD, Straus DJ, Testa MA, et al. Low-dose compared with standard-dose m-BACOD chemotherapy for non-Hodgkin's lymphoma associated with human immunodeficiency virus infection. National Institute of Allergy and Infectious Diseases AIDS Clinical Trials Group. N Engl J Med 1997;336:1641–8.

[19] Levine AM. Management of AIDS-related lymphoma. Curr Opin Oncol 2008;20:522–8.

[20] Sparano JA, Lee S, Chen MG, et al. Phase II trial of infusional cyclophosphamide, doxorubicin, and etoposide in patients with HIV-associated non-Hodgkin's lymphoma: an Eastern Cooperative Oncology Group Trial (E1494). J Clin Oncol 2004;22:1491–500.

[21] Little RF, Pittaluga S, Grant N, et al. Highly effective treatment of acquired immunodeficiency syndrome-related lymphoma with dose-adjusted EPOCH: impact of antiretroviral therapy suspension and tumor biology. Blood 2003;101:4653–9.

[22] Coiffier B, Lepage E, Briere J, et al. CHOP chemotherapy plus rituximab compared with CHOP alone in elderly patients with diffuse large-B-cell lymphoma. N Engl J Med 2002;346:235–42.

[23] Kaplan LD, Lee JY, Ambinder RF, et al. Rituximab does not improve clinical outcome in a randomized phase 3 trial of CHOP with or without rituximab in patients with HIV-associated non-Hodgkin lymphoma: AIDS-Malignancy Consortium Trial 010. Blood 2005;106:1538–43.

[24] Sparano JA, Lee JY, Kaplan LD, et al. Rituximab plus concurrent infusional EPOCH chemotherapy is highly effective in HIV-associated B-cell non-Hodgkin's lymphoma. Blood 2010;115:3008–16.

[25] Krishnan A, Molina A, Zaia J, et al. Durable remissions with autologous stem cell transplantation for high-risk HIV-associated lymphomas. Blood 2005;105:874–8.

[26] Gabarre J, Marcelin AG, Azar N, et al. High-dose therapy plus autologous hematopoietic stem cell transplantation for human immunodeficiency virus (HIV)-related lymphoma: results and impact on HIV disease. Haematologica 2004;89:1100–8.

[27] Re A, Michieli M, Casari S, et al. High-dose therapy and autologous

peripheral blood stem cell transplantation as salvage treatment for AIDS-related lymphoma: long-term results of the Italian Cooperative Group on AIDS and Tumors (GICAT) study with analysis of prognostic factors. Blood 2009;114:1306–13.

[28] Balsalobre P, Diez-Martin JL, Re A, et al. Autologous stem-cell transplantation in patients with HIV-related lymphoma. J Clin Oncol 2009;27:2192–8.

[29] Spitzer TR, Ambinder RF, Lee JY, et al. Dose-reduced busulfan, cyclophosphamide and autologous stem cell transplantation for HIV-associated lymphoma: AIDS Malignancy Consortium study 020. Biol Blood Marrow Transplant 2008;14:59–66.

[30] Diez-Martin J, Balsalobre P, Re A, et al. Comparable survival between HIV positive and HIV negative non-Hodgkin and Hodgkin lymphoma patients undergoing autologous peripheral blood stem cell transplantation. Blood 2009;113:6011–14.

[31] Krishnan A, Forman SJ. Hematopoietic stem cell transplantation for AIDS-related malignancies. Curr Opin Oncol 2010;22:456–60.

[32] De Luca A, Antinori A, Cingolani A, et al. Evaluation of cerebrospinal fluid EBV-DNA and IL-10 as markers for in vivo diagnosis of AIDS-related primary central nervous system lymphoma. Br J Haematol 1995;90:844–9.

[33] Bossolasco S, Cinque P, Ponzoni M, et al. Epstein–Barr virus DNA load in cerebrospinal fluid and plasma of patients with AIDS-related lymphoma. J Neurovirol 2002;8:432–8.

[34] Antinori A, De Rossi G, Ammassari A, et al. Value of combined approach with thallium-201 single-photon emission computed tomography and Epstein–Barr virus DNA polymerase chain reaction in CSF for the diagnosis of AIDS-related primary CNS lymphoma. J Clin Oncol 1999;17:554–60.

[35] Jacomet C, Girard PM, Lebrette MG, et al. Intravenous methotrexate for primary central nervous system non-Hodgkin's lymphoma in AIDS. AIDS 1997;11:1725–30.

[36] Newell ME, Hoy JF, Cooper SG, et al. Human immunodeficiency virus-related primary central nervous system lymphoma: factors influencing survival in 111 patients. Cancer 2004;100:2627–36.

[37] Spina M, Carbone A, Gioghini A, et al. Hodgkin's disease in patients with HIV infection. Adv Hematol 2010; Epub 2010 Sept 23..

[38] Berenguer J, Miralles P, Ribera JM, et al. Characteristics and outcome of AIDS-related Hodgkin lymphoma before and after the introduction of highly active antiretroviral therapy. J Acquir Immune Defic Syndr 2008;47:422–8.

[39] Levine AM. Hodgkin lymphoma: to the HAART of the matter. Blood 2006;108:3630.

[40] Thompson LD, Fisher SI, Chu WS, et al. HIV-associated Hodgkin lymphoma: a clinicopathologic and immunophenotypic study of 45 cases. Am J Clin Pathol 2004;121:727–38.

[41] Levine AM, Li P, Cheung T, et al. Chemotherapy consisting of doxorubicin, bleomycin, vinblastine and dacarbazine with granulocyte colony stimulating factor in HIV infected patients with newly diagnosed Hodgkin's disease: a prospective multi-institutional AIDS Clinical Trials Group Study (ACTG 149). J Acquir Immune Defic Syndr 2000;24:444–50.

[42] Gerard L, Galicier L, Boulanger E, et al. Improved survival in HIV-related Hodgkin's lymphoma since the introduction of highly active antiretroviral therapy. AIDS 2003;17:81–7.

[43] Hoffmann C, Chow KU, Wolf E, et al. Strong impact of highly active antiretroviral therapy on survival in patients with human immunodeficiency virus-associated Hodgkin's disease. Br J Haematol 2004;125:455–62.

[44] Hartmann P, Rehwald U, Salzberger B, et al. BEACOPP therapeutic regimen for patients with Hodgkin's disease and HIV infection. Ann Oncol 2003;14:1562–9.

[45] Spina M, Gabarre J, Rossi G, et al. Stanford V regimen and concomitant HAART in 59 patients with Hodgkin disease and HIV infection. Blood 2002;100:1984–8.

[46] Boulanger E, Gerard L, Gabarre J, et al. Prognostic factors and outcome of human herpes virus 8-associated primary effusion lymphoma in patients with AIDS. J Clin Oncol 2005;23:4372–90.

[47] Delecluse HJ, Anagnostopoulos I, Dallenbach F, et al. Plasmablastic lymphomas of the oral cavity: a new entity associated with the human immunodeficiency virus infection. Blood 1997;89:1413–20.

[48] Castilla JJ, Winer ES, Stachurski D, et al. Prognostic factors in chemotherapy-treated patients with HIV-associated plasmablastic lymphoma. Oncologist 2010;15:293–9.

[49] Castillo JJ, Reagan JL. Plasmablastic lymphoma: a systematic review. Scientific WorldJournal 2011;11:687–96.

[50] Van Rhee F, Stone K, Szmenia , et al. Castleman's disease in the 21st century; an update on diagnosis, assessment and therapy. Clin Adv Hematol Oncol 2010;8:486–98.

[51] Oksenhendler E, Carcelain G, Aoki Y, et al. High levels of human herpesvirus 8 viral load, human interleukin-6, interleukin-10, and C reactive protein correlate with exacerbation of multicentric Castleman disease in HIV-infected patients. Blood 2000;96: 2069–73.

[52] Cesarman E. The role of Kaposi's sarcoma-associated herpesvirus (KSHV/HHV-8) in lymphoproliferative diseases. Recent Results Cancer Res 2002;159:27–37.

[53] Bower M, How I treat HIV-associated multicentric Castleman disease. Blood 2010;116:4415–21.

[54] Berezne A, Agbalika F, Oksenhendler E. Failure of cidofovir in HIV-associated multicentric

Castleman disease. Blood 2004;103:4368–9.

[55] Marcelin AG, Aaron L, Mateus C, et al. Rituximab therapy for HIV-associated Castleman disease. Blood 2003;102:2786–8.

[56] Stebbing J, Pantanowitz L, Dayyani F, et al. HIV-associated multicentric Castleman disease. Am J Hematol 2008;83:498–503.

[57] Andrea E, Maloisel F. Interferon-alpha as first-line therapy for treatment of multicentric Castleman's disease. Ann Oncol 2000;11:1613–14.

[58] Martin JN, Ganem DE, Osmond DH, et al. Sexual transmission and the natural history of human herpesvirus 8 infection. N Engl J Med 1998;338:948–54.

[59] Ganem D. KSHV and the pathogenesis of Kaposi's sarcoma: listening to human biology and medicine. J Clin Invest 2010;120:939–49.

[60] Mesri EA, Cesarman E, Boshoff C. Kaposi's sarcoma and its associated herpesvirus. Nat Rev Cancer 2010;10:707–19.

[61] Dupont C, Vasseur E, Beauchet A, et al. Long-term efficacy on Kaposi's sarcoma of highly active antiretroviral therapy in a cohort of HIV-positive patients. CISIH 92. Centre d'information et de soins de l'immunodeficience humaine. AIDS 2000;14:987–93.

[62] Pellet C, Chevret S, Blum L, et al. Virologic and immunologic parameters that predict clinical response of AIDS-associated Kaposi's sarcoma to highly active antiretroviral therapy. J Invest Dermatol 2001;117:858–63.

[63] Cattelan AM, Calabro ML, De Rossi A, et al. Long-term clinical outcome of AIDS-related Kaposi's sarcoma during highly active antiretroviral therapy. Int J Oncol 2005;27:779–85.

[64] Martin-Carbonero L, Barrios A, Saballs P, et al. Pegylated liposomal doxorubicin plus highly active antiretroviral therapy versus highly active antiretroviral therapy alone in

HIV patients with Kaposi's sarcoma. AIDS 2004;18:1737–40.

[65] Kirova YM, Belembaogo E, Frikha H, et al. Radiotherapy in the management of epidemic Kaposi's sarcoma: a retrospective study of 643 cases. Radiother Oncol 1998;46:19–22.

[66] Bodsworth NJ, Bloch M, Bower M, et al. Phase III vehicle-controlled, multi-centered study of topical alitretinoin gel 0.1% in cutaneous AIDS-related Kaposi's sarcoma. Am J Clin Dermatol 2001;2:77–87.

[67] Northfelt DW, Dezube BJ, Thommes JA, et al. Pegylated-liposomal doxorubicin versus doxorubicin, bleomycin, and vincristine in the treatment of AIDS-related Kaposi's sarcoma: results of a randomized phase III clinical trial. J Clin Oncol 1998;16:2445–51.

[68] Gill PS, Tulpule A, Espina BM, et al. Paclitaxel is safe and effective in the treatment of advanced AIDS-related Kaposi's sarcoma. J Clin Oncol 1999;17:1876–83.

[69] Sprinz E, Caldas AP, Mans DR, et al. Fractionated doses of oral etoposide in the treatment of patients with AIDS-related Kaposi sarcoma: a clinical and pharmacologic study to improve therapeutic index. Am J Clin Oncol 2001;24:177–84.

[70] Olweny CL, Borok M, Gudza I, et al. Treatment of AIDS-associated Kaposi's sarcoma in Zimbabwe: results of a randomized quality of life focused clinical trial. Int J Cancer 2005;113:632–9.

[71] Nasti G, Errante D, Talamini R, et al. Vinorelbine is an effective and safe drug for AIDS-related Kaposi's sarcoma: results of a phase II study. J Clin Oncol 2000;18:1550–7.

[72] Strother RM, Gregory KM, Pastakia SD, et al. Retrospective analysis of the efficacy of gencitabine for previously treated AIDS-associated Kaposi's sarcoma in western Kenya. Oncology 2010;78:5–11.

[73] Krown SE, Li P, Von Roenn JH, et al. Efficacy of low-dose interferon with antiretroviral therapy in Kaposi's sarcoma: a randomized phase II

AIDS clinical trials group study. J Interferon Cytokine Res 2002;22:295–303.

[74] Dittmer DP, Krown SE. Targeted therapy for Kaposi's sarcoma and KS-associated herpesvirus. Curr Opin Oncol 2007; 19:452–7.

[75] Sullivan RJ, Pantanowitz L, Dezube BJ. Targeted therapy for Kaposi's sarcoma. BioDrugs 2009;23:69–75.

[76] Einstein MH, Phaeton R. Issues in cervical cancer: incidence and treatment in HIV. Curr Opin Oncol 2010;22:449–55.

[77] Engels EA, Biggar RJ, Hall HI, et al. Cancer risks in people infected with HIV in the United States. Int J Cancer 2008;123:187–94.

[78] Adler DH. The impact of HAART on HPV-related cervical disease. Curr HIV Res 2010;8:493–7.

[79] Garland SM, Hernandez-Avila M, Wheeler CM, et al. Quadrivalent vaccine against human papillomavirus to prevent anogenital diseases. N Engl J Med 2007;356:1928–43.

[80] Kahn JA. HPV vaccination for the prevention of cervical intraepithelial neoplasia. N Engl J Med 2009;361:271–8.

[81] ACOG Committee on Practice Bulletins—Gynecology. ACOG practice bulletin No. 117: Gynecologic care for women with human immunodeficiency virus. Obstet Gynecol 2010;116:1492–509.

[82] Sahasrabuddha VV, Bhosale RA, Kavatkar AN, et al. Comparison of visual inspection with acetic acid (VIA) and cervical cytology to detect high grade cervical neoplasia among HIV-infected women in India. Int J Cancer 2011; Feb 3. doi:10.1002/ijc.25971.

[83] Denny L, Kuhn L, H. CC, et al. Human papillomavirus-based cervical cancer prevention: long-term results of a randomized screening trial. J Natl Cancer Inst 2010;102:1557–67.

[84] Palefsky J. Human papillomavirus-related disease in people with HIV. Curr Opin HIV AIDS 2009;4:52–6.

[85] Stier E, Baranoski AS. HPV-related disease in HIV-infected individuals. Curr Opin Oncol 2008;20:541–6.

[86] Berry JM, Palefsky JM, Jay N, et al. Performance characteristics of anal cytology and HPV testing in patients with high-resolution anoscopy-guided biopsy of high-grade anal intraepithelial neoplasia. Dis Colon Rectum 2009;52:239–47.

[87] Cranston RD, Hirschowitz SL, Corina G, Moe AA. A retrospective clinical study of the treatment of high-grade anal dysplasia by infrared coagulation in a population of HIV-positive men who have sex with men. Int J STD AIDS 2008;19:118–20.

[88] Hauerstock D, Ennis RD, Grossbard M, Evans A. Efficacy and toxicity of chemoradiation in the treatment of HIV-associated anal cancer. Clin Colorectal Cancer 2010;9:238–42.

[89] Franceschi S, Lise M, Clifford GM, et al. Changing patterns of cancer incidence in the early- and late-HAART periods: the Swiss HIV cohort study. Br J Cancer 2010;103:416–22.

[90] Lanoy E, Spano JP, Bonnet F, et al. The spectrum of malignancies in HIV-infected patients in 2006 in France: the ONCOVIH study. Int J Cancer 2011;129: 467–75.

Chapter | 36 |

STDs and syphilis

Elysia Larson, Jeffrey D. Klausner

INTRODUCTION

Sexually transmitted infections like syphilis, herpes, gonorrhea, chlamydia and trichomoniasis have circulated for thousands of years, long before the emergence of HIV. The areas currently most affected by STDs are South and Southeast Asia and sub-Saharan Africa. Infections can lead to acute symptoms ranging from ulcers and abrasions to painful urination. Long-term outcomes are more severe, including infertility, ectopic pregnancy, and other adverse pregnancy outcomes. Because some sexually transmitted diseases (such as chlamydia and herpes) may be asymptomatic during acute infection, they are unknowingly spread and may lead to serious complications if they remain undetected.

As sexual transmission is the primary mode for the spread of HIV infection, individuals at risk for STDs are also at risk for HIV infection. Approximately one in five HIV-infected individuals worldwide is co-infected with a second sexually transmitted infection [1]. Additionally, the presence of untreated STDs has been shown to increase the acquisition and transmission of HIV. Therefore, all individuals infected with STDs should be treated and tested for HIV infection. Furthermore, recognition of a new STD in an HIV-infected patient is an indication of unprotected sex with the potential for HIV transmission in the community.

SYPHILIS

Epidemiology

About 90% of syphilis cases worldwide are in low-income countries, with sub-Saharan Africa and South and Southeast Asia carrying most of the burden (9.6 and 9.2 million

cases, respectively, in 1999) [2]. Every year over 2 million pregnant women are diagnosed with syphilis [3]. In North America, Western Europe, and Australia, a majority of new syphilis cases are among men, particularly men who have sex with men [4, 5].

Because syphilis may facilitate HIV acquisition and transmission, and because syphilis and HIV have similar modes of transmission, co-infection is common. In the United States approximately 10-20% of syphilis patients are co-infected with HIV; in Rwanda the prevalence of syphilis in HIV-infected women was almost twice as high as in HIV-uninfected women [6]. All patients with syphilis should therefore be tested for HIV infection, and HIV-infected patients should be screened at their initial visit and regularly thereafter with the frequency dependent on risk behavior.

Natural history, pathogenesis, and pathology

Syphilis is caused by infection with *Treponema pallidum pallidum*. The primary mode of transmission is through sexual contact. Syphilis is readily transmissible by oral sex and through vaginal and anal intercourse. Syphilis can also be transmitted vertically (*in utero* and at delivery) and less frequently by blood transfusion [5].

Syphilis occurs in three distinct stages: primary, secondary, and tertiary. Once infected, there is an approximately three-week incubation period before the initial lesion of primary syphilis develops. Primary syphilis lasts from a few days to several months and may overlap with the signs and symptoms of secondary syphilis in about one-third of patients (this increases to up to three-fourths among HIV co-infected patients.) Secondary syphilis presents between 1 to 3 months after infection and is followed by latent syphilis. Without therapeutic cure, approximately a third of patients will progress to tertiary syphilis [7].

Because syphilis is readily treatable with antibiotics, the natural history has not been well-studied. However, the Oslo syphilis natural history study conducted from 1891 to 1951 found a mortality rate of 15% for men and 8% for women [8].

Clinical features

Syphilis is a systemic disease that has symptomatic periods that alternate with periods of clinical latency. Primary syphilis is characterized by an ulcer or chancre at the site of inoculation (see Fig. 36.1). Usually the lesion is solitary, but HIV co-infected patients are more likely to have several lesions that may be larger and deeper than those in HIV-uninfected patients. Approximately 80% of patients also develop unilateral lymphadenopathy near the site of the lesion [5, 7].

Secondary syphilis typically presents as a diffuse non-pruritic rash consisting of many 3- to 10-mm pink, red, or copper-colored flat lesions or macules. The rash most often affects the trunk and limbs, and raised circular lesions (papulosquamous) with fine circumferential scaling are found on the palms and soles in some cases (see Fig. 36.2). In addition to the rash, 5–10% of patients may experience patchy hair loss. Some patients may experience diffuse lymphadenopathy, pharyngitis, or fever [5, 7].

Although the symptoms of secondary syphilis will abate even in the absence of treatment, up to 25% of patients will experience a recurrence of secondary syphilis, usually within the first year. The period during which no symptoms are present is termed latent syphilis, and although sexual transmission during latency is unlikely, the possibility of mother-to-child transmission remains [7].

Up to a third of patients with untreated syphilis will develop tertiary syphilis. Characterized by a broad range of long-term complications, tertiary syphilis is generally divided into three sub categories: cardiovascular syphilis, gummatous (late benign) syphilis, and late neurosyphilis. Cardiovascular syphilis is the most common manifestation, although it is on the decline, probably as a result of the

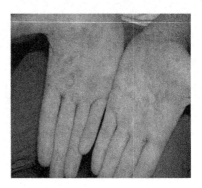

Figure 36.2 Palmar rash.
Courtesy of San Francisco City Clinic.

widespread use of antibiotics. The most common complication is disease of the aorta resulting in aortic regurgitation or aortic aneurysm, usually of the ascending arch. Gummatous syphilis is named for the granulomatous-like lesion most commonly found in the skin, bone, and liver. Although rarely physically debilitating, those lesions can present in any organ and can therefore cause complications. Incidence peaks approximately 15 years post infection [5, 7, 9].

Neurosyphilis is caused by invasion of the cerebrospinal fluid (CSF) by *T. pallidum* and can occur at any stage of disease. Most patients who experience early treponemal invasion of CSF will have spontaneous resolution. For others, early neurosyphilis is characterized by meningovascular disease, acute and subacute myelopathy, brainstem or cranial nerve abnormalities, or vestibular and ocular abnormalities [10]. Partial loss of movement and muscle weakness and abnormal physical sensations are classic late-stage neurosyphilis syndromes as well as dementia [5, 7].

Patient evaluation, diagnosis, and differential diagnosis

The diagnosis of a patient with suspected syphilis must begin with a detailed history (including sexual behavior, a risk assessment for HIV and other STDs and questioning regarding symptoms) and a physical examination (including examination of the skin, scalp, oropharynx, genital and anal area and a targeted neurological examination). In certain settings, direct darkfield microscopy or fluorescent antibody testing of lesion exudates can be performed. Serological testing is used to confirm the diagnosis in those with signs and symptoms or as a screening test in those who are asymptomatic. Non-treponemal testing (rapid plasma reagin [RPR], venereal disease research laboratory [VDRL], toluidine red unheated serum test [TRUST]) is used as the initial screen followed by a treponemal test (treponemal pallidum particle agglutination [TP-PA]) to confirm an initial reactive non-treponemal test. Increasingly in the United States and in other countries, due to the

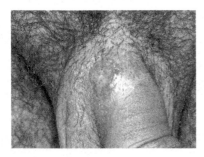

Figure 36.1 Penile chancre.
Courtesy of San Francisco City Clinic.

automation of treponemal testing using enzyme immuno-assays, a treponemal antibody test is used as the initial syphilis screening test. Since treponemal antibodies persist for life in most patients with syphilis, the clinician cannot determine based on a positive treponemal test the duration of infection. A second non-treponemal test is then used and, if positive, the patient is diagnosed with recent syphilis infection. In some cases, however, the initial treponemal test will be reactive and the second non-treponemal test will be negative, making the determination of active infection difficult. If a patient has no history of syphilis treatment, most national guidelines recommend treatment in that setting for latent infection. Interpretation of all serological tests should be the same for both HIV-infected and HIV-uninfected patients [11]. In low-resource settings rapid treponemal tests are often used as the single assay. Persons with a reactive test are treated without determination of the serological titer and staged by history and clinical findings. Those with symptoms are categorized as early syphilis (primary or secondary) and those without symptoms as latent syphilis. If syphilis exposure is likely to have occurred within the past 12 months, the patient is managed as early syphilis; if the exposure was more than 12 months or unknown, the patient is managed as late syphilis.

In patients with genital ulcerative lesions consistent with syphilis, other causes might include herpes simplex virus infection and chancroid. Rarely granuloma inguinale (*Klebsiella granulomatis*) is a cause of genital ulcer disease. Raised genital lesions of secondary syphilis (see Fig. 36.3) might also be confused with external genital warts Drug reactions, trauma, pyogenic bacterial infections, and malignancy might also be included in the differential diagnosis of early symptomatic syphilis. Because syphilis is curable, all patients with such genital lesions should be tested for syphilis [12, 13].

As congenital syphilis can be almost entirely avoided by early detection and treatment of maternal infections, all pregnant women should undergo syphilis screening at the first antenatal care visit [3]. Pregnant women with a reactive serology should be treated for latent syphilis if asymptomatic and early syphilis if there are clinical signs of disease. Male partners of pregnant women with syphilis should be treated presumptively to reduce the risk of maternal re-infection. Routine and frequent testing of syphilis in high-risk populations has been shown to be associated with a reduction in syphilis incidence in the target population [4].

Patients with signs or symptoms of neurologic involvement (e.g. cranial nerve palsies, motor or sensory defects) should undergo lumbar puncture and CSF examination to exclude neurosyphilis. Neurosyphilis is diagnosed on the basis of elevated cerebrospinal fluid total white cell count ([5-10] 10 cells/mm^3 for HIV-uninfected patients and [10-20] 20 cells/mm^3 for HIV-infected), abnormal protein or reactive VDRL or flourescent treponemal antibody-absorption test. Other indications for CSF analysis in patients with syphilis are suspected treatment failure or evidence of tertiary syphilis. HIV co-infection is not an indication for CSF analysis [11]. Because intramuscular penicillin G benzathine does not reach adequate levels in the brain to be treponemocidal, patients with neurosyphilis must be treated with intravenous penicillin G.

Treatment

Both HIV-infected and HIV-uninfected patients should undergo the same treatment: intramuscular benzathine penicillin G (see Table 36.1). The efficacy of benzathine penicillin G in the treatment of syphilis has been supported by decades of clinical experience and numerous case series, observational studies, and clinical trials. Patients should be informed about the Jarisch–Herxheimer reaction—fever, headache, chills, and rigors—which is an acute febrile reaction that usually occurs within the first 24 hours after syphilis treatment. It most often occurs among patients who have early syphilis and is more frequent among HIV-infected patients [7]. Pretreatment with acetaminophen (paracetamol) can reduce the severity of that reaction. In many countries, it is recommended that the treatment of pregnant women occurs in a hospital setting because the Jarisch–Herxheimer reaction is associated with premature labor and fetal loss.

Some efficacy has been demonstrated with other antibiotics in patients who have true penicillin allergies; for example, doxycycline, 100 mg orally twice a day for 14 days. However, tetracyclines are contraindicated in pregnant women and children < 8 years of age. Pregnant women with penicillin allergies should be desensitized and treated with penicillin [11]. A series of congenital syphilis cases was reported among pregnant women with syphilis in China treated with azithromycin [14]. A randomized controlled trial comparing intravenous ceftriaxone to intravenous penicillin G in HIV-infected patients with neurosyphilis found similar improvements clinically and in laboratory measures such as the CSF VDRL titer, CSF white blood cell count, and CSF protein concentration for the two groups [15].

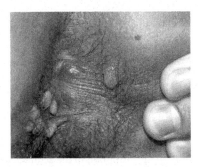

Figure 36.3 Anal condylomata lata of syphilis.
Courtesy of San Francisco City Clinic.

Table 36.1 Recommended treatment regimens for syphilis patients [11, 12]

POPULATION	RECOMMENDED REGIMENS	COMMENTS
Primary, secondary, and early latent syphilis (first year of latent syphilis)	Benzathine penicillin G 2.4 million units administered intramuscularly (IM) as a single dose	Routine penicillin allergy screening with injectable penicillin in or under the skin prior to treatment administration is not recommended
Late latent syphilis, latent syphilis of unknown duration, or tertiary syphilis without CNS involvement	Benzathine penicillin G 2.4 million units administered IM at 1-week intervals for three weeks for a total of 7.2 million units	Pregnant women who miss any dose must repeat the full course of therapy. In the general population if more than 14 days lapse between doses then the full course of therapy should be repeated [3]
Neurosyphilis or syphilitic eye disease	Intraveneous aqueous crystalline penicillin G 3–4 million units every 4 hours or continuous infusion for 10–14 days (total 18–24 million units per day) followed by at least one dose of benzathine penicillin G IM, 2.4 million units	
Children[a] with primary, secondary, or early latent syphilis	Benzathine penicillin G 50,000 units/kg IM, up to the adult dose of 2.4 million units	For children ≥ 1 month with acquired primary or secondary syphilis conduct an evaluation through consultation with child-protection services and a CSF examination for detection of asymptomatic neurosyphilis
Children with late latent syphilis or latent syphilis of unknown duration	Benzathine penicillin G 50,000 units/kg IM, up to the adult dose of 2.4 million units, administered at -week intervals for three weeks (3 doses in total)	

[a]Treatment for congenital syphilis is more complex and beyond the scope of this chapter.

Treatment success for both HIV-uninfected and HIV-infected persons is defined as a four fold decrease in non-treponemal titers at 6 to 12 months post treatment in early syphilis and 12 to 24 months post treatment in late syphilis. HIV-infected patients should be re-evaluated every 3 months for a year after initial treatment [11]. When considering treatment failure, the possibility of re-infection should be considered, as this simply requires retreatment. In the absence of evidence of re-infection, CSF analysis should be performed to rule out neurosyphilis, and a 3-week course of treatment should be initiated [4, 7]. If neurosyphilis cannot be excluded, the patient must be treated for neurosyphlis with intravenous penicillin G.

GENITAL HERPES

Epidemiology

Both herpes simplex virus type 1 (HSV-1) and type 2 (HSV-2) are prevalent worldwide. Most persons are infected with HSV-1 in childhood; however, HSV-2 infection is usually transmitted sexually and risk factors are thus similar to those of other sexually transmitted diseases: the number of lifetime sex partners, young age at sexual debut, and previous history of STDs [16]. HSV-1 seroprevalence in adults approaches 70% in developed countries and 100% in developing countries. Sub-Saharan Africa has the highest burden of HSV-2 infection, ranging from 20–80% in low-risk adults and about 40–90% in high-risk adults, with slightly lower prevalence in West Africa than the other regions. Similar prevalence of HSV-2 infection is found in Central and South America and the Middle East, ranging from about 30% to 50%. Although data are sparse from countries in Asia, available data suggest a lower HSV-2 prevalence [17].

Across the globe HSV-2 infection is more prevalent among women than men, and prevalence increases with age [17]. The burden of HSV-2 infection is consistently higher in HIV-infected individuals than in HIV-uninfected individuals. There is a wealth of epidemiologic evidence demonstrating that prevalent HSV-2 is associated with a two- to eight-fold increase in incident HIV-1 infection, even when adjusted for sexual behavior [18, 19]. Because HSV-2 infection leads to the disruption of the genital mucosa and an influx of CD4-bearing T cell lymphocytes, it is biologically plausible that HSV-2 infection could lead to increased risk of HIV-1 acquisition [18]. It has also been suggested that persons co-infected with HSV-2 and HIV-1 are more likely to transmit HIV-1; however, recent studies have found similar rates of HIV-1 transmission between HSV-2 infected and uninfected individuals [18]. Several clinical trials to treat HSV-2 infection were recently completed that demonstrated no impact of HSV-2 treatment on HIV acquisition or transmission [20, 21]. Treatment of HSV-2 infection in HSV-2/HIV co-infected patients, however, was associated with a delay in HIV disease progression [22].

Natural history, pathogenesis, and pathology

A person becomes infected with HSV after exposure to virus that is shed from the genital tract or skin of an HSV-infected individual. While most HSV-1 infection usually occurs from oral contact (kissing) in childhood, in many countries HSV-1 is increasingly being acquired from oral-genital contact in adolescence [23]. HSV-2 acquisition almost always occurs through sexual contact. Once infected, the virus replicates at the site of infection. The virus then spreads through the lymphatic system to the sensory nervous system, where it persists. HSV is cleared from the cells at the site of infection; however, recurrences at this and other sites can occur after HSV reactivation and transport back down the nerves to the dermis, skin, or mucous membranes. Reactivation of HSV leads to viral shedding, even in the absence of symptoms. Because most infections are asymptomatic, sexual transmission of herpes usually occurs from persons who are unaware they are infected [9, 16].

Clinical features

HSV infection is often asymptomatic. In a true primary first episode (a first episode in a person who was previously not infected with either HSV-1 or HSV-2), small fluid-filled erythematous papules or vesicles will usually appear after an incubation period of 1–14 days and quickly evolve into small, painful, itchy ulcers (see Figs. 36.4A and 4B) [9]. Although lesions primarily arise on the external genitalia, they can also appear in the vagina and on the cervix, in the anus and rectum, in the perianal region, on the buttocks or on the upper thighs. When the lesions are present approximately 80% of women report dysuria, and 40% of men and 70% of women report flu-like symptoms, including headache and fever [16]. In about 10% of newly infected patients, clinical symptoms and signs consistent with aseptic meningitis may develop [16, 24]. Primary HSV infection should always be included in the differential diagnosis of meningitis. The lesions take about 1–2 weeks to heal. During that period most patients develop new lesions. In the first year after a symptomatic first episode of genital herpes, 70–90% of HSV-2 -infected individuals and 20–50% of HSV-1-infected individuals will have a recurrent episode [16]. Recurrences, which occur approximately four times per year, decrease in frequency and severity over time. Some patients have prodromal symptoms, such as tingling, itching, and pain, which occur 6-24 hours before the lesions develop [9].

HIV-infected individuals are more likely to have HSV-2 reactivation than HIV-uninfected individuals; however, most reactivation is subclinical in both groups. Antiretroviral therapy with immune restoration can reduce the frequency of recurrent outbreaks in HIV/HSV-2 co-infected individuals [18].

Patient evaluation, diagnosis, and differential diagnosis

Because most patients are asymptomatic, and those with lesions have varying symptoms, clinical diagnosis is neither sensitive nor specific. Clinical diagnosis should ideally be confirmed by laboratory tests. Those tests should be type-specific, as the frequency of clinical recurrences is dependent on viral type.

When there are vesicles or ulcers, it is possible to diagnose infection and viral type with viral antigen assays,

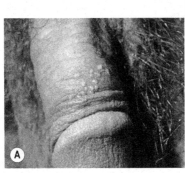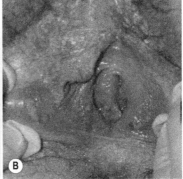

Figure 36.4 (A) Penile vesicles and (B) labial ulcerations.
Collection of Dr. Jeffrey Klausner.

including PCR and culture [11]. However, as the lesions begin to heal, viral detection becomes more difficult. The best means to detect virus during infection is to unroof the vesicle and swab the base of the ulcer. If the patient is asymptomatic or if the lesions have begun to crust over, it is necessary to perform serum antibody testing [16]. Type-specific HSV-1 or HSV-2 IgG antibody testing is readily available in many countries. However, antibody testing is limited as it is not a marker of disease and cannot be used to determine the duration of infection. Persons with prior history of infection may have a positive antibody assay, but the current genital lesion may or may not be related to HSV infection.

Treatment

Although treatment for genital herpes cannot eliminate latent virus or affect the frequency of recurrence once discontinued, antiviral treatment can reduce the symptoms of a recurrence, and if taken early enough during the prodrome (described above), can even abort the recurrence completely. Treatment depends on the type of clinical episode, the frequency of previous episodes, and the individual's HIV serostatus. Multiple clinical trials have demonstrated that acyclovir, valacyclovir, and famciclovir provide clinical benefit (see Table 36.2 for treatment guidelines). As symptoms are often systemic, currently available topical creams or ointments are not effective and thus not recommended. Chronic daily suppressive treatment with valacyclovir has been shown to reduce the transmission of HSV-2 infection to susceptible partners [25].

The transmission of herpes from mother to infant occurs most often around the time of delivery. While the likelihood of HSV transmission is greatest from an infection acquired during the third trimester before the development of protective maternal antibodies, most cases of neonatal herpes occur from asymptomatic genital HSV-2 reactivation and viral- shedding. Neonatal herpes is a devastating disease, with about 50% mortality and long term neurologic morbidity in those who survive [26]. Unfortunately there is limited experience with strategies to prevent neonatal herpes when HSV-2 infection is not identified in the mother [26].

GONORRHEA

Epidemiology

The global burden of gonorrhea was estimated at 62 million cases in 1999, with the highest incidence in South and Southeast Asia, at an estimated 27.2 million new cases. Sub-Saharan Africa and Latin America/Caribbean have the next highest burden. Asymptomatic gonorrhea is common, ranging between 67% and 100% of those with infection in the general population and 9–40% of those reporting to a genitourinary medicine clinic [2, 27].

Gonorrhea is more prevalent among women than men, among youth (aged 18–24 years old), persons who have never married, and persons who have had more than one partner in the previous 3 months [28].

Quinolone-resistant *Neisseria gonorrhoeae* is common among many populations worldwide and affects treatment decisions (see Treatment section). The prevalence of quinolone-resistant *N. gonorrhoeae* has been reported as greater than 40%, even reaching 98%, in South Africa as well as many countries in the Middle East, Asia,

Table 36.2 Recommended treatment for herpes simplex virus infection [11, 12]

POPULATION	ACYCLOVIR	FAMCICLOVIR	VALACYCLOVIR
First clinical episode of genital herpes	400 mg orally 3 times daily for 7–10 days OR 200 mg orally 5 times a day for 7–10 days	250 mg orally 3 times daily for 7–10 days	1 g orally twice daily for 7–10 days
Recurrent episode	400 mg orally 3 times daily for 5 days OR 800 mg orally twice daily for 5 days OR 800 mg orally three times daily for 2 days	125 mg orally twice daily for 5 days OR 1000 mg orally twice daily for 1 day	500 mg orally twice daily for 3 days OR 1.0 g orally once a day for 5 days
Suppressive therapy	400 mg orally twice daily	250 mg orally twice daily	500 mg orally once daily OR 1.0 g orally once daily
HIV-infected persons			
Recurrent episode	400 mg orally 3 times daily for 5–10 days	500 mg orally twice daily for 5–10 days	1.0 g orally twice daily for 5–10 days
Suppressive therapy	400–800 mg orally twice or 3 times daily	500 mg orally twice daily	500 mg orally twice daily

Central Asia, and the South Pacific [29]. Surveillance for antimicrobial resistance is essential to continue making informed treatment decisions.

Natural history, pathogenesis, and pathology

Gonorrhea is caused by infection with the bacterium *N. gonorrhoeae*. Once exposed, the gonococci colonize mucosal cells. Due to anatomical differences between men and women, infection is more easily transmitted from an infected man to a woman (50–73% probability) than from an infected woman to a man (20–35% probability) [30]. After infection there is an incubation period lasting approximately 1–2 days in men and 5–10 days in women before the onset of clinical symptoms [30]. Untreated infection may resolve within 6 months in men, whereas untreated infection in women may result in upper genital tract infection in about 15% of women [31].

Re-infection is common in both women and men (about 10–15% and 5–10%, respectively). Re-infection is more common in younger individuals. Treating partners or providing medications for infected patients to deliver to their partners significantly decreases the risk of reinfection [31, 32].

Clinical features

In men with symptomatic gonococcal infection, pain with urination usually precedes urethral discharge. Symptoms in women include pain during urination or intercourse, vaginal discharge, abnormal menstrual bleeding, and genital discomfort. If left untreated, local infection can ascend, causing pelvic inflammatory disease or upper reproductive tract infection that may lead to chronic pelvic pain, ectopic pregnancy or infertility [9, 30].

With rectal infections symptoms may range from mild rectal itchiness and discharge to frank proctitis with rectal bleeding and pain. Although oral infection is asymptomatic in a majority of cases, it may cause pharyngitis and rarely tonsillar abscess [9].

Patient evaluation, diagnosis and differential diagnosis

Definitive diagnosis can be made by Gram stain, culture, nucleic acid hybridization tests, or nucleic acid amplification tests (NAATs) of a clinical specimen (urethral, cervical, vaginal, rectal or pharyngeal swab) depending on the site of infection and resources available. A Gram stain to identify Gram-negative intracellular diplococci can be used with male urethral specimens (see Fig. 36.5). In asymptomatic cases culture or nucleic acid tests are required to increase sensitivity. Culture and nucleic acid tests are highly specific and can be used with various clinical specimens. However, because of the rigorous collection, storage, and transport

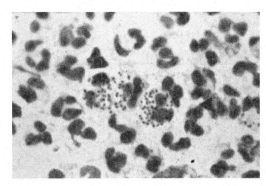

Figure 36.5 Gram stain of urethral exudate from patient with gonorrhea.
Courtesy of San Francisco City Clinic.

requirements, culture may not be the best choice in some low-resource settings. NAATs are becoming a popular choice for diagnosis, as they can be used with urine and endocervical or urethral swabs, vaginal swabs (self-collected), and rectal and pharyngeal swabs. NAATs are more sensitive and as specific as culture [11]. Some NAATs can be used to diagnose co-infection with chlamydia, but as NAATs differ by manufacturer, it is important that clinicians be aware of the performance characteristics of the particular NAAT being used. While culture is still the gold standard for antimicrobial susceptibility testing, novel methods have been used to describe specific gene mutations in *N. gonorrhoeae* associated with antimicrobial resistance and may soon replace culture in the monitoring of resistance [9, 11, 33]. Because asymptomatic infection is common, high-risk individuals, especially young women, should be screened for gonorrhea. Because re-infection is common, infected individuals should be re-screened 3 months after treatment [31, 32].

The differential diagnosis of urethral or cervico-vaginal discharge usually includes gonorrhea, chlamydia, and trichomoniasis, along with bacterial vaginosis and candidiasis in females. Other pathogens, such as *Mycoplasma* species, HSV, and oral bacterial flora or respiratory viruses (adenoviruses) may also cause urethral infection [12].

Treatment

With an increase in quinolone-resistant *N. gonorrhoeae* infections, treatment decisions for gonorrhea must be made within the context of local rates of antimicrobial resistance (see Table 36.3). If resistance to a drug is greater than 5% in a population, then that drug should no longer be used in that population. Infected individuals should also be asked about their recent travel history to exclude possible exposure to antimicrobial resistant infections elsewhere [29].

Because of the frequency of gonococcal and chlamydial co-infection, patients with gonorrhea should be co-treated

Table 36.3 Recommended treatment for gonorrhea [11, 12, 29]

POPULATION	RECOMMENDED REGIMENS

Uncomplicated infections of the cervix, urethra, and rectum	Ceftriaxone 250 mg IM as a single dose
	OR
	Cefixime 400 mg orally as a single dose
	OR
	Ciprofloxacin* 500 mg orally as a single dose
	PLUS
	    azithromycin 1 g orally as a single dose
	    OR
	    doxycycline 100 mg orally twice a day for 7 days

Uncomplicated infections of the pharynx	Ceftriaxone 250 mg IM as a single dose
	PLUS
	    Azithromycin 1 g orally as a single dose
	    OR
	    Doxycycline 100 mg orally twice a day for 7 days

Pregnant women	Ceftriaxone 250 mg IM as a
	single dose
	PLUS
	    Azithromycin 1 g orally as a single dose
	    OR if cannot tolerate cephalosporin,
	    azithromycin 2 g orally as a single dose

Gonococcal conjunctivitis	Ceftriaxone 1 g IM as a single dose
Disseminated gonococcal infection All regimens should be continued for 24-48 hours after improvement begins, then switched to one of the following oral antimicrobial regimens for at least an additional week	Recommended: Ceftriaxone 1 g IM or IV every 24 h OR Alternative Regimens: Cefotaxime 1 g IV every 8 hours OR Ceftizoxime 1 g every 8 hours Cefixime 400 mg orally twice daily
For prophylaxis in infants born to mothers with gonococcal infection or for infants with ophthalmia neonatorum	Ceftriaxone 25–50 mg/kg IV or IM as a single dose, not to exceed 125 mg
Ophthalmia neonatorum prophylaxis	Erythromycin (0.5%) ophthalmic ointment in each eye in a single application
For infants with disseminated gonococcal infection and scalp abscesses	Ceftriaxone 25–50 mg/kg/day IV or IM as a single daily dose, not to exceed 125 mg a day for 7 days; treat for 10–14 days if meningitis is documented OR Cefotaxime 25 mg/kg IV or IM every 12 hours for 7 days; treat for 10–14 days if meningitis is documented

*Ciprofloxacin in geographic areas where surveillance data show quinolone resistance is < 5%.

for uncomplicated genital chlamydial infection. Co-treatment might also slow the development of drug resistance in gonorrhea and is increasingly recommended. HIV-infected patients should receive the same treatment for gonorrhea as HIV-uninfected patients [11].

CHLAMYDIA

Epidemiology

Chlamydia is the most commonly reported sexually transmitted disease worldwide, with an estimated 92 million new cases in 1999. Following a similar geographic distribution as gonorrhea, the area with the most incident cases in 1999 was South and Southeast Asia (42.9 million cases) followed by sub-Saharan Africa and Latin America/Caribbean (15.9 and 9.3 million cases, respectively) [2]. Despite education and awareness campaigns, recent trends have shown increases in the prevalence of chlamydia. However, it is not clear if those increases are due at least in part to increased screening [34, 35].

Chlamydia is generally more prevalent among women and younger individuals (18–24 years), as well as persons who have multiple sex partners [28]. Asymptomatic infection is common among both women and men, accounting for over 75% of infections in many populations [2, 28].

Natural history, pathogenesis, and pathology

Chlamydia is caused by infection with the bacterium *Chlamydia trachomatis*. The bacteria infect epithelial cells and undergo intracellular replication. The clinical incubation period is about 7 to 21 days. It is likely that chlamydia is more readily transmitted from men to women than from women to men [35]. Studies have shown that re-infection is common in both women and men (approximately 10–20%) [31, 32]. Providing medications for infected patients' partners (expedited partner therapy) significantly decreases the risk of re-infection.

Clinical features

Men with clinical symptoms may present with painful urination, increased frequency of urination, thin mucoid urethral discharge, and penile itching or discomfort (see Fig. 36.6). Symptoms in women may include painful urination, increased frequency of urination, vaginal discharge, abnormal menstrual bleeding, lower abdominal pain, and/or pain during intercourse [9]. If infection is left untreated in women, more serious complications may include pelvic inflammatory disease, chronic pelvic pain, and ectopic pregnancy. In both men and women infertility may result [9]. Increasingly *C. trachomatis* has been recognized as a cause of rectal infection and proctitis. Patients may be asymptomatic or have symptoms ranging from mild rectal itching to discharge and proctitis with rectal bleeding. Some proportion of rectal chlamydial infection may be due to the *C. trachomatis* serovars L1–L3 traditionally associated with lymphogranuloma venereum.

Patient evaluation, diagnosis, and differential diagnosis

Even in persons with symptomatic chlamydial infection, the symptoms are not specific enough for a diagnosis, so it is necessary to perform diagnostic assays. Diagnosis

Figure 36.6 Non-gonococcal urethritis.
Courtesy of Dr Kenneth Katz.

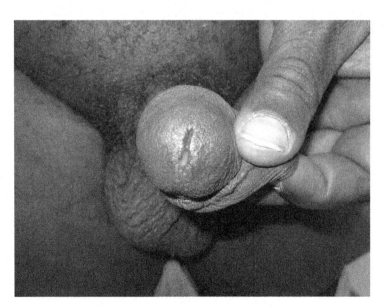

can be made from urine or swabs collected from the endocervix or vagina (in women), the urethra (in men), or the rectum (to detect rectal infection in persons with a history of receptive anal intercourse). Culture, direct fluorescent antibody tests, enzyme immunoassays, nucleic acid hybridization tests, and NAATs can all be used for testing swab specimens, but only NAATs can be used with urine. NAATs provide the most sensitive results, and because they can be used with urine samples, they can be used in non-clinical settings. NAATs are therefore recommended for use when available [11, 35]. Because co-infection with *N. gonorrhoeae* is common, patients should undergo testing for both chlamydia and gonorrhea.

The differential diagnosis of urethral or cervico-vaginal discharge usually includes gonorrhea, chlamydia and trichomoniasis, along with bacterial vaginosis and candidiasis in females. Other pathogens like *Mycoplasma* species, HSV, and oral bacterial flora or respiratory viruses (adenoviruses) may also cause urethral infection [12].

Treatment

Treatment of patients with chlamydia not only cures the infection and relieves symptoms, but also is important to prevent the further transmission to sex partners (Table 36.4). In pregnant women treatment generally prevents mother-to-child transmission of *C. trachomatis*. HIV-infected patients should receive the same treatment for chlamydia as HIV-uninfected patients [11].

Although doxycycline costs less than azithromycin, azithromycin should be used in patients for whom compliance with a multi-day regimen is uncertain. Patients remain infectious for 7 days after the start of treatment and should be advised to abstain from sex for that period. To prevent re-infection patients should be advised to ensure all their sex partners have been treated; providing patients additional treatment to give to sex partners should be considered. Retesting of pregnant women, infants, and children three weeks after treatment completion is recommended to confirm cure [11].

The optimal treatment of rectal chlamydial infection is unknown. For non-lymphogranuloma venereum sub-type or asymptomatic rectal chlamydial infection the recommended treatment is azithromycin 1 g once or doxycycline 100 mg orally twice daily for 7 days. Because in most settings the bacterial sub-type of rectal chlamydial infection cannot be determined, in symptomatic patients some experts recommend a 3-week course of treatment (doxycycline 100 mg orally twice daily for 21 days or azithromycin 1 g orally weekly for 3 weeks) [11].

TRICHOMONIASIS

Epidemiology

Although it is not a reportable infectious disease, trichomoniasis is the most common STD worldwide, with the highest incidence in South and Southeast Asia, followed by sub-Saharan Africa. Prevalence of *Trichomonas vaginalis* infection increases with age. While trichomoniasis is a common cause of vaginal and urethral discharge, up to one-third

Table 36.4 Recommended treatment for chlamydia [11, 12]

POPULATION	RECOMMENDED REGIMENS	ALTERNATIVE REGIMENS
Adults	Azithromycin 1 g orally as a single dose OR Doxycycline 100 mg orally twice daily for 7 days	Erythromycin base 500 mg orally four times a day for 7 days OR Ofloxacin 300 mg orally twice daily for 7 days
Women who are pregnant or lactating	Amoxicillin 500 mg orally three times daily for 7 days	Erythromycin base 500 mg orally four times daily for 7 days OR Erythromycin base 250 mg orally four times daily for 14 days
Neonatal chlamydial conjunctivitis, neonatal pneumonia, or children < 45 kg	Erythromycin base 50 mg/kg orally per day, divided into four doses daily for 14 days[a]	
Children ≥ 45 kg	Azithromycin 1 g orally in a single dose	For children >8 years old doxycycline 100 mg orally twice daily for 7 days

[a]Infants should be watched for signs of infantile hypertrophic pyloric stenosis.

of infected women and a majority of men are asymptomatic [36]. Asymptomatic infection results in long-standing chronic infection and continued transmission of infection. *Trichomonas* infection has been associated with increased acquisition of HIV due to vaginal inflammation, increased genital HIV viral replication in men and women, and vaginal mucosal micro-ulcerations [37].

Natural history, pathogenesis, and pathology

Trichomoniasis is caused when the parasite *T. vaginalis* infects the squamous epithelium of the vagina or urethra. The infection causes an inflammatory response, resulting in symptoms in about half of all women and a somewhat lower proportion of men [9]. Infection may persist asymptomatically for years.

Clinical features

Symptomatic women generally present with vaginal discharge (frothy and yellowish-green in appearance), irritation, itching, and sometimes lower abdominal pain and pain during urination. Those symptoms might be more common in HIV co-infected women than HIV-uninfected women [9, 36]. Long-term complications of untreated infection in women can include pelvic inflammatory disease and adverse birth outcomes [38]. Men may present with symptoms of urethritis and rarely chronic prostatitis [36].

Patient evaluation, diagnosis, and differential diagnosis

Where tests are available, women presenting with vaginal discharge should be tested for *trichomonas* infection. Culture is the most sensitive and specific diagnostic technique for *T. vaginalis*, but wet mount microscopy of vaginal secretions (sensitivity of about 60–70%) is commonly used. Point-of-care antigen detection tests have recently been developed. The sensitivity and specificity of those assays compared with culture are about 83 and 97%, respectively. Testing of oral and rectal specimens is not recommended, as rectal infection in men who have sex with men is rare, and *T. vaginalis* is not known to infect the oropharynx [11].

The differential diagnosis of vaginal discharge in women includes *Candida* vaginitis and bacterial vaginosis. If there is cervicitis, then chlamydia and gonorrhea should be considered. In men the differential diagnosis of urethral discharge includes gonorrhea and chlamydia along with other bacterial pathogens like *Mycoplasma* species, HSV, and oral bacterial flora or respiratory viruses (adenoviruses) [12].

Treatment

Both the WHO and CDC recommend treating trichomoniasis with either 2 g metronidazole orally in a single dose or 2 g tinidazole orally in a single dose. Pregnant women should be treated with metronidazole. If symptoms persist after 7 days and re-infection has been excluded, patients can be treated with 500 mg metronidazole orally twice daily for 7 days. HIV-infected patients should be treated with the same regimen as HIV-uninfected patients. Sex partners should also be treated in order to prevent reinfection [11, 12, 36]. There have been rare cases of metronidazole-resistant trichomoniasis. Usually treatment failure may be overcome with higher doses of metronidazole for a longer duration (e.g. 500 mg orally twice daily for 7 days or 2 g orally a day for 5–7 days). Persistent treatment failure in which re-infection has been excluded should be treated in consultation with an infectious disease specialist [11].

SYNDROMIC MANAGEMENT

Introduction

Unfortunately, the diagnostic tests described in the previous sections are not available in many settings, making definitive, specific diagnosis of symptomatic individuals impossible. In those instances it is necessary to provide individuals with treatment based on their symptoms. In addition to the benefits in individuals, syndromic management can lead to a reduction in the prevalence of curable sexually transmitted diseases that tend to become symptomatic [39].

When providing syndromic management clinicians should take into account the patient's sexual history and the local epidemiology of sexually transmitted diseases. All patients treated for sexually transmitted disease should undergo counseling and testing for HIV infection as well as counseling for safe sex practices.

Genital ulcers (Fig. 36.7A)

Because HSV-2 has become the leading cause of genital ulcer disease globally and syphilis is highly curable, when an ulcer is present (with no clear vesicles), the patient should be treated with acyclovir for 7 days for HSV infection and penicillin for syphilis [13]. If clear vesicles are present, treatment for HSV infection alone is recommended, unless the patient is RPR positive and has not been treated for syphilis recently. The WHO recommends treatment for chancroid as well (e.g. azithromycin 1 g orally as a single dose), but given the rarity of chancroid many national programs do not include that recommendation. If the ulcer has not healed after 7 days of treatment, treatments for other causes of genital ulcers, such as chancroid, should be considered [12].

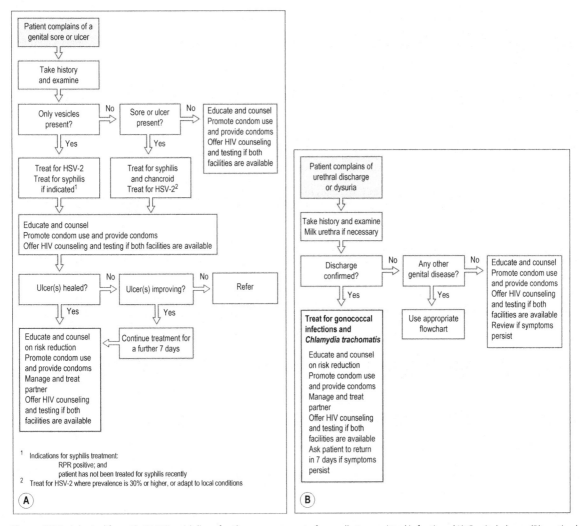

Figure 36.7 Adapted from the WHO guidelines for the management of sexually transmitted infection. (A) Genital ulcers, (B) urethral discharge,

Continued

Urethral discharge (Figs. 36.7B and 36.7C)

For men who present with complaints of pain on urination or urethral discharge, clinicians should investigate for evidence of discharge. If none is observed, the penis should be milked or massaged from the base to the tip in an attempt to produce discharge. If there is still none, and there is no other evidence of discharge (stained underwear or tissue) the patient should be counseled about safer sex and asked to return if symptoms persist. If there is evidence of discharge, then patients should be treated for both chlamydia and gonorrhea as these conditions are the primary

causes of male urethral discharge, accounting for 98% of cases in one recent South African study [40]. Whenever possible, single-dose regimens are preferred to encourage adherence. In the case of persistent or recurrent discharge, a medical and sexual history should be taken to rule out non-adherence with the treatment regimen or re-infection before other pathogens or drug resistance is considered. Other causes of urethral discharge include *Mycoplasma spp.*, *T. vaginalis*, and HSV infections [9, 12]. Given the frequency of *T. vaginalis* in some settings, the WHO recommends treatment for trichomoniasis as part of the urethral discharge management algorithm. National guidelines vary.

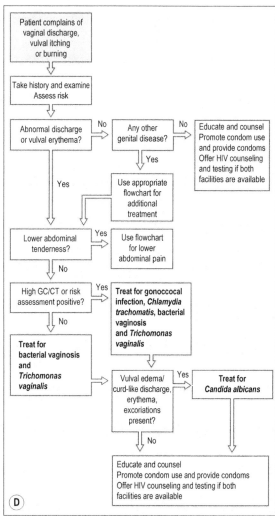

Figure 36.7, cont'd (C) persistent/recurrent urethral discharge, (D) vaginal discharge.
From Guidelines for the management of sexually transmitted infections. Geneva: World Health Organization; 2003.

Vaginal discharge (Fig. 36.7D)

Complaints of vaginal discharge are highly indicative of vaginal infection as opposed to cervical infection. In women of reproductive age, vaginal discharge is most often caused by *T. vaginalis*, *Candida albicans*, or bacterial vaginosis. The WHO recommends that patients be treated for all three conditions: metronidazole 400 or 500 mg orally twice daily for 7 days to treat *T. vaginalis* and bacterial vaginosis, AND miconazole or clotrimazole 200 mg intravaginally daily for 3 days (OR clotrimazole 500 mg intravaginally as a single dose OR 150 mg fluconazole orally as a single dose) to treat candidiasis [12]. In the absence of laboratory testing, treatment for chlamydia or gonorrhea should be given only if the infection appears to be cervical, if the woman has a high risk profile, or if the epidemiologic profile of the region suggests high incidence of chlamydia or gonorrhea in women presenting with vaginal discharge. Although symptoms may appear minor, it is important to properly treat women, as cervico-vaginal infections and abnormal vaginal flora are associated with adverse pregnancy outcomes and increased risk of HIV acquisition [41].

REFERENCES

[1] Kalichman SC, Pellowski J, Turner C. Prevalence of sexually transmitted co-infections in people living with HIV/AIDS: systematic review with implications for using HIV treatments for prevention. Sex Transm Infect 2011;87:183–90.

[2] WHO. Global prevalence and incidence of selected curable sexually transmitted infection. Geneva: WHO; 2001.

[3] Kamb ML, Newman LM, Riley PL, et al. A road map for the global elimination of congenital syphilis. Obstet Gynecol Int 2010; pii: 312798. Epub 2010 Jul 14.

[4] Drummond F, Guy R, Kaldor JM, Donovan B. The intersection between HIV and syphilis in men who have sex with men: some fresh perspectives. HIV Therapy 2010;4 (6):661–73.

[5] Kent ME, Romanelli F. Reexamining syphilis: an update on epidemiology, clinical manifestations, and management. Ann Pharmacother 2008;42:226–36.

[6] Goh BT. Syphilis in adults. Sex Transm Infect 2005;81:448–52.

[7] Zetola NM, Engelman J, Jensen TP, Klausner JD. Syphilis in the United States: an update for clinicians with an emphasis on HIV coinfection. Mayo Clin Proc 2007;82 (9):1091–102.

[8] Clark EG, Danbolt N. The Oslo Study of the natural history of untreated syphilis: an epidemiologic investigation based on a restudy of the Boeck-Bruusgaard material. J Chronic Dis 1955;2(3):311–44.

[9] Klausner JD, Hook III JD, (eds). Current Diagnosis and Treatment of Sexually Transmitted Diseases. New York: McGraw-Hill; 2007.

[10] Flood JM, Weinstock HS, Guroy ME, et al. Neurosyphilis during the AIDS epidemic, San Fransisco, 1985–1992. J Infect Dis 1998;177:931–40.

[11] Sexually Transmitted Diseases Treatment Guidelines, 2010. Centers for Disease Control and Prevention; 2010 Contract No.: RR-12.

[12] WHO. Guidelines for the management of sexually transmitted infections. Geneva: WHO; 2003.

[13] Corbell C, Stergachis A, Ndowa F, et al. Genital ulcer disease treatment policies and access to acyclovir in eight sub-Saharan African countries. Sex Transm Dis 2010;37:488–93.

[14] Zhou P, Qian Y, Xu J, et al. Occurence of congenital syphilis after maternal treatment with azithromycin during pregnancy. Sex Transm Dis 2007;34(7):472–4.

[15] Marra CM, Boutin P, McArthur JC. A pilot study evaluating ceftriaxone and penicillin G as treatment agents for neurosyphilis in human immunodeficiency virus-infected individuals. Clin Infect Dis 2000;30:540–4.

[16] Gupta R, Warren T, Wald A. Genital herpes. Lancet 2007;370:2127–37.

[17] Weiss H. Epidemiology of herpes simplex virus type 2 infection in the developing world. Herpes 2004;11 (Suppl. 1):24A–35A.

[18] Corey L, Wald A, Celum CL, Quinn TC. The effects of herpes simplex virus-2 on HIV-2 acquisition and transmission: a review of two overlapping epidemics. J Acquir Immune Defic Syndr 2004;35(5):435–45.

[19] Glynn JR, Biraro S, Weiss HA. Herpes simplex virus type 2: a key role in HIV incidence. AIDS 2009;23:1595–8.

[20] Celum C, Wald A, Hughes J, et al. Effect of aciclovir on HIV-1 acquisition in herpes simplex virus 2 seropositive women and men who have sex with men: a randomised, double-blind, placebo-controlled trial. Lancet 2008;371:2109–19.

[21] Celum C, Wald A, Lingappa JR, Magaret AS, et al. Acyclovir and transmission of HIV-1 from persons infected with HIV-1 and HSV-2. N Engl J Med 2010;362(5):427–39.

[22] Lingappa JR, Baeten JM, Wald A, et al. Daily acyclovir for HIV-1 disease progression in people dually infected with HIV-1 and herpes simplex virus type 2: a randomised placebo-controlled trial. Lancet 2010;375(9717):824–33.

[23] Roberts CM. Genital herpes in young adults: changing sexual behaviours, epidemiology and management. Herpes 2005;12 (1):10–14.

[24] Corey L, Adams HG, Brown ZA, Holmes KK. Genital herpes simplex virus infections: clinical manifestations, course, and complications. Ann Intern Med 1983;98:958–72.

[25] Corey L, Wald A, Patel R, et al. Once-daily valacyclovir to reduce the risk of transmission of genital herpes. N Engl J Med 2004;350(1):11–20.

[26] Donoval BA, Passaro DJ, Klausner JD. The public health imperative for a neonatal herpes simplex virus infection surveillance system. Sex Transm Dis 2006;33(3):170–4.

[27] Bozicevic I, Fenton KA, Martin IMC, et al. Epidemiological correlates of asymptomatic gonorrhea. Sex Transm Dis 2006;33(5):289–95.

[28] Detels R, Green AM, Klausner JD, et al. The incidence and correlates of symptomatic and asymptomatic C. trachomatis and N. gonorrhoeae infections in selected populations in five countries. Sex Transm Dis submitted.

[29] Newman LM, Moran JS, Workowski KA. Update on the management of gonorrhea in adults in the United States. Clin Infect Dis 2007;44(Suppl. 3):S84–101.

[30] Edwards JL, Apicella MA. The molecular mechanisms used by Neisseria gonorrhoeae to initiate infection differ between men and women. Clin Microbiol Rev 2004;17(4):965–81.

[31] Hosenfeld CB, Workowski KA, Berman S, et al. Repeat infection with chlamydia and gonorrhea among females: a systematic review of the literature. Sex Transm Dis 2009;36(8):478–89.

[32] Fung M, Scott KC, Kent CK, Klausner JD. Chlamydial and gonococcal reinfection among men: a systematic review of data to evaluate the need for retesting. Sex Transm Infect 2007;83:304–9.

[33] Klausner JD, Bernstein KT, Pandori M, et al. Clinic-based

testing for rectal and pharyngeal *Neisseria gonorrhoeae* and *Chlamydia trachomatis* infections by community-based organizations— five cities, United States, 2007: Centers for Disease Control and Prevention; 2009: Contract No. 26.

[34] Miller WC. Epidemiology of chlamydial infection: are we losing ground? Sex Transm Infect 2008;84:82–6.

[35] Stamm WE. *Chlamydia trachomatis*— the persistent pathogen. Sex Transm Dis 2001;28(12):684–9.

[36] Johnston VJ, Mabey DC. Global epidemiology and control of *Trichomonas vaginalis*. Curr Opin Infect Dis 2008;21:56–64.

[37] McClelland RS, Sangare L, Hassan WM, et al. Infection with *Trichomonas vaginalis* increases the risk of HIV-1 acquisition. J Infect Dis 2007;195:698–702.

[38] Pol BVD, Williams JA, Orr Dp, et al. Prevalence, incidence, natural history, and response to treatment of *Trichomonas vaginalis* infection among adolescent women. J Infect Dis 2005;192:2039–44.

[39] Johnson LF, Dorrington RE, Bradshaw D, Coetzee DJ. The effect of syndromic management interventions on the prevalence of sexually transmitted infections in South Africa. Sex Reprod Healthc 2011;2(1):13–20.

[40] Mhlongo S, Magooa P, Muller EE, et al. Etiology and STI/HIV coinfections among patients with urethral and vaginal discharge syndromes in South Africa. Sex Transm Dis 2010;37(9):566–70.

[41] Moodley P, Connolly C, Sturm AW. Interrelationships among human immunodeficiency virus type 1 infection, bacterial vaginosis, trichomoniasis, and the presence of yeasts. J Infect Dis 2002;185:69–73.

Section | 4 |

Prevention and management

Chapter | **37** |

Prevention of mother-to-child transmission of HIV-1

Lynne M. Mofenson

INTRODUCTION

Globally, mother-to-child transmission (MTCT) is the primary mode of HIV-1 acquisition in children. Prior to the development of effective interventions to reduce MTCT, estimated transmission rates ranged from 15–25% in non-breastfeeding populations in the USA and Europe to 25–40% in breastfeeding populations in resource-constrained countries.

An estimated 370,000 children were infected with HIV-1 worldwide in 2009 [1]. Although this represents a 24% decrease from 2001, over 1,000 infections continue to occur in children daily. Over 90% of these infections occurred in sub-Saharan Africa, where HIV-1 acquisition through breast milk accounts for at least 40% of infections.

In well-resourced health systems in the USA and Europe, virtual elimination of perinatal HIV-1 infection is within reach. Early identification of infection among pregnant women through routine, opt-out antenatal HIV-1 testing, immediate assessment of infected pregnant women to determine their need for treatment, and provision of antiretroviral therapy when needed or antiretroviral prophylaxis if therapy is not yet required has substantially reduced the risk of infant infection during pregnancy and delivery. When combined with elective cesarean delivery and complete avoidance of breastfeeding, these interventions have reduced MTCT rates to 1–2% [2].

However, in resource-constrained countries, where most HIV-1-infected women reside, control of the perinatal epidemic continues to be challenging. Clinical trials have identified simple, less expensive, effective antiretroviral prophylaxis regimens more relevant to these countries that can reduce transmission during pregnancy and delivery. However, implementation has been slow, as the existing limited maternal–child healthcare infrastructure has had difficulty supporting the addition of antenatal HIV-1 testing and antiretroviral programs [3]. Postnatal transmission remains a significant problem in these settings, where breastfeeding is a cornerstone of infant survival [4]. Recent clinical trials have demonstrated that antiretroviral prophylaxis of the breastfeeding infant or the lactating mother can significantly decrease postnatal HIV-1 acquisition, offering new hope for prevention in these settings [5].

This chapter will discuss risk factors for MTCT; review progress in prevention of MTCT, concentrating on antiretroviral interventions; and discuss guidelines related to prevention of MTCT in resource-rich and resource-constrained settings.

RISK FACTORS FOR HIV-1 MTCT

HIV-1 can be transmitted during pregnancy, labor, and through breast milk. While different risk factors may influence transmission during each of these periods, maternal HIV-1 viral load has consistently been a strong independent predictor of transmission, regardless of timing of transmission [6, 7]. Hence, interventions that reduce viral load might be expected to influence transmission during each of these periods.

In utero and intrapartum transmission

In the absence of breastfeeding and antiretroviral prophylaxis, *in utero* transmission proportionally accounts for 25–30% and intrapartum transmission 65–70% of MTCT. During pregnancy the placenta provides a physical and immune barrier between maternal and fetal circulations and also against *in utero* HIV-1 infection, as the absolute rate of *in utero* transmission is only 5–10%. Although the exact mechanisms of *in utero* transmission have not been elucidated, factors that disrupt placental integrity, such as chorioamnionitis, might be expected to play a role. Genetic factors (e.g. HLA type, CCR5 genotype) and viral characteristics, such as viral subtype, have been reported to influence *in utero* transmission.

Intrapartum transmission can occur through access of cell-free or cell-associated virus to the infant systemic circulation by maternal–fetal transfusions during uterine contractions in labor, or through the infant swallowing HIV-1 present in genital fluids during delivery, with resultant viral passage through the gastrointestinal mucosa to underlying lymphoid cells, followed by systemic dissemination. The proven efficacy of interventions restricted to the peripartum period, such as elective cesarean section performed prior to labor and rupture of membranes or antiretroviral prophylaxis administered only around the time of delivery, illustrates the importance of the intrapartum period in MTCT [8–12].

Risk factors for transmission during the antepartum and peripartum periods were examined in 3,396 infants with known infection status born between 2002 and 2006 in New York State [13]. On multivariable analysis, maternal HIV diagnosis at or after delivery, maternal acquisition of HIV during pregnancy, illicit substance use during pregnancy, having 0–2 prenatal care visits, and neonatal birth weight < 2,500 g were associated with MTCT.

Postnatal transmission

Breastfeeding substantially increases MTCT and can account for 30–50% of all transmission in breastfeeding populations. Postnatal transmission results in a significant diminution of the efficacy of antiretroviral interventions that prevent *in utero* and intrapartum transmission [11, 14, 15]. Thus, for optimal prevention of MTCT in a breastfeeding setting, additional interventions are needed to reduce postnatal transmission.

Determining the timing of breast milk transmission has been complicated by the difficulty in distinguishing between intrapartum and early breast milk transmission; thus, most studies have focused on postnatal transmission occurring after age 1 month. The Breastfeeding and HIV International Transmission Study was an individual patient meta-analysis involving 4,085 children in 9 clinical trials in breastfeeding populations [16]. Of 539 children with known timing of infection, 225 (42%) had late postnatal transmission (occurring after age 1 month). Overall, late postnatal transmission risk was 8.9 infections per 100 child-years of breastfeeding, with a generally constant risk throughout the breastfeeding period (~0.17%/week); the cumulative probability of late postnatal infection at age 18 months was 9.3%. Almost identical results were reported from the Zimbabwe Vitamin A for Mothers and

Babies (ZVITAMBO) trial, which enrolled infants born to 4,495 women with chronic HIV-1 infection [17].

Although the risk of HIV-1 transmission through breast milk persists for the duration of breastfeeding, the early breastfeeding period (first 1–2 months) may be the period of highest risk. This is illustrated by the SAINT trial, in which all women and infants received effective prophylaxis against intrapartum transmission (zidovudine [AZT]/lamivudine [3TC] or single-dose nevirapine [NVP]) [18]. The trial included formula and breastfed infants; breastfeeding was the most significant risk factor for MTCT. By age 8 weeks, breastfeeding accounted for an absolute 6% increase in MTCT compared to formula-feeding. Postnatal transmission was also highest in the first few weeks of life in the control arm of the Breastfeeding and Nutrition (BAN) study (receiving single-dose NVP and 1 week postnatal AZT/3TC): postnatal transmission was 0.5%/week between 2 and 6 weeks, 0.3%/week between 7 and 12 weeks, and 0.1%/week thereafter [5, 19].

In addition to duration of breastfeeding, postnatal transmission risk factors include high plasma and maternal viral load; low CD4 count; breast milk immunologic factors; breast pathology including clinical and subclinical mastitis, nipple bleeding, cracked nipples, or breast abscess; and infant pathology that disrupts mucosal integrity, such as thrush [7, 20]. Several studies have suggested that exclusive breastfeeding is associated with lower risk of transmission than mixed feeding including breast milk and non-human milk, fluids, or other foods [20–22]. In the Zambia Exclusive Breastfeeding Study, early postnatal transmission before age 4 months was 2.7-fold higher in infants who did not exclusively breastfeed compared to those who did, adjusted for maternal CD4 count and viral load, syphilis, and low birth weight [23]. Finally, primary infection during breastfeeding has been shown to substantially increase the risk of postnatal transmission [17, 24, 25].

ANTIRETROVIRAL INTERVENTIONS TO PREVENT HIV-1 MTCT

In 1994, the PACTG 076 clinical trial first demonstrated that an antiretroviral drug, AZT, given during pregnancy, intravenously during labor, and to the newborn for 6 weeks significantly reduces *in utero* and intrapartum HIV-1 transmission [26]. In resource-rich countries, this relatively complex regimen was rapidly adopted as standard of care for HIV-infected pregnant women and their infants, with subsequent decline in overall population-based MTCT rates [27]. As new antiretroviral drugs became available, treatment with combination drug regimens (initially dual and then triple regimens) became standard of care, including for treatment of pregnant women. Although there were no randomized clinical trials, observational data suggested that use of combination regimens during pregnancy further reduced MTCT compared to AZT alone, at least in women requiring therapy for their own health [2, 27]. Thus, in resource-rich countries, combination regimens that include 3 or more antiretroviral drugs are currently given during pregnancy to HIV-infected women. In women who meet treatment criteria, these drugs are continued postpartum; in women who do not yet require treatment for their own health, the drugs may be discontinued postpartum.

However, in resource-constrained countries, the PACTG 076 regimen was considered too complex and expensive to implement following the 1994 trial, and researchers explored the development of shorter, less expensive prophylactic regimens more applicable to these settings. Studies initially focused on shortened AZT-alone prophylaxis regimens, and moved to evaluating whether combination regimens, such as short-course AZT plus 3TC, might have better efficacy than AZT alone. Studies also evaluated whether even simpler, less expensive, single-drug regimens, such as single-dose intrapartum/neonatal NVP, would be effective, and whether combining single-dose NVP with other short-course regimens might result in improved efficacy.

The overall results from these international trials, as well as open-label and observational studies, demonstrate that a number of different regimens have efficacy in preventing *in utero* and intrapartum transmission, but that efficacy is diminished in breastfeeding populations due to postnatal HIV acquisition through breast milk. More recent trials have demonstrated that antiretroviral prophylaxis of the lactating woman or her breastfeeding infant is a safe and effective way to reduce postnatal transmission in settings where feeding with breast milk alternatives is not safe, acceptable, feasible, affordable, and sustainable.

Mechanisms of action of antiretroviral prophylaxis

Antiretroviral drugs can reduce *in utero* and intrapartum MTCT by several different mechanisms, including: decreasing maternal viral load in blood and genital secretions; provision of pre-exposure prophylaxis to the infant through drug administration to the mother during labor, resulting in systemic drug levels in the infant at a time of intensive exposure of the infant to HIV-1 during delivery; and provision of post-exposure prophylaxis through drug administration to the infant after birth to protect against cell-free or cell-associated virus that entered the circulation during uterine contractions or is passed through the mucosa of the infant during delivery.

Efficacy is likely multifactorial. In women with high viral loads, it is likely that lowering viral levels with antenatal antiretroviral drugs is a critical component of protection. However, antiretroviral drugs have been shown to reduce the risk of transmission even among women with very low viral levels [28]. The HIV RNA level (viral load) at

delivery and receipt of antenatal antiretroviral drugs are each independently associated with transmission, suggesting that antiretroviral prophylaxis does not work solely through viral load reduction [27].

Studies have demonstrated that the quantity of cell-free and cell-associated virus in cervico-vaginal secretions is associated with MTCT, independent of plasma viral load [29]. Thus, providing prophylaxis to the infant immediately before and after extensive viral exposure during labor and delivery is an additional important mechanism of efficacy and results of clinical trials (discussed below) have demonstrated that intrapartum/postpartum antiretroviral regimens, without any maternal antenatal drug component, can significantly decrease MTCT [10–12].

Clinical trials for prevention of HIV-1 MTCT

Early international trials to prevent MTCT largely focused on antiretroviral drug use solely for prevention of transmission, without consideration of maternal treatment, because antiretroviral therapy was not generally available in resource-constrained countries at the time the studies were performed. However, treatment is now available in these settings; a key issue in decisions on which antiretroviral regimen to choose for an HIV-infected pregnant woman (or a postpartum lactating woman) is whether the drugs are being provided for treatment (in which case combination antiretroviral therapy should be provided and continued for life) or solely for MTCT prophylaxis (in which case less intensive regimens may be equally effective and antiretroviral drugs could stop when transmission risk has ceased). In resource-constrained countries, guidelines recommend that pregnant women with CD4 < 350 cells/mm^3 or World Health Organization (WHO) stage III or IV disease should start on life-long combination antiretroviral therapy [30]. In a study of 3,736 HIV-1-infected pregnant women in 13 clinical programs in 8 African countries and Thailand, 52% met WHO treatment criteria and 48% did not [31]. Current research is focused on what prophylactic regimen would be most efficacious and cost-effective for the subgroup of women who don't require therapy.

Tables 37.1–37.3 summarize results of randomized clinical trials of antiretroviral interventions for prevention of MTCT. Table 37.1 summarizes early trials of AZT, AZT/3TC, and single-dose NVP; Table 37.2 summarizes trials combining single-dose NVP with various antepartum regimens; and Table 37.3 summarizes more recent trials evaluating regimens to prevent postnatal transmission. These trials have built sequentially on each other and identified a number of simple regimens effective in reducing MTCT. Direct comparison between trials is difficult, as they enrolled patient populations from different geographic areas, infected with different viral subtypes, and having different infant feeding practices. However, some general conclusions can

Table 37.1 Clinical trials of antiretroviral drugs for prevention of mother-to-child HIV-1 transmission—zidovudine, zidovudine/lamivudine, single-dose nevirapine

STUDY/ LOCATION	INFANT FEEDING	REGIMEN	ANTENATAL/ INTRAPARTUM	POSTPARTUM	EFFICACY
PACTG 076 USA, France [26]	Formula	AZT vs placebo	Long (from 14 weeks), Intravenous IP	Long (6 weeks) (Infant only)	MTCT at 18 months, 7.6% AZT vs 22.6% placebo (68% efficacy)
Bangkok Short-Course AZT Trial Thailand [32]	Formula	AZT vs placebo	Short (from 36 weeks) Oral IP	None	MTCT at 6 months, 9.4% AZT vs 18.9% placebo (50.1% efficacy)
Thai Perinatal HIV Prevention Trial (PHPT-1) Thailand [33]	Formula	AZT different length AP and infant PP regimens, no placebo	Long (from 28 weeks) Short (from 36 weeks) Oral IP	Long (for 6 weeks) Short (for 3 days) (Infant only)	Short-Short stopped early due to significantly higher MTCT (10.5%). MTCT at 6 months, 6.5% Long-Long vs 4.7% Long-Short vs 8.6% Short-Long (statistical equivalence). However, *in utero* transmission significantly lower with Long vs Short maternal AP AZT (1.6% vs 5.1%)
Ivory Coast Short-Course AZT Trial Ivory Coast [14]	Breastfeeding	AZT vs placebo	Short (from 36 weeks) Oral IP	None	MTCT at 3 months, 15.7% AZT vs 24.9% placebo (37% efficacy)
DITRAME / ANRS 049a Ivory Coast / Burkina Faso [15]	Breastfeeding	AZT vs placebo	Short (from 36 weeks) Oral IP	Short (1 week) (Mother only)	MTCT at 6 months, 18.0% AZT vs 27.5% placebo (38% efficacy); MTCT at 15 months, 21.5% vs 30.6% (30% efficacy). MTCT at 24 months (pooled analysis with other Ivory Coast trial), 22.5% vs 30.2% (26% efficacy)
PETRA South Africa, Tanzania, and Uganda [10]	Breastfeeding	AZT+3TC in 3 regimens (3-part AP/IP/PP; 2-part IP/ PP; IP alone) vs placebo	Short (from 36 weeks) Oral IP	Short (7 days) (Mother and Infant)	MTCT at 6 weeks, 5.7% 3-part (63% efficacy) vs 8.9% 2-part (42% efficacy) vs 14.2% IP alone vs 15.3% placebo. MTCT at 18 months, 14.9% 3-part vs 18.1% 2-part vs 20% IP alone vs 22.2% placebo

STUDY/LOCATION	INFANT FEEDING	REGIMEN	ANTENATAL/INTRAPARTUM	POSTPARTUM	EFFICACY
HIVNET 012 Uganda [11]	Breastfeeding	IP/PP NVP vs AZT	No AP ARV Oral IP: Single-dose oral NVP 200 mg vs AZT	Single-dose NVP 2 mg/kg within 72 h of birth vs short AZT (7 days) (Infant only)	MTCT 15.7% in NVP arm versus 25.8% in AZT arm (41% efficacy) at 18 months
SAINT South Africa [18]	Breastfeeding (42%) and formula feeding	IP/PP NVP versus AZT+3TC	No AP ARV Oral IP: Single-dose NVP 200 mg vs AZT+3TC	Single-NVP dose within 48 h of birth vs short AZT+3TC (7 days) (Mother and Infant)	MTCT at 8 weeks, 12.3% NVP vs 9.3% AZT+3TC

3TC = lamivudine; ARV = antiretroviral; AP = antepartum; AZT = zidovudine; IP = intrapartum; MTCT = mother-to-child transmission; NVP = nevirapine; PP= postpartum.

Table 37.2 Clinical trials of antiretroviral drugs for prevention of mother-to-child HIV-1 transmission—zidovudine or zidovudine/lamivudine combined with single-dose nevirapine

STUDY/LOCATION	INFANT FEEDING	REGIMEN	ANTENATAL/INTRAPARTUM	POSTPARTUM	EFFICACY
Thai Perinatal HIV Prevention Trial-2 (PHPT-2) Thailand [34]	Formula	AZT vs AZT + maternal/infant single-dose NVP vs AZT+ maternal single-dose NVP only	Long (AZT from 28 weeks) IP: Oral AZT + single-dose NVP or placebo	1 week AZT alone vs 1 week AZT + single-dose NVP (infant only)	AZT alone arm stopped early due to significantly higher MTCT: MTCT at 6 months, 6.3% AZT alone vs 1.1% with AZT plus maternal/infant NVP vs 2.1% with AZT plus maternal NVP alone. Final analysis, MTCT at 6 months, 2.8% with AZT plus maternal NVP only vs 1.9% with AZT plus maternal/infant NVP
DITRAME PLUS / ANRS 1201.0 Abidjan, Cote d'Ivoire [36]	Breastfeeding (54%) and formula feeding	Open label, AZT+ maternal/infant single-dose NVP	Short (from 36 weeks) Oral IP: Single-dose NVP 200 mg + AZT	Single-dose NVP + 1 week AZT (Infant only)	MTCT at 6 weeks, 6.5% (95% CI, 3.9–9.1%) Compared to MTCT in historical control AZT alone (1995–2000) 12.8% (in AZT alone group, breastfeeding rate was 97.6%)

Continued

Table 37.2 Clinical trials of antiretroviral drugs for prevention of mother-to-child HIV-1 transmission—zidovudine or zidovudine/lamivudine combined with single-dose nevirapine—cont'd

STUDY/ LOCATION	INFANT FEEDING	REGIMEN	ANTENATAL/ INTRAPARTUM	POSTPARTUM	EFFICACY
DITRAME PLUS / ANRS 1201.1 Abidjan, Cote d'Ivoire [36]	Breastfeeding (66%) and formula feeding	Open label, AZT+3TC boosted by IP/PP NVP	Short (from 32 weeks) Oral IP: Single-dose NVP 200 mg + AZT+3TC	AZT+3TC for 3 days (Mother only) Single-dose NVP + one week AZT (Infant only)	MTCT at 6 weeks, 4.7% (95% CI, 2.4–7.0%) MTCT not significantly different than observed with DITRAME 1201.0 regimen AZT + single dose NVP ($p = 0.34$)
PACTG 316 USA, Europe, Brazil, Bahamas [37]	Formula	IP/PP NVP vs placebo in women already receiving AZT or AZT plus other ARV (77% on combination drugs)	Non-study AP ARV Oral IP: Single-dose NVP 200 mg + intravenous AZT	Single-dose NVP 2 mg/kg within 72 h of birth + 6 weeks AZT (Infant only)	Trial stopped early due to very low MTCT in both arms. MTCT at 6 months, 1.4% NVP versus 1.6% placebo
NVAZ-1 Malawi [12]	Breastfeeding	Neonatal single-dose NVP only vs NVP+AZT	No ARV AP or IP (late presenters)	Single-dose NVP immediately after birth + AZT twice daily for one week (Infant only)	Overall MTCT at 6–8 weeks, 15.3% NVP+AZT vs 20.9% NVP only MTCT at 6–8 weeks in babies who were uninfected at birth, 7.7% NVP+AZT vs 12.1% NVP only (36% efficacy)
NVAZ-2 Malawi [38]	Breastfeeding	Neonatal single-dose NVP only vs NVP+AZT	No ARV AP Oral IP: Single-dose NVP to mother	Single-dose NVP immediately after birth + AZT twice daily for one week (Infant only)	Overall MTCT at 6–8 weeks, 16.3% NVP+AZT vs 14.1% NVP only MTCT at 6–8 weeks in babies who were uninfected at birth, 6.9% NVP+AZT vs 6.5% NVP only
Mashi Botswana [35]	Breastfeeding and formula feeding (randomized)	Factorial design, randomized to mode of infant feeding and maternal/infant single-dose NVP vs placebo Infant placebo discontinued 08/02 (after PHPT-2 results), study modified to maternal NVP vs placebo, with all infants receiving single-dose NVP	Short (AZT from 34 weeks) Oral IP: AZT + single-dose NVP or placebo (infant only)	Single-dose NVP + 1 month AZT if formula feeding Single-dose NVP + 6 months AZT if breastfeeding (infant only)	*Original study* (maternal/infant NVP vs placebo): NVP provides added efficacy in formula-fed but not breastfed infants. MTCT at 1 month, formula-fed infants, 2.4% NVP/NVP vs 8.3% placebo/placebo; breastfed infants, 8.4% NVP/NVP vs 4.1% placebo/placebo *Revised study* (maternal NVP vs placebo, all infant NVP): No added efficacy from maternal NVP

Study	Infant feeding	Description	Regimen	Outcomes
				regardless of infant feeding mode. MTCT at 1 month, 4.3% NVP/NVP vs 3.7% placebo/NVP. *Infant feeding:* Breastfeeding + AZT higher transmission than formula. MTCT at 7 months, 9.1% breastfeeding + AZT vs 5.6% formula. However, higher infant mortality with formula at 7 months, 9.3% formula vs 4.9% breastfeeding + AZT. Incremental risk of postnatal MTCT between 1 and 7 months, 4.5% (comparable to postnatal MTCT in BHITS meta-analysis between 1 and 6 months, 4.2%, with no infant prophylaxis). HIV-free survival at 18 months did not differ between arms. MTCT or death at 18 months, 14.2% formula (33 infected, 46 deaths) vs 15.6% breastfed + AZT (54 infected, 34 deaths)
NICHD/HPTN 040 USA, Brazil, South Africa [39]	Formula feeding	Compares 3 different infant prophylaxis regimens when mothers do not receive AP drugs	No AP drugs. IP regimen (if presents early enough): Intravenous AZT. *Arm 1 (control):* Infant AZT for 6 weeks. *Arm 2:* Control as above + 3 doses of NVP in first week. *Arm 3:* Control as above + daily 3TC and nelfinavir for first 2 weeks (infants only)	Total *in utero* transmission was 5.7%, and not significantly different between arms. Total *intrapartum* transmission rate was 3.2%: 4.9% (95% CI: 3.3–7.2) in control Arm 1; 2.2% (95% CI: 1.2–4.0) in Arm 2 ($p = 0.045$ compared to control); AZT + NVP 2.2%, (95% CI: 1.2–4.0, $p = 0.045$ compared to control); 2..5% (95% CI: 1.4–4.3) in Arm 3 ($p = 0.045$ compared to control). More neutropenia seen in Arm 3.

3TC = lamivudine; ARV = antiretroviral; AP = antepartum; AZT = zidovudine; IP = intrapartum; MTCT = mother-to-child transmission; NVP = nevirapine; PP = postpartum.

Table 37.3 Clinical trials of antiretroviral drugs for prevention of postnatal breast milk mother-to-child HIV-1 transmission

STUDY/ LOCATION	INFANT FEEDING	REGIMEN	ANTENATAL/ INTRAPARTUM	POSTPARTUM	EFFICACY
SWEN (Six Week Extended-Dose Nevirapine) Uganda, Ethiopia, India [56]	Breastfeeding	Infant prophylaxis: Single-dose maternal/infant NVP vs extended 6 weeks infant NVP	No ARV AP Oral IP: Single-dose NVP to mother	Single-dose NVP vs single-dose NVP + 6 weeks daily NVP (infant only)	Postnatal infection in infants uninfected at birth: • MTCT at 6 weeks was 5.3% in single-dose NVP arm vs 2.5% in extended NVP arm (risk ratio 0.54, $p = 0.009$) • MTCT at 6 months was 9.0% in single-dose NVP arm vs 6.9% in extended NVP arm (risk ratio 0.80, $p = 0.16$) • HIV-free survival significantly better in extended NVP arm at both 6 weeks and 6 months
PEPI trial Malawi [55]	Breastfeeding	Infant prophylaxis: Single-dose NVP vs 14 weeks extended infant regimen	No ARV AP Oral IP: Single-dose NVP to mother (if presents in time to receive)	Infant single-dose NVP + AZT for 1 week (control) vs control + NVP for 14 weeks vs control + NVP/ AZT for 14 weeks (infant only)	Postnatal infection in infants uninfected at birth: • MTCT at 6 weeks was 5.1% in control vs 1.7% in extended NVP (67% efficacy) and 1.6% in extended NVP/AZT arms (69% efficacy) • MTCT at 9 months was 10.6% in control vs 5.2% in extended NVP (51% efficacy) and 6.4% in extended NVP/AZT arms (40% efficacy) • No significant difference in MTCT between the extended prophylaxis arms; however, more hematologic toxicity with NVP/AZT
HPTN 046 Uganda, Zimbabwe,	Breastfeeding	Infant prophylaxis: Compares 6 months and 6 weeks daily infant NVP to prevent postnatal infection	AP: Provided outside of study	All infants receive 6 weeks of daily infant NVP starting at birth Randomized at 6 weeks: *Arm 1 (control)*: Daily placebo	Postnatal infection at 6 months in infants uninfected at age 6 weeks:

Study	Feeding	Intervention	Timing	Regimen detail	Results
Tanzania, South Africa [57]			from 6 weeks to 6 months Arm 2: Daily NVP from 6 weeks to 6 months (infant only)		• Overall MTCT was 2.4% (95% CI, 1.3–3.6) in placebo Arm 1 and 1.1% (95% CI, 0.3–1.8%) in NVP Arm 2 ($p = 0.048$) • In mothers on ART at randomization, overall MTCT was 0.2% (0% placebo Arm 1 and 0.5% NVP Arm 2); in women not on ARV treatment, overall MTCT was 2.4% (3.4% placebo Arm 1 and 1.4% NVP Arm 2, $p = 0.027$) • In mothers *not* on ARV treatment, if CD4 was <350, MTCT not significantly different between arms (8.1% placebo Arm 1 and 4.8% NVP Arm 2, $p = 0.44$); however, if CD4 was ≥ 350, MTCT significantly less with extended NVP and similar to that seen in women on ARV treatment (2.8% placebo Arm 1 and 0.7% NVP Arm 2, $p = 0.014$)
Mma Bana Botswana [47]	Breastfeeding	Maternal prophylaxis: Maternal triple-drug prophylaxis (compares 2 regimens) in women with CD4 >200	*Arm 1:* AZT/3TC/ABC *Arm 2:* AZT/3TC/LPV/r From 26 weeks through labor	*Arm 1:* Maternal AZT/3TC/ABC for 6 months; infant single-dose NVP + AZT for 4 weeks *Arm 2:* Maternal AZT/3TC/LPV/r for 6 months; infant single-dose NVP + AZT for 4 weeks	MTCT at 6 months overall was 1.3%: 2.1% in AZT/3TC/ABC Arm 1 and 0.4% in AZT/3TC/LPV/r Arm 2 ($p = 0.53$)
Kesho Bora Multi-African [63]	Breastfeeding and formula feeding	Maternal prophylaxis: AP AZT/single-dose NVP with no postnatal prophylaxis vs maternal triple-drug prophylaxis in women with CD4 between 200 and 500	*Arm 1:* AZT/LPV/r *Arm 2:* AZT + single-dose NVP From 28 weeks through labor	*Arm 1:* Maternal AZT/3TC/LPV/r for 6 months; infant single-dose NVP + AZT for 1 week *Arm 2:* Maternal AZT/3TC for 1 week (no further postnatal prophylaxis); infant single-dose NVP + AZT for 1 week (no further postnatal prophylaxis)	MTCT at birth was 1.8% with maternal triple-drug prophylaxis Arm 1 and 2.5% with AZT/single-dose NVP Arm 2, *not* significantly different. MTCT at 12 months was 5.4% with maternal triple-drug prophylaxis Arm 1 and 9.5% with AZT/single-dose NVP (with no further postnatal prophylaxis after 1 week) Arm 2 ($p = 0.029$).

Continued

Table 37.3 Clinical trials of antiretroviral drugs for prevention of postnatal breast milk mother-to-child HIV-1 transmission—cont'd

STUDY/ LOCATION	INFANT FEEDING	REGIMEN	ANTENATAL/ INTRAPARTUM	POSTPARTUM	EFFICACY
BAN Malawi [5]	Breastfeeding	Infant vs maternal prophylaxis: Postpartum maternal triple-drug prophylaxis vs infant NVP in women with CD4 ≥250	No AP drugs Oral IP regimens: *Arm 1 (control):* AZT/3TC + single-dose NVP *Arm 2:* AZT/3TC + single-dose NVP *Arm 3:* AZT/3TC + single-dose NVP	*Arm 1 (control):* Maternal AZT/3TC for 1 week; infant single-dose NVP + AZT/3TC for 1 week *Arm 2:* Control as above, then maternal AZT/3TC/LPV/r for 6 months *Arm 3:* Control as above, then infant NVP for 6 months	Postnatal infection in infants uninfected at 2 weeks: • MTCT at 28 weeks was 5.7% in control Arm 1; 2.9% in maternal triple-drug prophylaxis Arm 2 ($p = 0.009$ vs control); 1.7% in infant NVP Arm 3 (<0.001 vs control) No significant difference between maternal triple-drug prophylaxis Arm 2 and infant NVP Arm 3 ($p = 0.12$)

3TC = lamivudine; ABC = abacavir; ARV = antiretroviral; AP = antepartum; AZT = zidovudine; ddI = didanosine; IP = intrapartum; LPV/r = lopinavir/ritonavir; MTCT = mother-to-child transmission; NVP = nevirapine; PP= postpartum.

be drawn regarding antiretroviral drug use for prevention of MTCT that are relevant to both resource-constrained and resource-rich countries.

Short-term efficacy has been demonstrated for regimens with AZT alone; AZT plus 3TC; single-dose NVP; and combining single-dose NVP with either short-course AZT or AZT/3TC. Combination regimens, such as short-course AZT plus single-dose NVP, are more effective than single-drug regimens in reducing MTCT, and a longer antenatal/intrapartum/postpartum regimen is superior in preventing MTCT than a shorter 2-part antepartum/intrapartum or intrapartum/postpartum regimen.

Almost all trials have included an intrapartum prophylaxis component, with varying durations of maternal antenatal and/or infant (and sometimes maternal) postpartum prophylaxis. Regimens with antenatal components starting as late as 36 weeks' gestation and lacking infant prophylaxis can reduce transmission [32]; however, longer duration of antenatal therapy starting at 28 weeks is more effective than shorter [33]. Observational data from the European National Study of HIV in Pregnancy and Childhood have shown even longer antenatal drug duration (starting before 28 weeks' gestation) further reduces MTCT; each additional week of drug corresponded to a 10% reduction in transmission after adjusting for viral load, mode of delivery, and infant sex [2]. More prolonged post-exposure prophylaxis of the infant does not substitute for longer duration of maternal therapy [33].

Regimens that include no antenatal prophylaxis but include intrapartum and postpartum drug administration are also effective (Table 37.1) [10, 11]. However, the PETRA study demonstrated that intrapartum pre-exposure prophylaxis alone, without continued post-exposure prophylaxis of the infant, is not effective [10]. The SAINT trial demonstrated that the two proven effective intrapartum/postpartum regimens (AZT/3TC or single-dose NVP) were similar in efficacy and safety [18].

In an attempt to improve the efficacy of short-course regimens but retain a regimen that remains appropriate to the cost limitations in resource-constrained countries, researchers evaluated whether the addition of a potent intrapartum intervention—the single-dose NVP regimen—to short-course antepartum regimens might increase efficacy (Table 37.2). In the setting of short-course AZT alone or AZT/3TC regimens, the Perinatal HIV Prevention Trial (PHPT)-2 study in non-breastfeeding women in Thailand, the Mashi study in Botswana (in the formula-fed strata), and the DITRAME studies in a partly breastfeeding population in the Cote d'Ivoire, demonstrated that the addition of single-dose NVP did significantly increase efficacy [34–36]. However, a clinical trial conducted in resource-rich countries, PACTG 316, demonstrated that the addition of single-dose NVP did not appear to offer significant benefit in the setting of potent combination antiretroviral therapy throughout pregnancy and very low viral load at the time of delivery [37]. The relative importance of the maternal and infant components of single-dose NVP

remains unclear. The Thailand PHPT-2 study suggested that the infant NVP dose may not be necessary when maternal NVP is provided, and the Botswana Mashi study suggested that maternal NVP may not be necessary when infant single-dose NVP is provided at birth [34, 35].

In some countries, a significant proportion of women lack antenatal care and present to the healthcare system during labor. A trial was conducted in a breastfeeding population in Malawi to define the optimal infant prophylaxis regimen in resource-constrained settings when no antenatal maternal therapy was received (Table 37.2). The addition of one week of AZT to infant single-dose NVP reduced the risk of transmission by 36% compared to infant single-dose NVP alone (12). However, when maternal intrapartum NVP was received, thereby providing pre-exposure in addition to post-exposure prophylaxis, infant single-dose NVP alone was as effective as the combined NVP/AZT infant post-exposure prophylaxis regimen (38).

In resource-rich countries, standard infant prophylaxis in the absence of maternal antenatal antiretroviral drugs is 6 weeks of AZT. NICHD/HPTN 040 was designed to determine the optimal infant prophylaxis regimen in formula-fed infants born to women who did not receive antepartum therapy (Table 37.2). The trial compared standard 6-week infant AZT prophylaxis to 6 weeks of AZT combined with either 3 NVP doses during the first week of life or 2 weeks of nelfinavir and 3TC. Both combination regimens reduced intrapartum MTCT compared to AZT alone by approximately 50%: intrapartum MTCT was 4.9% with AZT alone versus 2.2% with AZT/NVP and 2.5% with AZT/3TC/nelfinavir [39].

In breastfeeding populations, the impact of short-course antiretroviral prophylaxis regimens on long-term risk of infant infection is diminished due to the continued transmission during the breastfeeding period. Several trials have assessed the effect of antiretroviral prophylaxis provided to the mother during lactation or to the breastfeeding infant (Table 37.3) and are reviewed in detail elsewhere [40]. It is not possible to directly compare MTCT rates in these studies. The patient populations significantly differ; all the infant prophylaxis studies except one (BAN) enrolled women regardless of CD4 count, whereas the 3 randomized trials of maternal prophylaxis restricted enrollment to women with CD4 counts > 200–250 cells/mm^3 (Table 37.3). Antepartum antiretroviral drug administration and duration significantly differ: the infant prophylaxis studies enrolled women who had not received any antepartum drugs while all the maternal prophylaxis studies except one (BAN) provided antepartum drugs (of different durations, starting at 25 to 36 weeks' gestation). Additionally, the postnatal prophylaxis duration differs between studies, with 2 infant prophylaxis studies providing only 6 to 14 weeks of postnatal prophylaxis while all of the maternal prophylaxis studies provided 6 months of postnatal prophylaxis.

Despite these differences, currently available data suggest that both infant and maternal prophylaxis are effective in reducing postnatal infection in women who don't require therapy for their own health, and may have similar efficacy when compared during similar periods of prophylaxis [5, 40]. This is best illustrated by the BAN study, the only trial that included both infant and maternal prophylaxis arms (Table 37.3) [5]. Given two presumably similarly effective interventions, the choice of intervention to prevent MTCT for breastfeeding women who do not require treatment for their own health will involve weighing a number of different considerations, including relative costs, feasibility, and risks and benefits of the interventions.

SHORT- AND LONG-TERM SAFETY OF ANTIRETROVIRAL EXPOSURE FOR INFANTS AND WOMEN

Infant

The short-course antiretroviral regimens studied in clinical trials in resource-constrained settings have been associated with minimal short-term infant toxicity; antiretroviral exposure is associated with transient, mild hematologic abnormalities that resolve following completion of prophylaxis [41, 42]. However, longer-term outcome data in infants exposed to the more complex and prolonged maternal antiretroviral prophylaxis regimens used in resource-rich countries are still limited.

Current data indicate no increase in congenital abnormalities among offspring of women with first trimester use of most antiretroviral drugs [43]. However, there remain concerns related to efavirenz (EFV). In a primate study, prenatal EFV exposure was associated with central nervous system defects in infant monkeys and the Antiretroviral Pregnancy Registry has received six retrospective reports of central nervous system defects (e.g. meningomyelocoele) in human infants after first trimester exposure [43]. However, a meta-analysis of observational data from 1,132 women with first trimester EFV exposure from 9 prospective cohorts (including the Antiretroviral Pregnancy Registry) found no increased risk of overall birth defects compared with exposure to other antiretroviral drugs [44]. Across 11 cohorts including 1,256 live births with first trimester EFV exposure, one neural tube defect was observed, giving a prevalence of 0.08% [44]. Although these data are reassuring, the low neural tube defect incidence in the general population means that larger exposure numbers are needed to definitively rule out an increased risk of this specific defect. EFV should be avoided in the first trimester of pregnancy (although second/third trimester use may be considered). Women of childbearing potential should undergo pregnancy testing before initiating EFV therapy, and be counseled about the potential risk to the fetus and provided with adequate contraception [45].

Data are conflicting on whether combination antiretroviral drug use during pregnancy is associated with preterm delivery. A pooled analysis of 19,585 singleton births from 4 European and US observational cohorts concluded that a 3-drug regimen conferred a 1.5-fold increased adjusted odds of preterm delivery compared with a 2-drug regimen [46]. A randomized trial comparing two different combination regimens found a higher preterm delivery rate in women receiving a protease inhibitor-based compared to a triple nucleoside regimen [47]. In contrast, a US study of 777 HIV-1-infected pregnant women who were not receiving antiretroviral drugs at conception found no association of combination drugs with preterm delivery [48]. However, only 21% had received drugs during the first trimester; some studies suggest that preterm delivery is more likely to be associated with drug use early in pregnancy (e.g. first trimester or at conception) [49].

Some data suggest that short-term toxicity may be greater with combination regimens than single-drug regimens. Higher rates of anemia and neutropenia in the first few months of life were observed in uninfected infants born to mothers receiving 3-drug regimens during pregnancy compared to those exposed only to single or dual drugs, but this resolved by age 6 months [50, 51]. Additionally, uninfected infants exposed to maternal 3-drug regimens had lower birth weight and length than those exposed only to AZT, although this difference resolved (weight) or narrowed (height) by age 6 months [52].

Longer-term data are limited. Pre-clinical data indicate that some nucleoside analogue reverse transcriptase inhibitor (NRTI) drugs are carcinogenic *in vitro* and can be associated with mitochondrial toxicity. No increase in overall cancer risk has been observed in >9,000 uninfected NRTI-exposed children followed to median age 5.4 years [53]. However, French researchers have reported rare occurrence of mitochondrial dysfunction in uninfected infants with *in utero* antiretroviral exposure, with higher risk among those exposed to combination regimens. In a cohort of 4,392 uninfected HIV-1-exposed children, evidence of mitochondrial dysfunction was identified in 12 children (with 2 deaths), yielding an 18-month incidence of 0.26% [54]. All children presented with neurologic symptoms, often with abnormal magnetic resonance imaging and/or a significant episode of hyperlactatemia, and all had an identified deficit in one of the mitochondrial respiratory chain complexes and/or abnormal muscle biopsy histology.

While continued follow-up of infants exposed to antiretroviral drugs for potential adverse long-term effects is critical, current data indicate that if such toxicity is observed, it is relatively rare, and potential risks of antiretroviral exposure for the infant need to be placed in perspective with the proven benefit of antiretroviral therapy for the health of the mother and in reducing HIV-1 MTCT by up to 70%.

Extended daily infant NVP prophylaxis can prevent breast milk MTCT [5, 55–57]. Extended NVP used for up to 6 months has been studied in over 4,500 infants in the SWEN, PEPI—Malawi, HPTN 046, and BAN trials (Table 37.3); the regimen appears safe compared to control interventions, with the exception of higher number of rashes in the BAN study (however, grade 3 or 4 rash in BAN was <2%) [5]. Daily AZT/NVP infant prophylaxis was associated with higher rates of hematologic toxicity than daily NVP [55].

Pregnant woman

Minimal toxicity has been seen in women receiving the short-course regimens studied in trials in resource-constrained settings. Toxicity has been primarily confined to women receiving longer, more complex, combination regimens; primary toxicity concerns include lactic acidosis with NRTI drugs; rash and hepatic toxicity with NVP; and potential for hyperglycemia with protease inhibitors [45].

It is unclear if pregnancy augments the incidence of the lactic acidosis/hepatic steatosis syndrome reported in non-pregnant individuals receiving NRTI drugs. Cases of lactic acidosis, including maternal and fetal fatalities, have been reported in HIV-1-infected pregnant women receiving prolonged therapy with NRTIs, with symptoms presenting in late pregnancy. Physicians caring for HIV-infected pregnant women receiving NRTIs need to be alert for the early diagnosis of this syndrome [45].

Severe symptomatic, and rarely fatal, hepatic toxicity associated with chronic NVP therapy is more frequent in females. Some but not all studies suggest increased risk in pregnant women with CD4 count $>250/mm^3$ or elevated transaminases at the start of treatment [58, 59]. Hepatic toxicity has not been observed in women receiving single-dose NVP. Women who experience clinical hepatotoxicity or rash while receiving NVP should have the drug discontinued and should not receive NVP in the future.

Protease inhibitors can be associated with metabolic abnormalities, including hyperglycemia and new-onset diabetes. Data are conflicting regarding whether there is an increase in gestational hyperglycemia in HIV-1-infected pregnant women and its association with protease inhibitor use [60, 61]. This complication may be increased in HIV-1-infected pregnant women co-infected with hepatitis C virus [62].

The use of antepartum and extended postpartum maternal 3-drug prophylaxis to prevent breast milk MTCT, studied in over 1,800 mother/infant pairs in the Kesho Bora, BAN and Mma Bana trials (Table 37.3), appears safe for the mother compared to control interventions, with the exception of maternal neutropenia; in the BAN trial significantly more neutropenia was observed in women receiving triple drugs [5, 47, 63].

There are only limited data on the safety of stopping 3-drug regimens used solely for prevention of MTCT in women who do not need therapy for their own health [64, 65]. This is being assessed in a large randomized trial (Promoting Maternal Child Health Everywhere, PROMISE—Clinical trial NCT00955968).

ANTIRETROVIRAL DRUG RESISTANCE

Short-course antiretroviral drug regimens used to prevent MTCT that do not fully suppress viral replication may be associated with antiretroviral drug resistance. This is most likely to occur with prophylaxis regimens using drugs for which a single point mutation can confer drug resistance, such as NVP or 3TC.

Genotypic resistance to 3TC was observed in pregnant women receiving 3TC with AZT as a dual NRTI regimen to prevent MTCT. In a study in France, 3TC was added to AZT after 32 weeks' gestation; 39% of 132 women had detectable high-level resistance (M184V) to 3TC at 6 weeks, postpartum [66]. Resistance was only detected in women who had received 3TC for ≥4 weeks during pregnancy. Despite the high prevalence of 3TC resistance, the MTCT rate was low, 1.6%. Whether the presence of 3TC drug resistance following prophylaxis is associated with diminished virologic response to subsequent 3TC-based therapy is unknown.

Resistance mutation selection in infected women and infants following single-dose NVP is well documented. NVP has a long half-life, and hence persists for a prolonged period, and a single mutation in the viral codon confers drug resistance. Resistance rates vary by maternal CD4 count and viral load at the time of exposure, viral subtype, whether other antiretroviral drugs were given, the type of resistance assay, and for infants, whether the mother received single-dose NVP [67, 68]. Women who require treatment for their own health are also those at greatest risk for resistance following single-dose NVP; identification of such women and initiation of lifelong combination antiretroviral therapy during pregnancy will avoid the development of resistance in this high-risk group [68].

While resistance is frequent in the first few weeks–months following exposure, detection decreases with time, although low levels of virus with resistance mutations can persist for prolonged periods and in some cases can remain present in latently infected cells. Current data suggest that protease inhibitor-based therapy is superior to NNRTI-based therapy in women starting treatment within 12–24 months of single-dose NVP exposure and in infants infected despite use of single-dose NVP [69, 70].

Antiretroviral drug administration for a short period following single-dose NVP (use of a "tail") can reduce resistance incidence to very low levels. Regimens studied for prevention of resistance include AZT/3TC given for 4 to 7 days following single-dose NVP; tenofovir/emtricitabine as a single-dose during labor or for 7 days postpartum; AZT/didanosine (ddI)/lopinavir-ritonavir for 7 or 30 days; and administration of AZT/ddI for 30 days [67]. NNRTI resistance rates of 0 to 7% at 2 to 6 weeks' postpartum using ultrasensitive assays have been reported with some of these tail regimens. Thus, administration of a minimum 7-day tail following use of single-dose NVP as MTCT prophylaxis is recommended to reduce resistance in women.

Very high NVP resistance rates are observed in infants infected despite extended infant NVP prophylaxis of breast milk transmission. In the SWEN study of 6 weeks of infant NVP prophylaxis, 92% of infants infected during the first 6 weeks of life (the period of NVP prophylaxis) had NNRTI resistance compared to 38% in the control single-dose NVP arm [71]. However, NNRTI resistance among infants who became infected after prophylaxis had ceased (after age 6 weeks) was similar, 15%, to the single-dose NVP control. Co-administration of NVP and AZT in PEPI—Malawi trial decreased NVP resistance but resistance was still frequent (62%) [72].

Antiretroviral drug resistance has also been observed in infants infected despite maternal triple-drug prophylaxis. Some antiretroviral drugs are known to enter breast milk. 3TC appears to concentrate in breast milk, and is present at levels 3–5 times that in maternal plasma, while AZT appears to be present at levels similar to or somewhat less than maternal plasma [73]. NVP levels are only about 60–75% of maternal plasma, and the protease inhibitors that have been studied have had very limited penetration into milk [74]. Thus, breastfeeding infants of mothers receiving triple-drug prophylaxis who become infected may be ingesting sub-therapeutic levels of antiretroviral drugs present in breast milk and therefore develop drug-resistant virus. Three studies have now identified multi-class drug resistance (mutations conferring resistance to NRTIs as well as to NNRTIs) in breastfeeding infants who have become infected despite maternal triple-drug prophylaxis [75–77].

NON-ANTIRETROVIRAL INTERVENTIONS

In general, with the exception of elective cesarean delivery, the results of non-antiretroviral interventions to prevent MTCT have been disappointing. Approaches have included treatment/prophylaxis of chorioamnionitis, vaginal virucidal cleansing, and nutritional supplementation, none of which have proven effective for prevention of MTCT and hence will not be discussed here.

Elective cesarean delivery

Prolonged duration of membrane rupture is associated with MTCT; elective cesarean delivery (performed prior to labor and membrane rupture) has been shown to reduce MTCT in an individual patient data meta-analysis including 8,533 non-breastfeeding mother–child pairs from 15 prospective US and international cohort studies, and a randomized clinical trial [8, 9]. Non-elective cesarean delivery performed *after* onset of labor or rupture of membranes did not reduce MTCT compared with vaginal delivery.

It is unclear if benefit would be observed in women on receiving potent combination drugs who have undetectable virus [78, 79]; in this situation, the risk of MTCT is very low and the risk of operative delivery to the mother may outweigh the potential benefit in reducing MTCT.

CURRENT GUIDELINES FOR PREVENTION OF MTCT FOR THE UNITED STATES

Current guidelines for antiretroviral therapy and elective cesarean delivery for the USA [45] are shown in Table 37.4 (see http://AIDSInfo.nih.gov for more details). Based on observational studies indicating that MTCT rates are extremely low in women receiving antiretroviral drugs who have very low or undetectable HIV RNA levels, combination antiretroviral drug regimens are recommended for all pregnant women. Additionally, elective cesarean delivery is recommended if HIV RNA levels remain $\geq 1,000$ copies/mL near delivery.

Based on efficacy studies in preventing transmission and large safety experience with use in pregnancy, the preferred NRTI combination for antiretroviral-naïve pregnant women is AZT/3TC. The alternative NRTI combination regimen if AZT/3TC is not tolerated (e.g. anemia) is tenofovir with 3TC or emtricitabine. There is less experience with tenofovir in pregnancy. The Antiretroviral Pregnancy Registry has not reported an increase in overall birth defects in 879 pregnancies with first trimester exposure, but a primate study has suggested the potential for decreased fetal growth and reduction in fetal bone porosity with *in utero* exposure, and studies in infected children on chronic tenofovir-based therapy has shown bone demineralization in some children. Therefore, tenofovir is considered an alternative NRTI during pregnancy for naïve women. However, for pregnant women with HIV/hepatitis B co-infection, tenofovir with 3TC or emtricitabine would be the preferred NRTI combination. In addition to the two NRTIs, either an NNRTI or PI would be preferred for combination regimens in antiretroviral-naïve pregnant women. Efavirenz is not recommended for use in the first trimester of pregnancy due to concerns related to birth defects, as discussed earlier. Use of efavirenz after the first trimester of pregnancy may be considered based on clinical indication, although current data are limited. Nevirapine would be the preferred NNRTI for antiretroviral naïve pregnant women with CD4 count less than 250 cells/mm^3, and may be continued in an antiretroviral experienced woman already receiving a nevirapine-based regimen regardless of CD4 count. Lopinavir/ritonavir is the preferred protease inhibitor for antiretroviral-naïve pregnant women

Table 37.4 Recommendations for antiretroviral drug use by pregnant HIV-1-infected women and prevention of mother-to-child transmission in the USA[a]

CLINICAL SITUATION	RECOMMENDATION
HIV-1-infected women of childbearing potential and indications for initiating antiretroviral therapy	• Combination treatment as per adult treatment guidelines. Use one or more NRTI with good placental passage as a component of the antiretroviral regimen when feasible. • Avoid drugs with teratogenic potential (e.g. efavirenz) if the woman is trying to conceive or is not using adequate contraception. Exclude pregnancy before starting treatment with efavirenz and assure access to effective contraception.
HIV-infected women with indications for antiretroviral therapy, are receiving treatment, and become pregnant	***Woman:*** • In general, if woman requires treatment, antiretroviral drugs should not be stopped during the first trimester or during pregnancy. • Continue current combination antiretroviral therapy regimen if successfully suppressing viremia; however, avoid use of efavirenz or other potentially teratogenic drugs in the first trimester and drugs with known adverse potential for mother throughout the pregnancy. • Perform HIV antiretroviral drug resistance testing if the woman has detectable viremia on therapy. • Continue combination antiretroviral therapy regimen during intrapartum period (AZT given as continuous infusion during labor while other antiretroviral agents are continued orally) and postpartum. • Schedule cesarean delivery at 38 weeks' gestation if plasma HIV RNA remains > 1,000 copies/mL near the time of delivery. ***Infant:*** • AZT for six weeks.

HIV-infected pregnant women who are antiretroviral naïve and have indications for therapy	***Woman:***
	• Perform HIV antiretroviral drug resistance testing prior to initiating combination antiretroviral drug therapy and repeat after initiating therapy if viral suppression is suboptimal.
	• Initiate combination antiretroviral regimen.
	  - Avoid use of efavirenz or other potentially teratogenic drugs in the first trimester and drugs with known adverse potential for mother (e.g. combination stavudine/didanosine).
	  - Use one or more NRTI with good placental passage as a component of the antiretroviral regimen when feasible.
	  - Use NVP as a component of the antiretroviral regimen only if the woman has CD4 count $\leq$250 cells/mm^3. If the woman has CD4 count >250 cells/mm^3, use NVP as a component of therapy only if the benefit clearly outweighs the risk due to an increased risk of severe hepatic toxicity.
	• If woman requires initiation of therapy for her own health, initiate treatment as soon as possible, including in the first trimester.
	• Continue combination antiretroviral therapy regimen during intrapartum period (AZT given as continuous infusion during labor while other antiretroviral agents are continued orally) and postpartum.
	• Schedule cesarean delivery at 38 weeks' gestation if plasma HIV RNA remains > 1,000 copies/mL near the time of delivery.
	
	Infant:
	• AZT for 6 weeks.

Continued

Table 37.4 Recommendations for antiretroviral drug use by pregnant HIV-1-infected women and prevention of mother-to-child transmission in the USA—cont'd

CLINICAL SITUATION	RECOMMENDATION

HIV-infected pregnant women who are antiretroviral naïve and do not require treatment for their own health	**Woman:**
	• Perform HIV antiretroviral drug resistance testing prior to initiating combination antiretroviral drug therapy and repeat after initiation of therapy if viral suppression is suboptimal.
	• Prescribe a combination antiretroviral drug prophylaxis regimen (i.e. at least 3 drugs) for prophylaxis of perinatal transmission.
	  - For women who are receiving antiretroviral drugs solely for prevention of perinatal transmission, delaying initiation of prophylaxis until after the first trimester of pregnancy may be considered, but earlier initiation of prophylaxis may be more effective in reducing perinatal transmission of HIV.
	  - Avoid use of efavirenz or other potentially teratogenic drugs in the first trimester and drugs with known adverse potential for mother (e.g. combination stavudine/didanosine).
	  - Use one or more NRTIs with good placental passage as a component of the antiretroviral regimen when feasible.
	  - If the woman has CD4 count >250 cells/mm^3 use NVP as a component of therapy only if the benefit clearly outweighs the risk due to an increased risk of severe hepatic toxicity.
	• Continue antiretroviral prophylaxis regimen during intrapartum period (AZT given as continuous infusion during labor while other antiretroviral agents are continued orally).
	• Evaluate need for continuing the combination regimen postpartum; following delivery, considerations regarding continuation of the antiretroviral regimen for maternal therapeutic indications are the same as for other non-pregnant individuals. If stopping and the regimen includes drug with long half-life like NNRTI, consider stopping NRTIs at least 7 days after stopping NNRTI.
	• Schedule cesarean delivery at 38 weeks' gestation if plasma HIV RNA remains >1,000 copies/mL near the time of delivery.
	
	Infant:
	• AZT for six weeks.

HIV-infected women who have received no antiretroviral therapy prior to labor	**Woman:** • Give AZT as continuous infusion during labor. **Infant:** • AZT given for 6 weeks, + 3 doses of NVP: first dose by 48 h of age; second dose 48 h after first dose; third dose 96 h after second dose (e.g. 2, 4, and 7 days of age). **OR** • AZT given for 6 weeks, + 3TC and nelfinavir daily from birth to 14 days of age.
Infant born to HIV-infected woman who has received no antiretroviral therapy prior to or during labor	**Infant:** • AZT given for 6 weeks, + 3 doses of NVP: first dose by 48 h of age; second dose 48 h after first dose; third dose 96 h after second dose (e.g. 2, 4, and 7 days of age). **OR** • AZT given for 6 weeks, + 3TC and nelfinavir twice daily from birth to 14 days of age.

[a]Adapted from Panel on Treatment of HIV-Infected Pregnant Women and Prevention of Perinatal Transmission [45].
3TC = lamivudine; AZT = Zidovudine; NRTI = nucleoside analogue reverse transcriptase inhibitor; NNRTI = non-nucleoside reverse transcriptase inhibitor; NVP = nevirapine.

because of efficacy studies in adults and experience with use in pregnancy [45]. The alternative protease inhibitor if lopinavir/ritonavir is not tolerated would be atazanavir/ritonavir. Data on use in pregnancy for darunavir, fosamprenavir, and tipranavir are too limited to recommend routine use in pregnancy, although these drugs can be used in antiretroviral-experienced women when resistance or intolerance prevents use of a preferred regimen. When pregnancy is identified in HIV-infected women already receiving antiretroviral therapy for their own health, continuation of therapy is recommended, with the exception being if a woman is receiving efavirenz and her pregnancy is recognized during the first trimester, an alternative antiretroviral drug should be substituted when possible. More detailed discussion can be found in *Recommendations for Use of Antiretroviral Drugs in Pregnant HIV-1-Infected Women for Maternal Health and Interventions to Reduce Perinatal HIV Transmission in the United States* [45].

Because antiretroviral prophylaxis is beneficial in reducing perinatal transmission even among infected pregnant women with HIV RNA < 1,000 copies/mL, use of prophylaxis is recommended for all pregnant women regardless of antenatal HIV RNA level. Following delivery, considerations regarding continuation of the antiretroviral regimen for maternal therapeutic indications are the same as for non-pregnant individuals. When used solely to prevent perinatal transmission, it is not known what impact discontinuing combination antiretroviral drug regimens postpartum will have on the short- and long-term health of the mother. However, so far, studies of pregnant women with relatively high CD4 counts who stop therapy after delivery have not shown a risk for increased disease progression. As noted earlier, the risks versus benefits of stopping therapy postpartum in women with high CD4 counts is being evaluated in an ongoing trial. Breastfeeding is not recommended for HIV-1-infected women in the USA because breast milk transmission can occur even in women receiving combination antiretroviral regimens and safe and affordable infant formula is available. When no antenatal drugs are received, intravenous intrapartum AZT is recommended for the mother if there is adequate time. Given the recent results of the NICHD/HPTN 040 study (Table 37.2) [39], when the mother has not received antepartum drugs, combining the standard 6-week infant AZT regimen with NVP given at birth and days 3 and 7 of life or with 2 weeks of 3TC/nelfinavir is recommended (Table 37.4).

CURRENT GUIDELINES FOR PREVENTION OF MTCT FOR RESOURCE-CONSTRAINED SETTINGS

WHO guidelines for antiretroviral therapy for pregnant women and preventing MTCT were updated in July 2010 (Table 37.5) [30]. For women who meet WHO criteria

for initiation therapy for their own health (CD4 count < 350 cells/mm^3 or WHO stage III or IV disease), starting a standard combination therapy regimen is recommended, which should be continued postpartum for life. For women who lack indications for therapy for their own health, two options are available, started as early as 14 weeks, gestation. Option A includes maternal antepartum AZT with intrapartum single-dose NVP and AZT/3TC continued for 7 days postpartum, plus daily infant NVP from birth until the end of the breastfeeding period. Option B includes a three-drug regimen given to the mother during pregnancy until the end of the breastfeeding period; the infant then receives 6 weeks of infant prophylaxis (either AZT or NVP). If the infant is not breastfeeding, then 6 weeks of infant prophylaxis (either AZT or NVP) would be given for either Option A or B (see Table 37.5).

Infant feeding guidelines have also been revised to recommend that national public health authorities should decide whether health services will principally counsel mothers to either breastfeed and receive maternal or infant antiretroviral interventions or avoid all breastfeeding, as the strategy that will most likely give infants the greatest chance of HIV-free survival [80]. If breastfeeding, exclusive breastfeeding for the first 6 months of life with continued breastfeeding through age 12 months with introduction of complementary foods is recommended. Breastfeeding should stop only once a nutritionally adequate and safe diet without breast milk can be provided. Gradual weaning over the course of 1 month is recommended, with infant or maternal antiretroviral prophylaxis continued until 1 week after breastfeeding is fully stopped.

SUMMARY

There has been dramatic progress in reducing HIV MTCT in both resource-rich and resource-constrained settings in recent years. In resource-rich countries, new pediatric infections are nearly eliminated. In resource-constrained settings, when services are available and accessible, MTCT can be reduced to less than 5% in breastfeeding populations with current interventions. However, while there has been impressive improvement in access to services in low- and middle-income countries since 2004, only 26% of pregnant women were tested for HIV, and 53% of pregnant women living with HIV received any antiretroviral drugs to prevent MTCT in 2009 (up from 7 and 10%, respectively, in 2004–2005). In 2010, UNAIDS called for the virtual elimination of mother-to-child transmission globally by 2015, promoting a comprehensive approach including primary prevention of HIV infection among, women of childbearing age; preventing unintended pregnancies among women living with HIV; preventing transmission from an HIV-positive woman to her infant; and providing appropriate treatment, care, and support

Table 37.5 World Health Organization recommendations for antiretroviral drug use in HIV-1-infected pregnant women in resource-limited settings[a]

CLINICAL SITUATION	RECOMMENDATION

HIV-1-infected women with childbearing potential and indications for starting therapy	• Treatment regimen choice should follow WHO recommendations (all women with CD4 $\leq$ 350 cell/mm^3 irrespective of clinical staging or WHO clinical stage III or IV, irrespective of CD4 count)
	First-line regimens for childbearing-age women:[b]
	  - AZT + 3TC + NVP or
	  - AZT + 3TC + EFV or
	  - TDF + 3TC (or FTC) + NVP
	  - TDF + 3TC (or FTC) + EFV
	• Exclude pregnancy before starting treatment with efavirenz and provide adequate contraception

HIV-1-infected women with indications for antiretroviral therapy, are receiving treatment, and become pregnant	***Woman:*** • Continue current regimen except discontinue drugs during the first trimester that have teratogenic potential (efavirenz) (women who are receiving efavirenz and are in the second or third trimester can continue the current regimen). • Continue combination regimen during intrapartum period and postpartum ***Infant:*** • Once-daily NVP or twice-daily AZT from birth until 4–6 weeks of age (irrespective of mode of infant feeding)

Women first diagnosed with HIV-1 infection during pregnancy with clinical indications for antiretroviral therapy	***Woman:***
	• Treatment should be provided to:
	  ○ All women with CD4 $\leq$ 350 cell/mm^3, irrespective of clinical staging, and all women with clinical stage III or IV, irrespective of CD4 count
	• Treatment regimen choice should follow WHO recommendations
	  ○ First-line regimens for childbearing-age women:[b]
	    - AZT + 3TC + NVP or
	    - AZT + 3TC + EFV or
	    - TDF + 3TC (or FTC) + NVP
	    - TDF + 3TC (or FTC) + EFV
	• Avoid drugs with teratogenic potential in women of childbearing age (efavirenz) the first trimester
	• Start treatment as soon as possible, including the first trimester.
	• Continue combination regimen during intrapartum period and postpartum
	
	Infant:
	• Once-daily NVP or twice-daily AZT from birth until 4–6 weeks of age (irrespective of mode of infant feeding)

Pregnant HIV-1-infected women without indication for treatment for their own health	***Woman:*** • Start antiretroviral prophylaxis as early as 14 weeks' gestation. *Option A: maternal AZT* • AZT during pregnancy plus • Single-dose NVP + AZT/3TC during labor and delivery plus • AZT/3TC x 7 days postpartum

Table 37.5 World Health Organization recommendations for antiretroviral drug use in HIV-1-infected pregnant women in resource-limited settings—cont'd

CLINICAL SITUATION	RECOMMENDATION
	OR *Option B: triple antiretroviral drug prophylaxis until one week after all exposure to breast milk has ended* • AZT + 3TC + LPV/r or • AZT + 3TC + ABC or • AZT + 3TC + EFV • TDF + 3TC (or FTC) + EFV ***Infant:*** *Option A* *Breastfeeding infants:* • Once-daily NVP from birth till 1 week after all exposure to breastfeeding *Non-breastfeeding infants:* • Once-daily NVP or single-dose NVP + twice-daily AZT from birth until 4–6 weeks of age OR *Option B* • Once-daily NVP or twice-daily AZT from birth until 4–6 weeks of age
Pregnant women of unknown HIV infection status at time of labor or HIV-infected pregnant women who have not received antepartum antiretroviral drugs	• If there is time, counsel and offer HIV-1 rapid test; if positive, initiate intrapartum prophylaxis. If insufficient time to obtain HIV-1 test result while in labor, offer HIV-1 test as soon as possible after delivery, and follow the recommendations in next scenario *Option A (infant antiretroviral drug prophylaxis):[c]* • Mother: single-dose NVP at start of labor and AZT/3TC twice daily for 1 week • Infant (if breastfeeding): Once-daily NVP from birth until 1 week after all exposure to breast milk has ended, or for 4–6 weeks if breastfeeding ceases prior to 6 weeks. • Infant (not breastfeeding): Single-dose NVP plus twice-daily AZT or once-daily NVP from birth until 4–6 weeks of age. *Option B (maternal triple antiretroviral drug prophylaxis, relevant only if breastfeeding)[d]:* • Mother: Triple-drug prophylaxis during labor until one week after all exposure to breast milk has ended. • Infant: Daily NVP from birth until 6 weeks of age (since infant is breastfeeding and immediate protection is desirable, NVP would be the preferred infant prophylaxis and given for a full 6 weeks)
Infants born to HIV-infected women who have not received antepartum and intrapartum antiretroviral drugs	*Option A (infant antiretroviral drug prophylaxis):[c]* • Infant (if breastfeeding): Daily NVP from birth until 1 week after all exposure to breast milk has ended, or for 4–6 weeks if breastfeeding ceases prior to 6 weeks • Infant (not breastfeeding): single-dose NVP + twice-daily AZT or once-daily NVP from birth until 4 to 6 weeks of age.

Continued

Table 37.5 World Health Organization recommendations for antiretroviral drug use in HIV-1-infected pregnant women in resource-limited settings—cont'd

CLINICAL SITUATION	RECOMMENDATION
	Option B (maternal triple antiretroviral drug prophylaxis, relevant only if breastfeeding):[d] • Mother: Triple-drug prophylaxis until 1 week after all exposure to breast milk has ended, or for 4–6 weeks if breastfeeding ceases prior to 6 weeks • Infant: Daily NVP from birth until 4–6 weeks of age
Related infant feeding recommendation for breastfeeding HIV-infected women	National authorities should decide whether health services will principally counsel mothers to either breastfeed and receive ARV interventions or avoid all breastfeeding, as the strategy that will most likely give infants the greatest chance of HIV-free survival. If breastfeeding recommended: • Exclusively breastfeed for the first 6 months, introduce appropriate complementary food thereafter, and continue breastfeeding for 12 months • Wean gradually within 1 month

[a]Adapted from World Health Organization [30].
[b]If exposed to single-dose NVP within past 12 months, then AZT + 3TC + LPV/r recommended for first-line.
[c]A clinical assessment should be done postpartum and CD4 count drawn. Women who are found to require treatment for their own health should be started on an appropriate lifelong treatment regimen.
[d]A clinical assessment should be done postpartum and CD4 count drawn. Women who are found to require treatment for their own health should not discontinue their triple-drug regimen but continue on an appropriate lifelong treatment regimen.
3TC = lamivudine; ABC = abacavir; AZT = zidovudine; EFV = efavirenz; FTC = emtricitabine; LPV/r = lopinavir/ritonavir; NVP = nevirapine.

to mothers living with HIV and their children and families (WHOPMTCT10).

Although debate continues over the optimal intervention to reduce MTCT in women who don't require treatment for their own health, and results from new clinical trials are eagerly awaited, tools are now available that will have a significant impact on the HIV epidemic in children globally. The ability to implement such programs is now tied less to the choice of regimen or regimen cost than to the development and support of the required maternal–child health infrastructure.

REFERENCES

[1] Joint United Nations Programme on HIV/AIDS (UNAIDS). Global Report: UNAIDS report on the global AIDS epidemic, 2010, Geneva, Switzerland: UNAIDS/WHO; 2010. URL: http://www.unaids.org/globalreport/Global_report.htm.

[2] Townsend CL, Cortina-Boria M, Peckham CS, et al. Low rates of mother-to-child transmission of HIV following effective pregnancy interventions in the United Kingdom and Ireland, 2000–2006. AIDS 2008;22:973–81.

[3] Barker PM, Mphatswe W, Rollins N. Antiretroviral drugs in the cupboard are not enough: the impact of health systems' performance on mother to child transmission of HIV. J Acquir Immune Defic Syndr 2011;56: e45–48.

[4] Humphrey JH. The risks of not breastfeeding. J Acquir Immune Defic Syndr 2010; 53:1–4.

[5] Chasela CS, Hudgens MG, Jamieson DJ, et al., BAN Study Group. Maternal or infant antiretroviral drugs to reduce HIV-1 transmission. N Engl J Med 2010;362:2271–81.

[6] Magder LS, Mofenson L, Paul ME, et al. Risk factors for in utero and intrapartum transmission of HIV.

J Acquir Immune Defic Syndr 2005;38:87–95.

[7] Shapiro RL, Smeaton L, Lockman S, et al. Risk factors for early and late transmission of HIV via breastfeeding among infants born to HIV-infected women in a randomized clinical trial in Botswana. J Infect Dis 2009;199:1–5.

[8] The International Perinatal HIV Group. The mode of delivery and the risk of vertical transmission of human immunodeficiency virus type 1: a meta-analysis of 15 prospective studies. N Engl J Med 1999;340:977–87.

[9] The European Mode of Delivery Collaboration. Elective cesarean-section versus vaginal delivery in prevention of vertical HIV-1 transmission: a randomized clinical trial. Lancet 1999;353:1035–9.

[10] The Petra Study Team. Efficacy of three short-course regimens of zidovudine and lamivudine in preventing early and late transmission of HIV-1 from mother to child in Tanzania, South Africa, and Uganda (Petra study): a randomised, double-blind, placebo-controlled trial. Lancet 2002;359:1178–86.

[11] Jackson JB, Musoke P, Fleming T, et al. Intrapartum and neonatal single-dose nevirapine compared with zidovudine for prevention of mother to child transmission of HIV-1 in Kampala, Uganda: 18 month follow-up of the HIVNET 012 randomised trial. Lancet 2003;362:859–68.

[12] Taha TE, Kumwenda NI, Gibbons A, et al. Short postexposure prophylaxis in newborn babies to reduce mother to child transmission of HIV-1: NVAZ randomized clinical trial. Lancet 2003;362:1171–7.

[13] Birkhead GS, Pulver WP, Warren BL, et al. Acquiring human immunodeficiency virus during pregnancy and mother-to-child transmission in New York: 2002–2006. Obstet Gynecol 2010;115:1247–55.

[14] Wiktor S, Ekpini E, Karon J, et al. Short-course oral zidovudine for prevention of mother-to-child transmission of HIV-1 in Abidjan, Cote d'Ivoire: a randomised trial. Lancet 1999;353:781–5.

[15] Leroy V, Karon JM, Alioum A, et al. Twenty-four month efficacy of a maternal short-course zidovudine regimen to prevent mother to child transmission of HIV-1 in West Africa. AIDS 2002;16:631–41.

[16] The Breastfeeding and HIV International Transmission Study Group. Late postnatal transmission of HIV-1 in breast-fed children: an independent patient data meta-analysis. J Infect Dis 2004;189:2154–66.

[17] Humphrey JH, Marinda E, Mutasa K, et al. Mother to child transmission of HIV among Zimbabwean women who seroconverted postnatally: prospective cohort study. Br Med J 2010;341:c6580.

[18] Moodley D, Moodley J, Coovadia H, et al. The South African Intrapartum Nevirapine Trial (SAINT) Investigators. A multicenter, randomized, controlled trial of nevirapine compared to a combination of zidovudine and lamivudine to reduce intrapartum and early postpartum mother-to-child transmission of human immunodeficiency virus type-1. J Infect Dis 2003;187:725–35.

[19] Mofenson LM. Protecting the next generation—eliminating perinatal HIV-1 infection. N Engl J Med 2010;362:2316–18.

[20] John-Stewart G, Mbori-Ngacha D, Ekpini R, et al. Breastfeeding and transmission of HIV-1. J Acquir Immune Defic Syndr 2004;35:196–202.

[21] Kuhn L. Milk mysteries: why are women who exclusively breast-feed less likely to transmit HIV during breast-feeding? Clin Infect Dis 2010;50:770–2.

[22] Lunney KM, Iliff P, Mutasa K, et al. Associations between breast milk viral load, mastitis, exclusive breast-feeding, and postnatal transmission of HIV. Clin Infect Dis 2010;50:762–9.

[23] Kuhn L, Sinkala M, Kankasa C, et al. High uptake of exclusive breastfeeding and reduced early post-natal HIV transmission. PLoS ONE 2007;2:e1363.

[24] Liang K, Gui X, Zhang Y-Z, et al. A case series of 104 women infected with HIV-1 via blood transfusion postnatally: high rate of HIV-1 transmission to infants through breastfeeding. J Infect Dis 2009;200:682–6.

[25] Lockman S, Creek T. Acute maternal HIV infection during pregnancy and breastfeeding: substantial risk to infants. J Infect Dis 2009;200:667–9.

[26] Connor EM, Sperling RS, Gelber R, et al. Reduction of maternal-infant transmission of human immunodeficiency virus type 1 with zidovudine treatment. N Engl J Med 1994;3312:1173–80.

[27] Cooper ER, Charurat M, Mofenson L, et al. Combination antiretroviral strategies for treatment of pregnant HIV-1-infected women and prevention of perinatal HIV-1 transmission. J Acquir Immune Defic Syndr 2002;29:484–94.

[28] Ioannidis JPA, Abrams EJ, Ammann A, et al. Perinatal transmission of human immunodeficiency virus type 1 by pregnant women with RNA virus loads < 1000 copies/mL. J Infect Dis 2001;183:539–45.

[29] Tuomala RE, O'Driscoll PT, Bremer JW, et al. Cell-associated genital tract virus and vertical transmission of human immunodeficiency virus type 1 in antiretroviral-experienced women. J Infect Dis 2003;187:375–84.

[30] World Health Organization. Antiretroviral drugs for treating pregnant women and preventing HIV infections in infants: recommendations for a public health approach 2010, Geneva: World Health Organization; 2010. Available at http://whqlibdoc.who.int/publications/2010/9789241599818_eng.pdf.

[31] Carter RJ, Dugan K, El-Sadar WM, et al. CD4+ cell count testing more effective than HIV disease clinical staging in identifying pregnant and postpartum women eligible for antiretroviral therapy in resource-limited settings. J Acquir Immune Defic Syndr 2010;55:404–10.

[32] Shaffer N, Chuachoowong PA, Mock C, et al. Short-course zidovudine for perinatal HIV-1 transmission in Bangkok, Thailand: a randomized controlled trial. Lancet 1999;353:773–80.

[33] Lallemant M, Jourdain G, Le Coeur S, et al. A trial of shortened zidovudine regimens to prevent mother-to-child transmission of human immunodeficiency virus type 1. N Engl J Med 2000;343:982–91.

[34] Lallemant M, Jourdain G, Le Coeur S, et al. Single-dose perinatal nevirapine plus standard

zidovudine to prevent mother to child transmission of HIV-1 in Thailand. N Engl J Med 2004;351:217–28.

[35] Shapiro RL, Thior I, Gilbert PB, et al. Maternal single-dose nevirapine versus placebo as part of an antiretroviral strategy to prevent mother-to-child HIV transmission in Botswana. AIDS 2006;20:1281–8.

[36] ANRS 1201/1202 DITRAME PLUS Study Group. Field efficacy of zidovudine, lamivudine and single-dose nevirapine to prevent peripartum HIV transmission. AIDS 2005;19:309–18.

[37] Dorenbaum A, Cunningham CK, Gelber RD, et al. Two-dose intrapartum/newborn nevirapine and standard antiretroviral therapy to reduce perinatal HIV-1 transmission: a randomized trial. JAMA 2002;288:189–98.

[38] Taha TE, Kumwenda NI, Hoover DR, et al. Nevirapine and zidovudine at birth to reduce perinatal transmission of HIV in an African setting: a randomized controlled trial. JAMA 2004;292:202–9.

[39] Nielsen-Saines K, Watts DH, Santos VV, et al., NICHD HPTN 040/PACTG 1043 Protocol Team. Phase III randomized trial of the safety and efficacy of three neonatal antiretroviral regimens for preventing intrapartum HIV-1 transmission (NICHD HPTN 040/ PACTG 1043). In: 18th Conference on Retroviruses and Opportunistic Infections. Boston, MA, February 27–March 2; 2011 (Abstract 214LB).

[40] Mofenson LM. Antiretroviral drugs to prevent breastfeeding HIV transmission. Antivir Ther 2010;15:537–53.

[41] Taha TE, Kumwenda N, Gibbons A, et al. Effect of HIV-1 antiretroviral prophylaxis on hepatic and hematological parameters of African infants. AIDS 2002;16:851–8.

[42] Taha TE, Kumwenda N, Kafulafula G, et al. Haematological changes in African children who received short-term prophylaxis with nevirapine and zidovudine at birth. Ann Trop Paediatr 2004;24:301–9.

[43] Antiretroviral Pregnancy Registry Steering Committee. Antiretroviral Pregnancy Registry International Interim Report for 1 January 1989 through 31 January 2011. Wilmington, NC: Registry Coordinating Center; 2011. Available from URL: http://www.apregistry.com.

[44] Ford N, Mofenson L, Kranzer K, et al. Safety of efavirenz in first-trimester of pregnancy: a systematic review and meta-analysis of outcomes from observational cohorts. AIDS 2010;24:1461–70.

[45] Panel on Treatment of HIV-Infected Pregnant Women and Prevention of Perinatal Transmission. Recommendations for Use of Antiretroviral Drugs in Pregnant HIV-1-Infected Women for Maternal Health and Interventions to Reduce Perinatal HIV Transmission in the United States. September 14, 2011. pp. 1–117. Available at http://www.aidsinfo.nih.gov/ContentFiles/PerinatalGL.pdf [accessed 10.11.11].

[46] Townsend C, Schulte J, Thorne C, et al. Antiretroviral therapy and preterm delivery—a pooled analysis of data from the United States and Europe. Br J Obstet Gynaecol 2010;117:1399–410.

[47] Shapiro RL, Hughes MD, Ogwu A, et al. Antiretroviral regimens in pregnancy and breast-feeding in Botswana. N Engl J Med 2010;362:2282–94.

[48] Patel K, Shapior DE, Brogley SB, et al. Prenatal protease inhibitor use and risk of preterm birth among HIV-infected women initiating antiretroviral drugs during pregnancy. J Infect Dis 2010;201:1035–44.

[49] Machado ES, Hofer CB, Costa TT, et al. Pregnancy outcome in women infected with HIV-1 receiving combination antiretroviral therapy before versus after conception. Sex Transm Infect 2009;85:82–7.

[50] Dryden-Peterson S, Shapiro RL, Hughes MD, et al. Increased risk of severe infant anemia following exposure to maternal HAART. Botswana. J Acquir Immune Defic Syndr 2011; 56:428–36.

[51] Feiterna-Sperling C, Weizsaecker K, et al. Hematologic effects of maternal antiretroviral therapy and

[52] Powis KM, Smeaton L, Ogwu A, et al. Effects of in utero antiretroviral exposure on longitudinal growth of HIV-exposed uninfected infants in Botswana. J Acquir Immune Defic Syndr 2011;56:131–8.

[53] Benhammou V, Warszawski J, Bellec S, et al. Incidence of cancer in children perinatally exposed to nucleoside reverse transcriptase inhibitors. AIDS 2008;22:2165–77.

[54] Barrett B, Tardieu M, Rustin P, et al. Persistent mitochondrial dysfunction in HIV-1-exposed but uninfected infants: clinical screening in a large prospective cohort. AIDS 2003;17:1769–85.

[55] Kumwenda NI, Hoover DR, Mofenson LM, et al. Extended antiretroviral prophylaxis to reduce breast-milk HIV-1 transmission. N Engl J Med 2008;359:119–29.

[56] Six Week Extended-Dose Nevirapine (SWEN) Study Team, et al. Extended-dose nevirapine to 6 weeks of age for infants to prevent HIV transmission via breastfeeding in Ethiopia, India, and Uganda: an analysis of three randomised controlled trials. Lancet 2008;372:300–13.

[57] Coovadia H, Brown E, Maldonado Y, et al. HPTN 046: efficacy of extended daily infant nevirapine (extNVP) through age 6 months compared to 6 weeks for prevention of postnatal mother-to-child transmission (MTCT) of HIV through breastfeeding (BF). In: 18th Conference on Retroviruses and Opportunistic Infections. Boston, MA, February 27-March 2; 2011 (abstract 123 LB).

[58] Peters PJ, Stringer J, McConnell MS, et al. Nevirapine-associated hepatotoxicity was not predicted by CD4 count ≥ 250 cells/μL among women in Zambia, Thailand and Kenya. HIV Med 2010;11:650–60.

[59] Ouyang DW, Brogley SB, Lu M, et al. Lack of increased hepatotoxicity in HIV-infected pregnant women receiving nevirapine compared to other antiretrovirals. AIDS 2010;24:109–14.

[60] Hitti J, Andersen J, McComsey G, et al., AIDS Clinical Trials Group 5084 Study Team. Protease inhibitor-based antiretroviral therapy and glucose tolerance in pregnancy: AIDS Clinical Trials Group A5084. Am J Obstet Gynecol 2007;196(331):e1–7.

[61] González-Tomé MI, Ramos Amador JT, Guillen S, et al. Spanish cohort of HIV-infected mother–infant pairs. Gestational diabetes mellitus in a cohort of HIV-1 infected women. HIV Med 2008;9:868–74.

[62] Pinnetti C, Floridia M, Cingolani A, et al. Effect of HCV infection on glucose metabolism in pregnant women with HIV receiving HAART. HIV Clin Trials 2009;10:403–12.

[63] The Kesho Bora Study Group. Triple antiretroviral compared with zidovudine and single-dose nevirapine prophylaxis during pregnancy and breastfeeding for prevention of mother-to-child transmission of HIV-1 (Kesho Bora study): a randomised controlled trial. Lancet Infect Dis 2011; 11:171–80.

[64] Watts DH, Lu M, Thompson B, et al. Treatment interruption after pregnancy: effects on disease progression and laboratory findings. Infect Dis Obstet Gynecol 2009;2009:456717.

[65] Shapiro R, Kitch D, Hughes M, et al. Increased maternal and infant mortality following completion of HAART and breastfeeding at 6 months postpartum in a randomized PMTCT trial: Botswana, the Mma Bana Study. In: 18th Conference on Retroviruses and Opportunistic Infections. Boston, MA; 27 February–2 March; 2011.

[66] Mandelbrot L, Landreau-Mascaro A, Rekacewicz C, et al. Lamivudine-zidovudine combination for prevention of maternal–infant transmission of HIV-1. JAMA 2001;285:2083–93.

[67] Mofenson LM. Prevention in neglected subpopulations: prevention of mother-to-child transmission of HIV infection. Clin Infect Dis 2010;50(Suppl. 3): S130–48.

[68] Dorton B, Mulindwa J, Li M, et al. CD4 cell count and risk for antiretroviral drug resistance among women using peripartum nevirapine for perinatal HIV prevention. BJOG 2011;118:495–9.

[69] Lockman S, Hughes MD, McIntyre J, et al. Antiretroviral therapies in women after single-dose nevirapine exposure. N Engl J Med 2010;363:1499–509.

[70] Palumbo P, Lindsey J, Hughes M, et al. Treatment strategies for HIV-infected children previously exposed to nevirapine: the P1060 nevirapine versus lopinavir-ritonavir trial. N Engl J Med 2010;363:1510–20.

[71] Moorthy A, Gupta A, Bhosale R, et al. Nevirapine resistance and breast-milk HIV transmission: effects of single and extended-dose nevirapine prophylaxis in subtype C HIV-infected infants. PLoS ONE 2009;4:e4096.

[72] Lidstrom J, Li Q, Hoover DR, et al. Addition of extended zidovudine to extended nevirapine prophylaxis reduces nevirapine resistance in infants who were HIV-infected in utero. AIDS 2010;24:381–6.

[73] Mirochnick M, Thomas T, Capparelli E, et al. Antiretroviral concentrations in breastfeeding infants of mothers receiving highly active antiretroviral therapy. Antimicrob Agents Chemother 2009;53:1170–6.

[74] Colebunders R, Hodossy B, Burger D, et al. The effect of highly active antiretroviral treatment on viral load and antiretroviral drug levels in breast milk. AIDS 2005;19:1912–15.

[75] Zeh C, Weidle P, Nafisa L, et al. HIV-1 drug resistance emergence among breastfeeding infants born to HIV-infected mothers during a single-arm trial of triple-antiretroviral prophylaxis for prevention of mother-to-child transmission: a secondary analysis. PLoS Med 2011;8(3):e1000430.

[76] Lidstrom J, Guay L, Musoke P, et al. Multi-class drug resistance arises frequently in HIV-infected breastfeeding infants whose mothers initiate HAART postpartum, In: 17th Conference on Retroviruses and Opportunistic Infections. San Francisco, CA, February 16–19; 2010 (Abs. 920).

[77] Fogel J, Li Q, Taha TE, et al. Initiation of antiretroviral treatment in women after delivery can induce multi-class drug resistance in breastfeeding HIV-infected infants. Clin Infect Dis 2011;52 (8):1069–76.

[78] Legardy-Williams JK, Jamieson DJ, Read JS. Prevention of mother-to-child transmission of HIV-1: the role of cesarean delivery. Clin Perinatol 2010;37:777–85.

[79] European Collaborative Study, Boer K, England K, Godfried MH, Thorne C. Mode of delivery in HIV-infected pregnant women and prevention of mother-to-child transmission: changing practices in Western Europe. HIV Med 2010;11:368–78.

[80] World Health Organization. Guidelines on HIV and infant feeding 2010—principles and recommendations for infant feeding in the context of HIV and a summary of evidence. Geneva: World Health Organization; 2010.

[81] World Health Organization. PMTCT Strategic Vision 2010-2015: preventing mother to child transmission of HIV to reach the UNGASS and Millennium Development Goals. Geneva: World Health Organization; 2010.

Chapter | **38** |

Managing HIV infection in children and adolescents

Elizabeth H. Doby, Andrew T. Pavia

EPIDEMIOLOGY

The epidemiology of HIV disease in children in developed countries has changed substantially. These changes have been driven by the evolving epidemiology of HIV infection in women, the ability to prevent mother-to-child transmission, the dramatic increases in survival for children treated with combination antiretroviral therapy (cART) [1–3], and the evolution of drug resistance. Women constitute a significant proportion of AIDS cases and new HIV infections. Women account for 27% of new HIV infections in the United States [4]; this has remained stable over the last 5 years. However, women account for 25% of the estimated 1 million people living with HIV in the United States, suggesting that 250,000 women are infected [4, 5]. In 2005, the Centers for Disease Control (CDC) estimated that 6,000–7,000 infants were born to HIV-infected women each year in the USA [6]; however, only 141 new perinatal infections were reported in 2008 [5].

Since 1992, the number of children younger than 13 years diagnosed with AIDS in developed countries has decreased dramatically, representing one of the remarkable successes in the fight against HIV. In the USA, the estimated number of children younger than 13 diagnosed with AIDS decreased from 952 in 1992, to 34 in 2008 [5]. This likely represents improvements in clinical care and survival, but this has led to a larger population of surviving children. By the end of 2008, an estimated 908 children were living with AIDS in the USA and its territories, and an additional 2,919 children were reported to be living with HIV infection (not AIDS) from the 37 states with name-based reporting [5]. No accurate data are available regarding the number of HIV-infected immigrants, refugees, and adopted children living in the United States. However, foreign-born children may represent a significant portion of HIV-infected children entering care, and they may face unique challenges.

Thus, a large number of children are living with HIV/AIDS, but few new infections are occurring. Many older children have been infected for years, and usually have received prolonged antiretroviral therapy and may have complex resistance patterns. Many are, or soon will be, adolescents. The major challenges of treatment now revolve around managing viral resistance, complications of therapy, and the psychological and social impact of HIV infection rather than when to start therapy.

NATURAL HISTORY

Timing of infection

HIV progresses more rapidly in children with perinatal infection than among children infected at an older age or among adults. It has long been recognized that there was a bimodal distribution of clinical progression following perinatal infection [7–9]. About 20% of children had early onset of symptoms before the advent of effective therapy. These children have a rapid downhill course in the first 12 months of life, marked by rapid decline in CD4 count, and development of category C disease, often with pneumonia due to *Pneumocystis jiroveci* (formerly *P. carinii* pneumonia), or death.

There appear to be a number of predictors of rapid progression, including severe maternal disease [10], evidence of *in utero* transmission (positive PCR at birth), early hepatosplenomegaly [11], and higher viral loads after 1 month of life [12, 13]. CD4 and CD8 counts below the fifth percentile in infancy were associated with rapid progression

Table 38.1 1994 revised human immunodeficiency virus pediatric classification system: Immune categories based on age-specific CD4 count and percentage

IMMUNE CATEGORY	< 12 MONTHS No./mL (%)	1–5 YEARS No./mL (%)	6–12 YEARS No./mL (%)
Category 1: No suppression	>1,500 (>25%)	>1,000 (>25%)	>500 (>25%)
Category 2: Moderate suppression	750–1499 (15–24%)	500–999 (15–24%)	200–499 (15–24%)
Category 3: Severe suppression	<750 (<15%)	<500 (<15%)	<200 (<15%)

From Centers for Disease Control and Prevention; 1994 revised classification system for human immunodeficiency virus infection in children less than 13 years of age. MMWR 1994; 43 (RR-12):1–10.

among babies infected *in utero* in one study [14], perhaps reflecting early destruction of the thymus.

The natural history of HIV among adolescents who have acquired infection through adult behaviors generally parallels adults. However, younger age at infection for those with non-perinatally acquired HIV is associated with significantly slower progression in the absence of antiretroviral therapy (ART) [15, 16].

Declining CD4 count and CD4% are the hallmarks of HIV disease progression in children. CD4 count normally declines with age in young children, making interpretation somewhat difficult. CD4% is less age-dependent and is also useful in disease staging (Table 38.1) [17]. The revised CDC, PENTA, and WHO classifications use both immunologic status and clinical status for staging. Growth failure is a sensitive indicator of disease activity, and improved growth is a marker of successful ART.

Predicting progression

Quantitative measurement of plasma viral RNA revolutionized the management of HIV in adults; similar data in children required a few more years to accumulate [13, 18, 19]. The kinetics of plasma HIV RNA in children differs from adults in several ways. First, children tend to have higher viral loads, with median peak values between 100,000 and 1,000,000 copies. Second, after primary infection, the viral load slowly declines during the first year of life, in contrast to the rapid 2–3 log drop in adults. Third, although viral load is consistently associated with prognosis,

it has been difficult to establish specific levels that are sensitive and specific for high risk [20]. These differences may reflect a greater number of target cells and a limited ability to mount an immune response by the immature immune system. Children infected *in utero* tend to have modest viral loads at birth, but the peak value at 1–2 months is higher than those with presumed intrapartum infection.

A pivotal meta-analysis of survival data on 3,941 European and American children with HIV infection in the pre-HAART era demonstrated that CD4% and viral load were independent predictors of progression to AIDS or death over the next 12 months. CD4% was the strongest short-term predictor (Fig. 38.1) [20]. The risk of progression at a given CD4 level or viral load varied by age. Importantly, among children < 12 months, the risk of progression remained moderately elevated even when the CD4% was high or the viral load was low. A recent analysis of the same cohorts concluded that CD4 count may be more useful than CD4% in determining treatment initiation, particularly if only one has crossed a threshold [17].

With the advent of three-drug combination ART for children, survival has increased dramatically. In a cohort of 1,000 children in the UK, there was an 80% decline in mortality and a 50% decline in progression to AIDS between 1997 and 2002, along with a 80% decline in hospital admission rates between 1996 and 2002 [21].

EARLY DIAGNOSIS AND MANAGEMENT OF THE EXPOSED INFANT

Diagnosis of HIV infection

Currently, the diagnosis of HIV infection in children born to HIV-infected mothers can be made in most infants by 2–4 weeks of age using methods that directly detect virus. Detection of virus by HIV DNA PCR of the infants' peripheral blood mononuclear cells (PBMCs) or HIV RNA in plasma is presumptive evidence of infection but *must* be confirmed by repeat testing.

Viral culture is no longer used for diagnosis of HIV in infants. Currently, either detection of DNA or RNA by PCR is the test of choice. HIV DNA PCR is only moderately sensitive in the first 48 hours of life (38%–90% confidence interval [CI], 29–46%). Sensitivity rises rapidly during the second week; 93% of infected children (90% CI, 76–97%) were PCR positive by 14 days of age. Quantitative RNA PCR is at least as sensitive and specific as DNA PCR, and offers the advantages of using smaller blood volumes, providing important prognostic data [22, 23], and being more sensitive for detecting non-clade B strains [24]. False positives can occur; levels <5,000 copies/mL should be considered suspect. Measurement of p24 antigen, either conventionally or with immune dissociation,

Figure 38.1 Probability of developing AIDS in the next 12 months by age group. (A) By CD4%; age groups (top to bottom) = 6 months, 1 year, 2 years, 5 years, 10 years.
Adapted from Dunn [20]. (B) By CD4 count; age groups = 6 months, 1 year, 2 years, 3 years, 4 years, 10 years.
Adapted from HIV Paediatric Prognostic Markers Collaborative Study [35].

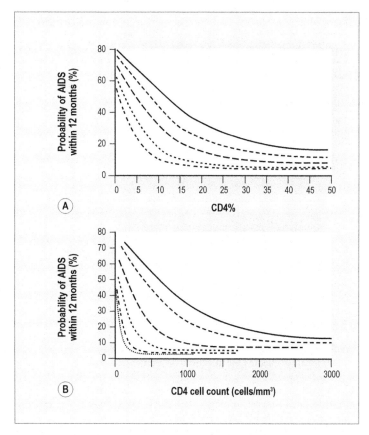

is not recommended for the diagnosis of neonatal HIV infection because it is less sensitive and specific than PCR.

Many experts recommend obtaining a first sample for DNA or RNA PCR during the first 48 hours of life, especially if the infant is at higher risk of infection. Cord blood should not be used because of the possibility of contamination with maternal blood. A positive viral test in the first 48 hours of life presumptively identifies children infected *in utero* who may have a more rapid disease course. However, plasma RNA measurement after the first month of life may be more prognostic than time of first positive test.

For infants with an initial negative test or who are not tested at birth, testing should be repeated at 14–21 days of life. Testing at 14 days offers the potential to stop zidovudine monotherapy for patients with presumed infection and begin combination therapy during the period of acute infection. For infants with initial negative tests, testing should be repeated again at 1–2 months of age. An infant with two negative virologic tests, one at ≥ 14 days and one at ≥ 1 month of age, can be viewed as *presumptively* uninfected. Thus, one does not need to initiate PCP prophylaxis. Testing should be repeated at 4–6 months of age for definitive exclusion of HIV infection.

Any positive test should be confirmed immediately by testing of a separate blood sample. Two positive tests should be considered diagnostic of infection. Many experts recommend checking HIV antibody at 12 months to document the clearance of maternal antibody. If antibody is still detectable, testing should be repeated until antibody becomes undetectable.

Monitoring in the HIV-exposed or HIV-infected infant

Infants born to HIV-infected women should receive oral AZT during the first 6 weeks of life, based on the PACTG 076 protocol. Myelosuppression is common with both AZT and trimethoprim-sulfamethoxazole, and the complete blood count should be monitored. Plasma viral RNA and CD4 count and percentage should be monitored immediately once the diagnosis of HIV is established, and followed every 3–4 months. When starting ART, plasma viral RNA and CD4 count should be measured at baseline, after 1 and 2 months, and every 3–4 months thereafter. A suggested monitoring scheme is shown in (Table 38.2).

Table 38.2 Suggested schedule for routine monitoring of HIV-exposed and infected infants

INTERVENTION	BIRTH	14–21 DAYS	1–2 MONTHS	4–6 MONTHS	1 YEAR
AZT	X	X	Through week 6		
PCP prophylaxis[a]			X[a]		
CBC with differential	X	X	X	X	
HIV plasma RNA or HIV DNA PCR[b]	X	X	X	X	
CD4 absolute and %[c]					
HIV antibody					X

[a]PCP prophylaxis is continued until HIV is excluded or for the first 12 months of life in children who are infected or whose infection status is unknown.
[b]See text for use of HIV plasma RNA PCR or HIV DNA PCR. HIV plasma RNA should be measured immediately if infection is detected based on a positive HIV DNA PCR. If no treatment is initiated, plasma RNA should be monitored every 3–4 months in infected children. If treatment is initiated or changed, plasma RNA should be monitored 4 and 8 weeks after changing therapy and every 3–4 months thereafter.
[c]CD4 counts should be repeated every 3–4 months in children who are infected.

Vaccination

Timely vaccination is important for HIV-infected children. Guidelines are available [25]. Inactivated vaccines (hepatitis B, *Haemophilus influenzae* type B, diphtheria-tetanus-pertussis, IPV) are given according to the schedule recommended for all children. Measles, mumps, and rubella (MMR) and varicella vaccines are live-attenuated, which pose a theoretical risk to severely immunocompromised children. The vaccines should not be given to those with CD4% less than 15%. HIV-infected children without immunosuppression should receive their first dose of MMR as soon as possible after the first birthday. The second dose does not need to be delayed until school entry; it can be given as soon as 1 month after the first dose. Annual immunization against influenza is recommended for all HIV-infected children. Initially, two doses are given, separated by at least 1 month.

Since infections with encapsulated bacteria are prominent among HIV-infected children, the potential benefit of pneumococcal vaccine is large. Unfortunately, children < 2 years old respond poorly to polysaccharide vaccines. In February 2010, a new 13-valent pneumococcal conjugate vaccine (PCV-13) was approved by the FDA, which offers expanded coverage of the serotypes causing the majority of invasive pneumococcal disease (IPD) in children. PCV-13 is recommended for all children younger than 72 months with an underlying medical condition, including HIV. In addition, children aged 6–18 years may receive one dose of PCV-13. A single dose of PCV-13 should be given to children younger than 6 years who were previously vaccinated with PCV-7. After completion of the PCV-13 series, the 23-valent pneumococcal vaccine (PPSV23) should also be given after 24 months of age. Re-vaccination should be offered 5 years after the first dose of PPSV23 [26].

Vaccination is also important for HIV-infected adolescents. They should receive pneumococcal and annual influenza vaccinations. Their immunization status to hepatitis A, hepatitis B, and measles should be reviewed and updated. Meningococcal conjugate vaccine and tetanus diphtheria acellular pertussis (Tdap) are recommended for all adolescents. Human papillomavirus vaccine is licensed for use in both females and males; however, no specific recommendations exist regarding its use in HIV-infected children and adolescents [4, 27]. Given the increased risk of HPV-related disease among HIV-infected persons, HPV vaccine (HPV4) should be strongly considered for both female and male HIV-infected adolescents.

ANTIVIRAL THERAPY

Principles of therapy

The goal of ART in children, as in adults, is to suppress viral replication to extremely low levels to prevent loss of CD4 cells and to allow immune reconstitution. If viral replication continues in the face of antiretroviral agents, ongoing mutation will lead to drug resistance. Combination therapy with three or more agents offers the greatest opportunity to achieve maximal suppression. The ability to adhere to a regimen is a key determinant of continued viral suppression. The complexity of HIV therapy in children and adolescents and the rapidly changing evidence base suggest that children with HIV should receive care from physicians with substantial expertise in HIV and in conjunction with multidisciplinary teams. Whenever possible, children should be offered the opportunity to participate in clinical trials.

It is important, however, to appreciate ways in which children differ from adults. The majority of HIV-infected children are infected around the time of delivery, and therapy can potentially be started during primary infection. Theoretically, this offers children an advantage that is rare in adults. Intact thymic architecture offers the potential for greater immune reconstitution, and in one study, thymic volume on CT scan correlated with completeness of immune reconstitution [28].

However, many of the differences lead to challenges. In general, clinical trial data in children are limited and pharmacokinetic studies may be inadequate. The disposition of drugs changes during growth and development, changing from infancy into childhood, and again during adolescence. In general, volume of distribution is larger, and clearance is faster, which may require more frequent dosing. In general, rates of viral suppression below the limits of quantification have been lower in trials among children and adolescents than among adults. The developing central nervous system of children appears to be more vulnerable to damage by HIV. Regimens, therefore, should be highly active in the CNS. Young children usually require liquid formulations, which may be unpalatable or unavailable. Young children are dependent on the caregiver's ability to give medications consistently, on schedule, and despite protests. Older children may be concerned about taking antiviral therapy in public, at school, or at friends' houses. The social problems which are common in families with HIV-infected children (poverty, homelessness, parents who may be ill or absent, substance abuse, mental illness, isolation, fear of disclosure) compound the problems of complex regimens, unpleasant tasting medicine, and sometimes resistance from the child or adolescent. Thus, problems with adherence can be daunting.

When to start

Recommendations on starting therapy and preferred regimens have been formulated by the Panel on Antiretroviral Therapy and Medical Management of HIV-Infected Children in the US and the Paediatric European Network for Treatment of AIDS (PENTA) (Table 38.3) [24, 29]. These guidelines are generally concordant but have subtle differences. The decision to start therapy balances the probability of developing severe clinical disease in the near term and the risk of irreversible damage to the immune system or developing organs with the known difficulties of maintaining suppression in children, short-term side effects, the risk of developing drug resistance, and the possibility of running out of effective agents. In addition, uncertainty remains about the importance and frequency of long-term toxicities in children, including abnormalities of lipid, glucose, and bone metabolism.

Historically, the decision to initiate ART in children was based on myriad factors, including age, clinical status, CD4 count, and CD4 percentage. A meta-analysis of 3,345 children in 17 cohort studies and randomized trials from 1983 to 2002 showed that CD4 percentage had little or no additional prognostic value over CD4 cell count, regardless of age [17]. These data are reflected in the new treatment guidelines: both the European and WHO no longer use CD4 percentages for treatment initiation decisions. The US guidelines continue to use CD4 percentage thresholds for children < 5 years of age.

Prompt initiation of ART for all HIV-infected infants < 12 months of age is now universally recommended. The Children with HIV Early Antiretroviral Therapy (CHER) randomized trial in South Africa showed a 76% reduction in early infant mortality and a 75% reduction in HIV progression in those infants receiving immediate ART with a lopinavir-ritonavir-based regimen, as compared to infants randomized to defer therapy until they met clinical or immunologic criteria [30]. The benefits of early initiation of ART for infants were confirmed in a resource-rich setting by the European Infant Collaboration (EIC) cohort study [31]. Even with demonstrable improvements in mortality and morbidity, early initiation of ART can be challenging. Complete virologic suppression often is not achieved or takes longer in younger children and likely is associated with higher rates of genotypic resistance mutations [32]. In addition, administering drugs and ensuring adherence can be challenging in infants.

In children with category C and most category B disease, treatment always should be started, as well as in those with severe immunosuppression, as defined by age-related CD4 markers (Table 38.1). Treatment for children older than 1 year with limited or no symptoms is more problematic. For those with preserved immune function, one approach would be to treat all children. This is consistent with evolving data favoring earlier treatment in adults [33]. The aggressive approach can be considered when the family or caregivers are committed to therapy, there is adequate medical and social support, and there is a high likelihood of good adherence.

An alternative approach is to defer therapy in older children who have limited symptoms, have no evidence of immune dysfunction, and are at low risk of rapid progression based on HIV RNA. However, the optimal thresholds remain unknown. The risk of progression increases when the CD4 percentage is < 25%, especially in younger children. In these cases, therapy should be considered. Viral loads > 100,000 copies/mL are associated with higher rates of progression or death [18, 20, 34, 35], and treatment is recommended. Patients in whom deferral of therapy might be preferred are older children with minimal symptoms, well-preserved CD4 levels, and low viral loads. Perhaps the most important consideration, and one which requires thoughtful clinical judgment, is whether to defer therapy in low- and intermediate-risk patients in whom the risk of poor adherence and development of resistance is felt to be very high and might outweigh the benefit of immediate therapy. If ART is deferred, close monitoring is essential. Therapy should be initiated if new symptoms develop, or if the CD4 cell count is falling rapidly (confirmed by repeated measures).

Table 38.3 When to start therapy: Comparison of DHHS 2011, PENTA 2009, and WHO 2010 recommendations

AGE GROUP	DHHS 2011	PENTA 2009	WHO 2010
< 12 months	**Treat** All (AI)	**Treat** All	**Treat** All

12–<24 months	**Treat**
	• CDC stage B* or C (AI)
	• CD4 <25% (AII)
	• Asymptomatic or mild symptoms and
	  • CD4 ≥25% *and*
	  • HIV RNA ≥100,000 copies /mL (BII)
	Consider or defer
	• Asymptomatic or mild symptoms *and*
	  • CD4 ≥25% *and*
	  • HIV RNA <100,000 copies/mL (CIII)
		Treat
		• CDC stage B or C
		• WHO stage 3 or 4
		• CD4 < 1000 cells/mm³
		• CD4 < 25%
		Consider
		• HIV RNA ≥100,000 copies/mL	

24–<36 months 36 months–<5 years		**Treat** • CDC stage B or C • WHO stage 3 or 4 • CD4 < 500 cells/mm³ • CD4% < 20% **Consider** • HIV RNA ≥100,000 copies/mL	**Treat** • WHO stage 3 or 4 • CD4 < 750 cells/mm³ • CD4% < 25%

> 5 years	**Treat**
	• CDC stage Bᵃ or C (A1)
	• CD4 < 350 cells/mm³ (A1)
	• CD4 ≥ 350–500 cells/mm³ (B11)
	• Asymptomatic or mild symptoms *and*
	  • CD4 ≥350 cells/mm³ *and*
	  • HIV RNA ≥100,000 copies/mL (BII)
	Consider or defer
	• Asymptomatic or mild symptoms *and*
	  • CD4 ≥350 cells/mm³ *and*
	  • HIV RNA <100,000 copies/mL (CIII)
		Treat
		• CDC stage B or C
		• WHO stage 3 or 4
		• CD4 < 350 cells/mm³
		Consider
		• HIV RNA ≥100,000 copies/mL
			Treat
			• WHO stage 3 or 4
			• CD4 < 350 cells/mm³

DHHS: Panel on Antiretroviral Therapy and Medical Management of HIV-Infected Children. Guidelines for the Use of Antiretroviral Agents in Pediatric HIV Infection. August 11, 2011. Available at http://aidsinfo.nih.gov/ContentFiles/PediatricGuidelines.pdf
PENTA: PENTA Steering Committee. PENTA 2009 guidelines for the use of antiretroviral therapy in paediatric HIV-1 infection. HIV Medicine (2009), 10, 591–613
WHO: WHO. Antiretroviral therapy of HIV infection in infants and children: towards universal access: recommendations for a public health approach — 2010 revision. Available at http://www.who.int/hiv/pub/paediatric/infants2010/en/index.html
(The strength of the recommendation [A–C] and the strength of the evidence [I–III] is shown for the DHHS recommendations)
ᵃExcludes LIP or single episode of serious bacterial infection.

Initial therapy

When therapy is begun for children, combination therapy with at least three drugs, including two nucleoside reverse transcriptase inhibitors and either a non-nucleoside reverse transcriptase inhibitor or a potent protease inhibitor, is preferred. Monotherapy or the use of two nucleoside analogs is no longer considered adequate therapy.

Selection of appropriate drugs is complicated by the limited availability of adequate pharmacokinetic data to allow appropriate drug exposure, the availability and palatability of liquid formulations or smaller pills, and the availability of clinical efficacy data. In the US Guidelines, the combination of two nucleoside analogs plus either lopinavir/ritonavir, atazanavir with low dose ritonavir (for children ≥ 6) efavirenz (or nevirapine for children <3 or who cannot swallow capsules) is designated as preferred (Table 38.4). NNRTI-based regimens should not be used in infants exposed to perinatal nevirapine, even if baseline resistance testing does not show significant NNRTI resistance mutations [36–38]. A recent pediatric trial, PENPACT-1, suggests that among children without perinatal exposure to nevirapine, long-term outcomes are similar for children initiating therapy with PI compared with NNRTI-containing regimens [39]. Preferred dual-NRTI backbones include either lamivudine or emtricitabine in combination with abacavir (after testing for HLA B*5701), zidovudine, or tenofovir (in postpubertal adolescents). Because the data from the PENTA-5 trial show improved viral suppression and growth [40], the European guidelines recommend abacavir and lamivudine as the initial dual-NRTI backbone in HLA-B 5701 negative children [29]. Alternative ritonavir-boosted PI-based regimens include darunavir, and fosamprenavir for children aged 6 years and older. Regimens are designated as alternative regimens either because data are limited or suggest lower efficacy or because of toxicity. Data were insufficient to make recommendations for several drugs and regimens that have important potential roles, including raltegravir, etravirine, rilpivirine maraviroc, enfuvirtide, and triple-class regimens.

Initial studies demonstrated that rates of viral suppression to <400 copies/mL were substantially lower than among adults. However, more recent trials show rates of suppression among antiretroviral-naïve children of 65–84% [39, 41].

When to change

In children, the decision to change therapy must balance the need to better control viral replication and the higher likelihood of control with earlier switching against the limited number of active drugs and the problems of cross-resistance. In children who may need therapy for decades, it is important not to exhaust the limited options. When there is major toxicity, the regimen must be changed. For minor clinical or laboratory toxicities, it is worth trying to manage the symptoms.

When therapy appears to be failing, the issues are more complex. When the initial regimen is failing in a child over 6 years, there may be several acceptable treatment options. In children younger than 6 and those with extensive drug resistance mutations, there may be limited opportunities to design an effective regimen.

Before changing therapy, it is essential to carefully assess potential problems with dosing, absorption, and adherence and to try and solve adherence problems. Otherwise, the new regimen is doomed to fail.

There are three broad indicators of drug failure: virologic, immunologic, and clinical [24] Virologic indicators have the advantage of being easily quantifiable and often correlate with the emergence of drug-resistant virus. RNA measurements should be repeated before deciding to change therapy. Failure to achieve 1.0 log decrease in viral load after 8–12 weeks should prompt a change. The repeated detection of viral RNA (especially levels $> 1,000$ copies/mL) after a period falling below limits of quantification indicates failure. Failure to achieve a viral load of <400 copies/mL 6 months after beginning an aggressive initial regimen is an inadequate response. Recent data suggest that therapy switch should be considered at lower viral loads ($1,000$ copies/mL) with NNRTI-based regimens because more major NRTI mutations developed when therapy switch was triggered at higher viral loads among children compared to PI-based regimens [39].

Virologic failure may not predict immediate clinical or immunologic failure. The decision to change therapy should weigh the ability to achieve adherence, available options, and the CD4 response. Stable or increasing CD4 counts in the face of continued viral replication among children who remain on therapy are common, as in adults [42].

Immunologic progression is an indicator of increased risk of death. Therefore, therapy should be changed in the face of immunologic progression and detectable virus. CD4% is less affected by age, but absolute CD4 counts may be used in children at 5 years of age and older. A change to a new immunologic category, a sustained decline in CD4% by 5 percentiles at any age, or decline to below pre-therapy CD4 counts in children 5 years of age and older are clear indicators of immunologic progression. However, rate of change should also be considered.

Certain types of clinical progression are ominous and should prompt change in therapy. Growth failure, severe or recurrent infections, and progressive neurodevelopmental decline are clear indicators of disease progression. Although definitive data on the clinical efficacy are lacking, agents that achieve good antiretroviral activity in the CSF should be used. These include AZT, d4T, 3TC, FTC, and nevirapine.

The choice of agents for 'salvage' therapy is difficult, and there are few clear guidelines. Strategies recommended in adults also make sense for children. However, fewer antiretrovirals are available for children due to limited pharmacokinetic data and pediatric formulations. The availability of additional agents in the future must be considered. For

Table 38.4 Options for initial antiretroviral therapy in children with HIV infection (DHHS 2011)

Protease inhibitor-based regimens	
Preferred regimen	Two NRTIs[a] *plus* lopinavir/ritonavir or atazanavir plus low dose ritonavir (children ≥6 years)
Alternative regimen	Two NRTIs[a] *plus* fosamprenavir with low-dose ritonavir, or darunavir with low-dose ritonavir (children ≥ 6 years)
Non-nucleoside reverse transcriptase inhibitor-based regimens	
Preferred regimen	Two NRTIs[a] *plus* efavirenz[b] (children ≥ 3 years)
Alternative regimen	Two NRTIs[a] *plus* nevirapine[b,c]
Use in special circumstances	Two NRTIs[a] *plus* atazanavir unboosted (for treatment-naïve adolescents ≥ 13 years of age and > 39 kg; not for use with tenofovir) Two NRTIs[a] *plus* fosamprenavir unboosted (children ≥ 2 years of age) Two NRTIs[a] *plus* nelfinavir (children > 2 years of age) Zidovudine *plus* lamivudine *plus* abacavir
Regimens that are not recommended as *initial* therapy for children	Etravirine-containing regimens Raltegravir-containing regimens Efavirenz-containing regimens for children < 3 years of age Tipranavir-, saquinavir-, or indinavir-containing regimens Dual (full-dose) PI regimens Full-dose ritonavir or use of ritonavir as the sole PI Unboosted atazanavir-containing regimens in children < 13 years of age and/or < 39 kg Nelfinavir-containing regimens for children < 2 years old Triple-NRTI regimens other than abacavir *plus* zidovudine *plus* lamivudine Triple-class regimens, including NRTI plus NNRTI plus PI Regimens with dual-NRTI backbones of abacavir *plus* didanosine, abacavir *plus* tenofovir, didanosine *plus* tenofovir, and didanosine *plus* stavudine Tenofovir-containing regimens in children in Tanner stages 1–3 Enfuvirtide (T-20)- or maraviroc-containing regimens
Regimens that should never be used in children	Monotherapy Two NRTIs alone Certain two-NRTI combinations as part of a regimen (lamivudine *plus* emtricitabine due to similar resistance pattern and no additive benefit; and zidovudine *plus* stavudine due to virologic antagonism) Dual-NNRTI combinations Unboosted saquinavir, darunavir, or tiprinavir Atazanavir *plus* indinavir Certain NRTI-only regimens (tenofovir *plus* didanosine *plus* lamivudine *or* emtricitabine; or tenofovir *plus* abacavir *plus* lamivudine *or* emtricitabine)

[a]Dual NRTI combinations:
- Preferred choices: abacavir (screen for HLA-B*5701) *plus* lamivudine *or* emtricitabine; tenofovir *plus* lamivudine *or* emtricitabine (for Tanner stage 4 or postpubertal adolescents only); zidovudine *plus* lamivudine *or* emtricitabine. Of note, the 2009 PENTA guidelines recommend abacavir *plus* lamivudine (if HLA-B*5701 negative), and zidovudine *plus* lamivudine (if HLA-B*5701 positive)
- Alternative choices: zidovudine *plus* abacavir; zidovudine *plus* didanosine; didanosine plus lamivudine or emtricitabine
- Use in special circumstances: stavudine *plus* lamivudine *or* emtricitabine
- Not recommended: abacavir *plus* didanosine; abacavir *plus* tenofovir; didanosine *plus* tenofovir; and didanosine *plus* stavudine.

[b]Efavirenz currently available only in capsule form, although liquid formulation is under study. Nevirapine is preferred NNRTI for children < 3 years because of liquid formulation and well. established PK.

[c]Nevirapine-based therapy should not be used in infants exposed to peripartum nevirapine for prevention of maternal-to-child transmission.

example, additional active agents may be available for use when a child reaches 6 years of age. When available, enrollment in clinical trials can provide more options. Prior to changing therapy, barriers to adherence must be addressed, and resistance testing should be performed. Ideally, all drugs should be changed in a failing first-line regimen. At least two fully active antiretroviral agents (preferably three) should be used. The addition or substitution of a single new drug should be avoided.

Resistance testing

Recent data demonstrate that the prevalence of resistance among newly diagnosed HIV-infected children is similar to the 12–24% prevalence among recently infected adults [24, 43–45]. In children born in countries where single-dose nevirapine is used for prevention of peripartum transmission, the prevalence of NNRTI resistance may be high. Resistance testing should be obtained before beginning therapy in all treatment-naïve children. In addition, resistance testing is necessary to guide selection of new regimens for children with virologic failure. Of note, the absence of resistance mutations in a child who is failing therapy likely indicates poor adherence.

Therapeutic drug monitoring

The patient-to-patient variability of bioavailability, drug metabolism, and drug levels is generally larger for children than adults. Complex drug interactions may make it difficult to predict drug levels. To date, however, there are no prospective data that demonstrate that therapeutic drug monitoring improves treatment outcomes in children. In the absence of prospective data, it is reasonable to consider therapeutic drug monitoring for children in certain circumstances. These circumstances might include children on regimens for which dosing recommendations are based on limited data, children on unusual combinations or with complex drug–drug interactions, those who might have difficulty with drug absorption, or those whose clinical response varies from that which is expected [24, 46].

USE OF PCP PROPHYLAXIS

Pneumocystis jiroveci pneumonia occurs most often between 3 and 6 months of age in perinatally infected children. Disease may develop before HIV infection is confirmed or before a drop in CD4 counts has been documented. Because of continuing mortality with CD4-based guidelines for prophylaxis, the CDC published revised guidelines in 1999 that recommended that PCP prophylaxis should be considered at 4–6 weeks of life in HIV-exposed infants if HIV infection cannot be excluded (see above) [25]. Prophylaxis should be continued until 12 months of age in all infected

infants. After that age, prophylaxis is recommended for all children with severe immunosuppression (CDC category 3). Trimethoprim-sulfamethoxazole is the preferred drug. The recommended dose is 150 mg/m^2 per day in divided doses on three consecutive days each week, but there are several acceptable alternatives [25].

Prophylaxis of other opportunistic infections

The primary prevention of specific opportunistic infections is extremely important for children with advanced immunosuppression. Guidelines are available which categorize the advisability of prophylaxis, the CD4 levels, and the agents of choice [47].

The safety of stopping primary prophylaxis in adults after immune reconstitution has been clearly established. Recently, the PACTG 1008 clinical trial established the safety of discontinuing *Pneumocystis jiroveci* (PJP) and *Mycobacterium avium* complex (MAC) prophylaxis in children with stable immune reconstitution [48].

Lifelong suppression (secondary prevention) has been the standard of care for children with many opportunistic infections, including PJP, *Toxoplasma gondii* infection, and *Mycobacterium avium* complex. However, secondary prevention can, in some cases, be discontinued once stable immune reconstitution has occurred, based upon adult data and the PACTG 1008 trial. This issue merits further study in children.

MANAGEMENT

Comprehensive management of the HIV-infected child is beyond the scope of this chapter. Optimal care requires a multidisciplinary approach, and if possible, a dedicated team. Careful attention must be given to nutrition, developmental assessment, psychosocial issues, and education. Teaching about HIV and multiple strategies to support adherence are critical. Medical care of the mother is important to the child's health as well as the mother's. If possible, HIV services for mother and child should be available at the same site and should be coordinated. Periodic case management meetings to coordinate issues among providers and agencies are extremely useful.

ADOLESCENTS

Adolescents infected with HIV pose unique challenges. The needs of perinatally infected children who have survived into adolescence are different from those infected during adolescence. They have demonstrated slow disease progression, but often have advanced disease and may have been extensively pre-treated. They have often outlived their parents. Most adolescents who are recently infected were infected through sexual activity. HIV infection through sexual abuse occurs, and can be recognized only if there is awareness and careful investigation. Adolescent behavior problems, including drug use or having run away, are relatively common, and there is a high prevalence of mental illness among adolescents living with HIV [49]. Screening instruments for depression may be helpful. The clinical course of disease for adolescents infected sexually or through drug use is more similar to adults; adult treatment guidelines are appropriate.

Some issues are common among adolescents. Disclosure of infection status is a difficult issue. Ideally, disclosure is a progressive process that should begin well before adolescence. Rapid growth, changes in metabolism, and increases in muscle mass in males and in fat for women affect drug metabolism. Adolescents in early puberty (Tanner stage I and II) should be dosed as children. Those in late puberty (Tanner V) should be dosed as adults. There are no clear guidelines for those at intermediate stages. Puberty may be delayed in those with long-standing HIV infection, and delayed growth may be an additional stressor. Contraception is extremely important, both to prevent HIV transmission and unintended pregnancies. However, oral contraceptives and antiretrovirals have potential interactions, which can result in less effective contraception or increased hormone-related side effects. Hormonal contraception is optimally managed by an obstetrician/gynecologist with expertise in the care of HIV-affected women; condom use remains essential.

Adherence with medical care and ART is particularly difficult for adolescents. Autonomy, distrust of authority, embarrassment, lack of support, chaotic lives, and low self-esteem may contribute to poor adherence. Adolescents are often unable to grasp long-term risks and consequences. Medical care

and medications may make the adolescent feel different and, at times, vulnerable. Multidisciplinary teams, including mental health, social work, educators, and peer-to-peer counseling, may be helpful. In some adolescents at moderate risk of progression or with treatment failure due to adherence, it may be wise to delay ART until adherence is more likely.

UNANSWERED QUESTIONS

Despite the important gains in antiviral therapy and the promise of further improvement, frustrating gaps remain in our knowledge and our ability to deliver antiviral therapy to children. Early diagnosis of HIV-infected children and early treatment with fully suppressive regimens hold enormous promise. However, we need to learn much more about the pharmacology of antiretroviral drugs in all stages of growth. Delays in the availability of newer drugs can be life threatening; agents must be studied in infants and children during the early phase of development. The optimal combinations and sequences of drugs and the best way to ensure adherence to difficult and complex regimens remain unknown. The long-term consequences of changes in lipid, glucose, and bone metabolism may be more complex and potentially more serious in children over decades of treatment [50].

The prevention of perinatal transmission is the ultimate answer to controlling pediatric AIDS. In developed countries, it is possible to virtually eliminate perinatal transmission of HIV through universal screening of pregnant women, use of effective antiviral regimens during pregnancy and delivery, and optimal obstetrical management.

REFERENCES

[1] Berk DR, Falkovitz-Halpern MS, Hill DW, et al. Temporal trends in early clinical manifestations of perinatal HIV infection in a population-based cohort. JAMA 2005;293(18):2221–31.

[2] de Martino M, Tovo PA, Balducci M, et al. Reduction in mortality with availability of antiretroviral therapy for children with perinatal HIV-1 infection. Italian Register for HIV Infection in Children and the Italian National AIDS Registry. JAMA 2000;284(2):190–7.

[3] McConnell MS, Byers RH, Frederick T, et al. Trends in antiretroviral therapy use and survival rates for a large cohort of HIV-infected children and adolescents in the United

States, 1989–2001. J Acquir Immune Defic Syndr 2005;38 (4):488–94.

[4] Centers for Disease Control and Prevention. HIV in the United States. MMWR 2010; July 2010 (7 February 2011).

[5] Centers for Disease Control and Prevention. HIV Surveillance Report, 2008. June 2010; 20.

[6] Centers for Disease Control and Prevention. HIV/AIDS: Pregnancy and Childbirth. Atlanta, GA; [updated October 10, 2007; February 12, 2011]; Available from: http://www.cdc.gov/hiv/topics/perinatal/.

[7] Blanche S, Newell ML, Mayaux MJ, et al. Morbidity and mortality in European children vertically

infected by HIV-1. The French Pediatric HIV Infection Study Group and European Collaborative Study. J Acquir Immune Defic Syndr Hum Retrovirol 1997;14(5):442–50.

[8] De Rossi A, Chieco-Bianchi L, Zacchello F, et al. The European Collaborative Study: natural history of vertically acquired human immunodeficiency virus-1 infection. Pediatrics 1994;94:815–19.

[9] Barnhart HX, Caldwell MB, Thomas P, et al. Natural history of human immunodeficiency virus disease in perinatally infected children: an analysis from the Pediatric Spectrum of Disease Project. Pediatrics 1996;97 (5):710–16.

[10] Ioannidis JP, Tatsioni A, Abrams EJ, et al. Maternal viral load and rate of disease progression among vertically HIV-1-infected children: an international meta-analysis. AIDS 2004;18(1):99–108.

[11] Mayaux MJ, Burgard M, Teglas JP, et al. Neonatal characteristics in rapidly progressive perinatally acquired HIV-1 disease. The French Pediatric HIV Infection Study Group. JAMA 1996;275(8):606–10.

[12] Rich KC, Fowler MG, Mofenson LM, et al. Maternal and infant factors predicting disease progression in human immunodeficiency virus type 1-infected infants. Women and Infants Transmission Study Group. Pediatrics 2000;105 (1):e8.

[13] Shearer WT, Quinn TC, LaRussa P, et al. Viral load and disease progression in infants infected with human immunodeficiency virus type 1. Women and Infants Transmission Study Group. N Engl J Med 1997;336(19):1337–42.

[14] Nahmias AJ, Clark WS, Kourtis AP, et al. Thymic dysfunction and time of infection predict mortality in human immunodeficiency virus-infected infants. J Infect Dis 1998;178:680–5.

[15] Carre N, Deveau C, Belanger F, et al. Effect of age and exposure group on the onset of AIDS in heterosexual and homosexual HIV-infected patients. SEROCO Study Group. AIDS 1994;8(6):797–802.

[16] Rosenberg PS, Goedert JJ, Biggar RJ. Effect of age at seroconversion on the natural AIDS incubation distribution. Multicenter Hemophilia Cohort Study and the International Registry of Seroconverters. AIDS 1994;8 (6):803–10.

[17] Boyd K, Dunn DT, Castro H, et al. Discordance between CD4 cell count and CD4 cell percentage: implications for when to start antiretroviral therapy in HIV-1 infected children. AIDS 2010;24 (8):1213–17.

[18] Palumbo PE, Raskino C, Fiscus S, et al. Predictive value of quantitative plasma HIV RNA and CD4+ lymphocyte count in HIV-infected infants and children. JAMA 1998;279(10):756–61.

[19] Dickover RE, Dillon M, Leung KM, et al. Early prognostic indicators in primary perinatal human immunodeficiency virus type 1 infection: importance of viral RNA and the timing of transmission on long-term outcome. J Infect Dis 1998;178(2):375–87.

[20] Dunn D. HIV Paediatric Prognostic Markers Collaborative Study Group. Short-term risk of disease progression in HIV-1-infected children receiving no antiretroviral therapy or zidovudine monotherapy: a meta-analysis. Lancet 2003;362:1605–11.

[21] Gibb DM, Duong T, Tookey PA, et al. Decline in mortality, AIDS, and hospital admissions in perinatally HIV-1 infected children in the United Kingdom and Ireland. BMJ 2003;327(7422):1019.

[22] Nesheim S, Palumbo P, Sullivan K, et al. Quantitative RNA testing for diagnosis of HIV-infected infants. J Acquir Immune Defic Syndr 2003;32(2):192–5.

[23] Young NL, Shaffer N, Chaowanachan T, et al. Early diagnosis of HIV-1-infected infants in Thailand using RNA and DNA PCR assays sensitive to non-B subtypes. J Acquir Immune Defic Syndr ?2000;24(5):401–7.

[24] Guidelines for the Use of Antiretroviral Agents in Pediatric HIV Infection, August 11 [database on the Internet] 2011. Available from: http://aidsinfo.nih.gov/ ContentFiles/PediatricGuidelines. pdf. 2010.

[25] Mofenson LM, Brady MT, Danner SP, et al. Guidelines for the Prevention and Treatment of Opportunistic Infections among HIV-exposed and HIV-infected children: recommendations from CDC, the National Institutes of Health, the HIV Medicine Association of the Infectious Diseases Society of America, the Pediatric Infectious Diseases Society, and the American Academy of Pediatrics. MMWR Recomm Rep 2009;58(RR-11):1–166.

[26] Nuorti JP, Whitney CG. Prevention of pneumococcal disease among infants and children — use of

13-valent pneumococcal conjugate vaccine and 23-valent pneumococcal polysaccharide vaccine — recommendations of the Advisory Committee on Immunization Practices (ACIP). MMWR Recomm Rep 2010;59(RR-11):1–18.

[27] Centers for Disease Control and Prevention. FDA Licensure of Quadrivalent Human Papillomavirus Vaccine (HPV4, Gardasil) for Use in Males and Guidance from the Advisory Committee on Immunization Practices (ACIP). MMWR 2010;59 (20):630–2.

[28] Vigano A, Vella S, Saresella M, et al. Early immune reconstitution after potent antiretroviral therapy in HIV-infected children correlates with the increase in thymus volume. AIDS 2000;14(3):251–61.

[29] Welch S, Sharland M, Lyall EG, et al. PENTA 2009 guidelines for the use of antiretroviral therapy in paediatric HIV-1 infection. HIV Med 2009;10(10):591–613.

[30] Violari A, Cotton MF, Gibb DM, et al. Early antiretroviral therapy and mortality among HIV-infected infants. N Engl J Med 2008;359 (21):2233–44.

[31] Goetghebuer T, Haelterman E, Le Chenadec J, et al. Effect of early antiretroviral therapy on the risk of AIDS/death in HIV-infected infants. AIDS 2009;23(5): 597–604.

[32] Aboulker JP, Babiker A, Chaix ML, et al. Highly active antiretroviral therapy started in infants under 3 months of age: 72-week follow-up for CD4 cell count, viral load and drug resistance outcome. AIDS 2004;18(2):237–45.

[33] Kitahata MM, Gange SJ, Abraham AG, et al. Effect of early versus deferred antiretroviral therapy for HIV on survival. N Engl J Med 2009;360(18):1815–26.

[34] Mofenson LM, Korelitz J, Meyer 3rd WA, et al. The relationship between serum human; immunodeficiency virus type 1 (HIV-1) RNA level, CD4 lymphocyte percent, and long-term mortality risk in HIV-1-infected children. National Institute of Child Health and Human Development Intravenous Immunoglobulin

Clinical Trial Study Group. J Infect Dis 1997;175(5):1029–38.

[35] HIV Paediatric Prognostic Markers Collaborative Study. Predictive value of absolute CD4 cell count for disease progression in untreated HIV-1-infected children. AIDS 2006;20(9):1289–94.

[36] MacLeod IJ, Rowley CF, Thior I, et al. Minor resistant variants in nevirapine-exposed infants may predict virologic failure on nevirapine-containing ART. J Clin Virol 2010;48(3):162–7.

[37] Lockman S, Hughes MD, McIntyre J, et al. Antiretroviral therapies in women after single-dose nevirapine exposure. N Engl J Med 2010;363 (16):1499–509.

[38] Palumbo P, Lindsey JC, Hughes MD, et al. Antiretroviral treatment for children with peripartum nevirapine exposure. N Engl J Med 2010;363(16):1510–20.

[39] PENPACT-1 Study Team. Babiker A, Castro nee Green H, et al. First-line antiretroviral therapy with a protease inhibitor versus non-nucleoside reverse transcriptase inhibitor and switch at higher versus low viral load in HIV-infected children: an open-label, randomised phase 2/3 trial. Lancet Infect Dis 2011; 11:273–83.

[40] Green H, Gibb DM, Walker AS, et al. Lamivudine/abacavir maintains virological superiority over zidovudine/lamivudine and zidovudine/abacavir beyond 5 years in children. AIDS 2007;21 (8):947–55.

[41] Chadwick EG, Yogev R, Alvero CG, et al. Long-term outcomes for HIV-infected infants less than 6 months of age at initiation of lopinavir/ritonavir combination antiretroviral therapy. AIDS 2011;25:643–9.

[42] Deeks SG, Barbour JD, Grant RM, Martin JN. Duration and predictors of CD4 T-cell gains in patients who continue combination therapy despite detectable plasma viremia. AIDS 2002;16(2):201–7.

[43] Karchava M, Pulver W, Smith L, et al. Prevalence of drug-resistance mutations and non-subtype B strains among HIV-infected infants from New York State. J Acquir Immune Defic Syndr 2006;42 (5):614–19.

[44] Parker MM, Wade N, Lloyd Jr RM, et al. Prevalence of genotypic drug resistance among a cohort of HIV-infected newborns. J Acquir Immune Defic Syndr 2003;32 (3):292–7.

[45] Persaud D, Palumbo P, Ziemniak C, et al. Early archiving and predominance of nonnucleoside reverse transcriptase inhibitor-resistant HIV-1 among recently infected infants born in the United States. J Infect Dis 2007;195 (10):1402–10.

[46] Fraaij PL, van Kampen JJ, Burger DM, de Groot R. Pharmacokinetics of antiretroviral therapy in HIV-1-infected children. Clin Pharmacokinet 2005;44 (9):935–56.

[47] Centers for Disease Control and Prevention. Guidelines for the Prevention and Treatment of Opportunistic Infections Among HIV-Exposed and HIV-Infected Children; recommendations from CDC, the National Institutes of Health, the HIV Medicine Association of the Infectious Diseases Society of America, the Pediatric Infectious Diseases Society, and the American Academy of Pediatrics. MMWR 2009;58(No. RR-11).

[48] Nachman S, Gona P, Dankner W, et al. The rate of serious bacterial infections among HIV-infected children with immune reconstitution who have discontinued opportunistic infection prophylaxis. Pediatrics 2005;115(4):e488–e94.

[49] Gaughan DM, Hughes MD, Oleske JM, et al. Psychiatric hospitalizations among children and youths with human immunodeficiency virus infection. Pediatrics 2004;113(6):e544–51.

[50] McComsey GA, Leonard E. Metabolic complications of HIV therapy in children. AIDS 2004;18 (13):1753–68.

Chapter | **39** |

Special issues regarding women with HIV infection

Ruth M. Greenblatt, Monica Gandhi

NATURE OF THE HIV EPIDEMIC AMONG WOMEN

Globally, about half the cases of HIV infection (or roughly 16.8 million) occur in women and girls, with the majority (12 million) occurring in females in sub-Saharan Africa [1]. Indeed, a recent report released by the World Health Organization lists the most common cause of death and disability in women of reproductive age worldwide to be HIV/AIDS [2]. Although HIV infection among women is not as common in the developed world, rates have increased in this group over the last 30 years. Currently, the number of cases of HIV infection among women in developed countries is comparable to those of many other chronic diseases. As of the last UNAIDS global update on the epidemic in 2009, 240,000 women were reported to be living with HIV in Western and Central Europe and 390,000 in North America [1]. In the USA, as reported in the 2009 surveillance report, 75% of HIV cases were in males and 25% in females [3]. The number of cases among males increased 10% between 2005 and 2008, but case numbers among women remained flat; these data contrast with expectations that the number of recognized HIV infections among US women would substantially increase if testing became more routine. Regardless of the sex ratio, the average rate of HIV infections among US women is currently 179 cases per 100,000 women, with some states reporting rates up to 460 per 100,000. Racial disparities in rates of HIV infection among US women are prominent: although only 14% of US women are African American [4], this group comprises 67% of all cases. Figure 39.1 shows the percentages of HIV/AIDS cases in US women by race/ethnicity compared to those in US men as of the latest CDC surveillance report [3]. Although HIV/AIDS does affect racial and ethnic minorities disproportionally in men as well, this disparity is even more stark among US women.

AIDS is among the 10 most frequently reported causes of death among African American and Hispanic adolescent and adult women (Fig. 39.2) [5]; this figure is likely to underestimate the contribution of HIV to mortality among these groups because it is limited to cases in which HIV infection was recognized, and only includes cases in which AIDS was reported to be a cause of death. Not only is HIV infection more common among African American women at all age ranges but also rates of death in this community from HIV/AIDS are disproportionately higher than mortality rates from the infection in other groups of American women. Moreover, although the most common causes of death at all ranges are malignancy and cardiovascular disease or strokes, undiagnosed HIV infection could contribute to any of these causes of death. Indeed, HIV infection, even when treated, is associated with excess deaths due to cancer, pneumonia, cardiovascular and neurovascular disease, diabetes, liver disease, and renal dysfunction. Therefore, HIV, whether undiagnosed or treated, could contribute to excess death and to morbidity in minority women that may not be registered in mortality statistics. Even when treated, the contribution of HIV to other forms of chronic morbidity and to mortality is expected to only increase as HIV-infected individuals on combination antiretroviral therapies (cART) survive for longer periods of time. Women living with HIV infection, therefore, require careful clinical assessment and treatment, including special attention to these chronic conditions that result directly from HIV-mediated immune activation.

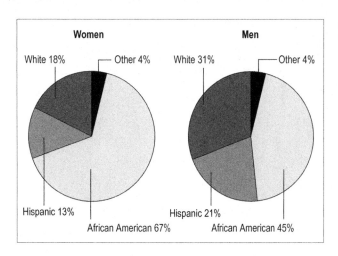

Figure 39.1 US epidemic affects minorities disproportionally in women.

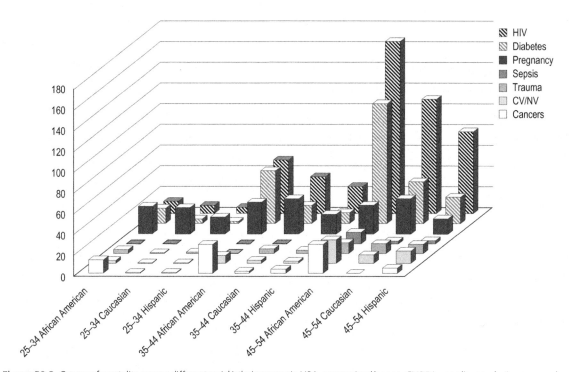

Figure 39.2 Causes of mortality among different racial/ethnic groups in USA, categorized by age. CV/NV = cardiovascular/neurovascular.

TRANSMISSION OF HIV TO WOMEN

Most transmission of HIV to women occurs during sexual contact and sexual risk may coincide with risks from injection needle use, making the precise determination of the mode of transmission in women with dual risk factors difficult. Because exposure events are frequently not recognized (the presence of HIV infection in sexual or needle-sharing partners is frequently unknown), women with HIV infection may deny any known risk factor. For large populations, the predominance of heterosexual transmission is imputed, and likely to be correct. The key concept here is that risk factors for HIV acquisition are frequently not recognized among women, so that assessment of risk is not a sensitive or useful means of triggering testing in women. Routine screening for HIV infection in medical settings is now recommended for all individuals aged 13 to 64 years in the USA;

this strategy is likely to be cost-effective [6] and may be of particular value to case identification in women.

Transmission rates per heterosexual coital act are very low but likely to be highly variable within sexual pairs (discussed in Chapter 36) [7]. Estimates of the rates of transmission for single male-to-female sexual acts range from 0.02 to 0.43 depending on geographic location (rates are higher in low-income countries), and whether the sex was transactional (transmission rates are lower with commercial sex) [8]. Even though single sex acts confer minimal risk, sex is a common behavior, so the ongoing sexual transmission of HIV to women on a global basis has been sustained. Several factors are known to influence infectiousness or susceptibility to HIV infection, and other factors are biologically plausible but unproven. Table 39.1 summarizes the factors that may modify the susceptibility of women to HIV acquisition during heterosexual sex and further detail on how these factors influence risk is provided below:

- **HIV viral load in partner:** Greater HIV RNA copy numbers (viral load) in blood or genital secretions is an important predictor of infectivity from males to females [3]. Factors that reduce viremia, such as receipt of cART, are associated with decreases in HIV transmission [9]. Consistent use of cART on the population level should result in decreased HIV

transmission rates [10, 11]. Indeed, the HIV Prevention Trials Network (HPTN) 052 trial, terminated early due to positive results, showed that the risk of transmission from HIV-infected to HIV-uninfected partners is reduced by 96% with the early use of cART, regardless of CD4 cell count [12]. In individual couples, consistent use of cART may not completely eliminate transmission, but massively reduces the risk [13].

- **Acute HIV infection:** The period of time surrounding acquisition of new HIV infection is an important window of increased infectivity likely related to relatively uncontrolled viral replication with minimal host immune responses leading to high levels of viremia and genital shedding [14]. Non-specific symptoms of the acute seroconversion syndrome limit the efficacy of strategies that involve counseling individuals to avoid sexual contact with acutely infected persons. If the substantial challenge of improving the detection of cases of early HIV infection was paired with safer sex or treatment interventions, a significant reduction in the incidence of HIV infection could be achieved [15]. The risk of transmission is also heightened in late-stage untreated HIV infection when HIV viral loads rise.

Table 39.1 Factors that modify the susceptibility to HIV acquisition in women

FACTOR	AFFECT	IMPACT	REFERENCE
High viral load in partner's blood	Increase	Major	[9–13]
Viral shedding in partner's genital fluids	Increase	Major	[9]
Acute HIV Infection in partners	Increase	Major	[14, 15]
Number of male partners	Variable	Moderate	[16]
Commercial sex work	Variable	Minor	[17]
Genital tract infections in partner	Increase	Minor–moderate	[18]
Genital tract infections in woman	Increase	Minor–moderate	[18]
Pregnancy	Possibly increase	Minor–moderate	[21–23]
Hormonal contraceptives	Possible increase	Moderate	[25–29]
Male or female condoms	Decrease	Major	
Use of vaginal irritants	Increase	Moderate	[39]
Pre-exposure prophylaxis	Decrease, presumably	Major	[30–38]
Tenofovir vaginal gel	Decrease	Major	[43]
Male circumcision	No effect	Moderate	[44]
Disempowerment of women	Increase	Major	[45]

- **Number of sex partners:** A larger number of male sexual partners is consistently associated with increased rates of infection [16], but infections are also commonplace in women with a single sexual partner.
- **Commercial sex work:** Exchanging sex for money, drugs or other items is associated with increased risk of HIV infection, though commercial sex workers in developing regions have demonstrated a lower per sexual contact risk than other women, perhaps due to greater use of condoms in this high-risk population over time [17].
- **Genital tract infections:** Genital infections have been found to be associated with HIV transmission in numerous studies [18]. The findings are based on studies of a wide variety of pathogens ranging from viruses to protozoans, and clinical manifestations including cervicitis/urethritis, vaginitis, genital warts, and ulcers. Each of the implicated diseases produces localized inflammation and/or immune activation, which could increase susceptibility to HIV. Genital ulcerative diseases are of particular import, having the most consistent association with an increased prevalence of HIV infection. Of these conditions, genital herpes is a key pathogen due to its high prevalence and recurrence rate. Another important pathogen implicated in the spread of HIV infection in developing world settings is *Haemophilus ducreyi*, the agent of chancroid, a bacterial infection that is prevalent in regions with high-intensity HIV epidemics. Genital ulcers result in loss of epidermal or mucosal barrier functions in addition to producing local inflammation, which may be a particularly potent combination in terms of augmenting HIV transmission. However, the extent of the interactions between sexually transmitted diseases (STDs) and HIV transmission is, for the most part, relatively modest, and intervention studies designed to control STDs as a means of preventing HIV infection have not been consistently successful [19, 20]. Regardless of the precise biological interaction between STDs and HIV, the occurrence of STDs is an indicator of the risk of HIV, and the prevalence of STDs in a given population is a good predictor of the intensity of the HIV epidemic in that setting.
- **Pregnancy:** Overall research findings indicate that pregnancy increases susceptibility to sexual HIV transmission [21, 22]; however, study results are not entirely consistent [23]. Findings from studies in sub-Saharan African women are most consistent, perhaps because the large number of transmission events supports adequate study power. Pregnancy could influence susceptibility to HIV infection in several ways, including increased fragility of genital tract tissues and alteration in host immunity during pregnancy, increasing the susceptibility to some infections. Incident infection with HIV during pregnancy is associated with an increased risk of mother-to-child transmission [24] and may be missed if HIV testing is only performed in the first trimester.

Therefore, the CDC routine testing guidelines recommend repeat HIV testing during the third trimester if risk factors are present or if the prevalence of HIV infection in the surrounding community is high. Finally, since acute infection with HIV late in pregnancy could be missed prior to delivery with an HIV antibody test alone, testing should be extended to the postpartum period in high-risk individuals.

- **Hormonal contraceptives:** Several studies have found that the use of hormonal contraceptives increases susceptibility to HIV infection [25, 26], but not all studies support this association [27, 29]. A variety of hormonal contraceptive formulations are commonly used, and the existing studies have often grouped them in assessing their effect on susceptibility to HIV. Since the specific sex steroid composition of these drugs may influence immunologic and genital tissue effects, mixing of formulations in studies may tend to obfuscate underlying associations. Current studies indicate that of the contraceptive sex steroids, depo medroxyprogesterone acetate (depo MPA) has the closest association with HIV transmission, but further study is needed to confirm this given the tremendous utility of this injectable contraceptive in resource-rich and resource-poor settings.
- **Pre-exposure prophylaxis (PrEP)** in the form of daily use of tenofovir/emtricitabine (TFV/FTC) has been recently demonstrated to reduce rates of HIV acquisition among men who have sex with men (MSM)[30]. Two other recent studies (Partners-PrEP and the Botswana TDF2 HIV Prevention Study [31, 32]) demonstrated the efficacy of TFV/FTC as pre-exposure prophylaxis in both men and women in stable serodiscordant heterosexual couples. The FEM-PrEP trial, however, designed to assess the efficacy of TFV/FTC in high-risk African women for PrEP, was terminated early (on April 18, 2011) after interim analysis showed equal rates of infection in each group [33]. The ongoing VOICE study (Vaginal and Oral Interventions to Control the Epidemic) is a 5-arm placebo-controlled trial assessing the effectiveness and safety of daily oral TFV-based products or vaginal TFV gel in preventing HIV acquisition in African women. The five arms of the trial were originally established to compare daily oral TFV, oral TFV/FTC, vaginal 1% TFV gel to the appropriate placebo products in preventing HIV acquisition on women. On September 16, 2011, the TFV-only arm of VOICE was closed for futility, although the arm evaluating the efficacy of TFV/FTC is continuing. Although data are not yet available on the reasons for these disparate efficacy results for PrEP in MSM, heterosexual women in stable serodiscordant partnerships, and high-risk African women, postulated reasons include differences in adherence to study product, differences in trial designs in terms of the use of hormonal contraceptives, and differences in the degree of penetration of oral tenofovir into the rectal mucosa versus the vaginal mucosa (i.e. rectal penetration higher

than vaginal). Ongoing data analyses of these trials and ongoing arms of PrEP trials in heterosexual women should further refine the utility, frequency, timing, route of administration, and specific populations who will benefit most from TFV-based prevention.

- **Topical spermicides and genital preparations** have been proposed as prevention interventions for HIV that would have special relevance for HIV-infected women. Nonoxynol-9, a commonly used detergent that serves as a spermicide, is virucidal in the test tube, but resulted in paradoxical increases in HIV transmission in humans [39]. Follow-up studies demonstrated that nonokynol-9 produced inflammation of the vaginal mucosa, a finding that may explain this apparent promotion of HIV transmission. Several other topic vaginal microbicides demonstrated no efficacy in preventing HIV transmission [40–42]. A recent trial demonstrated that vaginal application of 1% tenofovir gel twelve hours before and after each coital episode was effective in reducing the incidence of HIV infection among women in South Africa. The CAPRISA 004 trial found that vaginal 1% TFV gel reduced HIV infection rates by 39%, with a 54% reduction in "high adherers" (>80%) defined by self-report or applicator counts [43]. However, the vaginal 1% tenofovir gel arm of the VOICE trial was recently halted (on November 17, 2011) when the data safety and monitoring board concluded that the gel applied daily was ineffective in preventing HIV acquisition in VOICE trial participants. Ongoing studies of strategies to administer vaginal 1% TFV gel in women as an HIV prevention measure will hopefully clarify the utility of this product. Moreover, additional HIV-specific products formulated as microbicides to prevent HIV acquisition in women are currently under study.
- **Male and female condom use** is highly effective in the prevention of HIV transmission to and from women.
- **Male circumcision:** While male circumcision is highly effective in reducing the risk of sexual acquisition of HIV infection in men, it has little effect on transmission from an infected male to his female sexual partner [44]. However, population effects by which male circumcision will promote reduced prevalence of HIV infection among sexually active males will eventually lead to reduced exposure to the infection among female partners.

While biological factors are undoubtedly important determinates of HIV transmission in populations, additional characteristics likely influence the chances that an individual woman will acquire HIV infection, including many social factors that may determine whether she encounters an infected male partner and is capable of effectively engaging in risk-reduction behaviors. These social factors include income, education, employment, family size, mental health, cognitive function, and the presence of substance use. The social factors may produce vulnerabilities in individual women that are ultimately mediated through a loss of sexual autonomy [45].

THE NATURAL HISTORY OF HIV IN WOMEN

While the similarities in the course of HIV infection among women and men outnumber the differences [46, 47], the differences are important to understand. Women have higher rates of many autoimmune diseases than men, reflecting, in part, a pattern of more robust immune responses in females. Women also tend to respond more vigorously to vaccination and to clear some infections more frequently than men. Females have higher absolute CD4 cell counts than males (approximately 100 cells/mm^3), a difference that is found across age and racial groups, and a difference that persists in HIV infection [48, 49].

Women have viral loads approximately 0.2 to 0.8 log$_{10}$ lower than men during early HIV infection, when CD4 cell counts are greater than 400 cells/mm^3 (Fig. 39.3) [48, 50–63]. As CD4 cell counts decline, the sex discordancy in viral load lessens and disappears. Since viral load is predictive of the rate of disease progression, longer disease-free survival might be expected for women, but this has not been observed. Time to clinical progression is equal between the sexes, so women actually progress more rapidly to AIDS per a given viral load. Recent research has provided some clues to this seeming paradox. Women pay a price in heightened immune activation for their early control of viral replication, and this heightened immune activation may eventually lead to more rapid loss of CD4 cells [64]. Additionally, women produce more IL-7, a regulator of CD4 cell production, at a given CD4 cell count than men [49]. IL-7 also stimulates HIV replication, so the greater response to CD4 depletion that females demonstrate could also result in the generation of more HIV viral particles.

CD4 cell counts and immune functions in general are influenced by sex steroids. Women in the third trimester of pregnancy, when estrogen and progestin levels are very high, demonstrate transiently reduced peripheral blood CD4 cell counts. Menopause, which is characterized by significant and permanent decreases in estrogen and progestin levels, may also influence immune function, and interact with other immune perturbations of aging. As HIV infection or antiretroviral therapy results in increased aging in the HIV population, information regarding the effects of menopause on the course of HIV infection and related conditions of aging will be useful.

In the USA the chances of progression to clinical AIDS among HIV seroconverting women is heavily influenced by race and geographic location, with the highest rates of clinical AIDS occurring among African American and Southern women [48]. Women with HIV infection have lower blood hemoglobin and albumin levels, which are indicators of overall and non-AIDS-related survival, but women experience similar increases in these values to men after initiation of cART [65].

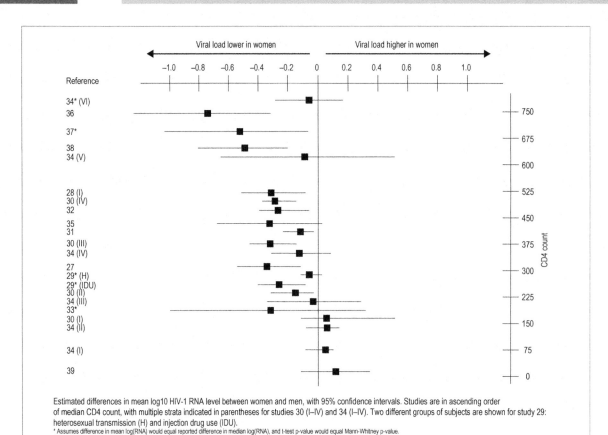

Figure 39.3 Comparisons of HIV viral loads by sex and CD4 count.
Adapted from Gandhi et al. [50].

In terms of clinical progression rates of chronically infected individuals on therapy (see Antiretroviral Treatment of Women section), earlier studies showed that women seemed to have higher rates of progression to AIDS or death than men [66], likely due to differential access to care or ART, or increased rates of substance abuse. Later studies that correct for these factors show no differences in rates of progression by sex [67], with some more recent studies suggesting better clinical outcomes in women versus men when adjusting for other relevant factors [68]. Hypotheses around these sex disparities are presented below.

CLINICAL MANIFESTATIONS OF HIV IN WOMEN

The symptoms of HIV, either acute or chronic infection, among women are comparable to those in men, and in general fairly non-specific. Sex differences in the occurrence or course of certain conditions exist and are summarized below.

Acute infection

A recent paper evaluated race and sex differences in outcomes of primary HIV infection in the Acute Infection and Early Disease Research Program (AIEDRP), a multicenter, observational cohort of more than 2,000 patients diagnosed with acute and recent HIV infection during the cART era [48]. At enrollment into AIEDRP, women averaged 0.40 $\log_{10}$ fewer copies/mL of HIV-1 RNA ($p < 0.001$) and 66 more CD4 cells (cells/mm^3) ($p = 0.006$) than men, consistent with reports from chronically infected individuals [49, 50]. In terms of differences unrelated to biology, initiation of cART was less likely at any time point by nonwhite women and men compared to white men ($p < 0.005$). Sex (and race) did not affect responses to ART after 6 months on therapy, but women were 2.17-fold more likely than men to experience more than one HIV/AIDS-related event ($p < 0.001$). Therefore, despite more favorable clinical parameters initially, female HIV-1-seroconverters had worse outcomes than did male seroconverters and these differences were exacerbated in non-white individuals.

Cancer

In the cART era, HIV-infected men and women both continue to experience cancer rates that are on an average 3–4 times that of the general population, although one recent analysis of cancer cases among HIV patients in France indicates that peak age of the highest relative risk of cancer is lower among women than men (under 40 versus under 50 years) [69]. These data likely reflect the small number of cases of malignancy in older individuals; more precise estimates of the cancer rate in older groups of HIV-infected persons will become available with increasing survival rates due to treatment and subsequently larger populations of older HIV-infected adults. In a large study of cancer cases among HIV-infected individuals in Belgium, rates of non-AIDS-defining malignancies were comparable between men and women, but survival of the women, many of whom were immigrants from sub-Saharan Africa, was significantly shorter than for the men (an average of 14 versus 32 months) [70]. The section below on women-specific conditions discusses cancers (e.g. breast, cervical, anal) that are more likely to demonstrate disparities by sex.

Hepatitis C

Hepatitis C virus (HCV) infection is common among HIV-infected women. Clinicians should be aware that spontaneous clearance of this co-infection occurs more frequently among women than men [71]. Furthermore, women with HCV are less likely to be viremic and tend to have lower hepatic transaminase levels with higher platelet counts than men at similar stages of HCV infection [71, 72]. However, data on sex differences in HCV infection mainly exist for the mono-infected population and further studies on the impact of sex on HCV progression in HIV-infected individuals are indicated [73].

Body habitus and metabolic changes

Sex differences in the distribution of body fat in HIV-uninfected adults are quite evident, and these differences persist in HIV-infected men and women. However, although HIV-infected women have smaller amounts of subcutaneous fat and total body fat than uninfected women [74], both HIV-infected and HIV-uninfected women have higher measurements of body fat than men [75]. The decreases in body fat (most prominent in the limbs) associated with HIV infection are smaller among women than men [75]. HIV infection in women is associated with higher blood levels of triglycerides and insulin, as well as lower levels of HDL, than observed in HIV-uninfected women [76]. Menopause influences blood lipids and triglycerides, such that LDL and triglyceride levels increase after menopause in HIV-uninfected women [77]. Therefore, careful evaluation of lipids in HIV-infected women, with greater attention in the postmenopausal period, is warranted.

Osteopenia and osteoporosis

Inadequate bone mineralization is a significant concern for women (and men) with HIV infection [78], both in the pre- or postmenopausal periods [79]. HIV-infected postmenopausal women have significantly lower T scores on dual-energy X-ray absorptiometry (DXA) scanning in the spine, hip, and femoral neck and greater levels of bone turnover markers, which could lead to an increased risk of serious fracture [80]. However, current data, which tends to be focused on premenopausal women, do not indicate that HIV infection is independently associated with increased fracture rates in women [81]. Nonetheless, as the HIV-infected population continues to age and, as cART is increasingly linked with higher rates of bone loss in the treated population [82, 83], careful attention to screening for osteopenia and osteoporosis in HIV-infected women (especially after menopause) is warranted [79].

Thyroid dysfunction

Autoimmune thyroiditis (including Hashimoto's thyroiditis and Graves disease) and hypothyroidism are significantly more common in women than men [84, 85]. Recurrences of clinical thyroiditis, hyperthyroidism, or new-onset hypothyroidism have all been reported after initiation of cART, likely as a late manifestation of immune reconstitution [86, 87]. Follow-up thyroid function testing should be performed after cART initiation in individuals with a history of previous thyroid dysfunction, particularly in patients with clinical AIDS or if nadir CD4 cell counts were <350 cells/mm^3. Clinicians should also be aware that new-onset thyroiditis can occur after the initiation of cART. Thyroid tenderness and the presence of antithyroid peroxidase and antithyroid stimulating hormone receptor antibodies can provide clues to this diagnosis [88].

Cardiovascular and cerebrovascular disease

Women have longer QT intervals than men on electrocardiograms (EKGs), and are therefore more susceptible to drug-induced torsade de pointes [89, 90], though less frequently experience arrhythmias in the setting of myocardial ischemia. The disparity in duration of the intervals recorded on EKGs is related to the relatively lower levels of testosterone in women, and, to a lesser extent, cyclic variability in progestin and estrogen levels [90]. This difference is pertinent to HIV since some antiretrovirals, including ritonavir, can prolong the QT interval, as does methadone, potentially increasing the risk of torsades in women being treated for HIV and/or opioid addiction [91, 92].

The incidence of coronary artery disease (CAD) is much lower among women under the age of 60 than among men. After age 60 the incidence of CAD in women increases steadily until it reaches that of men around the age of 80 [93].

The incidence of cerebrovascular incidents follows the same pattern. Sex steroids influence cardiovascular (and likely cerebrovascular) risk in a sex-dependent manner [94]. The role of exogenous estrogen treatment to reduce rates of vascular disease is controversial, and given the prothromotic and inflammatory milieu that is associated with HIV infection, the potentially adverse effects of estrogen treatment may be increased even more in this population. The cardiovascular effects of androgens are influenced by sex and concomitant levels of other sex steroids [95]. Higher androgen levels in both premenopausal women with polycystic ovary syndrome and in postmenopausal women are associated with increased LDL levels and increased rates of cardiovascular disease. However, the cardiovascular effects of androgen supplementation are currently not clear, and likely depend on other sex steroids and underlying host genetic traits [96]. Until more definitive studies can be done, the potentially adverse effects of androgen supplementation in women with HIV infection must be carefully considered. The impact of the pro-inflammatory state that is present in treated and untreated HIV infection on CAD and cerebrovascular disease rates in younger women is currently not known, but actively under investigation. Clinicians should follow ongoing observational and interventional research studies that will eventually determine diagnostic and preventive strategies for CAD in premenopausal and postmenopausal HIV-infected women.

WOMAN-SPECIFIC CONDITIONS AND HIV

Cervical cancer and genital epithelial dysplasia

HIV infection is associated with the detection of human papillomavirus (HPV) and epithelial dysplasia in cervical and anal tissues in women. HIV infection is also associated with the detection of a wider range of HPV types than is found in HIV-uninfected women; although HPV type 16 predominates in high-grade cervical dysplasia in HIV-uninfected women, HIV-infected women often have multiple HPV types contributing to the dysplastic lesions [97]. Greater CD4 cell depletion results in more HPV replication and integration of oncogenic HPV DNA (e.g. from HPV types 16 and 18) into cervical cells, an event that is closely associated with the occurrence of epithelial dysplasia [12, 98]. Cervical HPV infection also tends to persist longer in HIV-infected versus HIV-uninfected women [99]. Finally, the presence of HIV proteins themselves may also contribute to the development of dysplasia beyond the effect of HPV [100].

The severity of cervical dysplasia and rate of recurrence after excisional treatment are both greater in HIV-infected women and are proportionate to the extent of immunological injury [101, 102]. Current recommendations for screening of HIV-uninfected women stipulate that the Pap test should be repeated every 3 years if normal cytology is seen. Current recommendations for HIV-infected women call for cervical cytologic screening twice in the first year after HIV infection is diagnosed, and then annually thereafter if the Pap smear is normal. Consensus recommendations for tissue assessment and treatment following abnormal cytology do not currently differ by HIV status [103]. Milder forms of dysplasia (either low-grade squamous intraepithelial lesions [LSIL] or atypical squamous cells of undetermined significance [ASCUS] are the most common types of lesions reported. The optimal clinical management of these milder levels of dysplasia is unclear. The US Centers for Disease Control currently recommends magnified examination of the cervix or colposcopy in HIV-infected women with ASC-US or any higher grade cytologic abnormality with the goal of identifying other higher-grade lesions. HIV infection may not influence the risk of progression of low-grade lesions to higher-grade lesions. However, HIV infection is associated with reduced disease-free survival when invasive cervical cancer occurs, arguing for the role of circumspect preventive care.

Since the sensitivity of HPV testing as a means of detecting or predicting dysplasia is variable, the benefits of more costly HPV detection testing remains to be established. Fortunately, HIV-infected women who receive regular cytological screening and recommended treatment are not at increased risk for invasive cervical cancer when compared to HIV-uninfected women [103]. Recurrence after excisional or ablative treatment of cervical lesions is associated with persistent HPV detection [104]. Moreover, even after hysterectomy, HIV-infected women with high-grade cervical lesions experience increased rates of vaginal and vulvar abnormalities compared with HIV-uninfected women [105, 106]. Therefore, the current guidelines for the prevention and treatment of opportunistic infections in HIV-infected adults and adolescents stress the importance of careful inspection of the vaginal and vulvar areas during examinations [107].

Adherent cART use is associated with reductions in detection and quantity of oncogenic HPV types in cervical cells [108] and the clearance of oncogenic HPV-related cervical lesions [109]. However, the risk of dysplasia and response to treatment remain diminished in the context of HIV infection, despite antiretroviral therapy [102]. HIV-infected women, whether on or off cART, are at high risk for cervical dysplasia and incomplete responses to treatment, so routine cytologic testing is crucial.

Anal cancer

The anal canal has a transitional zone between keratinized and columnar epithelium that is roughly analogous to that of the cervix. The anus is susceptible to infections with ongogenic HPV types which are linked to anal epithelial dysplasia and anal cancer. HIV infection is associated with abnormal anal cytology in women with HPV infections. Depletion of CD4 cells and higher levels of HIV viremia are both linked to shedding of HPV and the occurrence of dysplasia [110]. Cytologic screening can detect significant dysplasia before invasive disease occurs. However, anal cancer is rare, and since cytologic screening of the anus is an imperfect tool, screening of HIV-infected women for anal cancer, as currently practiced in many centers, may not be cost-effective [111].

No national recommendations exist for routine screening for anal cancer. The 2010 STD treatment guidelines from the CDC have determined that evidence is still limited concerning the natural history of anal intraepithelial neoplasias, the reliability of screening methods, and the safety and efficacy of treatment. Therefore, specialists at large HIV treatment centers vary in their approach to screening for dysplasia in the anal canal. Some centers recommend just an annual digital rectal examination to evaluate for masses and others have instituted routine anal cytologic screening for HIV-seropositive men and women along the lines of the cervical cancer screening guidelines above.

Other gynecological conditions

Candidal vaginitis occurs more frequently among HIV-infected women in relation to the extent of CD4 cell depletion; this condition is therefore similar to other mucosal candidal infections in immuno compromised individuals. Among women with CD4 counts of 350 cells/mm^3 and above, topical or oral therapies can be used for candidal vaginitis similar to the HIV-uninfected population. For women who are significantly immunocompromised, oral fluconazole in two 150 mg doses 3 days apart [103], or a short course of daily 100 mg treatment, may be more effective than topical treatment. Suppressive prophylactic azole treatment has been advocated by some, but it is of unproven benefit, and may risk the development of azole-resistant *C. albicans* strains or other *Candida* species.

While certain sexually transmitted infections, such as genital herpes and syphilis, can have altered manifestations in the setting of HIV infection, these are not female specific. Current guidelines for the diagnosis and treatment of these infections are available from the Centers for Disease Control [112].

Breast cancer

Breast cancer was less frequently reported among HIV-infected women than HIV-uninfected women prior to the availability of cART [113]. Since the advent of cART, breast cancer rates rose to meet those of HIV-uninfected women, but have not exceeded baseline rates [114]. This increase in breast cancer rates among HIV-infected women may be attributable to increased survival related to effective antiretroviral treatment. Recently an interesting interaction between the HIV virus and possible protection from some breast cancers was reported [115]. Women who had detectable X4-tropic HIV in their blood were significantly less likely to develop breast cancer, a finding that may be explained by the expression of the CXCR4 receptor in some breast cancer cells. While this finding may provide new directions

for breast cancer care, HIV-infected women should receive the same diagnostic surveillance frequency for breast cancer as HIV-uninfected women.

Menopause

As noted previously, the menopausal transition is likely to be particularly important for the care of HIV-infected women because menopause is associated with:

- Significant immunologic changes that may have a bearing on HIV disease progression and treatment responses (more research is needed to define these effects).
- Changes in lipid metabolism and vascular endothelial function that can influence risks for vascular, cardiovascular, renal, and cerebrovascular diseases, which may then interact with the proinflammatory and prothrombotic milieu of HIV infection.
- Acceleration of loss of bone mineral density that can then result in fracture and disability that may also interact with other morbidities of HIV infection.

Menopause is clinically defined as the cessation of menses for 12 months when no underlying etiology is present. This definition has limited applicability to the setting of chronic illness in which a variety of factors may lead to menstrual irregularity and amenorrhea (including weight loss, use of a range of medications, co-infections, and central nervous system conditions). Irregular menses and amenorrhea are common in both HIV-infected and HIV-uninfected women [116], but overall amenorrhea is associated with HIV infection [117]. Greater rates of viremia and CD4 cell depletion are associated with cycle irregularity [118]. Self-reporting menopause, followed by a resumption of regular menses after cART initiation, is not uncommon. Irregular menstrual cycles are associated with the use of medications and recreational drugs [119], which is an important consideration in the evaluation of an HIV-infected woman.

While the effects of menopause on the course of HIV infection and related conditions are still an open question, a range of studies have focused on whether HIV influences the course of menopause. The average age at menopause in the United States is 51 years. Several studies cite menopause occurring at a younger age among HIV-infected women [120], with the average age reported as below 50 years [120, 121]. More definitive determination of whether HIV infection affects the timing of menopause awaits studies that enroll a broader age range of women, and an optimally matched HIV-uninfected group. Since aging is a strong predictor of more rapid HIV progression, it will be important to dissect out the effects of somatic aging from gonadal aging on HIV progression in women.

Many symptoms are attributed to menopause, but research findings consistently demonstrate that vasomotor symptoms (including facial flushing and night sweats), vaginal dryness and irritation, and sleep disruptions are associated with the menopausal transition. Night sweats and sleep disruptions are common in HIV infection regardless of menopausal status, however. Some studies have found that HIV-infected women are more likely to have meno-pausal symptoms than HIV-uninfected women, but this disparity could be explained by differences in demographics between the two groups [120]. Furthermore, menopausal symptoms can be more pronounced in women who experience social stress, a factor that is highly prevalent among HIV-infected women living in resource-rich environments. Thus it can be difficult to determine whether symptoms often attributed to menstrual irregularities are related or not related to menopause.

Menopause coincides with depletion of ovarian follicles, and result in characteristic patterns in gonadotropins that are related to ovarian depletion. Levels of sex steroids and gonadotropins are often used as biomarkers of menopause. However, ovarian cycling occurs during early perimenopause when gonadotropic follicular stimulation can produce elevated levels of estradiol. Blood levels of the most commonly used biomarkers of ovarian aging, estradiol, follicle stimulating hormone (FSH), and inhibin B, all vary significantly with the ovarian cycle phase. Optimal interpretation of levels requires collection during the early follicular phase, which occurs during days 2–5 of the menstrual cycle. However, determining the phase of the cycle in women with irregular menses can be difficult. Moreover, FSH levels themselves are influenced by medications and tobacco smoking. Therefore, the most commonly used laboratory tests to detect ovarian aging in clinical practice all have limitations, particularly for women with chronic illness. Measurement of anti-Müllerian hormone (AMH) may provide a better measure of menopausal status and studies of this test in the context of HIV infection are underway in large observational studies. Until then, HIV-infected women, particularly if under age 50 and particularly in the context of cART initiation, should be cautioned that their menses and consequent fertility may resume once they regain health.

ANTIRETROVIRAL TREATMENT OF WOMEN

While most studies of the efficacy of cART regimens are underpowered for the detection of sex differences [67], the aggregate data suggest that men and women experience comparable responses to cART in terms of CD4 cell gain, rates of virologic suppression, and gains in survival [122]. The studies that do show sex differences often feature male and female groups with significant differences in timing of treatment initiation, adherence, concurrent conditions, and drug use [123]. For example, one European/Canadian multicohort assessment of seroconverters found that since the introduction of cART, women have lower rates of progression to AIDS, death without AIDS, dementia, tuberculosis, Kaposi's sarcoma, and lymphoma than men; injection drug use was significantly more prevalent among the male versus female seroconverters [68].

However, despite this apparent improvement in rates of clinical progression to AIDS or death seen in women compared to men across studies over time (Fig. 39.4), women have higher rates of discontinuation of cART therapy than men [124], a phenomenon observed with even newer ART components [125, 126] and multiple different regimen types that include protease inhibitors (PI) [127] or non-nucleoside reverse transcriptase inhibitors (NNRTIs) [128]. Moreover, in a meta-analysis comparing the frequency of adverse effects on cART in women compared to men,

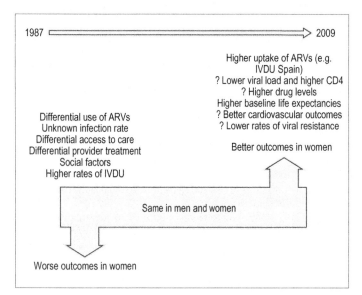

Figure 39.4 Clinical progression or mortality: trends of observational studies across time.

Figure 39.5 Sex differences in antiretroviral pharmacokinetics.

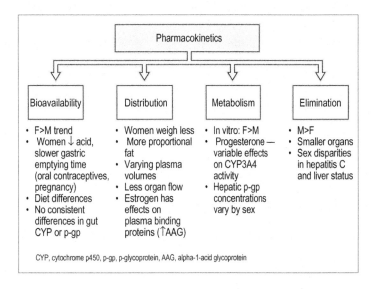

women were consistently more likely to experience toxicities of antiretroviral therapy at higher rates than men [67]. The most likely explanation of these discrepancies—where women experience improved clinical outcomes on cART with a higher frequency of adverse effects—is pharmacokinetic differences in antiretroviral drug levels by sex [129]. Although women may have higher drug levels of the antiretrovirals (ARVs) than men for a number of different reasons related to absorption, metabolism, distribution, and elimination (Fig. 39.5), ARV dosing does not typically take sex differences into account. Many experts in the research and care of HIV-infected women are advocating for larger studies that stratify outcomes by sex, examine sex-based differences in the pharmacokinetic and pharmacodynamic differences of ARVs, and explore dose adjustment as a means to maintain good treatment outcomes for women on ARVs while minimizing the development of adverse effects.

CONCLUSIONS

Although significant similarities in the progression and pathogenesis of HIV infection exist among HIV-infected women and men, some key differences in transmission risk factors, co-infections, and complications, and women-specific conditions are outlined in this chapter. Moreover, although combination antiretroviral treatment is the defining component of improved morbidity and mortality outcomes in patients living with HIV disease, differences in pharmacokinetics by sex may lead to early and frequent discontinuation of regimens in women compared to men. The 30th year commemoration of HIV/AIDS mandates greater attention to sex differences in HIV disease to accommodate the growing impact of this infection in women worldwide.

REFERENCES

[1] UNAIDS. UNAIDS report on the global AIDS epidemic 2011. Geneva: United Nations Global Programme on AIDS; 2011.

[2] Brubaker S, Bukusi EA, Odoyo J, et al. Pregnancy and HIV transmission among HIV-discordant couples in a clinical trial in Kisumu, Kenya. HIV Med 2011;12:316–21.

[3] Department of Health and Human Services and Henry J. Kaiser Family Foundation living document. Guidelines for the use of antiretroviral agents in HIV-infected adolescents and adults. http://www.hivatis.org/guidelines/adult. Updated October 29, 2004.

[4] Wawer MJ, Tobian AA, Kigozi G, et al. Effect of circumcision of HIV-negative men on transmission of human papillomavirus to HIV-negative women: a randomised trial in Rakai, Uganda. Lancet 2011;377:209–18.

[5] Statistics NCfH. Leading causes of death by age group, Women, United States, 2004. In. Atlanta: Health and Human Services, Centers for Disease Control and Prevention; 2009.

[6] Long EF, Brandeau ML, Owens DK. The cost-effectiveness and population outcomes of expanded HIV screening and antiretroviral treatment in the United States. Ann Intern Med 2010;153:778–89.

[7] Powers KA, Poole C, Pettifor AE, Cohen MS. Rethinking the heterosexual infectivity of HIV-1: a systematic review and meta-analysis. Lancet Infect Dis 2008;8:553–63.

[8] Boily MC, Baggaley RF, Wang L, et al. Heterosexual risk of HIV-1 infection per sexual act: systematic review and meta-analysis of observational studies. Lancet Infect Dis 2009;9:118–29.

[9] Attia S, Egger M, Muller M, et al. Sexual transmission of HIV according to viral load and antiretroviral therapy: systematic review and meta-analysis. AIDS 2009;23:1397–404.

[10] Granich RM, Gilks CF, Dye C, et al. Universal voluntary HIV testing with immediate antiretroviral therapy as a strategy for elimination of HIV transmission: a mathematical model. Lancet 2009;373:48–57.

[11] Charlebois ED, Das M, Porco TC, Havlir DV. The effect of expanded antiretroviral treatment strategies on the HIV epidemic among men who have sex with men in San Francisco. Clin Infect Dis 2011;52:1046–9.

[12] Canadas MP, Darwich L, Sirera G, et al. Human papillomavirus 16 integration and risk factors associated in anal samples of HIV-1 infected men. Sex Transm Dis 2010;37:311–15.

[13] Donnell D, Baeten JM, Kiarie J, et al. Heterosexual HIV-1 transmission after initiation of antiretroviral therapy: a prospective cohort analysis. Lancet 2010;375:2092–8.

[14] Fox J, Fidler S. Sexual transmission of HIV-1. Antiviral Res 2010;85:276–85.

[15] Miller WC, Rosenberg NE, Rutstein SE, Powers KA. Role of acute and early HIV infection in the sexual transmission of HIV. Curr Opin HIV AIDS 2010;5:277–82.

[16] Kaiser R, Bunnell R, Hightower A, et al. Factors associated with HIV infection in married or cohabitating couples in Kenya: results from a nationally representative study. PLoS ONE 2011;6:e17842.

[17] Gorbach PM, Sopheab H, Chhorvann C, et al. Changing behaviors and patterns among Cambodian sex workers: 1997–2003. J Acquir Immune Defic Syndr 2006;42:242–7.

[18] Mayer KH, Venkatesh KK. Interactions of HIV, other sexually transmitted diseases, and genital tract inflammation facilitating local pathogen transmission and acquisition. Am J Reprod Immunol 2011;65:308–16.

[19] Watson-Jones D, Weiss HA, Rusizoka M, et al. Effect of herpes simplex suppression on incidence of HIV among women in Tanzania. N Engl J Med 2008;358:1560–71.

[20] Celum C, Wald A, Lingappa JR, et al. Acyclovir and transmission of HIV-1 from persons infected with HIV-1 and HSV-2. N Engl J Med 2010;362:427–39.

[21] Gray RH, Li X, Kigozi G, et al. Increased risk of incident HIV during pregnancy in Rakai, Uganda: a prospective study. Lancet 2005;366:1182–8.

[22] Brubaker SG, Bukusi EA, Odoyo J, et al. Pregnancy and HIV transmission among HIV-discordant couples in a clinical trial in Kisumu, Kenya. HIV Med 2011;12:316–21.

[23] Morrison CS, Wang J, Van Der Pol B, et al. Pregnancy and the risk of HIV-1 acquisition among women in Uganda and Zimbabwe. AIDS 2007;21:1027–34.

[24] Moodley D, Esterhuizen T, Reddy L, et al. Incident HIV infection in pregnant and lactating women and its effect on mother-to-child Transmission in South Africa. J Infect Dis 2011;203:1231–4.

[25] Wang CC, Reilly M, Kreiss JK. Risk of HIV infection in oral contraceptive pill users: a meta-analysis. J Acquir Immune Defic Syndr 1999;21:51–8.

[26] Baeten JM, Benki S, Chohan V, et al. Hormonal contraceptive use, herpes simplex virus infection, and risk of HIV-1 acquisition among Kenyan women. AIDS 2007;21:1771–7.

[27] Morrison CS, Richardson BA, Mmiro F, et al. Hormonal contraception and the risk of HIV acquisition. AIDS 2007;21:85–95.

[28] Blish CA, Baeten JM. Hormonal contraception and HIV-1 transmission. Am J Reprod Immunol 2011;65:302–7.

[29] Heffron R, Donnell D, Rees H, et al.; for the Partners in Prevention HSV/HIV Transmission Study Team. Use of hormonal contraceptives and risk of HIV-1 transmission: a prospective cohort study. Lancet Infect Dis. 2012 12(1):19–26. Epub 2011 Oct 3.

[30] Grant RM, Lama JR, Anderson PL, et al. Preexposure chemoprophylaxis for HIV prevention in men who have sex with men. N Engl J Med 2010;363:2587–99.

[31] Baeten J, Celum C. Antiretroviral Pre-Exposure Prophylaxis for HIV-1 prevention among heterosexual African men and women: the Partners PrEP Study. Paper MOAX0106. 6th IAS Conference on HIV Pathogenesis, Treatment and Prevention. Rome, Italy. July 2011.

[32] Thigpen M, et al. Daily oral antiretroviral use for the prevention of HIV infection in heterosexually active young adults in Botswana: results from the TDF2 study. Paper WELBC01. 6th IAS Conference on HIV Pathogenesis, Treatment and Prevention. Rome, Italy. July 2011.

[33] Miller AM, Alcaraz Ruiz A, Borrayo Sanchez G, et al. Metabolic syndrome: clinical and angiographic impact on patients with acute coronary syndrome. Cir Cir 2010;78:113–20.

[34] Choi SO, Rezk N, Kim JS, Kashuba AD. Development of an LC-MS method for measuring TNF in human vaginal tissue. J Chromatogr Sci 2010;48:219–23.

[35] Patterson KB, Dumond JB, Prince H, et al. Pharmacokinetics of TDF in blood plasma and cervicovaginal fluid of HIV+ post-menopausal compared with pre-menopausal women. In: 18th Conference on Retroviruses and Opportunistic Infections (CROI). Boston, MA. Paper 32; 2011.

[36] Dumond JB, Yeh RF, Patterson KB, et al. Antiretroviral drug exposure in the female genital tract: implications for oral pre- and post-exposure prophylaxis. AIDS 2007;21:1899–907.

[37] Vourvahis M, Tappouni HL, Patterson KB, et al. The pharmacokinetics and viral activity of tenofovir in the male genital tract. J Acquir Immune Defic Syndr 2008;47:329–33.

[38] Anderson PL, Kiser JJ, Gardner EM, et al. Pharmacological considerations for tenofovir and emtricitabine to prevent HIV infection. J Antimicrob Chemother 2011;66:240–50.

[39] Van Damme L, Chandeying V, Ramjee G, et al. Safety of multiple daily applications of COL-1492, a nonoxynol-9 vaginal gel, among female sex workers. COL-1492 Phase II Study Group. AIDS 2000;14:85–8.

[40] Skoler-Karpoff S, Ramjee G, Ahmed K, et al. Efficacy of Carraguard for prevention of HIV infection in women in South Africa: a randomised, double-blind, placebo-controlled trial. Lancet 2008;372:1977–87.

[41] McCormack S, Ramjee G, Kamali A, et al. PRO2000 vaginal gel for prevention of HIV-1 infection (Microbicides Development Programme 301): a phase 3, randomised, double-blind, parallel-group trial. Lancet 2010;376:1329–37.

[42] Van Damme L, Govinden R, Mirembe FM, et al. CS Study Group. Lack of effectiveness of cellulose sulfate gel for the prevention of vaginal HIV transmission. N Engl J Med. 2008 31;359(5):463–72.

[43] Abdool Karim Q, Abdool Karim SS, Frohlich JA, et al. Effectiveness and safety of tenofovir gel, an antiretroviral microbicide, for the prevention of HIV infection in women. Science 2010;329:1168–74.

[44] Weiss HA, Hankins CA, Dickson K. Male circumcision and risk of HIV infection in women: a systematic review and meta-analysis. Lancet Infect Dis 2009;9:669–77.

[45] Higgins JA, Hoffman S, Dworkin SL. Rethinking gender, heterosexual men, and women's vulnerability to HIV/AIDS. Am J Public Health 2010;100:435–45.

[46] Hall HI, McDavid K, Ling Q, Sloggett A. Determinants of progression to AIDS or death after HIV diagnosis, United States, 1996 to 2001. Ann Epidemiol 2006;16:824–33.

[47] Prins M, Meyer L, Hessol NA. Sex and the course of HIV infection in the pre- and highly active antiretroviral therapy eras. AIDS 2005;19:357–70.

[48] Meditz AL, MaWhinney S, Allshouse A, et al. Sex, race, and geographic region influence clinical outcomes following primary HIV-1 infection. J Infect Dis 2011;203:442–51.

[49] Napolitano LA, Burt TD, Bacchetti P, et al. Increased circulating interleukin-7 levels in HIV-1-infected women. J Acquir Immune Defic Syndr 2005;40:581–4.

[50] Gandhi M, Bacchetti P, Miotti P, et al. Does patient sex affect human immunodeficiency virus levels? Clin Infect Dis 2002;35:313–22.

[51] Moore R, Cheever L, Keruly J, Chaisson R. Lack of sex difference in CD4 to HIV-1 RNA viral load ratio. Lancet 1999;353:463–4.

[52] Sterling T, Lyles C, Vlahov D, et al. Sex differences in longitudinal human immunodeficiency virus type 1 RNA levels among seroconverters. J Infect Dis 1999;180:666–72.

[53] Evans J, Nims T, Cooley J, et al. Serum levels of virus burden in early-stage human immunodeficiency virus type 1 disease in women. J Infect Dis 1997;175:795–800.

[54] Sterling TR, Vlahov D, Astemborski J, et al. Initial plasma HIV-1 RNA levels and progression to AIDS in women and men. N Engl J Med 2001;344:720–5.

[55] Farzadegan H, Hoover D, Astemborski J, et al. Sex differences in HIV-1 viral load and progression to AIDS. Lancet 1998;352:1510–14.

[56] Anastos K, Gange SJ, Lau B, et al. Association of race and gender with HIV-1 RNA levels and immunologic progression. J Acquir Immune Defic Syndr 2000;24:218–26.

[57] Rezza G, Lepri AC, d'Arminio Monforte A, et al. Plasma viral load concentrations in women and men from different exposure categories and with known duration of HIV infection. I.CO.N.A. Study Group. J Acquir Immune Defic Syndr 2000;25:56–62.

[58] Lyles C, Dorrucci M, Vlahov D, et al. Longitudinal human immunodeficiency virus type 1 load in the Italian Seroconversion Study: correlates and temporal trends of virus load. J Infect Dis 1999;180:1018–24.

[59] Moroni M. Sex differences in HIV-1 viral load and progression to AIDS. ICONA Study Group. Italian cohort of HIV-1 positive individuals [letter; comment]. Lancet 1999;353:589–90; discussion 590–1.

[60] Katzenstein D, Hammer S, Hughes M, et al. The relation of virologic and immunologic markers to clinical outcomes after nucleoside therapy in HIV-infected adults with 200 to 500 CD4 cells per cubic millimeter. N Engl J Med 1996;335:1091–8.

[61] Junghans C, Ledergerber B, Chan P, et al. Sex differences in HIV-1 viral load and progression to AIDS. Lancet 1999;353:589.

[62] Bush C, Donovan R, Markowitz N, et al. Gender is not a factor in serum human immunodeficiency virus type 1 RNA levels in patients with viremia. J Clin Microbiol 1996;34:970–2.

[63] Kalish LA, Collier AC, Flanigan TP, Kumar PN. Plasma human immunodeficiency virus (HIV) type 1 RNA load in men and women with advanced HIV-1 disease. J Infect Dis 2000;182:603–6.

[64] Meier A, Chang JJ, Chan ES, et al. Sex differences in the Toll-like receptor-mediated response of plasmacytoid dendritic cells to HIV-1. Nat Med 2009;15:955–9.

[65] Shah S, Smith CJ, Lampe F, et al. Haemoglobin and albumin as markers of HIV disease progression in the highly active antiretroviral therapy era: relationships with gender. HIV Med 2007;8:38–45.

[66] Melnick S, Sherer R, Louis T, et al. Survival and disease progression according to gender of patients with HIV infection. The Terry Beirn Community Programs for Clinical Research on AIDS. JAMA 1994;272:1915–21.

[67] Nicastri E, Leone S, Angeletti C, et al. Sex issues in HIV-1-infected persons during highly active antiretroviral therapy: a systematic review. J Antimicrob Chemother 2007;60:724–32.

[68] Jarrin I, Geskus R, Bhaskaran K, et al. Gender differences in HIV progression to AIDS and death in industrialized countries: slower disease progression following HIV seroconversion in women. Am J Epidemiol 2008;168: 532–40.

[69] Lanoy E, Spano JP, Bonnet F, et al. The spectrum of malignancies in HIV-infected patients in 2006 in France: the ONCOVIH study. Int J Cancer 2011;129(2):467–75.

[70] Dauby N, De Wit S, Delforge M, et al. Characteristics of non-AIDS-defining malignancies in the HAART era: a clinico-epidemiological study. J Int AIDS Soc 2011;14:16.

[71] Narciso-Schiavon JL, Schiavon LL, Carvalho-Filho RJ, et al. Anti-hepatitis C virus-positive blood donors: are women any different? Transfus Med 2008;18:175–83.

[72] Thio CL. Host genetic factors and antiviral immune responses to hepatitis C virus. Clin Liver Dis 2008;12:713–26, xi.

[73] Langohr K, Sanvisens A, Fuster D, et al. Liver enzyme alterations in HCV-monoinfected and HCV/HIV-coinfected patients. Open AIDS J 2008;2:82–8.

[74] Tien PC, Cole SR, Williams CM, et al. Incidence of lipoatrophy and lipohypertrophy in the women's interagency HIV study. J Acquir Immune Defic Syndr 2003;34:461–6.

[75] Scherzer R, Shen W, Bacchetti P, et al. Simple anthropometric measures correlate with metabolic risk indicators as strongly as magnetic resonance imaging-measured adipose tissue depots in both HIV-infected and control subjects. Am J Clin Nutr 2008;87:1809–17.

[76] Currier J, Scherzer R, Bacchetti P, et al. Regional adipose tissue and lipid and lipoprotein levels in HIV-infected women. J Acquir Immune Defic Syndr 2008;48:35–43.

[77] AbouRjaili G, Shtaynberg N, Wetz R, et al. Current concepts in triglyceride metabolism, pathophysiology, and treatment. Metabolism 2010;59:1210–20.

[78] Brown TT, McComsey GA. Osteopenia and osteoporosis in patients with HIV: a review of current concepts. Curr Infect Dis Rep 2006;8:162–70.

[79] McComsey GA, Tebas P, Shane E, et al. Bone disease in HIV infection: a practical review and recommendations for HIV care providers. Clin Infect Dis 2010;51:937–46.

[80] Yin MT, McMahon DJ, Ferris DC, et al. Low bone mass and high bone turnover in postmenopausal human immunodeficiency virus-infected women. J Clin Endocrinol Metab 2010;95:620–9.

[81] Yin MT, Shi Q, Hoover DR, et al. Fracture incidence in HIV-infected women: results from the Women's Interagency HIV Study. AIDS 2010;24:2679–86.

[82] Bonjoch A, Figueras M, Estany C, et al. High prevalence of and progression to low bone mineral density in HIV-infected patients: a longitudinal cohort study. AIDS 2010;24:2827–33.

[83] Brown TT, McComsey GA, King MS, et al. Loss of bone mineral density after antiretroviral therapy initiation, independent of antiretroviral regimen. J Acquir Immune Defic Syndr 2009;51:554–61.

[84] McCombe PA, Greer JM, Mackay IR. Sexual dimorphism in autoimmune disease. Curr Mol Med 2009;9:1058–79.

[85] Aoki Y, Belin RM, Clickner R, et al. Serum TSH and total T4 in the United States population and their association with participant characteristics: National Health and Nutrition Examination Survey (NHANES 1999–2002). Thyroid 2007;17:1211–23.

[86] Madeddu G, Spanu A, Chessa F, et al. Thyroid function in human immunodeficiency virus patients treated with highly active antiretroviral therapy (HAART): a longitudinal study. Clin Endocrinol (Oxf) 2006;64:375–83.

[87] Knysz B, Bolanowski M, Klimczak M, et al. Graves' disease as an immune reconstitution syndrome in an HIV-1-positive patient commencing effective antiretroviral therapy: case report

and literature review. Viral Immunol 2006;19:102–7.

[88] Jubault V, Penfornis A, Schillo F, et al. Sequential occurrence of thyroid autoantibodies and Graves' disease after immune restoration in severely immunocompromised human immunodeficiency virus-1-infected patients. J Clin Endocrinol Metab 2000;85:4254–7.

[89] Ebert SN, Liu XK, Woosley RL. Female gender as a risk factor for drug-induced cardiac arrhythmias: evaluation of clinical and experimental evidence. J Womens Health 1998;7:547–57.

[90] Jonsson MK, Vos MA, Duker G, et al. Gender disparity in cardiac electrophysiology: implications for cardiac safety pharmacology. Pharmacol Ther 2010;127:9–18.

[91] Petrosillo N, Lisena FP, Chinello P. QTc prolongation in human immunodeficiency virus-infected persons. Arch Intern Med 2006; 166:2288–9; author reply 2289–90.

[92] Baker JR, Best AM, Pade PA, et al. Effect of buprenorphine and antiretroviral agents on the QT interval in opioid-dependent patients. Ann Pharmacother 2006;40:392–6.

[93] Blum A, Blum N. Coronary artery disease: Are men and women created equal? Gend Med 2009;6:410–18.

[94] Siegel C, Turtzo C, McCullough LD. Sex differences in cerebral ischemia: possible molecular mechanisms. J Neurosci Res 2010;88:2765–74.

[95] Vitale C, Mendelsohn ME, Rosano GM. Gender differences in the cardiovascular effect of sex hormones. Nat Rev Cardiol 2009;6:532–42.

[96] Miller VM. Sex-based differences in vascular function. Womens Health (Lond Engl) 2010;6:737–52.

[97] Clifford GM, Goncalves MA, Franceschi S. Human papillomavirus types among women infected with HIV: a meta-analysis. AIDS 2006;20:2337–44.

[98] Harris TG, Burk RD, Xue X, et al. Association of cutaneous anergy with human papillomavirus and cervical neoplasia in HIV-seropositive and seronegative women. AIDS 2007;21:1933–41.

[99] Strickler HD, Burk RD, Fazzari M, et al. Natural history and possible reactivation of human papillomavirus in human immunodeficiency virus-positive women. J Natl Cancer Inst 2005;97:577–86.

[100] Nicol AF, Nuovo GJ, Salomao-Estevez A, et al. Immune factors involved in the cervical immune response in the HIV/HPV co-infection. J Clin Pathol 2008;61:84–8.

[101] Nappi L, Carriero C, Bettocchi S, et al. Cervical squamous intraepithelial lesions of low-grade in HIV-infected women: recurrence, persistence, and progression, in treated and untreated women. Eur J Obstet Gynecol Reprod Biol 2005;121:226–32.

[102] De Vuyst H, Lillo F, Broutet N, Smith JS. HIV, human papillomavirus, and cervical neoplasia and cancer in the era of highly active antiretroviral therapy. Eur J Cancer Prev 2008;17:545–54.

[103] Miller ME, Bonds DE, Gerstein HC, et al. The effects of baseline characteristics, glycaemia treatment approach, and glycated haemoglobin concentration on the risk of severe hypoglycaemia: post hoc epidemiological analysis of the ACCORD study. BMJ 2010;340: b5444.

[104] Lodi CT, Michelin MA, Lima MI, et al. Factors associated with recurrence of cervical intraepithelial neoplasia after conization in HIV-infected and noninfected women. Arch Gynecol Obstet 2011;284:191–7.

[105] Elit L, Voruganti S, Simunovic M. Invasive vulvar cancer in a woman with human immunodeficiency virus: case report and review of the literature. Gynecol Oncol 2005;98:151–4.

[106] Paramsothy P, Duerr A, Heilig CM, et al. Abnormal vaginal cytology in HIV-infected and at-risk women after hysterectomy. J Acquir Immune Defic Syndr 2004;35:484–91.

[107] Department of Health and Human Services living document. Guidelines for Prevention and Treatment of Opportunistic Infections in HIV-Infected Adults and Adolescents. http://www. aidsinfo.nih.gov/guidelines. Updated 4/10/2009.

[108] Lillo FB, Lodini S, Ferrari D, et al. Determination of human papillomavirus (HPV) load and type in high-grade cervical lesions surgically resected from HIV-infected women during follow-up of HPV infection. Clin Infect Dis 2005;40:451–7.

[109] Minkoff H, Zhong Y, Burk RD, et al. Influence of adherent and effective antiretroviral therapy use on human papillomavirus infection and squamous intraepithelial lesions in human immunodeficiency virus-positive women. J Infect Dis 2010;201:681–90.

[110] Holly EA, Ralston ML, Darragh TM, et al. Prevalence and risk factors for anal squamous intraepithelial lesions in women. J Natl Cancer Inst 2001;93:843–9.

[111] Czoski-Murray C, Karnon J, Jones R, et al. Cost-effectiveness of screening high-risk HIV-positive men who have sex with men (MSM) and HIV-positive women for anal cancer. Health Technol Assess 2010;14:iii–iv, ix–x,1–101.

[112] Workowski KA, Berman S. Sexually transmitted diseases treatment guidelines, 2010. MMWR Recomm Rep 2010;59:1–110.

[113] Goedert JJ, Schairer C, McNeel TS, et al. Risk of breast, ovary, and uterine corpus cancers among 85,268 women with AIDS. Br J Cancer 2006;95:642–8.

[114] Shiels MS, Pfeiffer RM, Engels EA. Age at cancer diagnosis among persons with AIDS in the United States. Ann Intern Med 2010;153:452–60.

[115] Hessol NA, Napolitano LA, Smith D, et al. HIV tropism and decreased risk of breast cancer. PLoS ONE 2010;5:e14349.

[116] Ellerbrock T, Wright T, Bush T, et al. Characteristics of menstruation in women infected with human immunodeficiency virus. Obstet Gynecol 1996;87:1030–4.

[117] Cejtin HE, Kalinowski A, Bacchetti P, et al. Effects of human immunodeficiency virus on protracted amenorrhea and ovarian dysfunction. Obstet Gynecol 2006;108:1423–31.

[118] Harlow S, Schuman P, Cohen M, et al. Effect of HIV infection on menstrual cycle length. J Acquir Immune Defic Syndr 2000;24:68–75.

[119] Harlow SD, Cohen M, Ohmit SE, et al. Substance use and psychotherapeutic medications: a likely contributor to menstrual disorders in women who are seropositive for human immunodeficiency virus. Am J Obstet Gynecol 2003;188:881–6.

[120] Ferreira CE, Pinto-Neto AM, Conde DM, et al. Menopause symptoms in women infected with HIV: prevalence and associated factors. Gynecol Endocrinol 2007;23:198–205.

[121] Schoenbaum EE, Hartel D, Lo Y, et al. HIV infection, drug use and onset of natural menopause. Clin Infect Dis 2005;41:1517–24.

[122] Nicastri E, Angeletti C, Palmisano L, et al. Gender differences in clinical progression of HIV-1-infected individuals during long-term highly active antiretroviral therapy. AIDS 2005;19:577–83.

[123] Perez-Hoyos S, Ferreros I, Hernan MA. Marginal structural models application to estimate the effects of antiretroviral therapy in 5 cohorts of HIV seroconverters. Gac Sanit 2007;21:76–83.

[124] Murri R, Lepri AC, Phillips AN, et al. Access to antiretroviral treatment, incidence of sustained therapy interruptions, and risk of clinical events according to sex: evidence from the I.Co.N.A. Study. J Acquir Immune Defic Syndr 2003;34:184–90.

[125] Touloumi G, Pantazis N, Antoniou A, et al. Highly active antiretroviral therapy interruption: predictors and virological and immunologic consequences. J Acquir Immune Defic Syndr 2006;42:554–61.

[126] Elzi L, Marzolini C, Furrer H, et al. Treatment modification in human immunodeficiency virus-infected

individuals starting combination antiretroviral therapy between 2005 and 2008. Arch Intern Med 2010;170:57–65.

[127] Currier J, Averitt Bridge D, Hagins D, et al. Sex-based outcomes of darunavir-ritonavir therapy: a single-group trial. Ann Intern Med 2010;153:349–57.

[128] Smith CJ, Sabin CA, Youle MS, et al. Response to efavirenz-containing regimens in previously antiretroviral-naive HIV-positive patients: the role of gender. J Acquir Immune Defic Syndr 2007;46:62–7.

[129] Gandhi M, Aweeka F, Greenblatt RM, Blaschke TF. Sex differences in pharmacokinetics and pharmacodynamics. Annu Rev Pharmacol Toxicol 2004;44:499–523.

Chapter | 40 |

HIV disease among substance users: treatment issues

R. Douglas Bruce, Frederick L. Altice, Gerald Friedland

EPIDEMIOLOGY

HIV/AIDS and illicit drug use adversely impact tens of millions of people, with explosive epidemics of both described worldwide. Non-injection drug use such as alcohol and stimulant use (e.g. cocaine and methamphetamines) contribute to risky sexual behaviors leading to HIV acquisition [1]. Injection drug use (IDU), largely of opioids, has been reported in 136 countries and 114 of these have reported HIV cases [2]. The link between drug use, particularly IDU, and HIV has been well described since the beginning of the HIV pandemic [3]. The world's most volatile and emerging HIV epidemics are in areas that are fueled by illicit drug use, particularly heroin. New IDU epidemics continue to emerge with some of the newest in Kenya and Tanzania. Recently, HIV seroprevalence of 42% has been reported among 534 male and female injectors in Dar es Salaam, Tanzania [4]. Particularly troubling is that many of these epidemics are among individuals younger than 30 and within the most densely populated regions of the world. Injection drug use is especially important in the HIV/AIDS epidemic among women and children.

In light of the increasingly central role of drug use, particularly IDU, in the global HIV/AIDS epidemic, issues of HIV clinical care and therapeutics in this population are of great importance. Of particular relevance are the special clinical features of HIV disease in drug-dependent patients, the treatment of HIV disease itself in this population, the special difficulties in providing care to drug users and the treatment of drug addiction and special issues of HIV prevention [5].

HIV DISEASE IN DRUG USERS

The natural history of HIV disease among drug users has been demonstrated to be similar to that in other transmission risk categories [6]. Drug users are, however, at an increased risk for a number of other infections compared with other risk categories. Although most of these infections and other complications were common among drug users prior to the HIV epidemic, their incidence and severity have been accentuated, and clinical presentation affected by HIV infection. In both inpatient and outpatient settings, these are more common than the designated AIDS indicator diseases or specific HIV-related complications and often confound both diagnosis and treatment [5].

Multiple features of injection drug use that contribute to the increased risk of infection are summarized in Box 40.1, A detailed discussion of these infections and their management is beyond the focus of this chapter. Table 40.1 offers a summary of substance use-related complications in HIV-infected injection drug users. This chapter will address specific issues for co-managing and treating HIV infection itself among users of illicit drugs.

TREATMENT OF HIV INFECTION IN DRUG USERS

Combination antiretroviral therapy (cART) has resulted in impressive benefit for people living with HIV/AIDS, including decreasing morbidity, mortality, and hospitalization,

Box 40.1 **Features of injection drug use (IDU) contributing to the infectious diseases listed in Table 40.1**

1. Increased rates of skin, mucous membrane, and nasopharyngeal carriage of pathogenic organisms.
2. Unsterile injection techniques.
3. Contamination of injection equipment or drugs with microorganisms that may be present in residual blood in shared injection equipment.
4. Humoral, cell-mediated, and phagocyte defects induced by HIV infection and/or drug use.
5. Poor dental hygiene.
6. Impairment of gag and cough reflexes due to intoxication resulting in increased risk for pneumonia.
7. Alteration of the normal microbial flora by self-administered antibiotic use.
8. Increased prevalence of exposure to certain pathogens (notably *Mycobacterium tuberculosis*).
9. Concomitant behaviors such as cigarette smoking (i.e. increased susceptibility to pulmonary infections), alcohol use (i.e. increased progression of hepatic fibrosis for HCV-infected drug users), or exchange of sex for drugs or money (i.e. exposure to sexually transmitted infections).
10. Decreased access to and/or lack of appropriate use of preventive and primary healthcare services.

and has been demonstrated from a societal perspective to be cost-effective [7]. Despite the widespread availability of antiretroviral medications in resource-rich settings, IDUs have derived less benefit than other populations. This disparity in benefit among IDUs has been and will likely continue to be experienced in resource-limited settings even as cART becomes increasingly available for adults and children with HIV disease. The reasons for the disparity are multifactorial.

In many societies worldwide, both HIV and illicit drug use are stigmatized such that either or both conditions are often cloaked in secrecy and may result in a lack of detection and treatment [8]. Drug users are among the most socially marginalized populations and often hidden by circumstances and/or choice from mainstream medical care. Even when available, healthcare services are often constructed in ways that are difficult for many drug users to access, either by their absence in communities with high prevalence of drug use or by their organization that does not accommodate the chaotic and sometimes unpredictable use of services characteristic of drug-using populations. In addition, clinical care for drug users with HIV disease is often challenging and stressful for clinicians and other healthcare workers as a result of the complex array of substance misuse-related medical, psychological and social problems. The frequent co-morbid underlying psychiatric disease often contributes to these difficulties. Substance misusers may also have increased difficulties with adherence to cART, which may be compounded by their underlying co-morbid diseases, increased side effects, and drug interactions.

Table 40.1 A summary of drug use-related complications in HIV-infected injection drug users

LOCATION	DISEASE	ORGANISMS	TREATMENT	COMMENTS
Skin and soft tissue	Cellulitis	Group A and other streptococci, *Staphylococcus aureus*	Anti-staphylococcal agents Same as for cellulitis Parenteral antibiotics to cover both Gram (+) and (−) organisms	Consider hospitalization Consider MRSA
	Abscess Necrotizing fasciitis Septic thrombophlebitis	Same as for cellulitis Polymicrobial *Staphylococcus aureus*	Anti-staphylococcal agents	Incision and drainage Consider if crepitus noted; immediate surgical consultation required Surgical exploration and vein ligation
Cardiovascular	Endocarditis	*Staphylococcus aureus,* streptococci, enteric Gram (−) rods	Anti-staphylococcal agents until cultures grow Treat for 4–6 weeks	Consider if (a) regurgitant murmur, (b) presence of peripheral or pulmonary emboli, (c) blood culture (+), (d) echocardiogram Consider MRSA
Pulmonary	Community-acquired pneumonia Septic emboli	*S. pneumoniae, H. influenzae,* atypical organisms Tuberculosis Opportunistic	PCN, cephalosporin, macrolide Isoniazid, rifampin, pryzinamide, ethambutol	Consider even with normal chest X-ray Consider rifabutin due to PI interactions. Rifampin has strong methadone interaction

Table 40.1 A summary of drug use-related complications in HIV-infected injection drug users—cont'd

LOCATION	DISEASE	ORGANISMS	TREATMENT	COMMENTS
		infection PCP *Staphylococcus aureus,* streptococci, enteric Gram (−) rods	Bactrim Anti-staphylococcal agents until cultures grow	Common complication, consider with pleuritic chest pain
Liver	Hepatitis	Hepatitis B	Interferon, lamivudine, adefovir, entecavir, telbivudine	HBsAg positive HCV antibody positive with detectable RNA
		Hepatitis C	Pegylated interferon (PEG) + ribavirin (RBV) Telaprevir + PEG + RBV Boceprevir + PEG + RBV	
Neurology	Altered mental status Neuropathy Cerebrovascular accident	Substance-induced, dementia head trauma Metabolic, opportunistic infection Substance-induced (cocaine or amphetamines) brain abscess Hemorrhage due to emboli	Amitriptyline, Gabapentin Same as for endocarditis	Consider urine toxicology Consider pattern and tempo of event (slowly progressive or sudden onset)
Renal	Heroin or HIV nephropathy	Both present with nephritic syndrome	Renal biopsy to establish diagnosis. Electron microscopy distinguishes diagnosis	Focal and segmental glomerular sclerosis (FSGS) with progression to renal failure in weeks to months

There is often mutual suspicion between drug users and healthcare providers. Clinicians tend to have stereotypic views of drug users and may harbor negative feelings about their social worth. As with other "difficult" patients, physicians may come to view drug users as manipulative, unmotivated, and undeserving of care. The chronic relapsing nature of addiction as a medical disease is often not appreciated by clinicians, nor is the fact that drug users may be quite diverse and heterogeneous. Many physicians assume that drug users' antisocial behavior and drug use indicate a lifelong lack of concern for others and indifference to their own well-being, rather than a consequence of addiction. Conversely, drug users often are mistrustful of the healthcare system and harbor expectations that they will be treated punitively. Drug users often conceal their continuing drug use from healthcare professionals out of fear of rejection prompted by previous difficult encounters with the healthcare system. In turn, clinicians are sometimes reluctant to confront patients with their suspicions about ongoing drug use, fearing that the confrontation will compromise their relationship. The failure to acknowledge ongoing drug use itself, however, can compromise the clinician–patient relationship since one of the most important aspects of the patient's health is off-limits for discussion.

Because the life of a patient struggling with substance use disorders (SUDs) is often chaotically organized around their substance use needs, successful programs for this population have developed some or all of the following characteristics: (1) pharmacologic (e.g. methadone and buprenorphine programs) and/or non-pharmacological treatment (e.g. 12 steps) for SUDs; (2) flexible outpatient and community care settings (e.g. walk-in clinics, mobile healthcare programs); (3) low-threshold sites to engage active users (e.g. syringe exchange sites); (4) modified directly observed therapy; (5) intensive outreach and case management services; or (6) treatment during incarceration [5].

Clinicians involved in the care of drug users with HIV, should be aware of several key principles, which include the following: (1) Become educated about substance abuse and its wide array of treatment options. (2) Establish a multidisciplinary team of individuals with expertise in managing HIV, substance abuse, and mental illness, and broadened to include social work, nursing, case management, and community outreach. Identify a single provider to maximize consistency. (3) Obtain a thorough history of the patient's substance abuse history, practices, needle and syringe source, drug abuse complications, and treatment history. Non-judgmental, clinical assessment of this information is essential. Non-judgmental discussion of the adverse health and social consequences of drug use and the benefits of abstinence may increase the patient's understanding of his or her disease and interest in change. (4) Be aware of pharmacological drug interactions between HIV therapies and substance abuse therapies and provide simplified, low pill burden regimens to improve treatment adherence. (5) Link HIV and substance abuse treatment goals such that success in one arena is linked to improved outcomes in the other. (6) Establish a relationship of mutual respect. Avoid moral condemnation or attribution of addiction to moral or behavioral weakness. Acknowledge that SUDs are medical diseases, compounded by psychological and social circumstances. As such, they should be treated using evidence-based guidelines with a combination of pharmacological and behavioral interventions. Reducing or stopping drug use is difficult, as is sustaining abstinence. Success may require several attempts and relapse is common. Complete abstinence may not be a realistic goal for many substance-misusing patients. Rather, increasing the proportion of days, weeks, and months free from mind-altering substances is an acceptable goal. (7) Work closely with a drug treatment program. (8) Define and agree on the roles and responsibilities of both the healthcare team and the patient. Establish a formal treatment contract that specifies the services to be provided to the patient, the caregiver's expectations about the patient's behavior, and periodic urine toxicology for substances, and delineate the consequences of behaviors that violates the contract. Such a contract should be agreeable to both parties, and not simply a contract of the physician's expectations. (9) Set appropriate limits and respond consistently to behavior that violates those limits. These should be imposed in a professional manner that reflects the aim of enhancing patients' well-being, and not in an atmosphere of blame or judgment. (10) Carefully evaluate pain syndromes and provide sufficient analgesia as medically indicated. (11) Always consider acute substance ingestion when evaluating behavior change and neurologic disease. Use urine toxicology testing to evaluate behavioral changes and to discourage illicit drug use by HIV-infected injection drug users during hospital stay.

(12) Work consistently as a team. Do not make agreements about treatment decisions until the entire team has become involved. This will avoid 'splitting' behaviors that often unravel the fabric of a multidisciplinary team. (13) Consider integrating drug treatment into the HIV clinical care settings or HIV clinical care into a drug treatment setting (e.g., a methadone program). While there are no specific recommendations for accomplishing this goal, a number of key approaches have been described. These include complete integration where all clinicians are stakeholders in the treatment of both conditions, the integration of a specialized addiction specialist team or a hybrid model where both are implemented [9].

COMMONLY USED DRUGS

The illicit drugs most closely associated with the acquisition of HIV infection globally are heroin, cocaine, and methamphetamine use. Each of these can be administered by a variety of routes. Injection with shared contaminated needles and syringes or other injection paraphernalia carry the greatest risk for HIV transmission and other complications. Non-injection use of cocaine and methamphetamine, however, increasingly facilitates HIV transmission through its association with the exchange of drugs for sex or money or as a result of intoxication. It is important to be aware of local patterns of drug availability and routes of use.

Heroin

There are a number of illicit opioid and prescribed medications with abuse potential. Heroin is a short-acting, semi-synthetic opioid produced from opium. It may be smoked, inhaled, or injected; peak heroin euphoria begins shortly after injection and lasts approximately 1 h, followed by 1–4 h of sedation. Withdrawal symptoms commence several hours later. As a consequence, most heroin-dependent individuals inject 2–4 times per day. Many heroin users will mediate the sedating effects of heroin by injecting a small amount of cocaine, or other stimulant, with heroin, a mixture known as a "speedball." In some areas, smoking a heat-stable form of cocaine ("crack") produces the same rapid effect as injecting cocaine and is, in effect, a more modern version of a speedball. The unsterile method of use, unpredictable concentrations in street samples, adulterants in the injection mixture, and the lifestyle necessary to procure drugs are responsible for most heroin-associated medical complications.

Cocaine

Cocaine is available as a water-soluble hydrochloride salt that is injected or taken by nasal inhalation, "snorted." Although cocaine hydrochloride is heat labile, it may be chemically converted to a heat-stable basic form (crack), which can be smoked. Pulmonary absorption of crack is as rapid as intravenous injection. Cocaine's half-life is short, resulting in the need for frequent administration. Active cocaine users may inject or inhale cocaine as many as 20 times a day. Cocaine induces feelings of elation, omnipotence and invincibility and with rapid development of psychological dependence. The multiple psychological and physical effects of cocaine can increase HIV transmission and acquisition risk and markedly disrupt clinical care. As such, programs that are non-judgmental are essential to continue to engage these patients in care rather than risk losing them to follow-up and diminish the likelihood of risk-reduction interventions.

Methamphetamine

Methamphetamine is a psychostimulant that is similar in chemical structure to amphetamine but has more profound effects on the central nervous system. It can be smoked, snorted, injected or administered rectally. Like cocaine, methamphetamine ingestion produces stimulation and similar feelings of euphoria; however, methamphetamine has a longer duration of action (6–8 h after a single dose). Tolerance develops rapidly and escalation of dose and frequency is required. As is the case with cocaine, methamphetamine use is associated with high-risk sexual behavior and subsequent HIV acquisition [10].

Alcohol

Although not illicit in most societies, the widespread use and medical and psychological importance of alcohol is associated with many adverse HIV effects. HIV-infected patients have a higher prevalence of alcohol consumption than the general population [11]. Alcohol use ranges from hazardous drinking (i.e. drinking at a level that could be hazardous to the individual's health) to alcoholism. Alcohol use can result in ongoing risky sexual behaviors that can lead to the transmission of HIV [12, 13]. Alcohol use, in addition, can compromise cART by influencing both access and adherence to ARVs. In addition to HIV, alcohol has well-known negative effects upon the course of hepatitis C (HCV) treatment and HIV/HCV co-infected patients with hazardous drinking are of special concern [14]. As in all chemical dependencies, a comprehensive approach to the treatment of alcoholism integrates psychosocial treatment with pharmacologic treatments [5]. In the physiologically dependent patient, a structured withdrawal utilizing benzodiazepines or barbiturates is also necessary and typically occurs on an inpatient unit. Afterwards, a combination of pharmacological and psychosocial treatments (e.g. 12 steps) should be utilized to maintain abstinence and can be prescribed by a primary care provider.

MEDICATION-ASSISTED THERAPIES

Drug dependence is a chronic, relapsing, and treatable disease, characterized by compulsive drug-seeking and drug use. Although exposure to addictive substances is widespread in society, high vulnerability to addiction is more limited and is the product of biologic, psychological, and environmental influences. Thus, identification of addictive disease and referral to appropriate treatment services is an essential part of the clinical care of HIV-infected patients. Indeed, successful treatment of HIV disease in drug users often requires attention to and treatment of SUDs. Recent data confirm that effective and sustained treatment of SUDs improves HIV treatment outcomes [15]. There is a wide variety of treatment modalities. Selection of the appropriate program is an individual decision based in part upon the drug used, the length and pattern of the patient's drug use, personal psychosocial characteristics, and local availability (Table 40.2) [16]. Resources are limited in many communities, substantially limiting options for referral.

The most effective treatment for opioid dependence for patients with long-standing dependence, particularly injection drug users, is pharmacological therapy with methadone or buprenorphine [17, 18].

Medically supervised opioid withdrawal

Withdrawal from opioids involves the gradual reduction of dosage over a period of time. A hallmark of drug dependence is the patient's inability to reduce consumption of the drug over time without any external assistance. Although patients can be withdrawn using the drug to which they are addicted, in most instances it is easier to use methadone or buprenorphine. It is usually not possible to know with certainty how much drug the patient has been taking, though self-reports can be reliable. Regardless of the amount, myalgias, diarrhea, and insomnia and irritability associated with withdrawal can be reduced with a daily oral dose of 25–30 mg of methadone or 16 mg of buprenorphine. This dose of methadone, however, will not fully eliminate drug craving, whereas 16 mg of buprenorphine will often eliminate craving [19]. Decreasing the methadone dose by 10–20% every few days after the withdrawal syndrome is suppressed should maintain patient comfort. Buprenorphine, due to its longer half-life, can be tapered more rapidly. The decision to medically supervise opioid withdrawal or to recommend chronic maintenance therapy depends on a number of factors. In general, supervised opioid withdrawal should be reserved for short-term opioid users (<6 months), young adults, and non-injectors. Otherwise, relapse to drug use among chronic opioid users exceeds 85% when patients undergo supervised

Table 40.2 Modalities of substance abuse treatment

TREATMENT	BENEFITS	LIMITATIONS	APPROPRIATE FOR WHOM?	INAPPROPRIATE FOR WHOM?	LOCATION
Therapeutic community	Can address polysubstance abuse	Low retention rates	Highly motivated individuals	Individuals with family/work commitments	Community settings
Methadone	Reduces crime, transmission of infectious diseases, high retention rates	Does not address other drug use; potential for diversion	Heavy use of opioids	Non-opioid-dependent patients; individuals abusing other sedatives (e.g. benzodiazepines)	Requires a more restrictive infrastructure
Buprenorphine	Reduces crime, transmission of infectious diseases, high retention rates	Does not address other drug use; possibly less potential for diversion than methadone	Opioid-dependent patients. Improved safety profile compared with methadone	Non-opioid-dependent patients; individuals abusing other sedatives (e.g. benzodiazepines)	Due to improved safety profile, may be more widely accessible and available in primary care settings
Naltrexone	Effective among very motivated individuals	Lacking high motivation, treatment is ineffective	Individuals with high levels of social support and motivation	Individuals with low social support and/or motivation	Not a narcotic and so less regulation

Adapted with permission from Smith-Rohrberg et al. [16]

withdrawal without chronic maintenance therapy with buprenorphine or methadone [20].

Treatment of opioid dependence

The treatment of choice for the patient who is opioid-dependent and has HIV disease is chronic maintenance with an opioid agonist such as methadone or buprenorphine. In addition to agonist therapy, the patient should be enrolled in a comprehensive drug treatment program designed to prevent the abuse of other drugs and promote rehabilitation [21]. Agonist treatment of opioid addiction is particularly important for the patient with co-morbid HIV infection because effective treatment enhances HIV treatment and may decrease risk-taking behaviors [22].

Methadone, a semisynthetic, long-acting opioid analgesic, is particularly valuable for its oral bioavailability, long half-life of 24–36 h, and the consistent plasma levels that are obtained with regular administration. A single daily dose is given to maintain stable plasma levels. As a result, tolerance develops and regular methadone users do not experience the euphoria of the heroin cycle [23]. Drug-seeking behavior decreases, creating the possibility for the development of more constructive behaviors and relationships.

Methadone maintenance remains a well-validated, evidenced-based treatment for opioid addiction [24]. Methadone has been shown to decrease the injection of opioids

and therefore to moderate this HIV risk-taking behavior [17, 18]. Chronic maintenance with methadone prevents relapse to opioid injection-related behavior and maintains patients in treatment [20]. Methadone maintenance has been shown to be effective in decreasing psychosocial and medical morbidity associated with opioid addiction, including increasing access to and retention on ARV and other therapies. Furthermore, in addition to its benefit in decreasing the spread of HIV among injection drug users, it improves overall health status, and is associated with decreased criminal activity and improved social functioning. Methadone, therefore, is effective for primary and secondary HIV prevention [25] and is cost-effective to society [26].

There is no optimal dose of methadone for treatment of opioid-dependent patients who must be assessed *individually* for treatment response. Generally, doses of 30–60 mg daily will block opioid withdrawal symptoms, but higher doses in the 100–150 mg daily range are needed to reduce opioid craving and decrease illicit drug use. These higher doses are also associated with greater retention in treatment [27]. In the first 6 months of treatment, however, some patients may experience side effects common to other opioids, but tolerance to the majority of these effects develops rapidly. Persistent side effects include diaphoresis, constipation, and amenorrhea (the majority of women experience the return of menses after 12–18 months of therapy).

Buprenorphine, unlike methadone, which is a full agonist, is a partial μ-receptor agonist. As a partial agonist, there is a plateau of its agonist effects at higher doses which improves its safety profile compared with methadone and may reduce its likelihood for medication diversion. The plateau includes an upper limit on the severity of side effects associated with overdose, such as respiratory depression [28]. Buprenorphine has a higher binding affinity for the μ-receptor than heroin or methadone [29]. Because buprenorphine dissociates slowly from the μ-receptor, alternate day dosing is possible [30]. Buprenorphine has been prescribed in France since 1996 and resulted in dramatic improvements in the treatment of opioid addiction there. Buprenorphine was approved for use in the USA in 2002 and population outcome data have recently been reported among HIV-infected patients [15]. Worldwide, it is becoming increasingly more available [31]. Integration of buprenorphine is now being incorporated into HIV clinical care settings for HIV prevention and stabilization to initiate cART and using various different models of care prevention [32]. Unlike methadone, which typically is limited to specialized treatment settings, buprenorphine, due to its enhanced safety profile, can be utilized in primary and HIV clinical care in some countries. Buprenorphine's cost, however, limits its availability worldwide. Methadone remains, gram for gram, the cheapest and most effective pharmacological treatment for any opioid addiction [24]. Although buprenorphine and methadone are comparable in many ways, methadone tends to retain patients in treatment longer than buprenorphine [27].

Naltrexone, an opioid receptor antagonist, can also be used in the treatment of opioid addiction. Naltrexone has demonstrated efficacy in highly motivated populations [33]. Its use among HIV-infected drug users is discouraged, as methadone and buprenorphine have higher retention rates and allow for engagement when less motivation for treatment exists. In the primary care setting where methadone cannot currently be prescribed for opioid addiction, buprenorphine remains the best option for the treatment of opioid addiction as it has been shown to be superior to oral naltrexone in a recent randomized controlled trial [34].

HIV-infected drug users must have as their treatment plan an evidence-based approach to provide appropriate and adequate treatment for substance abuse in order to improve the psychological and physiological disruptions that perpetuate the often unstable life of a person struggling with addiction.

Treatment for cocaine dependence

Disulfiram remains the most promising therapeutic agent for cocaine addiction to date. Six randomized controlled trials have now shown the efficacy of disulfiram in treating cocaine addiction [35]. The goal of pharmacological therapy for cocaine is to relieve the craving for dopamine by maintaining stable, elevated levels. Taking cocaine in addition to disulfiram frequently results in a less rewarding, dysphoric response caused by excessive amounts of dopamine.

Pharmacological interactions are possible with HIV therapies as disulfiram is bioactivated by CYP3A4 [36]. As with many treatments in addiction medicine, adherence remains a problem with disulfiram. Treatment works well for motivated patients and for patients receiving disulfiram as directly observed therapy with methadone maintenance.

Treatment for methamphetamine dependence

Unlike the case of opioid addiction, studies seeking an effective and evidence-based pharmacological treatment for methamphetamine addiction have been disappointing [37]. The lack of successful, standardized treatment strategies for methamphetamine users is a significant problem as the epidemic of methamphetamine use grows and is now an international problem. In the absence of effective pharmacological treatments for methamphetamine use, HIV care providers may feel helpless and frustrated. Counseling is the only treatment modality shown to decrease use of methamphetamine [38]. Referral to a substance abuse treatment program, if available, is essential.

Treatment for alcohol use disorders and alcoholism

Naltrexone, the opioid receptor antagonist discussed earlier, remains the most studied and consistently most effective pharmacotherapy for alcohol dependence [39]. The extended release formulation is the most effective treatment currently available. Alcohol stimulates receptor-mediated dopamine release through a complex mechanism involving gamma-aminobutyric acid activation and the opioid receptor system [40]. By blocking the mu-opioid receptor, naltrexone acts to decrease the dopamine reward. Patients consume less alcohol while receiving naltrexone and those who are sober while receiving treatment tend to have relapses of reduced severity [41]. The currently recommended dosage is 100 mg/day, and vigilance for hepatotoxicity must be maintained (as indicated by the drug's black box warning). Expert opinion suggests that even lower doses of naltrexone may be effective in the treatment of alcohol dependence; therefore, medical providers should consider starting patients at even lower doses (e.g. 25 mg/day) and titrating to effect. Although acamprosate and disulfiram are also approved for treatment of alcohol dependence, both have been demonstrated to be inferior to naltrexone and should be considered in those who are unable to take naltrexone [39].

MENTAL ILLNESS AND ILLICIT DRUG USE

A thorough discussion of mental illness as it relates to sub-stance misuse and HIV is outside the scope of this chapter and the reader is referred to the literature for more on this topic [42]. It must be noted, however, that substance misuse and mental illness are closely interrelated with HIV. Individuals with all three diagnoses are likely to engage in high-risk behaviors [43], and when untreated, they continue to fuel the HIV epidemic by engaging in risk behaviors and ongoing transmission of HIV. These three diagnoses should be viewed as overlapping spheres of influence, with each diagnosis affecting the others. Conceptually, this is important because successful therapy requires screening, diagnosis, and treatment of all three spheres of influence rather than ignoring any one single area. For this reason, it is essential to ensure a comprehensive and integrated approach to managing these three co-morbid conditions [42].

DRUG INTERACTIONS WITH HIV THERAPEUTICS

With the proliferation of medications to treat HIV and other medical conditions, drug–drug interactions are becoming more common and more complicated. It is essential to be familiar with the current state-of-the-art data on drug metabolism and expected or actual pharmacokinetic interactions between HIV therapeutics and the pharmacological treatment for addiction (Table 40.3 summarizes the key interactions for the practitioner) [44]. This understanding is critical as medication-assisted treatment with methadone or buprenorphine may alter metabolism of antiretroviral medications, resulting in increased toxicity or reduced efficacy. Alternatively, antiretroviral medications may alter the levels of medication-assisted treatment, resulting in clinical opioid withdrawal or overdose.

The currently approved nucleoside reverse transcriptase inhibitors (NRTIs) do not affect methadone levels in a

Table 40.3 Interactions between antiretrovirals and methadone, and buprenorphine

MEDICATION	EFFECT ON METHADONE	EFFECT ON BUP	ARV	COMMENTS
NRTI				
Abacavir (ABC)[a]	↑ clearance	Not studied	↓ C_{max}	No dose change required for METH
Didanosine (ddI)	No clinical effect	No clinical effect	METH ↓ ddI AUC by 57% for buffered tablet, partially corrected by EC capsule. No BUP effect on ddI	No dose adjustments necessary when EC capsule used with METH patients
Emtriva (FTC)	Not studied	Not studied	Not studied	
Festinavir	Not studied	Not studied	Not studied	
Lamivudine (3TC)	No clinical effect	No clinical effect	No effect of BUP on 3TC	AZT/3TC co-formulation studied only with METH. No dose adjustments necessary
Stavudine (d4T)	No clinical effect	Not studied	↓ d4T AUC_{12h} by 23% and C_{max} by 44%	No dose adjustments necessary
Tenofovir (TDF)	No clinical effect	No clinical effect	No significant effect on TDF by BUP	No dose adjustments necessary
Zalcitabine (ddC)	Not studied	Not studied	Not studied	
Zidovudine (AZT)	No clinical effect	No clinical effect	↑ AZT AUC by 40%	Watch for AZT-related toxicity (symptoms and laboratory). Dose reductions of AZT may be required

Table 40.3 Interactions between antiretrovirals and methadone, and buprenorphine—cont'd				
MEDICATION	**EFFECT ON METHADONE**	**EFFECT ON BUP**	**ARV**	**COMMENTS**
NNRTI				
Delavirdine (DLV)	↑ AUC by 19%; ↑C_{max} by 10%	↑ AUC by 400%, without clinical effect	No clinical effect	No dose adjustments necessary; however, should be used with caution as long-term effects (>7 days) are unknown
Efavirenz (EFV)	↓ AUC by 57%	No clinical effect	No clinical effect	Opioid withdrawal from METH common. METH dose increase likely to be necessary
Etravirine (ETV)	No clinical effect (only 100 b.i.d. of etravirine studied)	Not studied	No clinical effect	No dose adjustments necessary
Lersivirine	No clinical effect	Not studied	Not studied	No dose adjustments necessary
Nevirapine (NVP)	↓ AUC by 46%	No clinical effect	No clinical effect	Opioid withdrawal from METH common. METH dose increase likely to be necessary
Rilpivirine (TMC278)	↓ AUC by 22%	Not studied	No clinical effect	Monitoring for symptoms of METH withdrawal is recommended
PI				
Amprenavir (AMP)	↓ AUC of R-METH by 13%	Not studied	↓ AUC by 30%	No dose adjustments necessary
Atazanavir (ATV)	No effect	↑ AUC by 167%	No effect	Some individuals may experience oversedation. Slower titration upwards of BUP may be advisable
Darunavir	↓ S-METH AUC by 36% and ↓ R-METH AUC by 15%	↑ norBUP AUC by 46%	No clinical effect	No ARV dose change when combined with METH or BUP. Four subjects out of 16 in METH study reported mild opioid withdrawal, but no dose adjustments were needed.
Fosamprenavir (fAMP)	↓ AUC R-METH by 18%	Not studied	No clinical effect	No dose adjustments necessary
Indinavir (IND)	No clinical effect	Not studied	↓ C_{max} between 16% and 28% and ↑ C_{min} between 50% and 100%	Differences do not appear to be clinically significant.
Lopinavir/ritonavir (LPV/r)	↓ AUC by 26–36%	No clinical effect	Not studied	↓ AUC of METH caused by lopinavir. One study reported opioid withdrawal symptoms in 27% of patients. METH dose increase may be necessary in some patients

Continued

Table 40.3 Interactions between antiretrovirals and methadone, and buprenorphine—cont'd

MEDICATION	EFFECT ON METHADONE	EFFECT ON BUP	ARV	COMMENTS
PI—cont'd				
Nelfinavir	↓ AUC by 40%	No clinical effect	↓ AUC of active M8 metabolite by 48%	Despite ↓ METH AUC, clinical withdrawal is usually absent and a priori dosage adjustments are not needed. Decrease in AUC of M8 unlikely to be clinically significant.
Ritonavir (RTV)	↓ AUC by 37% in one study and no effect in another (see text)	↑ AUC by 157%	Not studied	No dosage adjustments necessary
Saquinavir (SQV)	↓ AUC by 20–32%	Not studied	Not studied	Saquinavir boosted with ritonavir studied. Despite ↓ METH AUC, clinical withdrawal was not reported
Tipranavir (TPV)	↓ by 50%[a]	↓ norBUP ACU by 80%	No ARV dose change when combined with METH. TPV/r AUC and C_{max} decreased 19% and 25%, respectively, compared to historical controls in the presence of BUP	METH dose may need to be increased. TPV may be less effective with BUP, but no dosage adjustments necessary in BUP
Integrase				
Elvitegravir	Not studied	Not studied	Not studied	
Raltegravir (RAL)	No clinical effect	No clinical effect	No ARV dose adjustments necessary	
Entry Inhibitors				
Maraviroc	Not studied	Not studied	Not studied	
Enfurvitide	Not studied	Not studied	Not studied	

[a]Decrease in methadone not specified as AUC or C_{max}.
NRTI, nucleoside reverse transcriptase inhibitor; NNRTI, non-nucleoside reverse transcriptase inhibitor; PI, protease inhibitor; AUC, area under curve; METH, methadone; BUP, buprenorphine; norBUP, norbuprenorphine.
Adapted with permission from Bruce et al. [45].

clinically significant manner. Methadone, however, affects zidovudine significantly. Methadone increased zidovudine drug levels by approximately 40%. As a result, patients may experience symptoms associated with excessive zidovudine plasma levels that may be confused with symptoms of opioid withdrawal.

Zidovudine, lamivudine, didanosine, and tenofovir are the NRTIs that have been studied in combination with buprenorphine. Buprenorphine did not alter the pharmacokinetics of these NRTI in any clinically meaningful manner [45].

Nevirapine and efavirenz markedly reduce methadone levels and precipitate clinical opioid withdrawal [46].

Although efavirenz and nevirapine significantly reduce buprenorphine levels, this reduction is not associated with symptoms of opioid withdrawal [47, 48]. Newer NNRTIs have been recently studied and are summarized in Table 40.3.

Most protease inhibitors (PIs) studied do not appear to have clinically meaningful effects upon methadone levels with the following exceptions: One study of the co-formulated capsule of lopinavir/ritonavir administration with methadone reported that 27% of subjects co-administered lopinavir/ritonavir and methadone experienced clinical opioid withdrawal symptoms [49]. The package insert for tipranavir reports that standard dosing of tipranavir/ritonavir (500/200 mg b.i.d.) may result in a decrease in methadone levels requiring an increase in methadone dose. Darunavir has also been reported to potentially lead to opioid withdrawal in the methadone-maintained patient [50, 51].

Most PIs studied do not appear to have clinically meaningful effects upon buprenorphine levels with the following exceptions: Buprenorphine, appears to have a potential pharmacodynamic interaction with atazanavir that can lead to oversedation in some individuals [52]. Buprenorphine can be used with atazanavir, but slower upward titration of dosing is advised with monitoring. In a recent study, however, a lack of a pharamcodynamic effect was seen in a prospective cohort of HIV-infected opioid-dependent patients on buprenorphine [53]. This study, however, occurred after the previous publications cautioning providers on the rate of build-up and it is unclear if the lack of a pharmacodynamic effect was the result of a slower upward titration. Tipranavir alters the disposition of buprenorphine without producing a pharmacodyamic effect. More importantly, buprenorphine has been shown to reduce the AUC of tipranavir. The clinical significance of this is unknown; however, providers are cautioned to follow patients closely if the two are co-administered [54].

Raltegravir, the first available integrase inhibitor, has been studied in methadone- and buprenorphine-maintained patients with the finding that no dose modification of the methadone was necessary.

Several medications used to treat or prevent opportunistic infections in HIV-infected individuals deserve brief comment. Rifampin, a potent inducer of cytochrome P450, produces rapid and profound reductions in methadone levels and development of opioid withdrawal; as such, rifampin should be changed to rifabutin or methadone doses increased rapidly and dramatically to avoid opioid withdrawal and discontinuation of all medications [55]. A recent study of buprenorphine and rifampin has demonstrated that rifampin precipitates opioid withdrawal in buprenorphine-maintained patients [56]. Patients receiving both medications should be observed closely for opioid withdrawal and increases in buprenorphine may be required. Fluconazole, a known inhibitor of cytochrome P450 metabolism, increases methadone exposure, and methadone dosage may need to be reduced [57].

SPECIAL ISSUES IN PREVENTION

Risk reduction

The relapsing pattern of drug use and the wide array of serious infectious and other medical consequences require the development of preventive risk-reduction strategies. Risk reduction does not promote injection drug use, but seeks to decrease the frequency of adverse events that are related to this practice. Risk reduction is based on the underlying principle that injection drug use is a chronic and relapsing disease which may not be cured in the individual or eliminated from society but can be conducted in a way that minimizes harm to the user and others. While complete cessation of drug use remains a laudable goal, reduction in drug use frequency and safer injection practices is more realistic for many drug users until abstinence can be achieved. Risk-reduction strategies have been effectively incorporated into some drug treatment programs, syringe exchange programs and safe injection rooms [58]. There are several practical components inherent to risk-reduction strategies. Education about and provision of drug use paraphernalia (e.g. needles and syringes) for more hygienic injection practices for the prevention of infectious complications of injection are essential. In addition to the distribution or exchange of injection equipment, these programs typically include HIV/AIDS education, condom distribution, and referral or enrollment in a variety of drug treatment, medical, and social services [59]. Specifically, some programs provide onsite medical and drug treatment, resulting in reductions in emergency department use by IDUs.

Provision of primary medical care services linked to drug-abuse treatment is a way to promote preventive therapies to enhance harm reduction. In this and all other clinical settings, in addition to the treatment of HIV disease and prevention of complications, injection drug users should be routinely screened for hepatitis B and C, latent *M. tuberculosis* infection, syphilis, and other sexually transmitted disease. They should be offered pneumococcal, influenza, tetanus, and hepatitis A and B immunization and, if lately infected with *M. tuberculosis*, chemoprophylaxis with isoniazid.

The ultimate goal of risk-reduction strategies should be the reduction or prevention of illicit drug use itself, the development of strategies that will minimize the serious medical consequences of drug misuse, and the development of strategies that will eliminate drug misuse and its root causes. Until we are successful in this arena, we stand little chance of limiting the spread and consequences of HIV disease in this and related populations.

REFERENCES

[1] Morojele NK, Brook JS, Kachieng'a MA. Perceptions of sexual risk behaviours and substance abuse among adolescents in South Africa: a qualitative investigation. AIDS Care 2006;18:215–19.

[2] UNAIDS. Report on the Global HIV/AIDS Epidemic. In: UNAIDS, editor. United Nations. 2002.

[3] Hart GJ, Sonnex C, Petherick A, et al. Risk behaviours for HIV infection among injecting drug users attending a drug dependency clinic. BMJ 1989;298:1081–3.

[4] Williams ML, McCurdy SA, Bowen AM, et al. HIV seroprevalence in a sample of Tanzanian intravenous drug users. AIDS Educ Prev 2009;21:474–83.

[5] Altice FL, Kamarulzaman A, Soriano VV, et al. Treatment of medical, psychiatric, and substance-use comorbidities in people infected with HIV who use drugs. Lancet 2010;376:59–79.

[6] Alcabes P, Friedland GH. Injection drug use and human immunodeficiency virus infection. Clin Infect Dis 1995;20:1467–79.

[7] Anis AH, Guh D, Hogg RS, et al. The cost effectiveness of antiretroviral regimens for the treatment of HIV/AIDS. Pharmacoeconomics 2000;18:393–404.

[8] Kaplan AH, Scheyett A, Golin CE. HIV and stigma: analysis and research program. Curr HIV/AIDS Rep 2005;2:184–8.

[9] Kresina TF, Eldred L, Bruce RD, Francis H. Integration of pharmacotherapy for opioid addiction into HIV primary care for HIV/hepatitis C virus-co-infected patients. AIDS 2005;19(Suppl. 3): S221–6.

[10] Urbina A, Jones K. Crystal methamphetamine, its analogues, and HIV infection: medical and psychiatric aspects of a new epidemic. Clin Infect Dis 2004;38:890–4.

[11] Chander G, Himelhoch S, Moore RD. Substance abuse and psychiatric disorders in HIV-positive patients: epidemiology and impact on antiretroviral therapy. Drugs 2006;66:769–89.

[12] Morojele NK, Kachieng'a MA, Mokoko E, et al. Alcohol use and sexual behaviour among risky drinkers and bar and shebeen patrons in Gauteng province, South Africa. Soc Sci Med 2006;62:217–27.

[13] Hendershot CS, Stoner SA, George WH, Norris J. Alcohol use, expectancies, and sexual sensation seeking as correlates of HIV risk behavior in heterosexual young adults. Psychol Addict Behav 2007;21:365–72.

[14] Azar MM, Springer SA, Meyer JP, Altice FL. A systematic review of the impact of alcohol use disorders on HIV treatment outcomes, adherence to antiretroviral therapy and health care utilization. Drug Alcohol Depend 2010;112:178–93.

[15] Altice FL, Bruce RD, Lucas GM, et al. HIV treatment outcomes among HIV-infected, opioid-dependent patients receiving buprenorphine/naloxone treatment within HIV clinical care settings: results from a multisite study. J Acquir Immune Defic Syndr 2011;56(Suppl. 1): S22–32.

[16] Smith-Rohrberg D, Bruce RD, Altice FL. Review of corrections based therapy for opiate-dependent patients: implications for buprenorphine treatment among correctional populations. J Drug Issues 2004;34:451–80.

[17] Dolan K, Hall W, Wodak A. Methadone maintenance reduces injecting in prison. BMJ 1996;312:1162.

[18] Donny E, Walsh S, Bigelow G, et al. High-dose methadone produces superior opioid blockade and comparable withdrawal suppression to lower doses in opioid-dependent humans. Psychopharmacology 2002;161:202–12.

[19] Fudala PJ, Bridge TP, Herbert S, et al. Office-based treatment of opiate addiction with a sublingual-tablet formulation of buprenorphine and naloxone. N Engl J Med 2003;349:949–58.

[20] Murray JB. Effectiveness of methadone maintenance for heroin addiction. Psychol Rep 1998;83:295–302.

[21] Metzger DS, Woody GE, O'Brien CP. Drug treatment as HIV prevention: a research update. J Acquir Immune Defic Syndr 2010;55(Suppl. 1): S32–6.

[22] Metzger DS, Woody GE, McLellan AT, et al. Human immunodeficiency virus seroconversion among intravenous drug users in- and out-of-treatment: an 18-month prospective follow-up. J Acquir Immune Defic Syndr 1993;6:1049–56.

[23] Dole VP, Nyswander M. A medical treatment for diacetylmorphine (heroin) addiction. A clinical trial with methadone hydrochloride. JAMA 1965;193:646–50.

[24] Bruce RD. Methadone as HIV prevention: high volume methadone sites to decrease HIV incidence rates in resource limited settings. Int J Drug Policy 2010;21:122–4.

[25] Kerr T, Wodak A, Elliott R, et al. Opioid substitution and HIV/AIDS treatment and prevention. Lancet 2004;364:1918–19.

[26] Doran CM, Shanahan M, Mattick RP, et al. Buprenorphine versus methadone maintenance: a cost-effectiveness analysis. Drug Alcohol Depend 2003;71:295–302.

[27] Johnson RE, Chutuape MA, Strain EC, et al. A comparison of levomethadyl acetate, buprenorphine, and methadone for opioid dependence. N Engl J Med 2000;343:1290–7.

[28] Liguori A, Morse WH, Bergman J. Respiratory effects of opioid full and partial agonists in rhesus monkeys. J Pharmacol Exp Ther 1996;277:462–72.

[29] Clark N, Lintzeris N, Gijsbers A, et al. LAAM maintenance vs methadone maintenance for heroin dependence. Cochrane Database Syst Rev 2002: CD002210.

[30] Johnson RE, Eissenberg T, Stitzer ML, et al. Buprenorphine treatment of opioid dependence: clinical trial of daily versus alternate-day dosing. Drug Alcohol Depend 1995;40:27–35.

[31] Bruce RD, Dvoryak S, Sylla L, Altice FL. HIV treatment access and scale-up for delivery of opiate substitution therapy with buprenorphine for IDUs in Ukraine—programme description and policy implications. Int J Drug Policy 2007;18:326–8.

[32] Basu S, Smith-Rohrberg D, Bruce RD, Altice FL. Models for integrating buprenorphine therapy into the primary HIV care setting. Clin Infect Dis 2006;42:716–21.

[33] Greenstein RA, Evans BD, McLellan AT, O'Brien CP. Predictors of favorable outcome following naltrexone treatment. Drug Alcohol Depend 1983;12:173–80.

[34] Schottenfeld RS, Chawarski MC, Mazlan M. Maintenance treatment with buprenorphine and naltrexone for heroin dependence in Malaysia: a randomised, double-blind, placebo-controlled trial. Lancet 2008;371:2192–200.

[35] Petrakis IL, Carroll KM, Nich C, et al. Disulfiram treatment for cocaine dependence in methadone-maintained opioid addicts. Addiction 2000;95:219–28.

[36] Madan A, Parkinson A, Faiman MD. Identification of the human P-450 enzymes responsible for the sulfoxidation and thiono-oxidation of diethyldithiocarbamate methyl ester: role of P-450 enzymes in disulfiram bioactivation. Alcohol Clin Exp Res 1998;22:1212–19.

[37] Shoptaw S, Huber A, Peck J, et al. Randomized, placebo-controlled trial of sertraline and contingency management for the treatment of methamphetamine dependence. Drug Alcohol Depend 2006;85:12–18.

[38] Peck JA, Reback CJ, Yang X, et al. Sustained reductions in drug use and depression symptoms from treatment for drug abuse in methamphetamine-dependent gay and bisexual men. J Urban Health 2005;82:i100–8.

[39] Anton RF, O'Malley SS, Ciraulo DA, et al. Combined pharmacotherapies and behavioral interventions for alcohol dependence: the COMBINE study: a randomized controlled trial. JAMA 2006;295:2003–17.

[40] Town T, Schinka J, Tan J, Mullan M. The opioid receptor system and alcoholism: a genetic perspective. Eur J Pharmacol 2000;410:243–8.

[41] O'Malley SS, Jaffe AJ, Chang G, et al. Naltrexone and coping skills therapy for alcohol dependence. A controlled study. Arch Gen Psychiatry 1992;49:881–7.

[42] Basu S, Chwastiak LA, Bruce RD. Clinical management of depression and anxiety in HIV-infected adults. AIDS 2005;19:2057–67.

[43] Kalichman SC, Rompa D. HIV treatment adherence and unprotected sex practices in people receiving antiretroviral therapy. Sex Transm Infect 2003;79:59–61.

[44] Bruce RD, Altice FL, Gourevitch MN, Friedland GH. Pharmacokinetic drug interactions between opioid agonist therapy and antiretroviral medications: implications and management for clinical practice. J Acquir Immune Defic Syndr 2006;41:563–72.

[45] McCance-Katz EF, Rainey PM, Friedland G, et al. Effect of opioid dependence pharmacotherapies on zidovudine disposition. Am J Addict 2001;10:296–307.

[46] Clarke SM, Mulcahy FM, Tjia J, et al. The pharmacokinetics of methadone in HIV-positive patients receiving the non-nucleoside reverse transcriptase inhibitor efavirenz. Br J Clin Pharmacol 2001;51:213–17.

[47] McCance-Katz EF, Pade P, Friedland G, et al. Efavirenz is not associated with opiate withdrawal in buprenorphine-maintained individuals. In: 12th Conference on Retroviruses and Opportunistic Infections. Boston, MA: Foundation for Retrovirology and Human Health; 2005.

[48] McCance-Katz EF, Moody DE, Morse GD, et al. Lack of clinically significant drug interactions between nevirapine and buprenorphine. Am J Addict 2010;19:30–7.

[49] Clarke S, Mulcahy F, Bergin C, et al. Absence of opioid withdrawal symptoms in patients receiving methadone and the protease inhibitor lopinavir-ritonavir. Clin Infect Dis 2002;34:1143–5.

[50] McCance-katz EF, Rainey PM, Friedland G, Jatlow P. The protease inhibitor lopinavir/ritonavir may produce opiate withdrawal in methadone-maintained patients. Clinical infections Diseases 2003;37:476–82.

[51] Sekar V, Tomaka F, Lefebvre E, et al. Pharmacokinetic interactions between darunavir/ritonavir and opioid maintenance therapy using methadone or buprenorphine/naloxone. J Clin Pharmacol 2011;51:271–8.

[52] McCance-Katz E, Pade P, Morse GD, et al. Interaction between buprenorphine and atazanavir. In: College on Problems of Drug Dependence. Scottsdale, AZ; 2006.

[53] Vergara-Rodriguez P, Tozzi MJ, Botsko M, et al. Hepatic safety and lack of antiretroviral interactions with buprenorphine/naloxone in HIV-infected opioid-dependent patients. J Acquir Immune Defic Syndr 2011;56 (Suppl. 1):S62–7.

[54] Bruce RD, Altice FL, Moody DE, et al. Pharmacokinetic interactions between buprenorphine/naloxone and tipranavir ritonavir in HIV-negative subjects chronically receiving buprenorphine/naloxone. Drug Alcohol Depend 2009;105: 234–9.

[55] Kreek MJ, Garfield JW, Gutjahr CL, Giusti LM. Rifampin-induced methadone withdrawal. N Engl J Med 1976;294:1104–6.

[56] McCance-Katz EF, Moody DE, Prathikanti S, et al. Rifampin, but not rifabutin, may produce opiate withdrawal in buprenorphine-maintained patients. Drug Alcohol Depend 2011. [Epub ahead of print].

[57] Cobb MN, Desai J, Brown Jr. LS, et al. The effect of fluconazole on the clinical pharmacokinetics of methadone. Clin Pharmacol Ther 1998;63:655–62.

[58] Broadhead R, Borch C, van Hulst Y, et al. Safer injection sites in New York City: a utilization survey of injection drug users. J Drug Issues 2003;33:533–8.

[59] Centers for Disease Control and Prevention. Compendium of HIV prevention interventions with evidence of effectiveness. National Center for HIV, STD and TB Prevention; 2001.

Chapter | 41 |

The HIV-infected international traveler

Malcolm John

INTRODUCTION

The advent of (ART) has led to significant decreases in human immunodeficiency virus type 1 (HIV-1)-related morbidity and mortality, with concomitant improved immunocompetence [1–5]. Despite this, the HIV-infected traveler is still at increased risk for opportunistic infections and other complications compared with HIV-uninfected travelers. This is especially true for those with low CD4 counts and those traveling to developing countries. Nonetheless, pre-travel health advice is often underutilized [6, 7].

One study of patients at an HIV clinic in a North American tertiary care hospital found that 46% of 290 surveyed individuals had traveled internationally within the previous 5 years. Yet, only 44% sought health advice before traveling [7]. Of those seeking pre-travel advice, only half told the provider that they were HIV-infected. International travel was associated with poor adherence to antiretrovirals (ARVs) and to risky sexual activity in these patients. A total of 93% of the 75 individuals not seeking pre-travel health advice believed such consultations were unnecessary. Such data are disturbing, given that international travel increased steadily throughout the 1990s and early twenty-first century [8]. Indeed, outbound overseas travel from the USA climbed to a high of almost 27 million by 2000 with travel to Asia, South America, and the Middle East growing by 93, 130, and 159%, respectively [7]. During this period, incident infections in returning international travelers continued to rise [9]. Post-9/11, US-international overseas travel increased to a new high of 47.7 million bidirectional visits in 2004. Countries within Eastern Europe and the Caribbean experienced the fastest growth from 2000 to 2004 (25 and 15%, respectively) [10].

There has also been increasing numbers of immigrants to developed countries who visit their countries of origin and return that are a population at high risk for tropical infections including tuberculosis (TB), malaria, food- and water-borne illnesses, hepatitis A, and sexually transmitted infections (STIs) [11]. It is therefore important that persons living with HIV/AIDS and their pre-travel providers stay informed about preparations and precautions that should be taken by the HIV-infected person when traveling internationally today.

GENERAL CONSIDERATIONS

The quality of pre-travel health advice can vary greatly; thus, consultation with a travel medicine specialist is advisable. A study from the United Kingdom (UK) of 215 clinicians serving higher education establishments in the UK showed that practitioners often gave good advice with respect to immunizations and malaria prophylaxis, but little on HIV and other risks [12]. Training in travel medicine was associated with more appropriate pre-travel health advice.

Pre-travel health advice for the HIV-infected international traveler should be sought as soon as possible. Consultation at least 6–8 weeks before travel is recommended to allow time for development of adequate responses to any necessary vaccinations. Use of resources such as travel clinics and travel-related websites before traveling is appropriate. Detailed counseling and evaluation of the risks and benefits of preventive prophylaxis and vaccinations are essential.

Pre-travel advice should include a discussion of immunizations, malaria prophylaxis, traveler's diarrhea management, supplemental health insurance, accidents and injuries, motion sickness, jet lag, extremes of temperature and sun exposure, food and water safety, use of an emergency medical bracelet, list of medical services abroad, and possible arrangement of visits with physicians who speak the traveler's language [13]. The last issue is especially important for extended visits, so that adequate medical follow-up and medication supplies are maintained. Emphasis on maintaining adherence to ARV regimens is important as there is evidence that adherence is more difficult abroad [14]. Strategies such as keeping antiretroviral medications in carry-on baggage should be reviewed. A discussion of behavioral risk reduction while traveling is also essential. Boxes 41.1 and 41.2 summarize advice on items to take while traveling and what to do while traveling that should be part of a pre-travel consultation.

It is wise to reassess the stage of HIV prior to travel as low CD4 counts are the biggest predictor of risk of opportunistic infections (OIs) when traveling. However, changing antiretroviral medications just prior to travel is not encouraged in order to avoid complications from the ARVs occurring while traveling. The Centers for Disease Control and Prevention (CDC) suggest that to minimize the risk of infection, treatment naïve HIV-infected individuals with CD4 counts below $200/mm^3$ should delay travel if possible until CD4 T cell reconstitution with ART occurs.

Box 41.1 What to take when traveling

- Adequate supply of medications (1–2 weeks' extra supply is advisable) and prophylactic agents (e.g. for malaria) for shorter trips, along with copies of prescriptions; attention should be given to any need for refrigeration of medications.
- Documentation of vaccinations.
- Medications for traveler's diarrhea, e.g. ciprofloxacin for 3- to 7-day courses of treatment or daily prophylaxis up to 3 weeks' duration; trimethoprim-sulfamethoxazole (TMP-SMX) recommended for children and pregnant women.
- Mosquito netting (preferably treated with permethrin).

- Insect repellent that contains <30% DEET (N,N-diethylmetatoluamide).
- Medications for sinusitis and jet lag.
- Condoms and other safe-sex items.
- First-aid kit, including topical antibiotics.
- Consider bringing own equipment for boiling water, purifying water by iodine treatment, and/or filtration of water using commercial filters with 1 μm or smaller filters.
- Consider need for fluconazole, itraconazole, and isoniazid prophylaxis if CD4 count <100 cells/mm^3.

Box 41.2 What to do when traveling

- Take steps to maintain adherence to medication regimen.
- Carry securely basic medical information, e.g. medical conditions, medications, allergies.
- Know how to access local health care (general care and HIV-specific care)
- Avoid behaviors that increase risk of new infections or complications:
  - "Boil it, peel it, cook it, or forget it", and WASH HANDS.
  - Avoid raw vegetables, fruit you have not peeled yourself, unpasteurized dairy products, cooked food not served steaming hot, and tap water, including ice; meat should be well-cooked, as undercooked beef, pork, or fish can be a source of tapeworms.
  - Purify water in high-risk areas—boiling water is the best method of purification; tincture of iodine or tetraglycine hydroperiodide tablets is an alternative but the water must be used within a few weeks and the method cannot be relied on to kill Cryptosporidium unless the water is allowed to sit for 15 h before it is drunk; filtering water produces variable results, especially for small bacteria or viruses, and proper selection, operation, care, and maintenance of water filters are essential.

  - Avoid walking barefoot in areas with high risk of soil pathogens.
  - Avoid swimming in bodies of water that may be contaminated by other people and from sewage, animal wastes, and wastewater run-off; avoid swallowing water when swimming, even chlorinated water, which may contain live organisms (e.g. Cryptosporidium, Giardia, hepatitis A virus, and Norwalk virus), and which have moderate to very high resistance to chlorine; avoid swimming in areas of endemic schistosomiasis or water at risk of contamination from animals carrying Leptospira.
  - Use safe-sex practices to avoid risks from acquiring sexually transmitted diseases. These risks include increased severity and complications (e.g. herpes outbreaks more prolonged and severe), risks related to acquiring new HIV strains (e.g. non-nucleoside reverse transcriptase inhibitors are not active against HIV-2).
  - Avoid blood exposures (e.g. acupuncture, tattoos, injections with possibly unsterile needles, sharing razors, manicures and pedicures) that can lead to acquiring hepatitis C as hepatitis C-related cirrhosis is accelerated in those co-infected with HIV.

The CDC also warns that some countries screen for HIV and deny entry to those who have AIDS or test positive for HIV (usually those entering for extended periods, e.g. for work or study). Some countries further deny entry to those carrying antiretroviral medications. Placing ARVs in an empty vitamin or other medication container is one means of avoiding problems in such situations. More specific information is best obtained from the consular officials of the individual nations. See Box 41.3 for a list of travel resources.

Vaccinations

Concerns over vaccinating HIV-infected persons because of documented elevations in HIV viral loads have not borne out. Such viral load elevations are transient, resolving within 4–6 weeks and sooner if on ART without any documented long-term deleterious effects [15]. All HIV-infected travelers should therefore be uptodate on routinely recommended vaccines and those routinely recommended for HIV-infected individuals. Additional vaccines should be given based on the specific travel risk exposures to endemic infections. It should be noted that vaccine responses are generally inadequate if the patient's CD4 count is < 100 cells/mm^3; best results are obtained if the CD4 count is > 350 cells/mm^3 [16]. The CDC's *Yellow Book* states that antiretroviral drug-induced increased CD4 counts, and not nadir counts, should be used to categorize HIV-infected persons and that waiting 3 months post-immune reconstitution before immunization is advisable.

In general, inactivated vaccines are safe to administer and should be initiated 6–8 weeks before travel. Live vaccines, including BCG, should be avoided with two exceptions (Table 41.1):

- Live measles vaccine is recommended for non-immune travelers whose CD4 counts are > 200 cells/mm^3 as the clinical course of the disease is worse in those with HIV. Non-immune travelers with CD4 counts < 200 cells/mm^3 should receive the immune globulin if traveling to endemic areas (CDC, *Yellow Book*).

Table 41.1 Summary of vaccination recommendations

ROUTINELY GIVEN	GIVEN IF TRAVEL INDICATES	CONTRAINDICATED
• Tetanus–diphtheria (Td or Tdap vaccines) • Hepatitis A • Hepatitis B • Influenza (inactivated) • Pneumococcal polysaccharide vaccine (*H. influenzae B* generally not recommended as HIV-infected adults are generally infected with non-typeable strains; children should be vaccinated)	• Japanese B encephalitis (many side effects not unique to HIV-infected persons; use if at high risk, e.g. >1 month in rural endemic area) • Measles (live vaccine should not be given if severe immunosuppression; use immunoglobulin if needed) • Meningococcal (consider either the polysaccharide or conjugate vaccine) • Polio, inactivated (IPV) • Rabies (safe; pre-exposure prophylaxis generally not indicated) • Tick-borne encephalitis (only if high risk, e.g. forested endemic areas and drinking unpasteurized milk products) • Typhoid Vi (inactivated, Vi) • Yellow fever (live vaccine should not be given if severe immunosuppression, instruct how to avoid mosquito bites and provide a vaccination waiver letter)	• BCG • Polio, live • Typhoid, live • Influenza, live attenuated (LAIV) • Varicella-zoster virus (VZV; can consider if CD4 count > 200 cells/mm^3) (cholera vaccine no longer recommended or required)

- Yellow fever vaccine is of unknown risk and benefit to HIV-infected individuals; however, it should be offered to asymptomatic HIV-infected individuals with minimal immunosuppression (avoid if CD4 counts <200 cells/mm^3) who cannot avoid potential exposure to the yellow fever virus. Those at risk who defer immunization should be instructed in methods to avoid mosquito bites and provided a vaccination waiver letter understanding that such a letter may not be accepted by some countries (CDC, http://www.cdc.gov/travel/hivtrav.htm).

Prophylaxis considerations

Prophylaxis should be given for malaria to those at risk. Empiric treatment for traveler's diarrhea (TD) rather than primary prophylaxis is generally recommended. However, primary prophylaxis for TD can be considered for those who cannot afford to get ill, e.g. those with severely depressed CD4 counts (see sections below on Malaria and Enteric Infections for details).

Consider prophylaxis for those with severe immunosuppression (e.g. CD4 counts <100 cells/mm^3) at risk for TB or disseminated infections from endemic mycoses such as *Penicillium marneffei, Coccidioides immitis, Histoplasma capsulatum,* and *Paracoccidioides brasiliensis* as well as *Cryptococcus neoformans* (see below).

SELECTED DISEASE-SPECIFIC ISSUES

HIV-infected travelers and their healthcare providers should review the risks of the following disorders and opportunistic infections to travelers to the developing world, especially to those with low CD4 counts:

- Enteric infections (e.g. *salmonella*) and wasting.
- TB, bacterial respiratory infections (e.g. *S. pneumoniae*).
- Malaria, leishmaniasis, Chagas disease, and other parasitic infections.
- Penicilliosis and other disseminated endemic mycoses.
- Other, e.g. new HIV infections, fevers.

Enteric infections

Etiologies of traveler's diarrhea (TD) in HIV-infected travelers

The main enteric bacterial pathogen to which HIV-infected individuals are at increased risk of acquiring is *Salmonella typhimurium* and other non-typhoidal *Salmonella* (NTS). HIV-infected patients have up to a 100-fold risk of infection compared with HIV-uninfected individuals in developing countries where NTS is the leading cause of diarrhea with fever [17]. Disease often relapses and can be difficult to treat effectively, leading to significant morbidity and

mortality. HIV-infected persons with *Salmonella* septicemia require chronic maintenance therapy to prevent recurrence.

Other common bacterial enteric infections in the HIV-infected traveler include enterotoxigenic *E. coli*, enteroaggregative *E. coli*, *Shigella*, and *Campylobacter*, especially among men who have sex with men. Other causes of TD include parasites, e.g. *Giardia, Isospora, CRYPTOSPORIDIUM,* and *Cyclospora,* especially in Central America. Despite the fact that parasitic diarrheal diseases occur in the HIV-infected traveler, there appears to be little evidence that HIV infection increases the risk of intestinal helminth infections [18, 19]. More rarely, one sees TD related to *Yersinia, Plesiomonas, Aeromonas* (more commonly in Southeast Asia), *Entamoeba,* and non-cholera *Vibrio* species. Rarely, cholera or polio is found. Viruses can cause TD in HIV-infected travelers as in HIV-uninfected persons although this may reflect infection prior to travel; rotavirus and Norwalk viruses are common agents in this group and have been implicated in outbreaks on cruise ships in the Caribbean. TD due to infection with hepatitis A can be avoided with proper immunization.

Prevention of TD in HIV-infected travelers

Some recommend empiric daily prophylaxis (e.g. ciprofloxacin 500 mg daily) for up to 3 weeks for those who must avoid TD [16, 18, 20]. This may include those with severely depressed CD4 counts and may be desired even if such travelers are already on trimethoprim-sulfamethoxazole (TMP/SMX) for *Pneumocystis carinii* pneumonia (PCP) prophylaxis given the high rates of TMP/SMX resistance in enteric pathogens worldwide. Antibiotics recommended by the Infectious Disease Society of America include ciprofloxacin, norfloxacin, rifaximin, and bismuth subsalicylate. Care should be taken to avoid contact with reptiles (e.g. snakes, lizards, iguanas, and turtles) as well as chicks and ducklings because of the risk for salmonellosis [20]. Travelers should avoid swallowing water during swimming and should not swim in water that might be contaminated with sewage or animal waste to avoid getting illnesses like cryptosporidiosis and giardiasis.

Prevention of enteric infections in the HIV-infected traveler is best accomplished by ensuring safe water for drinking, brushing teeth, and making ice cubes. Bottled beverages, hot coffee and tea, beer, and wine, are considered safe for drinking. All fruits and vegetables must be washed and peeled, preferably by the travelers themselves; all meats and other foods should be cooked thoroughly to steaming hot. Boiling water is the best method of water purification and should be done until at least 1 min (3 min at >2000 m altitude) of vigorous boiling has been achieved. Tincture of iodine or tetraglycine hydroperiodide tablets is an alternative, but the water must be used within a few weeks and the method cannot be relied on to kill *Cryptosporidium* unless the water is allowed to sit for 15 h before it is drunk. Filtering water produces variable results, especially for small bacteria or viruses.

Proper selection, operation, care, and maintenance of water filters is essential. Commercial filters should be labeled either "reverse osmosis," "absolute pore size of 1 micron or smaller," "tested and certified by NSF Standard 53 or NSF Standard 58 for cyst removal," or "tested and certified by NSF Standard 53 or NSF Standard 58 for cyst reduction." Reverse-osmosis filters provide broad protection but they are expensive, relatively large, and have small pores that are easily plugged by dirty water. Microstrainer filters with pore sizes in the range 0.1–0.3 μm do not remove viruses, so disinfection with iodine or chlorine is still necessary.

The importance of preventing diarrheal disease in the HIV-infected traveler is underscored by the fact that wasting syndrome ("slim disease") has been associated with international travel in a study carried out among 4,549 participants of the SWISS HIV Cohort Study [21]. Slim disease has been a major health problem in developing nations consisting of chronic diarrhea associated with wasting in HIV-infected patients. There is also evidence that chronic parasitic infections of the intestines may negatively influence the natural history of HIV infection and chronically increase HIV viral loads [22, 23]. Additional concerns include the risk of post TD irritable bowel syndrome which can occur in up to 14% of those with TD [24].

Treatment of TD in HIV-infected travelers

Empiric treatment for TD should be given at the onset of diarrhea. This consists of antiperistaltic agents (e.g. loperamide) for mild diarrhea (<2 loose stools/day), which should not be used if there is high fever, blood in the stool, or symptoms persisting >48 h on antiperistaltics. Antibiotics should be combined with antiperistaltic agents for more severe diarrhea or diarrhea with fevers or constitutional symptoms. Medical attention should be sought for fevers lasting beyond 10–14 days, high fevers, abdominal pain, bloody diarrhea, vomiting, or dehydration. Recommended antibiotics include ciprofloxacin 500 mg twice daily (or equivalent quinolone) for 3–7 days. Azithromycin 500 mg once daily for 3 days can be given for pregnant women, those in areas of increasing fluoroquinolone resistance (e.g. Thailand and Nepal), and children (5–10 mg/kg × 1). Single-dose regimens such as azithromycin 1000 mg once can be attempted when taken early in the course of infection and with milder symptoms. Rifaximin is a poorly absorbed rifamycin FDA approved for diarrhea from non-invasive strains of E. coli in persons ≥ 12 years old. It is a reasonable alternative to ciprofloxacin for afebrile, non-dysenteric TD. It may be useful in pregnant women and children as there is less interaction with ARVs than with the macrolides, but there are little data to support this. Rifaximin has been shown to be as effective as ciprofloxacin in the management of TD in Mexico and Jamaica, perhaps attributable to its activity against a wide range of enteric bacteria [25]. The usual dose of rifaximin is 200 mg three times per day for 3 days. Its use should be limited to areas outside of Asia where the predominant cause of

TD is *Campylobacter* rather than enterotoxigenic *E. coli* until further studies are done. Note that trimethoprim-sulfamethoxazole is no longer a first-line treatment due to increased resistance worldwide.

Respiratory infections

Bacterial pneumonia

Bacterial infections are increased in HIV-infected individuals and bacterial pneumonias may be acquired during travel [18]. *Streptococcus pneumoniae* infections in particular may be problematic given the increased rates of penicillin/β-lactam-resistant *S. pneumoniae* worldwide (often also resistant to TMP-SMX and macrolides). All travelers should be immunized with the 23-valent polysaccharide pneumococcal vaccine as part of their routine care. This may be repeated if not vaccinated within the previous 5 years [20].

Tuberculosis

HIV-infected travelers are at increased risk for primary TB or reactivation upon return from developing countries or other areas with a high prevalence of TB. Care should be taken to avoid conditions that promote TB transmission such as crowded situations and contact with hospital, prison, or homeless shelter populations. TB skin testing should be assessed prior to travel as part of routine care and again 3 months after returning from developing countries [26]. Travelers with negative TB skin tests prior to travel to high-risk areas are at increased risk for primary infection but efficacy of treatment among this group has not been demonstrated. Decisions concerning the use of chemoprophylaxis in these situations must be considered individually and latent TB infections treated according to treatment guidelines [20].

Other respiratory infections

PCP is not more common during travel and the incidence is lower in tropical areas than in North America. However, all at risk should be on appropriate chemoprophylaxis. HIV-infected travelers should note that the common cold and sinusitis are some of the more common health issues to affect all travelers and should bring along medications for symptomatic relief.

Emerging and re-emerging infections in HIV

Malaria

Despite mixed data in the past, it now appears that malaria interacts with HIV especially in advanced HIV disease and pregnancy, which has long been associated with more severe disease independent of HIV serostatus [22].

Malaria presentation changes with decreasing CD4 counts, with increased episodes of symptomatic parasitemia, increased density and duration of parasitemia, and prolonged fever and malaria can be more severe in areas of unstable disease transmission [27–29]. In addition, there is increased activation and replication of HIV during infection with malaria [27]. Changes in host–parasite interactions occur that may worsen malarial disease in HIV-infected persons on ART [22].

Prophylaxis for malaria should be given to those traveling to endemic areas. Some caution may be warranted as mefloquine has been shown to decrease ritonavir levels, a component of most protease-based ART regimens, in healthy volunteers [30]. The clinical relevance of this is unclear. There is also concern that ARVs with central nervous system effects such as efavirenz may worsen the neuropsychiatric effects of mefloquine. For this reason, doxycycline, chloroquine, atovaquones, and proguanil may be the preferred prophylaxis in travelers on ART, but there is no contraindication to mefloquine. Those on TMP-SMX for PCP prophylaxis will have some protection against malaria. Malaria prophylaxis should be started prior to travel to monitor for any side effects and to achieve adequate drug levels in the body before being exposed to infected mosquitoes. Use of the CDC's hotline (1-800-CDC-INFO/1-800-232-4636) or malaria website (http://www.cdc.gov/malaria) can help in assessing the risk of acquiring malaria and drug-resistant *P. falciparum* malaria.

Despite many pharmacological interactions, there appear to be little clinically significant interactions between antimalarials and HIV ARVs with two possible exceptions. Lumefantrine and halofantrine are extensively metabolized by CYP3A4; use with CYP3A4 inhibitors such as protease inhibitors is contraindicated in the manufacturer's documentation of halofantrine and should be used with caution with lumefantrine. Quinine and quinidine are also extensively metabolized by CYP3A4 and should be used with caution, if at all, with ritonavir-containing regimens.

Leishmaniasis

Visceral leishmaniasis (Kala-Azar) remains an emerging opportunistic infection among HIV-infected individuals. Co-infections with HIV and *Leishmania* have occurred at significant rates in Eastern Africa, India, Brazil, and Europe and have been reported in 35 countries [22]. In Brazil and southwestern Europe, HIV–*Leishmania* co-infection is promoted by the sharing of needles in intravenous drug use rather than the usual case of transmission by sandflies. When CD4 counts fall below 200–300 cells/µL, parasites spread to atypical sites, especially the gastrointestinal site. Only 50% of patients have fever and hepatosplenomegaly; cytopenias are very severe [31]. Diagnosis may be difficult as 50% of patients do not develop characteristic antibodies. Ultimately, diagnosis

from visualization of parasites in peripheral blood monocytes may be possible given the high parasite burden in HIV-infected patients [20, 22]. Polymerase chain reaction of the buffy coat of blood can yield the diagnosis in up to 100% of patients [22]. Treatment consists of stibogluconate or amphotericin B with 50–100% of patients responding. However, long-term suppressive treatment will be required, e.g. ART with intermittent liposomal amphotericin B every 21 days until CD4 >350 cells/mm^3 for 3–6 months [32].

Chagas disease

Trypanosoma cruzi infection (Chagas disease) is accelerated and more severe in HIV infection [22]. The chronic phase of infection is characterized by persistent reactivation of Chagas disease with high levels of parasitemia in co-infected individuals in contrast with low-level parasitemia in HIV-uninfected persons [33]. Fever, cutaneous eruptions, and myocarditis similar to that seen in acute Chagas disease is often seen in contrast to the cardiac and GI involvement characteristic of disease in HIV-uninfected persons. CNS involvement such as meningoencephalitis that can be fatal, CNS abscesses, and granulomatous encephalitis is usually present in co-infected patients while it is rarely seen in HIV-uninfected patients [22, 34]. Diagnosis in co-infected persons can be made by examination of the peripheral blood for spirochetes, PCR of the blood or tissue, or examination of tissue biopsies. Treatment for *T. cruzi* should be initiated earlier than usually done in HIV-uninfected persons, preferably in the asymptomatic phase of the disease. Lifelong treatment with benznidazole or nifurtimox may be needed [34].

Precautions should be taken to avoid infection if traveling in the Americas where the infection exists and is spread by the bite of the reduviid bug. The risk of infection is significant for those with extended stays; infections of tourists are uncommon. To minimize risk of infection, avoid sleeping in substandard houses, use mosquito nets, and use insect repellents at night.

Other parasitic infections

Few major interactions exist between HIV and other emerging parasitic infections in travelers. The propensity for disseminated strongyloidiasis is associated with HTLV-1 not HIV-1 infection. The egg burden in schistosomiasis may be higher in HIV-infected persons and the time until re-infection may be shorter [22]. Onchocerciasis does not appear to be significantly affected by HIV infection, although cellular immune responses may be depressed in HIV–*Onchocerca volvulus* co-infected individuals [22, 35]. There are little data on the impact of HIV on filariasis and loiasis [22].

Penicilliosis

Penicilliosis, disseminated infection with the fungus *Penicillium marneffei*, has become an important opportunistic infection in AIDS patients in southeast Asia (especially northern Thailand) and southern China. The disease usually occurs when CD4 counts fall below 50 cells/mm^3 [36]. Common presenting symptoms include fever, sweats, wasting, and skin lesions—often papules with central umbilication or nodules, but a wide range of skin eruptions are possible—in association with anemia, lymphadenopathy, and hepatomegaly. Diagnosis is often made by bone marrow examination or skin biopsy, and less reliably from blood cultures. Treatment consists of amphotericin B followed by itraconazole. Chronic maintenance therapy with itraconazole is needed as post-treatment relapse is common [37]. Untreated, mortality is over 75% [37]. Penicilliosis can occur in AIDS patients with a remote history of only brief travel to endemic areas. Soil exposure is a known risk factor and should be avoided in endemic areas, especially during the rainy season. Prophylactic itraconazole at 200 mg/day for AIDS patients traveling in high-risk parts of endemic areas may be considered, especially for those with CD4 counts < 100 cells/mm^3.

Other endemic mycoses

HIV-infected travelers with low CD4 counts are at risk for diseases from other endemic fungal infections. These include coccidioidomycosis in southwest USA, northern Mexico, and South America, histoplasmosis with a world-wide distribution but primarily in the Americas and Africa, and paracoccidioidomycosis in Central America. These disseminated diseases are more common in the immunocompromised host with decreased cell-mediated immunity such as HIV-infected travelers with low CD4 counts. Disease can reflect new infection, re-infection, or reactivation of previous infections.

Prophylaxis with itraconazole at 100 mg/day can be considered for travelers with CD4 counts < 100 cells/mm^3, who are at high risk for acquiring histoplasmosis because of occupational exposure or who travel to a community with a hyperendemic rate of histoplasmosis (> 10 cases/100 patient-years) although there has not been demonstrated survival benefit in doing this [20]. Severely immunocompromised travelers should avoid activities known to be associated with increased risk such as creating dust when working with surface soil; cleaning chicken coops that are heavily contaminated with droppings; disturbing soil beneath bird roosting sites; cleaning, remodeling, or demolishing old buildings; and exploring caves [20]. Prophylaxis for the other endemic mycoses is generally not recommended. Avoiding the agents of coccidioidomycosis and paracoccidioidomycosis is not entirely possible, but at-risk travelers should avoid activities associated with increased risk including those involving extensive exposure to disturbed native soil, e.g. dust storms [20].

Cryptococcus neoformans causes disseminated cryptococcosis, a common opportunistic infection worldwide in AIDS patients with CD4 counts < 50 cells/mm^3. *Cryptococcus neoformans* has been found in soil samples from around the world in areas frequented by birds, especially pigeons and chickens, but there has been no evidence linking exposure to pigeon droppings with an increased risk for acquiring cryptococcosis. Little can be done to avoid exposure to *C. neoformans*. Prophylaxis for those at risk is not commonly recommended but can be considered in the context of prophylaxis for other mycoses.

TRAVEL-RELATED SKIN DISORDERS

Dermatologic lesions in the returning traveler are common in the HIV-infected and HIV-uninfected traveler alike. One prospective study of 269 returning travelers with skin disorder found that the most common skin lesions were cutaneous larva migrans (25%); pyodermas (18%); pruritic arthropod-reactive dermatitis (10%); myiasis (9%); tungiasis (6%); urticaria (5%); fever and rash (4%); and cutaneous leishmaniasis (3%) [38].

The appearance of skin lesions can give clues to their etiology [9]:

- Papules, usually pruritic: consider insect bites, scabies, seabather's eruption for rashes confined to skin covered by bathing suits, cercarial dermatitis for rashes involving exposed skin, onchocerciasis in long-term travelers, and drug eruptions.
- Nodules: consider myiasis if painful boil-like lesions with central opening with intermittently visible fly larva, tungiasis (jiggers) especially if lesions mainly on soles of the feet and around toenails, loiasis if migratory areas of angioedema (Calabar swellings), acute East African trypanosomiasis and furuncles.
- Ulcers: consider pyoderma if lesions painful (frequently bite-related with secondary infection from *S. aureus* or group A streptococci), leishmaniasis if lesions painless, and rickettsial diseases if an eschar is present.
- Linear and migratory lesions: consider cutaneous larva migrans, larva currens due to strongyloidiasis if perianal cutaneous track present, and photodermatitis if painless, non-pruritic fixed linear streaks (from skin exposure to psoralen-containing products, e.g. limes).

OTHER ISSUES IN THE HIV-INFECTED TRAVELER

New HIV infections

In Western countries, where the B-subtype is predominant, there is a steep increase in non-B-subtypes and circulating recombinant forms, while new recombinants emerge worldwide. Travelers contribute to the spread of HIV-1 genetic diversity worldwide; in the developing world, migration of rural populations and civil war are additional contributing factors. The spreading of HIV-1 variants has implications for diagnostic, treatment (unknown clinical relevance at this time), and vaccine development [39].

Fever in the returning HIV-infected traveler

The evaluation of fever in the returning HIV-infected traveler should focus on the same etiologies as those in the HIV-uninfected traveler. Common causes are still most likely, such as sinusitis, pneumonia, urinary tract infection, and drug fever. Important infectious causes of non-specific fevers include malaria, dengue, rickettsial diseases (e.g. RMSF, scrub typhus), leptospirosis, typhoid fever, tuberculosis, acute schistosomiasis, East African trypanosomiasis, viral hepatitis, and traveler's diarrhea [9].

CONCLUSION

As individuals with HIV/AIDS continue to live longer in the era of ART, we can expect increased rates of international travel in this population, including those with depressed CD4 counts. Careful medical evaluation and appropriate pre-travel health advice will be increasingly important. Simple precautions and the use of a travel health expert can help minimize risks, enabling all HIV-infected travelers to have safer and more enjoyable international travel.

REFERENCES

[1] Palella F, Delaney K, Moorman A, et al. Declining morbidity and mortality among patients with advanced human immunodeficiency virus infection. N Engl J Med 1998;338:853–60.

[2] van Sighem AI, van de Wiel MA, Ghani AC, et al. Mortality and progression to AIDS after starting highly active antiretroviral therapy. AIDS 2003;17:2227–36.

[3] Autran B, Carcelain G, Debre P. Immune reconstitution after highly active anti-retroviral treatment of HIV infection. Adv Exp Med Biol 2001;495:205–12.

[4] Autran B, Carcelain G, Li TS, et al. Positive effects of combined antiretroviral therapy on CD4+ T cell homeostasis and function in advanced HIV disease. Science 1997;277:112–16.

[5] The Antiretroviral Therapy Cohort Collaboration. Life expectancy of individuals on combination antiretroviral therapy in high-income countries: a collaborative analysis of 14 cohort studies. Lancet 2008;372:293–9.

[6] Kemper CA, Linett A, Kane C, et al. Travels with HIV: the compliance and health of HIV-infected adults who travel. Int J STD AIDS 1997;8:44–9.

[7] Salit IE, Sano M, Boggild AK, et al. Travel patterns and risk behaviour of HIV-positive people travelling internationally. Can Med Assoc J 2005;172:884–8.

[8] Bureau of Transportation Statistics. US International Travel and Transportation Trends, BTS02–03. Washington, DC: US Department of Transportation; 2002.

[9] Ryan ET, Wilson ME, Kain KC. Illness after international travel. N Engl J Med 2002;347:505–16.

[10] US Department of Transportation Research and Innovative Technology Administration Bureau of Transportation Statistics US International Travel and Transportation Trends, September 2006. Washington, DC; 2006.

[11] Fulford M, Keystone JS. Health risks associated with visiting friends and relatives in developing countries. Curr Infect Dis Rep 2005;7:48–53.

[12] Porter JF, Knill-Jones RP. Quality of travel health advice in higher-education establishments in the United Kingdom and its relationship to the demographic background of the provider. J Travel Med 2004;11:347–53.

[13] Suh KN, Mileno MD. Challenging scenarios in a travel clinic: advising the complex traveler. Infect Dis Clin North Am 2005;19:15–47.

[14] Mahto M, Ponnusamy K, Schuhwerk M, et al. Knowledge, attitudes and health outcomes in HIV-infected travellers to the USA. HIV Med 2006;7:201–4.

[15] Glesby M, Hoover D, Farzedegan H, et al. The effect of influenza vaccination on human immunodeficiency virus type 1 load: a randomized, double-blinded, placebo-controlled study. J Infect Dis 1996;174:1332–6.

[16] Castelli F, Patroni A. The human immunodeficiency virus-infected traveler. Clin Infect Dis 2000;31:1403–8.

[17] Gruenewald R, Blum S, Chan J. Relationship between human immunodeficiency virus infection and salmonellosis in 20- to 59-year-old residents of New York City. Clin Infect Dis 1994;18:358–63.

[18] Mileno MD, Bia FJ. The compromised traveler. Infect Dis Clin North Am 1998;12:369–412.

[19] McCombs SB, Dworkin MS, Wan PC. Helminth infections in HIV-infected persons in the United States, 1990–1999. Clin Infect Dis 2000;30:241–2.

[20] Kaplan JE, Benson C, Holmes KH, et al. Guidelines for prevention and treatment of opportunistic infections in HIV-infected adults and adolescents: recommendations from CDC, the National Institutes of Health, and the HIV Medicine Association of the Infectious Diseases Society of America. MMWR Recomm Rep 2009;58 (RR-4):1–207.

[21] Furrer H, Chan P, Weber R, et al. Increased risk of wasting syndrome in HIV-infected travellers: prospective multicentre study. Trans

R Soc Trop Med Hyg 2001;95:484–6.

[22] Harms G, Feldmeier H. The impact of HIV infection on tropical diseases. Infect Dis Clin North Am 2005;19:121–35.

[23] Bentwich Z, Maartens G, Torten D, et al. Concurrent infections and HIV pathogenesis. AIDS 2000;14:2071–81.

[24] Stermer E, Lubezky A, Potasman I, et al. Is traveler's diarrhea a significant risk factor for the development of irritable bowel syndrome? A prospective study. Clin Infect Dis 2006;43: 898–901.

[25] DuPont HL, Jiang ZD, Ericsson CD, et al. Rifaximin versus ciprofloxacin for the treatment of traveler's diarrhea: a randomized, double-blind clinical trial. Clin Infect Dis 2001;33:1807–15.

[26] Ericsson CD. Travellers with pre-existing medical conditions. Int J Antimicrob Agents 2003;21:181–8.

[27] Whitworth J, Morgan D, Quigley M, et al. Effect of HIV-1 and increasing immunosuppression on malaria parasitaemia and clinical episodes in adults in rural Uganda: a cohort study. Lancet 2000;356:1051–6.

[28] French N, Nakiyingi J, Lugada E, et al. Increasing rates of malarial fever with deteriorating immune status in HIV-1-infected Ugandan adults. AIDS 2001;15:899–906.

[29] Grimwade K, French N, Mbatha DD, et al. HIV infection as a cofactor for severe falciparum malaria in adults living in a region of unstable malaria transmission in South Africa. AIDS 2004;18:547–54.

[30] Khaliq Y, Gallicano K, Tisdale C, et al. Pharmacokinetic interaction between mefloquine and ritonavir in healthy volunteers. Br J Clin Pharmacol 2001;51:591–600.

[31] Rosenthal E, Marty P, del Giudice P, et al. HIV and *Leishmania* coinfection: a review of 91 cases with focus on atypical locations of *Leishmania*. Clin Infect Dis 2000;31:1093–5.

[32] Lopez-Velez R, Videla S, Marquez M, et al. Amphotericin B lipid complex versus no treatment in the secondary prophylaxis of visceral leishmaniasis in HIV-infected patients. J Antimicrob Chemother 2004;53:540–3.

[33] Sartori AM, Neto JE, Nunes EV, et al. *Trypanosoma cruzi* parasitemia in chronic Chagas disease: comparison between human immunodeficiency virus (HIV)-positive and HIV-negative patients. J Infect Dis 2002;186:872–5.

[34] Ferreira MS, Nishioka Sde A, Silvestre MT, et al. Reactivation of Chagas' disease in patients with AIDS: report of three new cases and review of the literature. Clin Infect Dis 1997;25: 1397–400.

[35] Sentongo E, Rubaale T, Buttner DW, et al. T cell responses in coinfection with *Onchocerca volvulus* and the human immunodeficiency virus type 1. Parasite Immunol 1998;20:431–9.

[36] Clezy K, Sirisanthana T, Sirisanthana V, et al. Late manifestations of HIV in Asia and the Pacific. AIDS 1994;8:35–43.

[37] Supparatpinyo K, Khamwan C, Baosoung V, et al. Disseminated *Penicillium marneffei* infection in southeast Asia. Lancet 1994;344:110–13.

[38] Caumes E, Carriere J, Guermonprez G, et al. Dermatoses associated with travel to tropical countries: a prospective study of the diagnosis and management of 269 patients presenting to a tropical disease unit. Clin Infect Dis 1995;20:542–8.

[39] Perrin L, Kaiser L, Yerly S. Travel and the spread of HIV-1 genetic variants. Lancet Infect Dis 2003;3:22–7.

Index

Note: Page numbers followed by *b* indicate boxes, *f* indicate figures and *t* indicate tables.

CPSIA information can be obtained at www.ICGtesting.com
Printed in the USA
BVOW09s1937080216

436013BV00005B/9/P